Breast Disease

Adnan Aydiner • Abdullah İğci
Atilla Soran
Editors

Breast Disease

Management and Therapies

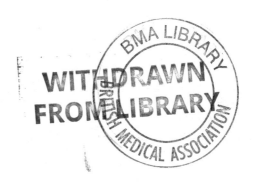
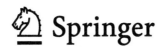 Springer

Editors
Adnan Aydiner
Institute of Oncology
Istanbul University
Istanbul
Turkey

Abdullah İğci
Institute of Oncology
Istanbul University
Istanbul
Turkey

Atilla Soran
Breast Surgery
Magee-Womens Hospital
Pittsburg
USA

ISBN 978-3-319-26010-5   ISBN 978-3-319-26012-9   (eBook)
DOI 10.1007/978-3-319-26012-9

Library of Congress Control Number: 2016934600

Printed on acid-free paper

This Springer imprint is published by Springer Nature
The registered company is Springer International Publishing AG Switzerland

Preface

The goal of *Breast Disease and Management and Therapies* is to provide a comprehensive, scholarly appraisal of contemporary therapy. We have attempted to provide useful and explicit recommendations on management, but we must stress that these recommendations are subject to change. Some of the recommendations are controversial and the subject of ongoing clinical trials. The gold standard for breast cancer care includes an integrated multidisciplinary team approach, comprising pathologists, radiologists, surgical oncologists, medical oncologists, radiation oncologists, oncology nurses, and plastic surgeons. This book is organized into 9 sections and 50 chapters, and we give a brief summary of its content below.

Diagnostic *breast biopsy* is one of the most common medical procedures, and a variety of methods have been developed in the last 30 years to augment classic surgical incisional and excisional biopsies. Fine-needle aspiration (FNA) has an important historical role and remains among the most cost-effective methods. However, this technique is limited by the weakness of current breast cytology to adequately reproduce all information provided by traditional histopathology. Core biopsies ranging from the use of simple needle cores to larger coring devices to remove spaghetti- to macaroni-sized pieces have become the mainstay of current biopsy techniques for most palpable and non-palpable lesions. Surgical incisional and excisional biopsies, which are classic standards, are reserved for a few exceptional circumstances, including the removal of symptomatic benign lesions or when coring biopsy tools fail to provide adequate diagnostic information and material.

After diagnosis, in the *evaluation of patients for metastases prior to surgery*, preoperative ultrasonography (US) and needle biopsy have emerged as effective methods for axillary staging for triaging women with breast cancer directly to axillary surgery for sentinel lymph node biopsy (SLNB) or axillary lymph node dissection (ALND) or to neoadjuvant chemotherapy (NCT) in those with axillary node-positive disease. However, no perfect modality is available to identify metastatic disease in breast cancer; every diagnostic test has its own advantages and limitations. The available evidence suggests routine evaluation for stage III and possibly stage II breast cancer using imaging techniques, including positron emission tomography–computerized tomography (PET-CT). The workup of abnormal findings in breast cancer patients is by patient signs and symptoms, including history and physical examination, laboratory tests, imaging, biopsy of suspicious finding in imaging studies, and monitoring serum markers.

Breast-conserving surgery (BCS) and mastectomy are two options for surgical treatment. SLNB has replaced *axillary lymph node dissection* (ALND) in clinically node-negative early-stage breast cancer patients. ALND is considered mandatory in sentinel node-positive patients, but recent data have demonstrated that BCS and radiotherapy are the equivalent of ALND for micro-/macrometastatic sentinel lymph nodes (SLNs). This approach reduces the morbidity of dissection without decreasing overall survival (OS).

Breast reconstruction provides closure to many women who have been treated for breast cancer by increasing their comfort in clothing and providing a psychological benefit. Patients who choose reconstruction must navigate a reconstructive pathway guided by their plastic surgeons that includes decisions regarding the timing, type, and extent of reconstruction.

After surgery, *adjuvant endocrine therapy* is a pivotal component of treatment for women with hormone receptor-positive early-stage breast cancer; this therapy delays local and distant relapse and prolongs survival. Patients with estrogen receptor (ER)- and/or progesterone receptor (PR)-positive invasive breast cancers should be considered for adjuvant endocrine therapy regardless of age, lymph node status, or adjuvant chemotherapy use. Features indicative of uncertain endocrine responsiveness include low levels of hormone receptor immunoreactivity, PR negativity, poor differentiation (grade 3), high Ki67 index, human epidermal growth factor receptor 2 (HER2) overexpression, and high gene recurrence score. Adjuvant hormonal manipulation is achieved by blocking the ER in breast tumor tissues with tamoxifen in premenopausal and postmenopausal women, lowering systemic estrogen levels with luteinizing hormone-releasing hormone agonists in premenopausal women, or blocking estrogen biosynthesis in non-ovarian tissues with aromatase inhibitors in postmenopausal women.

All patients with invasive breast cancer should be evaluated to assess the need for *adjuvant cytotoxic therapy*, trastuzumab therapy, and/or endocrine therapy. If patients must receive endocrine therapy (either tamoxifen or aromatase inhibitor) and cytotoxic therapy as adjuvant therapy, chemotherapy should precede endocrine therapy. Molecular subtypes of breast cancer can be distinguished by common pathological variables, including ER, PR, HER2, and Ki67 index. The inclusion of chemotherapy in the adjuvant regimen depends on the intrinsic subtype. Multigene expression array profiling is not always required for subtype definition after clinicopathological assessment. Young age, grade 3 disease, lymphovascular invasion, one to three positive nodes, and large tumor size are not adequate features to omit molecular diagnostics in the decision of adjuvant chemotherapy. Any lymph node positivity should not be a sole indication for adjuvant chemotherapy. However, patients with more than three involved lymph nodes, low hormone receptor positivity, positive HER2 status, triple-negative status, high 21-gene recurrence score (RS), and high-risk 70-gene scores should receive adjuvant chemotherapy. A high Ki67 proliferation index and histological grade 3 tumors are acceptable indications for adjuvant chemotherapy.

In patients with HER2-positive early-stage breast cancer, the monoclonal antibody trastuzumab has been approved as the first molecularly targeted agent for the adjuvant treatment. Current *adjuvant anti-HER2-therapies* must be refined for different patient subsets with HER2-positive tumors to provide personalized, effective, and minimally toxic treatment.

Mastectomy can remove any detectable macroscopic disease, but some tumor foci might remain in the locoregional tissue (i.e., chest wall or lymph nodes), potentially causing locoregional disease recurrence. *Postmastectomy adjuvant radiotherapy* (PMRT) has the potential to eliminate such microscopic disease. PMRT has been recommended for patients with ≥4 positive axillary lymph nodes but is not administered to most women with node-negative disease. Patients with one to three positive axillary lymph nodes constitute a gray zone.

Breast irradiation after BSC is an essential component of breast-conservation therapy for maximizing local control and overall survival. The optimal dose and fractionation schedule for radiation therapy after BCS has not yet been defined. There is renewed interest in hypofractionation for whole-breast irradiation, and this approach has important practical advantages and biological implications. Irradiating only the tumor-bearing quadrant of the breast instead of irradiating the entire breast after BCS has also increased in popularity in the last decade.

Preoperative systemic chemotherapy (PSC), also known as "neoadjuvant chemotherapy," is an important therapeutic option for most patients with breast cancer. PSC is becoming increasingly popular in the breast oncology community for the treatment of earlier-stage disease. PSC is a valuable research tool for identifying predictive molecular biomarkers and is a valid treatment option for patients with early-stage breast cancer.

The principles of *surgery after* PSC remain the same. Monitoring the response to therapy is important for surgical planning and prognostic information. Preoperative marking of the tumor is essential for guiding BCS after PSC and should be performed in all patients. Axillary staging can be performed prior to or after PSC, and both methods are associated with specific risks and benefits. Early literature supported the use of pre-PSC SLNB, but current literature suggests increased accuracy and decreased use of axillary dissection in patients who undergo SLNB after PSC.

Chemotherapy can be particularly toxic for elderly postmenopausal patients, and *neoadjuvant hormonal therapy* (NHT) is an alternative for patients with hormone receptor-positive, locally advanced, postmenopausal breast cancer. This treatment is also highly beneficial for patients with comorbidities and can comprise tamoxifen and steroidal or nonsteroidal aromatase inhibitors (AIs). The best activities in clinical trials have been observed with AIs. NHT produces good response rates and adequate down-staging of tumor size such that BCS may become an option. The optimal duration of such treatments should be at least 4 months and may be continued for as long as 8 months.

Neoadjuvant therapy is administered with the objective of improving surgical outcomes in patients with *locally advanced breast cancer* for whom a primary surgical approach is technically not feasible and for patients with operable breast cancer who desire breast conservation but for whom either a mastectomy is required or a partial mastectomy would result in a poor cosmetic outcome. Patients treated with *neoadjuvant chemotherapy* are significantly more likely to undergo BCS without a significant increase in local recurrence compared with patients who are treated with surgery first. In addition, neoadjuvant chemotherapy is appropriate for patients with HER2-positive or triple-negative breast cancer who are most likely to have a good locoregional response to treatment, regardless of the size of their breast cancer at presentation.

The decision to treat patients with *radiotherapy after preoperative chemotherapy* is still largely based on the initial clinical staging of the patients. The use of three-field radiotherapy, including the chest wall/breast and regional lymphatics, after surgery in locally advanced, node-positive patients receiving neoadjuvant systemic chemotherapy is well-established. A pooled analysis is the only prospective dataset that can assist radiotherapy decisions in the neoadjuvant setting. Well-designed randomized, controlled studies are urgently needed in this controversial area.

Inflammatory breast carcinoma (IBC) is the most aggressive, lethal, and rare form of breast cancer. IBC is characterized by the rapid development of erythema, edema, and peau d'orange over one-third or more of the skin of the breast due to the occlusion of dermal mammary lymphatics by tumor emboli. Plugging of the dermal lymphatics of the breast finding is not mandatory for diagnosis. The most striking progress in the management of IBC has been the sequential incorporation of preoperative systemic chemotherapy [an induction regimen containing an anthracycline and a taxane (plus trastuzumab in *HER2*-positive patients)] followed by surgery and radiation therapy.

Breast cancer risk increases with age, and life expectancy continues to increase; therefore, *breast cancer in older women* has become a significant public health concern. The basic principles of imaging, diagnosis, and treatment remain standard for all women with breast cancer. However, in the elderly population, comorbid conditions, life expectancy, and quality of life take on particular importance for the clinician to consider and balance with treatment decisions. Historically, older women have been poorly represented in breast cancer trials, and their surgical and adjuvant treatment often differs from that of younger women. *Breast cancer in young women* accounts for almost one-quarter of all breast cancer diagnoses in the USA. Young women with breast cancer exhibit a significantly worse prognosis than their postmenopausal counterparts. Differences in presentation, tumor phenotype, and options for therapy may explain some of the difference in outcome. *Breast cancer is observed in men* 100-fold less often than in women. Previous studies have shown that metastatic breast cancer (MBC) cases significantly differ from female cases, whereas new studies have reported that breast cancer has similar characteristics at the same stages in both genders.

Pregnancy-associated breast cancer is defined as breast cancer that is diagnosed during gestation, lactation, or the first postpartum year. Surgical treatment can be undertaken during any phase of the pregnancy. Chemotherapy can potentially be administered during the second or third trimester. Radiotherapy is reserved for the postpartum period.

Paget's disease of the breast is characterized by eczema-form changes accompanied with erosion and ulceration of the nipple and areolar epidermis. This condition is primarily correlated with ductal carcinoma in situ (DCIS); additionally, it can be accompanied by invasive ductal carcinoma (IDC). The diagnosis is determined upon the microscopic observation of Paget cells in a skin biopsy. The width of the lesion is evaluated via mammography and MRI in patients for whom breast-preserving surgery is planned. Depending on the extent of the lesion, SLNB and axillary curettage for those having axillary metastases are treatment alternatives to breast-preserving surgery or mastectomy.

Phyllodes tumors, also termed phylloides tumors or cytosarcoma phyllodes, are rare fibroepithelial neoplasms of the breast that remain challenging for both surgeons and pathologists. The World Health Organization (WHO) established the name phyllodes tumor and the following histological types: benign, borderline, and malignant. Breast imaging studies may fail to distinguish the phyllodes tumor from a fibroadenoma. A core needle biopsy is preferable to fine needle aspiration for tissue diagnosis. The common treatment for phyllodes tumors is wide local excision. Mastectomy is indicated for patients with a large lesion. The benefits of adjuvant chemotherapy and radiotherapy are controversial.

Breast sarcomas are rare clinical entities. Surgical excision with clear margins is the primary treatment for localized tumors. Lymph node sampling and dissection is not recommended. Adjuvant or neoadjuvant therapy should be considered for high-risk patients. Angiosarcomas are the most common sarcomas of the breast. These lesions can be associated with lymphedema or irradiation. Surgery is the primary treatment, and wide negative margins are essential for a long-term cure. Primary breast lymphoma is a rare entity that arises from the periductal and perilobular lymphatic tissue and intramammary lymph nodes. Surgery is limited to biopsy. Metastatic involvement of the breast most often originates from the contralateral site. The most common malignancy of the body that metastasizes to the breast is *malignant melanoma*. Hematological malignancies such as *leukemia and lymphoma* also frequently occur.

Reducing estrogen production and preventing estrogen from interacting with the ER pathway have been the focus of several preclinical and clinical trials and are commonly used *endocrine treatment* strategies for treating HR+ MBC. Because the ovaries are the main source of estrogen in premenopausal women, ovarian ablation or functional suppression is the primary means of decreasing circulating estrogen. In postmenopausal women, the peripheral conversion of androgens to estrogen is the predominant source of estrogen. Thus, the inhibition of the conversion of androgens by an AI or via the interaction of estrogen with its receptor is the most frequently used approach to treat postmenopausal women with HR+ breast cancer.

In ER-positive/*HER2-negative MBC*, endocrine therapy is preferred, even in the presence of visceral metastasis. Chemotherapy should be reserved for patients with combination chemotherapy indications or proven endocrine resistance. Regarding the use of chemotherapy, sequential monotherapy is the preferred choice for MBC. Combination chemotherapy should be reserved for patients with rapid clinical progression, life-threatening visceral metastases, or the need for rapid symptom and/or disease control. HER2-targeted therapies have radically altered the prognosis of *HER2-positive MBC*. However, resistance to these therapies frequently leads to treatment failure and new tumor progression. The most promising new anti-HER therapies are T-DM1 and pertuzumab, which has been evaluated in trastuzumab-resistant patients as well as in a first-line setting with trastuzumab. The dual blockage of HER appears to be a favorable approach for these patients; however, downstream signaling steps can be activated to overcome *tyrosine kinase inhibition*. Because tumor cells can adapt themselves by using alternative pathways to maintain proliferation, providing a sufficient treatment approach also requires the consideration of possible escape mechanisms in tumor cells.

Although antiangiogenic therapies, including anti-vascular endothelial growth factor (VEGF) antibodies and tyrosine kinase inhibitors, have become important components of the standard of care for the treatment of many solid tumors, the results of clinical trials investigating the efficacy of *antiangiogenic agents* in breast cancer are contradictory.

Breast cancer during pregnancy must be managed with a multidisciplinary approach that should follow standard protocols for nonpregnant patients as much as possible while considering the safety of the fetus. Various assisted reproductive technology approaches are available for breast cancer patients who wish to preserve fertility after cancer treatment. These approaches can be utilized before or after the initiation of adjuvant breast cancer treatment. Hence, adequate counseling should be provided to premenopausal breast cancer patients prior to cancer treatment.

Cancer is a chronic, life-threatening disease that greatly impacts all spheres of life. Cancer patients develop various and differing emotional, mental, and behavioral reactions regarding their illness during diagnosis, treatment, and the palliative period. Some of these reactions are normal and may even tend toward adaptation in some cases. The treatment team must understand such reactions and support them. Disordered or maladaptive reactions, however, require psychiatric evaluation and treatment. It is essential to encourage the patient to express her feelings, support the patient, and provide her with security. Health-care professionals should be aware of and respect women's coping strategies and encourage them to use these strategies to reduce psychological symptoms. Health-care professionals should also make family members and friends aware of their role in supporting and encouraging coping strategies.

We have summarized some important points of this book above. We would like to dedicate this book to postgraduate physicians in training to become breast cancer specialists. We hope this book stimulates today's young doctors to contribute to the basic and clinical research on which future books will be based.

Istanbul, Turkey   Adnan Aydiner, MD
Istanbul, Turkey   Abdullag Igci, MD
Pittsburgh, PA, USA   Atilla Soran, MD, MPH

Contents

Contributors

Nihat Aksakal, MD Breast Unit, Department of General Surgery, Istanbul University Istanbul Faculty of Medicine, Topkapi, Istanbul, Turkey

Isik Aslay, MD Department of Radiation Oncology, Acibadem Hospital, Istanbul, Turkey

Adnan Aydiner, MD Department of Medical Oncology, Istanbul University Istanbul Medical Faculty, Institute of Oncology, Istanbul, Turkey

Fatih Aydoğan, MD, FEBS Division of Breast Disease, Department of General Surgery, Cerrahpasa School of Medicine, Istanbul University, Istanbul, Turkey

Dana Farber/Brigham and Women's Cancer Center, Harvard Medical School, Boston, MA, USA

Division of Breast Disease, Department of Surgery, Istanbul University Cerrahpasa Medical School, Istanbul, Turkey

Tümay Aydoğan, MD Department of Medical Education, Biruni School of Medicine, Biruni University, Istanbul, Turkey

Comprehensive Breast Center, Hallmark Health Medical Associates, Stoneham, MA, USA

Gul Basaran, MD Medical Oncology Department, Medical Faculty, Acibadem University, Istanbul, Turkey

Ercan Bastu, MD Department of Obstetrics and Gynecology, Istanbul University School of Medicine, Istanbul, Turkey

Yusuf Bayrak, MD Department of Thoracic Surgery, Vehbi Koc Foundation, American Hospital, Istanbul, Turkey

Saveri Bhattacharya, DO Hematology/Oncology, University of Pittsburgh, Pittsburgh, PA, USA

Halil Buldu, MD Department of Orthopaedics and Traumatology, Memorial Hospital, Istanbul, Turkey

Nişantaşı Hospital, Istanbul, Turkey

Faruk Buyru, MD Obstetrics and Gynecology, Istanbul University, Istanbul Medical Faculty, Istanbul, Turkey

Department of Obstetrics and Gynecology, Istanbul University School of Medicine, Istanbul, Turkey

Neslihan Cabioğlu, MD, PhD Department of General Surgery, Breast Cancer Department, Istanbul Faculty of Medicine, University of Istanbul, Istanbul, Turkey

Department of Surgery, Istanbul Faculty of Medicine, Istanbul University, Istanbul, Turkey

Devrim Cabuk, MD Department of Medical Oncology, Kocaeli University Hospital, Kocaeli, Turkey

Burcu Cakar, MD Medical Oncology Unit, Yunus Emre State Hospital Tepebasi, Eskisehir, Turkey

Department of Medical Oncology, Tulay Aktaş Oncology Hospital, Ege University Medical Faculty, Izmir, Turkey

Gulbeyaz Can, RN, PhD Department of Medical Nursing, Istanbul University Florence Nightingale Nursing Faculty, Istanbul, Turkey

Varol Çelik, MD Division of Breast Disease, Department of General Surgery, Cerrahpasa School of Medicine, Istanbul University, Istanbul, Turkey

Irfan Cicin, MD Department of Medical Oncology, Faculty of Medicine, Balkan Oncology Hospital, Trakya University of Medicine, Edirne, Turkey

Trakya Üniversitesi Hastanesi Medikal Onkoloji Bilim Dalı, Edirne, Turkey

Nergiz Dagoglu, MD Department of Radiation Oncology, Istanbul University, Istanbul Faculty of Medicine, Istanbul, Turkey

Faysal Dane, MD Division of Medical Oncology, Department of Internal Medicine, Marmara University Medical School, Istanbul, Turkey

Department of Medical Oncology, Marmara University, School of Medicine, Istanbul, Turkey

Edward H. Davidson, MA (Cantab), MBBS Department of Plastic Surgery, University of Pittsburgh, Pittsburgh, PA, USA

Gokhan Demir, MD Medical Oncology Department, Medical Oncology, Acibadem University School of Medicine, Istanbul, Turkey

Sukru Dilege, MD General Thoracic Surgery, Koç University School of Medicine, Istanbul, Turkey

Maktav Dincer, MD Department of Radiation Oncology, Florence Nightingale Hospital, Istanbul, Turkey

William C. Dooley, MD, FACS Department of Surgery and OU Breast Institute, The University of Oklahoma Health Sciences Center, Oklahoma City, OK, USA

Levent Eralp, MD Department of Orthopaedics and Traumatology, University of Istanbul, Istanbul School of Medicine, Istanbul, Turkey

Yesim Eralp, MD Department of Medical Oncology, Istanbul University Institute of Oncology, Istanbul, Turkey

Bulent Erdogan, MD Department of Medical Oncology, Faculty of Medicine, Balkan Oncology Hospital, Trakya University of Medicine, Edirne, Turkey

Deniz Eren-Böler, MD Department of General Surgery, Acıbadem University Medical Faculty, Kerem Aydınlar Kampüsü, Istanbul, Turkey
Department of Surgery, Faculty of Medicine, Acibadem Univesity, Istanbul, Turkey

Merdan Fayda, MD Department of Radiation Oncology, Istanbul University Institute of Oncology, Istanbul, Turkey

Erdem Göker, MD Department of Medical Oncology, Tulay Aktaş Oncology Hospital, Ege University Medical Faculty, Izmir, Turkey

İlknur Bilkay Görken, MD Radiation Oncology, Dokuz Eylül University, İzmir, Turkey

Tara Grahovac, MD Division of Surgical Oncology, Department of Surgery, Breast Surgery Unit, Magee-Womens Hospital, University of Pittsburgh Medical Center, Pittsburgh, PA, USA

Jelena Grusina-Ujumaza, MD Department of Thoracic Surgery, Pauls Stradins Clinical University Hospital, Riga, Latvia
Paul Stradins University, Riga, Latvia

Nilüfer Güler, MD Retared Member of Department of Medical Oncology, Hacettepe University Medical Faculty, Sıhhiye, Ankara, Turkey

Lejla Hadzikadic Gusic, MD, MSc Division of Surgical Oncology, Department of Surgery, Levine Cancer Institute, Carolinas Medical Center, Charlotte, NC, USA
Department of Surgery, Carolinas Medical Center, Charlotte, NC, USA
Magee-Womens Hospital, UPMC, Pittsburgh, PA, USA

Nora Hansen, MD Department of Surgery, Feinberg School of Medicine, Northwestern University, Chicago, IL, USA

Abdullah İğci, MD, FACS Breast Unit, Department of General Surgery, Istanbul University Istanbul Medical Faculty, Istanbul, Turkey

Ronald Johnson, MD, FACS Breast Surgery Unit, Surgical Oncology, Magee-Womens Hospital, UPMC, Pittsburgh, PA, USA

Şule Karaman, MD Radiation Oncology Department, Istanbul University Institute of Oncology, Istanbul, Turkey

Hasan Karanlik, MD Department of Surgery, Istanbul University, Institute of Oncology, Istanbul, Turkey

Serkan Keskin, MD Department of Medical Oncology, Memorial Hospital, Istanbul, Turkey

Leyla Kilic, MD Department of Medical Oncology, Firat University Hospital, Elazig, Turkey

Seden Küçücük, MD Radiation Oncology Department, Istanbul University Institute of Oncology, Istanbul, Turkey

Maurício Magalhães Costa, MSC, MD, PhD Gynecology Service of the Clementino Fraga Filho Teaching Hospital (UFRJ), Universidade Federal of Rio de Janeiro (UFRJ), Rio de Janeiro, Brazil

Radiumhemmet – Karolinska Institute, Stockholm, Sweden

American Society of Breast Disease (ASBD), Warsaw, IN, USA

SIS Journal – the Electronic Journal of the Senologic International Society (SIS), Warsaw, Poland

Latin American Federation of Mastology, Rio de Janeiro, Brazil

Americas Medical City, Rio de Janeiro, Brazil

Gynecology – Mastology, Universidade Federal do Rio de Janeiro, Rio de Janeiro, Brazil

Lisa Groen Mager, MPT, CLT-LANA, WCS Physical Therapy, Centers for Rehab Services UPMC, Cranberry Twp, PA, USA

University of Pittsburgh Medical Center, Pittsburgh, PA, USA

Anand Mahadevan, MBBS, MD, FRCS, FRCR Department of Radiation Oncology, Beth Israel Deaconess Medical Center, Harvard Medical School, Boston, MA, USA

Nil Molinas Mandel, MD Department of Medical Oncology, VKV American Hospital, Istanbul, Turkey

Department of Medical Oncology, Koc University Medical Faculty, Topkapi/Istanbul, Turkey

Kandace P. McGuire, MD, FACS Department of Surgery, Division of Surgical Oncology, University of North Carolina, Chapel Hill, NC, USA

Ebru Menekse, MD Surgical Oncology Department, Breast Surgery Unit, Magee-Womens Hospital, University of Pittsburgh School of Medicine, Pittsburgh, PA, USA

Division of Surgical Oncology, Department of Surgery, Magee-Womens Hospital, University of Pittsburgh School of Medicine, Pittsburgh, PA, USA

Denise Monahan, MD Department of Surgery, John H. Stroger, Jr. Hospital of Cook County and Rush University Medical Center, Chicago, IL, USA

Mahmut Müslümanoğlu, MD Department of General Surgery, Istanbul University Medical Faculty, Istanbul Medical School, Istanbul, Turkey

Surgery Department, Istanbul Medical Faculty, Topkapı, Istanbul, Turkey

Vu T. Nguyen, MD Department of Plastic Surgery, University of Pittsburg, Pittsburgh, PA, USA

Kerem Okutur, MD Medical Oncology Department, Istanbul Bilim University School of Medicine, Istanbul, Turkey

Medical Oncology Department, Medical Oncology, Acibadem University School of Medicine, Istanbul, Turkey

Serdar Ozbas, MD Breast and Endocrine Surgery Unit, Anakra Guven Hospital, Ankara, Turkey

Mine Özkan, MD Department of Psychiatry, Institute of Oncology, University of Istanbul, Istanbul Faculty of Medicine, Istanbul, Turkey

Department of Consultation Liaison Psychiatry, University of Istanbul, Istanbul Faculty of Medicine, Istanbul, Turkey

Enver Özkurt, MD Department of General Surgery, Istanbul Medical Faculty, Istanbul University, Istanbul, Turkey

Vahit Ozmen, MD, FACS Department of General Surgery, Istanbul Medical Faculty, Istanbul University, Istanbul, Turkey

Department of the Breast Surgery, Istanbul Medical Faculty, Turkish Federation of Breast Diseases Societies, Istanbul, Turkey

Ayfer Kamali Polat, MD, FACS General Surgery Department, Ondokuz Mayis University, Samsun, Turkey

University of Pittsburgh Medical Center, Pittsburgh, PA, USA

Shannon L. Puhalla, MD Division of Hematology/Oncology, Magee-Womens Hospital of UPMC, University of Pittsburgh School of Medicine, Pittsburgh, PA, USA

Breast Cancer Clinical Research Program, Magee Womens Cancer Program, University of Pittsburgh Cancer Institute, Pittsburgh, PA, USA

Yasuaki Sagara, MD Dana Farber/Brigham and Women's Cancer Center, Harvard Medical School, Boston, MA, USA

Pinar Saip, MD Department of Medical Oncology, Institute of Oncology, Istanbul University, Istanbul, Turkey

Paula Saldanha, MD Clínica Maurício Magalhães Costa, Rio de Janeiro, Brazil

Clementino Fraga Filho University Hospital (UFRJ), Rio de Janeiro, Brazil

Fatih Selcukbiricik, MD Department of Medical Oncology, Koc University Medical Faculty, Topkapi/Istanbul, Turkey

Fatma Sen, MD Department of Medical Oncology, Istanbul University Istanbul Medical Faculty, Institute of Oncology, Istanbul, Turkey

Kenneth C. Shestak, MD Department of Plastic Surgery, University of Pittsburgh, Pittsburgh, PA, USA

Atilla Soran, MD, MPH, FACS Division of Surgical Oncology, Department of Surgery, University of Pittsburgh School of Medicine, Magee-Womens Hospital, University of Pittsburgh Medical Center, Pittsburgh, PA, USA

Ozlem Soran, MD, MPH, FACC, FESC Heart and Vascular Institute, University of Pittsburgh, Pittsburgh, PA, USA

Gürsel Remzi Soybir, MD, FALS Department of General Surgery, Istanbul Memorial Hospital, Istanbul, Turkey

Serhan Tanju, MD Thoracic Surgery, Koç University School of Medicine, Istanbul, Turkey

Yunus Taşçı, MD Department of General Surgery, Bezmialem Vakif University Medical Faculty, Istanbul University, Istanbul, Turkey

Fusun Tokatlı, MD Radiation Oncology, Medicana International Hospital, Istanbul, Turkey

Alper Toker, MD Department of Thoracic Surgery, Istanbul Medical School, Istanbul University, Istanbul, Turkey

Department of Thoracic Surgery, Group Florence Nightingale Hospitals, Istanbul, Turkey

Mustafa Tükenmez, MD Department of General Surgery, Istanbul Medical Faculty, Istanbul University, Istanbul, Turkey

Nazim Serdar Turhal Medical Oncology, Anadolu Medical Center, Kocaeli, Turkey

Department of Medical Oncology, Marmara University, School of Medicine, Istanbul, Turkey

Bulent Unal, MD Department of Surgery, Turgut Ozal Medical Center, Inonu University Faculty of Medicine, Malatya, Turkey

Nejdet Fatih Yaşar, MD Department of General Surgery, Osmangazi Medical School, Eskişehir Osmangazi University, Eskisehir, Turkey

Ibrahim Yildiz, MD Department of Medical Oncology, Medical Faculty, Acibadem University, Istanbul, Turkey

Mehmet Halit Yılmaz, MD Department of Radiology, Cerrahpasa School of Medicine, Istanbul University, Istanbul, Turkey

Part I

Invasive Breast Cancer

Biopsy Techniques in Non-palpable or Palpable Breast Lesions

1

William C. Dooley

Abstract

Diagnostic breast biopsy is one of the most common medical procedures, and a variety of methods have been developed in the last 30 years to augment classic surgical incisional and excisional biopsies. Fine-needle aspiration (FNA) has an important historical role and remains among the most cost-effective methods but is limited by the weakness of current breast cytology to adequately reproduce all information provided by traditional histopathology. FNA continues to play an important role in assessing risk. Core biopsies ranging from the use of simple needle cores to larger coring devices to remove spaghetti- to macaroni-sized pieces have become the mainstay of current biopsy techniques for most palpable and non-palpable lesions. Surgical incisional and excisional biopsies, which are the classic standards, are reserved for a few exceptional circumstances, including the removal of symptomatic benign lesions or when coring biopsy tools fail to provide adequate diagnostic information and material. Ductoscopy, which was initially developed as a tool to investigate pathological nipple discharge, is an evolving technology that may have an increasing role in research and prevention as tools and techniques become more refined. Failure of biopsy to accurately diagnose breast problem remains a small but persistent problem requiring the diligent methodical use of biopsy methods and the careful consideration of issues such as sample bias when the entire lesion is not removed and there is discordance between clinical expectations and biopsy pathology.

Keywords

Breast biopsy • Breast cancer • Core biopsy • FNA • Surgical breast biopsy • Breast cytology • Ductoscopy • Mammoscopy • Breast diagnosis

W.C. Dooley, MD, FACS
Department of Surgery and OU Breast Institute,
The University of Oklahoma Health Sciences Center,
G. Rainey Williams Pavilion, Suite 2290, 920 Stanton
L. Young Blvd., Oklahoma City, OK 73103, USA
e-mail: william-dooley@ouhsc.edu

© Springer International Publishing Switzerland 2016
A. Aydiner et al. (eds.), *Breast Disease: Management and Therapies*,
DOI 10.1007/978-3-319-26012-9_1

Fine-Needle Aspiration Biopsy–Core Needle Biopsy

Fine-Needle Aspiration (FNA) Biopsy

Fine-needle aspiration has a long history in breast cancer diagnosis. It has been popularized as a part of the "triple test" for the evaluation of palpable abnormalities preceding the modern mammographic screening era [1]. FNA is a common tool in many European clinics where breast cytology is a more refined and practiced art. One of the inherent weaknesses of breast cytology is the substantial overlap in cytological appearance of many very early lesions and malignant, premalignant, and common benign lesions [2]. Further, if cancerous cells are observed, FNA cannot be used alone with cytology to definitively determine if the lesion is in situ or invasive [3, 4]. These critical issues have limited its use in the USA in favor of coring needle techniques. Globally, however, FNA remains a cost-effective tool with much value and efficiency.

FNA is typically performed to evaluate palpable abnormalities and asymmetric breast tissue in a perceived high-risk situation, to screen high-risk patients for biological markers indicative of current active proliferation to evaluate temporal breast cancer risk, or to monitor trials of prevention agents. FNA is typically performed with a 22–25 G needle on a 10 cc syringe. Local anesthesia is induced by dermal injection and installation into the region of biopsy. Rigorous rapid jiggling of the biopsy needle in and out under vacuum and releasing the vacuum before extracting the needle provides the best specimen and can be rapidly mastered by the immediate evaluation of specimen cellularity by the operator (Fig. 1.1). Initially, air-dried smears were prepared, but increasingly, the aspirate material is injected into a liquid transport fixative such as those used for cervical cytology. The cellular architecture is often less disrupted in liquid media [5]. Occasionally, the pH of the local anesthesia may impact the cellular appearance. This can be minimized by buffering the initial local anesthetic immediately prior to injection. The specimens can be adequate for routine cytology, immunohistochemistry, and molecular techniques in both clinical and research settings. Usually, FNA results are considered highly specific but variably sensitive.

The use of FNA for non-palpable abnormalities is more complex. When aspirating under image guidance, there is a slightly increased risk of parallax issues in which the aspiration is immediately in front or behind the target lesion. Because this leads to insufficient removal of the target for image confirmation, much hope is placed on the initial accuracy of the first few

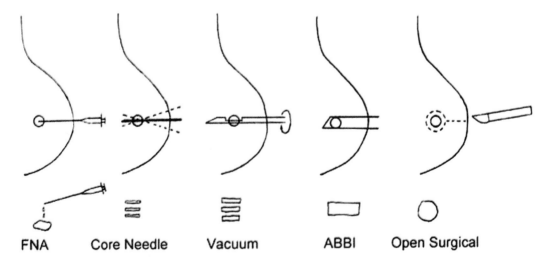

FNA   Core Needle   Vacuum   ABBI   Open Surgical

Fig. 1.1 Different types of biopsies (Reproduced with kind permission from Imaginis, Copyright 2000, Imaginis.com)

needle passes. The local anesthesia and hematoma from the biopsy typically rapidly interfere with imaging quality as the FNA continues. The results for non-palpable lesions are always confounded by these issues.

The most important use of FNA remains as a part of the triple test [1]. This technique has stood the test of time as highly reliable predating mammographic screening through the current plethora of new imaging technologies to evaluate palpable breast lesions. Most palpable breast lesions will have imageable lesions, which are then amenable to coring biopsy techniques. However, there are always some patients with odd asymmetric thickening, regionally focused reproducibility, worrisome history, or other factors that make the breast clinician suspicious of a significant abnormality in spite of negative breast imaging [6]. In this situation, the use of FNA as the third and final arm of a triple test is well justified by the medical literature and is considered highly accurate. Under this circumstance, the goal of screening is to confirm the presence or absence of significant glandular proliferation. If proliferative cells are not observed in an adequate cellular specimen, the probability of breast cancer is exceedingly low. If, however, proliferative ductal epithelial cells are observed, open surgical biopsy of the region is required to exclude an image-occult neoplastic change.

Core Needle Biopsy

Core needle biopsies were developed as a limited method of performing an incisional biopsy for diagnosis. Early coring needle technologies were cumbersome and were often used primarily for tiny biopsies of solid organs, such as the liver and kidney. In the late 1980s, the technology improved substantially with the introduction of automated coring needles. These needles typically cored 14 G, 16 G, or 18 G samples approximately 1–2 cm in length [7]. With improving mammographic imaging and increased facility with breast ultrasound, these new coring needles were applied to breast diagnostic work in the early 1990s. A series of trials demonstrated that these mini incisional biopsies

by needle under image guidance could accurately diagnose many breast lesions. Because of the small diameter and rapid fixation of these biopsies, the time from biopsy to diagnosis began to decrease rapidly [8]. Establishing the diagnosis prior to the initial surgical procedure dramatically improved the chances of obtaining surgically clear margins during the initial operation and expanded the use of breast conservation dramatically. This was a crucial event in the evolution of the diagnostic process for breast cancer [9, 10].

Core biopsy methods vary slightly in specific needle design and the imaging used to direct the biopsy. As the popularity of core biopsy has increased, this method is now used not only for non-palpable lesions but also for palpable lesions combined with imaging to ensure biopsy of the center of the target lesion. After pressing a button or trigger, each of the coring needles usually throws out a coring section up to 2 cm in length and then rapidly covers the entire coring section and tissue core with a larger hollow needle of the final core size. This basic mechanism underlies many of the shortcomings of this method. The rapid-fire mechanism can allow a hard lesion in the midst of soft breast tissue to bounce off, and thus, the core will be of the tissue side of the target and not the target itself. Similarly, the cores are relatively small in the imaged lesions, and imaging is usually inadequate to visualize the actual hole or tract after needle removal. This introduces two possibilities: that the target bounced off the needle or that the parallax issues of imaging led to a false assurance of central target biopsy. A single core in the center of the target should be histologically adequate for nearly all lesions except borderline atypia vs. in situ disease. Clearly, early experience demonstrated that one core was not adequate, and multiple cores are now obtained to reduce the possibility of underdiagnosis due to sampling bias [11–13]. Based on specific histologies and imaging characteristics, 4–15 cores to assure an adequate diagnosis are common [14] (Figs. 1.2, 1.3, 1.4, 1.5, 1.6, 1.7, 1.8, 1.9, 1.10, 1.11, and 1.12). However, when substantial proliferative changes, such as atypia and papillary changes,

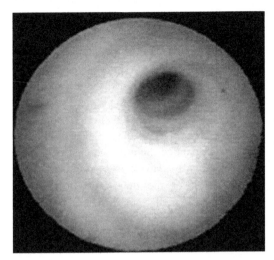

Fig. 1.2 Clean duct

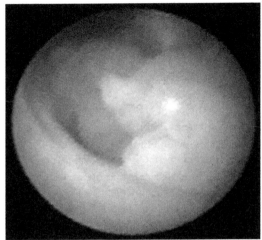

Fig. 1.5 Papillomas

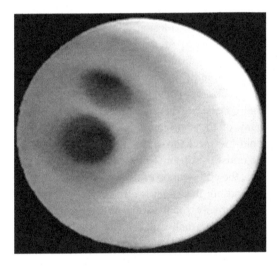

Fig. 1.3 Bifurcation

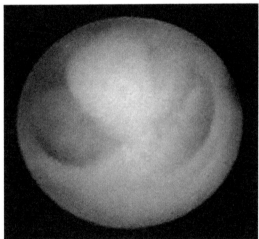

Fig. 1.6 Papillomas

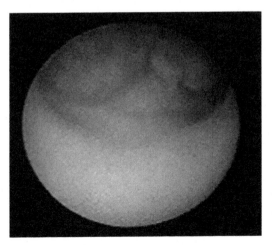

Fig. 1.4 Papilloma

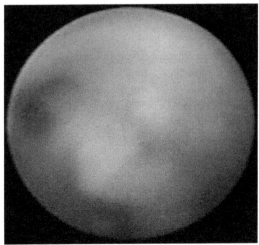

Fig. 1.7 DCIS

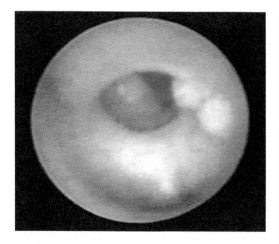

Fig. 1.8 Low-grade DCIS

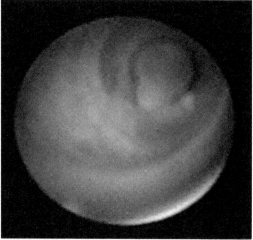

Fig. 1.11 DCIS

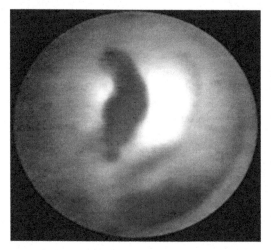

Fig. 1.9 High-grade DCIS

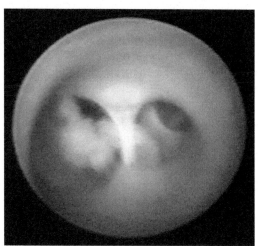

Fig. 1.12 High-grade DCIS

are observed, the core diagnosis is not reliable and requires open surgical excisional biopsy.

Core biopsy needles today are usually used in larger and advanced tumors where issues of sample bias are markedly diminished. Their importance in the evolution of modern breast diagnostic biopsy cannot, however, be understated. Reducing the number of breast cancers diagnosed by surgical biopsy has dramatically increased successful breast conservation and revolutionized the last two decades of breast cancer care in North America and Europe [15].

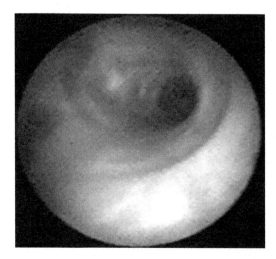

Fig. 1.10 DCIS

Vacuum-Assisted Breast Biopsy, Rotating Core Biopsy, and Radiofrequency Minimal Access Incisional Biopsy

The problem of throwing cores limited the safe use of older core needles to the axilla close to vessels or close to the chest wall. A new generation of coring devices have been developed to address the movement of the coring needle during biopsy to allow visualization of the biopsy in real time and increase the volume of tissue removed, thereby reducing the number of cores required to make a diagnosis and increasing the percentage of cores with actual pieces of the target lesion [12] (Fig. 1.12). The first versions were 10 G or larger solid-appearing needles inserted into the breast. Once inserted into or beside the target lesion, a trap door opens, allowing suction to be applied to pull tissue into the center of the needle. A rotating core inside the needle is then deployed to remove a larger core of tissue. Most of these needles allow the outer needle shaft to be left in place as cores are pulled out and new cores are taken. Reduced movement of the coring needle clearly reduces issues of biopsy pain but also allows sufficient excision of tissue in one location to confirm the adequacy of sampling by imaging before needle withdrawal.

This technique works well, but some of the hardest lesions within the softest breast tissue still cannot be sucked into the vacuum section of the needle. Alternatives, such as the insertion of a 19 G cold core needle into the lesion, followed by freezing of the lesion with liquid CO_2 and removal of a larger rotating core around the central needle within the ice ball, enable the biopsy of even the hardest lesions. Another approach to small hard lesions is to use radiofrequency (cautery) with an excision device introduced thru a large needle with a hole 5–8 mm in diameter. Rings of RF wire are deployed from the tip of such devices and under image control can be used to excise pieces of tissue up to 2 cm in diameter. Such techniques approach minimal access surgical incisional biopsy. Early enthusiasts believed that surgical lumpectomy might be accomplished on small subcentimeter lesions;

success of this type has been limited, which likely reflects the joint technical limitations of the RF devices and real-time imaging in 3-D during the biopsy.

These techniques have dramatically reduced the number of cores required for diagnostic accuracy. However, more than one core is still required in the majority of cases, and when there is histological atypia or worrisome changes, wide excision of the region surgically is required to prevent missed cancers. All of these techniques can be performed stereotactically with mammography or MRI. Because of their complexity and logistical setup issues and positioning, using mammography or MRI extends the duration of each biopsy procedure to 40–60 min, with multiple staff to support the equipment and patient needs. As ultrasound imaging has improved, the majority of image non-palpable lesions can be observed sufficiently well to direct one of these coring techniques without difficult patient positioning and minimal additional staff. The vast majority of breast biopsies today of palpable or non-palpable lesions are ultrasound-directed and continuously imaged vacuum core biopsies. Although small lesions less than 1 cm may be completely removed, imaging cannot be used to adequately predict which patients have received adequate histological excision without actually examining the exterior margin of an intact en bloc resection or its equivalent.

Surgical Biopsy: Incisional Biopsy– Excisional Biopsy

Excisional surgical biopsy of palpable or non-palpable image-visible lesions will always be considered the gold standard. Even when surgical excision occurs, the missed cancer rate is approximately 2 % or 1/50. Because breast biopsy is one of the most common medical procedures, this rate translates into many missed cancers. Even when the palpable lesion is obvious or the image lesion is clearly observed in specimen radiography, it is always necessary to ensure all potential abnormal targets are identified. In the case of palpable lesions, this requires adequate pre- and postoperative imaging to ensure any allied lesions are removed and never assuming that the imaged lesion is the palpable lesion without adequate proof. In the case of imaged lesions, the surgeon must carefully bimanually palpate the surrounding breast tissue to ensure all abnormalities have been identified. Similarly, postoperative imaging within 6 months or sooner revealing no additional lesions or residual lesions is needed.

Surgical incisional biopsy has been commonly used for more than a century for the diagnosis of large breast lesions and lesions that involve the skin [15]. Coring tools can often replace formal open surgical biopsies. There are circumstances in which incisions are still required, such as a mass coexistent with an abscess for which diagnostic biopsy can be accomplished by incision of the wall of the abscess during abscess drainage. Inflammatory breast cancer is a clinical diagnosis, but it is occasionally useful for clinical practice or research stratification to determine the involvement of dermal lymphatics. Such involvement was typically determined with an incision in a small region of inflamed skin. Today, 3–5-mm dermal punch core biopsy tools allow a "needle-like" approach to these diagnostic biopsies. Because a smaller sample is taken, sample bias is introduced, as with needle core biopsies. The region most likely to have dermal lymphatic involvement is the skin at the areolar edge in the same quadrant as the inflammatory lesion. Small core biopsies in this region can avoid the removal of skin requiring suturing required in older times. Similarly, these same dermal cores can be used to assess lesions of the nipple papilla for both Paget's disease and nipple adenomas.

Surgical excisional biopsy can be directed by palpation or use of an imaging adjunct. Ultrasound provides an almost direct extension of physical exam and can often localize well the majority of non-palpable abnormalities. For years, the ultrasound equipment available in imaging suites has had much greater resolution than those available in operating rooms. As more surgeons become adequately trained to use ultrasound equipment, intraoperative imaging with the highest quality devices has transformed breast surgery and especially added to our ability to achieve adequate

margins during the initial therapeutic operation. When the target lesion is not clearly visible by ultrasound or palpable, we must resort to some marking of the target region that can be used by the surgeon because excision between plates of a mammogram device or in the magnet of an MRI is difficult. The core biopsy world has introduced a series of markers to leave behind for future imaging post biopsy. Any of these markers can be used in this circumstance, the most useful of which are ultrasound-visible post-core markers that can be intraoperatively imaged with ultrasound during the surgical procedure. The classic method, however, has been to deploy a wire, needle, and/or dye injection into the target region under image guidance for the surgeon to use to find the lesion in question. In the case of malignant core biopsies, this has even evolved into leaving a small radioactive bead in the biopsy cavity to guide later wide excision lumpectomy. Whichever method is used, imaging the extracted tissue or the residual breast immediately post-procedure is the best but not an absolutely infallible method to assure the excision of the correct tissue target. The most efficient method is to either ultrasound the specimen or radiograph the specimen in the operating room. Using this immediate image information, the surgeon can most likely identify and remove the target lesion even if the first specimen was inadequate.

Ductoscopy

Mammary ductoscopy has evolved from initial experimentation in Japan, where pathological nipple discharge is a more common symptom of early-stage breast cancer [16]. American innovations in submillimeter endoscopes and the recognition of the safety and improved endoscopic potential when saline distension is used have prompted new interest in this technique to identify some of the earliest lesions in situ long before traditional imaging would allow detection. It is now possible to find nearly all lesions intraductally that give rise to bloody nipple discharge, atypical cells in nipple fluid, or extensive intraductal carcinoma around small early-stage breast cancers [17–22]. Biopsy tools and scope modifications that can allow biopsy under direct vision are being developed. Currently, clinically clear indications are relatively restricted. However, researchers now have a method that will repeatedly allow access to the ductal epithelium in high-risk patients. As molecular markers begin to replace traditional cytology, which has limitations as discussed before with FNA, we can expect anatomic mapping of the field defects of genetic changes that predispose to cancer and a crucial new understanding of how anatomy and molecular events interact in breast carcinogenesis [23–28]. These new understandings will hopefully shape the future of breast cancer prevention, which is beginning to replace our current standards of screening and treatment.

The most common indication for mammary ductoscopy is solitary duct spontaneous bloody nipple discharge. Occasionally, high-risk women produce abundant nipple fluid. Some prior research trials have indicated that there is increased risk if a non-lactating female is easily producing fluid [26, 29, 30]. If these high-risk women have nipple fluid cytology that is suspicious, this may appear sinister even in the absence of any imaging findings. The ducts that are producing fluid are usually quite large and can be easily cannulated with lachrymal duct probes and/or sutured with 22–24 G angiocaths. First, the duct is anesthetized and dilated by topical local anesthesia distention. Ductoscopy is readily performed with any available submillimeter endoscope. Most series of pathological nipple discharge reveal that 7–9 % are related to cancer [18, 19, 30].

Many stage 0–2 breast cancers (particularly if the invasive component is <2.5 cm) will have expressible nipple fluid [16, 28]. These ducts may produce less fluid, but if identified, can usually be used to locate the cancer and its allied proliferative changes in the region. Core biopsies performed on the nipple side of the target lesion usually disrupt the ducts making fluid, so if ductoscopy is of interest, it is important that diagnostic biopsies be performed from the deep non-nipple side of the target lesion. With some practice, ductoscopy at the time of therapeutic lumpectomy can be an important adjunct to achieving clear margins and can theoretically aid the selection of patients with limited region disease that may be ideal for partial-breast irradiation techniques.

Final Considerations

It is important to remember the 2 % miss rate of diagnostic breast biopsy in the USA. No biopsy procedure should be considered complete without a metachronous physical exam and repeat imaging after healing of the biopsy procedure. These procedures are usually performed after 6 months, and scientific data suggest that there is no decrease in survival if missed lesions are identified and removed within that initial 6-month period. This is of most crucial importance in image-guided non-palpable lesion biopsies. Any smaller incisional technique that yields pathological information that is unexpected or discordant with clinical expectations requires immediate confirmation by surgical excisional biopsy. Any surgical excision that does not clearly contain the lesion on specimen radiograph is difficult to resolve. Immediate postoperative (within the first month) imaging can be used, but edema and healing changes may substantially interfere with accurate target detection. If the pathology is concordant in these cases, 6-month imaging and exam follow-up seem prudent.

References

1. Nagar S, Iacco A, Riggs T, Kestenberg W, Keidan R. An analysis of fine needle aspiration versus core needle biopsy in clinically palpable breast lesions: a report on the predictive values and a cost comparison. Am J Surg. 2012;204(2):193–8.
2. Weigner J, Zardawi I, Braye S. The true nature of atypical breast cytology. Acta Cytol. 2013;57(5):464–72.
3. Fung AD, Collins JA, Campassi C, Ioffe OB, Staats PN. Performance characteristics of ultrasound-guided fine-needle aspiration of axillary lymph nodes for metastatic breast cancer employing rapid on-site evaluation of adequacy: analysis of 136 cases and review of the literature. Cancer Cytopathol. 2014;122(4):282–91.

4. Laucirica R, Bentz JS, Khalbuss WE, Clayton AC, Souers RJ, Moriarty AT. Performance characteristics of mucinous (colloid) carcinoma of the breast in fine-needle aspirates: observations from the College of American Pathologists Interlaboratory Comparison Program in Nongynecologic Cytopathology. Arch Pathol Lab Med. 2011;135(12):1533–8.

5. Konofaos P, Kontzoglou K, Parakeva P, Kittas C, Margari N, Giaxnaki E, Pouliakis M, Kouraklis G, Karakitsos P. The role of ThinPrep cytology in the investigation of ki-67 index, p53 and HER-2 detection in fine-needle aspirates of breast tumors. J BUON. 2013;18(2):352.

6. Georgieva RD, Obdeijn IM, Jager A, Hooning MJ, Tilanus-Linthorst MM, van Deurzen CH. Breast fine-needle aspiration cytology performance in the high-risk screening population: a study of BRCA1/BRCA2 mutation carriers. Cancer Cytopathol. 2013;121(10):561–7.

7. Lai HW, Wu HK, Kuo SJ, Chen ST, Tseng HS, Tseng LM, et al. Differences in accuracy and underestimation rates for 14- versus 16-gauge core needle biopsies in ultrasound-detectable breast lesions. Asian J Surg. 2013;36(2):83–8.

8. Gadgil PV, Korourian S, Malak S, Ochoa D, Lipschitz R, Henry-Tillman R, et al. Surgeon-performed touch preparation of breast core needle biopsies may provide accurate same-day diagnosis and expedite treatment planning. Ann Surg Oncol. 2014;21(4):1215–21.

9. Koca B, Kuru B, Yuruker S, Gokgul B, Ozen N. Factors affecting surgical margin positivity in invasive ductal breast cancer patients who underwent breast-conserving surgery after preoperative core biopsy diagnosis. J Kor Surg Soc. 2013;84(3):154–9.

10. Polat AV, Soran A, Andacoglu O, Kamali Polat A, McGuire K, Diego E, et al. The importance of preoperative needle core breast biopsy results on resected tissue volume, margin status, and cosmesis. J BUON. 2013;18(3):601–7.

11. D'Alfonso TM, Wang K, Chiu YL, Shin SJ. Pathologic upgrade rates on subsequent excision when lobular carcinoma in situ is the primary diagnosis in the needle core biopsy with special attention to the radiographic target. Arch Pathol Lab Med. 2013;137(7):927–35.

12. Polom K, Murawa D, Kurzawa P, Michalak M, Murawa P. Underestimation of cancer in case of diagnosis of atypical ductal hyperplasia (ADH) by vacuum assisted core needle biopsy. Rep Pract Oncol Radiother. 2012;17(3):129–33.

13. Buckley ES, Webster F, Hiller JE, Roder DM, Farshid G. A systematic review of surgical biopsy for LCIS found at core needle biopsy – do we have the answer yet? Eur J Surg Oncol. 2014;122(4):282–91.

14. Lee SK, Yang JH, Woo SY, Lee JE, Nam SJ. Nomogram for predicting invasion in patients with a preoperative diagnosis of ductal carcinoma in situ of the breast. Br J Surg. 2013;100(13):1756–63.

15. Soot L, Weerasinghe R, Wang L, Nelson HD. Rates and indications for surgical breast biopsies in a community-based health system. Am J Surg. 2014;207(4):499–503.

16. Dooley WC. Breast ductoscopy and the evolution of the intra-ductal approach to breast cancer. Breast J. 2009;15 Suppl 1:S90–4.

17. Kamali S, Bender O, Kamali GH, Aydin MT, Karatepe O, Yuney E. Diagnostic and therapeutic value of ductoscopy in nipple discharge and intraductal proliferations compared with standard methods. Breast Cancer. 2014;21(2):154–61.

18. Fisher CS, Margenthaler JA. A look into the ductoscope: its role in pathologic nipple discharge. Ann Surg Oncol. 2011;18(11):3187–91.

19. Dubowy A, Raubach M, Topalidis T, Lange T, Eulenstein S, Hünerbein M. Breast duct endoscopy: ductoscopy from a diagnostic to an interventional procedure and its future perspective. Acta Chir Belg. 2011;111(3):142–5.

20. Cyr AE, Margenthaler JA, Conway J, Rastelli AL, Davila RM, Gao F, et al. Correlation of ductal lavage cytology with ductoscopy-directed duct excision histology in women at high risk for developing breast cancer: a prospective, single-institution trial. Ann Surg Oncol. 2011;18(11):3192–7.

21. Tang SS, Twelves DJ, Isacke CM, Gui GP. Mammary ductoscopy in the current management of breast disease. Surg Endosc. 2011;25(6):1712–22.

22. Rose C, Bojahr B, Grunwald S, Frese H, Jäger B, Ohlinger R. Ductoscopy-based descriptors of intraductal lesions and their histopathologic correlates. Onkologie. 2010;33(6):307–12.

23. Zhu W, Qin W, Zhang K, Rottinghaus GE, Chen YC, Kliethermes B, et al. Trans-resveratrol alters mammary promoter hypermethylation in women at increased risk for breast cancer. Nutr Cancer. 2012;64(3):393–400.

24. Yamamoto D, Tsubota Y, Yoshida H, Kanematsu S, Sueoka N, Uemura Y, Tanaka K, Kwon AH. Endoscopic appearance and clinicopathological character of breast cancer. Anticancer Res. 2011;31(10):3517–20.

25. Feng XZ, Song YH, Zhang FX, Jiang CW, Mei H, Zhao B. Diagnostic accuracy of fiberoptic ductoscopy plus in vivo iodine staining for intraductal proliferative lesions. Chin Med J (Engl). 2013;126(16):3124–9.

26. Sauter ER, Klein-Szanto A, Macgibbon B, Ehya H. Nipple aspirate fluid and ductoscopy to detect breast cancer. Diagn Cytopathol. 2010;38(4):244–51.

27. Vaughan A, Crowe JP, Brainard J, Dawson A, Kim J, Dietz JR. Mammary ductoscopy and ductal washings for the evaluation of patients with pathologic nipple discharge. Breast J. 2009;15(3):254–60.

28. Hünerbein M, Raubach M, Dai K, Schlag PM. Ductoscopy of intraductal neoplasia of the breast. Recent Results Cancer Res. 2009;173:129–36.

29. Montroni I, Santini D, Zucchini G, Fiacchi M, Zanotti S, Ugolini G, et al. Nipple discharge: is its significance as a risk factor for breast cancer fully understood? Observational study including 915 consecutive patients who underwent selective duct excision. Breast Cancer Res Treat. 2010;123(3):895–900.

30. Kamali S, Bender O, Aydin MT, Yuney E, Kamali G. Ductoscopy in the evaluation and management of nipple discharge. Ann Surg Oncol. 2010;17(3):778–83.

Evaluation of Patients for Metastases Prior to Primary Therapy

2

Deniz Eren-Böler and Neslihan Cabioğlu

Abstract

For axillary staging, preoperative US and needle biopsy have emerged as effective methods for triaging women with breast cancer directly to axillary surgery for SLNB or ALND or to neoadjuvant chemotherapy in those with axillary node-positive disease. However, there is no perfect modality to identify metastatic disease in breast cancer; every diagnostic test has its own advantages and limitations. The available evidence suggests routine evaluation for stage III and possibly stage II breast cancer using imaging techniques including FDG PET/CT. The workup of abnormal findings in breast cancer patients is by patient signs and symptoms including history and physical examination, laboratory tests, imaging, biopsy of suspicious finding in imaging studies, and monitoring serum markers.

Keywords

Staging of breast cancer • Axillary staging • PET/CT

Introduction

Diagnostic and therapeutic modalities for breast cancer continue to improve, and the ultimate goal of achieving disease-free and long-term survival is increasingly feasible. Tumor-node-metastasis (TNM) staging, which quantifies the physical extent of disease, has been the mainstay of prognosis prediction [1]. The accurate staging of breast cancer is crucial for clinical decision-making because the extent of the disease has a direct impact on the patient's prognosis and consequently alters therapeutic choices, e.g., locoregional versus systemic therapy [2].

D. Eren-Böler, MD (✉)
Department of General Surgery,
Acıbadem University Medical Faculty,
Kerem Aydınlar Kampüsü,
Istanbul, Turkey
e-mail: denniseren@yahoo.com

N. Cabioğlu
Department of Surgery, Istanbul University
Istanbul Faculty of Medicine, Istanbul, Turkey

© Springer International Publishing Switzerland 2016
A. Aydiner et al. (eds.), *Breast Disease: Management and Therapies*,
DOI 10.1007/978-3-319-26012-9_2

As with any patient, a comprehensive history and systemic physical examination are essential to identify metastasis, and the examination should focus on the chest wall, skin, contralateral breast, regional and distant lymph nodes, skeletal system, lungs, liver, and central nervous system. Laboratory testing should include complete blood count (CBC), serum calcium, and alkaline phosphatase, as well as liver and renal function tests. Diagnostic tests and staging procedures are selected based on the organ sites that are most frequently involved in metastatic breast cancer and patient signs and symptoms.

The preoperative assessment should aim to predict the N stage (lymph node metastases) and M stage (distant metastases).

Workup for Axillary Metastases

Axillary lymph node status has long been considered the most important prognostic indicator of recurrence and survival for newly diagnosed breast cancer patients [3–5]. The accurate prediction of axillary lymph node status is the primary objective of physical examination and imaging and is essential in developing a treatment plan, which may include neoadjuvant chemotherapy, immediate reconstruction, and/or intraoperative accelerated partial-breast radiotherapy [5].

Physical examination is a primitive and rudimentary method for the detection of axillary metastasis. Although the palpation of enlarged lymph nodes in the axilla may indicate metastasis, differentiating a metastatic lymph node from an inflamed or reactive one by physical examination is extremely difficult. The sensitivity is very low ranging from 25 % to 39 % in various reports [6–9]. Imaging techniques are required to evaluate the axillary lymph node status before surgery.

The standard imaging method for the detection of breast cancer is mammography (MMG). Although the imaging of axillary lymph nodes is not consistent, lymph nodes in the lower part of the axilla can be visualized [10]. Valente et al. have reported a high likelihood of malignancy if suspicious nodes are identified in the axilla, with 99.5 % specificity [8]. As a complement to MMG, axillary ultrasound (US) is a simple test that has been increasingly used in the preoperative setting

to detect axillary metastases. Fine-needle aspiration biopsy (FNAB) or core biopsy (CB) of the suspicious lymph node has also been suggested to decrease the number of patients undergoing sentinel lymph node biopsy (SLNB) and subsequent axillary lymph node dissection (ALND) and, consequently, reduce healthcare costs [11].

The criteria to label a lymph node as suspicious in US evaluation include size, cortical thickening (>3 mm), a multilobulated cortex, the absence of the fatty hilum, and the presence of nonhilar blood flow (which reflects increased vascularity) [12–16]. Because lymph flows through the cortex toward the hilum in a normal lymph node, malignant cells are first deposited in the cortex and cause early architectural destruction that can be observed by US, followed by changes in the hilum [15]. Moore et al. have reported that cortical abnormalities are most predictive of N1a disease, whereas the loss or compression of the hyperechoic region or cortical hilum along with abnormal lymph node shape is more commonly observed in N2-N3 disease [16].

However, US alone is insufficient to accurately stage the axilla and is therefore combined with either FNAB or CB of the suspicious lymph node. The reported sensitivity and specificity of axillary US and percutaneous biopsy range from 45.2–86.2 % to 40.5–99 %, respectively [15–19]. This variability may be due to the application of nonuniform morphological criteria across different studies and the heterogeneity of study designs. In a systematic review conducted by Alvarez et al., the average sensitivity of US was 68 %, whereas the average specificity was 75.2 % if size (<5 mm or visible nodes on US) was used as the only criterion for malignant involvement [12]. However, the average sensitivity was 71 % with 96 % specificity when morphological criteria were used. In patients with nonpalpable axillary lymph nodes, sensitivity and specificity were 60.9 % and 75.2 %, respectively, when size was the only parameter. The corresponding values when morphological criteria were used were 43.9 % and 92.4 %, respectively.

In a meta-analysis of 21 studies by Houssami et al., the median US sensitivity and specificity were 61.4 % [with an interquartile range (IQR) of 51.2–79.4 %] and 82 % [IQR 76.9–89 %], respectively. In these studies, for the subset of 1,733 subjects who then were selected for US-guided needle biopsy based on US features, the median sensitivity and specificity were 79.4 % and 100 %, respectively [20, 21]. The authors suggested that preoperative US and needle biopsy could be used to effectively triage women with breast cancer directly to axillary surgery.

Diepstraten et al. conducted a meta-analysis of pooled data from 31 studies to estimate the false-negative rate of US and percutaneous biopsy; this rate was defined as the proportion of women with a negative US with or without aspiration biopsy in whom axillary nodal metastases were detected at SLNB [22]. For 50 % of the breast cancer patients with metastasis in the axilla, axillary involvement could be identified preoperatively by axillary US-guided FNAB or CB. However, 25 % of the patients (one in four women) with a negative US and biopsy result had axillary metastases at subsequent SLNB. Thus, a negative US and biopsy result for metastasis cannot preclude an operative intervention in the axilla for precise staging.

New techniques have been evaluated to increase the sensitivity and specificity of axillary US. Sever et al. [23] have demonstrated that contrast-enhanced US can be used to identify the sentinel lymph node, thus enabling targeted biopsy, which may reduce the false-negative rate. US elastography for the detection of metastatic lymph nodes by measuring stiffness on US examination has shown promise for increasing the sensitivity of conventional US, although reports are limited in number and patient sample size [24, 25].

MRI has been the best method to show the anatomy in relation to pathology [8]. Level 1–2 axillary lymph nodes as well as internal mammary and level III lymph nodes are visualized. The reported sensitivity of MRI is 36–78 %, with higher specificity (93–100 %) [7, 26, 27]. However, some studies have failed to demonstrate the superiority of MRI over axillary US; the sensitivity of MRI for axillary lymph node metastases was <40 %, whereas accuracy was similar to axillary US for the detection of axillary metastasis [8, 28].

Valente et al. have reported a trade-off in sensitivity and specificity for the prediction of lymph node involvement in breast cancer patients using a combination of physical examination, MMG, US, and MRI. If any of these modalities is suspicious, there is a 56 % chance of metastatic disease in the patient, which increases to nearly 100 % if three or four modalities are suspicious for metastatic disease [8]. The major flaw in combining various modalities is that the specific axillary lymph nodes detected by different imaging modalities cannot be correlated when the modality that initially detected the suspicious lymph node cannot be used as a guide to perform percutaneous biopsy of the suspicious node.

The methods for sampling and pathological assessment of the sample retrieved by percutaneous biopsy are also subject to limitations. Percutaneous FNAB only samples a portion of the node, and a negative FNAB or CB result does not exclude axillary metastasis. In a comparison of FNAB and CB in a series of 178 patients, Rautiainen et al. observed a sensitivity of 72.5 % and 88.2 %, respectively, and a specificity of 100 % for both methods [29]. The overall accuracy in this study was 78.8 % for FNAB and 90.9 % for CB. Additional histopathological examination was tested to improve the accuracy of CB of the morphologically abnormal lymph node but failed to provide a benefit [30]. Despite attempts to decrease the number of patients referred to the operating room for SLNB by increasing the accuracy of US and percutaneous biopsy, one major issue remains—the correlation of the suspicious lymph nodes with the sentinel nodes is only 64–78.3 % in perioperative frozen sections [14, 31].

The ACOSOG Z0011 trial recently provided insights into the management of the axilla in patients with T1-2N0 breast cancer by demonstrating that ALND can be omitted in patients with one or two positive sentinel lymph nodes (SLNs) without negative impact on disease-free survival or disease recurrence [32, 33]. In this group of patients, the value of US and percutaneous biopsy becomes questionable because the presence of ITCs or micrometastases in SLN core biopsy specimens may not correlate with the actual size of the LN metastatic disease on final surgical histology [34]. Therefore, the ACOSOG Z0011 trial casts doubt on the desirability of US-guided percutaneous biopsy in cT1-2N0 patients. However, US-guided percutaneous biopsy might be helpful to exclude patients with a higher lymph node ratio (LNR; defined as the number of positive nodes/number of nodes dissected), and additional studies are needed.

FDG PET/CT is a recently evolving technique used to stage patients pre- and postoperatively. Several studies have reported variable sensitivities of FDG PET/CT of 37–95 % for the detection of axillary metastases [35–39]. The accuracy decreases for small (<10 mm) metastatic lymph nodes and micrometastatic disease. Other studies have reported high sensitivity and specificity in detecting axillary metastasis and that FDG PET/CT could modify the TNM staging in 47 % of patients with breast cancer [35, 36]. The specificity and positive predictive value of FDG PET/CT are better (96 % and 88 %, respectively) for the prediction of axillary disease and correlates well with SLNB. However, the relatively poor sensitivity of FDG PET/CT must be considered in treatment planning [36, 39].

In a meta-analysis, Cooper et al. [40] reported that a high false-negative rate precludes the recommendation of FDG PET/CT for routine application in cases of clinically negative axilla. The clinical value of false-negative axilla has not been established because reported involvement has been limited to the sentinel node, some of which were micrometastases [41].

The sensitivity of FDG PET/CT for assessing the primary lesion and axilla may be increased by performing the examination in a prone position. In a prone position, the tumor can be more clearly distinguished from adjacent structures, enabling a more extensive evaluation of the axillary fat and its lymph nodes. More studies are needed to assess the efficacy of these protocols in increasing the sensitivity of FDG PET/CT in detecting axillary disease (Fig. 2.1a) [42].

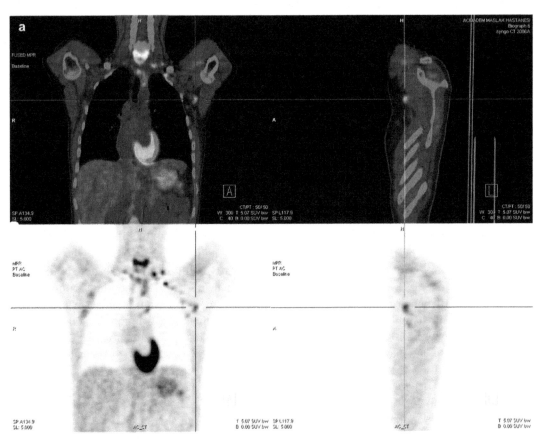

Fig. 2.1 (**a**) FDG PET/CT of a patient with increased SUV in the left axillary lymph nodes suspicious for metastases. (**b**) FDG PET/CT of a patient with increased SUV in the right axillary lymph nodes and the right pulmonary nodule suspicious for metastases. (**c**) FDG PET/CT of a patient with increased SUV in the left internal mammary lymph nodes suspicious for metastases. (**d**) NAF PET/CT of a patient with disseminated bone metastases in the calvarium, ribs, spine, pelvis, right humerus, and right femur suspicious for metastases

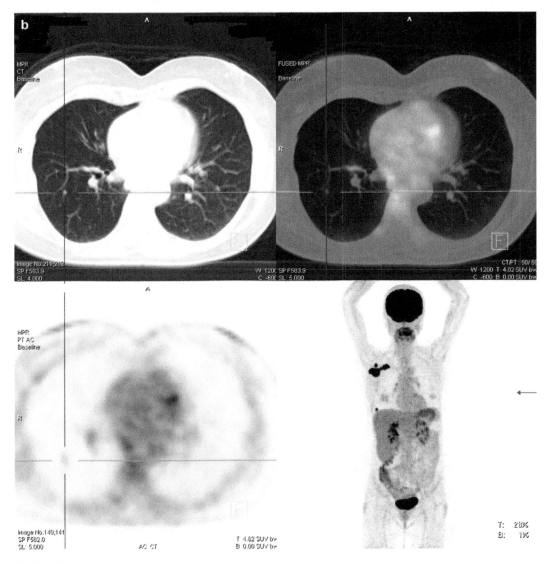

Fig. 2.1 (continued)

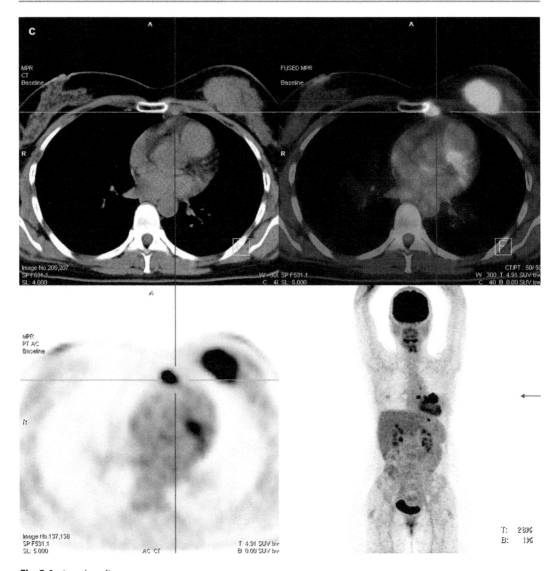

Fig. 2.1 (continued)

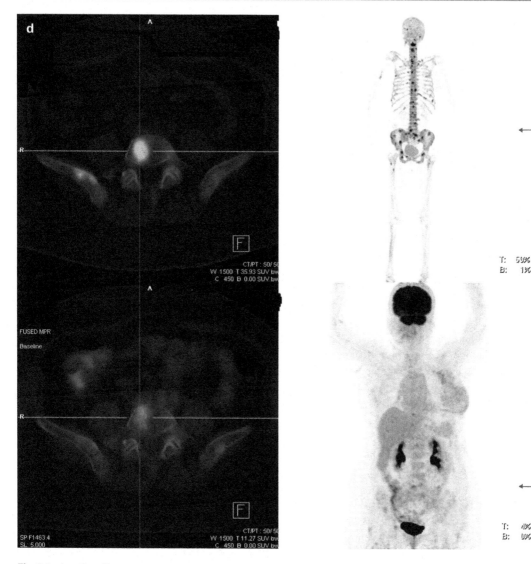

Fig. 2.1   (continued)

A tumor burden threshold must be met to detect metastatic lymph nodes using current imaging modalities, particularly FDG PET/CT. The ability to detect microscopic metastases prior to surgery and the correlation of these data with disease-free survival and/or overall survival in clinical practice remain to be established. At present, there is no imaging modality or combination of modalities that can reach the accuracy of and replace SLNB. In addition, there is also no modality that can be used to preclude SLNB where it is found to be negative in a subset of patients.

Workup for Distant Metastases

The presence of distant metastases is an adverse prognostic factor for survival [43]. The identification of unexpected distant metastases in a patient with a newly diagnosed breast cancer usually alters the management strategy. Approximately 4 % of patients with a diagnosis of breast cancer will have distant metastases at the time of presentation, and the majority of these will have signs and symptoms of metastasis [44]; 10 % of these patients have multiple lesions at multiple sites [45].

Noninvasive radiological workup targets the most common sites of distant metastasis: the bones, lungs, and liver [46]. The commonly employed tests are bone scan, chest radiography (which is replaced by diagnostic chest CT), and liver US. The sensitivity of these tests has been questioned in several studies that report inappropriateness in the subgroup of patients with small tumors and absent or minimal involvement of the axillary lymph nodes [46–48]. NCCN guidelines recommend CBC, liver function tests, alkaline phosphatase, bilateral mammography, and US/MRI (as needed) for all patients, whereas additional tests are required in the presence of specific signs or symptoms for stages I–II B [49]. However, for stage IIIA disease (T3N1M0) or locally advanced breast cancer, chest CT, abdominal ± pelvic CT or MRI, bone scan or sodium fluoride (NaF) PET/CT (optional), or FDG PET/CT (optional) are suggested.

As the number of early breast cancer patients has increased, the detection of possible distant metastasis remains to be addressed. Guidelines lack consensus about whom to evaluate and how to evaluate patients with primary operable breast cancer [46–48, 50, 51]. It is crucial to define a subgroup of patients in whom positive findings on staging tests would alter the treatment plan and provide more efficient local and systemic treatment to save healthcare costs and ensure optimal use of resources. Unnecessary examinations constitute physical, psychosocial, and financial burdens for both the patient and the healthcare providers.

The presence of detectable metastatic disease in breast cancer patients at the time of primary diagnosis is exceedingly low and increases from stage I to stage III [46, 47]. Bone is the most common site of metastasis; according to a systematic review by Myers, the incidence of positive bone scan across studies is 0.9–40 % for all stages, with the lowest incidence in stage I patients (0.5 %, 95 % confidence interval 0.1–0.9) and highest in stage III patients (8.3 %, 95 % CI 6.7–9.9) [47]. The incidences of liver and lung metastasis are even lower than that of bone metastasis. The incidence of liver metastasis is 0 %, 0.4 %, and 2 % for stage I, II, and III

diseases, respectively. The detection of lung metastases by chest X-ray is similar, with incidences of 0.1 %, 0.2 %, and 1.7 % for stage I, II, and III disease, respectively. Chen et al. found a prevalence of lung metastasis of 0.099 % in early breast cancer patients who were upstaged to stage IV by chest X-ray in a series of 1,493 subjects [52]. Puglisi found no pulmonary or liver metastases but only bone metastases in only 5 % of 516 patients using traditional modalities (i.e., bone scan, liver US, and chest X-ray) [46].

As radiological modalities have evolved and are more commonly applied in general practice, chest X-ray has been replaced by diagnostic chest CT. However, the clinical value of preoperative chest CT in clinically operable and asymptomatic patients has not been established. Recently, Kim and colleagues investigated the clinical value of preoperative chest CT in 1,703 patients and detected abnormal CT findings, including suspected metastases and indeterminate nodules in the lung or liver, in 266 patients (15.6 %) [53]. Among these, 1.5 % of all patients and 9.8 % of patients with abnormal CT findings had true metastases, including 17 lung, 3 liver, and 6 lung plus liver metastases. True metastases were detected in 0.2 %, 0 %, and 6 % of patients with stage I, II, and III disease, respectively. The authors concluded that in the absence of symptoms/signs suggestive of metastatic disease, the incidence of metastases is low, and false-positive findings are more common than true-positive findings, thus failing to compensate the high cost and exposure to ionizing radiation.

FDG PET/CT is an alternative technique that is becoming more widely used to encompass all diagnostic staging in a single study. Data for its use in staging primary breast cancer are accumulating, and recent studies have addressed the added value of FDG PET/CT over conventional techniques for staging primary breast cancer (Fig. 2.1b) [42, 54–56]. In several studies, FDG PET/CT has been reported to be more effective than conventional imaging methods in detecting occult distant metastases [35, 36, 57].

FDG PET/CT is important in the detection of extra-axillary involvement, such as supraclavicular, internal mammary, and mediastinal lymph nodes [35, 58]. Bernsdorf et al. reported that FDG PET/CT alone detected 6 cases of distant metastases and 12 cases of extra-axillary LN involvement in a comparison with conventional imaging of early breast cancer larger than 2 cm [59]. The detection of internal mammary lymph node metastases may have significant prognostic and therapeutic value because these patients are likely to have worse prognosis than those without malignant involvement of these nodes (Fig. 2.1c). Similarly, in a study by Garami et al. of 115 breast cancer patients for whom traditional diagnostic modalities showed no signs of distant metastases or extensive axillary and/or extra-axillary lymphatic spread, FDG PET/CT indicated nine distant metastases that were confirmed by direct sampling in eight patients [36]. The total yield was 7–8 % and was particularly relevant for stage II disease.

FDG PET/CT can also be used to detect bone metastases. Some authors have reported that FDG PET/CT is more efficient than bone scintigraphy in detecting lytic and mixed bone metastases and bone marrow involvement but may lack sensitivity for sclerotic bone metastases, and a multimodality approach is suggested [57, 60]. NaF PET/CT is another scintigraphic imaging technique that was reported to have superior image quality and ability to evaluate skeletal disease extent compared to FDG PET/CT and 99mTc-MDP in a pilot study (Fig. 2.1d) [61].

Another issue for the routine use of FDG PET/CT for staging is low specificity. Active granulomatous infections such as tuberculosis and sarcoidosis can exhibit increased FDG uptake [62, 63]. Functional ovaries in premenopausal women can also lead to false-positive results. Increased FDG uptake represents ovarian malignancy in postmenopausal patients, whereas the results should be handled carefully in premenopausal patients, in whom the uptake may be functional or malignant [35, 62, 63].

However, the sensitivity of FDG PET/CT is limited and decreased in small and/or low-grade tumors, particularly when the tumor size is <1–2 cm [35, 36]. At this time, FDG PET/CT is not a routine imaging modality for early breast cancer staging; instead, it is recommended as an adjunctive method to evaluate distant metastasis

and regional lymph nodes in advanced breast cancer [35, 49]. FDG PET/CT is an important adjunct to conventional studies when the results are equivocal or suspicious, particularly in locally advanced or metastatic disease. However, its use has been increasing widely over bone scan and liver US in early-stage breast cancer, particularly in patients with lobular histology and receptor-negative tumors [64].

The genetic heterogeneity and subsequent different clinical courses of breast cancer have been revealed by molecular subtype classification, a breakthrough in breast cancer research [65–67]. Different subtypes have different clinical courses and responses to treatment, which means that the clinician should consider distinct subtypes before selecting appropriate therapeutic strategies. Major molecular subtypes in breast cancer differ in their ability to metastasize to distant organ(s) and share biological features and pathways with their preferred distant metastatic sites [68]. Moreover, recent studies have found that the molecular subtypes of breast cancer may change at relapse [69, 70]. The correlation of the molecular characteristics of the tumor with baseline staging tests was addressed by Chen et al., who suggested preoperative baseline staging tests for every stage III cancer but limited tests for stage II patients based on histological subtypes [71]. They recommended bone scans for HER-2-positive luminal B, nonluminal HER-2 overexpressing, and basal-like subtypes; preoperative liver US for Her-2-positive luminal B and nonluminal HER-2-overexpressing subtypes; and chest X-ray for basal-like subtypes for the early detection of distant metastases.

Summary

For axillary staging, preoperative US and needle biopsy have emerged as effective methods for triaging women with breast cancer directly to axillary surgery for SLNB or ALND or to neoadjuvant chemotherapy in those with axillary node-positive disease.

However, by now, there is no perfect modality to identify metastatic disease in breast cancer;

every diagnostic test has its own advantages and limitations. The available evidence suggests routine evaluation for stage III and possibly stage II breast cancer using imaging techniques including FDG PET/CT. The development and validation of new molecular markers in the future may be beneficial to the diagnostic and therapeutic workup of patients with breast cancer.

References

1. Carter CL, Allen C, Henson DE. Relation of tumor size, lymph node status and survival in 24,740 breast cancer cases. Cancer. 1989;63:181–7.
2. Mauri D, Pavlidis N, Ioannidis JP. Neoadjuvant versus adjuvant systemic treatment in breast cancer: a meta-analysis. J Natl Cancer Inst. 2005;97:188–94.
3. Fisher B, Bauer M, Wickerham DL, Redmond CK, Fisher ER, Cruz AB, et al. Relation of number of positive axillary nodes to the prognosis of patients with primary breast cancer. A NSABP update. Cancer. 1983;52:1551–7.
4. Clayton F, Hopkins CL. Pathologic correlates of prognosis is lymph node-positive breast carcinomas. Cancer. 1993;71:1780–90.
5. Wilking N, Rutqvist LE, Carstensen J, Mattsson A, Skoog L. Prognostic significance of axillary nodal status in primary breast cancer in relation to the number of resected nodes. Stocholm Breast Cancer Study Group. Acta Oncol. 1992;31:29–35.
6. Pamilo M, Soiva M, Lavast EM. Real-time ultrasound, axillary mammography, and clinical examination in the detection of axillary lymph node metastases in breast cancer patients. J Ultrasound Med. 1989;8:115–20.
7. Kvistad KA, Rydland J, Smethurst HB, Lundgren S, Fjosne HE, Haraldseth O. Axillary lymph node metastases in breast cancer: preoperative detection with dynamic contrast-enhanced MRI. Eur Radiol. 2000;10:1464–71.
8. Valente SA, Levine GM, Silverstein MJ, Rayhanabad JA, Weng-Grumley JG, Ji L, Holmes DR, Sposto R, Sener S. Accuracy of predicting axillary lymph node positivity by physical examination, mammography, ultrasonography and magnetic resonance imaging. Ann Surg Oncol. 2012;19:1825–30.
9. Sacre RA. Clinical evaluation of axillar lymph nodes compared to surgical and pathological findings. Eur J Surg Oncol. 1986;12:169–73.
10. Shetty MK, Carpenter WS. Sonographic evaluation of isolated abnormal axillary lymph nodes identified on mammograms. J Ultrasound Med. 2004;23:63–71.
11. Boughey JC, Moriarty JP, Degnim AC, Gregg MS, Egginton JS, Long KH. Cost modeling of preoperative axillary ultrasound and fine-needle aspiration to guide surgery for invasive breast cancer. Ann Surg Oncol. 2010;17:953–8.
12. Alvarez S, Anorbe E, Alcorta P, Lopez F, Alonso I, Cortes J. Role of sonography in the diagnosis of axillary lymph node metastases in breast cancer: a systematic review. Am J Roentgenol. 2006;186:1342–8.
13. Bedi DG, Krishnamurthy R, Krishnamurthy S, Edeikan BS, Le-Petross H, Fornage BD, et al. Cortical morphologic features of axillary lymph nodes as a predictor of metastasis in breast cancer: in vitro sonographic study. Am J Roentgenol. 2008;191:646–52.
14. Britton PD, Goud A, Godward S, Barter S, Freeman A, O'Donovan M, et al. Use of ultrasound-guided axillary node core biopsy in staging of early breast cancer. Eur Radiol. 2009;19:561–9.
15. Elmore LC, Appleton CM, Zhou G, Margenthaler JA. Axillary ultrasound in patients with clinically node-negative breast cancer: which features are predictive of disease? J Surg Res. 2013;184:234–40.
16. Moore A, Hester M, Nam MW, Brill YM, McGrath P, Wright H, et al. Distinct lymph nodal sonographic characteristics in breast cancer patients at high risk for axillary metastases correlate with the final axillary stage. Br J Radiol. 2008;81:630–6.
17. Nori J, Vanzi E, Bazzocchi M, Bufalini FN, Distante V, Branconi F, et al. Role of axillary ultrasound in the selection of breast cancer patients for sentinel node biopsy. Am J Surg. 2007;193:16–20.
18. Lee MC, Eatrides J, Chau A, Han G, Kiluk JV, Kahkpour N, et al. Consequences of axillary ultrasound in patients with T2 or greater invasive breast cancers. Ann Surg Oncol. 2011;18:72–7.
19. Park SH, Kim MJ, Park BW, Moon HJ, Kwak JY, Kim EK. Impact of preoperative ultrasonography and fine-needle aspiration of axillary lymph nodes on surgical management of primary breast cancer. Ann Surg Oncol. 2011;18:738–44.
20. Houssami N, Ciatto S, Turner RM, Cody III HS, Macaskill P. Preoperative ultrasound-guided needle biopsy of axillary nodes in invasive breast cancer: meta-analysis of its accuracy and utility in staging the axilla. Ann Surg. 2011;254:243–51.
21. Houssami N, Diepstraten SCE, Cody III HS, Turner RM, Sever AR. Clinical utility of ultrasound-needle biopsy for preoperative staging of the axilla in invasive breast cancer. Anticancer Res. 2014;34:1187–98.
22. Diepstraten SCE, Sever AR, Buckens CFM, Veldhuis WB, van Dalen T, van den Bosch MAAJ, et al. Value of preoperative ultrasound-guided axillary lymph node biopsy for preventing completion axillary lymph node dissection in breast cancer: a systematic review and meta-analysis. Ann Surg Oncol. 2014;21:51–9.
23. Sever AR, Mills P, Jones SE, Cox K, Weeks J, Fish D, et al. Preoperative sentinel node identification with ultrasound using microbubbles in patients with breast cancer. Am J Roentgenol. 2011;196:251–6.
24. Taylor K, O'Keeffe S, Britton PD, Wallis MG, Treece GM, Housden J, et al. Ultrasound elastography as an adjuvant to conventional ultrasound in the preoperative assessment of axillary lymph nodes in suspected breast cancer: a pilot study. Clin Radiol. 2011;66:1064–71.

25. Choi JJ, Kang BJ, Kim SH, Lee JH, Jeong SH, Yim HW, et al. Role of sonographic elastography in the differential diagnosis of axillary lymph nodes in breast cancer. J Ultrasound Med. 2011;30:429–36.
26. García Fernández A, Fraile M, Giménez N, Reñe A, Torras M, Canales L, et al. Use of axillary ultrasound, ultrasound-fine needle aspiration biopsy and magnetic resonance imaging in the preoperative triage of breast cancer patients considered for sentinel node biopsy. Ultrasound Med Biol. 2011;37:16–22.
27. Yoshimura G, Sakuraii T, Oura S, Suzuma T, Tamaki T, Umemura T, et al. Evaluation of axillary lymph node status in breast cancer with MRI. Breast Cancer. 1999;6:249–58.
28. Luciani A, Dao TH, Lapeyre M, Schwarzinger M, Debaecque C, Lantieri L, et al. Simultaneous bilateral breast and high-resolution axillary MRI of patients with breast cancer: preliminary results. AJR Am J Roentgenol. 2004;182:1059–67.
29. Rautianen S, Masarwah A, Sudah M, Sutela A, Pelkonen O, Joukaninen S, et al. Axillary lymph node biopsy in newly diagnosed invasive breast cancer: comparative accuracy of fine-needle aspiration biopsy versus core-needle biopsy. Radiology. 2013;269: 54–60.
30. Mullen R, Purdie CA, Jordan LB, McLean D, Whelehan P, Vinnicombe S, et al. Can additional histopathological examination of ultrasound-guided axillary lymph node core biopsies improve preoperative diagnosis of primary breast cancer nodal metastasis? Clin Radiol. 2013;68:704–7.
31. Nathanson SD, Burke M, Slater R, Kapke A. Preoperative identification of the sentinel lymph node in breast cancer. Ann Surg Oncol. 2007;14: 3102–210.
32. Giuliano AE, Hunt KK, Ballman KV, Beitsch PD, Whitworth PW, Blumencranz PW, et al. Axillary dissection vs no axillary dissection in women with invasive breast cancer and sentinel node metastasis: a randomized clinical trial. JAMA. 2011;305:569–75.
33. Giuliano AE, McCall L, Beitsch P, Whitworth PW, Blumencranz P, Leitch AM, et al. Locoregional recurrence after sentinel lymph node dissection with or without axillary dissection in patients with sentinel lymph node metastases: the American College of Surgeons Oncology Group Z0011 randomized trial. Ann Surg. 2010;252:426–32. Discussion 432–43.
34. Cox K, Sever A, Jones S, Weeks J, Mills P, Devalina H, et al. Validation of a technique suing microbubbles and contrast enhanced ultrasound (CEUS) to biopsy sentinel lymph nodes (SLN) in pre-operative breast cancer patients with a normal grey-scale axillary ultrasound. Eur J Surg Oncol. 2013;39:760–5.
35. Choi YJ, Shin YD, Kang YH, Lee MS, Lee MK, Cho BS, et al. The effects of preoperative ^{18}F-FDG PET/CT in breast cancer patients in comparison to the conventional imaging study. J Breast Cancer. 2012;15:441–8.
36. Garami Z, Hascsi Z, Varga J, Dinya T, Tanyi M, Garai I, et al. The value of 18-FDG PET/CT in early stage breast cancer compared to traditional diagnostic modalities with an emphasis on changes in disease stage designation and treatment plan. Eur J Surg Oncol. 2012;38:31–7.
37. Danforth Jr DN, Aloj L, Carrasquillo JA, Bacharach SL, Chow C, Zujewski J, et al. The role of 18F-FDG-PET in the local/regional evaluation of women with breast cancer. Breast Cancer Res Treat. 2002;75:135–46.
38. Veronesi U, De Cicco C, Galimberti VE, Fernandez JR, Rotmensz N, Viale G, et al. A comparative study on the value of FDG-PET and senti- nel node biopsy to identify occult axillary metastases. Ann Oncol. 2007;18:473–8.
39. Robertson IJ, Hand F, Kell MR. FDG-PET/CT in the staging of local/ regional metastases in breast cancer. Breast. 2011;20:491–4.
40. Cooper KL, Harnan S, Meng Y, Ward SE, Fitzgerald P, Papaioannou D, et al. Positron emission tomography (PET) for assessment of axillary lymph node status in early breast cancer: a systematic review and meta-analysis. Eur J Surg Oncol. 2011;37:187–98.
41. Zornoza G, Garcia-Velloso MJ, Sola J, Regueira FM, Pina L, Beorlegni C. 18F-FDG Pet complemented with sentinel lymph node biopsy in the detection of axillary involvement in breast cancer. Eur J Surg Oncol. 2004;30:15–9.
42. Heusner TA, Freudenberg LS, Kuehl H, Hauth EA, Veit-Haibach P, Forsting M, et al. Whole-body PET/CT-mammography for staging breast cancer: initial results. Br J Radiol. 2008;81:743–8.
43. Mahner S, Schirrmacher S, Brenner W, Jenicke L, Habermann CR, Avril N, et al. Comparison between positron emission tomography using 2-[fluorine-18] fluoro-2-deoksy-D-glucose, conventional imaging and computed tomography for staging of breast cancer. Ann Oncol. 2008;19:1249–54.
44. Ravaioli A, Pasini G, Polselli A, Papi M, Tassinari D, Arcangeli V, et al. Staging of breast cancer: new recommended standard procedure. Breast Cancer Res Treat. 2002;72:53–60.
45. Patanaphan V, Salazar OM, Risco R. Breast cancer: metastatic patterns and their prognosis. South Med J. 1988;81:1109–12.
46. Puglisi F, Follador A, Minisini AM, Cardellino GG, Russo S, Andreetta C, et al. Baseline staging tests after a new diagnosis of breast cancer: further evidence of their limited indications. Ann Oncol. 2005;16:263–6.
47. Myers RE, Johnston M, Pritchard K, Levine M, Oliver T, Breast Cancer Disease Site Group of the Cancer Care Ontario Practice Guidelines Initiative. Baseline staging tests in primary breast cancer: a practice guideline. Can Med Assoc J. 2001;164:1439–44.
48. Gerber B, Seitz E, Muller H, Krause A, Reimer T, Kundt G, et al. Perioperative metastatic disease is not indicated in patients with primary breast cancer and no clinical signs of tumor spread. Breast Cancer Res Treat. 2003;82:29–37.
49. National Comprehensive Cancer Network Clinical Practice Guidelines in Oncology, Breast Cancer. Version 2.2015. http://www.nccn.org/. Published 03.11.2015.

50. Kasem AR, Desai A, Daniell S, Sinha P. Bone scan and liver ultrasound scan in the preoperative staging for primary breast cancer. Breast J. 2006;12:544–8.

51. Tennant S, Evans A, Macmillan D, Lee A, Cornford E, James J, et al. CT staging of loco-regional breast cancer recurrence: a worthwhile practice? Clin Radiol. 2009;64:885–90.

52. Chen A, Carlson GA, Coughlin BF, Reed Jr WP, Garb JL, Frank JL. Routine chest roentgenography is unnecessary in the work-up of stage I and II breast cancer. J Clin Oncol. 2000;18:3503–6.

53. Kim H, Han W, Moon HG, Min J, Ahn SK, Kim TY, et al. The value of preoperative staging chest computed tomography to detect asymptomatic lung and liver metastasis in patients with primary breast carcinoma. Breast Cancer Res Treat. 2011;126:637–41.

54. Kumar R, Zhuang H, Schnall M, Conant E, Damia S, Weinstein S, et al. FDG PET positive lymph nodes are highly predictive of metastasis in breast cancer. Nucl Med Commun. 2006;27:231–6.

55. Yang SN, Liang JA, Lin FJ, Kao CH, Lin CC, Lee CC. Comparing whole body (18) F-2-deoxyglucose positron emission tomography and technetium-99m methylene diphosphonate bone scan to detect bone metastases in patients with breast cancer. J Cancer Res Clin Oncol. 2002;128:325–8.

56. Ueda S, Saeki T, Shigekawa T, Omata J, Moriya T, Yamamoto J, et al. 18F-fluorodeoxyglucose positron emission tomography optimizes neoadjuvant chemotherapy for primary breast cancer to achieve pathological complete response. Int J Clin Oncol. 2012;17:276–82.

57. Fuster D, Duch J, Paredes P, Velasco M, Muñoz M, Santamaria G, et al. Preoperative staging of large primary breast cancer with [18F]fluorodeoxyglucose positron emission tomography/computed tomography compared with conventional imaging procedures. J Clin Oncol. 2008;26:4746–51.

58. Eubank WB, Mankoff DA, Takasugi J, Vesselle H, Eary JF, Shanley TJ, et al. 18 fluorodeoxyglucose positron emission tomography to detect mediastinal or internal mammary metastases in breast cancer. J Clin Oncol. 2001;19:3516–23.

59. Bernsdorf M, Berthelsen AK, Wielenga VT, Kroman N, Teilum D, Binderup T, et al. Preoperative PET/CT in early-stage breast cancer. Ann Oncol. 2012;23:2277–82.

60. Ohta M, Tokuda Y, Suzuki Y, Kubota M, Makuuchi H, Tajima T, et al. Whole body PET for the evaluation of bony metastases in patients with breast cancer: comparison with 99Tcm-MDP bone scintigraphy. Nucl Med Commun. 2001;22:875–9.

61. Iagaru A, Young P, Mitra E, Dick DW, Herfkens R, Gambhir SS. Pilot prospective evaluation of 99mTc-MDP scintigraphy, 18F NaF PET/CT, 18F FDG PET/CT and whole-body MRI for detection of skeletal metastases. Clin Nucl Med. 2013;38(7): e290–6.

62. Kumar R, Halanaik D, Malhotra A. Clinical applications of positron emission tomography-computed tomography in oncology. Indian J Cancer. 2010;47:100–19.

63. Alkhawaldeh K, Bural G, Kumar R, Alavi A. Impact of dual-time-point (18)F-FDG PET imaging and partial volume correction in the assessment of solitary pulmonary nodules. Eur J Nucl Med Mol Imaging. 2008;35:246–52.

64. Crivello ML, Ruth K, Sigurdson ER, Egleston BR, Evers K, Wong YN, Boraas M, Bleicher RJ. Advanced imaging modalities in early stage breast cancer: preoperative use in the United States Medicare population. Ann Surg Oncol. 2013;20:102–10.

65. Goldhirsch A, Wood WC, Coates AS, Gelber RD, Thürlimann B, Senn HJ. Panel members. Strategies for subtypes–dealing with the diversity of breast cancer: highlights of the St. Gallen international expert consensus on the primary therapy of early breast cancer 2011. Ann Oncol. 2011;33:1736–47.

66. Nielsen TO, Hsu FD, Jensen K, Cheang M, Karaca G, Hu Z, Hernandez-Boussard T, Livasy C, Cowan D, Dressler L, Akslen LA, Ragaz J, Gown AM, Gilks CB, van de Rijn M, Perou CM. Immunohistochemical and clinical characterization of the basal-like subtype of invasive breast carcinoma. Clin Cancer Res. 2004;33:5367–74.

67. Cheang MC, Chia SK, Voduc D, Gao D, Leung S, Snider J, et al. Ki67 index, HER2 status, and prognosis of patients with luminal B breast cancer. J Natl Cancer Inst. 2009;33:736–50.

68. Kennecke H, Yerushalmi R, Woods R, Cheang MC, Voduc D, Speers CH, et al. Metastatic behavior of breast cancer subtypes. J Clin Oncol. 2010;33:3271–7.

69. Lindstrom LS, Karlsson E, Wilking UM, Johansson U, Hartman J, Lidbrink EK, et al. Clinically used breast cancer markers such as estrogen receptor, progesterone receptor, and human epidermal growth factor receptor 2 are unstable throughout tumor progression. J Clin Oncol. 2012;33:2601–8.

70. Broom RJ, Tang PA, Simmons C, Bordeleau L, Mulligan AM, O'Malley FP, et al. Changes in estrogen receptor, progesterone receptor and Her-2/neu status with time: discordance rates between primary and metastatic breast cancer. Anticancer Res. 2009;33:1557–62.

71. Chen X, Sun L, Cong Y, Zhang T, Lin Q, Meng Q, et al. Baseline staging tests based on molecular subtype is necessary for newly diagnosed breast cancer. J Exp Clin Cancer Res. 2014;33:28–42.

Staging of Breast Cancer

3

Neslihan Cabioglu

Abstract

The TNM staging system for breast cancer as described by the American Joint Committee on Cancer (AJCC) was introduced to act as a standard tool to assess the prognosis of patients with newly diagnosed breast cancer. In 2009, the 7th revised edition of the TNM system was published to reflect updates in technology and clinical evidence. In the new staging system, the presence of isolated tumor cells or micrometastases in the axillary lymph nodes was found to have little impact on survival. Furthermore, breast cancer therapy has evolved with the increasing application of neoadjuvant therapy, and therefore, additional pretreatment and posttreatment staging were incorporated into the new staging system to determine chemotherapy response and treatment efficacy. Rapid advances in both clinical and laboratory sciences along with translational research have raised questions about the feasibility of ongoing TNM staging to determine whether to apply systemic therapy based on anatomic prognosis. Although multigene expression assays, such as the 70-gene prognostic signature or Oncotype DX tests, may provide additional prognostic and predictive information beyond anatomic TNM staging and ER/PR and HER2 status, there might be difficulties in incorporating these biomarkers into the TNM system. With advances in personalized medicine, more molecular gene assays and new prognostic and predictive markers such as tumor-infiltrating lymphocytes might be incorporated into future staging systems.

Keywords

TNM staging • Invasive breast cancer • Carcinoma in situ • Prognostic signature

N. Cabioglu, MD, PhD
Department of General Surgery, Breast Cancer Department, Istanbul University Istanbul Medical Faculty, Capa, Istanbul 34390, Turkey
e-mail: ncabioglu@gmail.com

© Springer International Publishing Switzerland 2016
A. Aydiner et al. (eds.), *Breast Disease: Management and Therapies*,
DOI 10.1007/978-3-319-26012-9_3

Introduction

The TNM staging system for breast cancer described by the American Joint Committee on Cancer (AJCC) applies to invasive and in situ carcinomas with or without microinvasion. This classification system was introduced to reflect the risk of recurrence and to be used as a standard prognostic assessment tool for patients with newly diagnosed breast cancer. In 2009, the seventh revised edition of the TNM system was published; careful definitions of the primary tumor (T), the status of the surrounding lymph nodes (N), and the presence of distant metastases (M) were refined to reflect updates in technology and clinical evidence [1] (Table 3.1).

In recent decades, remarkable progress in the surgical and systemic management of breast cancer has resulted in less radical surgery, moving away from radical mastectomies to breast-conserving therapies and from axillary dissections to sentinel lymph node biopsies.

Table 3.1 Definitions of TNM (2009)

T – Primary tumor
Tx – Primary tumor cannot be assessed
T_0 – No evidence of primary tumor
Tis – Carcinoma in situ
Tis (DCIS): Ductal carcinoma in situ
Tis (LCIS): Lobular carcinoma in situ
Tis (Paget): Paget's disease of the nipple (without a primary tumor)
T1 – T ≤2 cm
T1mic ≤0.1 cm microinvasive tumor
Tla ≤0.1 cm, <0.5 cm
Tlb >0.5 cm, ≤1 cm
Tlc >1 cm, ≤2 cm
T2 >2 cm, ≤5 cm
T3 T>5 cm
T4 Regardless of the size of the tumor: (a) involvement of the thoracic wall: *cots, intercostal muscles, and serratus muscles.* (b) skin involvement
T4a extension to the chest wall including m. pectoralis major
T4b edema, peau d'orange, ulceration, satellite skin nodules in the ipsilateral breast
T4c a+b
T4d inflammatory breast cancer

Furthermore, the increased use of antihormonal drugs and chemotherapeutics has been found to reduce recurrence and mortality. An improved understanding of prognostic and predictive biological markers, such as estrogen receptor (ER) and HER2 overexpression, has been used to predict the response to systemic therapies (antiestrogen, anti-HER2-neu "trastuzumab") [2, 3]. Therefore, rapid advances in both clinical and laboratory sciences along with translational research have raised questions about the feasibility of TNM staging as a guide to determine whether to apply systemic therapy based on anatomic prognosis. The use of these factors as predictive rather than prognostic markers is fundamentally important in the management of patients with newly diagnosed breast cancer, but there might be difficulties incorporating these biomarkers into the TNM system.

TNM Classification

Clinical Staging

Clinical staging involves physical examination, including inspection and palpation of the skin, mammary glands, and lymph nodes (axillary, supraclavicular, and cervical), imaging evaluation within 4 months of diagnosis in the absence of disease progression, and pathologic examination such as a core biopsy of the breast or of other tissues to diagnose any metastasis. These imaging findings include the size of the primary invasive cancer and the presence of any regional or systemic metastases. Imaging and clinical findings following neoadjuvant chemotherapy, hormonal therapy, immunotherapy, or radiation therapy should be recorded using the prefix "yc."

Pathologic Staging

Pathologic staging includes data from the pathologic examination of the primary carcinoma or regional lymph nodes after surgery and data regarding core biopsies obtained during surgery at metastatic sites (if applicable) with no macroscopic tumor involvement in any surgical margin along with clinical staging data. A cancer can be classified pT for pathologic staging if there is only microscopic involvement of the margin. If there is a transection in the tumor margin by macroscopic examination, the accurate pathologic size of the tumor should be the sum of the size of multiple resected pieces of the tumor.

Pathologic stage grouping includes the following two combinations of pathologic and clinical classifications: pT pN pM or pT pN cM. If surgery occurs after neoadjuvant chemotherapy, hormonal therapy, immunotherapy, or radiation therapy, the prefix "yp" should be used with the TNM classification, "ypTNM."

Determining Tumor Size

The size of a primary tumor (T) can be determined based on clinical findings, including physical examination and imaging modalities such as mammography, ultrasound, and MRI; these measurements define the clinical tumor size (cT). The pathologic tumor size (pT) is estimated based on measuring *only the invasive component*. The microscopic measurement is the most accurate method for small invasive tumors submitted in one section/paraffin block, whereas gross measurement is the preferred method for a large invasive tumor to determine pT. In cases with prior vacuum or core biopsy, however, the original invasive cancer size should be verified along with imaging, gross, and microscopic histologic findings. For patients who receive neoadjuvant systemic or radiation therapy, pretreatment T is defined as cT. Therefore, pretreatment staging is based on clinical findings from physical examination and imaging (cT), whereas posttreatment (ypT) size should be determined according to the imaging, gross, and microscopic pathologic findings.

Tis Classification

Pure carcinoma in situ is classified as Tis with an additional parenthetical subclassification including three subtypes: ductal carcinoma in situ (or intraductal carcinoma) (DCIS), lobular carcinoma in situ (LCIS), and Paget's disease of the nipple with no underlying invasive cancer. These are categorized as Tis (DCIS), Tis (LCIS), and Tis (Paget's), respectively. "Ductal intraepithelial neoplasia" (DIN) is an uncommonly used terminology for both DCIS and atypical ductal hyperplasia (ADH), and only cases referred to as DIN containing DCIS (±ADH) should be classified as Tis (DCIS) [4, 5]. Similarly, "lobular intraepithelial neoplasia" (LIN) is an uncommon terminology for both atypical lobular hyperplasia (ALH) and LCIS. If DCIS and LCIS are both present, the tumor should be classified as Tis (DCIS) (http://www.cap.org) [6].

Paget's disease is characterized by an exudate or crust of the nipple-areola complex caused by infiltration of the epidermis by noninvasive breast cancer epithelial cells. It presents in one of the following three conditions [7]:

1. Associated with an underlying invasive carcinoma with T classification according to the size of the invasive disease
2. Associated with an underlying noninvasive carcinoma, usually DCIS but rarely LCIS with a T classification based on the underlying tumor as Tis (DCIS) or Tis (LCIS), respectively
3. Not associated with an identified underlying invasive or noninvasive cancer classified as Tis (Paget's)

Microinvasive Carcinoma

Microinvasive carcinoma is defined as an invasive carcinoma with no focus larger than 1 mm encountered in a setting of DCIS where small foci of tumor cells have invaded through the basement membrane into the surrounding stroma. In cases with multiple foci, an estimate of the number or a note that the number of foci of microinvasion is too numerous to quantify should be provided. Microinvasive carcinoma is nearly always encountered. The prognosis of microinvasive carcinoma is generally thought to be favorable, although the clinical impact of multifocal or multicentric microinvasive disease is not well known.

Multiple Simultaneous Ipsilateral Primary Carcinomas

Multiple simultaneous ipsilateral primary carcinomas are defined as multifocal if located in the same quadrant or multicentric carcinomas if located in different quadrants in the same breast; these tumors are macroscopically measurable using available clinical and pathologic techniques. In these cases with multiple foci, T stage classification should be based only on the largest tumor, not on the sum of the sizes. The presence and sizes of the smaller tumor(s) should be recorded using the "(m)" modifier. In a recent analysis of patients enrolled in the MA.12 clinical trial, worse outcome findings were obtained if the largest single dimension was considered as the T size rather than the sum of the largest dimensions [8]. Therefore, the current method of T staging, as outlined in the 7th edition of the AJCC guidelines, appears to offer an equivalent prognostic assessment (Table 3.2).

When macroscopically apparently distinct tumors are very close (e.g., <5 mm) with similar histology, they are most often considered one tumor, and their T category should be based on the sum of the sizes. These criteria do not apply to one macroscopic carcinoma associated with multiple separate microscopic (satellite) foci.

In cases with simultaneous bilateral primary carcinomas, each carcinoma is staged as a separate primary carcinoma in a separate organ in its own category as specified in the TNM rules.

Inflammatory Carcinoma

Inflammatory carcinoma is a clinical-pathologic entity characterized by diffuse erythema and edema (peau d'orange) involving a third or more of the skin of the breast; this is classified as T4d [9]. If the skin alterations, however, involve less than one third of the skin, the cancer should be categorized as T4b or T4c. Locally advanced breast cancers directly invading the dermis or ulcerating the skin without clinical skin changes and tumor emboli in dermal lymphatics are not considered inflammatory carcinoma. On imaging, there may be a detectable mass and thickening of the skin over the breast. A skin biopsy may be required to demonstrate tumor emboli within the dermal lymphatics. A tissue diagnosis should be performed to demonstrate an invasive carcinoma in the underlying breast parenchyma or in the involved dermal lymphatics to assess the status of biological markers, such as estrogen receptor, progesterone receptor, and HER2, for planning the systemic therapy.

Table 3.2 Anatomic stage/prognostic groups (2009, 7th edition)

Stage 0	Tis	N0	M0
Stage IA	T1	N0	M0
Stage IB	T0-1	N1mi	M0
Stage IIa	T0	N1	M0
	T1	N1	M0
	T2	N0	M0
Stage IIb	T2	N1	M0
	T3	N0	M0
Stage IIIA	T0	N2	M0
	T1	N2	M0
	T2	N2	M0
	T3	N1	M0
	T3	N2	M0
Stage IIIB	T4	N0	M0
	T4	N1	M0
	T4	N2	M0
Stage IIIC	T1-4	N3	M0
Stage IV	T1-4	N0-3	M1

T1 included T1mi and M0 included M(i+)

Skin of the Breast

Skin changes such as dimpling of the skin and nipple retraction, except those clinical findings of T4b and T4d disease, may also be observed in T1, T2, or T3 disease without changing their T category.

Regional Lymph Nodes (N)

Nodes (N)

Small clusters of cells not greater than 0.2 mm, or nonconfluent or nearly confluent clusters of cells not exceeding 200 cells in a single histologic lymph node cross section, are defined as isolated tumor cells.

- Stage I breast cancer is subdivided into stage IA and stage IB; stage IB is defined as the presence of T1 tumors (Tl) with exclusively micrometastases in lymph nodes (Nlmi).
- The presence of pN3, regardless of primary tumor size, is classified as stage IIIC.

Macrometastases

Patients in which regional lymph nodes are not removed for pathologic examination are defined as Nx or pNx. Patients are classified as pN0 and/or cN0 if the regional lymph nodes are not involved. The classification criteria for clinically node-positive disease are defined in Table 3.3. If tumor involvement of lymph nodes is confirmed by a fine-needle aspirate or core biopsy, the lymph nodes are considered to contain macrometastases and labeled cN2a(f) by using the (f) modifier.

Axillary lymph nodes histopathologically examined by surgical excisional biopsy, sentinel lymph node biopsy (SLNB), or axillary lymph node dissection (ALND) are classified as described in Table 3.4. Patients with macrometa-

static disease in the lymph nodes must have at least one lymph node with a metastasis greater than 2 mm. For patients with SLNB, the additional designation (sn) for "sentinel node" should

Table 3.4 Pathologic classification of regional lymph nodes (pN)

pNx Regional lymph nodes cannot be assessed (e.g., previously removed or not removed for pathologic study)
pN0 No regional lymph node metastasis identified histologically
pN0 (i−) No regional lymph node metastases, immunohistochemistry (=IHC) (−)
pN0 (i+) Malignant cells in regional lymph nodes, no greater than 0.2 mm (detected by H&E or IHC including ITC)
pN0 (mol−) No regional lymph node metastasis, negative molecular findings: RT-PCR (−)
pN0 (mol+) Positive molecular findings: RT-PCR (+)
pN1
pN1mic Micrometastases >0.2 mm and/or >200 cells, ≤2 mm
pN1a Metastases in 1–3 axillary lymph nodes, at least one metastasis greater than 2 mm
pN1b Metastases in internal mammary nodes with micrometastasis or macrometastases detected by sentinel lymph node biopsy but not clinically or imaging detected
pN1c Metastases in 1–3 axillary lymph nodes and metastases in internal mammary nodes with micrometastasis or macrometastases detected by sentinel lymph node biopsy but not clinically or imaging detected
pN2
pN2a Metastases in 4–9 axillary lymph nodes (at least one tumor deposit is >2.0 mm)
pN2b Metastases in clinically/radiologically detected internal mammary lymph node metastases (except lymphoscintigraphy) in the absence of axillary lymph node metastases
pN3
pN3a 10 or more axillary lymph nodes (at least one tumor deposit >2.0 mm) or metastases to the infraclavicular lymph nodes (level 3)
pN3b Metastases in clinically/radiologically detected (except lymphoscintigraphy) ipsilateral internal mammary lymph nodes + at least one axillary lymph node metastasis, or: in more than 3 axillary lymph nodes and internal mammary lymph node micro- or macrometastases detected by SLNB (not clinically/radiologically)
pN3c Metastases in the ipsilateral supraclavicular lymph nodes

Table 3.3 Clinical classification of regional lymph nodes (cN)

cNx – Regional lymph nodes cannot be assessed (e.g., previously removed)
cN0 – No regional lymph node metastases
c N1 – Metastases movable ipsilateral level I, II axillary lymph nodes
N2 –
cN2a Metastases in the ipsilateral level I, II axillary lymph nodes fixed to one another (matted) or to other structures
cN2b Metastases only in imaging detected ipsilateral internal mammary nodes (excluding lymphoscintigraphy) in the absence of axillary metastases
cN3 –
cN3a Ipsilateral infraclavicular lymph node metastasis
cN3b Ipsilateral internal mammary lymph node metastasis with axillary lymph node(s) metastasis
cN3c Ipsilateral supraclavicular lymph node metastases

be used, e.g., pN1 (sn). Use of the (sn) modifier should be omitted when six or more sentinel nodes are identified on gross examination of pathologic specimens. For a case with a standard ALND followed by a positive SLNB, the classification is based on the total results of both SLNB and ALND. When the number of sentinel and nonsentinel nodes is less than six, the (sn) modifier should be used.

In pathologic evaluation, the entire lymph node is examined, whereas larger nodes should be bisected or thinly sliced ($\leq$2.0 mm). Certain techniques such as multilevel sectioning and immunohistochemistry may identify additional tumor deposits less than or equal to 2.0 mm [micrometastases and isolated tumor cell clusters (ITCs)].

Isolated Tumor Cells (ITCs) and Micrometastases

ITCs are defined as small clusters of cells not greater than 0.2 mm in largest dimension or single cells with little if any histologic stromal reaction by routine histology or immunohistochemistry (IHC). The lymph nodes should be categorized as pN0(i+) or pN0(i+)(sn) according to the surgery type.

The lymph nodes are more likely to have tumor deposits greater than 0.2 mm but not greater than 2.0 mm in largest dimension classified as micrometastases (pN1mi) or pN1mi (sn) if more than 200 individual tumor cells are counted as single dispersed cells or as a confluent focus in a single histologic section of a node. In cases with multiple tumor deposits in a lymph node, the size of only the largest tumor deposit should be considered to classify the node, not the sum of all tumor deposits. The number of involved nodes should be noted separately for ITCs and micrometastases.

If tumor cells are detected in histologically negative lymph nodes by molecular methods such as reverse transcriptase polymerase chain reaction (RT-PCR) using epithelial cell markers, the regional lymph nodes are classified as pN0(mol+) or pN0(mol+)(sn), as appropriate.

The prognostic significance of axillary metastases above a 2.0-mm threshold was confirmed by two studies reported over three decades ago [10, 11]. Following the first study, a subcategory

for micrometastases was added to the *Cancer Staging Manual*. The introduction of sentinel lymph node biopsy and the widespread use of immunohistochemistry facilitated the detection of minimal disease in axillary lymph nodes, and the sixth edition of the *Staging Manual* established a lower limit for micrometastases of >0.2 mm, thus creating a new category of minimal nodal disease. This limit was ten times smaller than the upper limit for micrometastases and had been tested in one retrospective study of occult metastases [12].

The 6th edition of TNM staging indicates that isolated tumor cell clusters should be distinguishable from micrometastases on the basis of metastatic characteristics, such as proliferation or stromal reaction [13, 14]. However, in the 7th edition, the Breast Cancer Task Force perceived that this distinction could be highly subjective and that achieving reproducibility among pathologists and institutions may be difficult. Therefore, for the seventh edition, the Breast Cancer Task Force continues to define isolated tumor cell clusters as not greater than 0.2 mm in diameter and micrometastases as greater than 2 mm but not greater than 2.0 mm in diameter. However, pathologists have had difficulty applying the size criterion when a large number of nonconfluent tumor cells are present in a lymph node such as may occur in some invasive lobular carcinomas [15]. For this reason, additional guidance has been incorporated in this edition. When more than 200 nonconfluent or nearly confluent tumor cells are present in a single histologic cross section of a lymph node, there is a high probability that more than 1,000 cells are present in the node and that the cumulative volume of these cells exceeds the volume of an ITC, and the node should be classified as containing a micrometastasis. The pathologist should use his/her judgment rather than an absolute cutoff of 0.2 mm or exactly 200 cells to determine the likelihood of whether the cluster of cells is an ITC or a true micrometastasis. Due to practical and economic constraints in the pathologic evaluation of lymph nodes and the absence of outcome data on the clinical significance of isolated tumor cell clusters and micrometastases *after* the systematic exclusion of macrometastases, the current thresholds in TNM classifications have not been changed.

An analysis published in the US Surveillance, Epidemiology, and End Results (SEER) national cancer database has demonstrated that when nodal tumor deposits no larger than 2.0 mm are the only finding in lymph nodes and the primary tumor is less than or equal to 2 cm (pTl), the incremental decrease in survival at 5 and 10 years was only 1 % compared to patients with no nodal metastases detected [16]. Among patients with pTl, the 10-year survival rate decreased from 78 % to 77 % and then to 73 % for pNO, pNlmi, and pNla, respectively. Therefore, in the 7th edition, pTl tumors with nodal micrometastases (pNlmi) are classified as stage IB to indicate the better prognosis of this particular patient subset. Furthermore, a recent report demonstrated that occult metastases were detected in 15.9 % of 3,887 patients with node-negative breast cancer by routine immunohistochemical staining for cytokeratin [17]. Log-rank tests indicated a significant difference between patients in whom occult metastases were detected and those in whom no occult metastases were detected with respect to overall survival (OS) ($P=0.03$), disease-free survival (DFS) ($P=0.02$), and distant DFS ($P=0.04$). The corresponding adjusted hazard ratios for death, any outcome event, and distant disease were 1.40 (95 % CI, 1.05–1.86), 1.31 (95 % CI, 1.07–1.60), and 1.30 (95 % CI, 1.02–1.66), respectively. The 5-year Kaplan-Meier estimates of overall survival among patients in whom occult metastases were detected and those without detectable metastases were 94.6 % and 95.8 %, respectively. Occult metastases were an independent prognostic variable in patients with negative sentinel lymph nodes on initial examination; however, the magnitude of the difference in outcome at 5 years was small (1.2 percentage points). Based on these data, a clinical benefit of additional evaluation, including immunohistochemical analysis, of initially negative sentinel lymph nodes in breast cancer patients could not be demonstrated. Interestingly, a recent analysis in T1 breast cancer further demonstrated that patients with micrometastases and negative nodes have shown similar survival outcomes, whereas the ER status and grade significantly stratified patients with respect to disease-specific survival (DSS) and OS [18]. These data indicate that tumor biology, including ER status and grade, are better discriminants of survival than the presence of small-volume nodal metastases.

The detection of isolated tumor cells and micrometastases has also become possible with the use of more sensitive molecular assays such as reverse transcriptase polymerase chain reaction (RT-PCR). Using this technique, epithelial markers such as cytokeratins were identified in a significant percentage of sentinel nodes that were negative for metastasis by both histologic and immunohistochemical stainings [19]. However, it seems unlikely that the minimal tumor burden would be as significant as macro- and micrometastases. Furthermore, because lymph node tissue is digested and consumed in preparation for RT-PCR, it is technically challenging to determine the exact size of the original metastatic involvement in the lymph node to justify the completion of axillary node dissection if the result of this assay is positive [20]. A lymph node that is exclusively positive by molecular assay (mol+) may contain isolated tumor cell clusters, micrometastases, and macrometastases, or it may be a false-positive result due to sampling, contamination, or features intrinsic to the assay [21]. Because the data are currently insufficient to suggest that RT-PCR assay of the lymph nodes should replace the traditional histologic evaluation of lymph nodes, the 7th edition of the *AJCC Cancer Staging* has classified any lesion identified by RT-PCR alone that is histologically negative for regional lymph node metastases as pN0 by using an appended designation (mol+). The first priority in evaluating lymph nodes should be the histologic identification of macrometastases (metastases larger than 2.0 mm) and the performance of N classification based on histologic findings and measurements.

Distant Metastases (M)

Patients without any distant metastases evaluated by clinical evaluation including physical examination and blood workup and/or radiographic methods are classified as cM0, whereas cases in which

Table 3.5 Distant metastases (M)

Mx Distant metastasis unknown
M0 No clinical or radiological evidence of distant metastases
M0 (i+) No clinical or radiological evidence of distant metastases, but deposits of molecularly or microscopically detected tumor cells in circulating blood, bone marrow, or other non-regional nodal tissue that are not larger than 0.2 mm in a patient without symptoms or signs of metastases
M1 Distant detectable metastases as determined by classic clinical and radiographic means and/or histologically proven larger than 0.2 mm

one or more distant metastases are detected by clinical and/or radiographic methods are defined as cM1 (Table 3.5). Patients with the subsequent development of recurrence in the form of new metastases should be considered as having recurrent stage IV disease even though the new metastases do not change the patients' initial staging.

The detection of metastatic disease by clinical examination should include a full physical examination based on evolving symptoms, radiographic findings, and/or laboratory findings. Because physical findings alone rarely provide the basis for M1 stage, radiographic studies are almost always required, and pathologic biopsy confirmation should be performed whenever feasible. All guidelines suggest that for symptomatic patients, as indicated by suspicious findings in the patient's history or physical examination and/or elevated serologic tests for liver or bone function, radiographic systemic imaging such as bone scintigraphy, PET-CT, or anatomic, cross-sectional imaging is required [22]. Likewise, staging is appropriate for patients with stage III disease (clinical or pathologic), whereas systemic radiographic staging for metastases is not warranted in asymptomatic patients with normal blood tests who have T1–2, N0 breast cancer [22]. However, no consensus has been reached regarding patients with T2N1 staging. The overuse of PET-CT may result in false-positive findings in patients with newly diagnosed breast cancer, which may result in unnecessary biopsies, thereby delaying the initiation of local or systemic therapies.

If the distant metastatic lesion has been confirmed by tissue biopsy, it is defined as pM1. The type of biopsy for a suspicious lesion should be determined by the location of the suspicious metastatic lesion along with patient preference, safety, and operator expertise. Fine-needle aspiration (FNA) may be adequate, especially for visceral lesions, if an experienced cytopathologist is available. Other biopsy techniques such as core needle or open surgical biopsy may be warranted for especially bony or scirrhous lesions. Histopathologic examination should include standard H&E staining and additional immunohistochemical staining (estrogen receptor, progesterone receptor, HER2, Ki67) as well as fluorescent in situ hybridization (FISH) techniques for HER2 in some cases with suspicious HER2 immunohistochemical staining. Biomarker staining is critical for the planning of systemic therapies for patients, especially if adequate biomarker data are not available from the primary tumor and discordance exists for biomarker staining results between the primary and metastatic sites. For patients in whom a tissue biopsy from the metastatic site may not be obtained for reasons such as safety risks related to performing the biopsy, follow-up studies after systemic therapy may be required to make the final decision, depending on whether the suspicious lesion that was present at the time of initial diagnosis has since disappeared.

Patients with abnormal liver function tests should undergo liver imaging, whereas those with elevated alkaline phosphatase or calcium levels or other suggestive symptoms should undergo bone imaging and/or scintigraphy. Anemia and other cytopenias require a full hematologic evaluation (e.g., examination of the peripheral smear, iron studies, B12/folate levels), and a bone marrow biopsy may be required during follow-up. The routine use of tumor markers, such as CA 15-3, CEA, Ca-125, and CA 27.29, during follow-up has not been shown to improve outcome.

Circulating Tumor Cells, Bone Marrow Micrometastases, and Disseminated Tumor Cells

Demonstrating the prognostic significance of circulating tumor cells in the peripheral blood and bone marrow of patients with both localized and metastatic breast cancers may allow for true biological breast cancer staging [23–26]. Circulating tumor cells (CTCs) and microscopic tumor cells detected in the bone marrow are collectively designated as DTCs. Several studies have shown a relationship between bone marrow DTCs and the recurrence risk and mortality in stage M0 breast cancer [23, 27, 28]. However, other reports could not demonstrate the prognostic significance of the presence of positive bone marrow micrometastases, possibly due to the different techniques used to detect bone marrow micrometastases such as immunofluorescence instead of immunohistochemistry [29, 30]. Similarly, the prognostic value of CTCs detected in breast cancer patients is currently under debate. Most of these studies were small with short follow-ups, were confounded by the effects of systemic therapy, and thus could not demonstrate a significant prognostic effect [31–34]. However, a recent meta-analysis conducted on 49 articles published between January 1990 and January 2012 including 6,825 patients showed that the presence of CTCs was significantly associated with shorter survival in the total population [35]. The prognostic value of CTCs was significant in both early (DFS: HR, 2.86; 95 % CI, 2.19–3.75; OS: HR, 2.78; 95 % CI, 2.22–3.48) and metastatic breast cancers (PFS: HR, 1.78; 95 % CI, 1.52–2.09; OS: HR, 2.33; 95 % CI, 2.09–2.60), irrespective of the CTC detection method and the time point of blood withdrawal.

In another recent study, CTCs were analyzed in 2,026 patients with early breast cancer before adjuvant chemotherapy and in 1,492 patients after chemotherapy using the CELLSEARCH System [36]. CTCs were detected in 21.5 % of patients ($n = 435$ of 2,026) before chemotherapy and in 22.1 % of patients ($n = 330$ of 1,493) after chemotherapy. The presence of CTCs was found to be an independent prognostic marker in multivariable analysis for DFS (hazard ratio [HR] = 2.11; 95 % confidence interval [CI] = 1.49–2.99; $P < 0.0001$) and OS (HR = 2.18; 95 % CI = 1.32–3.59; $P = 0.002$). The presence of persisting CTCs after chemotherapy negatively influenced DFS (HR = 1.12; 95 % CI = 1.02–1.25; $P = 0.02$) and OS (HR = 1.16; 95 % CI = 0.99–1.37;

$P = 0.06$) indicating the independent prognostic relevance of CTCs both before and after adjuvant chemotherapy in a large prospective trial of primary breast cancer patients. The worst prognosis for DFS and OS was found in patients with at least five CTCs per 30 cc's blood. Further studies are required to explore the clinical utility of CTCs in breast cancer.

In the presence of CTCs in the blood or micrometastases (<0.2 mm) in the bone marrow or other non-regional nodal tissues, the term M0(i+) has been used in the 7th edition TNM classification if other apparent clinical and/or radiographic findings corresponding to pathologic findings are absent. M0(i+) patients are staged according to T and N. In patients with overt metastases (M1), the presence and number of CTCs at the time of diagnosis are also prognostic for both disease progression and mortality [37–41]. Changes in CTCs after treatment are also predictive of the response to therapy and are prognostic for recurrence and mortality, although the American Society of Clinical Oncology Tumor Marker Guidelines Panel has not recommended routinely assessing CTCs in the management of metastatic breast cancer patients in 2008 because the utility of this assay in patient management decisions has not been demonstrated [24, 31, 37, 38]. Therefore, neither the presence nor the number of CTCs will change the overall classification of patients with M1 disease to further subclassify M1 staging.

In summary, many clinicians consider a palliative rather than curative intent for patients who are designated M1 (stage IV). However, no data suggest that the detection of DTCs in any tissue (bone marrow, blood) in the absence of clinical and/or radiographic findings confers incurability. Therefore, in the absence of overt metastases detected by clinical examination or imaging abnormalities, DTCs should not affect M staging, and the staging category should be M0(i+). For data collection purposes, however, the DTC designation should be expanded to include any cluster of malignant cells no greater than 0.2 mm found in any tissue outside of the breast and surrounding regional lymph nodes in the absence of clinical or radiographic signs of metastases (M0 disease).

Neoadjuvant Chemotherapy

The increasing importance of neoadjuvant therapy in breast cancer mandates that the staging system provide the information necessary to assess the prognosis in this diverse patient group. Outcomes after neoadjuvant systemic therapy, including either chemotherapy or endocrine therapy, differ among patients, and a staging system should reflect the potential prognosis [42–46]. Thus, in the 7th edition of the AJCC staging system, a post-therapy clinical or pathologic staging is recorded using the "yc" or "yp" prefix, respectively. Clinical staging (c) is defined by information gathered before neoadjuvant therapy or surgery, whereas pathologic staging (p) includes information gathered at surgery. However, no stage group is assigned if there is a complete pathologic response (pCR) to neoadjuvant therapy, e.g., ypT0ypN0cM0.

Furthermore, the use of fine-needle aspiration or sentinel lymph node biopsy before neoadjuvant therapy is defined with the subscript "f" or "sn," respectively. Nodal metastases detected by FNA or core biopsy are classified as macrometastases (Nl) regardless of the size of the tumor focus in the final pathologic specimen. For instance, a patient with an ultrasound-guided FNA biopsy of a nonpalpable axillary lymph node that is positive has been categorized as cNl (f) and considered as stage IIA. Similarly, a patient with a positive axillary sentinel node detected before neoadjuvant chemotherapy will be categorized as cNl (sn) (stage IIA).

Definition and Clinical Relevance of Complete Response

Pathologic complete response (pCR) has been associated with long-term outcome in several neoadjuvant studies and has therefore been a potential prognostic factor, whereas others comparing different neoadjuvant regimens have failed to show an association between the pCR rate and improved outcomes [43, 47, 48]. These discordant findings might mainly be due to the various definitions for pCR used in these studies. Some trials have applied the pCR definition to the breast tumor only, whereas others have also included the axillary lymph nodes [49, 50]. Furthermore, some studies have considered the presence of residual focal invasive cancer [51] or noninvasive cancer in their pCR definition [50], whereas others have defined pCR as the complete eradication of all invasive and noninvasive cancer [52]. Although an international expert panel proposed that a CR be defined as the absence of invasive and *noninvasive* tumor in the breast [43] in the 7th edition of the AJCC staging system, pCR has been defined as the absence of invasive carcinoma in the breast and the axillary nodes because the presence of DCIS was not a determinant of survival [1].

In a retrospective review from the MD Anderson Cancer Center, patients with a pCR with ($n = 199$) and without DCIS ($n = 78$) had similar outcomes but had significantly better survival rates than the patients with invasive cancer ($n = 2,025$) [53]. Similar findings were demonstrated by Jones et al. in a study of 435 patients [54]. However, in a study by Minckwitz et al. including 6,377 patients with primary breast cancer receiving neoadjuvant anthracycline-taxane-based chemotherapy, DFS was found to be significantly superior in patients with no invasive and no in situ residual disease in the breast or lymph nodes ($n = 955$) compared with patients with residual ductal carcinoma in situ only ($n = 309$), with no invasive residual disease in the breast but with involved nodes ($n = 186$), with only focal invasive disease in the breast ($n = 478$), and with gross invasive residual disease ($n = 4,449$; $P < 0.001$) [55].

Furthermore, the incidence and prognostic impact of pCR vary among breast cancer intrinsic subtypes [55, 56]. In a meta-analysis including 20 studies ($n = 8,095$), the pooled pCR% was 18.5 % (16.2–21.1 %) of patients receiving neoadjuvant chemotherapy for primary breast cancer. The subtype-specific pCR% was 8.3 % (6.7–10.2 %) in HR+/HER2− [OR 1/referent], 18.7 % (15.0–23.1 %) in HER2+/HR+, 38.9 % (33.2–44.9 %) in HER2+/HR− [OR 7.1], and 31.1 % (26.5–36.1 %) in triple negative (TN) [OR 5.0]; the pCR% was significantly higher for the HER2+/

HR− subtype compared with the TN subtype. Notably, the odds of achieving a pCR were highest for the TN and HER2+/HR− subtypes, with evidence that the inclusion of HER2-directed therapy with NAC influenced the pCR% in the HER2+/HR− subtype. In the study by Minckwitz et al., pCR was associated with improved DFS in luminal B/human epidermal growth factor receptor 2 (HER2)-negative ($P=0.005$), HER2-positive/nonluminal ($P<0.001$), and TN ($P<0.001$) tumors but not in luminal A ($P=0.39$) or luminal B/HER2-positive ($P=0.45$) breast cancer. Furthermore, pCR in HER2-positive (nonluminal) and TN tumors was associated with excellent prognosis. Therefore, the authors concluded that pCR defined as no invasive and no in situ residual disease in the breast and nodes can best distinguish patients with favorable outcomes from those with unfavorable outcomes. A pCR in patients overexpressing HER2 and treated with trastuzumab plus chemotherapy was associated with improved survival compared with those without a pCR [58, 59]. Similar findings were obtained in patients treated with trastuzumab plus a combination of pertuzumab and chemotherapy [60]. However, some other studies defining pCR as the absence of invasive cancer in breast and lymph nodes found no survival benefit in patients with a pCR [57].

To investigate the immunogenicity of HER2-positive and TN breast cancers (BCs), tumor-infiltrating lymphocytes (TILs), and their associations with pCR, tumors were evaluated for stromal TILs and lymphocyte-predominant breast cancer (LPBC) [61]. GeparSixto investigated the effect of adding carboplatin (Cb) to an anthracycline-plus-taxane combination (PM) on the pCR. Increased stromal TIL levels predicted a pCR in both univariate ($P<0.001$) and multivariate analyses ($P<0.001$). The pCR rate was 59.9 % in LPBC and 33.8 % for non-LPBC ($P<0.001$). pCR rates ≥75 % were observed in patients with LPBC tumors treated with PMCb. The presence of stromal TILs might be considered a predictive marker for pCR, especially in TN breast cancer.

The majority of the available data regarding the prognostic significance of pCR have been obtained from patients who received neoadjuvant chemotherapy; limited information is available regarding the prognostic significance of the response degree for neoadjuvant endocrine therapy. A pCR is rarely observed in patients receiving 3–4 months of neoadjuvant endocrine therapy, and its absence should not be considered as evidence of endocrine therapy resistance or a poor prognosis [62, 63]. Further studies including new targeted therapies are warranted to assess the relationship between response to systemic therapy and survival. Therefore, the collection of postneoadjuvant TNM data by the registrars has been suggested (Table 3.6).

Assessment of Neoadjuvant Therapy Response

An unresolved problem in defining the yp post-treatment stage is how to determine the best method for measuring tumor size after neoadjuvant chemotherapy. In the absence of a CR, the response assessment and tumor size measurement remain problematic. A partial response, in NSABP protocol B18 and in the grading system proposed by Chevillard et al., is defined by the presence of tumor cell nests in desmoplastic or fibrotic stroma [64, 65]. However, the Miller-Payne grading system and a system used at the MD Anderson Cancer Center rely upon the loss of cellularity to assess the degree of response [66, 67]. Concerns regarding reproducibility exist for all of these measures, and none of these methods have been found to predict outcomes. In the 7th edition of the TNM Staging System, the pathologic T size was defined by the largest contiguous tumor focus, with a suffix to alert the clinician when multiple scattered tumor foci are observed. When nests of tumor cells in fibrotic stroma are observed after treatment, the T should be determined based on the largest contiguous area of invasive carcinoma, excluding surrounding areas of fibrosis. This method of T measurement has been shown to correlate with survival, as reported by Carey et al. [68].

Patients who underwent primary surgery and lymph node evaluation and who have nodes with

Table 3.6 Postneoadjuvant therapy (yc or ypTNM)

In the setting of patients who received neoadjuvant therapy, the pretreatment clinical T (cT) should be based on clinical or imaging findings
Postneoadjuvant therapy T should be based on clinical or imaging (ycT) or pathologic findings (ypT)
A subscript will be added to the clinical N for both node-negative and node-positive patients to indicate whether the N was derived from clinical examination, fine-needle aspiration, core needle biopsy, or sentinel lymph node biopsy
The posttreatment ypT will be defined as the largest contiguous focus of invasive cancer defined histopathologically, with a subscript to indicate the presence of multiple tumor foci. Note: the definition of posttreatment ypT remains controversial and an area in transition
Posttreatment nodal metastases no greater than 0.2 mm are classified as ypN0(i+), as in patients who have not received neoadjuvant systemic therapy. However, patients with this status are not considered to have a pathologic complete response (pCR)
A description of the degree of response to neoadjuvant therapy (complete, partial, no response) will be collected by the registrar with the posttreatment ypTNM. The registrars are requested to describe how they defined the response [by physical examination, imaging techniques (mammogram, ultrasound, magnetic resonance imaging (MRI)), or pathologically]
If a patient presents with M1 prior to neoadjuvant systemic therapy, they are considered stage IV and remain stage IV regardless of their response to neoadjuvant therapy[a]
Post-neoadjuvant therapy is designated with the "yc" or "yp" prefix. Notably, no stage group is assigned if there is a pCR to neoadjuvant therapy, e.g., ypT0ypN0cM0

[a]The stage designation may be changed if postsurgical imaging studies reveal the presence of distant metastases, provided that the studies are conducted within 4 months of diagnosis in the absence of disease progression and provided that the patient has not received neoadjuvant therapy

ITCs are classified as pN0. However, in patients undergoing surgery after neoadjuvant therapy and presenting with ITCs in their lymph nodes, ITCs could represent the presence of minimal nodal disease at pretreatment that did not respond to therapy or the presence of residual tumor cells of macroscopic nodal disease, indicating a partial response. Until further data are available to address the prognostic significance of ITCs after treatment, those patients with ITCs after neoadjuvant chemotherapy are classified as ypN0(i+), indicating a complete response to therapy.

In the assessment of tumor responses to chemotherapy, modalities such as physical examination, mammography, ultrasound, and MRI, which may be used to determine the clinical tumor size, have been demonstrated to significantly overestimate and underestimate the extent of tumor compared with pathologic examination [69, 70]. However, a rough estimate of response should be determined by comparing posttreatment clinical, radiographic, and pathologic assessments with those made prior to the initiation of systemic therapy, and this should be recorded. In the 7th edition, the AJCC response criteria were defined

as follows: (1) complete response (CR), the absence of invasive carcinoma in the breast and nodes; (2) partial response (PR), a decrease in either or both the T or N stage; and (3) no response (NR), no change or increase in either or both the T or N stage.

The clinical usefulness of the AJCC response criteria was validated in a study by Keam et al. [71] that enrolled a total of 398 consecutive stage II or III breast cancer patients who received NAC. The 5-year RFS rates were 89.6 % with a CR, 74.1 % with a PR, and 62.6 % with NR ($P=0.002$). The 5-year OS rates were 97.4 % with a CR, 88.6 % with a PR, and 78.3 % with NR ($P=0.012$). When adjusting for potential prognostic factors, the AJCC response was independently associated with RFS and OS. The AJCC response criteria for NAC in breast cancer are clinically useful in evaluating the response to NAC as well as in predicting survival. The authors concluded that the AJCC response criteria could discriminate among patient subgroups with respect to survival.

Carey et al. demonstrated that the AJCC TNM posttreatment (yp) stage was a significant predictor of both 5-year disease-free and overall survival [68]. However, even in patients with a pCR, the clinical TNM stage at diagnosis provides valuable prognostic information. Of 226 patients at the MD Anderson Cancer Center with a pCR to neoadjuvant therapy, significant differences in the 10-year metastasis-free survival were found based on the initial stage at diagnosis before receiving neoadjuvant chemotherapy [44]. In a median follow-up of 63 months, the 10-year distant metastasis-free rate was 82 %. Multivariate Cox regression analysis using combined staging revealed that clinical stages IIIB, IIIC, and IBC (hazard ratio [HR], 4.24; 95 % CI, 1.96–9.18; $P<0.0001$) predicted for distant metastasis. The clinical relevance of the pretreatment stage, posttreatment stage, and degree of response in predicting survival remains to be defined. Therefore, in the 7th edition of the AJCC staging system, the pretreatment TNM data were not included in the calculation of posttreatment stage ("yp") unless the patient was Ml prior to the initiation of therapy. In this case, her M status is considered M1 regardless of response to therapy.

Other studies suggested the establishment of a novel means to assess the prognosis in patients treated with neoadjuvant chemotherapy using clinical and pathologic staging parameters along with biological tumor markers [72, 73]. This novel breast cancer staging system for assessing the prognosis after neoadjuvant chemotherapy was based on the pretreatment clinical stage (CS), estrogen receptor status (E), grade (G), and posttreatment pathologic stage (PS). The ability of the CPS + EG staging system, based on the assigned scores and summed points for each factor, to stratify outcomes was validated in the study by Mittendorf et al. Application of the CPS + EG staging system facilitated a more refined categorization of patients into prognostic subgroups by outcome rather than presenting the CS or final PS as defined by the AJCC staging system. The authors recommend that biological markers and treatment response be incorporated into revised versions of the AJCC staging system for patients receiving neoadjuvant chemotherapy. Future studies should focus on prospective validation of these scoring systems and refinement of the scoring systems by adding new biological markers.

Tumor Biology and Multigene Expression Assays

AJCC staging is used to assess the breast cancer prognosis, yet patient survival within each stage varies widely. Biological differences influence this variation, and the addition of biological markers to AJCC staging improves the assessment of prognosis. Increasingly in the modern era, many treatment decisions for patients with newly diagnosed breast cancer are based on multiple factors, including tumor biology and the TNM stage. In the 7th edition, the Task Force therefore added a "B" category for tumor biology, in which the ER, PR, and HER2 statuses and multigene expression profiles were incorporated into the stage grouping [1].

In a study by Yi et al., in a cohort of 3,728 patients who underwent primary surgery, the significance of adding grade (G), lymphovascular invasion (L), estrogen receptor (ER) status (E), progesterone receptor (PR) status, combined ER and PR status (EP), or combined ER, PR, and HER2 status (M) was tested by using a Cox proportional hazards model [74]. Values of 0–2 were assigned to these DSS-associated factors and assessed six different staging systems: PS, PS + G, PS + G L, PS + G E, PS + G EP, and PS + G M. The PS + G E status staging system was the most precise, with a low Akaike's information criterion (AIC) value (1,931.9) and the highest C-index (0.80). PS + G E status was confirmed to stratify outcomes in the analyzed patient cohorts. This staging system, which incorporates grade and ER status, has thus been suggested to improve the current AJCC system. The authors recommend that biological markers be incorporated into revised versions of the AJCC staging system.

In the last decade, breast cancer subtypes were identified by microarrays and immunohistochemistry, respectively, defined as luminal A, luminal B, nonluminal HER2-neu, and TN tumors [75, 76]. Of those, luminal A tumors have been associated with the most favorable clinical outcomes, whereas patients with TN invasive ductal cancer have shown the worst prognosis [76, 77]. In St. Gallen 2013, the breast cancer subtypes based on immunohistochemistry were defined as luminal A, luminal B, nonluminal HER2, and TN [76]. A useful surrogate definition distinguishing luminal A-like from luminal B-like disease could be made using a combination of ER, PgR, and Ki67 without requiring molecular diagnostics. The proliferation marker Ki67 is a promising prognostic and predictive breast cancer biomarker, but the best cutoff points remain under debate. The standardization of Ki67 remains relevant for diagnostic pathology as a prototype quantitative immunohistochemical biomarker. Several different cutoff points for Ki67 have been reported to be significant, and determining an evidence-based "optimal" cutoff point is very difficult. In the 2013 St. Gallen Breast Cancer Conference, the majority of the panel voted that a threshold of ≥ 20 % was clearly indicative of "high" Ki67 status; in 2015, this cutoff has increased to ≥ 35 % [77], supporting the view that Ki67 should be regarded as a continuous marker, reflecting continuous variation of the proliferation rate in different tumor types.

The prognostic relevance of the TNM staging system in regard to the intrinsic breast cancer subtype has been studied by Jung et al. [78]. In patients with primary surgery for stage I–III breast cancer ($n = 1,145$), the 5-year recurrence-free survival (RFS) in HR-positive and HER2-negative disease with a low Ki67 staining score (0–25 %) was 99 %. However, the 5-year RFS of patients with HER2-positive or TN breast cancer was 89 % and 83 %, respectively. In a multivariate analysis, advanced stage (II/III) and unfavorable biology (HER2 positive or TN) remained significant predictors of decreased RFS and OS. Additionally, patients with stage II or III disease but favorable tumor biology (HR positive, HER2 negative, and low Ki67) had better outcomes than those with stage I disease and unfavorable tumor biology in terms of RFS (99 % versus 92 %, P value = 0.011) and OS (99 % versus 96 %, P value = 0.03) at 5 years. These results suggest that the intrinsic subtype has a greater

prognostic impact in predicting clinical outcomes in patient subpopulations with stage I–III breast cancer who show discordance between stage and biological subtype.

Bagaria et al. investigated whether including the TN phenotype (TNP) could improve the prognostic accuracy of TNM staging for breast cancer [79]. Patients with invasive ductal breast cancer who underwent primary surgery ($n = 1,842$) were categorized by the TNM stage and by the presence or absence of TNP. Multivariable analysis has identified TNP status as a powerful prognostic factor, and the study demonstrated that the prognostic accuracy of the TNM staging system that incorporated the TNP was superior to the current TNM staging system ($P < 0.001$). A TNM staging system that incorporated the TNP reduced early-stage compression by 15 %. Similarly, whether the relevance of tumor biomarkers (ER/PR/HER2) in a recently proposed biological TNM (bTNM) classification system including the TN ER/PR/HER2 phenotype (TNP) could improve the prognostic accuracy of TNM has also been investigated by Orucevic et al. [79]. Of 782 patients with invasive ductal breast carcinoma, TNP significantly worsened survival only in more advanced TNM stages (stage III = HR 3.08, 95 % CI 1.88–5.04, stage IV = HR 24.36, 95 % CI 13.81–42.99), not in earlier stages (I and II). Therefore, all of these studies, along with others, suggest that incorporating nonanatomical factors such as ER, PR, and HER2 statuses according to luminal, TNP, and HER2 subtypes into the TNM staging system (bTNM) can improve the prognostic accuracy of the current breast cancer staging [78–81].

There is a growing consensus that multigene expression assays provide useful complementary information to tumor size and grade in ER-positive breast cancers. First-generation prognostic signatures such as MammaPrint and Oncotype Dx are substantially more accurate at predicting recurrence within the first 5 years than in later years. MammaPrint, the 70-gene prognostic signature developed by investigators from Amsterdam, has been used in women younger than 61 years with stage I or II node-negative breast cancer to "assess a patient's risk for distant metastases"

[82, 83]. In addition, a second multigene assay, based on RT-PCR analysis of the expression of 21 genes (designated as the "Oncotype Dx 21-gene recurrence score assay") can also be used to assess the prognosis in ER-positive breast cancer patients by assessing the benefit of chemotherapy in addition to hormonal treatment [84–86]. Newer tests (Prosigna, EndoPredict, Breast Cancer Index) appear to possess better prognostic value for late recurrences while also remaining predictive of early relapse [87]. Therefore, using genomic/gene expression arrays that incorporate additional prognostic/predictive biomarkers (e.g., the Oncotype Dx recurrence score) may provide additional prognostic and predictive information beyond anatomical TNM staging and ER/PR/HER2 statuses. Whether these multiparameter prognostic assays should be incorporated into the TNM staging system as an entirely new category related to predicting the benefit of chemotherapy regardless of TNM stage remains under debate.

Summary and Future Directions

In the final revised 7th edition of the AJCC staging system, molecular gene assays and markers were recognized in the management of newly diagnosed breast cancer. However, they have not been incorporated into the current staging system, which remains largely determined by anatomic findings. The presence of isolated tumor cells or micrometastases in axillary lymph nodes was found to have little impact on survival. However, the lymph node ratio (LNR), defined as the number of involved nodes divided by the total number of lymph nodes, was associated with OS independently of AJCC categorization and predicts OS independently of traditional clinicopathologic factors (tumor size, grade, ER, PR, and HER2 statuses) [88, 89]. Therefore, the LNR might be a surrogate marker of prognosis in an upcoming edition of the AJCC staging system. Furthermore, in patients with locally advanced breast cancer, chest wall invasion (T4) was defined in the 7th edition of the AJCC staging system as only direct extension to the ribs,

intercostal muscles, and serratus anterior muscle, excluding isolated pectoral muscle involvement. Due to the aggressive biology of T4 with muscle involvement, Murthy et al. suggested that T4 with a lower case letter "m" or "mus" be used to indicate pectoral muscle involvement in the next T stage revision [90]. Cancer therapy has evolved to include increasing applications for neoadjuvant therapy, requiring additional posttreatment staging to determine response and efficacy for this treatment approach. With evolving advances in personalized medicine, more molecular gene assays and new prognostic and predictive markers such as TILs and a new classification system regarding TN breast cancer, due to its dismal prognosis, might be incorporated into the future staging systems [78–81]. Notably, no clinically useful prognostic signatures exist for ER-negative cancers, and drug-specific treatment response predictors also remain elusive. Emerging areas of research involve the development of immune gene signatures that carry significant prognostic value independent of the proliferation and ER statuses and that represent candidate predictive markers for future immune-targeted therapies. Careful and complete staging on the part of physicians and cancer registrars will allow us to determine the outcomes for patients and to conduct more clinical research to improve the current staging system to increase the accuracy of staging schemes.

References

1. AJCC. In: Edge SB, Byrd DR, Compton CC, Fritz AG, Greene FL, Trotti A, editors. Cancer staging handbook. From the AJCC cancer staging manual. 7th ed. New York: Springer; 2010.
2. Hammond ME, Hayes DF, Dowsett M, Allred DC, Hagerty KL, Badve S, et al. American Society of Clinical Oncology/College of American Pathologists guideline recommendations for immunohistochemical testing of estrogen and progesterone receptors in breast cancer. J Clin Oncol. 2010;28:2784–95.
3. Wolff AC, Hammond ME, Hicks DG, Dowsett M, McShane LM, Allison KH, American Society of Clinical Oncology, College of American Pathologists, et al. Recommendations for human epidermal growth factor receptor 2 testing in breast cancer: American Society of Clinical Oncology/College of American

Pathologists clinical practice guideline update. J Clin Oncol. 2013;31:3997–4013.

4. Tavassoli FA. Ductal carcinoma in situ: introduction of the concept of ductal intraepithelial neoplasia. Mod Pathol. 1998;11:140–54.

5. Tavassoli FA. Breast pathology: rationale for adopting the ductal intraepithelial neoplasia (DIN) classification. Nat Clin Pract Oncol. 2005;2:116–7.

6. Lester SC, Bose S, Chen YY, et al. Protocol for the examination of specimens from patients with ductal carcinoma in situ of the breast. Arch Pathol Lab Med. 2009;133:15–25.

7. Chen CY, Sun LM, Anderson BO. Paget disease of the breast: changing patterns of incidence, clinical presentation, and treatment in the U.S. Cancer. 2006;107:1448–58.

8. Hilton JF, Bouganim N, Dong B, Chapman JW, Arnaout A, O'Malley F, et al. Do alternative methods of measuring tumor size, including consideration of multicentric/multifocal disease, enhance prognostic information beyond TNM staging in women with early stage breast cancer: an analysis of the NCIC CTG MA.5 and MA. 12 clinical trials. Breast Cancer Res Treat. 2013;142:143–51.

9. Walshe JM, Swain SM. Clinical aspects of inflammatory breast cancer. Breast Dis. 2005–2006; 22:35–44.

10. Huvos AG, Hutter RV, Berg JW. Significance of axillary macrometastases and micrometastases in mammary cancer. Ann Surg. 1971;173:44–6.

11. Fisher ER, Palekar A, Rockette H, et al. Pathologic findings from the National Surgical Adjuvant Breast Project (Protocol No. 4). V. Significance of axillary nodal micro- and macrometastases. Cancer. 1978;42:2032–8.

12. Nasser IA, Lee AK, Bosari S, et al. Occult axillary lymph node metastases in "node-negative" breast carcinoma. Hum Pathol. 1993;24:950–7.

13. Singletary SE, Allred C, Ashley P, et al. Revision of the American Joint Committee on Cancer staging system for breast cancer. J Clin Oncol. 2002;20:3628–36.

14. Hermanek P, Sobin LH, Wittekind C. How to improve the present TNM staging system. Cancer. 1999;86:2189–91.

15. Turner RR, Weaver DL, Cserni G, et al. Nodal stage classification for breast carcinoma: improving interobserver reproducibility through standardized histologic criteria and image-based training. J Clin Oncol. 2008;26:258–63.

16. Chen SL, Hoehne FM, Giuliano AE. The prognostic significance of micrometastases in breast cancer: a SEER population-based analysis. Ann Surg Oncol. 2007;14:3378–84.

17. Weaver DL, Ashikaga T, Krag DN, Skelly JM, Anderson SJ, Harlow SP, et al. Effect of occult metastases on survival in node-negative breast cancer. N Engl J Med. 2011;364:412–21.

18. Mittendorf EA, Ballman KV, McCall LM, Yi M, Sahin AA, Bedrosian I, et al. Evaluation of the stage IB designation of the American Joint Committee on Cancer staging system in breast cancer. J Clin Oncol. 2015;33:1119–27.

19. Min CJ, Tafra L, Verbanac KM. Identification of superior markers for polymerase chain reaction detection of breast cancer metastases in sentinel lymph nodes. Cancer Res. 1998;58:4581–4.

20. Blumencranz P, Whitworth PW, Deck K, et al. Scientific impact recognition award. Sentinel node staging for breast cancer: intraoperative molecular pathology overcomes conventional histologic sampling errors. Am J Surg. 2007;194:426–32.

21. Viale G, Dell'Orto P, Biasi MO, et al. Comparative evaluation of an extensive histopathologic examination and a real-time reverse-transcription- polymerase chain reaction assay for mammaglobin and cytokeratin 19 on axillary sentinel lymph nodes of breast carcinoma patients. Ann Surg. 2008;247:136–42.

22. National Comprehensive Cancer Network Clinical Practice Guidelines in Oncology, Breast Cancer. Version 2.2015. http://www.nccn.org/. Published 03.11.2015.

23. Braun S, Vogl FD, Naume B, Janni W, Osborne MP, Coombes RC, et al. A pooled analysis of bone marrow micrometastasis in breast cancer. N Engl J Med. 2005;353(8):793–802.

24. Dawood S, Broglio K, Valero V, Reuben J, Handy B, Islam R, et al. Circulating tumor cells in metastatic breast cancer: from prognostic stratification to modification of the staging system? Cancer. 2008;113:2422–30.

25. De Giorgi U, Valero V, Rohren E, Dawood S, Ueno NT, Miller MC, et al. Circulating tumor cells and [18F] fluorodeoxyglucose positron emission tomography/ computed tomography for outcome prediction in metastatic breast cancer. J Clin Oncol. 2009;27:3303–11.

26. Giordano A, Gao H, Anfossi S, Cohen E, Mego M, Lee BN, et al. Epithelial-mesenchymal transition and stem cell markers in patients with HER2-positive metastatic breast cancer. Mol Cancer Ther. 2012;11:2526–34.

27. Tjensvoll K, Oltedal S, Heikkilä R, Kvaløy JT, Gilje B, Reuben JM, et al. Persistent tumor cells in bone marrow of non-metastatic breast cancer patients after primary surgery are associated with inferior outcome. BMC Cancer. 2012;12:190–201.

28. Hartkopf AD, Taran FA, Wallwiener M, Hahn M, Becker S, Solomayer EF, et al. Prognostic relevance of disseminated tumour cells from the bone marrow of early stage breast cancer patients-results from a large single-centre analysis. Eur J Cancer. 2014;50:2550–9.

29. Falck AK, Bendahl PO, Inqvar C, Isola J, Jönsson PE, Lindblom P, et al. Analysis of and prognostic information from disseminated tumour cells in bone marrow in primary breast cancer: a prospective observational study. BMC Cancer. 2012;12:403.

30. Langer I, Guller U, Worni M, Berclaz G, Singer G, Schaer G, Swiss Multicenter Sentinel Lymph Node Study Group in Breast Cancer, et al. Bone marrow micrometastases do not impact disease-free and overall survival in early stage sentinel lymph node negative breast cancer patients. Ann Surg Oncol. 2014; 21:401–7.

31. Harris L, Fritsche H, Mennel R, et al. American Society of Clinical Oncology 2007 update of recommendations for the use of tumor markers in breast cancer. J Clin Oncol. 2007;25:5287–312.
32. Apostolaki S, Perraki M, Pallis A, et al. Circulating HER2 mRNA-positive cells in the peripheral blood of patients with stage I and II breast cancer after the administration of adjuvant chemotherapy: evaluation of their clinical relevance. Ann Oncol. 2007;18: 851–8.
33. Ignatiadis M, Kallergi G, Ntoulia M, et al. Prognostic value of the molecular detection of circulating tumor cells using a multimarker reverse transcrip- tion-PCR assay for cytokeratin 19, mammaglobin A, and HER2 in early breast cancer. Clin Cancer Res. 2008;14:2593–600.
34. Ignatiadis M, Xenidis N, Perraki M, et al. Different prognostic value of cytokeratin-19 mRNA positive circulating tumor cells according to estrogen receptor and HER2 status in early-stage breast cancer. J Clin Oncol. 2007;25:5194–202.
35. Zhanq L, Riethdorf S, Wu G, Wang T, Yang K, Penq G, et al. Meta-analysis of the prognostic value of circulating tumor cells in breast cancer. Clin Cancer Res. 2012;18:5701–10.
36. Rack B, Schündbeck C, Jückstock J, Andergassen U, Hepp P, Zwingers T, et al. Circulating tumor cells predict survival in early average-to-high risk breast cancer patients. J Natl Cancer Inst. 2014;106:1–11.
37. Cristofanilli M, Budd GT, Ellis MJ, et al. Circulating tumor cells, disease progression, and survival in metastatic breast cancer. N Engl J Med. 2004;351: 781–91.
38. Cristofanilli M, Hayes DF, Budd GT, et al. Circulating tumor cells: a novel prognostic factor for newly diagnosed metastatic breast cancer. J Clin Oncol. 2005;23:1420–30.
39. Budd GT, Cristofanilli M, Ellis MJ, et al. Circulating tumor cells versus imaging-predicting overall survival in metastatic breast cancer. Clin Cancer Res. 2006;12:6403–9.
40. Hayes DF, Cristofanilli M, Budd GT, et al. Circulating tumor cells at each follow-up time point during therapy of metastatic breast cancer patients predict progression-free and overall survival. Clin Cancer Res. 2006;12:4218–24.
41. Giordano A, Egleston BL, Hajage D, Bland J, Hortobagyi GN, Reuben JM, et al. Establishment and validation of circulating tumor cell-based prognostic nomograms in the first line metastatic breast cancer patients. Clin Cancer Res. 2013;19:1596–602.
42. Fisher B, Bryant J, Wolmark N, et al. Effect of preoperative chemotherapy on the outcome of women with operable breast cancer. J Clin Oncol. 1998;16: 2672–85.
43. Kaufmann M, Hortobagyi GN, Goldhirsch A, et al. Recommendations from an international expert panel on the use of neoadjuvant (primary) systemic treatment of operable breast cancer: an update. J Clin Oncol. 2006;24:1940–9.
44. Gonzalez-Angulo AM, McGuire SE, Buchholz TA, Tucker SL, Kuerer HM, Rouzier R, et al. Factors predictive of distant metastases in patients with breast cancer who have a pathologic complete response after neoadjuvant chemotherapy. J Clin Oncol. 2005;23:7098–8104.
45. Dawood S, Broglio K, Kau SW, Islam R, Symnans WF, Buchholz TA, et al. Prognostic value of initial clinical disease stage after achieving pathological complete response. Oncologist. 2008;13:6–15.
46. Eiermann W, Paepke S, Appfelstaedt J, et al. Preoperative treatment of postmenopausal breast cancer patients with letrozole: a randomized double blind multicenter study. Ann Oncol. 2001;12:1527–32.
47. Kuerer HM, Newman LA, Smith TM, et al. Clinical course of breast cancer patients with complete pathologic primary tumor and axillary lymph node response to doxorubicin-based neoadjuvant chemotherapy. J Clin Oncol. 1999;17:460–9.
48. Rastogi P, Anderson SJ, Bear HD, et al. Preoperative chemotherapy: updates of National Surgical Adjuvant Breast and Bowel Project Protocols B-18 and B-27. J Clin Oncol. 2008;26:778–85.
49. Bear HD, Anderson S, Brown A, et al. The effect on tumor response of adding sequential preoperative docetaxel to preoperative doxorubicin and cyclophosphamide: preliminary results from National Surgical Adjuvant Breast and Bowel Project Protocol B-27. J Clin Oncol. 2003;21:4165–74.
50. Green MC, Buzdar AU, Smith T, et al. Weekly paclitaxel improves pathologic complete remission in operable breast cancer when compared with paclitaxel once every 3 weeks. J Clin Oncol. 2005;23:5983–92.
51. Sataloff DM, Mason BA, Prestipino AJ, et al. Pathologic response to induction chemotherapy in locally advanced carcinoma of the breast: a determinant of outcome. J Am Coll Surg. 1995;180: 297–306.
52. von Minckwitz G, Rezai M, Loibl S, et al. Capecitabine in addition to anthracycline/taxane based neoadjuvant treatment in patients with primary breast cancer: the phase III GeparQuattro study. J Clin Oncol. 2010; 28:2015–23.
53. Mazouni C, Peintinger F, Wan-Kau S, et al. Residual ductal carcinoma in situ in patients with complete eradication of invasive breast cancer after neoadjuvant chemotherapy does not adversely affect patient outcome. J Clin Oncol. 2007;25:2650–5.
54. Jones RL, Lakhani SR, Ring AE, et al. Pathological complete response and residual DCIS following neoadjuvant chemotherapy for breast carcinoma. Br J Cancer. 2006;94:358–62.
55. von Minckwitz G, Untch M, Blohmer JU, Costa SD, Eidtmann H, Fasching PA, et al. Definition and impact of pathologic complete response on prognosis after neoadjuvant chemotherapy in various intrinsic breast cancer subtypes. J Clin Oncol. 2012;30:1796–804.
56. Houssami N, Macaskill P, von Minckwitz G, Marinovich ML, Mamounas E. Meta-analysis of the association of breast cancer subtype and pathologic

complete response to neoadjuvant chemotherapy. Eur J Cancer. 2012;48:3342–54.

57. Liedtke C, Mazouni C, Hess KR, et al. Response to neoadjuvant therapy and long-term survival in patients with triple-negative breast cancer. J Clin Oncol. 2008;26:1275–81.

58. Buzdar AU, Valero V, Ibrahim NK, Francis D, Broglio KR, Theriault RL, et al. Neoadjuvant therapy with paclitaxel followed by 5-fluorouracil, epirubicin, and cyclophosphamide chemotherapy and concurrent trastuzumab in human epidermal growth factor receptor 2-positive operable breast cancer: an update of the initial randomized study population and data of additional patients treated with the same regimen. Clin Cancer Res. 2007;13:228–33.

59. Kim MM, Allen P, Gonzalez-Angulo AM, Woodward WA, Meric-Bernstam F, Buzdar AU, et al. Pathologic complete response to neoadjuvant chemotherapy with trastuzumab predicts for improved survival in women with HER2-overexpressing breast cancer. Ann Oncol. 2013;24:1999–2004.

60. Swain SM, Baselga J, Kim SB, Ro J, Semiglazov V, Campone M, CLEOPATRA Study Group, et al. Pertuzumab, trastuzumab, and docetaxel in HER2-positive metastatic breast cancer. N Engl J Med. 2015;372:724–34.

61. Denkert C, von Minckwitz G, Brase JC, Sinn BV, Gade S, Kronenwett R, et al. Tumor-infiltrating lymphocytes and response to neoadjuvant chemotherapy with or without carboplatin in human epidermal growth factor receptor 2-positive and triple-negative primary breast cancers. J Clin Oncol. 2015;33:983–91.

62. Suman VJ, Hoog J, Lin L, Snider J, Prat A, Parker JS, et al. Randomized phase II neoadjuvant comparison between letrozole, anastrozole, and exemestane for postmenopausal women with estrogen receptor–rich stage 2 to 3 breast cancer: clinical and biomarker outcomes and predictive value of the baseline PAM50-based intrinsic subtype—ACOSOG Z1031. J Clin Oncol. 2011;29:2342–9.

63. Leal F, Liutti VT, Antunes Dos Santos VC, Novis de Figueiredo MA, Macedo LT, Rinck Junior JA, Sasse AD. Neoadjuvant endocrine therapy for resectable breast cancer: a systematic review and meta-analysis. Breast. 2015. doi:10.1016/j.breast.2015.03.004. Apr 6. pii: S0960-9776(15)00072-7.

64. Fisher ER, Wang J, Bryant J, et al. Pathobiology of preoperative chemotherapy: findings from the National Surgical Adjuvant Breast and Bowel (NSABP) protocol B-18. Cancer. 2002;95:681–95.

65. Chevillard S, Vielh P, Pouillart P. Tumor response of breast cancer patients treated by neaoadjuvant chemotherapy may be predicted by measuring the early level of MDR1 gene expression. Proc Am Soc Clin Oncol. 1993;12:59.

66. Ogston KN, Miller ID, Payne S, et al. A new histological grading system to assess response of breast cancers to primary chemotherapy: prognostic significance and survival. Breast. 2003;12:320–7.

67. Symmans WF, Peintinger F, Hatzis C, et al. Measurement of residual breast cancer burden to predict survival after neoadjuvant chemotherapy. J Clin Oncol. 2007;25:4414–22.

68. Carey LA, Metzger R, Dees EC, et al. American Joint Committee on cancer tumor-node-metastasis stage after neoadjuvant chemotherapy and breast cancer outcome. J Natl Cancer Inst. 2005;97:1137–42.

69. Berg WA, Gutierrez L, NessAiver MS, Berg WA, Gutierrez L, NessAiver MS, et al. Diagnostic accuracy of mammography, clinical examination, US, and MR imaging in preoperative assessment of breast cancer. Radiology. 2004;233:830–49.

70. Chagpar AB, Middleton LP, Sahin AA, Dempsey P, Buzdar AU, Mirza AN, et al. Accuracy of physical examination, ultrasonography, and mammography in predicting residual pathologic tumor size in patients treated with neoadjuvant chemotherapy. Ann Surg. 2006;243:257–64.

71. Keam B, Im SA, Lim Y, Han SW, Moon HG, Oh DY, et al. Clinical usefulness of AJCC response criteria for neoadjuvant chemotherapy in breast cancer. Ann Surg Oncol. 2013;20:2242–9.

72. Jeruss JS, Mittendorf EA, Tucker SL, Gonzalez-Angulo AM, Buchholz TA, Sahin AA, et al. Combined use of clinical and pathologic staging variables to define outcomes for breast cancer patients treated with neoadjuvant therapy. J Clin Oncol. 2008;26:246–52.

73. Mittendorf EA, Jeruss JS, Tucker SL, Kolli A, Newman LA, Gonzalez-Angulo AM, et al. Validation of a novel staging system for disease-specific survival in patients with breast cancer treated with neoadjuvant chemotherapy. J Clin Oncol. 2011;29:1956–62.

74. Yi M, Mittendorf EA, Cormier JN, Buchholz TA, Bilimoria K, Sahin AA, et al. Novel staging system for predicting disease-specific survival in patients with breast cancer treated with surgery as the first intervention: time to modify the current American Joint Committee on Cancer Staging System. J Clin Oncol. 2011;29:4654–61.

75. Sorlie T, Perou CM, Tibshirani R, et al. Gene expression patterns of breast carcinoma distinguish tumor subclasses with clinical implications. Proc Natl Acad Sci U S A. 2001;98:10869–74.

76. Goldhirsch A, Winer EP, Coates AS, Gelber RD, Piccart-Gebhart M, Thürlimann B, Panel members, et al. Personalizing the treatment of women with early breast cancer: highlights of the St Gallen International Expert Consensus on the Primary Therapy of Early Breast Cancer 2013. Ann Oncol. 2013;24:2206–23.

77. Esposito A, Criscitiello C, Curigliano G. Highlights from the 14th St Gallen International Breast Cancer Conference 2015 in Vienna: dealing with classification, prognostication, and prediction refinement to personalize the treatment of patients with early breast cancer. Ecancermedicalscience. 2015;9:518.

78. Jung HA, Park YH, Kim M, Kim S, Chang WJ, Choi MK, Hong JY, Kim SW, Kil WH, Lee JE, Nam SJ, Ahn JS, Im YH. Prognostic relevance of biological

subtype overrides that of TNM staging in breast cancer: discordance between stage and biology. Tumour Biol. 2015;36:1073–9.

79. Bagaria SP, Ray PS, Sim MS, Ye X, Shamonki JM, Cui X, Giuliano AE. Personalizing breast cancer staging by the inclusion of ER, PR, and HER2. JAMA Surg. 2014;149(2):125–9.

80. Orucevic A, Chen J, McLoughlin JM, Heidel RE, Panella T, Bell J. Is the TNM staging system for breast cancer still relevant in the era of biomarkers and emerging personalized medicine for breast cancer – an institution's 10-year experience. Breast J. 2015;21:147–54.

81. Murthy V, Chamberlain RS. Recommendation to revise the AJCC/UICC Breast Cancer Staging System for inclusion of proven prognostic factors: ER/PR receptor status and HER2 neu. Clin Breast Cancer. 2011;11:346–7.

82. Buyse M, Loi S, van't Veer L, Viale G, Delorenzi M, Glas AM, TRANSBIG Consortium, et al. Validation and clinical utility of a 70-gene prognostic signature for women with node-negative breast cancer. J Natl Cancer Inst. 2006;98:183–92.

83. Bueno-de-Mesquita JM, van Harten WH, Retel VP, van't Veer LJ, van Dam FS, Karsenberg K, et al. Use of 70-gene signature to predict prognosis of patients with node-negative breast cancer: a prospective community-based feasibility study (RASTER). Lancet Oncol. 2007;8:1079–87.

84. Paik S, Shak S, Tang G, et al. A multigene assay to predict recurrence of tamoxifen-treated, node-negative breast cancer. N Engl J Med. 2004;351:2817–26.

85. Tang G, Shak S, Paik S, Anderson SJ, Costantino JP, Geyer Jr CE, et al. Comparison of the prognostic and predictive utilities of the 21-gene recurrence score assay and adjuvant! for women with node-negative, ER-positive breast cancer: results from NSABP B-14 and NSABP B-20. Breast Cancer Res Treat. 2011;127:133–42.

86. Mamounas EP, Tang G, Fisher B, Paik S, Shak S, Costantino JP, et al. Association between the 21-gene recurrence score assay and risk of locoregional recurrence in node-negative, estrogen receptor–positive breast cancer: results from NSABP B-14 and NSABP B-20. J Clin Oncol. 2010;28:1677–83.

87. Győrffy B, Hatzis C, Sanft T, Hofstatter E, Aktas B, Pusztai L. Multigene prognostic tests in breast cancer: past, present, future. Breast Cancer Res. 2015; 17:11.

88. Chagpar A, Camp RL, Rimm DL. Lymph node ratio should be considered for incorporation into staging for breast cancer. Ann Surg Oncol. 2011;18:3143–8.

89. Schiffman SC, McMasters KM, Scoggins CR, Martin RC, Chagpar AB. Lymph node ratio: a proposed refinement of current axillary staging in breast cancer patients. J Am Coll Surg. 2011;213:45–53.

90. Murthy V, Chamberlain RS. Further expansion of the AJCC/UICC breast cancer staging system to encompass unique problems in the developing world. Ann Surg Oncol. 2011;18:S278–80.

Surgical Treatment of Early-Stage Breast Cancer

4

Vahit Ozmen

Abstract

Early-stage breast cancer is an issue of growing clinical importance due to ever-increasing rates of breast lesion detection. Wide population-based screening programs and improved visualization techniques are powerful tools for the early and more precise evaluation of breast tumors. Optimally timed and safe surgical approaches are needed to provide local control with satisfactorily high survival.

In this chapter, we attempt to define the entity of early breast cancer and the mainstream surgical approach in light of modern achievements in the surgical treatment of breast cancer.

Keywords

Breast-conserving surgery • Wound infection • Mastectomy • Surgical complications • Local recurrence • Lymphedema • Surgical border

Definition

The term "early-stage breast cancer" is quite controversial. Due to widespread screening with mammography and increased awareness of breast cancer, non-palpable breast cancers account for 75 % of all breast cancers. There is consequently a tendency to accept non-palpable breast cancers as early-stage breast cancer. However, the current generally accepted definition of early-stage breast cancer involves Stage I and Stage IIA breast cancer.

Clinical Staging

I would like to revise the staging for early-stage breast cancer in this section because the decision to start treatment with either surgery or chemotherapy is based on clinical staging [1].

V. Ozmen, MD, FACS
Department of Surgery, Istanbul University Istanbul Faculty of Medicine, Çapa, Istanbul, Turkey

Director, Breast Center, Istanbul Florence Nightingale Hospital, Sisli, Istanbul, Turkey
e-mail: vozmen@istanbul.edu.tr

© Springer International Publishing Switzerland 2016
A. Aydiner et al. (eds.), *Breast Disease: Management and Therapies*,
DOI 10.1007/978-3-319-26012-9_4

Primary Tumor

The diameter of a tumor can be measured via physical examination or radiological evaluation. Radiological evaluations permit more precise measurements.

T1: Defines tumors ≤2 cm and is further divided into four groups according to the diameter of the tumor:
   T1mic: ≤0.1 cm
   T1a: 0.1–0.5 cm
   T1b: 0.5–1 cm
   T1c: 1–2 cm
T2 defines tumors larger than 2 cm and smaller than 5 cm.

Regional Lymph Nodes

Clinical Evaluation

Regional lymph nodes are evaluated by physical examination.

NX: Regional lymph nodes cannot be evaluated (previously removed, etc.).
N0: There are no palpable regional lymph nodes.
N1: There are mobile and palpable lymph nodes in the axilla on the same side.
N2: There are fixed lymph nodes in the axilla on the same side, stuck together or to the surrounding tissue, or there are no palpable lymph nodes in the axilla, but there is a palpable internal mammary lymph node on the same side.

Distant Metastasis
M0: No distant metastasis.
M1: There is distant metastasis.

Stage I Breast Cancer
Defined as T1 N0 M0

Stage IIA Breast Cancer
Defined as T0 N1 M0, T1 N1 M0, or T2 N0 M0

Stage IIB Breast Cancer
Defined as T2 N1 M0 or T0 N2 M0 breast cancer

Because Stage IIB and Stage III breast cancer are regarded as locally advanced breast cancers, initial treatment with neoadjuvant chemotherapy is recommended in these cancers. Surgical treatment, such as breast-conserving surgery (BCS) or mastectomy, is initiated after this treatment.

If the tumor-to-breast volume ratio is appropriate in Stage IIB breast cancer patients (T2N1 = tumor size is 2–5 cm, axilla N1), treatment can be initiated with surgery, such as BCS or mastectomy. If the patient's axilla is rated N2, treatment should begin with chemotherapy.

For locally advanced breast cancer, BCS can be performed after neoadjuvant chemotherapy in selected cases. This topic is explained elsewhere in a separate section.

Preoperative Evaluation
Anamnesis, physical examination, chest X-ray, and routine laboratory work-up are sufficient for staging in early-stage breast cancer. Computed tomography of the thorax and abdomen, bone scintigraphy, and FDG PET-CT should be used for the evaluation of locally advanced breast cancer and only if the patient has complaints.

Evaluation of the Breast with Tumor
The breast with tumor should be examined in detail, particularly for BCS, because if the tumor is multicentric (tumor in more than one quadrant) in the same breast, BCS cannot be performed. In multifocal cancers (more than one tumor in the same quadrant), a large excision can be made if the tumor-to-breast volume ratio is appropriate. Careful physical examination and quality mammography should be performed primarily. Ultrasonography and magnetic resonance imaging (MRI) should be added if the patient is young and/or has high breast density. The presence of other tumors in the same quadrant (multifocal) or other quadrants (multicentric) will affect the extent of the treatment.

There are some studies suggesting digital mammography and tomosynthesis are better for the imaging of the breast and can successfully define other tumors and tumor size [2, 3]. In addition, ultrasonography is not needed with these techniques.

Using MRI routinely in BCS patients is controversial [4]. In a meta-analysis covering primary breast cancer patients, 16 % had multifocal/multicentric cancer by MRI prior to treatment [4]. However, the local recurrence rate in patients who have undergone BCS and radiotherapy is less than 10 %, even with 10-year surveillance. In a large retrospective study including patients who underwent BCS and radiotherapy, MRI made no contribution to treatment. MRI increases false positivity, leading to unnecessary biopsies and mastectomies. For this reason, it should only be performed in selected cases and when mandatory, and if possible, biopsies should be performed with MRI guidance to enable a histological diagnosis.

Evaluation of the Other Breast

Patients should also be reviewed carefully for the presence of cancer in the other breast. The probability of detecting synchronous bilateral breast cancer (cancer in the other breast within a year after the diagnosis of a primary tumor) is 1–3 % [5]. Ultrasonography and MRI can be useful if suspicious lesions are detected in the physical examination or by mammography.

Histopathological Diagnosis

If there is a suspicion of breast cancer based on anamnesis, physical examination, and radiological diagnostic methods, microscopic examination is essential for a definite diagnosis. Making the diagnosis prior to surgery aids the planning of the surgical treatment in cooperation with the patient.

Our most preferred method for biopsy today is a Tru-Cut (core) biopsy. This method yields adequate material for tissue determination and other required tests (determination of receptors, etc.). Excisional biopsy for diagnosis is not a preferred method for us because it makes determining surgical borders and performing BCS difficult in the next surgical intervention.

Surgical Procedures for Early-Stage Breast Cancer

1. Mastectomy
2. Breast-conserving surgery(BCS)

3. Skin-sparing mastectomy (explained in another section)
4. Subcutaneous mastectomy (sparing the nipple, areola, and breast skin) (explained in another section)

Mastectomy

History

Mastectomy was first defined and published by William Stewart Halsted and Meyer in the middle of the 1890s as a "radical mastectomy" [6, 7]. This surgical procedure involves en bloc resection of the breast together with the pectoral muscles and all tissues in the axilla. Because the breast skin is broadly excised, a free skin graft is used to close the defect in the thoracic wall. According to the Halsted hypothesis, because breast cancer is a local and regional disease, the excision of the breast together with regional lymphatics provides definitive treatment of the disease. At that time, when the 3-year local/regional recurrence and survival rates were greater than 50 % and approximately 20 %, respectively, Halsted listed these rates as 6 % and 40 % in his article published in 1907 [8]. These improvements in survival rates and local recurrence led to the performance of Halsted radical mastectomies for nearly a decade for the treatment of breast cancer [9, 10]. This surgical procedure has serious complications, such as thorax deformity, lymphedema, and motor and sensory loss. The addition of radiotherapy to radical mastectomy increases the complications and can also lead to brachial plexopathy (Fig. 4.1). Today, radical mastectomies for the surgical treatment of early-stage breast cancer are not performed. In cases when mastectomies are necessary, modified radical mastectomies that spare the pectoral muscles or BCS in appropriate patients are performed [10].

Although radical mastectomies provide excellent local regional control, due to the aforementioned high morbidity, modified radical mastectomies evolved in the 1940s. The aim of this surgical procedure was to conserve the

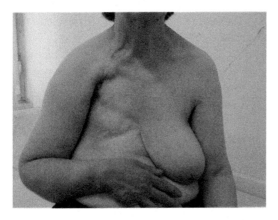

Fig. 4.1 Right arm edema and brachial plexopathy in a patient with pT1N0M0 who underwent radical mastectomy and radiotherapy 35 years ago

major pectoral muscles and, in particular, the long thoracic and thoracodorsal nerves. Patey and Dyson defined a surgical procedure preserving the major pectoral muscle but involving axillary dissection together with the minor muscle [11]. This procedure also helped preserve the medial and lateral pectoral nerves. Later, the technique that is accepted today as a modified radical mastectomy was defined by Auchincloss [12]. Level I and II axillary dissection were found to be satisfactory in this technique, and the major and minor pectoral muscles were preserved.

Modified Radical Mastectomy

Definition

Modified radical mastectomy is defined as the excision of the breast and the tumor together with the breast skin, the pectoral fascia, the lymph nodes in the axilla, and the soft tissue. If the tumor is close to the surface, the incision is adjusted accordingly, and the overlying skin is excised together with the tumor. If the pectoral fascia and/or major pectoral muscle are affected, the tumor-invaded muscle is excised locally to achieve a tumor-free, clean surgical border.

Indications

The generally preferred surgery in early-stage breast cancer is BCS. However, it is not always possible to conserve the breast, and some patients may also choose mastectomy:

1. Patients in which the obligatory radiotherapy after BCS is inapplicable or unfavorable: Patients with prior radiation to the thorax wall, first- or second-trimester pregnancy, collagen disease (scleroderma, active lupus erythematosus, etc.), or ataxia-telangiectasia. Radiotherapy may also not be preferred for social and economic reasons, or patients may refuse radiotherapy. Patients living in a location that is far from the radiotherapy center and patients who do not have sufficient funds for radiotherapy and its complications may also prefer mastectomy.

2. Patient desire: Patients generally accept the surgical treatment suggested by a doctor whom they trust. However, some patients prefer mastectomy to remove a breast which they believe is the reason in order to avoid radiotherapy or to complete the treatment in a short time. This desire is more commonly observed in patients who are old and calm and have low educational and economic status.

3. Presence of a multicentric tumor or diffuse ductal carcinoma in situ (DCIS) together with an invasive tumor: If there is cancer in more than one quadrant of the breast (multicentricity), BCS is not possible. In addition, even if the invasive tumor is small in size, the presence of diffuse ductal carcinoma in situ (DCIS) in its environment necessitates mastectomy. If the surgical border is found to be positive and the positivity remains in the recurrent excisions, mastectomy should be performed.

4. Inappropriate tumor-to-breast volume ratio: If the breast is small, conserving the breast can be difficult even if the tumor is small. The appearance of the remaining breast tissue after lumpectomy may not satisfy the patient or the surgeon. If the breast is very large or hanging loose, the application of radiotherapy to the

breast after lumpectomy can be difficult. Therefore, it is very important that breast cancer patients are discussed among all specialist physicians (breast surgeon, medical oncologist, radiation oncologist, etc.), and the treatment plan is prepared accordingly.

5. Patients who have previously undergone BCS with a diagnosis of breast cancer and who have recurrent cancer in the same breast: In patients who have local recurrence in the same breast after BCS, the suggested standard treatment is mastectomy. If axillary dissection was previously performed and there is no axillary recurrence at the time of diagnosis, there is no need for an axillary intervention. Performing sentinel lymph node biopsy (SLNB) in these patients is controversial.

6. Prophylactic mastectomy: For women who are positive for BRCA1 or BRCA2 genes or who are in a high-risk group and desire mastectomy, prophylactic mastectomy can be performed. This topic is explained in a different section.

Prophylactic Antibiotic Administration

Mastectomy incisions are classified as clean wounds because they are located remotely from systems that have high contamination risk, such as the gastrointestinal, genitourinary, and respiratory systems. Even so, wound infection rates after modified radical mastectomy are between 2 % and 15 % [13]. For this reason, breast surgeons favor the preoperative intravenous administration of single-dose cephalosporin or ampicillin-sulbactam, which has anti-staphylococcal activity. Single-dose prophylactic antibiotic administration decreases wound infections and, consequently, decreases prolonged wound healing and reduces the risk of delayed chemotherapy. However, other factors, such as increases in cost due to antibiotics, allergic reactions, and increases in bacterial resistance, should also be considered [14].

Surgical Techniques

Today, mastectomies in patients with positive axilla are performed as modified radical mastectomies and include the breast, pectoral fascia, axillary lymph nodes, and soft tissue. In patients with clinically negative axilla, sentinel lymph node biopsy should be performed primarily, and if there is no tumor, axillary dissection is not required. In mastectomies, the surgical borders are formed by the clavicle above, the upper insertion point of the anterior and posterior sheaths of the rectus muscle below, the sternum medially, and the latissimus dorsi muscle laterally.

Incision

In mastectomies, an elliptic Stewart incision is preferred as a standard procedure (Fig. 4.2). Making this incision in a mild oblique way is regarded as a modified Stewart incision, and it

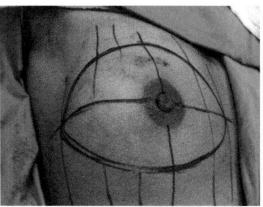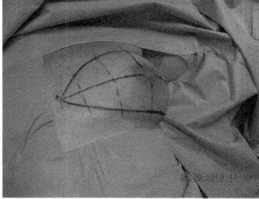

Fig. 4.2 Examples of transverse mastectomy incision (Stewart incision)

Table 4.1 Comparison of local recurrence and mean survival time of patients who had breast-conserving surgery (BCS) and mastectomy and were followed for 76 months (İstanbul Medical Faculty Breast Unit)

Stages of breast cancer	Number of patients	Follow-up time (months)	Tumor diameter (cm)	BCS surgical margin	RT boost	Local recurrence		Mean survival time	
						BCS (%)	Mastectomy (%)	(%) BCS	Mastectomy
Stage I	279 (37 %)	76	≤2 cm	Min 2 mm	Yes	6	5	91	91
Stage IIA	243 (32 %)	76	2–5 cm	Min 2 mm	Yes	6	5	89	89
Stage IIB	110 (15 %)	76	2–5 cm	Min 2 mm	Yes	6	4	82	86
Total	632	76	<5 cm	Min 2 mm	Yes	6	4	86	85

Modified from Karanlik et al. [16]

extends from the medial side of the sternum to the latissimus dorsi muscle. Some surgeons prefer Orr or modified Orr incisions. If early reconstruction is not performed, the skin should not be left loose. Leaving too much skin increases the risk of ischemia and necrosis, causes an irregular appearance on the thorax wall, and makes late reconstruction difficult. For the perfect alignment of skin flaps after mastectomy, lines that are perpendicular to the incision are drawn with a pen.

Dissection

The aim of a mastectomy is to remove as much of the breast tissue as possible such that no breast tissue is adhered subcutaneously. This minimizes the tumor recurrence rate on the mastectomized side. A retrospective clinical study led by Hartmann et al. at the Mayo Clinic from 1963 to 1990, which studied women who were in a high-risk group based on a positive family history and the Gail model and who underwent bilateral prophylactic mastectomy (BPM), revealed that BPM decreased breast cancer risk by 90 % in these women but did not totally eliminate it [15]. A study by Rebbeck et al. [17] of BRCA1 and BRCA2 carriers indicated that BPM reduces breast cancer risk by 90 %. These results indicate that despite mastectomy, breast cancer recurrence probability cannot be eliminated on the same side. This recurrence is also related to the amount of breast tissue left on cutaneous tissue. In our study conducted at the Istanbul Faculty of Medicine Breast Unit, the local recurrence rate was 4 % after 76 months of surveillance in

patients who had a mastectomy with a diagnosis of breast cancer (Table 4.1) [16].

After the incision of the cutaneous and subcutaneous tissue with a surgical blade, the superficial fascia overlying the breast parenchyma is exposed. Dissection should be continued along this cleavage between the thin subcutaneous tissue of the breast and the breast parenchyma. When the top and bottom flaps are being prepared, the skin and the underlying fat tissue and the vessels nourishing it should be protected to a thickness of approximately 5 cm. Electrocautery or a surgical blade can be used during dissection. The risk of ischemia and necrosis of the skin is slightly higher with electrocauterization. The technical skill and experience of the surgeon play a very important role in preparing a perfect flap. Some surgeons aim to facilitate the dissection and reduce blood loss by injecting a solution made of lactated Ringer's, lidocaine, and epinephrine into the subcutaneous tissue. However, it is unclear if this technique yields better results.

Flaps should be prepared reaching the clavicle above, the origin of the rectus muscle fascia below, the sternum on the inside, and the latissimus dorsi muscle outside. The whole breast tissue is dissected from the skin in this manner. Subsequently, proceeding laterally from the sternum, the fascia overlying the major pectoral muscle together with the breast tissue is skimmed from the muscle to the latissimus dorsi muscle. If axillary dissection is also performed, axillary tissues between the latissimus dorsi, the major pectoral muscle, and the

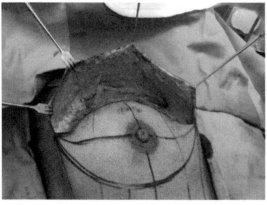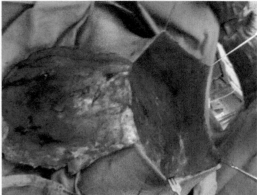

Fig. 4.3 Flap preparation in mastectomy

axillary vein should be removed en bloc together with the breast (Fig. 4.3).

Good hemostasis should be maintained during dissection. In particular, greater caution is required for anticoagulated patients to avoid hematoma under the flap despite subcutaneous drainage. The use of a surgical blade rather than electrocautery to dissect the pectoral fascia from the muscle helps to reduce necrosis and tissue loss in muscles due to coagulation. However, dissection with a surgical blade causes greater blood loss. In addition, using bipolar electrocautery for the hemorrhages over flaps and muscles reduces tissue loss to a minimum.

After the flaps are completely prepared, the breast gland is thoroughly removed, and the cavity is rinsed a few times with warm physiological serum, and hemostatic control is repeated. Regardless of axillary dissection, two 10-F Jackson-Pratt drains are placed under the top and bottom flaps and fixed to the skin with 2-0 silk sutures (Fig. 4.4).

Mastectomy incisions should be closed with subcutaneous and cutaneous sutures. Subcutaneous tissue is sutured with single sutures using 3-0 absorbable material (polyglactin 910 (Vicryl) or polydioxanone (PDS)). Cutaneous tissue is sutured with continuous intracutaneous sutures using 3-0 or 4-0 fast-absorbing material (Rapide Vicryl or PDS). Any excess skin at the medial or lateral end is excised with a triangular incision.

The closed mastectomy incision is covered vertically with thin Steri-Strips. Surgical gauzes

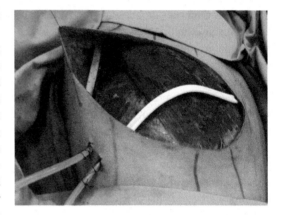

Fig. 4.4 Complete mastectomy and placement of drains

are placed around the drain and over the wound and taped with Hypafix. Because women have more sensitive skin, adhesive plasters should not be left on the skin for too long to avoid the rapid development of erosions and bullous lesions. For this reason, if wound dressings are desired, it can be bandaged in a figure of eight at the end of the day of surgery or the next day.

Complications of Mastectomy

Mastectomy has low mortality and morbidity and can be safely performed by a general surgeon. However, as with all surgical procedures, patients should be thoroughly evaluated prior to surgery, careful technique should be applied during surgery, good hemostatic control should be maintained, flaps should be prepared free of any breast tissue and to avoid compromising blood flow, and patients should be well followed after surgery. During the preoperative examination, patients should be evaluated for cardiac, respiratory, and other systems and for tolerance to general anesthesia, and medical issues, such as anemia, coagulopathy (particularly long-term anticoagulant usage), diabetes, and hypertension, should be corrected. Immunosuppressant (corticosteroids, antitumor medicine) use should be determined.

After mastectomy, rinsing the surgical site with physiological serum at body temperature is important to reveal any hemorrhages from previously clotted vessels and to remove unnecessary tissue. Bleeding sites on flaps and the major pectoral muscle should preferably be coagulated with bipolar cautery. Compared to monopolar cautery, bipolar cautery burns less tissue and thus reduces skin necrosis and pectoral muscle loss. Good hemostasis prevents the occurrence of hematoma at the surgical site and helps to reduce healing time and the timely initiation of other treatments.

Closed-suction drains (Jackson-Pratt or Blake) should be used to minimize seroma at the surgical site and to prevent hematoma after surgery. These are placed under the flap, conveyed out via a separate incision, and fixed with 2-0 nonabsorbable sutures. This incision should be close to the mastectomy incision and, keeping in mind that radiotherapy may be necessary, within the radiotherapy field. Closed-suction drains should be kept in place for 5–10 days. During that time, the catheters should be checked for any clots and fibrin remains and must be cleaned, and drainage should be maintained. Drains can be removed once the drained amount has decreased to 25 ml per 24 h.

After flaps are covered with a double tissue layer, closed, and adhered with strips, they are dressed with surgical gauze and taped. Tightly dressing the wound and bandaging with compression have no seroma-reducing or flap-adhering effects. However, when plasters are left on sensitive skin for too long, they cause erosions and bullous lesions; to keep dressings in place, bandages can be used instead of plaster at the end of the day of surgery or the next day.

We observed that patients generally use the operated extremity very little or sometimes not at all. Patients who are generally kept in the hospital for 1 day and then discharged should be advised about the activities they can participate in and their diet both orally and with written instructions at the time of discharge from the hospital. They should be advised that they must use the operated extremity for daily activities and that they should start the arm exercises they performed before the operation as soon as drains are removed. To restore arm/shoulder movements, they should receive support from physical therapy and rehabilitation polyclinics when necessary.

Wound Infection

Reported wound infection rates after modified radical mastectomy are 2–15 % [17]. Infection at the site of incision or in the arm is a cause of serious postoperative morbidity, delaying utilization of the extremity and increasing lymphedema.

Cellulitis is generally responsive to antibiotics. The resulting abscess should be drained early, the wound should be washed, debridement should be performed, and a closed-suction drainage system should be placed again. Antibiotic treatment should be administered according to antibiogram test results. When patient-related adverse factors (uncontrolled diabetes, advanced age, anemia, etc.) are combined with technical problems (flap not being well prepared, necrosis, ischemia, etc.), complications such as wound infection, necrosis, and abscess increase. The most common microorganisms causing wound infection are *Staphylococcus aureus* and *Staphylococcus epidermidis*.

Prophylactic antibiotic administration prior to surgery has become a routine procedure. However, some surgeons do not administer antibiotics if the patient is not in a high-risk group. We recommend the administration of a single dose of an anti-staphylococcal antibiotic before mastectomy.

Seroma

The term seroma denotes the accumulation of fluid at the surgical site. After mastectomy, the fluid accumulation rate under flaps in the dead space reaches up to 30 % despite drainage or after drainage [18]. Broad dissection of the breast disrupts lymphatics, vascular structures, and fatty tissue and causes lymphovascular fluid (transudate) to accumulate in the dead space. The surgical technique performed should aid in the preservation of the vascular nourishment of the flaps and cause less trauma to vascular and lymphatic structures. Seroma can be reduced in this way.

Seroma increases the risk of wound infection, which causes pain and a sensation of fullness at the operation site, delays wound healing, prolongs the hospital stay, and may delay the initiation of chemotherapy. For more than 30 years, the application of closed-suction drainage systems has significantly reduced seroma formation and related complications.

A high body mass index (>30), increased physical activity after the operation, the surgical technique, and improper closed-suction drainage system function are thought to be factors responsible for increasing seroma formation. In a study conducted by Tadych and Donegan [19] in which the amount of drainage was measured with a closed-suction drainage system daily and during the hospital stay, the relationship between the drainage volume and lymphedema formation was investigated. There was no relationship between the total volume drained and patient weight, but a high volume of drainage was directly related to edema in the arm on that side.

Beginning physical activity early after mastectomy is also considered a risk factor for seroma formation. A review of the literature by Shamley et al. revealed that the seroma formation was reduced with delayed physical activity [20].

Two mechanical methods were proposed to prevent seroma formation after mastectomy [18]. One is to apply pressure on the flaps from the outside. However, this method did not lead to reduced seroma formation and causes necrosis in the flaps due to pressure. The second method is fixation of the flaps to the thorax wall with absorbable sutures. It is suggested that this method reduces seroma and simplifies postoperative care and surgical dressing. However, careful surgical technique, good hemostasis, and not making the flaps larger than needed reduce seroma and thus eliminate the necessity of additional interventions.

Hemorrhage

Closed-suction drainage systems facilitate the early detection of hemorrhages and decrease hematomas. The reported hemorrhage rates after mastectomy are 1–4 % [21]. In hemorrhages that are noticed early, the reactivation of drains by cleaning and applying dressing to the surgical site with pressure may help stop bleeding. In moderate to severe bleeding, the wound should be opened in the operating room and irrigated, and the bleeding site should be detected and ligated or controlled with suturing. The dead space should then be drained with a closed-suction system. Serious hemorrhages are often due to perforation of branches of the thoracoacromial vessels or the internal mammary artery.

During mastectomy, to prepare the flaps quickly and without bleeding and to reduce postoperative complications, surgeons apply techniques such as monopolar electrocauterization, bipolar electrocauterization, cold blade, Shaw hot blade, laser coagulation, and fibrin filling [21, 22]. Studies do not indicate that any of these procedures are superior. The aim is to complete the surgery with careful technique and good hemostasis, observe the patient regularly, and prevent hematoma formation.

Pneumothorax

Pneumothorax is a rare complication. It is observed more often during radical mastectomy procedures when the major pectoral muscle is removed. Parietal pleura can be torn during the bleeding control of injuries to the intercostal perforating vessels and during dissection. In addition, pneumothorax can occur during the dissection of lymph nodes close to the sternum during internal mammary lymph node biopsy.

When pneumothorax occurs, torn pleura can be fixed and covered with muscle. Air in the pleural cavity is generally resorbed without intervention. If a serious pneumothorax is observed on the postoperative chest X-ray, a small tube can be placed through the second intercostal space to aspirate the air inside and is then connected to a closed-suction thorax drainage system. The thorax tube is removed once the lung fully expands.

Tissue Necrosis

When subcutaneous vascular structures are not preserved during broad dissection in mastectomy, skin necrosis occurs. Tissue necrosis also develops in uncontrolled seromas and infections. Debridement and wound care are sufficient to manage small necroses.

Current mastectomy techniques seldom require covering the mastectomy space with a free skin graft. However, reconstruction and repair with free pedicled skin grafts may be necessary for necrosis occurring in flaps after mastectomy, advanced-stage breast cancers that do not regress despite chemotherapy, recurrences in the thorax wall, and large breast sarcomas.

Local Recurrence Following Mastectomy

Rowell reviewed 22 studies including 18,863 patients. In these studies, 2.5 % of mastectomy materials from patients were found to be positive; there was a close surgical border in 8 % and pectoral fascia and/or muscle invasion in 7.2 % [23]. Some studies defined close surgical borders as 1 mm, some 2 mm, and others 4–10 mm.

In this meta-analysis, local recurrence rates in the studies varied between 4 % and 30 %. The most important risk factor was close surgical borders. The addition of radiotherapy to treatment was found to be imperative for the reduction of local/regional recurrence.

Local/regional recurrences after mastectomy were related to factors such as axillary involvement, the number of positive lymph nodes, extracapsular invasion, hormone receptor positivity, histological grade, tumor diameter, lymphovascular invasion, young age (40 years in some studies, 35 in others), and premenopausal status (Table 4.2) [23–26].

Naturally, one important factor for local/regional recurrence after mastectomy is the experience of the breast surgeon performing the operation. According

Table 4.2 Local recurrence factors in patients who undergo mastectomy

Mastectomy			
	Relationship with local recurrence		
Local recurrence factors	Strong (+++)	Fair (++)	Weak (+)
Axilla positivity and the number of nodules	+++		
No systemic treatment		++	
Surgical margin positivity		++	
Close surgical margin (<2 mm)			+
Tumor diameter			+
Age of the patient (<40 or <35)			+
Lymphovascular invasion (+)			+
Extracapsular invasion			+

+++ Relationship consistently reported in literature
++ Relationship frequently reported in literature
+ Relationship occasionally reported in literature

to "early diagnosis, screening and treatment guideline in breast cancer" published in the European Union in 2006, breast surgeons should be trained in a "breast unit" in which at least 150 breast cancer patients are treated annually and should be performing at least 50 breast cancer operations per year [27]. Surgeons performing less than this number may leave more breast tissue under the flaps, leading to more local recurrences [28].

Breast-Conserving Surgery

Definition

BCS is removal of the tumor (or tumors if multifocal) together with at least 10 mm of surrounding healthy breast tissue. This procedure is also called a lumpectomy, broad tumor excision, segmental mastectomy, and tylectomy. After tumor removal, the remaining breast should appear well and acceptable cosmetically.

History

High morbidity due to Halsted's radical mastectomy led surgeons to perform modified radical mastectomies first, preserving pectoral muscles. Thus, "radical mastectomy," which was first defined in the 1890s and was performed for nearly 100 years, gave way to "modified radical mastectomy" in the 1940s [6–10]. Fischer's hypothesis, which he developed after the results of studies conducted in the 1970s dictated that breast cancer was a systemic disease, led to surgery to conserve the breast in the treatment of breast cancer [29, 30].

The first prospective randomized clinical trial was conducted in Guy's Hospital (London, UK) and published in 1972 [31]. Because the radiation dose administered to patients in this trial (3,800 cGy) was below the standard treatment dosage (6,500 cGy), the local recurrence rate was higher in the BCS group.

In the 1970s, BCS was compared to mastectomy in several prospective clinical trials. In the six best known and accepted of these trials and in a meta-analysis of these trials, BCS was shown to yield similar survival rates to mastectomy and had acceptable local recurrence rates and cosmetic and functional results (Table 4.3) [32–38].

Although the results of 20 years of surveillance in the NSABP-B06 and Milan trials showed no significant difference in the mean survival rates in the BCS and mastectomy groups, local recurrence rates were significantly higher in the BCS group [32, 33]. In the NSABP-B06 trial, the BCS without radiotherapy group had a local recurrence rate of 39.2 %, and this ratio fell to 14.3 % in the BCS + radiotherapy group. This result demonstrated that radiotherapy should be a standard treatment after BCS.

In a study conducted by the EORTC Radiation Oncology Group, in addition to 50 Gy radiation applied to the breast, 16 Gy boost radiation applied to the tumor bed reduced local recurrence from 10.2 % to 6.2 % [39]. This study together with similar studies has indicated the importance of radiotherapy applied to the breast and a boost dose applied to the tumor cavity for reducing local recurrence after BCS [32–39].

The Milan study revealed that cosmetic results of quadrantectomy as BCS were satisfactory in only 60 % of patients [33]. Therefore, for patients who have broad tumor excision as BCS and when the cavity is very large, filling the cavity with breast tissue or with latissimus dorsi muscle (oncoplastic surgery) improves the cosmetic appearance.

Patient Selection

To achieve a low local recurrence rate and a good cosmetic appearance in BCS, patients should be carefully selected. After anamnesis, a careful physical examination and the necessary radiological examinations, patients should be prepared for BCS. In patients with dense breast texture and who are young, have higher local recurrence probability, and for whom radiotherapy is difficult due to economic or social reasons, mastectomy may be preferred.

For a low local recurrence rate after BCS, multiple tumors should be in the same quadrant (multifocal), surgical borders should be negative, and the appearance of breast should be cosmetically acceptable after lumpectomy.

Contraindications for BCS are summarized in Table 4.4. Multicentric cancers (two or more cancers in more than one quadrant), microcalcifications that show a tendency for diffuse pleomorphic cluster formation, a negative surgical border despite re-excisions, first- or second-trimester pregnancy, and prior radiotherapy to the thorax wall (Hodgkin's lymphoma, thymoma, etc.) all render BCS impossible.

Because the presence of collagen vascular disease in the patient (scleroderma, lupus erythematosus, etc.) will cause wound healing problems due to the application of radiotherapy in this region, care should be taken in these patients. In women who have low breast volume, the diminished breast after lumpectomy may disrupt its appearance cosmetically. Likewise, BCS may be difficult for cosmetic reasons in women who have a large tumor diameter.

Some patients find the breast with the tumor to be at fault, want to eliminate it, and desire mastectomy. In addition, if the patient is living in a location far from the center where radiotherapy will be administered and cannot travel for economic or other reasons, mastectomy is required.

Table 4.3 Modern prospective randomized clinical studies comparing breast-conserving surgery and mastectomy

Study	Number of patients	Follow-up time (years)	Tumor diameter (cm)	BCS surgical margin	RT boost	Local recurrence		Mean survival time	
						BCS (%)	Mastectomy (%)	(%) BCS	Mastectomy
NSABP [32]	1,851	20	<4	Without tumor	No	14.3	10.2	46.2	47.2
Milan [33]	701	20	<2	Far	Yes	8.8	2.3	41.7	41.2
NCI [34]	247	10	<5	Gross	Yes	18.0	10.0	77	75
EORTC [35]	903	8	<5	1 cm	Yes	15	10	60	64
Danish [36]	859	6	–	Gross	Yes	3	4	79	82
Gustav-Roussy [37]	179	14.5	<2	2 cm	Yes	11.4	11.0	72	65
EBCTCG [38]	3,100	10	All	Differs	+/–	5.9	6.2	50.1	48

NSABP National Surgical Adjuvant Breast Project, *NCI* National Cancer Institute, *EORTC* European Organization for Research and Treatment of Cancer, *EBCTCG* Early Breast Cancer Trialists' Collaborative Group

Table 4.4 Breast-conserving surgery (BCS) contraindications

Breast-conserving surgery
Absolute contraindications
Pregnancy (first and second trimesters)
Multicentricity
Microcalcifications with diffuse malignant appearances
Previous radiotherapy to the chest wall
Ongoing surgical margin positivity despite re-excisions
Relative contraindications
Incompliance of breast/tumor diameter
Collagen vascular diseases
Desire of the patient for mastectomy
Impossibility of radiotherapy treatment (economic reasons, distance from centers)

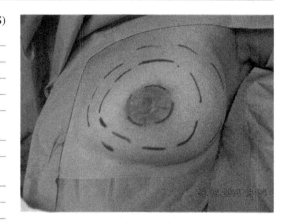

Fig. 4.5 Parallel incisions to the areola for breast-conserving surgery (BCS)

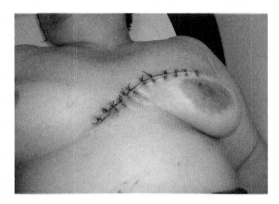

Fig. 4.6 An example of a bad and unacceptable incision in breast-conserving surgery

Surgical Technique

The aim of BCS is to completely remove the tumor from the breast, reduce local recurrence, and achieve a cosmetically acceptable appearance. Surgical treatment of breast cancer not only reduces local recurrence but also improves survival. In a meta-analysis conducted by the Early Breast Cancer Trialists' Collaborative Group (EBCTCG), BCS and radiotherapy improved survival by 5.3 % by the end of a 15-year period [24]. This rate was approximately 4.4 % with mastectomy and radiotherapy [24, 40].

Prophylactic Antibiotic Administration

Incisions in the breast and axilla make clean wounds and are considered to have a low risk of infection. However, studies have shown that wound infection rates after breast cancer surgery vary between 1 % and 15 % [41, 42]. This rate is low after lumpectomy (1–5 %) but higher after mastectomy (2–17 %) and reconstruction (6–15 %). For this reason, we recommend the administration of a single dose of a prophylactic antibiotic that is effective against *S. aureus* and *S. epidermidis* (cephalosporin, ampicillin-sulbactam, etc.).

Incision

Generally, circular incisions that are parallel to areola and in conformity with natural lines of Langer are preferred in BCS (Fig. 4.5). However, in some situations, a radial incision can be made for tumors localized at 3, 6, or 9 o'clock. Incisions starting from the sulcus of the other breast are a cause of poor cosmesis and should not be made (Fig. 4.6). Incisions should be made just over the tumor and should extend 1 cm proximal and 1 cm distal from the tumor for palpable tumors. If the tumor is close to the skin, it should be removed together with the skin. However, cosmetic appearance may deteriorate in this situation. For tumors located far from the areola, making an incision to the areola, creating a tunnel, and removing the tumor from this tunnel are strongly discouraged because tumor seeding may occur, and it is difficult to achieve a negative surgical border in this way.

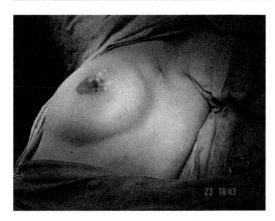

Fig. 4.7 Postoperative view of a patient who had BCS and sentinel lymph node biopsy (SLNB)

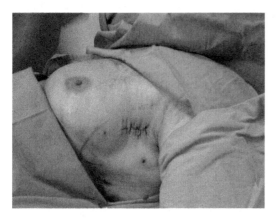

Fig. 4.8 An example of a bad incision in breast-conserving surgery. An incision oblique to the axilla was performed

To achieve a fine cosmetic result with BCS, for tumors localized in the upper lateral quadrant, separate incisions should be made for the dissection of the tumor and axilla (Fig. 4.7). Incisions that are made radially including the axilla could cause increased scar formation and subsequent deformity (Fig. 4.8).

Removal of the Tumor

The tumor should be removed together with the healthy breast tissue around it. Approximately 10 mm macroscopically is sufficient healthy tissue around the tumor. Microscopically, a border of 2 mm is generally accepted. The experience of the surgeon is important for identifying the healthy tissue around the tumor in palpable lesions and removing the tumor with an adequate border.

Morrow et al. investigated 2,030 patients who were treated for breast cancer in a population-based study [43]. Mastectomy was performed in 38 % of patients, with 9 % desiring a mastectomy from the beginning. In 13 %, a mastectomy was performed without any effort to perform a re-excision. Re-excision was necessary in 22 % of patients who had successful BCS. These results indicate that several factors related to the surgeon, the radiotherapist, and the patient play a role in performing BCS. A survey of "negative borders" was conducted among members of radiation oncology associations in North America and Europe. A total of 46 % of radiation oncologists in North America defined "negative" as tumors cells not in contact with the inked surface, 22 % as a 2-mm border, and 15 % as ≥5-mm border. Among European radiation oncologists, 28 % defined "negative" surgical borders as ink in the border, 9 % as 2 mm, and 45 % as ≥5 mm [44]. In a survey of 188 surgeons in the USA, 13 % found "surgically negative" borders adequate if ink in the border is not in contact with the tumor, 25 % if 2 mm or larger, and 55 % if larger than 5 mm [45].

The utilization of ultrasonography during surgery also helps to achieve a negative border. In a study conducted by Fine et al., performing lumpectomies in collaboration with intraoperative ultrasonography reduced the excised volume, decreased the length of the incision, and reduced re-excision due to border positivity [46].

In lumpectomies, there is an inverse relationship between the tissue volume excised during lumpectomy and cosmetic appearance, which is more evident in small-sized breasts. However, pathological multifocality and multicentricity rates are higher in tumors that have a diffuse intraductal component and in invasive lobular cancers, and broader excisions are necessary for these tumors.

If a tumor is not close to the overlying skin, the preservation of subcutaneous fat prevents retraction of the skin. In tumors that are close to the skin, tumors should be excised together with the overlying skin.

Evaluation of Surgical Borders

Borders should be marked before or after tumor removal. If different colored inks are used, every border is stained with a different color (Fig. 4.9). At least three borders of lumpectomy material, which is stained with only Indian ink, are marked with suturing materials in different lengths and colors (Fig. 4.10). Macroscopic (gross) evaluation of the removed specimen is essential for the adequate excision of the tumor. Close or positive surgical borders are re-excised and reevaluated. This procedure is repeated until a negative surgical border is obtained. If a negative surgical border cannot be achieved, a mastectomy should be performed. Therefore, patients should be

informed that the surgical border will be evaluated during the operation and that a mastectomy may be performed if necessary.

In some cases, it can be difficult to evaluate the surgical border; in these patients, the surgeons must wait for the results of the paraffin block, and a re-excision or mastectomy decision is made accordingly. Occasionally, a border that is diagnosed as negative in frozen sections is found positive after the evaluation of paraffin slides, and re-excision or mastectomy is necessary.

In tumors that are distant from the pectoral fascia, there is no need to go deep and remove the pectoral fascia.

After it is certain that the surgical borders are negative in the excised material, the walls of the cavity are marked with four or five metal clips for boost radiotherapy (Fig. 4.11).

In situations in which the cavity is too large after lumpectomy, the breast parenchyma close to the cavity wall can be shifted to the cavity following marking of the cavity with metal clips for boost radiotherapy. Therefore, the collapse of the cavity and an unwanted cosmetic result can be prevented.

Incision Closure

Very careful hemostasis should be applied to the walls of the lumpectomy cavity. For this hemostasis, bipolar cauterization should be used if possible to reduce the damage to breast parenchyma. Serious hematomas can develop if good hemostasis is not maintained, which prolongs

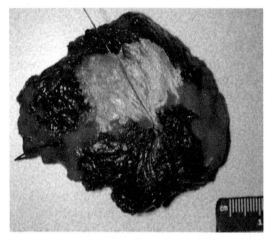

Fig. 4.9 Borders of lumpectomy material dyed with different colors

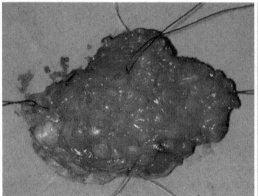
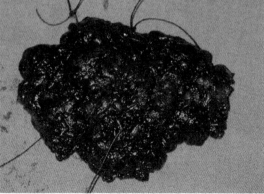

Fig. 4.10 Lumpectomy material marked with different-sized sutures (*left*) and dyed with one color (*right*)

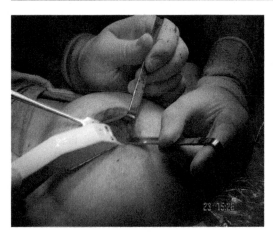

Fig. 4.11 Tumor cavity marked with a metal clip

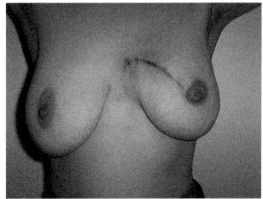

Fig. 4.12 Patient who underwent a quadrantectomy for a localized tumor in the left breast upper inner quadrant

wound healing, disrupts the cosmetic appearance, and delays adjuvant treatments.

For good cosmetic appearance, cavity walls should not be retracted with sutures, and drains should not be used. Subcutaneous tissue is sutured with single sutures using absorbable material (3-0–4-0). The skin is sutured with continuous sutures using thinner and absorbable material (3-0, 4-0, or 5-0) and then covered with thin strips.

Re-excision

Re-excision should be made if the surgical border is in contact with the ink or close to it (closer than 2 mm) by macroscopic evaluation. Re-excision is required in 20–30 % of patients who undergo BCS [38]. There is residual tumor in 40–70 % of re-excised patients. [37].

Quadrantectomy

Quadrantectomy is a method popularized by Veronesi et al. in Milan. In tumors smaller than 2 cm in diameter, the quadrant with the tumor is removed radially, including the surrounding 2–3 cm of tissue, the skin, and the pectoral fascia (Fig. 4.12). The axilla is also removed in tumors that are localized in the upper lateral quadrant. The excised volume was found to be inversely related to local recurrence in the Milan II study [47]. However, as stated previously, because broader excision yields a worse cosmetic appearance, this method is not preferred.

Local Recurrence Following Breast-Conserving Surgery

As stated earlier, the aim of BCS is to completely remove the tumor with negative surgical borders, reduce local recurrence, and achieve an acceptable cosmetic appearance. As mentioned earlier in the mastectomy section, the surgeon performing this procedure should be an experienced breast surgeon. It is essential that the breast surgeon discusses the patient with other breast specialists, such as the radiologist, pathologist, radiation oncologist, and medical oncologist in a "Weekly Tumor Council," and the patient's suitability for BCS should be determined. The pathologist should evaluate the excised material together with the surgeon, and re-excisions should be made when necessary. If the surgeon cannot ensure these conditions, he/she should not perform BCS.

To reduce local recurrence after BCS, apart from the experience of the surgeon, the patient should be evaluated carefully by physical examination and radiology prior to surgery, and the diffuseness of the tumor and its multifocality or multicentricity should be determined. The indications should not be forced according to the patient's desire.

Available imaging techniques detect a positive surgical border in 20–40 % of BCS cases. Risk factors for positive surgical border are related to tumor biology and patient-related

Table 4.5 Local recurrence factors in patients who undergo breast-conserving surgery

Breast-conserving surgery			
	Relationship with local recurrence		
Local recurrence factors	Strong (+++)	Fair (+++)	Weak (+++)
Surgical margin positivity	+++		
Age of the patient (<40 or <35)		++	
No systemic treatment		++	
Close surgical margin (<2 mm)			+
Lymphovascular invasion (+)			+
Axilla positivity			+

+++ Relationship consistently reported in literature
++ Relationship frequently reported in literature
+ Relationship occasionally reported in literature

factors. In a meta-analysis conducted by Pjleijhuis et al., local recurrence rates following BCS were 6–17 % [48]. In this study, close or positive surgical borders, tumor size, multifocal tumors, axilla positivity, excisional biopsy for diagnosis (compared with Tru-Cut and fine-needle aspiration biopsies), young patient age (<40 years or <35 years), diffuse intraductal component positivity, lobular histological type, presence of microcalcifications on mammography, and estrogen receptor negativity were related to local recurrence (Table 4.5).

Follow-Up of Patients After Breast-Conserving Surgery

Following BCS, there is an approximately 1–2 % risk of cancer development in the treated breast and the other breast [49]. Of local recurrences, 75 % are observed within 2 years, and 95 % are observed within 5 years. For this reason, follow-up of breast cancer patients is performed every 3 months during the first 3 years, every 6 months from 3 to 5 years, and annually after the fifth year with physical examination and necessary tests. Recent guidelines published by ASCO did not modify the current approach to follow-up after breast cancer treatment [50].

In patients who have had breast-conserving surgery and radiotherapy, a mammography of the treated breast is taken 6 months after radiotherapy. The patient is later followed with annual mammographies. Scar formation at the site of tumoral excision and its opacity in X-ray film can make the evaluation of this area difficult; Doppler ultrasonography may be helpful. However, gadolinium-contrasted MR imaging has proven to be very helpful in suspected cases for differential diagnosis. Although there is reduced contrast in scar tissue, there is increased vascularization together with increased contrast in recurrent tumoral tissue. If there is a suspicion of recurrence in radiological examinations, this mass should be reevaluated and biopsied.

Long-Term Complications of Breast-Conserving Treatment

The complications occurring in longer than 5-year surveillance of breast-conserving surgery and radiotherapy, which is the standard treatment for early-stage breast cancer, were edema in the arm, fibrosis in breast skin, limitations in shoulder movements, radiation pneumonia, neuropathy, fat necrosis, and costal fracture, in order of decreasing frequency. In 294 patients who had breast-conserving treatment and were followed for a mean average of 84 months at MD Anderson Cancer Center, the rate of grade 2 or higher complications was 9.9 % [51]. Of the 29 patients who had complications, the most common complications were edema of the arm in 13 patients (Fig. 4.13) and fibrosis of the breast skin in 12 patients. Severe fibrosis in the breast causes deformity in the breast (Fig. 4.14). Elderly patients represent the most-affected subpopulation of breast cancer survivors in terms of complications. In a study by de Glas NA et al., the odds ratio of postoperative morbidity was higher in older patients (OR 1.85, 95 % confidence interval (CI) 1.37–2.50, $p=0.001$) [52].

Fig. 4.13 Bilateral arm edema in a patient with breast cancer

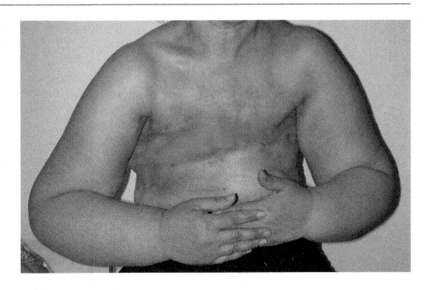

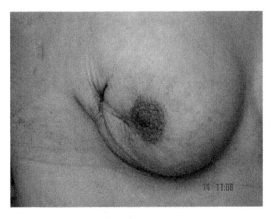

Fig. 4.14 A wider excision, radiotherapy, and fibrosis cause a worse cosmetic appearance

References

1. Singletary SE, Connolly JL. Breast cancer staging: working with the sixth edition of the AJCC Cancer Staging Manual. CA Cancer J Clin. 2006;56(1):37–47.
2. Hambly NM, Mc Nicholas MM, Phelan N, Hargaden GC, O'Doherty A, Flanagan FL. Comparison of digital mammography and screen-film mammography in breast cancer screening: a review in the Irish breast screening program. AJR Am J Roentgenol. 2009;193(4):1010–8.
3. Hakim CM, Chough DM, Ganott MA, Sumkin JH, Zuley ML, Gur D. Digital breast tomosynthesis in the diagnostic environment: a subjective side-by-side review. AJR Am J Roentgenol. 2010;195(2):W172–6.
4. Solin LJ. Counterview: pre-operative breast MRI (magnetic resonance imaging) is not recommended for all patients with newly diagnosed breast cancer. Breast. 2010;19(1):7–9.
5. Kheirelseid EA, Jumustafa H, Miller N, Curran C, Sweeney K, Malone C, et al. Bilateral breast cancer: analysis of incidence, outcome, survival and disease characteristics. Breast Cancer Res Treat. 2011;126(1):131–40.
6. Halsted WS. The results of operations for the cure of cancer of the breast performed at the Johns Hopkins Hospital from June 1889 to January 1894. Ann Surg. 1894;20:497–555.
7. Meyer W. An improved method of the radical operation for carcinoma of the breast. Med Rec NY. 1894;46:746.
8. Halsted WS. The results of radical operations for the cure of cancer of the breast. Tr Am S A. 1907;25:61.
9. Özmen V. Meme cerrahisinin tarihçesi ve cerrahi tekniklerin gelişimi. In: Topuz, editor. Meme Kanseri. İstanbul Üniversitesi Onkoloji Enstitüsü yayınları 3. 1997. p. 218–228.
10. Özmen V. Meme koruyucu cerrahide prospektif randomize klinik çalışmalar. In: Topuz E, Aydıner A, Dinçer M, editors. Meme Kanseri. Nobel Tıp Kitabevleri. 2003. p. 297–300.
11. Patey DH, Dyson WH. The prognosis of carcinoma of the breast in relation to the type of mastectomy performed. Br J Cancer. 1948;2:7–13.
12. Auchincloss H. Modified radical mastectomy: why not? Am J Surg. 1970;119(5):506–9.
13. Cunningham M, Bunn F, Handscomb K. Prophylactic antibiotics to prevent surgical site infection after breast cancer surgery. Cochrane Database Syst Rev. 2006;2, CD005360.
14. Throckmorton AD, Boughey JC, Boostrom SY, Holifield AC, Stobbs MM, Hoskin T, et al. Postoperative prophylactic antibiotics and surgical site infection rates in breast surgery patients. Ann Surg Oncol. 2009;16(9):2464–9.
15. Hartmann LC, Schaid DJ, Woods JE, Crotty TP, Myers JL, Arnold PG, et al. Efficacy of bilateral prophylactic mastectomy in women with a family history of breast cancer. N Engl J Med. 1999;340:77–84.

16. Karanlık H, Ozmen V, Asoglu O, İgci A, Keçer M, Tuzlali S, et al. Long term results of breast cancer surgery. J Breast Health. 2006;2:89–95.

17. Rebbeck TR, Freibel T, Lynch HT, Neuhausen SL, van 't Veer L, Garber JE, et al. Bilateral prophylactic mastectomy reduces breast cancer risk in BRCA1 and BRCA2 mutation carriers: the PROSE study group. J Clin Oncol. 2004;22:1055–62.

18. Kuroi K, Shimozuma K, Taguchi T, Imai H, Yamashiro H, Ohsumi S, et al. Effect of mechanical closure of dead space on seroma formation after breast surgery. Breast Cancer. 2006;13:260–5.

19. Tadych K, Donegan WL. Postmastectomy seromas and wound drainage. Surg Gynecol Obstet. 1987;165(6):483–7.

20. Shamley DR, Barker K, Simonite V, Beardshaw A. Delayed versus immediate exercises following surgery for breast cancer: a systematic review. Breast Cancer Res Treat. 2005;90(3):263–71.

21. Vitug AF, Newman LA. Complications in breast surgery. Surg Clin North Am. 2007;87(2):431–51.

22. Carless PA, Henry DA. Systematic review and meta-analysis of the use of fibrin sealant to prevent seroma formation after breast cancer surgery. Br J Surg. 2006;93(7):810–9.

23. Rowell NP. Are mastectomy resection margins of clinical relevance? A systematic review. Breast. 2010;19(1):14–22.

24. Clarke M, Collins R, Darby S, Davies C, Elphinstone P, Evans E, et al. Effects of radiotherapy and of differences in the extent of surgery for early breast cancer on local recurrence and 15-year survival: an overview of the randomised trials. Lancet. 2005;366: 2087–106.

25. Gruber G, Cole BF, Castiglione-Gertsch M, Holmberg SB, Lindtner J, Golouh R et al. International Breast Cancer Study Group. Extracapsular tumor spread and the risk of local, axillary and supraclavicular recurrence in node-positive, premenopausal patients with breast cancer. Ann Oncol. 2008;19(8):1393–401.

26. Elkhuizen PH, van Slooten HJ, Clahsen PC, Hermans J, van de Velde CJ, van den Broek LC, et al. High local recurrence risk after breast-conserving therapy in node-negative premenopausal breast cancer patients is greatly reduced by one course of perioperative chemotherapy: a European Organization for Research and Treatment of Cancer Breast Cancer Cooperative Group Study. J Clin Oncol. 2000; 18(5):1075–83.

27. http://ec.europa.eu/health/ph_projects/2002/cancer/fp.pdf. European guidelines for quality assurance of breast cancer screening, diagnosis, and treatment 4th edition, 2006.

28. Ozmen V. Meme hastalıklarının cerrahi tedavisinin kalitesi nasıl yükseltilebilir? Meme Sağlığı Dergisi. 2009;3:119–21.

29. Fisher B. The present status of tumor immunology. Adv Surg. 1971;5:189–254. Review.

30. Fisher B, Wolmark N, Fisher ER, Deutsch M. Lumpectomy and axillary dissection for breast cancer: surgical, pathological, and radiation considerations. World J Surg. 1985;9:692–8.

31. Atkins HJ, Hayward JL, Klugman DJ, Wayte AB. Treatment of early breast cancer. A report after ten years of clinical trial. Br MJ. 1972;2:423–9.

32. Fisher B, Anderson S, Bryant J, Margolese RG, Deutsch M, Fisher ER, et al. Twenty-year follow-up of a randomized trial comparing total mastectomy, lumpectomy, and lumpectomy plus irradiation for the treatment of invasive breast cancer. N Engl J Med. 2002;347(16):1233–41.

33. Veronesi U, Cascinelli N, Mariani L, Greco M, Saccozzi R, Luini A, et al. Twenty-year follow-up of a randomized study comparing breast-conserving surgery with radical mastectomy for early breast cancer. N Engl J Med. 2002;347(16):1227–32.

34. Jacobson JA, Danforth DN, Cowan KH, d'Angelo T, Steinberg SM, Pierce L, et al. Ten-year results of a comparison of conservation with mastectomy in the treatment of stage I and II breast cancer. N Engl J Med. 1995;332(14):907–11.

35. van Dongen JA, Bartelink H, Fentiman IS, Lerut T, Mignolet F, Olthuis G, et al. Randomized clinical trial to assess the value of breast-conserving therapy in stage I and II breast cancer, EORTC 10801 trial. J Natl Cancer Inst Monogr. 1992;11:15–8.

36. Blichert-Toft M, Rose C, Andersen JA, Overgaard M, Axelsson CK, Andersen KW, et al. Danish randomized trial comparing breast conservation therapy with mastectomy: six years of life-table analysis. Danish Breast Cancer Cooperative Group. J Natl Cancer Inst Monogr. 1992;11:19–25.

37. Arriagada R, Lê MG, Rochard F, Contesso G. Conservative treatment versus mastectomy in early breast cancer: patterns of failure with 15 years of follow-up data. Institut Gustave-Roussy Breast Cancer Group. J Clin Oncol. 1996;14(5):1558–64.

38. Early Breast Cancer Trialists' Collaborative Group. Effects of radiotherapy and surgery in early breast cancer: an overview of the randomized trials. N Eng J Med. 1995;333:1444.

39. Bartelink H, Horiot JC, Poortmans PM, Struikmans H, Van den Bogaert W, Fourquet A, et al. Impact of a higher radiation dose on local control and survival in breast-conserving therapy of early breast cancer: 10-year results of the randomized boost versus no boost EORTC 22881–10882 trial. J Clin Oncol. 2007;25(22):3259–65.

40. Punglia RS, Morrow M, Winer EP, Harris JR. Local therapy and survival in breast cancer. N Engl J Med. 2007;356(23):2399–405.

41. Olsen MA, Chu-Ongsakul S, Brandt KE, Dietz JR, Mayfield J, Fraser VJ. Hospital-associated costs due to surgical site infection after breast surgery. Arch Surg. 2008;143(1):53–60; discussion 61.

42. Indelicato D, Grobmyer SR, Newlin H, Morris CG, Haigh LS, Copeland 3rd EM, et al. Association between operative closure type and acute infection, local recurrence, and disease surveillance in patients undergoing breast conserving therapy for early-stage breast cancer. Surgery. 2007;141(5):645–53.

43. Morrow M, Hamilton AS, Katz SJ. Why do women get mastectomy? Results from a population based study. J Clin Oncol. 2007;25(18S):28S. Abstract 605.

44. Taghian A, Mohiuddin M, Jagsi R, Goldberg S, Ceilley E, Powell S. Current perceptions regarding surgical margin status after breast-conserving therapy: results of a survey. Ann Surg. 2005;241:629–39.

45. Morrow M. Margins in breast-conserving therapy: have we lost sight of the big picture? Expert Rev Anticancer Ther. 2008;8:1193–6.

46. Fine RE, Schwalke MA, Pellicane JV, Attai DJ. A novel ultrasound-guided electrosurgical loop device for intraoperative excision of breast lesions; an improvement in surgical technique. Am J Surg. 2009;198(2):283–6.

47. Veronesi U, Luini A, Galimberti V, Zurrida S. Conservation approaches for the management of stage I/II carcinoma of the breast: Milan Cancer Institute trials. World J Surg. 1994;18(1):70–5.

48. Pleijhuis RG, Graafland M, de Vries J, Bart J, de Jong JS, van Dam GM. Obtaining adequate surgical margins in breast-conserving therapy for patients with early-stage breast cancer: current modalities and future directions. Ann Surg Oncol. 2009;16(10): 2717–30.

49. Blair SL, Thompson K, Rococco J, Malcarne V, Beitsch PD, Ollila DW. Attaining negative margins in breast-conservation operations: is there a consensus among breast surgeons? J Am Coll Surg. 2009; 209(5):608–13.

50. Khatcheressian JL, Hurley P, Bantug E, Esserman LJ, Grunfeld E, Halberg F, et al. Breast cancer follow-up and management after primary treatment: American Society of Clinical Oncology clinical practice guideline update. American Society of Clinical Oncology. J Clin Oncol. 2013;31(7):961.

51. Meric F, Bucholz TA, Mirza NQ, Vlastos G, Ames FC, Ross MI, et al. Long-term complications associated with breast conserving surgery and radiotherapy. Ann Surg Oncol. 2002;9:543–9.

52. de Glas NA, Kiderlen M, Bastiaannet E, de Craen AJ, van de Water W, van de Velde CJ, et al. Postoperative complications and survival of elderly breast cancer patients: a FOCUS study analysis. Breast Cancer Res Treat. 2013;138(2):561–9.

Evaluation of Axillary Nodes

5

Mahmut Müslümanoğlu

Abstract

The choice of treatment plan depends on the TNM staging and biology of the tumor. Sentinel lymph node biopsy (SLNB) has replaced axillary lymph node dissection (ALND) in clinically node-negative early-stage breast cancer patients. ALND has been considered mandatory in sentinel node-positive patients, but recent data have demonstrated that breast-conserving surgery (BCS) and radiotherapy are equivalent to ALND of micro-/macro-metastatic sentinel lymph nodes (SLNs). This approach will reduce the morbidity of dissection without decreasing overall survival (OS).

Keywords

Sentinel lymph node • Micrometastasis • Axillary lymph node dissection • Neoadjuvant

Introduction

The choice of treatment plan in breast cancer depends on clinical staging, which determines the tumor load. Tumor diameter and axillary involvement are considered the most important major prognostic factors for predicting survival and selecting adjuvant treatment. Recent studies have demonstrated that tumor biology is more important than other factors in determining breast cancer prognosis, and treatments are planned based on the biological characteristics of the tumor. In this approach, tumor diameter and axillary involvement are of less significance. Although axillary evaluation (sentinel lymph node (SLN), ALND) does not have a profound effect on survival, the removal of metastatic lymph nodes from the axilla may contribute to locoregional control and improve quality of life.

Axillary staging was previously performed by complete axillary lymph node dissection (ALND) in clinically node-negative early-stage breast cancer patients; however, this method carries the risk of some morbidity. SLN biopsy (SLNB) is

M. Müslümanoğlu, MD
Department of General Surgery, Istanbul Medical Faculty, Istanbul Medical School, Topkapi, Istanbul 34390, Turkey

Surgery Department, Istanbul Medical Faculty, Istanbul, Turkey
e-mail: mahmutm@istanbul.edu.tr

equivalent to ALND in clinically node-negative patients in terms of staging, accuracy, disease-free survival (DFS), and OS. Consequently, ALND is not currently advised for patients able to undergo SLNB. SLNB examines the first lymph nodes; the lymphatics of the breast drain to these lymph nodes, which therefore are most likely to be the site reached by tumor cells. If there is no cancer metastasis in the SLN, the other lymph nodes are accepted to be clear (not containing cancer cells); thus, the technique of ALND has been abandoned.

Lymphatic Drainage of the Breast

The lymphatics of the breast comprise interconnected superficial and deep lymphatic vessels. The subdermal plexus in the retroareolar space, which is called *Sappey's plexus*, drains the lymphatics of the areola and nipple. The lymphatics of the interlobular connective tissue of the breast and the lymphatics of the walls of the lactiferous channels also drain to this plexus. Efferent lymphatic channels leaving this plexus trace along the lateral border of the major pectoral muscle, penetrate the clavipectoral fascia, and enter the axilla. Axillary lymph nodes collect nearly 75 % of the lymphatic drainage of the breast. The remaining lymphatics drain into the internal mammary (parasternal) lymph nodes (IMLNs) accompanying perforated branches of the internal mammary artery; this group generally receives drainage from the medial part of the breast.

Sentinel Lymph Node Biopsy

Sentinel means "sentry," and the SLN is the first lymph node at which cancer cells arrive via lymphatic channels starting from the primary tumor; multiple SLNs may exist. Because these lymph nodes are located on the lymphatic drainage course in breast cancer, they contain cancer cells when lymphatic metastasis has occurred. If metastasis is not detected in the pathological examination of the removed SLNs, the axilla is considered clear, and ALND is not performed.

Radioactive colloid and/or blue dye can be used to detect the SLN. SLNs that are identified by scintigraphic imaging in the preoperative phase can be detected intraoperatively using a gamma probe and/or by injecting blue dye into breast tissue; the dyed channel and lymph node can then be detected and removed surgically. There are different practices regarding the choice of agents used (blue dye, radioactive substance, or both), location of injection (periareolar, subareolar, peritumoral), and timing of scintigraphy (on the morning of the surgery or 1 day before). Furthermore, whether extra-axillary lymph nodes will be removed (internal mammary group) and whether any axillary approach will follow examination of the excised lymph nodes (ALND in presence of micrometastasis) are subjects of debate.

History

The blue dye method was first performed by Morl [1] in 1952 by injecting Indian ink into both breasts, and the drainage of all breast quadrants was observed to collect at the sternal lymph nodes. Haagensen [2] demonstrated in 1972 that blue dye drains to the axillary lymph nodes from the breast. The SLNB technique was first performed by Cabanas in 1972 to evaluate the metastasis of penile squamous cell carcinoma to inguinal lymph nodes [3]. In 1992, Morton demonstrated that unnecessary regional lymph node dissections could be avoided in early-stage melanoma patients using the SLNB technique [4]. Armando Giuliano first established SLNB using blue dye in breast cancer surgery by using a vital dye for mapping the lymphatic system in breast cancer in 1994 [5]. After injecting isosulfan blue around the tumor, he observed dyed lymph nodes in the axilla in 114 of 174 (65.5 %) breast cancer cases.

David Krag from Vermont University detected SLNs in 82 % of cases using Tc-sulfur colloid in 1993 [6]. Albertini et al. were the first to use a radioactive substance and blue dye together in 1996 [7].

Indications for SLNB

SLNB has been accepted as a standard treatment approach in all clinically node-negative (with physical examination and imaging techniques) breast cancer cases, regardless of tumor size and location. Today, many of the factors once thought to affect the accuracy of SLNB (large tumor, multifocal-multicentric tumor, etc.) have lost significance, and SLNB can be safely performed in nearly all patients.

Contraindications for SLNB

SLNB is contraindicated whenever a metastatic lymph node is clinically identified in the axilla or metastasis is detected in the lymph nodes by preoperative needle biopsy. In clinically N1 cases, tumor cells are assumed to infiltrate lymphatic channels and therefore will block the advance of dye or radiocolloid inside the channel. This blockage increases the false-negative rate because true positive SLNs could be missed due to lateral movement of the dye and detection of the next negative node.

Approximately 40 % of node-positive patients can be detected with preoperative ultrasonography and needle biopsy [8]. ALND should be performed directly in this case, or neoadjuvant chemotherapy may be recommended.

Whenever any suspicious lymph nodes (hard) are palpated during SLNB, they (non-SLNs) should also be removed independent of the SLNs and examined pathologically. If metastasis (particularly macrometastasis) is detected in SLNs or non-SLNs intraoperatively or during paraffin section examinations, ALND can be performed or left to the radiation therapy.

Allergic reactions are observed in approximately 1–3 % of cases and can cause serious anaphylactic reactions [9]. SLNB using dye is contraindicated in individuals who are known to be allergic to the dye. Blue dye is not used during pregnancy due to its potentially fatal effects [10]. Some studies indicate that radioactive substances in low doses can safely be used during pregnancy [11–13]; however, ALND is generally preferred. Another option in clinically

negative axillae is to wait for the completion of pregnancy and perform SLNB after delivery.

Diffuse blockage of lymphatic channels in locally advanced breast cancers manifests as inflammatory breast cancer and dermal edema and is another contraindication for SLNB.

SLNB in Specific Cases

Ductal Carcinoma In Situ

Ductal carcinoma in situ (DCIS) is a noninvasive breast carcinoma that is restricted to the ducts, with no stromal invasion. However, the detection of metastasis in 1–2 % of cases suggests that some DCIS cases can indeed be invasive and that failure to diagnose metastasis is due to a sampling error [14, 15]. The SLN metastasis detection rate is 7.4 % when a DCIS diagnosis is made by needle biopsy and 3.7 % when a DCIS diagnosis is made following excisional biopsy [16]. Because invasive foci can be detected in paraffin sections and SLNB is not associated with extensive complications, current practice is to perform SLNB in DCIS patients who have received a diagnosis by core biopsy or have grade III tumors, multifocal DCIS, comedo-type tumors, signs on palpation (tumor mass), or a large area of DCIS (calcified areas >2–3 cm) [10].

The axilla is also evaluated by SLNB in patients with an invasive or microinvasive focus detected by excisional biopsy. SLNB is also recommended for patients who plan to have a mastectomy because of the probability of detecting an invasive focus in the postoperative examination of the specimen [17].

Multicentric and Multifocal Breast Cancer

The detection of cancer foci in close proximity (less than 3–4 cm apart) in the same quadrant is defined as multifocal breast cancer. Multicentric breast cancer is defined as the presence of cancer in two different quadrants (further than 4 cm apart). SLNB can be safely performed in multifocal/multicentric breast cancers. However, an increase in the false-negative rate has been reported in some studies. Performing the procedure using a radioactive substance may increase the accuracy of SLN [18–21].

SLNB for Patients with Previous Axillary and Breast Surgery

It was previously thought that previous surgical operations performed on the breast and axilla could alter the lymphatic drainage tracts of the breast and prevent SLN detection. However, later studies have demonstrated that SLNs can be detected if superficial and deep lymphatic channels are not disrupted in breast cancer via excisional biopsy (particularly together with a large skin incision at the upper-lateral quadrant and if the deep pectoral fascia is not affected). However, in patients who have undergone breast-conserving surgery (BCS) and radiotherapy or have undergone ALND, the success rate is low due to altered lymphatics, and axillary SLNs cannot be detected in most cases. In these cases, lymphatic flow to internal mammary glands and contralateral axilla is observed, and these areas are considered the second region for SLNs. The detection of axillary SLNs for the second time in patients who previously underwent SLNB is a subject of research. SLN exploration during the early postoperative period (prior to adjuvant therapy to avoid ALND in cases with positive paraffin section results from SLNB) generally has low success rates. Because the lymphatic chanel has been established in patients who have completed their adjuvant therapy, axillary or extra-axillary SLNs can be successfully detected (95–99 %) at the second SLN exploration for recurrent breast cancer [22–25]. SLNB can be performed after aesthetic interventions and even mastectomy [26, 27]. Using tandem methods (blue dye lymphoscintigraphy) during SLNB in patients with previous operations increases the success rate [22].

Axillary Staging in Patients Treated with Neoadjuvant Chemotherapy

The axilla is clinically negative in approximately 40–50 % of patients who are planned to receive neoadjuvant chemotherapy. In cases with a posi-

tive axillary node, axillary downstaging occurs at a rate of 30–40 % with treatment [28, 29]. Research is ongoing to identify an approach that avoids unnecessary ALNDs in these two patient groups, but the method and timing of axillary staging remain controversial. In clinically axilla-negative cases, SLNB can be performed prior to neoadjuvant chemotherapy, and the need for ALND can be determined after treatment [30].

The opinion that alterations of the breast and lymphatic channels due to chemotherapeutic agents decrease the success rate of SLNB performed after chemotherapy and increase the false-negative rate has essentially been abandoned. In the NSABP-B27 trial, the SLN detection rate after neoadjuvant chemotherapy was 84.8 %, and the false-negative rate was 10.6 %. Recent trials showed that use of radiocolloid alone or together with blue dye significantly enhanced the accuracy, and SLNB was possible after neoadjuvant chemotherapy [31–33]. ALND should be performed whenever the SLN cannot be detected.

Male Breast Cancer

Breast cancer in males is rare and constitutes 1 % of all breast cancer cases. The disease is observed at older ages in males; clinically, the tumors are larger, and the prevalence and extent of axillary metastasis are greater. However, SLNB should be performed in clinically node-negative male breast cancer to avoid unnecessary ALNDs. SLNs can be detected at a rate of 97–100 %. Because male breast cancer is diagnosed at an older age than female breast cancer, SLN positivity is higher in male breast cancer, and non-SLN positivity is higher in the presence of positive SLNs. However, SLNB prevents unnecessary ALND in more than half of patients [33–36].

Elderly and Overweight

Although studies report high success rates of SLN detection in elderly and overweight patients, we observe that this patient group is more problematic in practice; it is particularly difficult to detect SLNs using blue dye alone. The utilization of lymphoscintigraphy along with blue dye in elderly and overweight patients increases the success rate.

SLNB Technique

Utilization of Radiocolloid and Lymphoscintigraphy

Lymphoscintigraphy is based on the detection of lymph nodes following drainage of the injected radiopharmaceutical agent to the regional lymph nodes via the lymphatic current. Regional lymphatic tracts are mapped using this method and whether an SLN is identified as axillary or extraaxillary using preoperative imaging techniques; during the operation, the SLN is detected by a gamma probe [37].

Colloidal gold, which was used during the initial practice of lymphoscintigraphy, is not used in routine practice due to its high gamma radiation [38]. The most frequently used radiopharmaceuticals today are 99mTc-sulfur colloid, 99mTc-nanocolloid, and 99mTc-antimony trisulfide colloid. Particle size is an important aspect of the radiopharmaceutical used in SLN imaging. The particles are not homogeneously distributed within the radiopharmaceutical agent; thus, to obtain a certain particle size, the agent may need to be filtered. Ideally, the radiopharmaceutical agent should quickly drain to the SLN and remain there. Particles smaller than 100 nm enter the lymphatics and drain into lymph nodes, followed by larger particles; however, particles that are 500–2,000 nm in size cannot move and remain in the injection area. However, very small particles (<4–5 nm) escape into the capillary flow and cannot be drained to the lymph nodes [39]. Small particles allow SLNB to be performed over the course of 2 h following the injection. For patients whose operations are planned for the next morning, larger particles should be included in the radiopharmaceutical agent.

While the pharmaceutical agent to be used depends on the facilities of the existing center, particle size can be adjusted according to the type of usage. Whereas 99mTc-sulfur colloid with particle sizes of 100–200 nm is used in the USA, 99mTc-nanocolloid albumin with particles sizes of 5–100 nm is used in Europe, and 99mTc-antimony trisulfide with particle sizes of 3–30 nm is used in Canada and Australia [10].

Another factor affecting the velocity of the radiopharmaceutical is the injection site. Intratumoral, peritumoral, subcutaneous, and intradermal injection routes have been defined; however, the fastest result is obtained via intradermal injection due to the rich lymphatic network [39].

Two to 3 h or 1 day prior to the operation, radiocolloid material is injected intradermally in superficial tumors, peritumorally in deeply located tumors, and into the cavity wall in patients who have had a previous excision. In the lymphoscintigraphy method, the SLN can be detected preoperatively or intraoperatively using a gamma camera. Lymphoscintigraphy is time consuming, more costly, and dependent on another unit; thus, it is not recommended in routine practice, except in complicated cases.

Technique

During the operation, the tumor mass, including the primary site of injection, is excised first to perform the count correctly and minimize background activity. While the gamma probe is scanned over the skin of the axilla, the site producing the highest activity count is determined, and a small incision is made to enter the axilla. The gamma probe is inserted through the incision, and the lymph node yielding the highest activity count is excised together with its surrounding fat tissue by fine dissection. The activity count of the excised tissue is assessed in a separate location, and after confirming that it is the SLN, the excised tissue is sent to pathology for examination. Then, the axilla is reevaluated using the probe. If there are any remaining sites producing high activity counts, other SLNs are excised until the activity count is less than 10 % that of the initial node.

Vital Stain

Blue dye injection is another method for visualizing the SLN. The vital stains used for this purpose include patent blue V, isosulfan blue (1 % lymphazurin), and methylene blue. Vital stains can alter oxygen saturation, and their utilization in pregnancy is associated with risks [10]. Isosulfan blue is the most frequently used agent; however, following injection, reactions ranging from a simple rash to serious anaphylaxis are observed with an incidence ratio of 1:1.1 % [40, 41]. Methylene blue is a less expensive alternative that does not bind to plasma proteins and causes less anaphylactic reactions. However, methylene blue can cause skin necrosis when intradermally administered, and a dilution ratio of 1:2 is recommended [42]. Studies have yielded similar mapping results using both dyes.

Technique

During the operation, approximately 2–5 ml of blue dye is injected by the surgeon via peritumoral (1 cm surrounding the tumor, in four quadrants) and subareolar routes; alternatively, in patients in whom excision has been performed, blue dye is injected into the cavity walls. Depending on the distance of the tumor to the axilla, the area is massaged toward the axilla for 2–5 min. Then, the axilla is entered using a 2–3 cm transverse incision just below the axillary hairline. After opening the clavipectoral fascia, the lateral thoracic vein, which extends toward the tail of the breast, is identified. The SLN is generally located where the intercostal nerve crosses this region (axilla, level 1). The blue-stained tract is identified via dissection. When traced either to the axilla or to the breast, a blue-stained lymph node or nodes can be observed. The blue-stained lymph node is removed together with the surrounding thin fat tissue and sent for pathological examination. The results obtained with blue dye are similar to those obtained using radioactive substances [43].

Combination of Vital Stains and Radioisotopic Methods

Many studies have reported that blue staining and radiocolloid use are complementary methods that enable the detection of additional SLNs when used together. Moreover, the addition of blue dye to the radiocolloid prevents unnecessary dissections. The SLN detection rate is 95–98 % using the radioisotope method [44] and is improved to 95–100 % using the combined method [10]. Adding the radioisotope method to the use of blue dye is beneficial; however, the reported contribution of adding blue dye to the radioisotope method is only 2 % [45]. Both methods have high success rates when performed alone, but combined methods should be used in select cases (elderly, overweight, patients who are undergoing SLNB for the second time). We use blue dye (isosulfan blue) in routine practice in our clinic. The addition of preoperative lymphoscintigraphy and intraoperative gamma probe utilization to the blue dye method enables the detection of SLNs and reduces false negativity in the extra-axillary region, particularly for patients who previously underwent breast surgery (to determine the intercostal space in which the incision will be made, including infra-/supraclavicular and contralateral axillary localization) [10].

In the combined method, the site of high activity count with the gamma probe is first marked. Blue dye is then injected via the preferred route of administration, and after 5–10 min, the axilla is entered via an incision over the marked area. The SLN is detected by tracing the blue tract and by assessing the activity count detected by the gamma probe.

Determining the Site of Injection

When blue dye was first used by Giuliano in breast cancer, it was injected using a peritumoral route or into the wall of the biopsy cavity [5]. In later studies, subdermal, intradermal, periareolar, and subareolar injection routes were employed. The lymphatic drainage routes of the breast parenchyma and breast skin are the same. Studies suggest that SLN detection is more successful via the intradermal or subareolar/periareolar routes; however, most studies indicate that the location of injection does not have an effect on SLN detection [44, 46, 47]. The importance of a combination of deep and superficial injection techniques (peritumoral and subareolar/periareolar or subdermal and peritumoral) to decrease false-negative rates has been emphasized [48, 49]. Each clinic should perform the technique it finds successful. We initially employed peritumoral injections but now prefer subareolar injections. In addition, we have been investigating deep pectoral injections for internal mammary drainage in tumors of the central and medial quadrants.

Number of SLNs

Frequently, one SLN is removed from the axilla. Metastatic lymph nodes may be missed when the number of lymph nodes to be removed is small; however, removing too many lymph nodes may cause increased morbidity, as in ALND. The false-negative rate is 10 % if a single SLN is removed but drops to 1 % when three or more SLNs are removed. However, no benefit is observed when more than four to five SLNs are removed [50–52]. When more than one blue ganglion is detected, removing all of lymph nodes decreases false-negative rates.

Behavior of Micrometastases

Detailed SLN examination (multiple sections with several ganglia) has enabled the detection of smaller metastases. Metastasis was identified in cases with previously negative axillary evaluation results (with single section), resulting in an increase in cancer stage. According to the new staging system, metastases smaller than 0.2 mm are defined as submicro-isolated tumor cells, metastases that are 0.2–2 mm in size are considered micrometastases, and those >2 mm are considered macrometastases. When isolated tumor cells are detected, the axilla is considered negative, and additional dissection is unnecessary. When micrometastasis is detected in SLNs, the rate of metastasis in non-SLNs is 10–40 %. In macrometastasis, this rate is even higher. Consequently, ALND is accepted as the gold standard procedure in patients with lymph node metastasis. ALND is believed to reduce local axillary recurrence and improve survival rates (although this link is controversial).

In a study of SLNB (+) patients, Viale et al. observed that the non-SLN metastasis rate was 3 % if the detected metastasis in SLNB had a sinusal localization but 29 % if the metastasis had an intranodal localization. In addition, in the presence of a metastasis <1 mm, the rate of detection of another metastasis was 8 %, whereas for a metastasis of 1–2 mm, this rate was 28 %.

Recent studies of patients with micrometastases in SLNs who did not undergo ALND did not observe a difference in locoregional recurrence between the group of patients who underwent dissection and those who did not at an average follow-up of 5 years. The results of the best study on this subject, a randomized trial in SLN+ patients conducted by the American College of Surgeons (Z0011), were published in 2010 [53]. This trial followed 446 patients who underwent SLNB and 445 patients who underwent SLNB + ALND. The proportion of patients who had three or more positive LNs was 5 % in the SLNB group and 17.6 % in the SLNB + ALND group ($p < 0.001$). After an average follow-up of 6.2 years, the 5-year breast recurrence rate was 2.1 % in the SLNB group and 3.7 % in the other group ($p = 0.16$). The 5-year lymph node (axilla) recurrence rate was 1.3 % in SLNB group and 0.6 % in the other group ($p = 0.44$). There was no difference in the rates of 5-year DFS and OS (DFS, 82.8 % vs 82.2 %; OS, 92.5 % vs 91.9 %). The general opinion that ALND improves survival rates in patients who undergo breast-conserving surgery and adjuvant radiotherapy as well as systemic therapy could not be confirmed by this study. In addition, according to this study, which was terminated due to difficulties in patient accrual and low recurrence rates, there was no benefit for the patients in the ALND group.

The detection of minimal disease (micrometastasis) in SLNs is sufficient to initiate adjuvant therapy. In all valid protocols used today, these patients receive adjuvant therapy similar to that used in axilla+ disease (N1a). Therefore, treatment for these patients is not incomplete.

The only difficulty in treating micrometastatic disease is determining the irradiation area for axillary and peripheral lymphatics. The number of involved axillary lymph nodes is a critical component of this decision. Given the availability of effective adjuvant treatment options and very low axillary recurrence rates (as in ALND), conservative decisions are now made on behalf of the patient when selecting a radiotherapy area; irradiating wide areas, as is done in Nx, appears to be overtreatment.

Locally Advanced Breast Cancer (LABC)-SLNB

In locally advanced breast cancer (LABC), the utilization of axilla-effective systemic treatment modalities (taxane, trastuzumab, etc.) in routine practice has led to increases in complete response rates (breast + axilla) from approximately 10 % to 39–70 %; for some specific patient groups (ER negative, PR negative, HER2 positive), higher rates of complete response have been achieved [54, 55]. ALND following chemotherapy is the standard axillary approach for LABC; SLNB is recommended in experienced centers if patients who were axillary positive prior to chemotherapy display complete clinical responses after chemotherapy. According to the results of two prospective randomized trials, if two to three lymph nodes are removed using both blue dye and lymphoscintigraphy, the false-negative rates are 14 %, and the detection rate is 98 %. For patients who underwent SLNB prior to neoadjuvant chemotherapy and had (+) results, the detection rate drops to 60 % when SLNB is performed again followed by CT. For this reason, SLNB should be delayed until after chemotherapy [54, 55].

Internal Mammary Lymph Node Biopsy (IMLNB)

A small percentage (10 %) of lymphatics drain into the IMLNs, particularly in centrally and medially located tumors. In the case of axillary involvement, the + or − status of IMLNs does not alter the adjuvant treatment policy. IMLNB may alter the treatment plan in 0.1 % of breast cancer patients, and thus, it is regarded as unnecessary. However, according to the new staging system, only IMLN positivity is classified as N1c, and therefore, IMLNB could change the stage for this group of patients. IMLN detection and sampling are necessary to make a decision regarding the adjuvant treatment policy in axilla-negative patients and to determine if IMLNs will be irradiated. For this reason, we recommend performing IMLNB when the axilla is negative in centrally or medially located tumors.

IMLNs are generally located in the second to third intercostal spaces. The only method demonstrating lymphatic drainage to this region is lymphoscintigraphy with the utilization of gamma probes. Blue dye does not reveal the space to which lymphatics are drained. To observe drainage, a colloid injection should be applied to the deep pectoral region. Our clinical experience suggests that colloid injection may not provide any benefit in patients with IMLN involvement (blocked lymphatic drainage). For this reason, the second to third intercostal space could be explored in selected axilla-negative cases.

The IMLNs are located just anteriorly to the pleura, around the internal mammary artery and vein. Consequently, complications such as pneumothorax and hemothorax have been reported due to pleural injury.

Examination of the SLN

It is important to retain a thin layer of fat tissue around the lymph node to evaluate perinodal fat invasion. Paraffin blocks are prepared, and slices are obtained in numbers and thicknesses defined by the laboratory protocol; these sections are then evaluated using hematoxylin and eosin (H&E) and immunohistochemical staining methods. Intraoperative evaluations can be performed using imprint and scrape cytology, frozen sections, and fast immunohistochemical methods to detect metastatic lymph nodes, allowing ALND to be performed within the same session. The imprint method is a simple and low-cost method that provides fast results. It is frequently used because it does not cause tissue loss. Due to ice crystal artifacts in frozen sections, subsequent paraffin evaluation may be impossible. In addition, freezing of sections causes tissue loss and prolongs the procedure. However, the use of frozen sections allows for the differentiation of micro- and macrometastases, and the pathologist does not need to have experience in cytology to perform this method [56]. False-negative rates of 9–52 % for frozen sections and 5–70 % for imprint cytology have been reported [57, 58]. Because of these high false-negative rates, some authors recommend intraoperative SLN evaluation only in the presence of clinical suspicion. Fast immunohistochemical methods are not commonly used due to their high cost. We use imprint cytology in our clinic for intraoperative evaluation (paraffin section examination is mentioned elsewhere in this book). Lymph nodes are sliced into 2-mm-thick macroscopic slices, two to four paraffin blocks are obtained from each slice, four to eight serial sections in sequence are prepared from each block, and one section is dyed with H&E. If metastasis is detected, the other sections are not processed; however, if there is a problem in determining the size, the second section is dyed with hematoxylin and eosin, the third section is dyed with pan-cytokeratin, and the fourth section is left unprocessed.

False Negativity

False negativity is defined as the detection of negative SLNs when axillary metastasis is indeed present. False-negative rates as high as 29 % have been reported in the literature. Some causes of false negativity include the surgical technique, examination technique in the pathology laboratory, and anatomical variations in the lymphatic channels.

There are some criteria for routinely performing SLNB without ALND: SLNs should be detected in at least 85 % of patients using the method of choice, and the false-negative rate should be less than 5 % [17]. Use of the blue dye and radiocolloid techniques in combination is recommended for surgeons in training to allow them to become familiar with the anatomy and decrease false negativity.

Axillary Lymph Node Dissection

Indications

ALND was once routinely practiced in breast cancer cases, but the indications for ALND have been reorganized as SLNB has become standard in early-stage (stage I, II) clinically N0 cases. Today, ALND is performed in LABC. For early-stage breast cancer, ALND should be performed when lymph node metastasis has been confirmed clinically, radiologically, or by biopsy at the time of patient assessment or when an SLN cannot be detected or is found to be positive.

Anatomy of the Axilla

The axilla is a pyramidal cavity through which the lymphatics originating from the ipsilateral thorax wall and arm pass before joining the systemic circulation. The medial borders of the axilla are the serratus anterior muscle and thoracic wall, the lateral border is the latissimus dorsi muscle, the superior border is the axillary vein, and the posterior borders are the subscapular muscle, teres major muscle, and partially the latissimus dorsi muscle. The axilla is covered by the clavipectoral fascia, and its apex is formed by the costoclavicular ligament (Halsted ligament) at the site where the axillary vein becomes the subscapular vein.

Lymph nodes in the axilla are categorized into six groups. Four to six lymph nodes located medially or posteriorly to the axillary vein form the *axillary vein group* and drain most of the lymphatics of the upper extremities. *The external mammary group*, which drains most of the lateral part of the breast, comprises approximately five to six lymph nodes that trace the lateral thoracic vessels along the lower border of the minor pectoral muscle. *The scapular group* comprises five to seven lymph nodes extending along the subscapular vessels at the posterior wall of the axilla and the lateral border of the scapula; it drains the inferior part of the neck and the posterior parts of the shoulder and trunk. These three lymph node groups drain into the central group, which comprises four to five lymph nodes buried inside the axillary fat tissue directly posteriorly to the minor pectoral muscle. This group also receives direct drainage from the breast. Because it is close to the skin, palpable metastatic nodes generally belong to this group. Between the minor and major pectoral muscles is the *interpectoral lymph node group* (Rotter), which comprises one to four lymph nodes; these nodes drain lymphatics directly from the breast. This group drains into the central and subclavicular lymph nodes. The subclavicular (apical) group drains all other groups and comprises 6–12 lymph nodes located superiorly to the upper border of the minor pectoral muscle.

These lymph node groups are categorized into three levels according to their orientation to the minor pectoral muscle for the surgeon's convenience. *Level 1* contains the external mammary and scapular groups and the axillary vein lateral to the lateral border of the minor pectoral muscle. The central and interpectoral groups, which are located between the medial and lateral borders of the minor pectoral muscle, form *level 2*. The subclavicular group, which is located medially or superiorly to the upper border of the minor pectoral muscle, is categorized as *level 3*.

At the axilla, the first holding station for the lymphatics of the breast is generally the IMLN group and, less frequently, the scapular group. The last station for lymphatics in the axilla is the subclavicular lymph node group. The trunk formed by the lymphatics originating from this location can drain directly to the internal jugular vein, the subclavian vein, or their joining site; however, it can also drain to the right lymphatic channel on the right and the thoracic duct to the left.

Axillary Structure

The axillary artery can be observed medially to the minor pectoral muscle. The second segment of the artery is located posteriorly to the muscle; the thoracoacromial and lateral thoracic arteries originate from here, as can be observed upon ALND. The thoracodorsal artery, which originates more distally, is the artery of the latissimus dorsi muscle and approaches the inferior thoracodorsal nerve. Veins accompany arteries.

The intercostal brachial and intercostal thoracic nerves are sensory nerves; they innervate the skin at the medial part of the upper arm and the posterior part of the axilla. They are named according to the number of the costa that they originate below. The intercostal brachial nerve originates from the second intercostal space; it is located approximately 1 cm inferiorly to the axillary vein, extends laterally, and passes through the axillary tissue. In case of an injury, it results in sensory loss at the corresponding skin area.

The long thoracic nerve, which innervates the serratus anterior muscle, is observed at the level of the second intercostal space, posterior to the intercostal brachial nerve. It originates from C5 to C7, extends inferiorly over the thoracic wall, branches at the level of the fourth to fifth intercostal space, and innervates the serratus anterior muscle. It is sometimes located more laterally, inside the axillary tissue, but is always posterior to the intercostal brachial nerve. Its injury causes a winged scapula defect. For this reason, it is important to identify and preserve the nerve during ALND.

The thoracodorsal nerve, which innervates the latissimus dorsi, originates from C6 to C8. It is located posteriorly to the lateral thoracic vein (thoracoepigastric vein). It extends inferolaterally, accompanies subscapular vessels over the subscapular muscle, and finally innervates the medial part of the latissimus dorsi muscle. Preservation of this nerve during dissection is important for subsequent reconstructive interventions.

The Rotter ganglia are in contact with the lateral pectoral pedicle, which is located posteriorly to the major pectoral muscle. *The lateral pectoral nerve*, which is located in this pedicle, innervates the medial part of the major pectoral muscle. It originates from the lateral chord of the brachial plexus (C5–C7) and is located medially to the minor pectoral muscle. Its injury results in atrophy of the major pectoral muscle.

The medial pectoral nerve innervates the inferolateral part of the major and minor pectoral muscles. The medial nerve is located anteriorly to the minor pectoral muscle at a distance of 1–2 cm, and the lateral nerve is located more laterally. It originates from the medial chord of the brachial plexus (C8–T1). Its injury results in the atrophy of both muscles.

Atrophy of the pectoral muscles does not cause problems at the early stage but results in cosmetic issues at the chest wall in the long term.

ALND Technique

It is now known that extended lymphatic resection does not provide any benefit for patient survival. Therefore, in routine ALNDs, only level 1 and level 2 lymph nodes are removed. When lymph nodes are confirmed as positive by preoperative examinations or detected intraoperatively via palpation, level 3 lymph nodes are also included in the dissection. With an efficient extraction, level 3 lymph nodes can be removed without sacrificing the minor pectoral muscle.

With the patient in the supine position, placing a guard on the head side of the patient and suspending the arm prevent exposure of the distal axillary vein and the upper portion of the latissimus dorsi muscle, making it difficult for the assistant to reach the surgical site. Therefore, it is preferable to move the arm to 80–90° of abduction without using a guard on the head side of the patient. In this approach, the surgeon stands between the patient's arm and trunk, while the assistant stands in the gap between the patient's arm and head.

Cleaning of the operative area is extended from the lateral chest wall to the elbow; the forearm can be left in the operative area after wrapping it. The incision should be made below the hairline to permit subsequent epilation and should not continue beyond the pectoral muscle anteriorly and the latissimus dorsi muscle posteriorly. Oblique transverse incisions, U-shaped incisions with the gap facing up, and reverse S incisions provide good exposure.

Using electrocautery, the surgeon extends the incision to the axillary fascia, and skin flaps are prepared at this level. Beginning to prepare flaps above this level could cause deep hollowness in the axilla. The major pectoral muscle border is reached medially; above it, the jugular vein is observed. This is the upper border of dissection. Laterally, the dissection extends to the lateral border of the latissimus dorsi muscle; inferiorly, the dissection is extended to the joining site of this muscle with the serratus anterior muscle (fourth to fifth costa). The procedure can be performed medially to laterally or laterally to medially, depending on the surgeon's choice.

When started medially, the major pectoral muscle is elevated with a retractor. Anterior to the minor pectoral muscle below, the medial pectoral pedicle can be observed 1–2 cm medial of its border. This pedicle should be preserved to avoid atrophy of the major pectoral muscle.

The lateral border of the minor pectoral muscle is freed from the chest wall. This incision is extended upward until the axillary vein is exposed. When continued toward the posterior side of the minor pectoral muscle over the chest wall, the intercostal brachial and intercostal thoracic nerves, which originate out of the fibrils of the serratus anterior muscle and pass transversely to the axilla, can be observed. In most cases, these nerves are sacrificed; however, with a fine dissection at T2 and T3 above, the nerves can be separated from the axillary tissue and preserved.

Then, the long thoracic nerve is again identified over the serratus anterior muscle but located deeper (more posterior) than these sensory nerves. This nerve enters the axilla from the medial part of the axillary vein; however, it should not be sought out at this entry site because it is susceptible to trauma here. At the level of the third intercostal nerve below, it can be found by caressing the serratus anterior muscle with an index finger. It is located inside the fascia of the muscle and should always be preserved. After its exposure, the axillary tissue is dissected laterally from the chest wall.

By retracting the major pectoral muscle, palpable lymph nodes are identified in the interpectoral region (Rotter ganglion). The few lymph nodes found here are removed without damaging the lateral pectoral pedicle, which extends anteriorly toward the major pectoral muscle.

There is no need to resect the minor pectoral muscle for a level 3 dissection. The pectoral muscles are elevated with a good retraction; the axillary sheath is traced medially to the minor pectoral muscle. The upper border is the Halsted ligament. Fatty tissue is skimmed off the vessel, marked separately, and sent for examination.

For a level 2 dissection, the surgeon should begin from the highest point posterior to the minor pectoral muscle. The surgeon should not extend the incision above the axillary vein; resection of the overlying fatty tissue increases the risk for lymphedema. Below the axillary vein, fatty tissue is skimmed off inferiorly from the chest wall. The dissection is continued inferiorly and laterally, and small branches emanating from the axillary vein are ligated. The lateral thoracic vein (thoracoepigastric vein), which originates from the direction of the axillary vein and enters the axillary tissue, is ligated. The thoracodorsal vein originates distally and posteriorly to the axillary vein and laterally to the lateral thoracic vein. The thoracodorsal nerve occasionally enters more medially, extends more deeply, and distally joins the thoracodorsal vessels. The thoracodorsal nerve can also be observed as a single pedicle adhered to the thoracodorsal vessels. However, it always enters the latissimus dorsi muscle from the medial side.

Fatty tissue between the long thoracic nerve and the thoracodorsal pedicle is skimmed off inferiorly from the axillary vein, and the subscapular muscle is exposed behind. Then, by placing an index finger on the long thoracic nerve, the nerve is traced until its entry site into the serratus anterior muscle (finger dissection); at this level, it is freed from the chest wall, preserving the nerve. Laterally, the thoracodorsal pedicle is traced until its entry site into the latissimus dorsi muscle; the small venous branches are ligated, and the specimen is removed during this procedure.

While approaching the axilla laterally to medially, the latissimus dorsi muscle is traced upward from its border; at the site where it becomes tendinous, the axillary vein is exposed. Dissection should be continued below to where the latissimus dorsi muscle joins the serratus anterior muscle.

Following removal of the piece, a suction drain is placed in the axillary cavity near the incision. The subcutaneous tissue is sutured with single sutures using an absorbable material, and the skin is closed with continuous subcutaneous sutures.

Complications of ALND

SLNB is now the method of choice to avoid short- and long-term morbidities caused by ALND. Unfortunately, ALND must still be performed in many cases. Educating patients about the problems that they may face after the operation can prevent many complications and make them more tolerable when they occur.

Neurovascular Injury

To avoid neurovascular injury, neurovascular structures in the axilla should be identified during the operation. The long thoracic nerve is located posteriorly; it extends inferiorly along the serratus anterior muscle and can occasionally bulge into the axillary tissue laterally. Injury of this nerve is caused by cutting, traction, or thermal damage; however, it is damaged in less than 1 % of cases. Winged scapula defect caused by its injury results in cosmetic problems. It should immediately be repaired if cut during surgery.

Injury to the thoracodorsal nerve innervating the latissimus dorsi muscle prevents the utilization of this muscle in later reconstruction. Because this does not cause a significant neurological deficit, this nerve can be excised to obtain a clean axilla if it is invaded by metastatic lymph nodes.

The intercostal brachial nerve, which transverses the axilla, is generally cut during ALND. This causes paresthesia at the medial half of the upper arm and adversely affects quality of life in women.

Injury to the medial pectoral nerve does not cause short-term problems but results in cosmetic problems due to atrophy of the major pectoral muscle.

The brachial plexus is located superior to the axillary vein; thus, there is no risk of injury as long as one does not extend the dissection above the axillary vein. Rarely, one of the fibers of the brachial plexus extends inferiorly along the axillary vein. For this reason, during ALND, all neural structures should be identified before they are cut. Brachial plexus injury due to patient positioning can heal when conservatively followed.

Seroma

Seroma is an expected situation following ALND. Seroma forms in nearly all cases to some extent and is thus not considered a surgical complication. However, prolonged seroma increases the risk of infection and delays adjuvant treatment. A low-pressure suction drain is placed during the operation to inhibit seroma formation. Prolonged placement of the drain increases the risk of infection due to retrograde movement of bacteria. Because prolonged seroma following removal of the drain is a source of infection, it should be emptied via percutaneous aspiration. Several techniques have been assessed to prevent seroma formation, including performing a precise dissection rather than electrocauterization during surgery, covering dead space surgically or with fibrin adhesives, and applying elastic bandages in the postoperative period; however, these techniques are not very effective. One effective method is delaying exercise and complete shoulder movements until after the fifth day following the operation. However, some arm and shoulder exercises should be started in the early stage to prevent shoulder problems due to a limited range of movement.

Chronic Pain and Limited Range of Movement

More than 50 % of women experience neuropathic pain, which is sometimes severe and interferes with sleep; this pain increases with movement; is localized to the chest wall, axilla, arm, and shoulder regions; and can continue after the third month postoperatively. These pains are thought to be due to nerve injury and to the addition of radiotherapy and/or chemotherapy to the treatment [57]. Patients who experience more pain with movement generally limit their shoulder movements, leading to frozen shoulder syndrome.

Starting arm movements at the early period postoperatively with the aid of adequate analgesia prevents these complications. In addition, intercostal nerve blockage before awakening of the patient may inhibit postoperative pain sensation. However, performing SLNB instead of conventional ALND results in less invasive surgery, largely eliminating neuropathic pain. To treat this pain, alternative methods such as acupuncture, massage, and biofeedback have also been used.

Lymphedema

The function of the lymphatics is to collect large particles such as proteins, bacteria, and blood cells that cannot enter venules due to their large size and therefore accumulate in gaps in tissues. Lymphatic fluid, which originates in small lymphatic channels, first drains into regional lymph nodes; it is then carried to the systemic circulation via efferent lymphatic channels and the main lymphatic duct. Any obstruction in these channels results in the development of lymphedema in the tissue that could not be drained.

Irradiation of the peripheral lymphatics is another factor that increases lymphedema. Recurrent attacks of lymphangitis and cellulitis also increase the risk for lymphedema in the arm. Lymphedema of up to 1–2 cm is considered mild and is observed in 20–30 % of patients with level 1–2 ALND. Larger swelling is considered a serious lymphedema and is observed in less than 5 % of patients. The risk of lymphedema in patients with level 3 ALND is 30 % and is therefore not performed without a valid reason. Mild lymphedema can be observed in 5 % of patients following SLNB.

Lymphedema can also occur in the late postoperative period (3–5 years); its development is usually independent of disease recurrence.

The aims are to educate patients and prevent lymphedema before it develops. Patients who have undergone ALND should be advised not to strain the affected arm, not to suspend the arm while working, and to avoid procedures that could increase the risk of lymphangitis (skin injury due to manicure, etc.); patients are also recommended not to gain weight.

When lymphedema develops, its severity is first assessed.

Stage 0: There is only dullness in the arm.
Stage 1: There is pitting edema (recoverable stage because there is no fibrosis).
Stage 2: Arm is stretched, and there is fibrosis.
Stage 3: Elephantiasis: skin signs such as fibrosis, sclerosis, and keratosis.

Treatment and Prevention

Regular trunk cleaning and massage, which is called manual lymphatic drainage, are applied to patients by trained physiotherapists, and bandaging is applied. In this procedure, lymphatic channels of the trunk are first emptied; the lymphatic current is then enabled from the lymphatics of the affected arm toward the trunk. In some countries, manual lymphatic drainage clothes powered by electricity that perform the same procedure automatically appropriate for home use are employed. If no response is obtained using these procedures and if fibrosis has begun in the arm, laser therapy (low-level laser therapy) can be attempted. Laser therapy resolves fibrotic scar tissue by acting on fibroblasts and stimulates lymphatic drainage. This method was demonstrated to have a lymphedema-reducing effect in 52 % of cases [59].

With reference to the hypothesis suggesting that the lymphatics of the breast and arm drain into different lymph nodes, Thompson et al. stated that the lymphatics of the upper extremities could be preserved in ALND, thereby enabling the prevention of lymphedema. The detection and preservation of lymphatics of the arm in the axilla using the injection of blue dye into the upper arm is called reverse axillary mapping. Research on this subject is ongoing [60].

References

1. Morl F. Importance of the sternal lymph vessels for metastases of cancer of the breast. Chirurg. 1952;23(7):298–300.
2. Haagensen CD, Feind KR, Herter FP, Slanetz CA, Weinberg JA. The lymphatics in cancer. Philadelphia: WB Saunders Company; 1972.
3. Cabanas RM. An approach for the treatment of penile carcinoma. Cancer. 1977;39(2):456–66.
4. Morton DL, Wen DR, Wong JH, Economou JS, Cagle LA, Storm FK, et al. Technical details of intraoperative lymphatic mapping for early stage melanoma. Arch Surg. 1992;127(4):392–9.
5. Giuliano AE, Kirgan DM, Guenther JM, Morton DL. Lymphatic mapping and sentinel lymphadenectomy for breast cancer. Ann Surg. 1994;220:391–8.
6. Krag DN, Weaver DL, Alex JC, Fairbank JT. Surgical resection and radio localization of the sentinel lymph node in breast cancer using a gamma probe. Surg Oncol. 1993;2:335–9.
7. Albertini JJ, Lyman GH, Cox C, Yeatman T, Balducci L, Ku N, et al. Lymphatic mapping and sentinel node biopsy in the patient with breast cancer. JAMA. 1996;276:1818–22.
8. Deurloo EE, Tanis PJ, Gilhuijs KG, Muller SH, Kröger R, Peterse JL, et al. Reduction in the number of sentinel lymph node procedures by preoperative ultrasonography of the axilla in breast cancer. Eur J Cancer. 2003;39:1068–73.
9. Raut CP, Hunt KK, Akins JS, Daley MD, Ross MI, Singletary SE, et al. Incidence of anaphylactoid reactions to isosulfan blue dye during breast carcinoma lymphatic mapping in patients treated with preoperative prophylaxis: results of a surgical prospective clinical practice protocol. Cancer. 2005;104:692–99. ChengG, KuritaS, TorigianDA, AlaviA. Current status of sentinel lymph node biopsy in patients with breast cancer. Eur J Nucl Med Mol Imaging. 2011 Mar;38(3):562–75. Vogt H, Schmidt M, Bares R, Brenner W, Grünwald F, Kopp J, et al. Procedure guideline for sentinel node diagnosis. Nuklear Med. 2010;49:167–72.
10. Gentilini O, Cremonesi M, Toesca A, Colombo N, Peccatori F, Sironi R, et al. Sentinel lymph node biopsy in pregnant patients with breast cancer. Eur J Nucl Med Mol Imaging. 2010;37:78–83.
11. Spanheimer PM, Graham MM, Sugg SL, Scott-Conner CE, Weigel RJ. Measurement of uterine radiation exposure from lymphoscintigraphy indicates safety of sentinel lymph node biopsy during pregnancy. Ann Surg Oncol. 2009;16:1143–7.
12. Sakr R, Bezu C, Raoust I, Antoine M, Ettore F, Darcourt J, et al. The sentinel lymph node procedure for patients with preoperative diagnosis of ductal carcinoma in situ: risk factors for unsuspected invasive disease and for metastatic sentinel lymph nodes. Int J Clin Pract. 2008;62:1730–5.
13. Sakr R, Antoine M, Barranger E, Dubernard G, Salem C, Darai E, et al. Value of sentinel lymph node biopsy in breast ductal carcinoma in situ upstaged to invasive carcinoma. Breast J. 2008;14:55–60.
14. Ansari B, Ogston SA, Purdie CA, Adamson DJ, Brown DC, Thompson AM. Meta- analysis of sentinel node biopsy in ductal carcinoma in situ of the breast. Br J Surg. 2008;95:547–54.
15. Lyman GH, Giuliano AE, Somerfield MR, Benson 3rd AB, Bodurka DC, Burstein HJ, et al. American Society of Clinical Oncology guideline recommendations for sentinel lymph node biopsy in early-stage breast cancer. J Clin Oncol. 2005;30:7703–20.
16. Kumar R, Jana S, Heiba SI, Dakhel M, Axelrod D, Siegel B, et al. Retrospective analysis of sentinel node localization in multifocal, multicentric, palpable or nonpalpable breast cancer. J Nucl Med. 2003; 44:7–10.
17. Knauer M, Konstantiniuk P, Haid A, Wenzl E, Riegler-Keilb M, Postlberger S, et al. Multicentric breast cancer: a new indication for sentinel node biopsy a multi-institutional validation study. J Clin Oncol. 2006;24:3374–80.
18. Goyal A, Newcombe RG, Mansel RE, Chetty U, Ell P, Fallowfield L, ALMANAC Trialists Group, et al. Sentinel lymph node biopsy in patients with multifocal breast cancer. Eur J Surg Oncol. 2004;30:475–9.

19. D'Eredita G, Giardina C, Ingravallo G, Rubini G, Lattanzio V, Berardi T. Sentinel lymph node biopsy in multiple breast cancer using subareolar injection of the tracer. Breast. 2007;16:316–22.

20. Port ER, Garcia-Etienne CA, Park J, Fey J, Borgen PI, Cody 3rd HS. Reoperative sentinel lymph node biopsy: a new frontier in the management of ipsilateral breast tumor recurrence. Ann Surg Oncol. 2007;14:2209–14.

21. Luini A, Galimberti V, Gatti G, Arnone P, Vento AR, Trifiro G, et al. The sentinel node biopsy after previous breast surgery: preliminary results on 543 patients treated at the European Institute of Oncology. Breast Cancer Res Treat. 2005;89:159–63.

22. Intra M, Trifiro G, Galimberti V, Gentilini O, Rotmensz N, Veronesi P. Second axillary sentinel node biopsy for ipsilateral breast tumor recurrence. Br J Surg. 2007;94:1216–9.

23. Koizumi M, Koyama M, Tada K, Nishimura S, Miyagi Y, Makita M, et al. The feasibility of sentinel node biopsy in the previously treated breast. Eur J Surg Oncol. 2008;34:365–8.

24. Rodriguez Fernandez J, Martella S, Trifiro G, Caliskan M, Chifu C, Brenelli F, et al. Sentinel node biopsy in patients with previous breast aesthetic surgery. Ann Surg Oncol. 2009;16:989–92.

25. Karam A, Stempel M, Cody 3rd HS, Port ER. Reoperative sentinel lymph node biopsy after previous mastectomy. J Am Coll Surg. 2008;207:543–8.

26. Filippakis GM, Zografos G. Contraindications of sentinel lymph node biopsy: are there any really? World J Surg Oncol. 2007;5:10.

27. Soran A. Uras C, Aydoğan F. In: Uras C, Aydogan F editors. Sentinel Lenf Nodu Biopsisi, 1. Baskı, İstanbul Medical Yayıncılık, Neoadjuvan kemoterapi alanlarda sentinel lenf nodu biyopsisi. 2007. p. 93–99.

28. Sabel MS, Schott AF, Kleer CG, Merajver S, Cimmino VM, Diehl KM, et al. Sentinel node biopsy prior to neoadjuvant chemotherapy. Am J Surg. 2003;186:102–5.

29. Mamounas EP, Brown A, Anderson S, Smith R, Julian T, Miller B, et al. Sentinel node biopsy after neoadjuvant chemotherapy in breast cancer: results from National Surgical Adjuvant Breast and Bowel Project Protocol B-27. J Clin Oncol. 2005;23:2694–702.

30. Xing Y, Foy M, Cox DD, Kuerer HM, Hunt KK, Cormier JN. Meta-analysis of sentinel lymph node biopsy after preoperative chemotherapy in patients with breast cancer. Br J Surg. 2006;93:539–46.

31. Kelly AM, Dwamena B, Cronin P, Carlos RC. Breast cancer sentinel node identification and classification after neoadjuvant chemotherapy-systematic review and meta-analysis. Acad Radiol. 2009;16:551–63.

32. Boughey JC, Bedrosian I, Meric-Bernstam F, Ross MI, Kuerer HM, Akins JS, et al. Comparative analysis of sentinel lymph node operation in male and female breast cancer patients. J Am Coll Surg. 2006;203: 475–80.

33. Gentilini O, Chagas E, Zurrida S, Intra M, De Cicco C, Gatti G, et al. Sentinel lymph node biopsy in male patients with early breast cancer. Oncologist. 2007;12:512–5.

34. Synn LW, Park J, Patil SM, Cody 3rd HS, Port ER. Sentinel lymph node biopsy is successful and accurate in male breast carcinoma. J Am Coll Surg. 2008;206:616–21.

35. Sayman HB. In: Uras C, Aydogan F editors, Sentinel Lenf Nodu Biopsisi, 1.Baskı, İstanbul Medical Yayıncılık, Sentinel lenf nodu biyopsisinde nükleer tıp teknikleri. Istanbul; 2007. p. 45–53.

36. Sherman AI, Ter-Pogossian M. Lymph-node concentration of radioactive colloidal gold following interstitial injection. Cancer. 1953;6:1238–40.

37. Wilhelm AJ, Mijnhout GS, Franssen EJ. Radiopharmaceuticals in sentinel lymph-node detection – an overview. Eur J Nucl Med. 1999;26:36–42.

38. Wilke LG, McCall LM, Posther KE, Whitwoth PW, Reintgen DS, Leitch AM, et al. Surgical complications associated with sentinel lymph node biopsy: results from a prospective international cooperative group trial. Ann Surg Oncol. 2006;13:491–500.

39. Albo D, Wayne JD, Hunt KK, Rahlfs TF, Singletary SE, Ames FC, et al. Anaphylactic reactions to isosulphane blue during sentinel lymph node biopsy for breast cancer. Am J Surg. 2001;182:393–8.

40. Stradling B, Aranha G, Gabram S. Adverse skin reactions after methylene blue injections for sentinel lymph node localization. Am J Surg. 2002;184:350–2.

41. Kargozaran H, Shah M, Li Y, Beckett L, Gandour-Edwards R, Schneider PD, et al. Concordance of peritumoral technetium 99m colloid and subareolar blue dye injection in Breast cancer sentinel lymph node biopsy. J Surg Res. 2007;143:126–9.

42. Rodier JF, Velten M, Wilt M, Martel P, Ferron G, Vaini-Elies V, et al. Prospective multicentric randomized study comparing periareolar and peritumoral injection of radiotracer and blue dye for the detection of sentinel lymph node in breast sparing procedures: Fransenode trial. J Clin Oncol. 2007;25:3664–9.

43. Derossis AM, Fey J, Yeung H, Yeh SD, Heerdt AS, Petrek J, et al. A trend analysis of the relative value of blue dye and isotope localization in 2,000 consecutive cases of sentinel node biopsy for breast cancer. J Am Coll Surg. 2001;193:473–8.

44. Bauer TW, Spitz FR, Callans LS, Alavi A, Mick R, Weinstein SP, et al. Subareolar and peritumoral injection identify similar sentinel nodes for breast cancer. Ann Surg Oncol. 2002;9:169–76.

45. Pelosi E, Baiocco C, Ala A, Gay E, Bello M, Varetto T, et al. Lymphatic mapping in early stage breast cancer: comparison between periareolar and subdermal injection. Nucl Med Commun. 2003;24:519–23.

46. Noguchi M, Inokuchi M, Zen Y. Complement of peritumoral and subareolar injection in breast cancer sentinel lymph node biopsy. J Surg Oncol. 2009;100: 100–5.

47. Argon AM, Duygun U, Acar E, Daglioz G, Yenjay L, Zekioglu O, et al. The use of periareolar intradermal Tc-99m tin colloid and peritumoral intraparenchymal isosulfan blue dye injections for determination of the sentinel lymph node. Clin Nucl Med. 2006;31: 795–800.

48. Goyal A, Newcombe RG, Mansel RE, Axillary Lymphatic Mapping Against Nodal axillary Clearance (ALMANAC) Trialists Group. Clinical relevance of multiple sentinel nodes in patients with breast cancer. Br J Surg. 2005;92:438–42.

49. Goyal A, Newcombe RG, Chhabra A, Mansel RE, ALMANAC Trialists Group. Factors affecting failed localization and false-negative rates of sentinel node biopsy in breast cancer: results of the ALMANAC validation phase. Breast Cancer Res Treat. 2006;99:203–8.

50. Schrenk P, Rehberger W, Shamiyeh A, Wayand W. Sentinel node biopsy for breast cancer: does the number of sentinel nodes removed have an impact on the accuracy of finding a positive node? J Surg Oncol. 2002;803:130–6.

51. Ilvan Ş. In: Uras C, Aydogan F editors, Sentinel Lenf Nodu Biopsisi, 1. Baskı, İstanbul Medikal Yayıncılık. Sentinel lenf nodlarının patolojik değerlendirmesi. 2007. p. 93–99.

52. Cserni G, Amendoeira I, Apostolikas N, Bellocq JP, Bianchi S, Bussolati G, et al. Pathological work-up of sentinel lymph node breast in cancer. Review of current data to be considered fort the formulation of guide lines. Eur J Cancer. 2003;39:1654–67.

53. Giuliano AE, Hunt KK, Ballman KV, Beitsch PD, Whitworth PW, Blumencranz PW, et al. Axillary dissection vs no axillary dissection in women with invasive breast cancer and sentinel node metastasis: a randomized clinical trial. JAMA. 2011;305(6):569–75.

54. Boughey JC, Suman VJ, Mittendorf EA, Ahrendt GM, Wilke LG, Taback B, et al. Sentinel lymph node surgery after neoadjuvant chemotherapy in patients with node-positive breast cancer: the ACOSOG Z1071 (Alliance) clinical trial. JAMA. 2013;310: 1455–61.

55. Kuehn T, Bauerfeind I, Fehm T, Fleige B, Hausschild M, Helms G, et al. Sentinel-lymph-node biopsy in patients with breast cancer before and after neoadjuvant chemotherapy (SENTINA): a prospective, multicentre cohort study. Lancet. 2013;14:609–18.

56. Sauer T, Engh V, Holck AM, Sørpebøl G, Heim M, Furu I, et al. Imprint cytology of sentinel lymph nodes in breast cancer. Experience with rapid, intraoperative diagnosis and primary screening by cytotechnologists. Acta Cytol. 2003;47:768–73.

57. Couceiro TC, Menezes TC, Valênça MM. Post mastectomy pain syndrome: the magnitude of the problem. Rev Bras Anestesiol. 2009;59:358–65.

58. Dirican A, Andacoglu O, Johnson R, McGuire K, Mager L, Soran A. The short-term effects of low-level laser therapy in the management of breast-cancer-related lymphedema. Support Care Cancer. 2011;19:685–90. Noguchi M. Axillary reverse mapping for breast cancer. Breast Cancer Res Treat. 2010;119:529–35.

59. Dirican A, Andacoglu O, Johnson R, McGuire K, Mager L, Soran A. The short-term effect laser therapy in the management of breast cancer related lymph edema. Support Care Cancer. 2011;19: 685–90.

60. Noguchi M. Axillary reverse mapping for breast cancer. Breast Cancer Res Treat. 2010;119:529–35.

Breast Reconstruction

6

Edward H. Davidson, Vu T. Nguyen,
and Kenneth C. Shestak

Abstract

Breast reconstruction provides closure to many women who have been treated for breast cancer by increasing their comfort in clothing and providing a psychological benefit. The role of the plastic surgeon is to guide the patient through the decision tree to select a reconstructive pathway that is safe and meets expectations. Patients who choose reconstruction must navigate a reconstructive pathway guided by their plastic surgeons that includes decisions regarding the timing, type, and extent of reconstruction. The gold standard for breast cancer care includes an integrated multidisciplinary team approach comprising surgical oncologists, medical oncologists, radiation oncologists, oncology nurses, and plastic surgeons.

Keywords

Breast reconstruction • Tissue expansion • Implant-based reconstruction • Latissimus flap • Free flap • Fat grafting • Nipple reconstruction

Introduction

Breast reconstruction provides closure to many women who have been treated for breast cancer by increasing their comfort in clothing and pro-

viding a psychological benefit [1, 2]. The role of the plastic surgeon is to guide the patient through the decision tree to select a reconstructive pathway that is safe and meets expectations (Fig. 6.1). The first decision many patients face is whether to embark upon breast reconstruction at all; limited provision of service, concerns regarding cost, and anxiety about the effect on cancer surveillance are commonly cited reasons for forgoing breast reconstruction. The reality, however, is that in the USA, the UK, and many countries in Europe and worldwide, breast reconstruction is part of a holistic approach to breast cancer treatment and hence is "covered"

E.H. Davidson, MA (Cantab), MBBS
K.C. Shestak, MD (✉) • V.T. Nguyen, MD
Department of Plastic Surgery,
University of Pittsburgh, Pittsburgh, PA, USA
e-mail: davidsoneh@upmc.edu;
shestakkc@upmc.edu; nguyenvt3@upmc.edu

© Springer International Publishing Switzerland 2016
A. Aydiner et al. (eds.), *Breast Disease: Management and Therapies*,
DOI 10.1007/978-3-319-26012-9_6

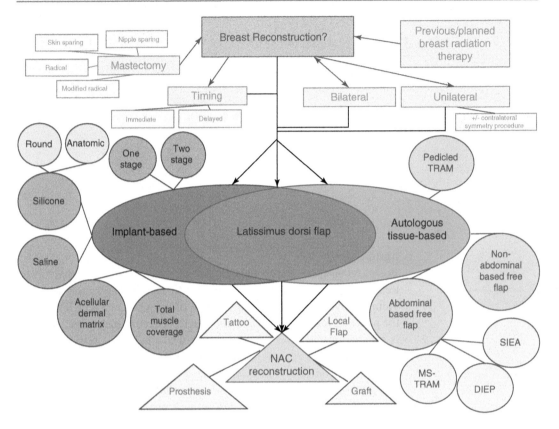

Fig. 6.1 The breast reconstruction decision tree

by insurance or under the public healthcare provision, thus imparting no financial burden on individual patients. Furthermore, no evidence suggests that any form of breast reconstruction increases the risk of recurrence or impairs oncological surveillance of the breast [3–10]. Patients who choose reconstruction must navigate a reconstructive pathway guided by their plastic surgeons that includes decisions regarding the timing, type, and extent of reconstruction. The gold standard for breast cancer care includes an integrated multidisciplinary team approach comprising surgical oncologists, medical oncologists, radiation oncologists, oncology nurses, and plastic surgeons. Decisions regarding radiation, chemotherapy, and oncological resection all impact the reconstructive approach; thus, the plastic surgery team should be involved as soon as possible rather than as an "afterthought" when oncological treatment is complete.

Type of Mastectomy and Impact on Breast Reconstruction

The determination of oncological resection is ultimately governed by the surgical oncologist with oncological treatment taking precedence over any reconstructive goals. However, within the confines of safe practice, various options should be considered at the time of mastectomy to ultimately optimize reconstruction.

Total Versus Skin-/Nipple-Sparing Mastectomy

Skin-sparing and now nipple-sparing mastectomies have become a safe clinical reality for many patients [7–9]. Skin-sparing mastectomy provides a reconstructive advantage for both implant-based and autologous reconstruction. Using a

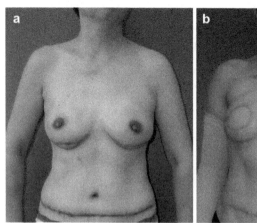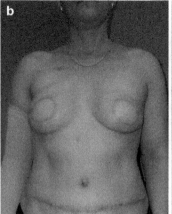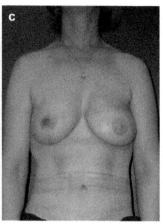

Fig. 6.2 Appearance of nipple-sparing, skin-sparing, and non-skin-sparing mastectomy with autologous reconstruction. (**a**) Early postoperative appearance of bilateral nipple-sparing mastectomy with abdominal-based free-flap reconstruction. The maintained envelope produces an optimal anatomic shape, and the nipple-areolar complex is preserved (note the free-flap skin paddle at the inframammary fold can later be resected but becomes less apparent as scars mature). (**b**) Early postoperative appearance of bilateral skin-sparing mastectomy with abdominal-based free-flap reconstruction prior to nipple-areolar reconstruction. The free-flap skin paddle appears at the center of the breast mound here. (**c**) Postoperative appearance of left mastectomy and delayed abdominal-based free-flap reconstruction with subsequent nipple-areolar reconstruction. Note the "stuck on" appearance of the breast with a scar across the superior pole

native skin envelope to house either a prosthetic or replacement tissue confers an aesthetic advantage by enabling more rapid expansion to the preferred size with the former and avoiding the "artificial construct" appearance of a free flap with the latter (Fig. 6.2).

The ideal candidate for nipple (or rather nipple and areolar)-sparing mastectomies is characterized by small, non-ptotic breasts; an ideal patient would wish to be the same size or slightly to moderately larger. If the patient is a suitable candidate, subsequent nipple-areolar reconstruction is unnecessary. Furthermore, maintenance of the envelope may enable an optimal anatomically shaped autologous reconstruction (Fig. 6.2). Alternatively, in the case of implant-based reconstruction, nipple-sparing mastectomy enables the "direct-to-implant" technique, bypassing the need for preceding expansion in some cases.

As more experience is gained with nipple-sparing mastectomy, pre-mastectomy nipple delay procedures are increasingly advocated for those at high risk of postmastectomy nipple necrosis (i.e., smokers and those with prior peri-areolar surgery). The nipple-areolar complex is surgically separated

from the underlying breast tissue to promote circumareolar blood flow to the nipple-areolar complex from the surrounding skin.

Bilateral Versus Unilateral Mastectomy

In addition to enhancing breast cancer prophylaxis, bilateral rather than unilateral mastectomy may also offer a reconstructive advantage; although not guaranteed, symmetry is easier to achieve when both sides are treated by the same method. However, nipple-sparing mastectomies can better maintain the natural appearance of the contralateral breast, reducing the benefit of bilateral mastectomy.

Delayed Versus Immediate Reconstruction

Breast reconstruction decisions can often be overwhelming for some patients, particularly when confronting the ramifications of a cancer diagnosis. A discussion of implants, the concept of a free flap, and the uncertainties and consequences of the need for radiation therapy can make it very challenging to formulate an informed reconstructive plan. Many patients wish to first focus on achieving oncological clearance prior to proceeding with reconstruction. Delaying reconstruction under these circumstances may be the preferred option. Deferring reconstruction to a later date is also preferred to avoid delaying oncological treatment of patients who are indecisive about reconstruction. Furthermore, when it is unclear if the patient will require postmastectomy radiation, which negatively impacts breast reconstruction, planning for reconstruction becomes easier and better informed after the need for postoperative radiation is determined. Some of this uncertainty can be eliminated if the surgical oncologist is willing to perform a pre-mastectomy sentinel lymph node biopsy ahead of time. In the case of postmastectomy radiation in the USA and other countries, the gold standard is to delay reconstruction until the radiation treatment is completed.

Implant-Based Breast Reconstruction

Breast reconstruction in all forms necessitates volume replacement of the removed breast parenchyma. Implant-based reconstructive methodologies rely on either a silicone or saline prosthetic to achieve volume replacement. Both "silicone" and "saline" implants utilize an outer elastomer shell (envelope) of silicone and either an internal silicone gel or saline fluid, respectively; each is available in different shapes and sizes. Although the discussion of implant-based reconstruction presented herein will focus on these two approaches, it should be recognized that breast implants will continue to evolve, and dozens of different implants and designs will ultimately be available, each championing the benefits of their candidate material and design. The silicone and saline implants discussed herein are the most vigorously tested and most widely used at this time.

The advantages and disadvantages of implant-based reconstruction, particularly compared to

Table 6.1 Advantages and disadvantages of implant-based reconstruction

Implant-based breast reconstruction	
Advantages	Disadvantages
Shorter initial surgery	Need for a prosthesis
	Multiple surgeries
Shorter hospital stay	Need for regular office visits for expansion[a]
	Longer time to achieve reconstruction[a]
Shorter recovery	More difficult to recreate a larger/pendulous breast
	Less compatible with radiation therapy
No donor site scar or morbidity	Risk of implant failure and/or capsular contracture
	Need for future replacement surgery

[a]For two-stage not one-stage implant-based breast reconstruction

tissue-based reconstruction discussed below, are summarized in Table 6.1. Implant-based reconstruction offers the advantage of relatively smaller individual steps, albeit a greater number of steps, to reconstruction, fewer major surgical procedures. a shorter hospital stay, and the avoidance of any secondary donor site morbidity. However, implant-based reconstruction is often contraindicated in the setting of previous or planned breast radiation therapy, may not permit an adequate symmetrical match to a larger pendulous breast if unilateral reconstruction is desired, and necessitates future replacement surgery because no implant is truly permanent. The most common pathway for implant-based reconstruction is a two-stage approach in which a "tissue expander" is first placed to promote subsequent expansion of the soft tissues to create the desired sized pocket for subsequent placement of the permanent implant (Fig. 6.2).

Two-Stage, Implant-Based Reconstruction

Expander Placement
The precise operative details are beyond the scope of this chapter. However, briefly, either immedi-

ately following mastectomy or at a delayed time point (after initially excising the existing scar) following skin-sparing mastectomy, a submuscular pocket for the tissue expander is created by dissecting laterally from the intersection of the pectoralis major muscle and serratus anterior muscle or by splitting the pectoralis major muscle to create a pocket, medially towards the sternum as well as inferiorly, superiorly, and laterally. Care must be taken not to violate the integrity of the pectoralis major superficially or the chest wall to the plane of dissection. Dissection is preferentially performed medially and inferiorly to ensure subsequent preferential expansion by the device. Inferior dissection proceeds to the level of the inframammary fold and medially to just lateral to the sternum. Completion of the pocket is subsequently dependent on whether "total muscular coverage" or acellular dermal matrix (ADM) is used. With the former, the lateral portion of the pocket is created by dissecting laterally deep to the serratus anterior. Some surgeons are proponents of the use of ADM, citing the advantages of a more malleable, naturally draped expander pocket. Opponents of this technique argue that ADM carries a greater infection risk. However, this is a contentious issue. The completion of the expander pocket when ADM is used is achieved by disinserting the inferior pectoralis major and recreating the IMF and lateral aspect of the pocket with a curved triangular sling of ADM sutured inferiorly and laterally to the deep tissues as well as superiorly (after placement of the expander) to the now inferior free edge of the pectoralis major. With either technique, the deflated expander is placed in the pocket. The pocket is then closed by suturing either the serratus anterior or the ADM to the pectoralis major as appropriate. Care must be taken to complete this suture line with direct vision to avoid puncturing the expander. Again, as with implants, a plethora of expanders are available on the market. The author's preference is a low-height anatomically shaped expander with an indwelling port. This expander preferentially expands the inferior pole. Alternatively, a medium-height device can be used. Once closure of the pocket is achieved, the expander is partially inflated. The amount of inflation is dictated by

the quality of the overlying tissue, both the muscle of the pocket and the overlying skin. Essentially, the expander is inflated as much as possible without causing undue tension to the overlying muscle or subsequent skin closure. Finally, the skin is then closed over a Jackson-Pratt drain. When using ADM, a drain is commonly placed both in the pocket and in the subcutaneous space due to the increased risk of seroma.

Serial Expansion

Following expander placement, our protocol involves inpatient admission overnight; however, same-day discharge is not inappropriate. Patients routinely receive perioperative antibiotics for 24 h; however, some advocate a longer course of antibiotics, particularly with the use of ADM. This issue is heavily debated and dependent on surgeon preference. Typically, drains are removed 1 week postoperatively if the output has been less than 30 ml/day for two consecutive 24-h periods. Expansion is then commenced 2 weeks postoperatively. A magnet is used to identify the location of the filling port. The skin is marked and prepped with Betadine, and saline is infused percutaneously. Arbitrarily, weekly expansion for 3 weeks is performed, and the time between expansions is subsequently increased with a 30–40 ml infusion at our institution. These smaller volume expansions appear to cause less thinning of the overlying soft tissues. Expansions are largely well tolerated without the need for analgesia. Excessive pain noted post expansion should be addressed by fluid removal.

The expansion protocol is flexible and accommodating to patient convenience and preference; larger more frequent expansions if tolerable and "expansion holidays" are permissible and do not impact the ultimate results. Expansion proceeds in this manner until an endpoint determined by the patient's target breast size is achieved for bilateral procedures or the contralateral size is achieved in the case of unilateral breast reconstruction. Following the completion of expansion, a 4- to 6-week period of recovery for the soft tissue envelope is provided prior to the exchange of the expander for the implant.

Expander to Implant Exchange

Once expansion is completed, and a further latency period of 4–6 weeks has elapsed to allow tissue recovery; the expander is exchanged for the implant, which remains in place for a lengthy period of time. No implant is permanent. Although extensive and conflicting data are available, patients should be informed that they will likely need to replace the implant at some point in the future as a result of implant failure or capsular contracture. The time frame of this need for replacement is highly variable, but an estimate of a 50 % replacement rate at 10 years appears to be easily understood and remembered by both patients and surgeons. Every implant induces periprosthetic capsule formation; over time, this capsule can contract and cause a firm, visibly deformed and even painful breast. The most extensive form of this problem is not frequently observed. Saline implant failure is immediately obvious in most cases due to deflation. Silicone implant failures are less easy to detect. In the USA, the Federal Drug Administration (FDA) advocates monitoring by MRI 3 years after initial placement and every other year thereafter [11]. The reality is that this advice is largely ignored due to cost issues. Certainly, an MRI is advisable following any trauma to the breast or with symptoms that warrant concern for possible failure.

The choice of either silicone or saline implant is fundamentally a patient decision. Silicone implants provide a more aesthetic reconstruction and a more natural feel to the reconstructed breast. By contrast, failure of saline implants is more easily detected. Patients are occasionally wary of silicone implants given the 14-year moratorium on their use for cosmetic augmentation by the FDA from 1992 to 2006. Details regarding this moratorium are best explored elsewhere, but, in short, the moratorium was in response to numerous reports attributing the incidence of different systemic medical issues to silicone prosthesis implantation. Extensive research was unable to identify any association between these ailments and the presence of the implants; thus, the availability of these implants was restored. Although the reputation of silicone implants frequently remains compromised, the extensive scrutiny of silicone implants has established them among the most tested and

safe prostheses across all surgical specialties. Notably, silicone implants were only banned in the USA, and this ban did not extend to implant use in reconstruction or research [12–16]. We inform all our patients that all medical evidence emphasizes that implants are safe, but some patients are deterred from their use despite reassurance.

Similar to expanders, silicone or saline implants are available in numerous shapes and sizes with different projection to volume ratios. If choosing silicone implants, the choice is further complicated by the option for newer, so-called fourth-generation anatomically shaped implants. These "teardrop"-shaped implants aim to offer greater projection preferentially at the lower pole and more natural takeoff from the chest wall. If a patient is amenable to fourth-generation implants, the surgeon will consider this option in the selection of an implant at the time of surgery based on the surgeon's judgment of what implant will produce the most aesthetic result. Implant choice is somewhat predetermined by the base width of the original expander pocket; however, the base width can be adjusted at the time of implant exchange and by the volume with which the expander has been infused. Using these two data points, it is prudent to order numerous implants with dimensions that closely resemble these criteria and correspondingly test "sizers" that can be assessed at the time of surgery. It is also wise to order at least two implants of each type of interest for a unilateral reconstruction as well as at least three implants for a bilateral reconstruction in case of iatrogenic implant failure.

The exchange from expander to implant may safely be performed as same-day surgery, and the patient is discharged without the need for an inpatient hospital stay. In brief, the previous intraoperative incision is opened, and the underlying muscle and capsule are incised. The expander is then deflated and removed. Antibiotic solution is used to irrigate the pocket. If necessary, a capsulotomy is performed, and the implant is placed using a minimal touch technique to mitigate infection risk. The placement of the final implant is often preceded by trial placements of reusable implant sizers. The patient sits up on the operating table to judge the aesthetic appearance until the ideal appearance is achieved. With saline implants, the implant shell is placed and then filled with saline. A saline-filled implant has more flexibility in terms of size because it may be under- or over-filled according to the manufacturer's guidelines. In fact, overfilling by 10–20 % reduces the risk of implant rippling and failure [17, 18]. The capsule and skin are then closed without the need for drain placement. Perioperative antibiotic practice is again practitioner dependent and contentious, as is instruction regarding return to activity. Wearing a surgical bra or a sports bra that is not overly tight and lacks an underwire in the case of an IMF incision (i.e., following nipple-sparing mastectomy as described below) and avoidance of strenuous activity for 4 weeks is probably advisable.

Single-Stage, Implant-Based Reconstruction

The technique is modified for a nipple-sparing mastectomy. Using an inframammary fold incision, which is the common practice at our institution, the pectoralis is disinserted from its inferior attachments, and the pocket is dissected for placement of the expander. The selected implant is then placed, and the pocket is closed using a sling of ADM to support the inferior pole and maintain the inframammary fold. Nipple-sparing mastectomy, as preciously alluded to, increases the possibility of single-stage direct implant placement and avoids the need for tissue expansion, assuming the patient does not desire a significantly larger cup size than that prior to mastectomy. The maintenance of the full skin envelope can often accommodate immediate implant placement. However, patients should be counseled that the high tension closure can complicate wound healing, and optimal aesthetic results often require a revision procedure.

Radiation and Implant-Based Breast Reconstruction

Previous or proposed breast radiation therapy significantly increases the risk of complications of implant-based reconstruction. For patients with any history of breast conservation treatment with lumpectomy and radiation or planned/completed postmastectomy radiation, the gold standard for reconstruction to date is autologous tissue-based reconstruction, which introduces new, well-vascularized tissue outside the breast to the area of radiation damage. Conversely, expanding radiated tissue carries a high risk of expander extrusion, infection, and dehiscence (Fig. 6.3). Even if radiated tissue is successfully expanded, the risk of wound breakdown following implant exchange is high.

However, implant-based reconstruction pathways and radiation therapy occasionally collide. For example, a patient may choose to proceed with implant-based reconstruction despite the risks, or unanticipated radiation therapy may be required after mastectomy and immediate tissue expander placement have been performed. Some of this uncertainty can be removed if the surgical oncologist is willing to perform a pre-mastectomy sentinel lymph node biopsy prior to the scheduled mastectomy. For patients adamantly opposed to autologous tissue reconstruction or patients with no available autologous options who are appropriately informed of the risks, implant-based reconstruction may be appropriate in individual circumstances. Some surgeons will refuse to proceed with such treatment. In the case of autologous tissue reconstruction, proceeding with implant-based reconstruction is not absolutely precluded if appropriate planning is made. Mitigation of risk can be achieved by avoiding radiation, if oncologically safe, until completion of active expansion. In some centers, particularly those in which adjuvant rather than neoadjuvant chemotherapy is practiced, a timeline of postmastectomy expansion concomitant with chemotherapy, expander-implant exchange, and subsequent radiation of the permanent implant has been championed (Fig. 6.4) [19]. Of course, radiation damage is largely permanent and impacts future implant replacement surgeries. In some clinical circumstances, radiation oncologists are unable to reliably offer adequate radiation therapy in the presence of an implant and may request its removal, representing a surgical "return to square one."

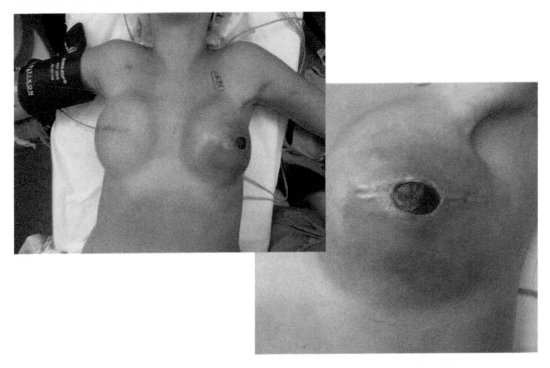

Fig. 6.3 Radiation and implant-based reconstruction; extrusion of a tissue expander in irradiated tissue

In the event of expander or implant extrusion or threatened extrusion in the context of radiation, the leading options involve salvaging implant-based reconstruction with the supplement of a pedicled latissimus dorsi flap under which an expansion and implant placement can be performed or abandoning implant-based reconstruction and proceeding with a delayed autologous tissue-based reconstruction (both discussed below).

Autologous Tissue-Based Breast Reconstruction

For autologous tissue-based breast reconstruction, volume replacement of the removed breast parenchyma is achieved by transfer of the patient's own tissues from an anatomic site distant from the breast. This procedure necessitates maintenance of the blood supply of the transferred replacement tissue either by preservation of a vascular leash or pedicle carrying the native arterial inflow and venous return or by dissection of a segment of native veins and arteries on the tissue to be transferred. This tissue is subsequently detached from the body, and these donor vessels are inserted in or anastomosed with similarly dissected recipient site arteries and veins to generate a "free flap."

The advantages and disadvantages of autologous tissue-based reconstruction compared to implant-based reconstruction are summarized in Table 6.2. Autologous tissue reconstruction enables definitive one-stage breast reconstruction, thus avoiding the need for protracted expansion protocols or future implant replacement surgeries. In the case of radiation therapy, this technique mitigates reconstructive complications with the provision of healthy well-vascularized tissues but requires major surgery and therefore the potential for major complications, requiring longer hospital stays and the risk of donor site morbidity.

Pedicled Transverse Rectus Abdominus Myocutaneous (Tram) Flap

Pedicle and free TRAM flaps were developed in the late 1970s and early 1980s. Proponents of the

Fig. 6.4 Timeline of two-stage expander-based reconstruction (*and with postmastectomy radiation)

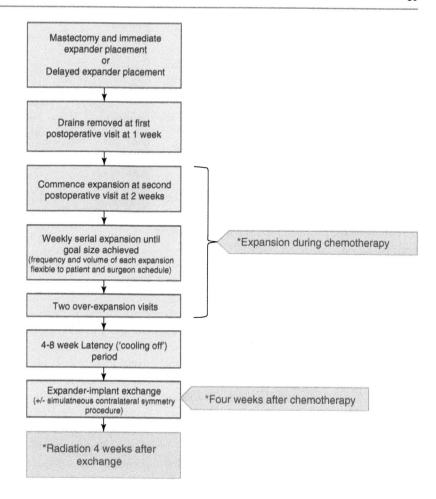

Table 6.2 Advantages and disadvantages of autologous tissue-based reconstruction

Autologous tissue-based breast reconstruction	
Advantages	Disadvantages
One-stage surgery	Longer surgery
No need for future replacement surgery	Longer hospital stay
Mitigates soft tissue injury from radiation	Longer recovery
Use of own tissue that mirror changes in body habitus	Donor site scar and risk of donor site morbidity

pedicled TRAM champion its reliability and reduced operative time and inpatient stay compared with free-tissue transfer and technical ease given the avoidance of microsurgery. The caveat to this technique is the increased risk of donor site morbidity, namely, abdominal wall bulge or hernia especially with bilateral reconstruction and segmental disruption of the inframammary fold.

Pedicled TRAM is based on superior epigastric vessels. A transverse ellipse of skin is marked in the lower abdomen from near the anterior superior iliac spine on one side to the other side. This region typically includes the umbilicus, which is ultimately transposed, similar to an abdominoplasty. Skin and subcutaneous tissues are incised down to the external oblique and rectus fascia muscles. The entire rectus or a strip of muscle with superior epigastric vessels, as identified with a 20-mHz handheld Doppler, is dissected off the abdomen either bilaterally or unilaterally as appropriate and tunneled superiorly into the postmastectomy skin envelope. Donor to recipient transfer may follow an ipsilateral or a contralateral path. At our institution, ipsilateral transfer is preferred. This decision is largely based on surgeon preference. The abdomen is closed via transposition of the umbilicus. Synthetic mesh reinforcement of the donor area is needed only if the closure is tight. The flap is inset.

Pedicled flaps do not require Doppler monitoring but rather are assessed based on the clinical appearance of any skin paddle. A healthy flap should appear the same color as the donor tissue, with comparable temperature and capillary refill. An arterially insufficient flap appears pale, may be cooler to touch, and exhibits prolonged capillary refill. Conversely, venous congested flaps exhibit a blue/purple hue and display rapid capillary refill. With venous congestion, an associated increase in dark red surgical drain output may be noted.

Following the pedicled TRAM flap procedure, patients at our institution typically undergo a two-night inpatient stay. Diet is advanced as tolerated postoperatively, and activity is advanced following initial bed rest overnight. On discharge, patients are counseled to maintain use of a surgical brassiere or loose sports brassiere without an underwire and an abdominal binder at all times for 4–6 weeks and to avoid strenuous activity for 6 weeks. Surgical drains in both the donor and recipient sites are sequentially removed in postoperative office visits at 1, 2, 4, and 12 weeks once output is less than 30 ml in two consecutive 24-h periods.

Some surgeons advocate a practice of flap "delay" to improve the vascularity of the flap; 10 days to 3 weeks prior to flap elevation and inset, which are performed as a short same-day surgery, the ipsilateral deep inferior epigastric vessels are ligated. This procedure has the benefit of increasing blood flow through the superior epigastric artery [20].

Abdominal-Based Free-Tissue Transfer

Although requiring comfort and proficiency with microvascular surgery techniques, abdominal-based free-tissue transfer obviates some of the donor site morbidity risk associated with the pedicled TRAM flap, particularly in higher-risk patients (i.e., those who are obese and/or smoke). There is a continuum of evolution in free-flap development from free TRAM to muscle-sparing free TRAM to deep inferior epigastric artery

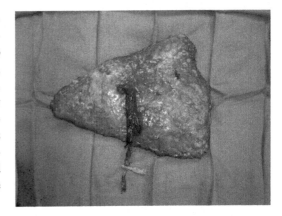

Fig. 6.5 Muscle-sparing TRAM (MS-TRAM); a cuff of rectus muscle with overlying subcutaneous tissue and skin based on the deep inferior epigastric artery and its branches

perforator (DIEP) to superficial inferior epigastric artery (SIEA) flaps. At the TRAM flap end of the spectrum, there is the advantage of a relatively more robust blood supply throughout the flap but a greater relative risk of abdominal wall morbidity. Conversely, the SIEA flap marks the most evolved form of abdominal-based, free-tissue transfer in terms of minimizing abdominal wall morbidity yet offering relatively less robust perfusion and subsequent increases in fat necrosis within the flap.

Free TRAM is characterized by harvesting of a full-length strip of rectus muscle. Alternatively, with muscle-sparing TRAM (MS-TRAM), a cuff of rectus muscle with overlying subcutaneous tissue and skin based on the deep inferior epigastric artery and its branches is more commonly harvested (Fig. 6.5). MS-TRAM is further subdivided into MS-I, in which the cuff is on the medial (MS-I-m) or lateral (MS-I-l) border of the rectus, and the more ideal MS-ii, in which a central cuff of muscle is obtained, preserving a lateral and medial band. To harvest a DIEP flap (occasionally referred to as MS-III), the dominant branches of the deep inferior epigastric artery that perforate through the rectus muscle are dissected out along with a minimal cuff of fascia around the perforating vessel. The SIEA flap utilizes the superficial inferior epigastric artery and vein, thus avoiding rectus muscle dissection and harvesting.

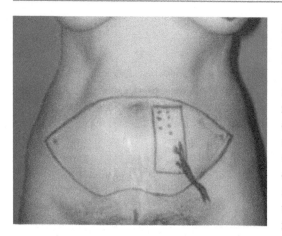

Fig. 6.6 Preoperative marking for abdominal-based free flap indicating the relative positions of skin incisions, strip of rectus muscle, and deep inferior epigastric vessels

At our institution, once a patient has opted for abdominal-based, free-tissue transfer reconstruction, a tentative operative plan is formulated based on a CT angiogram of the abdomen. Ultimately, the final decision regarding the type of flap vascularization is made at the time of surgery and is a balance between optimizing perfusion and minimizing abdominal wall morbidity based on each individual's vascular anatomy. If extended to also include the chest, the CT angiogram also enables preoperative assessment of the caliber of the internal mammary vessels. These vessels are our preferred recipients; however, thoracodorsal vessels are preferred by others. The advantage of the internal mammary is that the vessels are generally larger and their use obviates the need to work in a tunnel, in contrast to the use of the thoracodorsal vessels.

A transverse ellipse of skin is marked on the lower abdomen from near the anterior superior iliac spine on one side to the other side, similar in design to an abdominoplasty (Fig. 6.6). Flap elevation can proceed simultaneously to mastectomy if performed in the immediate setting and if acceptable to the surgical oncology team. The skin and subcutaneous tissue are incised down to the external oblique and rectus fascia muscles. Diligence in dissection through the subcutaneous tissues of the inferior incision is required to identify and preserve the SIEA and SIEV. Even if an SIEA flap is not an option, the SIEV is often

preserved as a "lifeboat" for a venous congested flap or as a secondary vein to "supercharge" outflow. Dissection of the subcutaneous tissue off the fascia proceeds laterally to medially with particular care given medial to the linear semilunaris. Perforating branches of the deep inferior epigastric artery are identified and preserved. If an SIEA is planned, the flap can simply be elevated off the fascia via cautery or ligation of all deep perforating branches. Dominant perforators are identified and dissected through the muscle until a pedicle that is sufficiently long to ease microvascular anastomosis is procured for a DIEP flap. Alternatively, the dominant perforator(s) may be harvested en masse with a strip of rectus muscle and a segment of the deep inferior epigastric vessels.

Depending on body habitus, desired flap side, and whether a unilateral or bilateral reconstruction is performed, the abdominal ellipse may be divided at the midline, with each hemi-flap requiring dissection of the donor blood vessels. Alternatively, if supported by the vascular tree, the entire ellipse may be used for a unilateral reconstruction if necessary. Preparation of the recipient vessels may proceed simultaneously to flap elevation, assuming mastectomy is complete. The abdomen is closed via transposition of the umbilicus. Mesh may be necessary only if substantial muscle is resected. Microvascular anastomosis is completed, and the flap is inset.

Free-flap monitoring is an extensive topic in itself. We commonly use an indwelling venous Doppler and an external handheld Doppler to monitor the arterial signal and clinically examine the appearance of any skin paddle. Postoperatively, patients are transferred to a unit with nursing staff trained in free-flap monitoring. Formal "flap checks," which assess venous and arterial signals as well as flap appearance, are performed by nursing staff every hour for the first 48 h and then every 2–4 h thereafter until discharge. Physician staff perform further checks every 6–12 h or immediately in response to any concern highlighted by the nursing staff. There is a low threshold for returning to the operating room to explore and attempt salvage as appropriate for any concern in flap signal or appearance, particularly within the first 48 h postoperatively because 80 % of flap jeopardizing complications occur during this time frame. Any intervention "resets" the clock. Patients are not permitted oral intake until flap assessments are completed and deemed satisfactory on the morning of postoperative day 1. At this time, only a clear liquid diet is permitted for a further 24 h. In the absence of any problems, diet and activity are advanced. Patients are confined to bed in the semi-Fowler's position for 24 h. Patients are then allowed out of bed to a chair for 24 h. After this time, patients are allowed out of bed and permitted to shower with assistance. If no complications are encountered, patients are discharged; this typically occurs on postoperative day 4. At discharge, patients are counseled to maintain use of a surgical brassiere or loose sports brassiere without an underwire and an abdominal binder at all times for 4–6 weeks and to avoid strenuous activity for 6–10 weeks. Surgical drains in both the donor and recipient sites are sequentially removed at postoperative office visits at 1, 2, 4, and 12 weeks once output is less than 30 ml in two consecutive 24-h periods.

Non-abdominal Tissue-Based Autologous Free Flaps

Abdominal tissue provides the workhorse flaps described above for autologous tissue-based breast reconstruction. However, microsurgical approaches have evolved such that flaps from other sites have been described and may be offered in certain circumstances. The reconstructive surgeon's willingness to offer options, such as superior or inferior gluteal artery perforator flaps or thigh flaps, is largely influenced by training bias and experience. In addition, options are typically only offered if a patient is not a candidate for abdominally based flap harvest due to prior surgery or they are adamantly opposed to any risk of abdominal wall morbidity. Typically, the risk of abdominal wall morbidity is traded for a flap that is technically more challenging to shape and one that confers a scar and contour deformity elsewhere, the conspicuity of which is dependent on surgical expertise and patient body habitus.

The Latissimus Dorsi Flap in Breast Reconstruction

The latissimus dorsi myocutaneous flap was the first flap used for breast reconstruction in the mid-1970s. Its popularity decreased with the introduction of abdominal wall flaps but has once again become popular given its significant utility in various settings.

A pedicled latissimus dorsi flap can serve as a "lifeboat" to salvage implant-based reconstruction complicated by radiation therapy. This flap may be used as an adjunct to implant-based reconstruction in providing a lower pole skin, subcutaneous tissue, and muscle sling to enable implant-based reconstruction of a pendulous breast. In addition, this flap may be an independent option for autologous tissue-based breast reconstruction.

When a tissue expander or permanent implant threatens extrusion or extrudes through radiation-damaged tissue, a pedicled latissimus dorsi flap provides well-vascularized, healthy tissue under which expansion can proceed.

A large pendulous or ptotic breast can be difficult to reconstruct using conventional implant-based methods as the vector of expansion, and therefore, the projection of the implant is horizontal from the chest. Expansion under a latissimus flap draping the inferior fold can recreate the ptotic breast.

An extended or volume-added latissimus has been described in which extensive subcutaneous tissue is harvested beyond that directly overlying the harvested muscle. In some reports, this method provides adequate volume to independently reconstruct an albeit small breast. Other researchers have reported further volume augmentation with supplemental autologous fat grafting (below).

Preoperatively marking the borders of the latissimus is performed with the patient standing. A tunnel through which the flap is passed anteriorly under the breast is also marked just inferior to the axilla. A "no man's land" area in which dissection is prohibited is also typically identified caudal to the tunnel to prevent violation of the lateral border of the breast. Either immediately following mastectomy or after scar excision and undermining of mastectomy flaps in a delayed fashion, the axillary tunnel is dissected with the patient in the supine position. The patient may then be turned prone or to the lateral decubitus position, and the flap is elevated. Sequentially, the skin paddle is incised, and dissection proceeds through the subcutaneous tissue with aggressive beveling to capture a volume of fat until muscle is encountered. The latissimus is traced to its medial, lateral, superior, and inferior borders and is released from its insertions. Care must be taken superomedially to not disrupt the trapezius muscle. The muscle is undermined in a caudal to cranial direction until it is sufficiently free to rotate through the tunnel on the pedicle of the thoracodorsal vessels that enter the undersurface of the muscle superiorly. The donor site skin may then be closed in layers over drains. The placement of at least two drains at the donor site is mandatory given the high risk of seroma. The patient is then turned supine once more, and the flap is inset as appropriate (Fig. 6.7).

Oncoplastic Breast Reduction Surgery

Oncoplastic breast reduction surgery offers something of an intermediate option between breast conservation therapy and breast reconstruction and is an option for a relatively smaller tumor in a relatively larger breast. Essentially, a reduction mammoplasty is performed bilaterally with resection of the tumor along with an adequate margin as part of the excision on the affected side (Fig. 6.8) [21].

Supplemental Symmetry Procedures

The limitations of reconstructive techniques to recapitulate the native breast in unilateral reconstruction can render an asymmetric mismatch. Asymmetry is typically the result of a smaller and/or less ptotic reconstructed breast compared to the native contralateral breast. A contralateral

mastopexy ("breast lift") or reduction mammoplasty can be performed at the time of expander-implant exchange following postoperative recovery after autologous-based reconstruction or at any later point in time. Some patients requiring mastectomy opt for a reconstruction larger than their native breast; thus, a subsequent contralateral augmentation may be offered as a matching procedure.

Nipple-Areolar Complex Reconstruction

For many women, reconstruction of the nipple-areolar complex is the final step of a long journey to overcoming breast cancer treatment. For some women, the restoration of breast parenchymal volume and a normal clothed appearance fulfils their breast reconstruction desires, but many patients opt for completion of breast reconstruction with pursuit of reconstruction of the nipple-areolar complex (NAC). As with restoration of breast volume, a multitude of variations and permutations are available for NAC recreation. Most of the common approaches involve the use of local flaps, skin grafts, or tattooing in isolation or in combination (Figs. 6.9 and 6.10) [22, 23].

Tattooing the nipple and/or areola has the advantage of being an essentially noninvasive, office-based procedure. Results can be variable; however, in skilled hands, this offers a remarkably natural appearance of both the nipple and areolar. The shortcoming is the lack of nipple projection.

To create a projected nipple, the following techniques are useful: grafts of the contralateral nipple, auricular tissue, and the use of prosthetics and local flaps. Initial overprojection should be considered with all of these options given the likelihood of loss of projection over time. Techniques for the creation of a projected nipple through local flaps are variants of a similar theme and include the skate flap, the bell flap, the C-V flap, and double-opposing periareolar flap. A caveat to projected nipple creation is that patients should be counseled regarding their constant projection

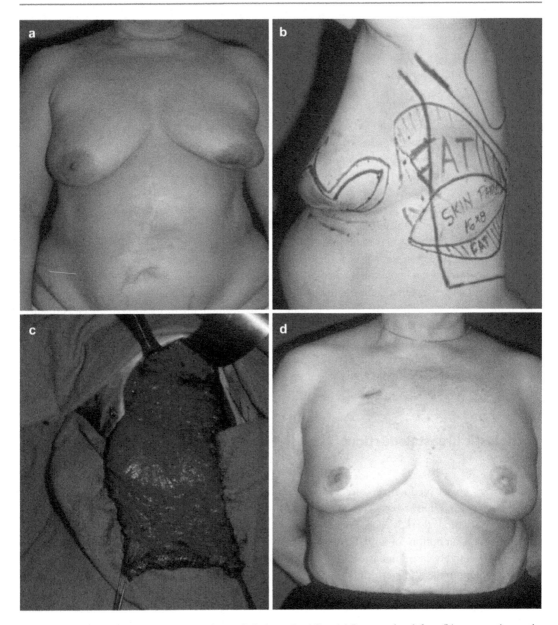

Fig. 6.7 Breast reconstruction with an autologous latissimus dorsi flap. (**a**) Preoperative defect, (**b**) preoperative marking, (**c**) intraoperative elevation of flap, (**d**) postoperative appearance at 2 years

rather than intermittent erection. In addition, these nipples offer no erogenous function.

The surgical solution for areola recreation is skin grafting, for which a plethora of donor sites have been described, including contralateral areola, thigh, groin, and labia.

Nipple preservation may be the premier choice. The nipple can be preserved either through nipple-areolar-sparing mastectomy, which confers the best aesthetics to a reconstructed breast, or in vivo or ex vivo tissue banking with delayed grafting if oncologically sound.

Some authors have advocated NAC reconstruction simultaneously with primary breast reconstruction procedures. NAC reconstruction is commonly delayed until the shape of the reconstructed breast has been achieved to ensure correct and symmetrical positioning.

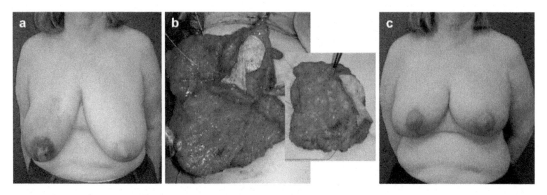

Fig. 6.8 Oncoplastic breast reduction surgery. (**a**) Preoperative appearance of bilateral macromastia with right unifocal breast cancer. (**b**) Intraoperative elevation of breast reduction flaps, resection, and removal of tumor with a large margin of surrounding normal tissue. (**c**) Postoperative appearance at 1 year with contralateral matching reduction mammoplasty

Fig. 6.9 Nipple reconstruction using a local flap method

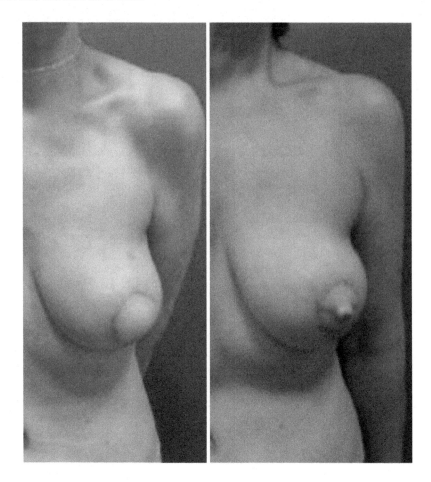

The Role of Autologous Fat Grafting in Breast Reconstruction

Autologous fat grafting is an evolving treatment modality in plastic surgery for both reconstructive and cosmetic means. Fat is typically harvested from the abdomen, thighs, or buttocks by suction or syringe-assisted lipoaspiration. Fat is subsequently processed by centrifugation or by rolling on absorbent gauze to remove the aqueous layer

Fig. 6.10 Nipple-
areolar complex
reconstruction with
tattooing

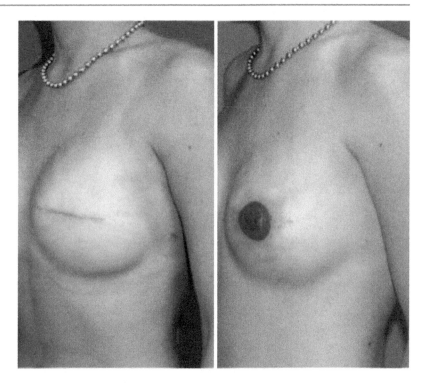

and oil. Fat is then transferred into small syringes and carefully injected into the recipient site in small aliquots in a layered lattice by multiple passes. Graft survival can be variable; thus, serial treatments are routinely needed.

In the context of breast reconstruction, this technique is useful for filling post lumpectomy defects, addressing contour abnormalities following autologous reconstruction (particularly in the upper pole, where the flap "takes off" from the chest wall) and camouflaging implants to hide rippling and the outline of the prosthesis (Fig. 6.11). Experimental and early clinical data support a role for fat grafting in protecting and rescuing skin from radiation injury. Fat grafting is also increasing in popularity for whole-breast reconstruction, with reports of successful cosmetic breast augmentation with fat grafting alone.

One additional adjunct to autologous fat-grafting techniques in breast reconstruction involves the development of external expansion, such as with the BRAVA device. Such devices, originally developed for cosmetic breast augmentation, are worn on the chest and exert negative pressure on the chest wall, causing chest wall edema. This edematous tissue not only creates a larger space for fat grafting but may also improve fat graft retention as a result of improved blood supply. Patients are instructed to wear the device as much as possible, typically approximately 12–14 h a day for 4 weeks and 24 h a day for 2–3 days prior to grafting. Patients then undergo fat grafting with a target of approximately 200 ml. The use of the device may be resumed 3 days post grafting, and three to six cycles of expansion and grafting are typically required to achieve an ideal result [24].

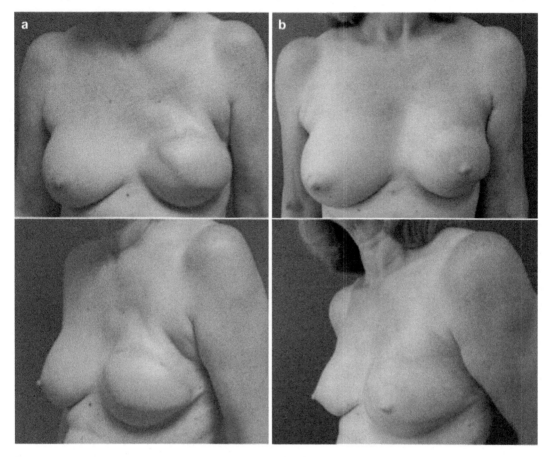

Fig. 6.11 Autologous fat grafting in breast reconstruction. (**a**) Preoperative appearance with significant left breast superior volume and contour deficit. (**b**) Correction with fat; grafting postoperative appearance at 22 months

References

1. Goin MK, Goin JM. Midlife reactions to mastectomy and subsequent breast reconstruction. Arch Gen Psychiatry. 1981;38(2):225–7.
2. Wellisch DK, Schain WS, Noone RB, Little 3rd JW. Psychosocial correlates of immediate versus delayed reconstruction of the breast. Plast Reconstr Surg. 1985;76(5):713–8.
3. Gieni M, Avram R, Dickson L, Farrokhyar F, Lovrics P, Faidi S, et al. Local breast cancer recurrence after mastectomy and immediate breast reconstruction for invasive cancer: a meta-analysis. Breast. 2012;21(3):230–6.
4. Mustonen P, Lepistö J, Papp A, Berg M, Pietiläinen T, Kataja V, et al. The surgical and oncological safety of immediate breast reconstruction. Eur J Surg Oncol. 2004;30(8):817–23.
5. Krumboeck A, Giovanoli P, Plock JA. Fat grafting and stem cell enhanced fat grafting to the breast under oncological aspects – recommendations for patient selection. Breast. 2013;22(5):579–84.
6. Ihrai T, Georgiou C, Machiavello JC, Chignon-Sicard B, Figl A, Raoust I, et al. Autologous fat grafting and breast cancer recurrences: retrospective analysis of a series of 100 procedures in 64 patients. J Plast Surg Hand Surg. 2013;47(4):273–5.
7. Boneti C, Yuen J, Santiago C, Diaz Z, Robertson Y, Korourian S, et al. Oncologic safety of nipple skin-sparing or total skin-sparing mastectomies with immediate reconstruction. J Am Coll Surg. 2011;212(4):686–93.
8. Mallon P, Feron JG, Couturaud B, Fitoussi A, Lemasurier P, Guihard T, et al. The role of nipple-sparing mastectomy in breast cancer: a comprehensive review of the literature. Plast Reconstr Surg. 2013;131(5):969–84.

9. Agrawal A, Sibbering DM, Courtney CA. Skin sparing mastectomy and immediate breast reconstruction: a review. Eur J Surg Oncol. 2013;39(4):320–8.

10. Petit JY, Lohsiriwat V, Clough KB, Sarfati I, Ihrai T, Rietjens M, et al. The oncologic outcome and immediate surgical complications of lipofilling in breast cancer patients: a multicenter study – Milan-Paris-Lyon experience of 646 lipofilling procedures. Plast Reconstr Surg. 2011;128(2):341–6.

11. McCarthy CM, Pusic AL, Kerrigan CL. Silicone breast implants and magnetic resonance imaging screening for rupture: do U.S. Food and Drug Administration recommendations reflect an evidence-based practice approach to patient care? Plast Reconstr Surg. 2008;121(4):1127–34.

12. Lipworth L, Tarone RE, McLaughlin JK. Silicone breast implants and connective tissue disease: an updated review of the epidemiologic evidence. Ann Plast Surg. 2004;52:598.

13. Lipworth L, Tarone RE, McLaughlin JK. Breast implants and fibromyalgia: a review of the epidemiologic evidence. Ann Plast Surg. 2004;52:284.

14. Rohrich RJ. Safety of silicone breast implants: scientific validation/vindication at last. Plast Reconstr Surg. 1999;104:1786.

15. Hulka BS, Kerkvliet NL, Tugwell P. Experience of a scientific panel formed to advise the federal judiciary on silicone breast implants. N Engl J Med. 2000;342:812.

16. Tugwell P, Wells G, Peterson J, Welch V, Page J, Davison C, et al. Do silicone breast implants cause rheumatologic disorders? A systematic review for a court-appointed national science panel. Arthritis Rheumatol. 2000;44:2477.

17. Al-Sabounchi S, De Mey AM, Eder H. Textured saline-filled breast implants for augmentation mammaplasty: does overfilling prevent deflation? A long-term follow-up. Plast Reconstr Surg. 2006;118(1):215–22.

18. Dowden RV. Breast implant overfill, optimal fill, and the standard of care. Plast Reconstr Surg. 1999;104(4):1185–6.

19. Cordeiro PG, Pusic AL, Disa JJ, Mc-Cormick B, VanZee K. Irradiation after immediate tissue expander/implant breast reconstruction: outcomes, complications, aesthetic results, and satisfaction in 156 patients. Plast Reconstr Surg. 2004;113:877–81.

20. Restifo RJ, Ward BA, Scoutt LM, Brown JM. Timing, magnitude, and utility of surgical delay in the TRAM flap: II. Clinical studies. Plastic and reconstructive. Surgery. 1997;99(4):1217–23.

21. Shestak KC, Johnson RR, Greco RJ, Williams SW. Partial mastectomy and breast reduction as a valuable treatment option for patients with macromastia and carcinoma of the breast. Surg Gynecol Obstet. 1993;177:54–6.

22. Shestak KC, Gabriel A, Landecker A, Peters S, Shestak A, Kim J. Assessment of long-term nipple projection: a comparison of three techniques. Plast Reconstr Surg. 2002;110(3):780–6.

23. Shestak KC, Nguyen TD. The double opposing periareola flap: a novel concept for nipple areola reconstruction. Plast Reconstr Surg. 2007;119(2):473–80.

24. Khouri R, Del Vecchio D. Breast reconstruction and augmentation using pre-expansion and autologous fat transplantation. Clin Plast Surg. 2009;36(2):269–80.

Adjuvant Systemic Therapy: Endocrine Therapy

7

Ibrahim Yildiz and Pinar Saip

Abstract

Estrogen receptor (ER)- and/or progesterone receptor (PR)-positive breast cancers are the most common types of breast cancer, accounting for 75 % of all breast cancers. Adjuvant endocrine therapy is a pivotal component of treatment for women with hormone receptor-positive early-stage breast cancer; it delays local and distant relapse and prolongs survival. Patients with ER- and/or PR-positive invasive breast cancers should be considered for adjuvant endocrine therapy regardless of age, lymph node status, or adjuvant chemotherapy use. Features indicative of uncertain endocrine responsiveness include low levels of hormone receptor immunoreactivity, PR negativity, poor differentiation (grade 3), high Ki-67 index, human epidermal growth factor receptor 2 overexpression, and high gene recurrence score. Adjuvant hormonal manipulation is achieved by blocking the ER in breast tumor tissues with tamoxifen in premenopausal and postmenopausal women, lowering systemic estrogen levels with luteinizing hormone-releasing hormone agonists in premenopausal women, or blocking estrogen biosynthesis in non-ovarian tissues with aromatase inhibitors in postmenopausal women.

Keywords

Breast cancer • Endocrine therapy • Adjuvant therapy

I. Yildiz, MD (✉)
Department of Medical Oncology, Medical Faculty,
Acibadem University, Istanbul, Turkey
e-mail: dr_ibrahim2000@yahoo.com

P. Saip, MD
Department of Medical Oncology, Institute of
Oncology, Istanbul University, Istanbul, Turkey
e-mail: pinarsaip@gmail.com

Principles of Adjuvant Endocrine Therapy

Adjuvant endocrine therapy (ET) is a major treatment modality for estrogen receptor (ER)-positive breast cancer. Among early-stage breast cancer patients, approximately 60 % require adjuvant ET after chemotherapy (CT), 20 % only

© Springer International Publishing Switzerland 2016
A. Aydiner et al. (eds.), *Breast Disease: Management and Therapies*,
DOI 10.1007/978-3-319-26012-9_7

require ET, and 20 % only require CT. The anti-estrogen drug tamoxifen was first introduced in the 1970s, and over the past 40 years, it has significantly improved overall survival (OS) in women with hormone receptor (HR)-positive early breast cancer. More recently, third-generation aromatase inhibitors (AIs) have been added to the repertoire of adjuvant ETs, and these inhibitors are superior to tamoxifen in reducing recurrence risk and improving OS in postmenopausal women.

Current ETs modulate or disrupt estrogen production or ER function/expression in breast cancer cells. In premenopausal women, the ovarian follicles are the main source of estrogen production. Ovarian estrogen production is regulated by the anterior pituitary gland, which produces luteinizing hormone (LH) and follicle-stimulating hormone (FSH). LH acts upon thecal cells to stimulate androgen synthesis, whereas FSH acts upon granulosa cells to stimulate the production of the enzyme aromatase, which converts testosterone and androstenedione to estradiol (E_2) and estrone, respectively, through aromatization. Pituitary LH and FSH production is in turn regulated by LH-releasing hormone (LHRH) (also known as gonadotropin-releasing hormone), which is produced in the hypothalamus. In postmenopausal women, estrogen production is dependent on peripheral aromatization, which predominantly occurs in the liver, adrenal glands, and adipose tissue. ET modulates or disrupts ER signaling by blocking pituitary LH/FSH production (LHRH agonists), blocking the ER (tamoxifen), degrading the ER (fulvestrant), or inhibiting peripheral estrogen production (AIs). Given their different modes of action, menopausal status is important in ET selection.

Rationale of Estrogen Receptor-Targeted Therapies

ERs belong to a family of nuclear steroid receptors that includes thyroid hormone, vitamin D, and retinoid receptors. ER phosphorylation, which occurs upon estrogen binding, induces a conformational change, resulting in receptor dimerization. The receptor complex binds to specific estrogen response elements in the promoters of target genes, resulting in the upregulation of target gene expression [1]. Two ERs, ERα and ERβ, have been described [2]. ERβ is broadly expressed in a variety of tissues, whereas ERα has a more restricted expression pattern (breast, ovary, uterus, and endometrium). The function and role of ERβ in breast cancer are not yet clear; thus, ER generally refers to ERα. The ER exerts both genomic and nongenomic effects in breast cancer. Genomic effects include the transcriptional activation of specific genes that are important for tumor cell growth and survival, whereas nongenomic effects include the activation of growth factor pathways, such as those of human epidermal growth factor receptor 2 (HER2), and insulin-like growth factor receptor, that enhance tumor growth. Growth factor receptor-linked kinases further activate the ER and its coactivators to augment ER-mediated transcriptional activity. This bidirectional crosstalk can cause ET resistance [3]. HR status is currently determined based on the immunohistochemical (IHC) expression of ER and progesterone receptor (PR). Tumors with any detectable (≥1 %) ER and/or PR expression are considered HR positive. ER expression correlates with slower tumor growth, better differentiation, and longer natural history. By contrast, the absence of both ER and PR expression is associated with poorer prognosis and reduced OS rate. A positive response to hormone therapy is correlated with higher HR protein and mRNA expression levels [4]. For example, 60 % of ER-positive/PR-positive patients were responsive to ET, compared with 30 % of ER-positive/PR-negative patients and <10 % of ER-negative/PR-negative patients. The updated results of the Early Breast Cancer Trialists' Collaborative Group (EBCTCG) clearly showed that the benefit of ET only occurs in ER-positive tumors and is strongest in tumors with high ER expression [5]. The benefit of adjuvant ET is very small in patients with HR-positive disease who have lymph node-negative cancers ≤0.5 cm or 0.6–1.0 cm in diameter with favorable prognostic features.

Determination of Endocrine Therapy Responsiveness

Endocrine-responsive breast cancer is a heterogeneous disease with a wide spectrum of clinical, pathologic, and molecular features. A variety of prognostic factors associated with recurrence risk in ER-positive breast cancer have emerged (Table 7.1). These factors provide information on the likelihood of tumor recurrence and on risk reduction with adjuvant ET. They may also help to estimate the absolute magnitude of treatment effects. However, to date, no single marker—aside from HR expression—is adequate for identifying patients who may benefit from adjuvant ET. Similarly, no single marker can identify the optimal ET for a given patient. Although molecular typing is an ideal method for assessing recurrence risk and treatment response, routine genetic profiling has not yet been established in clinical practice. IHC typing is still considered state of the art for assessing the risk of relapse and the potential benefits of specific therapies.

The evolving role of endocrine responsiveness in the selection of adjuvant breast cancer therapy is clearly seen in the consensus reports of the St. Gallen International Expert Consensus Meetings. In 2005, St. Gallen Conference panelists included endocrine responsiveness as the decisive criterion in adjuvant therapy selection [6]. Three categories (responsive, uncertain responsive, and unresponsive) were acknowledged and were later renamed as highly endocrine responsive, incompletely endocrine responsive, and endocrine nonresponsive [7]. The definitions of these categories rely mainly, but not exclusively, on the percentages of ER- and PR-positive tumor cells. High ER and PR expression and the absence of adverse biological factors (e.g., HER2 overexpression/amplification, high proliferation index, and high urokinase inhibitor type-1 level) denote highly endocrine-responsive tumors. Incompletely endocrine-responsive tumors are characterized by PR negativity, the presence of adverse biological factors, and extensive axillary lymph node invasion. At St. Gallen 2011, endocrine responsiveness was first linked to the intrinsic molecular breast cancer subtypes (Table 7.2) [8].

Gene Expression Profiling

Breast cancer is a heterogeneous disease with diverse morphologies, molecular characteristics, and clinical behaviors. Gene expression profiling studies have identified several distinct breast cancer subtypes that differ markedly in prognosis and therapy response [8–10]. A list of the intrinsic genes that are used to differentiate subtypes includes ER, HER2, and proliferation-related genes as well as a unique cluster of genes called the basal cluster. The molecular subtypes include the following: (1) luminal subtype (luminal A and B) expresses genes associated with luminal epithelial cells of normal breast tissue and overlaps with ER-positive breast cancers as defined by clinical assays, (2) HER2-enriched subtype comprises the majority of clinically

Table 7.1 Prognostic factors in HR-positive breast cancer

Tumor size
Nodal status
Tumor grade
Quantitative HR expression
HER2 status
Lymphovascular invasion
Proliferation status (e.g., Ki-67)
Multigene prognostic signatures (e.g., 21-gene recurrence score)

Table 7.2 Clinicopathologic definitions of the intrinsic subtypes according to the 2011 St. Gallen International Expert Consensus Meeting

Intrinsic subtype	Clinicopathologic definition
Luminal A	ER and/or PR positive
	HER2 negative
	Ki-67 low (<14 %)
Luminal B (HER2 negative)	ER and/or PR positive
	HER2 negative
	Ki-67 high
Luminal B (HER2 positive)	ER and/or PR positive
	HER2 positive
	Ki-67 any

Reprinted from Goldhirsch et al. [8] by permission of Oxford University Press

HER2-positive breast cancers, and (3) ER-negative subtype expresses low levels of HR-related genes.

The luminal A and luminal B subtypes comprise the majority of ER-positive breast cancers, with luminal A tumors being more common (40 % vs. 20 %, respectively, of all breast cancers). These subtypes have certain important molecular and prognostic distinctions. The clinicopathologic definitions of luminal A and B subtypes are shown below (Table 7.2). Luminal A tumors usually have high ER expression, low HER2 expression, and a low proliferation index (Ki-67). Compared with luminal A tumors, luminal B tumors have a lower ER expression, variable HER2 expression, and higher proliferation index. Luminal B tumors carry a worse prognosis than luminal A tumors.

Gene expression profiling has shed light on the complex molecular background of this disease and holds the potential for more accurate prognostication and patient stratification for therapy. Several genomic tests have been developed with the aim of improving prognostic information beyond that which is provided by classic clinicopathologic parameters [8–13]. Some of these tests are currently available in the clinic and are used to determine prognosis and, more importantly, to assist in determining the need for adjuvant chemotherapy, particularly in patients with ER-positive disease. The available data suggest that information generated from genomic tests has resulted in a change in decision making in approximately 25–30 % of cases. Molecular signatures, such as the 21-gene recurrence score (RS; Oncotype DX®) [11], the Amsterdam 70-gene prognostic profile (MammaPrint®) [12], and the Rotterdam/Veridex 76-gene signature [13], increase the prognostic value of conventional indicators in predicting breast cancer outcomes and treatment response. Oncotype DX is the most widely used of these assays. Oncotype DX can be performed using formalin-fixed paraffin-embedded tissue, whereas the other tests require fresh or frozen tissue. The predictive value of Oncotype DX has been validated in both premenopausal and postmenopausal women, and its use in node-negative, ER-positive breast cancer patients is suggested in the American Society of Clinical Oncology (ASCO) guidelines. MammaPrint and Oncotype DX have a similar predictive ability for clinical outcome [14]. The MammaPrint assay is approved by the Food and Drug Administration (FDA) for the assessment of recurrence risk in ER-positive and ER-negative breast cancer patients.

Currently, DNA microarray technologies only allow for the retrospective stratification of patients based on prognostic and predictive subsets. Prospective randomized clinical trials including TAILORx (the Trial Assigning Individualized Options for Treatment), MINDACT (Microarray In Node-negative and One to Three Positive Lymph Node Disease May Avoid Chemotherapy), and RxPONDER (Treatment for Positive Node, Endocrine Responsive Breast Cancer) are using gene-based assays to assess the additional benefit of adding adjuvant CT to ET in intermediate-risk patients with early-stage breast cancer.

21-Gene Recurrence Score in Lymph Node-Negative Patients Treated with Tamoxifen

The 21-gene assay includes 16 tumor-associated genes and 5 reference genes, which are used to compute an RS. Higher expression of favorable genes (e.g., *ER*, *glutathione S-transferase Mu 1*, and *BCL2-associated athanogene*) results in a lower RS because of a negative coefficient in the RS algorithm. Higher expression of unfavorable genes (CD68 and genes in the proliferation, HER2, and invasion groups) contributes to a higher RS because of a positive coefficient in the RS algorithm (Fig. 7.1). The 21-gene RS was validated in an independent dataset derived from 668 samples collected in the tamoxifen-treated arm of the National Surgical Adjuvant Breast and Bowel Project (NSABP) B-14 trial, a prospective randomized clinical trial that examined the benefit of adjuvant tamoxifen in HR-positive, node-negative breast cancer. Although this population had a generally good prognosis, the rates of distant recurrence at 10 years were 7 %, 14 %, and 31 % in patients with low (<18), intermediate [18–30], and high (>30) RSs, respectively (Table 7.3) [11]. The

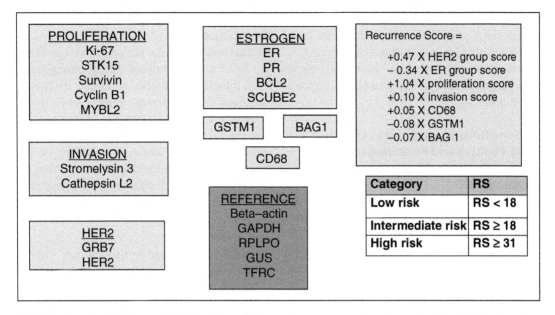

Fig. 7.1 Oncotype DX (Genomic Health, Redwood City, CA) recurrence score (*RS*): genes and algorithm. *HER* human epidermal growth factor, *ER* estrogen receptor, *PR* progesterone receptor. *BAG 1, BCL2* B-cell lymphoma 2, BCL2-associated athanogene, *ER* estrogen receptor, *HER2* epidermal growth factor receptor 2, *GAPDH* glyceraldehyde 3-phosphate dehydrogenase, *GRB7* growth factor receptor-bound protein 7, *GSTM1* glutatione S-transferase mu 1, *GUS* glucuronidase, *MYBL2* Myb-related protein B, *PR* progesterone receptor, *RPLPO* ribosomal large protein PO, *RS* recurrence score, *SCUBE2* signal peptide CUB domain EGF-like 2, *STK15* serine/threonine protein kinase 6, *TFRC* transferrin receptor

sensitivity of RS was 76.9 % (95 % CI 75.1–80.3), indicating that approximately 77 % of patients who developed distant recurrence had a high or intermediate RS. The specificity was 55.4 % (95 % CI 54.1–56.8), indicating that 55 % of patients with no recurrence had a low RS. The NSABP B-20 trial was performed to examine the benefit of concurrent tamoxifen and CT versus tamoxifen alone in node-negative, ER-positive breast cancer patients [15]. Tumor specimens from the tamoxifen-only arm were used as a training set for assay development [16]. In the tamoxifen-only arm, a high RS was almost five times more likely to occur in patients who developed distant recurrence at 10 years, whereas a low RS was five times more likely to occur in patients who did not develop distant recurrence at 10 years. RS sensitivity and specificity were 84 % (95 % CI 79–98) and 65 % (95 % CI 62.8–68.3), respectively. In a retrospective analysis of the NSABP B-14 and B-20 trials, RS was able to quantify recurrence risk as a continuous variable and predict tamoxifen and CMF responsiveness.

Table 7.3 Risk of distant recurrence at 10 years according to recurrence score in the NASBP B-14 validation study

Recurrence score	Risk group	n	10-year distant recurrence % (CI)
<18	Low	338	6.8 (4.0–9.6)
18–30	Intermediate	149	14.3 (8.3–20.3)
≥31	High	181	30.5 (23.6–37.4)

CI confidence interval

21-Gene Recurrence Score in Lymph Node-Positive Patients Treated with Tamoxifen

In the Southwest Oncology Group (SWOG)-8814 (North American Breast Cancer Intergroup (INT) 0100) study, 1477 postmenopausal women with HR-positive, node-positive disease were randomized to receive tamoxifen alone or cyclophosphamide, doxorubicin, and 5-fluorouracil (CAF) plus tamoxifen. For patients treated with tamoxifen alone, the 10-year disease-free survival (DFS) rates were 60 %, 49 %, and 43 % in the low, intermediate, and high RS groups, respectively. The continuous RS was prognostic for the first 5 years but not beyond 5 years [17]. Patients with high scores benefitted from CT, whereas those with low scores showed no benefit from CT regardless of the number of positive lymph nodes.

21-Gene Recurrence Score in Lymph Node-Positive and Node-Negative Patients Treated with Tamoxifen or Anastrozole

The Anastrozole, Tamoxifen, Alone or in Combination (ATAC) trial examined the predictive ability of RS for recurrence in CT-naive postmenopausal breast cancer patients with node-negative ($n=872$) or node-positive ($n=432$) disease. After combining the treatment arms, the 9-year distant recurrence rates were 4 %, 12 %, and 25 % and 17 %, 28 %, and 49 % for node-negative and node-positive patients in the low, intermediate, and high RS groups, respectively (both $p<0.001$).

Determination of Menopausal Status

Definitions of menopause-associated terms and biomarkers used to assess menopausal status are provided in Boxes 7.1 [18–20] and 7.2 [21, 22], respectively. Menopausal status is generally assessed using clinical features such as age, menstrual history, and menopausal symptoms, and it may be confirmed by serum FSH and E_2 levels within the menopausal range. Elevated FSH and reduced E_2 levels generally confirm the clinical diagnosis of menopause. However, the use of these biomarkers has several limitations. The transition toward menopause is highly variable, thus making it difficult to define diagnostic cutoff values for FSH/E_2. Therefore, single time point testing of FSH/E_2 levels is not sufficient to confirm menopause. Furthermore, FSH/estrogen levels are influenced by ETs. Tamoxifen increases circulating estrogens and decreases FSH levels [23]. AIs profoundly decrease estrogen levels and increase FSH levels in postmenopausal patients [23, 24]. Therefore, in these clinical settings, FSH/E_2 levels are not reliable surrogate markers of menopause.

Chemotherapy-Induced Amenorrhea/ Menopause

CT can cause significant changes in ovarian function by directly destroying the remaining functional follicles or indirectly promoting the loss of functional follicles through induction of ovarian fibrosis. CT can also lead to amenorrhea by inducing primary or hypergonadotropic hypogonadism [25]. CT is associated with the occurrence of POI. CT-induced POI results from an acceleration of the natural ovarian aging process caused by damage to the steroid-producing

---

Box 7.1. Definitions of Primary Ovarian Insufficiency, Amenorrhea, Menopause, Menopausal Transition, and Perimenopause

Primary ovarian insufficiency (POI): Amenorrhea for at least 3 months and serum FSH and E_2 concentrations of >40 IU/L and <10 pg/mL, respectively, obtained twice at least 1 month apart in a woman aged <40 years [18]. The cause of ovarian dysfunction is inherent in the ovary. In most cases, an unknown mechanism leads to premature exhaustion of the resting pool of primordial follicles. POI may also result from genetic defects, autoimmunity, surgery, radiotherapy, or cytotoxic CT.

Amenorrhea: The absence of menses on a permanent, intermittent, or temporary basis. Amenorrhea is classified as primary or secondary. Primary amenorrhea is the failure of menses to occur by age 16 years. Secondary amenorrhea is defined as the absence of menses for more than three cycles or 6 months in a woman with previously normal menses. Amenorrhea may be due to pregnancy or caused by infections, uncontrolled diabetes mellitus, malnutrition, hypothalamic or thyroid dysfunction, hyperprolactinemia, or polycystic ovary syndrome. Secondary amenorrhea in conjunction with increased FSH levels often indicates ovarian insufficiency. However, gonadotropin cutoff values suggestive of ovarian insufficiency onset have not been established, likely due to the intermittent and sometimes erratic decline in ovarian function [18].

Menopause: The permanent cessation of menses resulting from the loss of ovarian follicle activity. Natural menopause can only be retrospectively established after 12 consecutive months of spontaneous amenorrhea. The mean age of natural menopause is 51 years, with a range of 40–60 years [18]. Postmenopause is characterized by markedly high FSH levels, low E_2 levels, and very low or undetectable inhibin-B and anti-Müllerian hormone (AMH) [19]. Varying menopause definitions have been used in breast cancer clinical trials. According to the National Comprehensive Cancer Network (NCCN), menopause is defined as bilateral oophorectomy, age ≥ 60 years, or age <60 years with amenorrhea for ≥ 12 months in the absence of CT, tamoxifen, toremifene, or ovarian suppression and FSH and E_2 levels within postmenopausal range.

Menopausal transition: Menopausal transition typically begins in women in their mid-40s and precedes the final menses by 2–8 years (mean duration, 4 years). The endocrine changes underlying menopausal transition are predominantly the consequences of a marked decrease in ovarian follicle numbers. E_2 levels fall considerably, whereas estrone levels remain almost unchanged, reflecting peripheral aromatization of adrenal and ovarian androgens. The increase in FSH is greater than that of LH, presumably due to the loss of inhibins and estrogen feedback. Other significant changes include a decrease in inhibin-B levels during the early phase of the menstrual cycle and AMH levels.

Perimenopause: Perimenopause starts with menopausal transition and lasts throughout the 12 months of amenorrhea [20].

Box 7.2. Biomarkers for the Assessment of Menopausal Status

FSH: FSH is produced by the anterior pituitary gland in response to the pulsatile release of LHRH from the hypothalamus. FSH stimulates the growth of the small antral follicles and finally causes selection of the follicle with the most FSH receptors, which will become the dominant preovulatory follicle. Granulosa cells of the developing preovulatory follicles produce considerable amounts of E_2, which in turn exert negative feedback effect to decrease pituitary FSH secretion. The Stages of Reproductive Aging Workshop proposed FSH as the best predictive marker of menopause but did not establish a precise cutoff value to define menopausal status [21]. Elevated blood FSH levels reflect an age-dependent decrease in the follicle pool. FSH levels rise above 20 IU/L during the late perimenopausal phase; therefore, this level is often used as the cutoff value to determine ovarian reserve depletion. However, tamoxifen treatment in truly postmenopausal women may decrease FSH levels, even into the premenopausal range. Conversely, chemotherapy-induced amenorrhea (CIA) in premenopausal women may temporarily result in highly increased FSH levels; thus, folliculogenesis may resume later. Therefore, no absolute cutoff level of FSH can be provided above which folliculogenesis no longer occurs [22].

E_2: E_2 is mainly secreted by the late antral follicle and the ensuing corpus luteum. E_2 secretion is regulated by FSH and LH. Although E_2 levels <130 pmol/L are considered postmenopausal levels, values of 10–60 pmol/L have been reported. Furthermore, E_2 levels are higher in obese postmenopausal women because of the relatively high aromatase activity associated with the increased number of adipose cells. In contrast, E_2 levels are lower among smokers because nicotine and its metabolite cotinine are strong inhibitors of aromatase. In addition, hormone replacement therapy may lower FSH levels and increase E_2 levels up to 1 year after therapy cessation [22].

LH: LH levels increase with age, independent of E_2 levels, due to increased pituitary sensitivity to LHRH. During menopausal transition, LH increases slowly and reaches moderately elevated levels in postmenopause.

Antral follicle count (AFC), ovarian volume, and blood levels of FSH, E_2, inhibin-B, and AMH are used to evaluate ovarian reserve. AMH and AFC provide the most reliable assessment of the reproductive lifespan of the ovaries, fertility status, and risk of premature ovarian failure. Menstrual cycle irregularity, vasomotor symptoms, significantly elevated basal FSH, and undetectable inhibin-B levels are only short-term predictors of menopause (within 2 years) [24]. Low/undetectable AMH levels, low AFC, poor response to in vitro follicle stimulation, and rise in FSH during the early follicular phase indicate a limited ovarian reserve and risk of early menopause. However, these factors do not predict imminent menopause [24]. Although currently available enzyme-immunometric assays for AMH and FSH are highly sensitive (detection level, 0.05 ng/mL), the lowest level of detection is still not considered an absolute cutoff level to precisely mark menopause.

granulosa and theca cells and apoptotic death in a fraction of primordial follicles, which mainly impairs follicular development. The sensitivity of the ovaries to CT varies considerably (Table 7.4), with alkylating agents being the most commonly associated with permanent and irreversible gonadal damage [26]. The risk of CT-induced POI has been correlated with CT type, higher cumulative CT dose, and older age, and age >40 years is the strongest predictor of both CIA

and chemotherapy-induced menopause (CIM) [18, 20].

The estimated risk of CIA associated with single and combination CT regimens is shown in Table 7.4 [27]. Transient and prolonged amenorrhea are more frequently observed with CMF and cyclophosphamide, epirubicin, and 5-fluorouracil/CAF regimens compared with doxorubicin and cyclophosphamide, presumably

Table 7.4 Estimated risk of permanent amenorrhea associated with single-agent and combination adjuvant regimens in early breast cancer

	Single-agent therapy	Combination therapy
High risk (>80 %)	Cyclophosphamide	CMF, FEC, and FAC; six cycles in women aged ≥40 years
Intermediate risk	Cisplatin	CMF, FEC, and FAC; six cycles in women aged 30–39 years
	Carboplatin	AC and EC; four cycles in women aged ≥40 years
	Adriamycin	Taxane-containing combinations
	Taxanes	
Low risk (<20 %) or no risk	Methotrexate	CMF, FEC, and FAC; six cycles in women aged <30 years
	5-Fluorouracil	AC and EC; four cycles in women aged <40 years
To be determined	Trastuzumab	
To be determined	Lapatinib	

Adapted from Lee et al. [27] with permission from the American Society of Clinical Oncology
AC adriamycin and cyclophosphamide, *CMF* cyclophosphamide, methotrexate, and fluorouracil, *EC* epirubicin and cyclophosphamide, *FAC* fluorouracil, Adriamycin, and cyclophosphamide, *FEC* fluorouracil, epirubicin, and cyclophosphamide

due to the higher cumulative dose of cyclophosphamide received [25]. The addition of taxanes increases the risk of CIA in many individuals, particularly in the first year of use [20, 28]. Tamoxifen use following CT significantly increases the rate and/or duration of CIA and slightly but significantly increases the CIM risk [20, 25, 29]. However, the mechanism by which tamoxifen influences CIA/CIM remains unclear. Tamoxifen may increase plasma E_2 levels and interfere with the hypothalamic–ovarian feedback loop that regulates estrogen synthesis [20].

CIA complicates menopause assessment in premenopausal women with early breast cancer. In clinical practice, menopausal status in women with CIA may be determined only using hormonal evaluations and a nonvalidated pool of clinical data, including age, menstrual history, vasomotor symptoms, and the likelihood of gonadal toxicity from CT. The use of such criteria may lead to an inaccurate assessment of menopausal status. Furthermore, although many patients >40 years of age develop CIA, this type of ovarian failure may be temporary in a considerable number of patients. The percentage of women with CIA/oligomenorrhea who will later develop CIM is not yet known. Menstrual cycles and/or fertility may recover months to years after CT withdrawal. Resumption of menses is more likely to occur in younger women, those exposed to less gonadotoxic regimens, and those with a higher basal number of follicles. In fact, the remaining follicles may regrow from the primordial pool in 3–6 months, and gonadotropin levels may return to normal after CT withdrawal, especially in very young women [26]. However, individual CIM risk cannot be predicted. Thus, the use of both pre-CT and post-CT evaluations of ovarian reserve may better predict menopausal status.

Endocrine Therapy Selection According to Menopausal Status

Assessment of ovarian function is important in hormone-sensitive breast cancer patients who are eligible to receive adjuvant ET. Adjuvant AI treatment administered upfront or replacing tamoxifen is superior to tamoxifen alone in postmenopausal patients and has therefore become the standard of care in these patients. In contrast, adjuvant treatment with tamoxifen with or without ovarian suppression is recommended in premenopausal women. Tamoxifen can be safely given to premenopausal women; however, this is not the case for AIs. AIs interfere with androgen-to-estrogen conversion by blocking aromatase, thereby lowering E_2 levels in truly postmenopausal women. However, in the presence of functional ovaries, low levels of estrogen will enhance pituitary FSH production, thereby indirectly stimulating follicular aromatase production and subsequent E_2 production. Consequently, AI treatment in the absence of an LHRH agonist may be ineffective in postmenopausal women who were inaccurately classified as premenopausal. Moreover, in the case of CIA, AIs may promote recovery of ovarian function, leading to therapeutic failure and even to unwanted pregnancy.

The choice of adjuvant ET may be guided by age only in specific patient groups (Table 7.5). Women ≤40 years with CIA should not receive adjuvant ET with AIs alone. Estrogen depletion is the desired endocrine strategy in these patients. Their management should include oophorectomy or chemical ovarian suppression with combined LHRH agonist and tamoxifen. Serial monitoring of E_2 and gonadotropin levels should be performed in women 40–50 years of age with CIA. Women who have FSH and E_2 levels within the premenopausal range (≤40IU/L and ≥10 pmol/L, respectively) should receive tamoxifen alone or tamoxifen plus ovarian suppression. In patients with hormone levels indicative of postmenopausal status (FSH>40IU/L and E_2 <10 pmol/L), AMH assessment may be useful to detect any residual ovarian function. AI may be cautiously administered to patients whose AMH levels are below the lower limits of normal range. In addition, serial hormone monitoring should be performed (with a reasonable timing of 4 months between consecutive measurements) to achieve ongoing confirmation of menopausal status. For patients whose levels remain within the postmenopausal range, AI can be continued. Otherwise, tamoxifen alone or in combination with ovarian suppression is the appropriate ET. The same approach should be

Table 7.5 Suggested practical approaches to determine the appropriateness of adjuvant AI therapy in breast cancer patients with CIA or tamoxifen-induced amenorrhea

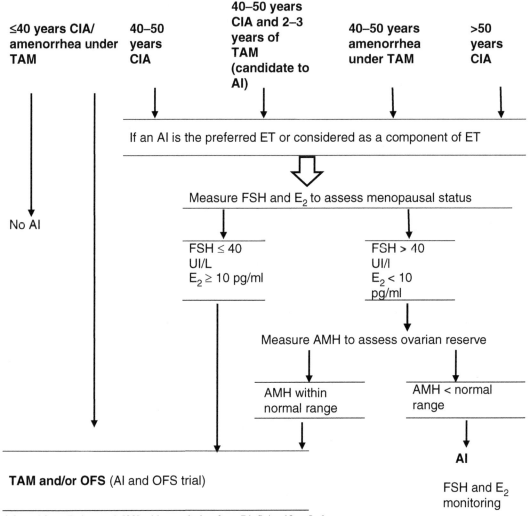

Adapted from Torino et al. [20] with permission from BioScientifica, Ltd.
AI aromatase inhibitor, AMH anti-Müllerian hormone, CIA chemotherapy-induced amenorrhea, E_2 estradiol, ET endocrine therapy, FSH follicle-stimulating hormone, OFS ovarian function suppression, TAM tamoxifen

used in premenopausal women >40 years of age with CIA who may start AI after 2–3 years of tamoxifen. Likewise, in women who develop tamoxifen-induced amenorrhea and are suitable candidates for switching to an AI, it is advisable to perform serial high-quality evaluations of E_2, FSH, and AMH. The switch can only be safely made in cases with confirmed menopausal status. Women >50 years of age at the time of CT with CIA lasting >6 months may receive AI if hormone assessment has provided enough certainty of menopausal status. However, tamoxifen should replace AI in patients whose E_2 levels continue to rise.

Adjuvant Endocrine Therapy for Premenopausal Women

Approximately 60 % of premenopausal breast cancers are ER positive. Adjuvant ET is an integral component of ER-positive breast cancer therapy. Patients with ER- and/or PR-positive invasive breast cancers should be considered for adjuvant ET regardless of age, lymph node status, or adjuvant CT use [30]. Features that are indicative of uncertain endocrine responsiveness include low levels of HR immunoreactivity, PR negativity, poor differentiation (grade 3), high proliferation index (Ki-67), HER2 overexpression, and high gene RS. In the absence of these features, tumors are considered highly endocrine responsive. Patients with tumors of different degrees of endocrine responsiveness may receive Et alone or in combination with CT. The type of treatment selected is determined by multiple factors, including ER and PR status, nodal status, histological grade, and peritumoral vascular invasion (Table 7.6) [31]. Patients with tumors of uncertain endocrine responsiveness are usually treated with a combination of ET and CT. Endocrine strategies in premenopausal women include ER blockade with tamoxifen, temporary ovarian suppression with LHRH agonists, or permanent ovarian suppression with oophorectomy or radiotherapy. Tamoxifen is the mainstay of ET in premenopausal women. The benefit of ovarian suppression has not been clearly demonstrated; however, prospective studies are currently ongoing. The use of AIs as single agents is contraindicated because the reduced feedback of estrogen to the hypothalamus and pituitary may increase gonadotropin secretion and stimulate the ovary, thereby leading to an increase in androgen substrates and aromatase. However, concurrent AI and ovarian suppression with an LHRH agonist, surgery, or radiotherapy may also be considered.

Tamoxifen

Until recently, tamoxifen has been the gold standard for the adjuvant treatment of ER-positive breast cancer in both premenopausal and postmenopausal women. The 2011 EBCTCG meta-analysis, which compared 5 years of tamoxifen treatment to no ET in premenopausal and postmenopausal women, was instrumental in establishing the efficacy of adjuvant tamoxifen [5]. Tamoxifen treatment resulted in a 39 % reduction

Table 7.6 Threshold for treatment modalities according to the 2009 St. Gallen Consensus Conference

Clinicopathologic feature	Relative indication for chemoendocrine therapy	Factor not useful for decision	Relative indication for endocrine therapy alone
ER and PR levels	Low		High
Histological grade	3	2	1
Proliferation index[a]	High	Intermediate	Low
Nodal status	Positive (≥4 involved nodes)	Positive (1–3 involved nodes)	Negative
PVI	Present		Absent
pT size, cm	>5	2.1–5	≤2
Patient preference	Use all available treatments		Avoid chemotherapy-related side effects
Multigene signature assay score[b]	High	Intermediate	Low

Adapted from Goldhirsch et al. [31] by permission of Oxford University Press

ER estrogen receptor, *HER2* epidermal growth factor receptor 2, *PR* progesterone receptor, *pT* pathological tumor size (i.e., size of the invasive component), *PVI* peritumoral vascular invasion

[a]Conventional measures of proliferation include assessment of the Ki-67 labeling index (low, ≤15 %; intermediate, 16–30 %; high, >30 %) and frequency of mitosis. The reliability of these measures will vary in different geographic settings. First-generation gene signatures consist of ER, HER2, and proliferation-related genes. A meta-analysis indicated that much of the prognostic information in these signatures resides in their sampling of proliferative genes, but their respective total scores may be the only form in which information is provided at present and are the only format that could be used in this component of assessment of relative indications for chemotherapy

[b]The European Society for Medical Oncology Panel agreed that validated multigene tests, if readily available, could assist in deciding whether to add chemotherapy in cases where its use was uncertain after consideration of conventional markers

in breast cancer recurrence compared with placebo (relative risk [RR] 0.61, 95 % CI 0.57–0.65), which translated into a 15-year absolute reduction of 13 % (33 % vs. 46 %, respectively). This outcome was observed in both node-negative and node-positive patients. Tamoxifen treatment also resulted in a 30 % reduction in breast cancer mortality risk (RR 0.70, 95 % CI 0.64–0.75), which translated into a 15-year absolute reduction of 9 % (24 % vs. 33 % in the placebo group). The magnitude of benefit was similar between women <45 and 55–69 years of age. Tamoxifen also reduced the risks of local recurrence (RR 0.54) and of contralateral breast cancer (RR 0.62).

Timing of Tamoxifen Therapy

Concurrent tamoxifen interferes with the cytotoxicity of CT in cancer cell lines in vitro [32, 33]. The SWOG-8814 (INT 0100) randomized trial investigated the timing of tamoxifen in 1558 patients receiving CT [34]. At a median follow-up of 9.94 years, CAF plus 5 years of tamoxifen was superior to tamoxifen alone, and CAF plus sequential tamoxifen was more effective than CAF plus concurrent tamoxifen. Based on these results, tamoxifen should be given sequentially and not concurrently with CT.

Duration of Tamoxifen Therapy

For decades, tamoxifen for 5 years has been the standard ET for premenopausal women [35]. Tamoxifen for more than 5 years has not been shown to be more beneficial than tamoxifen for 5 years in two North American and Scottish trials [36, 37]. However, the results of the ATLAS (Adjuvant Tamoxifen: Longer Against Shorter) and Adjuvant Tamoxifen—To Offer More (aTTom) trials have recently changed this paradigm. The ATLAS trial aimed to assess the further benefit of continuing tamoxifen for 10 years in women with HR-positive breast cancer who had completed 5 years of tamoxifen. Premenopausal and postmenopausal women ($n = 6846$) were randomly assigned to receive either 5 years of additional tamoxifen or no further therapy. Extended tamoxifen reduced breast cancer recurrence by 25 % (617 vs. 711 patients, respectively; $p < 0.01$) and breast cancer deaths

by 29 % (331 vs. 397 patients, respectively; $p = 0.001$), but it did not increase non-breast cancer mortality. These benefits were only observed after 10 years of tamoxifen use. In the extended tamoxifen arm, 1 % and 0.2 % increases in endometrial cancer incidence and related deaths, respectively, in women aged >50 years were observed [38]. In the aTTom trial, 6953 women with ER-positive ($n = 2755$) or ER-untested ($n = 4198$; estimated to be 80 % ER-positive) invasive breast cancer who had completed 5 years of tamoxifen were randomized to stop tamoxifen or continue tamoxifen to year 10. Extended tamoxifen reduced breast cancer recurrence (580/3468 vs. 672/3485; $p = 0.003$) in a time-dependent manner. The rate ratio was 0.99 (95 % CI 0.86–1.15), 0.84 (95 % CI 0.73–0.95), and 0.75 (0.66–0.86) during years 5–6, years 7–9, and later years, respectively. Longer treatment also reduced breast cancer recurrence-related mortality (392 vs. 443 deaths; $p = 0.05$) and overall mortality (849 vs. 910 deaths; $p = 0.1$). The rate ratios were 1.03 (95 % CI 0.84–1.27) during years 5–9 and 0.77 (95 % CI 0.64–0.92) during the later years for breast cancer recurrence-related mortality and 1.05 (95 % CI 0.90–1.22) during years 5–9 and 0.86 (95 % CI 0.75–0.97) during the later years for overall mortality. Non-breast cancer mortality was not significantly affected (457 vs. 467 deaths; rate ratio 0.94 [95 % CI 0.82–1.07]). However, extended tamoxifen treatment also increased the incidence of endometrial cancer (102 vs. 45 patients; rate ratio 2.20 [95 % CI 1.31–2.34]; $p < 0.0001$) and endometrial cancer-related deaths (37 [1.1 %] vs. 20 [0.6 %] deaths; absolute hazard ratio [HR] 0.5; $p = 0.02$) compared with 5 years of tamoxifen. The aTTom trial also demonstrated that, compared with 5 years tamoxifen, continuing tamoxifen to 10 years in patients with ER-positive disease yielded further reductions in recurrence from year 7 onward and breast cancer mortality after year 10.

In a recent meta-analysis of extended adjuvant tamoxifen in early breast cancer (eight trials including 29,138 patients), more than 5 years of tamoxifen significantly improved OS (odds ratio [OR] 0.89; 95 % CI 0.80–0.99; $p = 0.03$), breast cancer-specific survival (OR 0.78; 95 % CI 0.69–0.9; $p = 0.0003$), and recurrence-free survival (RFS; OR 0.72; 95 % CI 0.56–0.92; $p = 0.01$) compared with 5 years of tamoxifen. Locoregional and distant relapses were reduced by 36 % and 13 %, respectively. Compared with 5 years of tamoxifen, additional adjuvant ET reduced the risk of death and relapse in ER-positive breast cancer patients by 10 % and 30 %, respectively. Combining the results of the aTTom and ATLAS trials enhanced the significance of the recurrence ($p < 0.0001$), breast cancer mortality ($p = 0.002$), and OS ($p = 0.005$) benefits. Taken together, these studies indicate that, compared with tamoxifen for 5 years, 10 years of adjuvant tamoxifen reduces breast cancer mortality by approximately one-third in the first 10 years following diagnosis and by one-half in subsequent years [39].

The optimal duration of ET for premenopausal women to balance the potential benefits and side effects associated with treatment has yet to be determined. ET significantly affects reproductive options in premenopausal women because women are counseled not to become pregnant while undergoing adjuvant ET. Young women receiving ET may also experience menopausal symptoms, such as hot flashes, vaginal dryness, and sexual dysfunction. Tamoxifen is associated with an increased risk of thromboembolic events (1–2 % increased risk of deep venous thrombosis and threefold increased risk of pulmonary embolism), increased vaginal bleeding, and threefold increased risk of endometrial cancer. However, the absolute increase in endometrial cancer is <1 %, and almost all of the cancers that develop are stage I adenocarcinomas.

Tamoxifen Resistance

The expression of growth factor receptors, such as HER2, is associated with the development of tamoxifen resistance in breast cancer. Selected studies suggest that HER2-positive breast cancers may be less sensitive to some ETs, whereas other studies have failed to confirm this finding [40–43]. A retrospective analysis of tumor blocks collected in the ATAC trial indicated that HER2 amplification is a marker of relative endocrine resistance independent of ET type [44]. Some studies suggest that PR negativity in ER-positive tumors may be associated with increased growth factor expression, more aggressive tumor phenotype, and tamoxifen resistance. By contrast, higher levels of ER expression predict greater tamoxifen benefits. Other factors that may contribute to tamoxifen resistance include variable expression of ERα and ERβ isoforms, interference with coactivator and corepressor binding, alternative splicing of *ER* mRNA variants, modulators of ER expression (e.g., epidermal growth factor and its receptors, such as epidermal growth factor receptor 1 and HER2), and inherited drug-metabolizing *CYP2D6* genotypes. CYP2D6 converts tamoxifen to endoxifen, the major active tamoxifen metabolite. Over 100 allelic variants of *CYP2D6* have been reported. In the Breast International Group (BIG) 1-98 and ATAC trials, *CYP2D6* genotype status was shown to not influence breast cancer recurrence after tamoxifen use [45, 46]. Given the limited and conflicting evidence at this time, the NCCN Breast Cancer guidelines do not recommend CYP2D6 testing as a tool to determine the optimal adjuvant endocrine strategy.

Ovarian Suppression

The ovaries are the main site of estrogen production in premenopausal women. Therefore, ovarian ablation/suppression is an endocrine therapeutic option to consider in young women with ER-positive disease. Irreversible ovarian ablation may be accomplished by surgical oophorectomy or ovarian irradiation. Radiation is seldom used because of its side effects. Adjuvant CT frequently results in permanent amenorrhea and thus represents an indirect form of ovarian ablation. Chemical castration with LHRH is a reversible approach. Chemical ovarian suppression utilizes LHRH agonists to suppress LH and FSH release from the pituitary and reduce ovarian estrogen production. Goserelin, leuprolide, and triptorelin are also used for chemical ovarian suppression; however, only goserelin has been approved by the FDA. The advantage of chemical suppression is that it is a simple, reversible outpatient therapy. The disadvantages are restoration of estrogen production at the time of drug withdrawal, injection site reactions, and menopausal symptoms. The optimal form of ovarian suppression (surgical oophorectomy, ovarian irradiation, or chemical suppression) in the adjuvant setting is unknown because of the absence of direct comparison studies. Ovarian ablation therapy is the oldest type of breast cancer therapy. Beatson first reported its use in the palliation of young women with metastatic disease in 1896.

The role of adjuvant ovarian ablation/suppression in premenopausal women with HR-positive breast cancer remains undetermined. The combined analysis of the early studies in the 1995 overview from the EBCTCG demonstrated that ovarian ablation as a single intervention reduces breast cancer recurrence and increases survival in women <50 years of age [47]. Of the 12 randomized trials included in the analysis, 7 trials compared ovarian ablation and no CT, and 5 trials compared ovarian ablation combined with CT. By indirect comparison, the efficacy of ovarian ablation was similar to that of adjuvant CT and tamoxifen. The EBCTCG also performed a meta-analysis of randomized studies of ovarian ablation/suppression alone versus no adjuvant treatment in women >50 years. The annual odds of recurrence and death were reduced in favor of ovarian ablation/suppression over no adjuvant treatment. Reductions of 25 % and 29 % in recurrence and death rates, respectively, were observed in women <40 years of age, and a 29 % reduction in both recurrence rate and death rate was observed in women 40–49 years of age [48]. An analysis of ovarian suppression versus no adjuvant therapy showed no significant reductions in recurrence (HR reduction −28.4; 95 % CI −50.5–3.5; $p = 0.08$) or death (HR reduction −22; 95 % CI −44.1–6.4; $p = 0.11$) [49]. The following findings emerged from this meta-analysis. (1) As single agents, LHRH agonists such as goserelin, leuprolide, and triptorelin showed a trend toward a lower risk of breast cancer recurrence compared with no further systemic treatment (HR 0.72, 95 % CI 0.49–1.04). A trend toward a reduction in mortality was also observed (HR 0.82, 95 % CI 0.47–1.43), although the analysis was likely underpowered for this outcome. (2) The combination of LHRH agonist and tamoxifen showed a trend toward a lower risk of recurrence (HR 0.85, 95 % CI 0.67–1.09) and mortality (HR 0.84, 95 % CI 0.59–1.19) compared with tamoxifen alone. (3) The risks of recurrence (HR 1.04, 95 % CI 0.92–1.17) and mortality (HR 0.90, 95 % CI 0.79–1.10) did not differ between LHRH agonist plus non-anthracycline-containing adjuvant CT and adjuvant CT alone. These results suggest that LHRH agonists have limited efficacy in patients who receive non-anthracycline-based chemotherapy. This limitation is perhaps due to the high rate of treatment-induced suppression caused by CT regimens such as CMF. However, ovarian suppression may provide an additional benefit for women who are treated with contemporary anthracycline-based regimens. There is no definitive evidence of any additional benefit with the use of LHRH agonists administered as an alternative to or along with tamoxifen. LHRH agonists should be given for at least 2 years. However, the timing and optimal duration of treatment are still a matter of debate. Data comparing the efficacy of monthly and trimonthly formulations of LHRH agonists are lacking. However, monthly goserelin and trimonthly leuprolide have similar effects on E_2 and FSH levels [50]. Thus, to date, selected studies have suggested the benefits of ovarian ablation/suppression in the adjuvant treatment of premenopausal women with HR-positive breast cancer.

Ovarian suppression has also been studied with either tamoxifen or the AI exemestane in premenopausal patients in a combined analysis of the SOFT (Suppression of Ovarian Function Trial) and TEXT (Tamoxifen and Exemestane Trial) trials; exemestane use was associated with a significant reduction in the risk of recurrence compared with tamoxifen. In women who did not need chemotherapy, 5 years of tamoxifen was sufficient to reduce recurrence risk, and ovarian function suppression is not advised in this group. However, in the cohort that remained premenopausal after CT (average age, 40 years), ovarian suppression added to tamoxifen achieved a 22 % reduction in risk of recurrence versus tamoxifen alone. The combination of exemestane plus ovarian function suppression was even better, with a 35 % reduction in risk of recurrence versus tamoxifen alone. The 5-year event-free survival was 78 % for tamoxifen alone, 82.5 % for tamoxifen plus ovarian function suppression, and 85.7 % for exemestane plus ovarian function suppression [51].

In addition, randomized trials have shown that ovarian suppression with GnRH agonist therapy administered during adjuvant CT in premenopausal women with ER-negative tumors may preserve ovarian function and diminish the likelihood of CIA.

The abrupt interruption of ovarian function is a significant problem in young premenopausal patients. Adverse events may include severe menopause-related signs and symptoms, psychological distress, impaired quality of life, sexual dysfunction, changes in personal and family relationships, and bone loss. Ovarian ablation alone is not recommended as an alternative to any other form of systemic therapy, except in the specific cases of patients who are candidates for other forms of systemic therapy but who for some reason will not pursue other systemic therapies (e.g., patients who cannot tolerate other forms of systemic therapy or patients who choose no other form of systemic therapy).

Ovarian Ablation/Suppression Versus Chemotherapy

Studies of ovarian ablation/suppression alone versus CMF alone have generally demonstrated similar antitumor efficacy in premenopausal patients with HR-positive tumors, whereas superior outcomes were achieved with CMF in HR-negative patients (Table 7.7) [49, 52–59]. The benefits of ovarian suppression/ablation may be greater in younger premenopausal patients.

Ovarian Ablation/Suppression Plus Tamoxifen Versus Chemotherapy

In general, studies of ovarian ablation/suppression plus tamoxifen versus CT alone have shown no differences in recurrence or survival rates in premenopausal women (Table 7.7) [48, 60–62].

Chemotherapy Plus Ovarian Suppression/Ablation with or Without Tamoxifen

Clinical trials evaluating the efficacy of ovarian suppression as combination or sequential therapy in premenopausal women with HR-positive breast cancer are shown in Table 7.8 [52, 57, 63]. A large intergroup trial compared the efficacy of

Table 7.7 Randomized trials of adjuvant chemotherapy versus ovarian ablation/suppression with or without tamoxifen

Study	Patients	n	Treatment	Outcome
ZEBRA [54]	N+, HR+/-	1640	CMF × 6 vs. Z × 2 years	No difference in HR+; CMF better in HR-
IBCSG VIII [57]	N-, HR+/-	706	CMF × 6 vs. Z × 2 years	No difference in HR+; CMF better in HR-
Scottish Cancer Trial Breast Group [58]	N+/-	332	CMF × 6–8 vs. OA (XRT/surg)	No difference
TABLE [59]	N+, HR+	600	CMF × 6 vs. leuprorelin acetate × 2 years	No difference
GROCTA 02 [60]	N+, HR+	244	CMF × 6 vs. Z × 2 years + TAM × 5 years	No difference
FASG 06 [61]	N+, HR+	333	FEC × 6 vs. triptorelin × 3 years + TAM × 3 years	No difference
ABCSG 5 [62]	Stage I/II, HR+	1045	CMF × 6 vs. Z × 3 years + TAM × 5 years	DFS better with Z + TAM

ABCSG Austrian Breast Cancer Study Group, *CMF* cyclophosphamide, methotrexate, and fluorouracil, *FAC* fluorouracil, doxorubicin, and cyclophosphamide, *FASG* French Adjuvant Study Group, *FEC* fluorouracil, epirubicin, and cyclophosphamide, *GROCTA* Italian Breast Cancer Adjuvant Study Group, *HR+* hormone receptor positive, *HR-* hormone receptor negative, *IBCSG* International Breast Cancer Study Group, *N+* node positive, *N-* node negative, *OA* ovarian ablation, *surg* oophorectomy, *TABLE* Takeda Adjuvant Breast cancer study with Leuprorelin Acetate, *TAM* tamoxifen, *XRT* ovarian radiation, *Z* goserelin, *ZEBRA* Zoladex Early Breast Cancer Research Association

Table 7.8 Clinical trials evaluating the efficacy of ovarian suppression as combination or sequential therapy in premenopausal women with hormone receptor-positive breast cancer

Study	n	Treatment	Outcome
INT 0101 [52]	1503	CAF (6×)[a] vs. CAF (6×) → Z (5 years) vs. CAF (6×) → Z + TAM (both 5 years)	DFS, OS, TTR: CAF → Z + TAM > CAF → Z > CAF
IBCSG VIII [57]	1063	CMF (6×) vs. Z (24 months) vs. CMF (6 ×) → Z (18 months)	DFS (ER-negative tumors): CMF > Z, DFS (ER-positive tumors): CMF = Z CMF → Z > CMF CMF → Z > Z OS: no difference
ZIPP [63]	2710	After standard CT/RT Z vs. TAM vs. Z + TAM vs. No treatment	RFS and OS: Z > no Z

[a]Six cycles

CAF cyclophosphamide, doxorubicin, and 5-fluorouracil, *CMF* cyclophosphamide, methotrexate, and 5-fluorouracil, *CT* chemotherapy, *DFS* disease-free survival, *ER* estrogen receptor, *IBCSG* International Breast Cancer Study Group, *INT* North American Breast Cancer Intergroup, *OS* overall survival, *RFS* recurrence-free survival, *RT* radiotherapy, *TAM* tamoxifen, *TTR* time to recurrence, *Z* goserelin, *ZIPP* Zoladex in Premenopausal Patients

adjuvant CAF, CAF plus ovarian suppression with goserelin (CAF-Z), and CAF-Z plus tamoxifen (CAF-ZT) in premenopausal women with HR-positive, node-positive breast cancer [52]. Time to recurrence (TTR) and OS were similar between the CAF and CAF-Z groups. TTR (HR 0.73; 95 % CI 0.59–0.90; $p < 0.01$), but not OS, was improved in the CAF-Z group compared with the CAF-ZT group (HR 0.91; 95 % CI 0.71–1.15; $p = 0.21$). This study did not include a CAF plus tamoxifen arm; therefore, the contribution of goserelin to the improved TTR in the CAF-ZT arm could not be assessed. The addition of ovarian suppression/ablation has also been subjected to meta-analysis by the EBCTCG [48]. They found that the addition of ovarian suppression/ablation to CT did not result in significant reductions in annual recurrence or mortality rates in women <40 and 40–49 years of age.

Currently, there is no evidence that ovarian suppression/ablation is superior to tamoxifen, except perhaps in women who have not developed CIM. Ovarian ablation should not be routinely added to systemic CT, tamoxifen, or combined tamoxifen and CT. However, women <40 years of age and patients who do not become amenorrheic after CT may especially benefit from ovarian suppression with an LHRH agonist. The best use of LHRH agonists (concurrent or sequential with CT) is unknown. The combination of LHRH agonist plus AI or AI alone is not indicated in premenopausal patients outside clinical trials. Some women are offered treatment with ovarian suppression in association with AI therapy because of intolerance to or contraindications for tamoxifen.

Adjuvant Endocrine Therapy for Postmenopausal Women

In general, the following three groups of women can safely be considered postmenopausal: women >60 years of age, women who have undergone a bilateral ovariectomy, and women <60 years of age with intact uteri who are not using oral contraceptives or hormone replacement therapy and have been amenorrheic for at least 1 year prior to their breast cancer diagnosis. Women who experience regular menses without using oral contraceptives or hormone replacement therapy can be classified as premenopausal. Strictly stated, in all other cases, ovarian activity cannot be excluded and menopausal status is therefore considered uncertain. Approximately 75 % of breast cancers are diagnosed in postmenopausal women, and 80 % of these cancers are HR positive [64]. Third-generation AIs, including anastrozole, letrozole, and exemestane, block estrogen synthesis by inhibiting aromatase. Because these AIs do not block ovarian estrogen production, their use is limited to postmenopausal women.

A number of studies have compared AIs with tamoxifen in the adjuvant setting using either a head-to-head (i.e., randomly assigning patients to 5 years of either drug) or switched schedule approach (i.e., initial tamoxifen for 2–3 years followed by either an AI for 2–3 years or continued tamoxifen for a total of 5 years). The use of AIs in either approach reduces breast cancer recurrence rates compared with tamoxifen alone; however, the effect on survival is less clear [65]. Two large randomized studies showed no significant differences in recurrence or survival between upfront and switching AI therapy [66–68]. Randomized studies have also demonstrated that extended ET with 3–5 years of an AI following 5 years of tamoxifen decreases relapse rates and may improve survival, especially in women with nodal involvement [69–71]. Given the improved outcomes observed with the use of AIs compared with tamoxifen alone, both the ASCO and NCCN recommend the incorporation of AIs at some point in the treatment of postmenopausal women with HR-positive breast cancer [72]. Sequential rather than concurrent administration of cytotoxic and endocrine therapies should be used. The concurrent use of tamoxifen and anthracyclines has been shown to have detrimental effects, whereas the concurrent use of AIs and CT has not been investigated [8].

Several studies have evaluated AIs as initial adjuvant therapy, sequential therapy following 2–3 years of tamoxifen, and extended therapy following 4.5–6 years of tamoxifen in postmenopausal women with early-stage breast cancer (Table 7.9). Two prospective randomized clinical trials have provided evidence of an OS benefit in patients with early-stage breast cancer receiving initial adjuvant ET with tamoxifen followed by sequential anastrozole (HR 0.53; 95 % CI 0.28–0.99; $p=0.045$) or exemestane (HR 0.83; 95 % CI 0.69–1.00; $p=0.05$ [excluding patients with ER-negative disease]) compared with those receiving ET with tamoxifen alone [73, 74]. In addition, the National Cancer Institute of Canada Clinical Trials Group (NCIC-CTG) MA.17 trial demonstrated that, compared with placebo, extended letrozole therapy provided a survival advantage in women with axillary lymph node-positive, but not lymph node-negative, ER-positive breast cancer [69]. However, no survival differences have been reported for patients receiving initial adjuvant therapy with an AI versus first-line tamoxifen treatment [75, 76]. Tamoxifen and AIs have different side effect

Table 7.9 Major trials of AI adjuvant therapy in postmenopausal, early-stage, hormone receptor-positive breast cancer

	Study name	Schema	Total duration of therapy (years)	AI
Head-to-head	ATAC	TAM vs. AI vs. TAM + AI	5	ANA
	BIG 1-98	TAM → AI vs. AI → TAM vs. TAM vs. AI	5	LET
Switching AI therapy (after 2–3 years of TAM)	TEAM	AI vs. TAM → AI	5	EXE
	IES	TAM vs. TAM → AI	5	EXE
	ARNO 95 ABSCG 8	TAM vs. TAM → AI	5	ANA
	ITA			
Extended AI therapy (after 5 years of TAM)	NCIC-CTG MA.17	AI vs. placebo	10	LET
	ABCSG-6a	AI vs. placebo	8	ANA
	NSABP B-33	AI vs. placebo	10	EXE

ABSCG Austrian Breast Cancer Study Group, *AI* aromatase inhibitor, *ANA* anastrozole, *ARNO* Arimidex–Nolvadex, *ATAC* Anastrozole, Tamoxifen, Alone or in Combination, *BIG* Breast International Group, *EXE* exemestane, *IES* Intergroup Exemestane Study, *ITA* Italian Tamoxifen Anastrozole, *LET* letrozole, *NCIC-CTG* National Cancer Institute of Canada Clinical Trials Group, *NSABP* National Surgical Adjuvant Breast and Bowel Project, *TAM* tamoxifen, *TEAM* Tamoxifen Exemestane Adjuvant Multicenter

profiles, although both can cause hot flashes, night sweats, and vaginal dryness. AIs are more commonly associated with musculoskeletal symptoms, osteoporosis, and increased rates of bone fracture, whereas tamoxifen is associated with an increased risk of uterine cancer and deep venous thrombosis. However, randomized trials have demonstrated that bisphosphonates and denosumab, a receptor activator of nuclear factor kappa B ligand (RANKL) inhibitor, can ameliorate AI-associated bone loss [77, 78].

Upfront Aromatase Inhibitor Therapy

Two large randomized trials, the ATAC [75, 79] and BIG 1-98 [66, 76], compared initial adjuvant ET with either tamoxifen or an AI in postmenopausal breast cancer patients (Table 7.10). In these trials, randomization occurred before the initiation of adjuvant therapy, and analyses included all events during the 5-year period.

The double-blind, placebo-controlled ATAC trial evaluated the efficacy and safety of anastrozole, tamoxifen, or anastrozole plus tamoxifen as initial adjuvant therapy after surgery in 9366 postmenopausal women with localized HR-positive breast cancer. Anastrozole was superior to both tamoxifen and combined tamoxifen and anastro-

Table 7.10 Comparative efficacy of upfront aromatase inhibitor for 5 years versus tamoxifen for 5 years in early breast cancer

Study	ATAC [79]	BIG 1-98 [66]
Number of patients	6241	4922
Median follow-up, months	120	76
Disease-free survival		
HR	0.86[a]	0.88
p value	0.003[a]	0.03
Difference in 5-year disease-free survival, %	2.8	2.9
Time to distant recurrence		
HR	0.85[a]	0.85
p value	0.02[a]	0.05
Overall survival		
HR	0.95[a]	0.87
p value	0.4[a]	0.08

ATAC Anastrozole, Tamoxifen, Alone or in Combination, *BIG* Breast International Group; HR, hazard ratio
[a]ER-negative patients excluded

zole [79–81]. At a median follow-up of 120 months, fewer recurrences occurred in patients receiving anastrozole compared with those receiving tamoxifen [75, 79]. DFS, the primary endpoint, was also significantly longer in patients receiving anastrozole (HR 0.86; 95 % CI 0.78–0.95; $p=0.003$). No differences in survival were observed. Although the greatest relative reductions in DFS, TTR, and contralateral breast cancer were observed in the first 2 years of active therapy, these benefits were sustained throughout the entire follow-up period and after treatment completion. Patients in the combined tamoxifen and anastrozole group gained no additional benefit over those in the tamoxifen group, suggesting a possible deleterious effect from the weak estrogenic effect of tamoxifen in patients with near complete elimination of their endogenous estrogen levels [81]. The ATAC trial sub-protocols show a number of important findings, including a lesser effect of anastrozole compared with tamoxifen on endometrial tissue [82]; similar effects of anastrozole and tamoxifen on quality of life, with most patients reporting no significant impairment in overall quality of life [83]; a greater loss of bone mineral density with anastrozole [84]; a small pharmacokinetic interference of anastrozole in the presence of tamoxifen, with unclear significance [85]; and no evidence of an interaction between prior CT and anastrozole [86].

The BIG 1-98 trial, a phase III, double-blind, randomized trial, compared the efficacy of 5 years of tamoxifen, 5 years of letrozole, 2 years of tamoxifen followed by 3 years of letrozole, and 2 years of letrozole followed by 3 years of tamoxifen in 8010 postmenopausal women. An early analysis compared tamoxifen alone versus letrozole alone, including those patients in the sequential arms during their first 2 years of treatment only [76]. This analysis (25.8-month median follow-up) showed that 5 years of letrozole significantly improved DFS (HR 0.81; $p=0.003$) and distant DFS (DDFS) (HR 0.73; $p=0.001$) compared with 5 years of tamoxifen. These results led to the unblinding of the tamoxifen-alone arm, and 25.2 % of patients selectively crossed over to letrozole, which has complicated subsequent intention-to-treat analyses of the monotherapy arms. The updated report (76-month median follow-up) included both an intention-to-treat analysis and a censored weighted modeling analysis at the time of crossover [66]. Significant improvements in DFS and DDFS in favor of letrozole over tamoxifen and a nonsignificant improvement in OS (HR 0.87; 95 % CI 0.75–1.02; $p = 0.08$) were still observed. However, in an updated analysis of the BIG 1-98 trial that accounted for women who crossed over from tamoxifen to letrozole after study unblinding, a significant, although modest, improvement in survival was observed in the letrozole arm compared with the tamoxifen arm (HR 0.82, 95 % CI 0.70–0.95), resulting in an absolute difference of 1.4 % at 5 years [87]. The overall incidence of cardiac adverse events was similar between the letrozole and tamoxifen arms (4.8 % vs. 4.7 %, respectively). However, the incidence of grade 3–5 cardiac adverse events was significantly higher in the letrozole arm, whereas the overall incidences of all-grade and high-grade (grade 3–5) thromboembolic events were significantly higher in the tamoxifen arm [88]. In addition, a higher incidence of bone fractures was observed in the letrozole arm than in the tamoxifen arm (9.5 % vs. 6.5 %, respectively) [89].

The magnitude of any additional benefit from an AI may depend on the risk of relapse. Retrospective analyses of the BIG 1-98 trial suggest that patients with low-risk tumors (i.e., small, low-grade tumors without lymphatic vascular invasion or nodal involvement; strong positive HR expression; and low Ki-67) may do equally well on tamoxifen or an AI [90]; however, this outcome has not been established in a prospective trial. Thus, given the numerous randomized trials demonstrating superior outcomes with AI versus tamoxifen monotherapy, most patients should receive an AI during the first 5 years of adjuvant therapy when possible [91].

Switching from Tamoxifen to Aromatase Inhibitor Versus Continued Tamoxifen

Several trials (Table 7.11) have evaluated the efficacy of switching to an AI after 2–3 years of tamoxifen versus 5 years of tamoxifen alone in

Table 7.11 Comparative efficacy of 2–3 years of tamoxifen followed by 2–3 years of aromatase inhibitor versus 5 years of tamoxifen alone

Study	IES [92]	ARNO 95 [96]	ITA [93, 94]	ABCSG 8 [96]
Number of patients	4724	979	448	3714
Median follow-up, months	55.7	30.1	64	72
Disease-free survival				
HR	0.76	0.66	0.56	0.79
p value	0.0001	0.49	0.01	0.038
Overall survival				
HR	0.83	0.53	0.56	0.77
p value	0.05	0.045	0.1	0.025

ABCSG Austrian Breast Cancer Study Group, *ARNO* Arimidex–Nolvadex, *HR* hazard ratio, *IES* Intergroup Exemestane Study, *ITA* Italian Tamoxifen Anastrozole

an attempt to preempt the potential development of tamoxifen resistance and minimize the long-term side effects of 5-year AI and tamoxifen monotherapies. The largest of these studies, the Intergroup Exemestane Study (IES), compared the switch to exemestane after 2–3 years of tamoxifen versus 5 years of tamoxifen alone. Postmenopausal breast cancer patients who had completed a total of 2–3 years of tamoxifen ($n = 4724$) were randomized to receive either continued tamoxifen or exemestane to complete a total duration of 5 years of ET [92]. At a median follow-up of 55.7 months, sequential exemestane therapy was superior to tamoxifen alone in terms of DFS (HR 0.76; 95 % CI 0.66–0.88; $p = 0.0001$). A significant difference in OS was only found in patients with ER-positive tumors (HR 0.83; 95 % CI 0.69–1.00; log rank $p = 0.05$). In the most recent update (91-month median follow-up), the benefit in those patients who switched to exemestane has been sustained.

The Italian Tamoxifen Anastrozole (ITA) trial randomized 448 postmenopausal women with breast cancer who had completed 2–3 years of tamoxifen to either continue tamoxifen or switch to anastrozole to complete a total of 5 years of ET [93]. Updated results from this study showed that the HR for relapse-free survival was 0.56 (95 % CI 0.35–0.89; $p = 0.01$), and the p value for OS analysis remained at 0.1 [94]. A meta-analysis ($n=4006$) of the Austrian Breast and Colorectal Cancer Study Group (ABCSG) 8, Arimidex–Nolvadex (ARNO) 95, and ITA trials showed a significant improvement in OS (HR 0.71; $p=0.04$) with anastrozole switching therapy in postmenopausal women with hormone-sensitive disease [95, 96]. In the ARNO 95 and ITA trials, only patients who were relapse-free after 2–3 years of tamoxifen were randomized, whereas the ABCSG 8 study randomized patients at diagnosis. An additional meta-analysis of these studies ($n=9015$) demonstrated that AI switching therapy resulted in a significant 29 % proportional decrease in recurrence rate (absolute decrease of 3.1 % at 5 years and 3.6 % at 8 years), a significant 22 % proportional decrease in breast cancer mortality rate (absolute decrease of 0.7 % at 5 years and 1.7 % at 8 years), and a reduction in overall mortality rate (absolute decrease of 2.2 % at 8 years; $p=0.004$) [65]. An update of the ABCSG 8 trial (60-month median follow-up) showed a modest, statistically nonsignificant improvement in the primary endpoint of RFS and a significant improvement in the defined exploratory endpoint of distant relapse-free survival.

Switching from Tamoxifen to Aromatase Inhibitor Versus Upfront Aromatase Inhibitor

The use of upfront or switching AI therapy has been addressed in two large randomized trials, the Tamoxifen Exemestane Adjuvant Multicenter (TEAM) and the BIG 1-98 trials. The TEAM trial evaluated exemestane [68], and the BIG 1-98 trial evaluated letrozole [66, 67]. Neither trial demonstrated any significant difference in recurrence or survival rates between the upfront and switch arms. The TEAM trial compared exemestane alone versus 2.5–3 years of tamoxifen followed by exemestane to complete a total of 5 years of ET [68]. This trial was initially designed to compare 5 years of tamoxifen monotherapy to 5 years of exemestane monotherapy. However, based on the favorable results of the IES, the study design was changed to a switch trial consisting of 9229 postmenopausal patients. At the end of 5 years, 85 % of patients in the

sequential group versus 86 % of patients in the exemestane group were disease-free (HR 0.97; 95 % CI 0.88–1.08; $p=0.60$). This finding is consistent with data from the BIG 1-98 trial [66], in which tamoxifen followed by letrozole, letrozole followed by tamoxifen, and letrozole alone showed a similar efficacy at a 71-month median follow-up.

Extended Adjuvant Endocrine Therapy

Late recurrences are common in HR-positive breast cancer, and a continual risk of relapse exists throughout a 15-year time span despite 5 years of ET. Predictors of late recurrence remain poorly defined. The rationale for evaluating AI as extended adjuvant therapy is based on the observation that ER-positive patients continue to exhibit significant residual risk for recurrence and death long after the initial 5 years of tamoxifen therapy. Several trials, including the large MA.17 trial and the smaller ABCSG 6 and NSABP B-33 trials, have provided strong evidence of the benefit of extended adjuvant therapy with AIs following 5 years of tamoxifen (Table 7.12) [69, 71, 97]. The results of several established trials are currently awaited: (1) MA.17R, 5 versus 10 years of AI; (2) Secondary Adjuvant Long-term Study with

Table 7.12 Comparative efficacy of extended adjuvant therapy of 5 years of tamoxifen followed by 3–5 years of aromatase inhibitor versus 5 years of tamoxifen alone

Study	NCIC-CTG MA.17 [69]	ABCSG-6a [70]	NSABPB-33 [71]
Number of patients	5187	852	1562
Median follow-up, months	64	62	30
Disease-free survival			
HR	0.68	0.62	0.68
p value	0.0001	0.031	0.07
Overall survival			
HR	0.98	0.89	NR
p value	0.853	0.57	

ABCSG Austrian Breast Cancer Study Group, *HR* hazard ratio, *NCIC-CTG* National Cancer Institute of Canada Clinical Trials Group, *NR* not recorded, *NSABP* National Surgical Adjuvant Breast and Bowel Project

Arimidex, 2 versus 5 years of extended anastrozole treatment; (3) Gruppo Italiano Mammella Letrozole Adjuvant Therapy Duration, 2–3 years of tamoxifen followed by 2–3 or 5 years of letrozole to complete a total of 5 or 7–8 years of ET, respectively; (4) Different Durations of Anastrozole After Tamoxifen, 3 versus 6 years of anastrozole after 2–3 years of tamoxifen; (5) NSABP B-42, 5 years of extended letrozole versus placebo; and (6) Study of Letrozole Extension, continuous versus intermittent letrozole for 5 years after 4–6 years of ET.

The MA.17 trial evaluated the benefit of extended adjuvant ET with letrozole in postmenopausal patients who had completed 5 years of tamoxifen (Box 7.3). At a median follow-up of 2.5 years, extended letrozole treatment resulted in fewer recurrences and fewer new contralateral breast cancers (HR 0.58; 95 % CI 0.45–0.76; $p < 0.001$) compared with placebo. No difference in OS was demonstrated (HR 0.82; 95 % CI, 0.57–1.19; $p = 0.30$), although a survival advantage was observed in the subset of patients with axillary lymph node-positive disease (HR 0.61; 95 % CI 0.38–0.98; $p = 0.04$). However, in an updated analysis (64-month median follow-up) that adjusted for patients in the placebo arm who crossed over to letrozole after study unblinding, a significant 24–39 % proportional decrease in mortality was observed in patients who received letrozole after tamoxifen [69]. A formal quality-of-life analysis demonstrated reasonable preservation of life quality during extended ET, although some women experienced ongoing menopausal symptoms and loss of bone mineral density [98, 99]. In conclusion, the MA.17 study demonstrated that extended adjuvant treatment with letrozole after tamoxifen significantly improved DFS and distant metastasis-free survival in lymph node-positive and node-negative patients and extended OS in lymph node-positive patients.

Similar benefits in DFS have been reported with tamoxifen followed by 3 years of anastrozole and 5 years of exemestane [70, 71]. In the extension study of the ABCSG 6 trial, 852 HR-positive postmenopausal patients who were disease-free and received 5 years of adjuvant

---

Box 7.3 Evidence of the Efficacy of Adjuvant AI Therapy from the 2010 EBCTCG Meta-analysis and MA.17 Trial

Single-agent therapy—The 2010 EBCTCG meta-analysis compared adjuvant AI vs. tamoxifen in 9856 women (mean follow-up of 6 years). AI treatment resulted in (1) a reduction in recurrence risk within 5 years (rate ratio 0.77; $p < 0.001$), which translated into a 3 % absolute reduction in the 5-year recurrence risk (12 % vs. 15 %, respectively), and (2) a nonsignificant reduction in the risk of breast cancer death (rate ratio 0.89; $p > 0.1$), which translated into a 1 % absolute reduction in the 5-year breast cancer mortality rate (7 % vs. 8 %, respectively).

Switching therapy—A second analysis compared switching to AI vs. continued tamoxifen in 9015 women (mean follow-up of 4 years). After 2–3 years of tamoxifen, patients were randomly assigned to receive AI or continued tamoxifen to complete a total of 5 years of ET. Switching therapy resulted in (1) a reduction in recurrence risk at 6 years (8 % vs. 11 %, respectively; rate ratio 0.71; $p < 0.001$) and (2) a reduction in the 5-year breast cancer mortality rate (6 % vs. 8 %, respectively; rate ratio 0.79; $p = 0.004$).

Extended therapy—A third adjuvant AI strategy is to initiate a 5-year course of AI after the completion of 5 years of tamoxifen. Evidence to support extended therapy comes from the MA.17 trial. In this trial, 5187 postmenopausal women (node-positive, 46 %; ER-positive, 98 %) who had completed 5 years of adjuvant tamoxifen were randomly assigned to receive letrozole or placebo for 5 years. At a median follow-up of 64 months, letrozole improved DFS (HR 0.68, 95 % CI 0.45–0.61) and OS (HR 0.51, 95 % CI 0.42–0.61). Interestingly, women in the placebo arm who switched to letrozole after study unblinding still experienced an improvement in DFS despite the substantial interval between therapies (median, 2.8 years).

tamoxifen were randomized to 3 years of anastrozole ($n=387$) or no further therapy ($n=469$). At a median follow-up of 62.3 months, anastrozole significantly reduced the recurrence risk compared with no further treatment (HR 0.62; 95 % CI 0.40–0.96; $p=0.031$) [70]. The results of the ABCSG-6a trial confirmed the benefit of extended adjuvant anastrozole treatment, showing a 38 % decrease in recurrence risk. However, these findings should be viewed cautiously because of the limited statistical power and the lower than expected recruitment rate. Despite the limitations of the NSABP B-33 trial (premature closing and crossover from placebo to exemestane in some patients), the intention-to-treat analysis showed an improvement in DFS at 4 years with exemestane.

Biomarkers for Endocrine Therapy Selection

No single biomarker can reliably predict the optimal ET for use in a given patient. The prognostic significance of ER and PR levels, PR negativity, HER2 overexpression, Ki-67 level, and 21-gene RS has been examined. In the initial exploratory analysis of the ATAC trial, a greater benefit of anastrozole compared with tamoxifen in the PR-negative subgroup was suggested. A subsequent central analysis using 2006 of 5880 specimens showed that quantitative expression of ER, PR, and HER2 was not useful in identifying patients who would benefit from anastrozole. The TEAM trial showed that, in patients receiving exemestane, ER and PR expression levels predicted DFS, relative risk of relapse increased with decreased ER and PR expression, and PR status did not predict treatment response. In the BIG 1-98 trial, more relapses occurred in the first 2 years in women who received tamoxifen followed by letrozole than in those who received letrozole alone (4.4 % vs. 3.1 %, respectively). This increased risk of relapse was particularly evident in women with >3 involved nodes ($p<0.001$), tumors ≥2 cm in size ($p=0.001$), or vascular invasion ($p=0.02$). A retrospective analysis demonstrated that these factors in conjunction with ER and PR levels, Ki-67 labeling index, and HER2 status may be useful in guiding the selection of letrozole or tamoxifen [90]. IHC analysis of the nuclear antigen Ki-67 is used to estimate the proliferative activity of tumor cells. Studies have demonstrated the prognostic value of Ki-67 in predicting response and clinical outcomes [100]. One small study suggested that analyzing Ki-67 after short-term ET may be useful in selecting patients who are resistant to ET and may benefit from additional interventions [101]. However, these data require greater analytic and clinical validation. Patients at the highest risk of recurrence benefited the most from AI treatment for 5 years, whereas relapse rates in those at lowest risk did not differ among patients treated with tamoxifen, letrozole, or a switch approach [102]. A summary of the criteria used for adjuvant ET selection in postmenopausal women is shown in (Table 7.13).

Comparison of Letrozole, Anastrozole, and Exemestane Efficacy

According to the evidence to date, AIs exhibit very similar activity. Although letrozole leads to more complete aromatase inhibition [103] and lower serum estrogen levels [104] than anastrozole, the clinical importance of these findings is unclear. To date, indirect comparisons between adjuvant trials suggest that letrozole, anastrozole, and exemestane have similar benefits when compared with tamoxifen. In addition, a neoadjuvant study showed that letrozole, anastrozole, and exemestane similarly suppress the proliferation marker Ki-67 and preoperative endocrine prognostic index scores [105].

The NCIC-CGC MA.27 study compared the efficacy and safety of 5 years of exemestane, a steroidal AI that binds irreversibly to aromatase, to that of anastrozole, a nonsteroidal AI that forms reversible bonds, in 7576 postmenopausal women [106]. At a median follow-up of 4.1 years, the 4-year event-free survival was 91 % for exemestane and 91.2 % for anastrozole (stratified HR 1.02; 95 % CI, 0.87–1.18; $p=0.85$). The overall DDFS and disease-specific survival rates were also similar. In all, 31.6 % of patients discontinued treatment because of adverse effects, concomitant disease, or study refusal. Osteoporosis/osteopenia, hypertriglyceridemia, vaginal bleeding, and hypercholesterolemia were less frequent

Table 7.13 Criteria used for adjuvant endocrine therapy selection in postmenopausal women [102]

Adjuvant endocrine therapy	Criteria for therapy selection			
5 years of AI Preferred	1. Higher risk of early relapse (e.g., larger tumor size or several positive nodes) 2. History or risk of thromboembolic event 3. Patient on a CYP2D6 inhibitor	→	If muscle/joint discomfort or other adverse effects, use an alternative AI	If unable to tolerate AI, use tamoxifen to complete at least 5 years
Switch from tamoxifen (2–3 years) to AI (2–3 years) to complete a total of 5 years of endocrine therapy Preferred	1. Significant osteopenia/osteoporosis 2. Musculoskeletal and/or joint discomfort 3. Hypercholesterolemia/heart disease	→	AI may be continued up to 5 years if tolerated High proliferative rate (Ki-67) High grade Lower ER/PR level HER2 amplification Presence of LVI	
5 years of tamoxifen Less preferred	AI contraindicated or declined by patient	→	5 years of AI if appropriate or consider 5 years of tamoxifen if AI use is still not an option	

Reprinted from Tung [102] with permission from the American Society of Clinical Oncology)
AI aromatase inhibitor, *ER* estrogen receptor, *LVI* lymphovascular invasion, *PR* progesterone receptor

in response to exemestane, whereas mild liver function abnormalities and rare episodes of atrial fibrillation were less frequent in response to anastrozole. Vasomotor and musculoskeletal symptoms were similar between the arms. Compliance is a major issue for the use of all chronic medications, including adjuvant ET. Given the adverse effects of both tamoxifen and AIs and the uncertain survival benefit of any particular approach, the schedule that leads to better compliance is likely to have the most benefit. For some patients, a switch approach may offer the best balance between efficacy and toxicity [107]. The Femara versus Anastrozole Clinical Evaluation (NCT00248170) trial was established to assess the potential differences in efficacy and safety between the nonsteroidal AIs anastrozole and letrozole in postmenopausal women with HR-positive, node-positive breast cancer. The results of this study are currently awaited.

Optimal Timing of Aromatase Inhibitor Therapy

Studies have consistently demonstrated that the use of third-generation AIs as initial adjuvant therapy, sequential therapy, or extended therapy

lowers recurrence risk, including ipsilateral breast tumor recurrence, contralateral breast cancer, and distant metastatic disease, in postmenopausal women with HR-positive breast cancer. However, a direct comparison of these strategies is not possible given the differences in design and patient populations among studies. All three adjuvant strategies have shown similar antitumor efficacy and toxicity profiles in randomized studies. The benefit of upfront and switching adjuvant AI therapy was established in the 2010 EBCTCG meta-analysis. Two separate analyses were performed: (1) AI versus tamoxifen monotherapy and (2) switching to AI after 2–3 years of tamoxifen versus continued tamoxifen. The findings of this meta-analysis are summarized in Box 7.3. Upfront or switching AI therapy improved DFS compared with 5 years of tamoxifen. In contrast, AI-containing regimens had no clear impact on OS. However, a modest OS benefit was observed in all switching studies, yielding an absolute gain in survival at 8 years.

The current version of the NCCN Guideline recommends the following adjuvant ET options for postmenopausal women with early breast cancer: 5 years of AI as initial adjuvant therapy (category 1), 2–3 years of AI followed by tamoxifen to complete 5 years of adjuvant ET (category 1), 2–3 years of tamoxifen followed by an AI to complete 5 years (category 1) or 5 years of AI alone (category 2B), or 5 years of tamoxifen followed by 5 years of AI (category 1). The use of tamoxifen alone for 5 years or longer is limited to postmenopausal women who decline AI treatment or have a contraindication to AIs. Patients who experience intolerable adverse effects on the initial adjuvant AI therapy and switch to tamoxifen after 2 years have similar outcomes to those who complete 5 years of AI therapy [67]. Switching to a different AI is reasonable because 39 % of patients are able to tolerate an alternative AI [108].

In conclusion, AI use, either upfront or after 2–3 years of tamoxifen, should be recommended for the majority of breast cancer patients. When choosing between upfront and switch strategies, it is reasonable to weigh the potential added benefit of AIs in reducing early relapse in the patients who are most likely to suffer tamoxifen and AI toxicities [109]. Support from prospective studies for the preferential use of upfront AI in patients with greater tumor burdens or more aggressive tumor biology would be extremely useful [90].

Optimal Duration of Adjuvant Endocrine Therapy

Because of the chronic nature of HR-positive disease, the risk of recurrence remains after 5 years. The optimal duration of adjuvant ET is not yet known but should be more than 5 years. It is unclear how the results of the extended adjuvant ET trials, such as the MA.17, should be incorporated into practice because AIs are used at some point in the first 5 years of breast cancer therapy. Because 5 years of an AI is effective after 5 years of tamoxifen use and because recurrence is decreased every year of AI use, it is logical to assume that 5 years of an AI would also be effective after 2–3 years of tamoxifen. Therefore, up to 5 years of AI treatment is reasonable after switching from tamoxifen regardless of when the switch is made. However, current data firmly support a total of 5 years of ET when AIs are used after 2–3 years of tamoxifen. Currently, no efficacy or safety data exist to support the use of AIs beyond 5 years. Two important ongoing trials, the MA.17R and NSABP B-42, are evaluating the benefits of longer adjuvant AI therapy.

Conclusion

Adjuvant ET remains a mainstay of therapy for women with ER-positive breast cancer. A summary of the 2016 NCCN and ASCO recommendations regarding the use of AIs and tamoxifen in the adjuvant setting is provided in Boxs 7.4 and 7.5, respectively. Adjuvant ET has made a major contribution in reducing recurrence risk and improving OS in ER-positive disease. In premenopausal

---

Box 7.4 Summary of the 2016 NCCN Breast Cancer Panel Recommendations for Adjuvant Endocrine Therapy (NCCN Guidelines Version 1. 2016 Breast Cancer)

- Endocrine strategies in premenopausal women include ER blockade with tamoxifen, temporary ovarian suppression with LHRH agonists, or permanent ovarian suppression with oophorectomy or radiotherapy. Premenopausal women should not be given AIs as an initial adjuvant therapy outside the confines of a clinical trial. Women who are premenopausal at diagnosis and become amenorrheic after CT may have continued estrogen production from the ovaries without menses. Serial assessment of circulating LH, FSH, and E_2 levels to confirm postmenopausal status is mandatory in this subset of women if AI therapy is considered. Tamoxifen with or without ovarian suppression for 5 years has been the standard ET for premenopausal women (category 1). In women who are postmenopausal at the time of completion of 5 years of tamoxifen (including those who have become postmenopausal during the 5 years of tamoxifen therapy), extended therapy with continued tamoxifen for 5 years (category 2A) or an AI for up to 5 years (category 1) is recommended. For those who remain premenopausal after the initial 5 years of tamoxifen, continued tamoxifen therapy for up to 10 years is recommended based on the data from the ATLAS trial (category 2A). AI for 5 years + ovarian suppression may be considered as an alternative option based on the SOFT and TEXT clinical trial outcomes.

- The following adjuvant ET options are recommended for women who are postmenopausal at diagnosis: initial adjuvant therapy with an AI for 5 years (category 1), AI for 2–3 years followed by tamoxifen to complete a total of 5 years of adjuvant ET (category 1), tamoxifen for 2–3 years followed by an AI to complete a total of 5 years (category 1) or 5 years of an AI (category 2B), or tamoxifen for 4.5–6 years followed by 5 years of an AI (category 1) or consideration of tamoxifen for up to 10 years (category 2A). The use of tamoxifen alone for 5 years (category 1) or up to 10 years (category 2A) is limited to postmenopausal women who decline or have a contraindication to AIs.

- Small, HR-positive tumors (those less than 0.5 cm in greatest diameter that do not involve the lymph nodes) have such favorable prognoses that adjuvant ET is of minimal benefit (category 2B).

- IHC analysis of the nuclear antigen Ki-67 estimates the proliferative activity of tumor cells. Studies have demonstrated the prognostic value of Ki-67 in predicting response and clinical outcome. Standardization of tissue handling and processing is required for improving the reliability and prognostic value of Ki-67 analysis. To date, there is no conclusive evidence that Ki-67 alone, especially baseline Ki-67, is useful in ET selection. Therefore, Ki-67 assessment is not currently recommended.

- The cytochrome P-450 enzyme CYP2D6 converts tamoxifen to endoxifen. Because of the limited and conflicting evidence at this time, CYP2D6 testing for adjuvant ET selection is not recommended. When prescribing a selective serotonin reuptake inhibitor, it is reasonable to avoid potent and intermediate CYP2D6 inhibitors, particularly paroxetine and fluoxetine, if an appropriate alternative exists.

Box 7.5. Summary of the ASCO Recommendations Specific for Adjuvant Endocrine Therapy

1. *Treatment of choice in premenopausal patients with HR-positive early breast cancer*: Women with HR-positive breast cancer who are premenopausal or perimenopausal at the time of diagnosis should be offered adjuvant ET with tamoxifen for an initial duration of 5 years. After 5 years, women should receive additional therapy based on menopausal status. Premenopausal and perimenopausal women and those with unknown or undetermined menopausal status should be offered continued tamoxifen for a total duration of 10 years. Women who have become definitively postmenopausal should be offered the choice of continued tamoxifen for a total duration of 10 years or switching to up to 5 years of an AI to complete a total of up to 10 years of adjuvant ET.

2. *Optimal duration of tamoxifen*: Five trials have evaluated tamoxifen treatment for longer than 5 years; three showed positive results. The two largest studies

with the longest reported follow-up now show a breast cancer survival advantage with longer durations (10 years) of tamoxifen use. The beneficial effects of tamoxifen become more pronounced with longer duration. Thus, a minimum of 5 years of extended treatment (i.e., 10 years since diagnosis) is needed to observe clinical benefit. In addition to modest gains in survival, extended therapy with tamoxifen for 10 years was associated with lower risks of recurrence and of contralateral breast cancer compared with 5 years. Extended tamoxifen did not affect non-breast cancer mortality in the studies examined. Consistent with previous reports on the effects of adjuvant ET, only patients with ER-positive tumors appear to benefit from extended therapy with tamoxifen.

3. *What is the appropriate sequence of adjuvant ET in postmenopausal patients?* Postmenopausal women who are intolerant of either tamoxifen or AIs should be offered an alternative adjuvant ET. Women who have received an AI but discontinued treatment at less than 5 years may be offered tamoxifen for a total of 5 years. Women who have received tamoxifen for 2–3 years should be offered the option of switching to an AI for up to 5 years to complete a total of up to 7–8 years of adjuvant ET. Women who have received 5 years of tamoxifen as adjuvant ET should be offered additional adjuvant ET. Postmenopausal women should be offered continued tamoxifen for a total of up to 10 years or the option of switching to up to 5 years of an AI to complete a total of up to 10 years of adjuvant ET. Premenopausal and perimenopausal women and those with unknown or undetermined menopausal status should be offered an additional 5 years of tamoxifen to complete a total of 10 years of adjuvant ET.

4. *Determination of ET responsiveness*: Tumor size, nodal status, ER expression, PR expression, and HER2 expression are well-established predictors of breast cancer recurrence. However, robust biomarkers that are capable of predicting early versus late recurrence, the most appropriate ET (tamoxifen vs. AI), and the need for extended adjuvant ET are not available.

5. *Subsets of patients who are more likely to benefit from an AI versus tamoxifen*: Currently, no subgroups have been well identified as being more likely to benefit from an AI versus tamoxifen. Most analyses are retrospective and mix predictive and prognostic factors. Tamoxifen is recommended for male patients because of the lack of AI data. The predictive value of CYP2D6 for tamoxifen response is unknown. Thus, CYP2D6 genotype testing is not recommended for treatment selection. However, caution is needed in patients taking tamoxifen with CYP2D6-interacting agents. CYP2D6-interacting agents should not be used in combination with tamoxifen if alternative choices exist.

6. *Risks associated with adjuvant AI therapy*: Toxicity, the presence of comorbidities, and patient preference should be taken into account in treatment selection. Switching therapy should be considered if there is poor adherence or intolerable toxicity. Although serious adverse events are rare, these agents have different and unique toxicity profiles that should be considered when recommending a specific treatment. AI use is associated with increased risk of cardiovascular disease, bone disorders, hypercholesterolemia, and hypertension, whereas tamoxifen is more often

associated with gynecologic side effects, flushing, endometrial lesions, and venous thromboembolic events.

7. *Interchangeability of AIs*: There are no clinically relevant differences among AIs. Therefore, patients intolerant of one AI can be switched to another.

women, tamoxifen remains the standard treatment. Currently, up to 10 years of tamoxifen can be safely administered, especially in women who remain premenopausal. The addition of an LHRH agonist to tamoxifen treatment represents another choice. Patients who are considered to be perimenopausal should be initially treated like premenopausal patients. Depending on their serum hormone levels, these patients can be safely switched to an AI therapy once the E_2 and FSH levels prove the establishment of postmenopausal status. In postmenopausal women, several sequences of endocrine treatment are available. The AI therapy can be induced upfront or sequentially by switching from AI to TAM and vice versa. Because women with ER-positive breast cancer have a long-term risk of relapse, emerging data demonstrating further survival gains with extended adjuvant ET are particularly relevant and indicate that the full potential of currently available endocrine agents has not yet been realized. Ongoing AI studies will further help to define the benefit of extended ET. However, the benefit is likely to vary based on recurrence risk; thus, a move from a one-size-fits-all strategy to a risk-adaptive strategy is needed.

References

1. Osborne CK, Schiff R, Fuqua SA, Shou J. Estrogen receptor: current understanding of its activation and modulation. Clin Cancer Res. 2001;7:4338s–42; discussion 4411s–4412s.
2. Kumar R, Thompson EB. The structure of the nuclear hormone receptors. Steroids. 1999;64:310–9.
3. Shou J, Massarweh S, Osborne CK, Wakeling AE, Ali S, Weiss H, Schiff R. Mechanisms of tamoxifen resistance: increased estrogen receptor-HER2/neu cross-talk in ER/HER2-positive breast cancer. J Natl Cancer Inst. 2004;96:926–35.
4. Osborne CK, Yochmowitz MG, Knight 3rd WA, McGuire WL. The value of estrogen and progesterone receptors in the treatment of breast cancer. Cancer. 1980;46:2884–8.
5. Davies C, Godwin J, Gray R, Clarke M, Cutter D, Darby S, et al. Relevance of breast cancer hormone receptors and other factors to the efficacy of adjuvant tamoxifen: patient-level meta-analysis of randomised trials. Lancet. 2011;378:771–84.
6. Goldhirsch A, Coates AS, Gelber RD, Glick JH, Thürlimann B, Senn HJ, et al. First – select the target: better choice of adjuvant treatments for breast cancer patients. Ann Oncol. 2006;17:1772–6.
7. Goldhirsch A, Wood WC, Gelber RD, Coates AS, Thürlimann B, Senn HJ, 10th St. Gallen conference. Progress and promise: highlights of the international expert consensus on the primary therapy of early breast cancer 2007. Ann Oncol. 2007;18:1133–44.
8. Goldhirsch A, Wood WC, Coates AS, Gelber RD, Thürlimann B, Senn HJ, Panel members. Strategies for subtypes – dealing with the diversity of breast cancer: highlights of the St. Gallen International Expert Consensus on the Primary Therapy of Early Breast Cancer 2011. Ann Oncol. 2011;22:1736–47.
9. Perou CM, Sørlie T, Eisen MB, van de Rijn M, Jeffrey SS, Rees CA, et al. Molecular portraits of human breast tumours. Nature. 2000;406:747–52.
10. Sørlie T, Perou CM, Tibshirani R, Aas T, Geisler S, Johnsen H, et al. Gene expression patterns of breast carcinomas distinguish tumor subclasses with clinical implications. Proc Natl Acad Sci U S A. 2001;98:10869–74.
11. Paik S, Shak S, Tang G, Kim C, Baker J, Cronin M, et al. A multigene assay to predict recurrence of tamoxifen-treated, node-negative breast cancer. N Engl J Med. 2004;351:2817–26.
12. van de Vijver MJ, He YD, van't Veer LJ, Dai H, Hart AA, Voskuil DW, et al. A gene-expression signature as a predictor of survival in breast cancer. N Engl J Med. 2002;347:1999–2009.
13. Wang Y, Klijn JG, Zhang Y, et al. Gene-expression profiles to predict distant metastasis of lymphnode-negative primary breast cancer. Lancet. 2005;365:671–9.
14. Fan C, Oh DS, Wessels L, Weigelt B, Nuyten DS, Nobel AB, et al. Concordance among gene-expression-based predictors for breast cancer. N Engl J Med. 2006;355:560–9.
15. Fisher B, Redmond C. Systemic therapy in node-negative patients: updated findings from NSABP clinical trials. National Surgical Adjuvant Breast and Bowel Project. J Natl Cancer Inst Monogr. 1992;11:105–16.
16. Paik S, Tang G, Shak S, Kim C, Baker J, Kim W, et al. Gene expression and benefit of chemotherapy in

women with node-negative, estrogen receptor-positive breast cancer. J Clin Oncol. 2006;24:3726–34.

17. Albain KS, Barlow WE, Shak S, Hortobagyi GN, Livingston RB, Yeh IT, Breast Cancer Intergroup of North America, et al. Prognostic and predictive value of the 21-gene recurrence score assay in post-menopausal women with node-positive, oestrogen-receptor-positive breast cancer on chemotherapy: a retrospective analysis of a randomised trial. Lancet Oncol. 2010;11:55–65.

18. De Vos M, Devroey P, Fauser BC. Primary ovarian insufficiency. Lancet. 2010;376:911–21.

19. Knauff EA, Eijkemans MJ, Lambalk CB, ten Kate-Booij MJ, Hoek A, Beerendonk CC, Dutch Premature Ovarian Failure Consortium, et al. Anti-mullerian hormone, inhibin B, and antral follicle count in young women with ovarian failure. J Clin Endocrinol Metab. 2009;94:786–92.

20. Torino F, Barnabei A, De Vecchis L, Appetecchia M, Strigari L, Corsello SM. Recognizing meno-pause in women with amenorrhea induced by cytotoxic chemotherapy for endocrine-responsive early breast cancer. Endocr Relat Cancer. 2012;19: R21–33.

21. Soules MR, Sherman S, Parrott E, Rebar R, Santoro N, Utian W, et al. Stages of reproductive aging work-shop (STRAW). J Womens Health Gend Based Med. 2001;10:843–8.

22. De Vos FY, van Laarhoven HW, Laven JS, Themmen AP, Beex LV, Sweep CG, et al. Menopausal status and adjuvant hormonal therapy for breast can-cer patients: a practical guideline. Crit Rev Oncol Hematol. 2012;84:252–60.

23. Rossi E, Morabito A, Di Rella F, Esposito G, Gravina A, Labonia V, et al. Endocrine effects of adjuvant letrozole compared with tamoxifen in hormone-responsive postmenopausal patients with early breast cancer: the HOBOE trial. J Clin Oncol. 2009;27:3192–7.

24. Lambalk CB, van Disseldorp J, de Koning CH, Broekmans FJ. Testing ovarian reserve to predict age at menopause. Maturitas. 2009;63:280–91.

25. Bines J, Oleske DM, Cobleigh MA. Ovarian func-tion in premenopausal women treated with adju-vant chemotherapy for breast cancer. J Clin Oncol. 1996;14:1718–29.

26. Sonmezer M, Oktay K. Fertility preservation in young women undergoing breast cancer therapy. Oncologist. 2006;11:422–34.

27. Lee SJ, Schover LR, Partridge AH, Patrizio P, Wallace WH, Hagerty K, American Society of Clinical Oncology, et al. American Society of Clinical Oncology recommendations on fertility preservation in cancer patients. J Clin Oncol. 2006;24:2917–31.

28. Najafi S, Djavid GE, Mehrdad N, Rajaii E, Alavi N, Olfatbakhsh A, et al. Taxane-based regimens as a risk factor for chemotherapy-induced amenorrhea. Menopause. 2011;18:208–12.

29. Swain SM, Land SR, Ritter MW, Costantino JP, Cecchini RS, Mamounas EP, et al. Amenorrhea in premenopausal women on the doxorubicin-and-cyclophosphamide-followed-by-docetaxel arm of NSABP B-30 trial. Breast Cancer Res Treat. 2009;113:315–20.

30. Tamoxifen for early breast cancer: an overview of the randomised trials. Early Breast Cancer Trialists' Collaborative Group. Lancet. 1998; 351:1451–67.

31. Goldhirsch A, Ingle JN, Gelber RD, Coates AS, Thürlimann B, Senn HJ, Panel members, et al. Thresholds for therapies: highlights of the St Gallen International Expert Consensus on the primary therapy of early breast cancer 2009. Ann Oncol. 2009;20:1319–29.

32. Sutherland RL, Green MD, Hall RE, Reddel RR, Taylor IW. Tamoxifen induces accumulation of MCF 7 human mammary carcinoma cells in the G0/G1 phase of the cell cycle. Eur J Cancer Clin Oncol. 1983;19:615–21.

33. Hug V, Hortobagyi GN, Drewinko B, Finders M. Tamoxifen-citrate counteracts the antitumor effects of cytotoxic drugs in vitro. J Clin Oncol. 1985;3:1672–7.

34. Albain KS, Barlow WE, Ravdin PM, Farrar WB, Burton GV, Ketchel SJ, Breast Cancer Intergroup of North America, et al. Adjuvant chemotherapy and timing of tamoxifen in postmenopausal patients with endocrine-responsive, node-positive breast cancer: a phase 3, open-label, randomised controlled trial. Lancet. 2009;374:2055–63.

35. Lonning PE. Evolution of endocrine adjuvant ther-apy for early breast cancer. Expert Opin Investig Drugs. 2010;19 Suppl 1:S19–30.

36. Fisher B, Dignam J, Bryant J, DeCillis A, Wickerham DL, Wolmark N, Breast Cancer Intergroup of North America, et al. Five versus more than five years of tamoxifen therapy for breast cancer patients with negative lymph nodes and estrogen receptor-positive tumors. J Natl Cancer Inst. 1996;88:1529–42.

37. Stewart HJ, Forrest AP, Everington D, McDonald CC, Dewar JA, Hawkins RA, et al. Randomised comparison of 5 years of adjuvant tamoxifen with continuous therapy for operable breast cancer. The Scottish Cancer Trials Breast Group. Br J Cancer. 1996;74:297–9.

38. Davies C, Pan H, Godwin J, Gray R, Arriagada R, Raina V, Adjuvant Tamoxifen, Longer Against Shorter (ATLAS) Collaborative Group, et al. Long-term effects of continuing adjuvant tamoxifen to 10 years versus stopping at 5 years after diagnosis of oestrogen receptor-positive breast cancer: ATLAS, a randomised trial. Lancet. 2013;381:805–16.

39. Petrelli F, Coinu A, Cabiddu M, Ghilardi M, Lonati V, Barni S. Five or more years of adjuvant endocrine therapy in breast cancer: a meta-analysis of pub-lished randomised trials. Breast Cancer Res Treat. 2013;140:233–40.

40. Piccart MJ, Di Leo A, Hamilton A. HER2. a 'pre-dictive factor' ready to use in the daily manage-ment of breast cancer patients? Eur J Cancer. 2000;36:1755–61.

41. Arpino G, Green SJ, Allred DC, Lew D, Martino S, Osborne CK, et al. HER-2 amplification, HER-1 expression, and tamoxifen response in estrogen receptor-positive metastatic breast cancer: a southwest oncology group study. Clin Cancer Res. 2004;10:5670–6.

42. Berry DA, Muss HB, Thor AD, Dressler L, Liu ET, Broadwater G, et al. HER-2/neu and p53 expression versus tamoxifen resistance in estrogen receptor-positive, node-positive breast cancer. J Clin Oncol. 2000;18:3471–9.

43. Mass R. The role of HER-2 expression in predicting response to therapy in breast cancer. Semin Oncol. 2000;27:46–52; discussion 92–100.

44. Dowsett M, Allred C, Knox J, Quinn E, Salter J, Wale C, et al. Relationship between quantitative estrogen and progesterone receptor expression and human epidermal growth factor receptor 2 (HER-2) status with recurrence in the Arimidex, Tamoxifen, Alone or in Combination trial. J Clin Oncol. 2008;26:1059–65.

45. Regan MM, Leyland-Jones B, Bouzyk M, Pagani O, Tang W, Breast International Group (BIG) 1-98 Collaborative Group, et al. CYP2D6 genotype and tamoxifen response in postmenopausal women with endocrine-responsive breast cancer: the breast international group 1-98 trial. J Natl Cancer Inst. 2012;104:441–51.

46. Rae JM, Drury S, Hayes DF, Stearns V, Thibert JN, Haynes BP, ATAC trialists, et al. CYP2D6 and UGT2B7 genotype and risk of recurrence in tamoxifen-treated breast cancer patients. J Natl Cancer Inst. 2012;104:452–60.

47. Early Breast Cancer Trialists' Collaborative Group. Ovarian ablation in early breast cancer: overview of the randomised trials. Lancet. 1996;348:1189–96.

48. Puhalla S, Brufsky A, Davidson N. Adjuvant endocrine therapy for premenopausal women with breast cancer. Breast. 2009;18 Suppl 3:S122–30.

49. LHRH-agonists in Early Breast Cancer Overview group, Cuzick J, Ambroisine L, Davidson N, Jakesz R, Kaufmann M, Regan M, et al. Use of luteinising-hormone-releasing hormone agonists as adjuvant treatment in premenopausal patients with hormone-receptor-positive breast cancer: a meta-analysis of individual patient data from randomised adjuvant trials. Lancet. 2007;369:1711–23.

50. Aydiner A, Kilic L, Yildiz I, Keskin S, Sen F, Kucucuk S, et al. Two different formulations with equivalent effect? Comparison of serum estradiol suppression with monthly goserelin and trimonthly leuprolide in breast cancer patients. Med Oncol. 2013;30:354.

51. Pagani O, Regan MM, Walley BA, Fleming GF, Colleoni M, Láng I, TEXT and SOFT Investigators, International Breast Cancer Study Group, et al. Adjuvant exemestane with ovarian suppression in premenopausal breast cancer. N Engl J Med. 2014;371:107–18.

52. Davidson NE, O'Neill AM, Vukov AM, Osborne CK, Martino S, White DR, et al. Chemoendocrine

therapy for premenopausal women with axillary lymph node-positive, steroid hormone receptor-positive breast cancer: results from INT 0101 (E5188). J Clin Oncol. 2005;23:5973–82.

53. Ejlertsen B, Mouridsen HT, Jensen MB, Bengtsson NO, Bergh J, Cold S, et al. Similar efficacy for ovarian ablation compared with cyclophosphamide, methotrexate, and fluorouracil: from a randomized comparison of premenopausal patients with node-positive, hormone receptor-positive breast cancer. J Clin Oncol. 2006;24:4956–62.

54. Kaufmann M, Jonat W, Blamey R, Cuzick J, Namer M, Fogelman I, Zoladex Early Breast Cancer Research Association (ZEBRA) Trialists' Group, et al. Survival analyses from the ZEBRA study. goserelin (Zoladex) versus CMF in premenopausal women with node-positive breast cancer. Eur J Cancer. 2003;39:1711–7.

55. Schmid P, Untch M, Wallwiener D, Kossé V, Bondar G, Vassiljev L, TABLE-study (Takeda Adjuvant Breast cancer study with Leuprorelin Acetate), et al. Cyclophosphamide, methotrexate and fluorouracil (CMF) versus hormonal ablation with leuprorelin acetate as adjuvant treatment of node-positive, premenopausal breast cancer patients: preliminary results of the TABLE-study (Takeda Adjuvant Breast cancer study with Leuprorelin Acetate). Anticancer Res. 2002;22:2325–32.

56. von Minckwitz G, Graf E, Geberth M, Eiermann W, Jonat W, Conrad B, et al. CMF versus goserelin as adjuvant therapy for node-negative, hormone-receptor-positive breast cancer in premenopausal patients: a randomised trial (GABG trial IV-A-93). Eur J Cancer. 2006;42:1780–8.

57. International Breast Cancer Study Group (IBCSG), Castiglione-Gertsch M, O'Neill A, Price KN, Goldhirsch A, Coates AS, Colleoni M, et al. Adjuvant chemotherapy followed by goserelin versus either modality alone for premenopausal lymph node-negative breast cancer: a randomized trial. J Natl Cancer Inst. 2003;95:1833–46.

58. Adjuvant ovarian ablation versus CMF chemotherapy in premenopausal women with pathological stage II breast carcinoma: the Scottish trial. Scottish Cancer Trials Breast Group and ICRF Breast Unit, Guy's Hospital, London. Lancet. 1993;341:1293–98.

59. Schmid P, Untch M, Kossé V, Bondar G, Vassiljev L, Tarutinov V, et al. Leuprorelin acetate every-3-months depot versus cyclophosphamide, methotrexate, and fluorouracil as adjuvant treatment in premenopausal patients with node-positive breast cancer: the TABLE study. J Clin Oncol. 2007;25:2509–15.

60. Boccardo F, Rubagotti A, Amoroso D, Mesiti M, Romeo D, Sismondi P, et al. Cyclophosphamide, methotrexate, and fluorouracil versus tamoxifen plus ovarian suppression as adjuvant treatment of estrogen receptor-positive pre-/perimenopausal breast cancer patients: results of the Italian Breast Cancer Adjuvant Study Group 02 randomized trial. J Clin Oncol. 2000;18:2718–27.

61. Roché H, Kerbrat P, Bonneterre J, Fargeot P, Fumoleau P, Monnier A, et al. Complete hormonal blockade versus epirubicin-based chemotherapy in premenopausal, one to three node-positive, and hormone-receptor positive, early breast cancer patients: 7-year follow-up results of French Adjuvant Study Group 06 randomised trial. Ann Oncol. 2006;17:1221–7.

62. Jakesz R, Hausmaninger H, Kubista E, Gnant M, Menzel C, Bauernhofer T, Austrian Breast and Colorectal Cancer Study Group Trial 5, et al. Randomized adjuvant trial of tamoxifen and goserelin versus cyclophosphamide, methotrexate, and fluorouracil: evidence for the superiority of treatment with endocrine blockade in premenopausal patients with hormone-responsive breast cancer – Austrian Breast and Colorectal Cancer Study Group Trial 5. J Clin Oncol. 2002;20:4621–7.

63. Baum M, Hackshaw A, Houghton J, Rutqvist, Fornander T, Nordenskjold B, ZIPP International Collaborators Group, et al. Adjuvant goserelin in pre-menopausal patients with early breast cancer: results from the ZIPP study. Eur J Cancer. 2006;42:895–904.

64. Anderson WF, Chatterjee N, Ershler WB, Brawley OW. Estrogen receptor breast cancer phenotypes in the surveillance, epidemiology, and end results database. Breast Cancer Res Treat. 2002;76:27–36.

65. Dowsett M, Cuzick J, Ingle J, Coates A, Forbes J, Bliss J, et al. Meta-analysis of breast cancer outcomes in adjuvant trials of aromatase inhibitors versus tamoxifen. J Clin Oncol. 2010;28:509–18.

66. BIG 1-98 Collaborative Group, Mouridsen H, Giobbie-Hurder A, Goldhirsch A, Thürlimann B, Paridaens R, Smith I, et al. Letrozole therapy alone or in sequence with tamoxifen in women with breast cancer. N Engl J Med. 2009;361:766–76.

67. Regan MM, Neven P, Giobbie-Hurder A, Goldhirsch A, Ejlertsen B, Mauriac L, BIG 1-98 Collaborative Group, International Breast Cancer Study Group (IBCSG), et al. Assessment of letrozole and tamoxifen alone and in sequence for postmenopausal women with steroid hormone receptor-positive breast cancer: the BIG 1-98 randomised clinical trial at 8.1 years median follow-up. Lancet Oncol. 2011;12:1101–8.

68. van de Velde CJ, Rea D, Seynaeve C, Putter H, Hasenburg A, Vannetzel JM, et al. Adjuvant tamoxifen and exemestane in early breast cancer (TEAM): a randomised phase 3 trial. Lancet. 2011;377:321–31.

69. Goss PE, Ingle JN, Martino S, Robert NJ, Muss HB, Piccart MJ, et al. Randomized trial of letrozole following tamoxifen as extended adjuvant therapy in receptor-positive breast cancer: updated findings from NCIC CTG MA.17. J Natl Cancer Inst. 2005;97:1262–71.

70. Jakesz R, Greil R, Gnant M, Schmid M, Kwasny W, Kubista E, Austrian Breast and Colorectal Cancer Study Group, et al. Extended adjuvant therapy with anastrozole among postmenopausal breast can-

cer patients: results from the randomized Austrian Breast and Colorectal Cancer Study Group Trial 6a. J Natl Cancer Inst. 2007;99:1845–53.

71. Mamounas EP, Jeong JH, Wickerham DL, Smith RE, Ganz PA, Land SR, et al. Benefit from exemestane as extended adjuvant therapy after 5 years of adjuvant tamoxifen: intention-to-treat analysis of the National Surgical Adjuvant Breast And Bowel Project B-33 trial. J Clin Oncol. 2008;26:1965–71.

72. Burstein HJ, Prestrud AA, Seidenfeld J, Anderson H, Buchholz TA, Davidson NE, American Society of Clinical Oncology. American Society of Clinical Oncology clinical practice guideline: update on adjuvant endocrine therapy for women with hormone receptor-positive breast cancer. J Clin Oncol. 2010;28:3784–96.

73. Coombes RC, Kilburn LS, Snowdon CF, Paridaens R, Coleman RE, Jones SE, Intergroup Exemestane Study, et al. Survival and safety of exemestane versus tamoxifen after 2–3 years' tamoxifen treatment (Intergroup Exemestane Study): a randomised controlled trial. Lancet. 2007;369:559–70.

74. Kaufmann M, Jonat W, Hilfrich J, Eidtmann H, Gademann G, Zuna I, et al. Improved overall survival in postmenopausal women with early breast cancer after anastrozole initiated after treatment with tamoxifen compared with continued tamoxifen: the ARNO 95 Study. J Clin Oncol. 2007;25:2664–70.

75. Arimidex, Tamoxifen, Alone or in Combination (ATAC) Trialists' Group, Forbes JF, Cuzick J, Buzdar A, Howell A, Tobias JS, Baum M, et al. Effect of anastrozole and tamoxifen as adjuvant treatment for early-stage breast cancer: 100-month analysis of the ATAC trial. Lancet Oncol. 2008;9:45–53.

76. Breast International Group (BIG) 1-98 Collaborative Group, Thürlimann B, Keshaviah A, Coates AS, Mouridsen H, Mauriac L, Forbes JF, et al. A comparison of letrozole and tamoxifen in postmenopausal women with early breast cancer. N Engl J Med. 2005;353:2747–57.

77. Brufsky A, Harker WG, Beck JT, Carroll R, Tan-Chiu E, Seidler C, et al. Zoledronic acid inhibits adjuvant letrozole-induced bone loss in postmenopausal women with early breast cancer. J Clin Oncol. 2007;25:829–36.

78. Ellis GK, Bone HG, Chlebowski R, Paul D, Spadafora S, Smith J, et al. Randomized trial of denosumab in patients receiving adjuvant aromatase inhibitors for nonmetastatic breast cancer. J Clin Oncol. 2008;26:4875–82.

79. Cuzick J, Sestak I, Baum M, Buzdar A, Howell A, Dowsett M, ATAC/LATTE investigators, et al. Effect of anastrozole and tamoxifen as adjuvant treatment for early-stage breast cancer: 10-year analysis of the ATAC trial. Lancet Oncol. 2010;11:1135–41.

80. Baum M, Buzdar AU, Cuzick J, Forbes J, Houghton JH, Klijn JG, ATAC Trialists' Group, et al. Anastrozole alone or in combination with tamoxifen versus tamoxifen alone for adjuvant treatment of postmenopausal women with early breast cancer:

first results of the ATAC randomised trial. Lancet. 2002;359:2131–9.

81. Howell A, Cuzick J, Baum M, Buzdar A, Dowsett M, Forbes JF, ATAC Trialists' Group, et al. Results of the ATAC (Arimidex, Tamoxifen, Alone or in Combination) trial after completion of 5 years' adjuvant treatment for breast cancer. Lancet. 2005;365:60–2.

82. Duffy S, Jackson TL, Lansdown M, Philips K, Wells M, Pollard S, et al. The ATAC ('Arimidex', Tamoxifen, Alone or in Combination) adjuvant breast cancer trial: first results of the endometrial sub-protocol following 2 years of treatment. Hum Reprod. 2006;21:545–53.

83. Fallowfield L, Cella D, Cuzick J, Francis S, Locker G, Howell A. Quality of life of postmenopausal women in the Arimidex, Tamoxifen, Alone or in Combination (ATAC) Adjuvant Breast Cancer Trial. J Clin Oncol. 2004;22:4261–71.

84. Eastell R, Adams JE, Coleman RE, Howell A, Hannon RA, Cuzick J, et al. Effect of anastrozole on bone mineral density: 5-year results from the anastrozole, tamoxifen, alone or in combination trial 18233230. J Clin Oncol. 2008;26:1051–7.

85. Dowsett M, Cuzick J, Howell A, Jackson I. Pharmacokinetics of anastrozole and tamoxifen alone, and in combination, during adjuvant endocrine therapy for early breast cancer in postmenopausal women: a sub-protocol of the 'Arimidex and tamoxifen alone or in combination' (ATAC) trial. Br J Cancer. 2001;85:317–24.

86. Buzdar AU, Guastalla JP, Nabholtz JM, Cuzick J, ATAC Trialists' Group, et al. Impact of chemotherapy regimens prior to endocrine therapy: results from the ATAC (Anastrozole and Tamoxifen, Alone or in Combination) trial. Cancer. 2006;107:472–80.

87. Colleoni M, Giobbie-Hurder A, Regan MM, Thürlimann B, Mouridsen H, Mauriac L, et al. Analyses adjusting for selective crossover show improved overall survival with adjuvant letrozole compared with tamoxifen in the BIG 1-98 study. J Clin Oncol. 2011;29:1117–24.

88. Mouridsen H, Keshaviah A, Coates AS, Rabaglio M, Castiglione-Gertsch M, Sun Z, et al. Cardiovascular adverse events during adjuvant endocrine therapy for early breast cancer using letrozole or tamoxifen: safety analysis of BIG 1-98 trial. J Clin Oncol. 2007;25:5715–22.

89. Rabaglio M, Sun Z, Price KN, Castiglione-Gertsch M, Hawle H, Thürlimann B, BIG 1-98 Collaborative and International Breast Cancer Study Groups, et al. Bone fractures among postmenopausal patients with endocrine-responsive early breast cancer treated with 5 years of letrozole or tamoxifen in the BIG 1-98 trial. Ann Oncol. 2009;20:1489–98.

90. Viale G, Regan MM, Dell'Orto P, Mastropasqua MG, Maiorano E, Rasmussen BB, BIG 1-98 Collaborative and International Breast Cancer Study Groups, et al. Which patients benefit most from adjuvant aromatase inhibitors? Results using a composite measure of prognostic risk in the BIG 1-98 randomized trial. Ann Oncol. 2011;22:2201–7.

91. Aydiner A, Tas F. Meta-analysis of trials comparing anastrozole and tamoxifen for adjuvant treatment of postmenopausal women with early breast cancer. Trials. 2008;9:47.

92. Coombes RC, Hall E, Gibson LJ, Paridaens R, Jassem J, Delozier T, Intergroup Exemestane Study, et al. A randomized trial of exemestane after two to three years of tamoxifen therapy in postmenopausal women with primary breast cancer. N Engl J Med. 2004;350:1081–92.

93. Boccardo F, Rubagotti A, Puntoni M, Guglielmini P, Amoroso D, Fini A, et al. Switching to anastrozole versus continued tamoxifen treatment of early breast cancer: preliminary results of the Italian Tamoxifen Anastrozole Trial. J Clin Oncol. 2005;23:5138–47.

94. Boccardo F, Rubagotti A, Guglielmini P, Fini A, Paladini G, Mesiti M, et al. Switching to anastrozole versus continued tamoxifen treatment of early breast cancer. Updated results of the Italian tamoxifen anastrozole (ITA) trial. Ann Oncol. 2006;17 Suppl 7:vii10–4.

95. Jonat W, Gnant M, Boccardo F, Kaufmann M, Rubagotti A, Zuna I, et al. Effectiveness of switching from adjuvant tamoxifen to anastrozole in postmenopausal women with hormone-sensitive early-stage breast cancer: a meta-analysis. Lancet Oncol. 2006;7:991–6.

96. Jakesz R, Jonat W, Gnant M, Mittlboeck M, Greil R, Tausch C, ABCSG and the GABG, et al. Switching of postmenopausal women with endocrine-responsive early breast cancer to anastrozole after 2 years' adjuvant tamoxifen: combined results of ABCSG trial 8 and ARNO 95 trial. Lancet. 2005;366:455–62.

97. Jin H, Tu D, Zhao N, Shepherd LE, Goss PE. Longer-term outcomes of letrozole versus placebo after 5 years of tamoxifen in the NCIC CTG MA.17 trial: analyses adjusting for treatment crossover. J Clin Oncol. 2012;30:718–21.

98. Perez EA, Josse RG, Pritchard KI, Ingle JN, Martino S, Findlay BP, et al. Effect of letrozole versus placebo on bone mineral density in women with primary breast cancer completing 5 or more years of adjuvant tamoxifen: a companion study to NCIC CTG MA.17. J Clin Oncol. 2006;24:3629–35.

99. Whelan TJ, Goss PE, Ingle JN, Pater JL, Tu D, Pritchard K, et al. Assessment of quality of life in MA.17: a randomized, placebo-controlled trial of letrozole after 5 years of tamoxifen in postmenopausal women. J Clin Oncol. 2005;23:6931–40.

100. Dowsett M, Nielsen TO, A'Hern R, Bartlett J, Coombes RC, Cuzick J, International Ki-67 in Breast Cancer Working Group, et al. Assessment of Ki67 in breast cancer: recommendations from the International Ki67 in Breast Cancer working group. J Natl Cancer Inst. 2011;103:1656–64.

101. Dowsett M, Smith IE, Ebbs SR, Dixon JM, Skene A, A'Hern R, IMPACT Trialists Group, et al. Prognostic value of Ki67 expression after short-term presurgical

endocrine therapy for primary breast cancer. J Natl Cancer Inst. 2007;99:167–70.

102. Tung N. What is the optimal endocrine therapy for postmenopausal women with hormone receptor-positive early breast cancer? J Clin Oncol. 2013;31:1391–7.

103. Geisler J, Haynes B, Anker G, Dowsett M, Lønning PE. Influence of letrozole and anastrozole on total body aromatization and plasma estrogen levels in postmenopausal breast cancer patients evaluated in a randomized, cross-over study. J Clin Oncol. 2002;20:751–7.

104. Dixon JM, Renshaw L, Young O, Murray J, Macaskill EJ, McHugh M, et al. Letrozole suppresses plasma estradiol and estrone sulphate more completely than anastrozole in postmenopausal women with breast cancer. J Clin Oncol. 2008;26:1671–6.

105. Ellis MJ, Suman VJ, Hoog J, Lin L, Snider J, Prat A, et al. Randomized phase II neoadjuvant comparison between letrozole, anastrozole, and exemestane for postmenopausal women with estrogen receptor-rich stage 2 to 3 breast cancer: clinical and biomarker outcomes and predictive value of the baseline PAM50-based intrinsic subtype – ACOSOG Z1031. J Clin Oncol. 2011;29:2342–9.

106. Goss PE, Ingle JN, Pritchard KI, Ellis MJ, Sledge GW, Budd GT, et al. Exemestane versus anastrozole in postmenopausal women with early breast cancer: NCIC CTG MA.27 – a randomized controlled phase III trial. J Clin Oncol. 2013;31:1398–404.

107. Amir E, Seruga B, Niraula S, Carlsson L, Ocaña A. Toxicity of adjuvant endocrine therapy in postmenopausal breast cancer patients: a systematic review and meta-analysis. J Natl Cancer Inst. 2011;103:1299–309.

108. Henry NL, Azzouz F, Desta Z, Li L, Nguyen AT, Lemler S, et al. Predictors of aromatase inhibitor discontinuation as a result of treatment-emergent symptoms in early-stage breast cancer. J Clin Oncol. 2012;30:936–42.

109. Aydiner A. Meta-analysis of breast cancer outcome and toxicity in adjuvant trials of aromatase inhibitors in postmenopausal women. Breast. 2013;22:121–9.

Adjuvant Systemic Chemotherapy for HER2-Negative Disease

8

Leyla Kilic and Adnan Aydiner

Abstract

Breast cancer is a heterogeneous, phenotypically diverse disease comprising several biological subtypes with distinct behaviors and responses to therapy. All patients with invasive breast cancer should be evaluated to assess the need for adjuvant cytotoxic therapy, trastuzumab, and/or endocrine therapy. If patients must receive endocrine therapy (either tamoxifen or aromatase inhibitor) and cytotoxic therapy as adjuvant therapy, chemotherapy should precede endocrine therapy. The pathology report must provide uniform information about the tumor and should include at a minimum the parameters recommended in the ASCO-CAP guideline. Molecular subtypes of breast cancer can be distinguished by common pathological variables, including estrogen receptor (ER), progesterone receptor (PR), human epidermal growth factor receptor (HER2), and Ki67 index. The inclusion of chemotherapy in the adjuvant regimen depends on the intrinsic subtype. Multigene expression array profiling is not always required for subtype definition after clinicopathological assessment. Young age, grade 3 disease, lymphovascular invasion, one to three positive nodes, and large tumor size are not adequate features to omit molecular diagnostics in the decision of adjuvant chemotherapy. Any lymph node positivity should not be a sole indication for adjuvant chemotherapy. However, patients with more than three involved lymph nodes, low hormone receptor positivity, positive HER2 status, triple-negative status, high 21-gene RS (e.g., >25), and high-risk 70-gene scores should receive adjuvant chemotherapy.

L. Kilic, MD
Department of Medical Oncology,
Firat University Hospital, Elazig 23119, Turkey
e-mail: leylahmet@gmail.com

A. Aydiner, MD (✉)
Department of Medical Oncology,
Istanbul University Istanbul Medical Faculty,
Institute of Oncology, Capa, Istanbul 34390, Turkey
e-mail: adnanaydiner@superonline.com

© Springer International Publishing Switzerland 2016
A. Aydiner et al. (eds.), *Breast Disease: Management and Therapies*,
DOI 10.1007/978-3-319-26012-9_8

A high Ki67 proliferation index and histological grade 3 tumors are acceptable indications for adjuvant chemotherapy. For women desiring fertility preservation and for patients with certain comorbidities such as cardiovascular disease and diabetic neuropathy, specific chemotherapy regimens may be preferred.

Keywords

Adjuvant • Luminal A • Luminal B • Triple negative • Multigene • Basal-like • Ki67 • Grade • Chemotherapy • Oncotype DX • Immunohistochemistry • MammaPrint • PAM50 • Genomic grade index • Theros • EndoPredict • Elderly • Obese • Pregnancy

Introduction

Breast cancer is the most common type of cancer and the most common cause of cancer-related mortality among women worldwide [1]. Mammography screening and earlier diagnosis are responsible for at least half of the reduction in breast cancer-related mortality between 1990 and 2003. However, adjuvant systemic therapy accounts, at least in part, for the reduction in cause-specific mortality from breast cancer observed in almost every Western nation [2].

Breast cancer is a heterogeneous, phenotypically diverse disease composed of several biological subtypes that have distinct behaviors and responses to therapy. Chemotherapy probably offers potentially minimal benefits for the 5-year survival rate in women with small endocrine-responsive tumors, although there is considerable data suggesting improvements in both recurrence-free and overall survival for ER-positive or ER-negative tumors ≤1 cm in size [3]. Modest benefits are achieved when each patient is evaluated and grouped according to similar profiles utilizing standard pathological parameters (e.g., nodal status, tumor size, receptor status) and treated with similar available chemotherapeutic agents. However, these benefits are of great value when applied to large populations with breast cancer. Long-term follow-up from an Oxford overview demonstrated an absolute benefit from chemotherapy, irrespective of age and ER receptor status [4].

One of the current challenges in adjuvant chemotherapy is the selection of the subset of patients who might preferentially benefit from chemotherapy or be spared from adjuvant chemotherapy. Moreover, the chemotherapy dose and schedule must be optimized to achieve the best clinical results and minimize the side effects of treatment. This chapter will focus on these major subjects and the evolution of chemotherapeutic agents.

Indications for Chemotherapy

Estimating Risks and Benefits

The administration of adjuvant chemotherapy for human epidermal growth factor receptor (HER2)-negative breast cancer requires a consideration of major prognostic factors such as patient age, receptor status (expression of estrogen (ER) and/or progesterone (PR) receptors), tumor size, histology, and nodal involvement.

Algorithms have been published to estimate rates of recurrence, and a validated computer-based model (Adjuvant! Online (AOL); www.adjuvantonline.com) that incorporates all of the above prognostic factors except HER2 tumor status is available to estimate 10-year disease-free (DFS) and overall survival (OS) [5, 6]. These tools assist clinicians in predicting outcomes for local treatment only and the absolute benefits expected from systemic adjuvant endocrine therapy and chemotherapy.

Tumor Size

For patients with node-negative breast cancer, tumor size is a known independent prognostic factor [7, 8]. According to statistics from the American Cancer Society, the 5-year relative survival based on tumor size alone is 95, 82, and 63 % for tumors ≤2 cm, 2.1–5 cm, and >5 cm, respectively [7]. Additional evidence of tumor size as a risk factor for recurrence and death from breast cancer was provided by a European Organization for Research and Treatment of Cancer (EORTC) study involving over 1000 patients younger than 40 years. Pathological tumor size (>2 cm) was associated with both distant disease-free survival (DDFS; hazard ratio [HR] for recurrence 1.61, 95 % CI 1.14–2.25) and OS (HR for mortality 1.68, 95 % CI 1.12–2.52) [8]. For young, node-negative patients, tumor size was still a significant prognostic factor for both DFS and OS; however, in a multivariate analysis, molecular subtype was the only factor associated with overall survival ($p = 0.02$; basal subtype vs. luminal A subtype: HR 0.22, 95 % CI 0.08–0.60, $p = 0.003$) and distant metastasis-free survival (DMFS; $p = 0.08$; basal subtype vs. luminal A subtype: HR 0.46, 95 % CI 0.25–0.85, $p = 0.013$). According to this study, the established prognostic factors molecular subtype (including hormonal receptor status, histological grade, and HER2 receptor status), tumor size, and nodal status remain independent prognostic factors for disease outcome in young breast cancer patients.

Long-term outcomes and, the role of adjuvant therapy in patients with small (<1 cm), node-negative breast cancer remain unclear. Compared with patients with ER-positive tumors, patients with triple-negative tumors have a worse prognosis even when diagnosed at a very small tumor size. This was demonstrated in a study involving 421 breast cancer cases with tumor sizes ≤1 cm, of which 29 (7 %) were triple negative [9]. The recurrence rate was 11, 1, and 7 % among triple-negative, ER-positive, and HER2-positive patients, respectively. Patients with small, node-negative breast tumors usually have a good prognosis, but HER2-positive and triple-negative tumors appear to have a higher recurrence rate, warranting consideration of the broad use and optimization of systemic adjuvant treatments.

Nodal Status

The risk of breast cancer recurrence is substantially increased in patients with pathologically involved lymph nodes (defined as one or more nodes with greater than a 2-mm focus of cancer). Notably, although the staging system for breast cancer includes the presence of isolated tumor cells (a small cluster of cells within the node no greater than 0.2 mm) as node-positive disease, this condition is not clinically significant. However, micrometastases (tumor clusters >0.2 mm but no greater than 2.0 mm) may have a modest negative impact on breast cancer outcomes and are treated as pathologically node-positive breast cancer.

Compared with patients with localized disease (i.e., cancer confined to the breast only), those with regional disease (i.e., spread to the lymph nodes) have a lower rate of survival at 5 years (84 % vs. 99 %, respectively) [10].

Prognostic and Predictive Assays

Several molecular and immunohistochemical studies of early-stage breast cancer patients have yielded promising results regarding prognostic and predictive value. These assays have led to the determination of different subtypes within breast cancer and subtype-specific treatment planning. Intrinsic breast cancer subtypes and the clinical application of available prognostic and/or predictive assays are explained below.

Intrinsic Subtyping

The indication for chemotherapy has traditionally been based upon prognostic factors such as the stage, clinical, and histopathological tumor characteristics described above or algorithms defined by different consensus statements. However, risk stratification based on only clinicopathological parameters may be misleading and may cause over- or undertreatment. Most of the international guidelines (ESMO, ASCO,

St. Gallen) recommend the additional use of validated protein or gene expression tests that reflect intrinsic tumor characteristics. Progress in gene profiling techniques and hierarchical clustering has confirmed biological heterogeneity at a molecular level. In contrast to classification by immunohistochemistry techniques (IHC), at least six major breast cancer subtypes have been defined: luminal A, luminal B, HER2 enriched, basal-like, normal breast-like, and claudin low or mesenchymal-like [11, 12].

Representing approximately 60 % of all breast cancer subtypes, the two molecular luminal subtypes almost entirely comprise tumors expressing a variable degree of ER and/or PR. Luminal A tumors are characterized by the expression of estrogen-regulated genes such as solute-carrier family 39 (zinc transporter); the transcription factors GATA3, FOXA1, and XBP1; and luminal cytokeratins such as CK8 and CK18 [13, 14]. They exhibit relatively low mutation rates and are associated with better outcomes. However, luminal B tumors are characterized by a higher genomic grade, lower ER levels, varying degrees of HER2 gene cluster expression, and poorer outcomes [15, 16]. The luminal B subtype exhibits higher genomic instability and harbors mutations in *TP53* and PIK3CA (phosphatidylinositol-4,5-bisphosphate 3-kinase, catalytic subunit α) [17, 18].

Approximately 20–30 % of all malignant breast tumors are of the HER2-enriched subtype. They are associated with high expression of HER2/*neu* proliferation genes and low expression of luminal clusters. These tumors are usually but not always HER2 positive and ER/PR negative and typically exhibit high expression of genes associated with cell cycle progression [14].

The term "basal-like" breast cancer refers to the common gene expression patterns of normal basal/myoepithelial cells. Basal-like tumors are characterized by high expression of basal CK5 and CK17 and other genes typically expressed in basal/myoepithelial cells such as laminin γ1 (LAMC1) and cadherin 3 (CDH3) [13, 19]. These tumors do not express ER or other luminal epithelial genes and are negative for ERBB2. They often overexpress epidermal growth factor receptor (EGFR). This subtype constitutes approximately 15 % of all invasive breast cancers.

The normal breast-like subtype was named based on similarities in gene expression patterns with normal epithelial cells, adipose tissue, and other non-epithelial cell types [19]. These tumors do not express proliferation-associated genes and are supposed to have a low tumor cell percentage [14]. They share gene expression features with both the basal-like and luminal subtypes.

Claudin-low tumors are characterized by low expression of genes involved in cell–cell adhesion such as claudins 3, 4, and 7 (CLDN3, CLDN4, CLDN7) and E-cadherin (CDH1) [20]. These tumors represent a rare type of triple-negative breast cancer with mesenchymal features and high expression of immune system response genes. In contrast to basal-like tumors, they do not exhibit high expression of proliferation-associated genes [11].

Each intrinsic tumor subtype is associated with specific histological, clinical, epidemiological, and therapeutic characteristics [21]. The prognoses of the different intrinsic tumor types differ with respect to both short-term and long-term survival, and adjuvant therapy may affect prognosis in a subtype-specific manner [22]. Thus, future adjuvant treatment modalities should be designed with awareness of these intrinsic subtypes. Because of the limitations of hierarchical clustering for the classification of individual samples, investigators have developed single sample predictors (SSPs), which enable the subtyping of a single tumor based on microarray gene expression profiling (GEP) [16]. The SSPs have been further refined, and a classifier named prediction analysis of microarray (PAM) was developed using 50 genes to identify the four major intrinsic subtypes, namely, luminal A, luminal B, HER2 enriched, and basal-like [23]. This classifier was subsequently converted to a quantitative real-time PCR (qRT-PCR) assay that can be performed using RNA extracted from formalin-fixed, paraffin-embedded (FFPE) samples, thereby making it applicable to archival material. PAM50 is a standardized gene set based on the NanoString nCounter technology [24]. It was validated for intrinsic subtyping in a clinical trial involving 348 premenopausal women treated with tamoxifen [25]. The test also provides a prognostic score (referred to as the risk of recurrence score (ROR-S) for predicting recurrence of cancer over 10 years; this will be discussed in more detail below. PAM50 is considered a robust assay with high concordance between laboratories and was superior to IHC with respect to prognosis and the prediction of endocrine response in the previous study. However, this observation was not confirmed in an independent series of breast carcinomas. Given the similarities of the subtypes defined by gene expression profiling and IHC, surrogate IHC definitions were to be generated. However, the concordance between the two tests was not as expected; 31–59 % of cases with HER2 positivity as defined by IHC and/or in situ hybridization (ISH) are classified as an "intrinsic" subtype other than HER2 enriched [26, 27]. Conversely, up to 30 % of the HER2-enriched tumors are clinically HER2 negative [17]. The majority of basal-like breast cancers are of the triple-negative phenotype; however, 1–3 % of ER-positive tumors display a basal-like phenotype [13, 16].

The other commercial kit available for determining intrinsic breast cancer subtypes is MammaTyper®. It is based on the quantitative measurement of ER, PR, HER2, and Ki67 at the mRNA level instead of IHC. This test was developed based on the inadequacy of IHC for the discrimination of luminal A and luminal B tumors on the basis of Ki67 and tumor grade. MammaTyper® uses a cutoff definition of 75 % for HER2 and exhibited high concordance with central IHC assessment in a clinical trial [28]. The HER2 status defined at this cutoff level better predicts OS and DFS compared with the HER2 status determined with IHC. This test also provides continuous values of other parameters such as Ki67 in addition to subtype information. However, the MammaTyper results have not been systematically compared with PAM50 or IHC.

Clinical Application of Protein Markers and Genomic Assays

Recent studies among breast cancer patients have yielded increasing numbers of prognostic and predictive assays that can be routinely used for optimizing diagnosis and orientating treatment choices. Some of these are summarized below.

Urokinase Plasminogen Activator (uPA) and Plasminogen Activator Inhibitor (PAI-1)

Various proteolytic enzymes play a crucial role in tumor invasion and metastasis. The urokinase plasminogen activator (uPA) system involves multiple members that participate in fibrinolysis, cell migration, angiogenesis, tumor cell dissemination, and metastasis in a variety of solid tumors [29]. This system includes urokinase-type plasminogen activator (uPA), the glycolipid-anchored cell membrane receptor for uPA (uPAR), and plasminogen activator inhibitors (PAIs). uPA and uPAR are overexpressed in diverse human malignant tumors compared to normal tissue. The uPA system transforms inactive plasminogen to active plasmin, leading to the degradation and regeneration of the basement membrane and extracellular matrix (ECM) and thereby facilitating metastasis. The uPA system not only acts through ECM degradation but also promotes tumor metastasis by initiating the activation of matrix metalloproteinases (MMPs) [30]. Moreover, the binding of uPA to uPAR can activate the Ras–Raf–MEK–ERK pathway, resulting in the activation of several cell signaling events [31].

Studies of breast cancer patients have revealed that increased levels of uPA and/or PAI-1 in primary tumor tissues correlate with tumor aggressiveness and poor clinical outcomes. Patients with a high tumor tissue antigen content of uPA and/or PAI-1 have a worse probability of DFS and OS than patients with low levels of both biomarkers (uPA ≤3 ng/mg protein, PAI-1 ≤14 ng/mg protein) serving as prognostic markers [32]. Moreover, uPA appears to be an important independent variable that is stronger than most traditional prognostic factors, particularly in the node-negative subtype [33]. uPA and PAI-1 can classify approximately half of node-negative breast cancer patients as low risk; low levels indicate a very good prognosis, whereas high levels correlate with shortened DFS and reduced OS [34, 35]. For node-positive patients, the PAI-1 protein has a stronger prognostic impact than uPA [36].

In addition to being clinically useful prognostic factors that allow estimates of the course of disease in early-stage breast cancer, uPA and PAI-1 may also serve as factors that predict the response to systemic therapy. The prospective multicenter Chemo N0 trial included 556 node-negative early-stage breast cancer patients. High-risk patients identified by uPA and PAI-1 tumor tissue levels were randomized to chemotherapy or observation [37]. Initial interim analysis results suggested that high-risk patients in the chemotherapy group benefited, with a 43.8 % lower estimated probability of disease recurrence at 3 years than high-risk patients in the observation group (relative risk = 0.56; 95 % CI 0.25–1.28). Ten-year follow-up results confirmed the prognostic and predictive role of these protein markers. The actuarial 10-year recurrence rate (without any adjuvant systemic therapy) for high-uPA/PAI-1 observation group patients was 23.0 %, in contrast to the rate of 12.9 % for low-uPA/PAI-1 patients. High-risk patients randomized to receive cyclophosphamide–methotrexate–5-fluorouracil (CMF) therapy had a 26.0 % lower estimated probability of disease recurrence than those randomized for observation (HR: 0.74, 95 % CI 0.44–1.27). Similarly, the ongoing NNBC-3 trial aims to compare risk assessment by traditional clinicopathological factors and by uPA/PAI-1. It is also designed to evaluate the predictive value of these markers for benefit from sequential anthracycline–docetaxel regimen or anthracycline-based chemotherapy in high-risk node-negative breast cancer patients [38].

Data from the Chemo N0 trial has indicated that nearly half of node-negative breast cancer patients (with low concentrations of both proteins) could be spared from the side effects and costs of chemotherapy. Thus, the German Working Group for Gynecological Oncology (AGO) and ASCO [39] have recommended both biomarkers as risk–group–classification markers for routine clinical decision making in node-negative breast cancer, secondary to established clinical and histomorphological factors [www.ago-online.de]. However, probably due to the need for fresh-frozen tissue for analysis, these markers are not extensively used outside Germany.

Immunohistochemistry (IHC) Studies

Immunohistochemistry4 (IHC4)

As a surrogate for assessing RNA-based gene signatures, IHC techniques have been utilized to enable more economical and simplified assays. IHC4 is based on four routine IHC markers: ER, PR, HER2 (with fluorescent or calorimetric in situ hybridization), and Ki67. The retrospective TransATAC study, which included ER-positive chemo-naive breast cancer patients of the Arimidex, Tamoxifen, Alone or in Combination trial (ATAC), assessed the prognostic impact of IHC4 score. This 4-parameter IHC score was initially compared with the 21-gene General Health Recurrence Score (Oncotype DX®) using distant metastasis as the primary endpoint [40]. The results showed that the IHC score not only provided prognostic information independent of classic clinicopathological variables but also was similar in strength to Oncotype DX. The prognostic value of the IHC4 score was also validated in a second separate cohort of patients, and the results indicated that the amount of prognostic information provided by the four widely performed IHC assays is similar to that provided by Oncotype DX. By combining the IHC4 score with clinicopathological factors (tumor grade, size, nodal burden, patient age, and aromatase inhibitor treatment), another prognostic tool has been created, known as IHC4+C. This tool was utilized for the reclassification of 101 postmenopausal, hormone receptor-positive, early-stage breast cancer patients defined as intermediate risk by AOL and the Nottingham Prognostic Index (NPI) [41]. The NPI is based on operative pathological findings such as tumor size and nodal status and is calculated postoperatively for each patient. Fifteen of the 26 patients classified as intermediate risk by AoL were reallocated to a low-risk group by application of the IHC4+C score, and no patient was reclassified as high risk. Of the 59 patients classified as intermediate risk by the NPI, 24 were reallocated to a low-risk group and 13 to a high-risk group. The results suggested an improvement in decision making regarding adjuvant chemotherapy. However, there are quality assurance issues with the qualitative assessment of ER, PR, HER2, and Ki67 IHC due to the potential for interlaboratory variation in values. Although considerably less expensive than gene expression profiling tools, Ki67 in particular has caused apprehension due to variable assessment methods and heterogeneity in interlaboratory results. Recently, the impact of follow-up duration on the prognostic value of IHC4 and another IHC test, Mammostrat, revealed that their efficacy is restricted to the first 5 years after diagnosis [42]. However, this finding needs to be validated in further studies before being accepted as clear evidence.

Mammostrat®

A number of different statistical approaches have been used to identify minimal gene sets for prognostication or to predict response to therapy for early-stage breast cancer patients. The clinical development of gene expression-based assays has made impressive initial progress but suffers from the inherent limitation that application as a clinical tool will require specialized laboratories for quality assurance. Ring et al. [43] explored the possibility of developing IHC tests utilizing data from several gene studies. The authors investigated gene expression patterns in three patient cohorts and, using a stepwise process, identified a minimal set of five antisera reflecting the expression of five genes: p53, which is involved in cell cycle checkpoint control; SLC7A5, which is involved in nutrient transport; HTF9C, the expression of which oscillates during the cell cycle; NDRG1, a stress- and hypoxia-inducible gene; and CEACAM5, a carcinoembryonic differentiation antigen. These prognosticators were first used to predict outcomes in ER-positive breast cancer patients; however, the first study was underpowered in the node-negative (N0) subsets. Therefore, a second study was performed to further validate this five-antibody IHC test [44]. In the NSABP B-14 trial, a total of 837 patients were evaluated. This study was initiated to determine the benefit of adjuvant tamoxifen. The other patient cohort included 457 patients from the NSABP B-20 trial, which investigated the benefit of adjuvant chemotherapy added to tamoxifen. The test stratified patients into three groups: low, moderate, and high risk. Younger patients in the low-risk group identified by the test had a 20 % risk of disease progression that warranted the consideration of aggressive treatment strategies. By contrast, in elderly patients (≥60 years) in whom cytotoxic chemotherapy is currently used much more cautiously, the test identified high-risk patients with a 22 % risk of breast cancer-specific death compared with 6 % in low-risk patients. In addition, the high-risk patients in the B20 study had a 21 % decreased recurrence rate associated with the administration of adjuvant chemotherapy. However, stratification into age groups was not a prespecified analysis in the trial design and therefore must be cautiously interpreted.

Oncotype DX

One of the most widely used gene-based approaches is the 21-gene assay using reverse transcription polymerase chain reaction (RT-PCR) on RNA isolated from paraffin-embedded breast cancer tissues (Oncotype DX). The test was first developed to predict the likelihood of disease recurrence among hormonal receptor-positive, lymph node-negative, stage I or II breast cancer patients who had received tamoxifen for 5 years [45]. Through retrospective analysis of three independent clinical studies involving a total of 447 patients, including the tamoxifen-only group of the NSABP B-20 trial, the relationship between the expression of the 250 candidate genes and the recurrence of breast cancer was initially assessed [46, 47]. Oncotype DX is routinely performed on formalin-fixed, paraffin-embedded (FFPE) tissues. To select a panel of 16 cancer-related genes and 5 reference genes (Table 8.1), the results of the three studies were utilized to design an algorithm and to compute a recurrence score (RS) as a continuous variable between 0 and 100 for each tumor sample. Then, patients were classified into three categories based on their RS: low risk (RS <18), intermediate risk (RS 18–30), or high risk (RS >31). Low-risk groups had an estimated risk of

Table 8.1 Genes assessed in the Oncotype DX assay

Cancer-related genes	Reference genes
Estrogen genes	ACTB (β-actin)
ER, PR, BCL 2, SCUBE2	GAPDH
Invasion genes	RPLPO
MMP11 (stromelysin 3), CTSL2 (cathepsin L2)	GUS
Proliferation genes	TFRC
Ki67, STK15, survivin, CCNB1 (cyclin B1), MYBL2	

recurrence of less than 10 % at 10 years according to the NSABP-B20 results. The 16 cancer-related genes involved components of ER pathways (ER, PR, BCL2, SCUBE2), the HER2 amplicon (HER2, GRB7), proliferation-related genes (Ki67, STK15, survivin, CCNB1, MYBL2), invasion-related genes (MMP11, CTSL2), and GSTM1, BAG1, and CD68 [45]. Higher expression of the estrogen-related genes GSTM1 and BAG1 was associated with improved survival; by contrast, high invasion- or proliferation-related gene expression and HER2 expression were associated with a higher risk of recurrence and poor relapse-free survival.

Oncotype DX has been validated in large retrospective sets of trials. In the first study, tumor blocks were retrieved from the NSABP-B14 study, which was designed to evaluate the benefit of adjuvant tamoxifen among node-negative, ER-positive breast cancer patients. Clinically, a low-risk score (RS <18) was translated as a 10 % risk of distant metastasis at 10 years, and a high score (RS ≥31) was translated as a 20 % risk. The study identified 51 % of the patients as low risk, with 93.2 % 10-year distant relapse-free survival (DRFS), whereas 27 % of the patients were identified as high risk, with 69.5 % 10-year DRFS [45]. Subsequently, Oncotype DX was retrospectively evaluated in another trial, the NSABP-B20, which was designed to investigate the benefit of adding adjuvant chemotherapy to tamoxifen for node-negative, ER-positive (potentially including HER2-positive) invasive breast cancer patients. In this trial, patients received either non-anthracycline-based chemotherapy, cyclophosphamide, methotrexate, and 5-fluorouracil (CMF) or methotrexate and 5-fluorouracil (MF) plus concurrent tamoxifen or tamoxifen alone. Of 2299 patients, 670 patients' FFPE tumor tissues were available for analysis. The NSABP-B20 trial validated Oncotype DX as a prognostic and predictive test. On the basis of the data, 54 % of the patients had RS <18, whereas 25 % were classified in the high-risk group. The administration of adjuvant CT was associated with 27.6 % reduction in the risk of distant metastasis at 10 years in high-risk patients. However, the benefit of adjuvant CT in the low-risk group was quite low (3.78 % risk reduction) [48]. Those in the intermediate-risk group did not seem to experience a significant benefit from adjuvant CT, but a clinically significant benefit could not be excluded due to uncertainty in the estimate.

The prognostic and predictive value of the 21-gene RS was also evaluated among node-positive patients in the TransATAC (Arimidex, Tamoxifen, Alone or in Combination) study [49]. RNA was extracted from 1372 tumor blocks from postmenopausal patients with hormonal receptor-positive primary breast cancer in the monotherapy arms of ATAC. RSs were available for 1231 patients, of whom 306 had nodal involvement. Nine-year distant recurrence rates in the low (RS<18), intermediate (RS: 18–30), and high RS (RS ≥31) groups were 4 %, 12 %, and 25 %, respectively, in N0 patients and 17 %, 28 %, and 49 %, respectively, in N+ patients. However, the study failed to demonstrate a predictive effect for differential benefit between tamoxifen and anastrozole.

In clinical practice, physicians usually subjectively combine RS with pathological and clinical measures based on their individual experience. The evidence that RS and traditional measures provide independent prognostic information has encouraged investigators to develop a formal integration of RS and traditional pathological and clinical measures. The RS–pathology–clinical (RSPC) model by Tang et al. [50] included RS, age, tumor size, and grade. Patients in the NSABP B-14 and translational research cohort of the TransATAC studies ($n=647$ and $n=1088$, respectively) with assessable clinicopathological factors and ER-positive tumors who received hormonal monotherapy were included. RSPC had significantly more prognostic value for distant recurrence than did RS ($p=0.001$), with a better discrimination of risk in the study population. Moreover, RSPC classified fewer patients as intermediate risk (17.8 % vs. 26.7 %, $p=0.001$) and more patients as lower risk (63.8 % vs. 54.2 %, $p=0.001$) than RS. The study indicated that RSPC can provide greater accuracy in the assessment of distant recurrence risk, particularly when RS and clinicopathological measures are discordant.

The 21-gene RS assay was also assessed for the prediction of chemotherapy benefit among node-positive, postmenopausal HR + breast cancer patients within the study population of SWOG 8814 [51]. Because of the inferior efficacy of concurrent tamoxifen and CAF (cyclophosphamide, doxorubicin, 5-fluorouracil) in the parent trial, that arm was excluded. Thus, this analysis compared the sequential CAF-T group to the tamoxifen control group. RS was determined to be a strong predictive factor of CAF benefit for DFS, but the degree of CAF benefit depended on the RS. There was no apparent benefit for scores <18 ($p=0.97$; HR=1.02, 95 % CI 0.54–1.93) or 18–30 ($p=0.48$; HR=0.72, 95 % CI 0.39–1.31). However, there was a significant advantage for CAF-T compared with tamoxifen alone for patients with RS ≥31 ($p=0.033$; HR=0.59, 95 % CI 0.35–1.01).

The response to neoadjuvant chemotherapy has been determined to be a valid surrogate marker of survival, with significantly better survival in those patients whose tumors completely regress compared with all other responses. Several gene expression studies of human breast cancer have suggested that gene analyses can discriminate patients who are more likely to benefit from certain therapies such as anthracyclines or taxanes [52, 53]. The first study evaluating RS for predicting the response to neoadjuvant CT was performed by Gianni et al. [54]. They identified a set of genes for which the expression correlated with pathological complete response (pCR) to neoadjuvant doxorubicin and paclitaxel. Of 384 candidate genes tested by RT-PCR analysis, the expression of 86 genes significantly correlated with pCR ($p=0.05$). The RS strongly correlated with pCR, supporting the previous findings that patients with high RS values, who were thus most likely to experience recurrence, were most likely to receive the greatest clinical benefit from chemotherapy treatment. Similarly, Chang et al. [55] tested the utility of the 21-gene recurrence assay in the neoadjuvant setting to demonstrate that sufficient RNA could be obtained from core biopsies to directly examine the association of RS to neoadjuvant docetaxel and complete response (CR). CR was associated with lower expression of the ER gene group and higher expression of the proliferation gene group from the 21-gene assay. Moreover, CR was more likely with a high RS ($p=0.008$).

Although Oncotype DX is a useful and practical tool for prognostic and predictive purposes, like all biomarkers, it has limitations. In particular, the data from RT-PCR and IHC studies for HER2 status conflict. The US Food and Drug Administration (FDA) has approved two immunohistochemical assays and three fluorescent in situ hybridization (FISH) assays for HER2 assessment in the clinical laboratory. Although test platform preference among pathologists and oncologists remains controversial, both IHC and FISH remain independently validated tests in the clinical laboratory based on outcome data and response to trastuzumab. HER2 gene amplification is closely associated with mRNA overexpression and increased protein levels, and several studies have compared mRNA expression by reverse transcription PCR. The Oncotype DX test depends on mRNA extracted from FFPE tumors. A major study comparing the HER2 FISH assay and qRT-PCR technique indicated an overall 97 % concordance rate [56]. However, the results of another analysis that included 843 patients from three high-volume centers contradicted this finding. Of the 784 (93 %) patients classified as negative by IHC or FISH, 779 (99 %) were also classified as negative by the Oncotype DX RT-PCR assay. However, all 23 equivocal patient cases were reported as negative by Oncotype DX. Of the 36 positive cases, only 10 (28 %) were reported as positive, 12 (33 %) as equivocal, and 14 (39 %) as negative [57]. The results corresponded to >50 % false HER2 negativity by Oncotype DX RT-PCR technique. Similarly, another retrospective review evaluating concordance rates between hormonal receptor, HER2 FISH, and Oncotype DX RT-PCR assays revealed a positive percent agreement for HER2 of 0 % (0/2) and a negative percent agreement of 100 % (245/245). Of the three FISH HER2-amplified cases, two were negative, and one was equivocal, and all FISH HER2 equivocal cases ($n=3$) were negative by Oncotype DX [58]. Although the results demonstrated high concordance between IHC and Oncotype DX for ER and PR, the data indicated poor positive percent agreement for HER2. Patients who were FISH HER2 amplified and Oncotype DX HER2 negative did not receive trastuzumab, and information on the outcome of such patients in the general breast cancer population is lacking. Taken together, these data do not support the use of Oncotype DX as an assay for further clarification, particularly in cases of equivocal IHC and/or FISH results or discordance between FISH and IHC.

The underlying reason for these inconsistencies is unclear. A possible explanation for the discrepancy between IHC/FISH and Oncotype DX is that Oncotype DX utilizes RT-PCR, a molecular technique that disregards tissue morphology. Consequently, tumor mRNA may be contaminated with nonneoplastic tissue or biopsy cavity material [56, 59, 60]. Prior studies have documented that cellular stroma, inflammatory cells, or the presence of a biopsy cavity can influence Oncotype DX results [59, 60]. In addition, the extent of fragmentation of extracted FFPE tissue RNA significantly increases with archive storage time. However, probe and primer sets for RT-PCR assays based on amplicons that are both short and homogeneous in length enable effective reference gene-based data normalization for the cross comparison of specimens that substantially differ in age. Using RNA extracted from FFPE sections of archived breast cancer specimens, Cronin et al. [61] demonstrated that the RT-PCR and IHC results for ER, PR, and HER2 receptor status were concordant. Similarly, Cobleigh et al. [62] have demonstrated that RNA extraction from paraffin blocks of archived tissues, some more than 20 years old, may yield accurate information regarding the risk of distant recurrence, even among patients with ten or more metastatic lymph nodes.

Despite these limitations, a meta-analysis of 11 published decision-impact studies ($n=1154$) concluded that the 21-gene RS assay could spare some patients from the high cost of adjuvant chemotherapy. According to the analysis, 404 (49 %) of 820 patients were further assigned to a high-risk group with a further recommendation for chemoendocrine therapy. Moreover, 16 % ($n=99$) of the 632 patients initially recommended for endocrine therapy alone were offered chemoendocrine therapy. In total, the recommendations changed for 35 % of the patients ($n=515$). Oncotype DX has consistently resulted in a significant reduction in the number of patients who are prescribed chemotherapy; in addition, this assay can identify a smaller subset of patients who would benefit from chemotherapy among patients who would otherwise receive endocrine therapy alone. Such changes in treatment decisions are cost-effective for the health system [63]. However, long-term follow-up of these patients is lacking, and the effect of the decision-impact studies on survival has not been prospectively evaluated.

Concordantly, one of the major objectives of the TAILORx trial, which uses the Oncotype DX recurrence score to assign ER(+), HER2(−), node-negative patients to receive chemotherapy plus hormonal therapy vs. hormonal therapy alone, is to reduce chemotherapy overtreatment by integrating molecular diagnostic testing into the clinical decision-making process (Table 8.2) [64]. The TAILORx trial has enrolled more than 11,000 patients. Patients with an RS less than 11 are assigned to hormonal therapy only (arm A), those with an RS greater than 25 receive adjuvant chemotherapy plus hormonal therapy (arm D), and patients with an RS of 11 through 25 are randomized to hormonal therapy only (arm B) vs. chemotherapy plus hormonal therapy (arm C). In this trial, the RS scores used as cutoffs between these groups differ from those reported in the NSABP studies to minimize the potential

Table 8.2 Comparison of prospective trials utilizing multigene tests for prognostic and predictive factors

	TAILORx	MINDACT	RxPONDER
Tests	Oncotype DX	MammaPrint and Adjuvant! Online	Oncotype DX (RS ≤ 25)
Receptor status	ER (+), HER2 (−)	ER (+), HER2 (−)	ER (+), HER2 (−)
Lymph node status	Node negative	Node negative or N1	Node positive
Treatment arms	Arm A (RS < 11): HRT	Arm A (clinical and genomic high risk): CT and HRT	Arm A: CT and HRT
	Arm B (RS:11–25): HRT	Arm B (Low clinical and genomic risk): HRT	Arm B: HRT
	Arm C (RS:11–25): CT and HRT	Arm C (discordant risk factors): CT and HRT vs. HRT	
	Arm D (RS > 25): CT		
Stratification factor	(For arms B and C: tumor size, menopausal status, planned CT, planned RT	(For arm C: clinicopathological vs. genomic risk	RS < 14 vs. 14–25, menopausal status, axillary dissection vs. SN biopsy

CT chemotherapy, *HRT* hormonal therapy, *RT* radiotherapy, *RS* recurrence score, *SN* sentinel node

Table 8.3 Comparison of Oncotype DX, PAM50 and MammaPrint multigene tests

	Oncotype DX	PAM 50	MammaPrint
Number of genes	21	50 (+5 control genes)	70
Sample	Formalin-fixed, paraffin-embedded tissue	Formalin-fixed, paraffin-embedded tissue	Fresh-frozen tissue
Features	RS predicts the likelihood of recurrence at 10 years	Classifies intrinsic subtypes	Stratifies patients by good or poor prognostic signature
	Identifies low-risk patients to be spared from CT	Predicts DFS and the likelihood of recurrence at 10 years for ER (+) tamoxifen-treated patients	
		Identifies patients who benefit from neoadjuvant endocrine therapy or CT	

undertreatment of high-risk patients. The upper limit of the low-risk score was also reduced from 18 to 11 because RS <11 is correlated with a recurrence risk of 5–10 % for endocrine therapy alone, the minimum threshold for clinical justification of cytotoxic chemotherapy.

The 21-gene RS assay system is currently available to quantify the risk of distant recurrence as a continuous variable and to predict responsiveness to both tamoxifen and CMF or MF chemotherapy among ER-positive, stage I or II breast cancer patients of any age (Table 8.3). The test has been included in the ASCO and NCCN guidelines as a predictor of recurrence for ER-positive, lymph node-negative breast cancer patients.

MammaPrint

Several other approaches have been developed to estimate prognosis in breast cancer patients. The MammaPrint assay uses microarray technology to stratify early (T1 and T2) hormonal receptor-negative/receptor-positive breast cancer patients with node-negative (N0) and node-positive (N+) disease into high- and low-risk categories for distant recurrence. The functions of the 70 genes are mainly related to apoptosis, self-sufficiency in growth signals, insensitivity to anti-growth signals, limitless replicative capacity, tissue invasion, metastasis, and angiogenesis. These genes reflect the acquired malignant characteristics of a cancer cell along with tumor progression-related biological activities [65]. Researchers of the

Netherlands Cancer Institute (NKI) initially tested MammaPrint in 79 young (<55 years) N0 breast cancer patients [66] and then validated it in a second set of 295 frozen tissue specimens of both N0 and N+ patients [67]. Both of these studies demonstrated that MammaPrint outperformed standard clinical and histological predictors of patient prognosis. In the N0 group of the second study, 10-year distant metastasis-free survival (DMFS) for the low-risk group was 87 % vs. 44 % in the high-risk group. Multivariate analysis revealed that MammaPrint was the strongest prognostic factor, with an HR of 4.6 (95 % CI 2.3–9.2). However, both studies included very few chemotherapy-treated patients; thus, the results did not indicate the predictive utility of the test.

The next validation study included 302 patients from the TRANSBIG (Translational working group of Breast International Group) Consortium who had received only locoregional treatment with a median follow-up time of 13.6 years [68]. The 10-year DMFS rates were 88 % and 71 % for the low-risk and high-risk group, respectively. Multivariate analysis indicated that MammaPrint provided the most valuable prognostic information for N0 early-stage breast cancer patients compared with other clinicopathological criteria, including age, tumor size and grade, and hormonal receptor status. This study did not present any information about the predictive value of the test because none of the patients received adjuvant chemotherapy or endocrine therapy. Similarly, another trial including patients with pT1-T2N0 disease confirmed the prognostic applicability of MammaPrint [69]. High-risk patients, which constituted 48 % of the group, had a median 5-year OS rate of 82 %, while low-risk scores corresponded to a median OS of 97 %. When compared to the AOL risk scores, the clinical outcomes of discordant cases were most accurately predicted by MammaPrint. Of the high-risk patients classified by AOL, 34 % had a low-risk profile according to MammaPrint and thus could have avoided unnecessary chemotherapy. Conversely, 14 % of the low-risk group by AOL had a high-risk profile and required adjuvant treatment based on the current outcome data.

Another trial investigating the efficacy of MammaPrint as a prognostic tool for node-positive patients included frozen tumor samples from 241 patients with operable T1–T3 breast cancer and one to three positive axillary lymph nodes [70]. The 10-year DMFS and breast cancer-specific survival (BCSS) probabilities were 91 % and 96 %, respectively, for the good prognostic signature group and 76 % and 76 %, respectively, for the poor prognostic signature group. The 70-gene signature was significantly superior to traditional prognostic factors in predicting BCSS, with an HR of 7.17 (95 % CI 1.81–28.43; $p = 0.005$), thus accurately identifying patients with favorable disease outcome, even those with node-positive disease, who may be safely spared with adjuvant chemotherapy.

The predictive role of the assay is mainly based on retrospective evidence. Knauer et al. [71] evaluated 541 patients in a pooled study series who received either endocrine treatment (ET) or chemotherapy plus endocrine treatment (ET+CT). BCSS and DDFS at 5 years were assessed separately for the 70-gene high- and low-risk groups. The 70-gene signature classified 47 % of the patients as low risk and 53 % as high risk. In the low-risk group, BCSS was 97 % for the ET group and 99 % for the ET+CT group at 5 years (HR: 0.58, 95 % CI 0.07–4.98; $p = 0.62$). In the high-risk group, BCSS at 5 years was 81 % and 94 % for the ET and ET + CT groups, respectively (HR: 0.21 95 % CI 0.07–0.59; $p = 0.01$). Multivariate analysis yielded similar results and demonstrated that the low-risk group derived no significant survival benefit from CT added to ET. Notably, very few events were observed in this 70-gene low-risk patient group, irrespective of the type of adjuvant treatment, confirming their overall good outcome. One of the clear limitations of this study, in addition to the limited patient numbers and differences in chemotherapy regimens, is its retrospective design. The first study designed for the prospective evaluation of an adjuvant systemic treatment decision based on the 70-gene signature was the microarRAy-prognoSTics-in-breast-cancER (RASTER) study [72]. RASTER was a prospective, observational, community-based trial in which physicians were encouraged to use chemotherapy based on MammaPrint scores. The 5-year distant recurrence-free-interval (DRFI) probabilities were compared between subgroups based on the 70-gene signature and AOL. Of the 70-gene signature low-risk patients, 15 % received adjuvant chemotherapy (CT) vs. 81 % of the 70-gene signature high-risk patients. The 5-year DRFI probabilities for 70-gene signature low-risk ($n = 219$) and high-risk ($n = 208$) patients were 97.0 % and 91.7 %, respectively. For 70-gene signature low risk, AOL high-risk patients ($n = 124$), of whom 76 % ($n = 94$) had not received CT, the 5-year DRFI was 98.4 %. In the AOL high-risk group, 32 % (94/295) less patients would be eligible to receive adjuvan CT if the 70-gene signature was used. The omission of adjuvant chemotherapy as judged appropriate by doctors and patients and supported by a low-risk 70-gene signature result appeared not to compromise the outcome.

The predictive role of MammaPrint was also tested in the neoadjuvant setting [73]. To assess chemosensitivity, 167 stage II–III breast cancer patients were classified according to prognostic signatures prior to neoadjuvant therapy. Among 167 patients, none of the good prognostic signature patients ($n = 23$) achieved pCR, compared to 20 % of the poor prognostic signature patients ($p = 0.015$). Thus, tumors with a poor prognostic signature were assumed to be more sensitive to chemotherapy.

The survival data from ongoing randomized controlled trials such as the MINDACT trial should provide better insight for the predictive role of the 70-gene signature. The MINDACT trial uses MammaPrint and AOL for treatment arm assignments [74]. MINDACT has very broad eligibility criteria and two secondary randomizations for selecting chemotherapy and hormonal therapy regimens. The trial initially enrolled only node-negative patients but was amended in 2008 to include patients with one to three positive lymph nodes (N1 disease) [75, 76]. The findings from this trial will help determine the prognostic value of MammaPrint and the benefit of treating intermediate-risk patients with adjuvant chemotherapy.

Currently, the 70-gene assay is a prognostic test that provides a dichotomous test result for women <62 years of age who are N0 or N+ (one to three lymph nodes), regardless of their ER status. The results are reported as low risk (13 % chance of developing distant metastasis at 10 years without adjuvant therapy) or high risk (56 % chance of developing distant metastasis at 10 years without adjuvant therapy). Because MammaPrint is performed using a DNA microarray, it requires frozen breast cancer samples, which are difficult to obtain in many cancer centers. Several studies have addressed the limitations in the reproducibility and reliability of microarray measurements; however, strict adherence to standard operating procedures appears to resolve concerns about inter- and intralaboratory variations [77, 78].

PAM50

The PAM50 test is based on a qRT-PCR assay to classify ER-positive and ER-negative breast cancer patients into subtypes that could predict outcomes [79, 80]. It measures the expression of 50 classifier genes and 5 control genes, categorizes tumors into the 4 intrinsic subtypes (luminal A, luminal B, HER2 enriched, and basal-like), and provides a risk of recurrence (ROR) score to estimate the probability of relapse at 5 years [28]. ROR score was utilized to divide node-negative and node-positive tamoxifen-treated patients into low- and intermediate-risk groups and was found to be of greater prognostic value than standard clinicopathological criteria [81]. In the translational research cohort within the ATAC trial (TransATAC), the performance of the ROR score was compared with that of the RS and of IHC4 for distant recurrence in 1007 postmenopausal women. The results demonstrated that the ROR provided more prognostic information for endocrine-treated women with node-negative disease than the RS [82]. Similarly, the Austrian Breast and Colorectal Cancer Study Group 8 (ABCSG 8) trial demonstrated that the ROR score predicted the risk of distant recurrence in 1478 postmenopausal women with ER-positive early-stage breast cancer. To determine to what extent the ROR score could help predict late recurrence, Sestak et al. [83] combined the data from the TransATAC and ABCSG 8 trials and investigated the prognostic value of the ROR score for distant recurrence exclusively in 5–10 years after diagnosis. The authors compared the accuracy of the ROR score with the Clinical Treatment Score (CTS), which contains information on nodal status, tumor size, grade, age, and treatment and was developed using the TransATAC data set. A total of 2137 women who did not have recurrence 5 years after diagnosis were included in the analyses. The Clinical Treatment Score (CTS) was the strongest prognostic factor 5 years after diagnosis. The ROR score itself was significantly prognostic in 5–10 years. In the node-negative, HER2-negative subgroup, more prognostic value for late distant recurrence was provided by the ROR score compared with the CTS.

The predictive value of PAM50 was tested using tissue samples from patients involved in the MA.12 trial, which was designed to evaluate the efficacy of tamoxifen vs. placebo in premenopausal breast cancer patients [25]. Total RNA from 398 of 672 (59 %) patients was available for intrinsic subtyping with PAM50. A tissue microarray was also constructed from 492 of 672 (73 %) patients of the study population to assess a panel of six IHC antibodies to define the same intrinsic subtypes. Classification into intrinsic subtypes by the PAM50 assay was prognostic for both DFS and OS ($p = 0.0003$ and 0.0002, respectively), whereas classification by the IHC panel was not. Moreover, intrinsic subtype classification by the PAM50 assay was superior to IHC profiling for both prognosis and the prediction of benefit from adjuvant tamoxifen for both node-negative and node-positive diseases. Cheang et al. [22] classified the patients included in the NCIC.CTG MA.5 trial, which randomized premenopausal women with node-positive breast cancer to adjuvant CMF (cyclophosphamide–methotrexate–5-fluorouracil) vs. CEF (cyclophosphamide–epirubicin–fluorouracil) chemotherapy according to PAM50 intrinsic subtypes. The results revealed that intrinsic subtypes were associated with relapse-free survival (RFS) and OS ($p = 0.0005$, $p < 0.0001$, respectively). The data also demonstrated the predictive value of intrinsic subtyping for anthracycline benefit.

The HER2-enriched subtype exhibited the greatest benefit from CEF vs. CMF, with a 21 % gain in 5-year RFS and 20 % gain in 5-year OS. By contrast, no survival advantage for CEF over CMF was observed for basal-like tumors, with a reverse trend of a 10 % higher 5-year OS for the CMF arm. The multivariate analysis results suggested that patients with luminal B tumors trended toward better survival when treated with CEF, whereas luminal A tumors had a tendency for better survival when treated with CMF (RFS, $p = 0.25$; OS, $p = 0.11$). The predictive value of PAM50 subtypes was evaluated in 820 patients from the GEICAM/9906 randomized phase III trial comparing adjuvant FEC to FEC followed by weekly paclitaxel (FEC-P) [84]. In GEICAM/9906, the OS of the FEC-P arm was significantly superior compared to the FEC arm (HR = 0.693, $p = 0.013$). The individual PAM50 subtypes were not predictive of weekly paclitaxel efficacy. However, the PAM50 proliferation score signature, which is the average expression value of 11 proliferation-related genes, was predictive for a benefit of weekly paclitaxel in the adjuvant setting. The investigators did not specify a cutoff point for this signature, but the HR for OS in the low quartile group was very significant (unadjusted HR = 0.232, $p = 0.002$). This was an unexpected finding because it is generally assumed that chemotherapy is not effective in tumors with low proliferative activity.

The ongoing RxPONDER (SWOG S1007) trial primarily uses Oncotype DX and PAM50 as a secondary analysis among patients with ER+, HER2 breast cancer with one to three positive nodes [85]. The primary objective is to determine the effect of chemotherapy on patients with node-positive breast cancer who have an RS ≤25. The secondary objective of the study is to compare the RS with the PAM50 ROR to provide valuable information regarding the comparison of the two different gene assays.

In conclusion, PAM50 may offer useful information about intrinsic subtype classification, DDFS, and the risk of recurrence at 10 years for ER-positive patients. In addition, PAM50 may help predict the response to tamoxifen for both node-negative and node-positive breast cancer patients. The assay received approval in 2013 and is commercially available in the European Union and Israel.

Genomic Grade Index (MAPQUANT Dx)

The genomic grade index (GGI) is the first microarray-based molecular diagnostic test for measuring tumor grade as an indicator of proliferation, risk of metastasis, and response to chemotherapy. GGI is mainly based on 97 genes related to tumor differentiation and grade. Although histopathological tumor grading has been regarded as one of the most important prognostic indicators, grading currently suffers from the uncertainty of the G2 grade in the context of decision making in particular and from interobserver variability in general. To create more precise and objective grading criteria, the 97-gene signature was identified and validated in a cohort of 597 tumors from different subtypes [86]. The signature was found to be more closely associated with relapse-free survival compared with the histological grade. In addition, the GGI reclassified histological grade 2 tumors into two subgroups: high vs. low risk of recurrence (HR: 3.61, $p < 0.001$). The GGI was also shown to be predictor of relapses in postmenopausal patients treated with tamoxifen or letrozole within the BIG 1–98 trial [87]. One of the limitations of this assay was the need for fresh or frozen tissue. A formalin-fixed, paraffin-embedded (FFPE) tissue-based PCR genomic grade was developed to overcome this difficulty. Eight genes (four representative of GGI and four reference genes) were selected from the initial original set of 97 genes and validated in a consecutive series of 212 systemically treated early-stage breast cancer patients [88]. A significant correlation was observed between the microarray-derived GGI and the qRT-PCR assay using frozen (rho = 0.95) and FFPE material (rho = 0.89).

Theros Breast Cancer Gene Expression Ratio Assay

Theros was originally designed by Ma et al. as a qRT-PCR-based gene signature for FFPE tissue to identify the expression of three predictive genes: the homeobox gene HOXB13, interleukin 17B receptor (IL17BR), and EST AI240933 [89]. Ectopic expression of HOXB13 by breast epithelial cells enhances motility and invasion *in vitro*, and its expression is increased in both preinvasive and invasive primary breast cancers. The initial study involving ER-positive breast cancer patients treated with tamoxifen indicated that the HOXB13:IL17BR (H:I) expression ratio was highly associated with recurrence [89]. The two-gene ratio accurately classified both tamoxifen-treated and untreated patients into high- and low-risk groups [90, 91]. The prognostic value of this ratio was also tested in larger data sets ($n = 1252$) including ER-positive patients. A higher H:I ratio was associated with a more aggressive clinical course and consequently shorter disease-free and overall survival. Furthermore, it was a useful tool for predicting the response to tamoxifen [92]. Currently, the H:I ratio is considered a marker of recurrence in ER-positive and node-negative patients and is used to classify patients into low (10–27 %) or high (28 to >60 %) breast cancer recurrence risk at 5 years.

EndoPredict

In contrast to Oncotype DX, PAM50, and MammaPrint, the EndoPredict (EP) assay includes eight genes associated with tumor proliferation and hormonal receptor activity and four reference genes but not ER, PR, and HER2 status. An EP score ranging between 0 and 15 stratifies ER-positive, HER2-negative breast cancer patients to high- and low-risk groups, with a threshold of 5. The qRT-PCR technique allows the assay to be performed in FFPE tissue to estimate distant recurrence in luminal breast cancer patients treated with adjuvant endocrine therapy alone [93]. EPclin, which is a combined score of clinical risk factors (tumor size and nodal status) and the EP score, revealed significant differences in the 10-year recurrence rates for ABCSG 6 and ABCSG 8 patients. Both were randomized trials including only endocrine therapy. According to the analysis, approximately half of the patients were in the high-risk group and further required chemotherapy based on the current data [93]. The EPclin score was recently compared with purely clinical risk classifications and was found to be strikingly superior to known prognosticators such as St. Gallen, German S3, and NCCN [94].

In light of these studies involving protein markers and genomic assays, future treatment guidelines concerning breast cancer patients will likely be refined based on individual tumor characteristics, probably derived from translational research projects, rather than age, tumor size, or nodal status alone.

Selecting Patients for Adjuvant Chemotherapy

The decision regarding systemic adjuvant treatment should be based on the predicted sensitivity to treatment methods and the individual risk of relapse. The final decision should also consider the possible side effects and the patient's age, general health status, comorbidities, and preferences. Treatment should begin 2–8 weeks after surgery; a retrospective analysis of 2594 breast cancer patients revealed that RFS and OS are significantly compromised by delays of more than 12 weeks after definitive surgery (HR: 1.6, 95 % CI 1.2–2.3; $p=0.005$) [95]. A recent study by Gagliato et al. [96] evaluated the association between time to initiation of adjuvant chemotherapy and survival according to breast cancer subtype and stage at diagnosis. The initiation of chemotherapy ≥61 days after surgery was associated with adverse outcomes among patients with stage II and stage III disease. Patients with triple-negative breast cancer (TNBC) tumors and those with HER2-positive tumors treated with trastuzumab who started chemotherapy ≥61 days after surgery had worse survival (HR: 1.54, 95 % CI 1.09–2.18 and HR: 3.09, 95 % CI 1.49–6.39, respectively) than those whose treatment was initiated in the first 30 days after surgery. Thus, particularly for stage II and III breast cancer, TNBC and HER2-positive tumors, avoiding postponing the initiation of adjuvant chemotherapy should be prioritized and may lead to an improvement in outcomes for these patient subsets.

The absolute benefit derived from adjuvant chemotherapy varies substantially with the risk of the individual patient, which is determined by the biology and the burden of the disease (e.g., the absolute benefit of adjuvant chemotherapy for a low-burden luminal A-like breast cancer is extremely small and must be balanced against the known short- and long-term side effects). Algorithms, validated computer-based models such as AOL, and the genetic assays mentioned above may help determine the benefits and detrimental effects of a planned treatment schedule.

When multigene assays are readily available, clinical practice has developed to rely on their results to guide decisions about the inclusion of chemotherapy in the treatment of patients with ER-positive, HER2-negative disease. The 70-gene assay returns a dichotomous result, whereas the 21-gene RS is continuous. A subject of debate is the level of RS that should justify cytotoxic therapy: only high RS values (>31) were significantly associated with chemotherapy benefit in prospective/retrospective studies [48, 51], whereas substantially lower values are being investigated in ongoing prospective trials and used in clinical practice. In many regions of the world, the cost of these multigene assays remains prohibitive.

According to the 2013 St. Gallen guidelines, the decision regarding systemic adjuvant therapies should be based on the surrogate intrinsic phenotype determined by ER/PR, HER2, and Ki67 assessment with the selective help of genomic tests such as MammaPrint® or Oncotype DX® for luminal cases with unclear chemotherapy indications [97]. The clinicopathological surrogate definition for luminal A-like disease includes the existence of positive ER and PR, negative HER2, and low Ki-67. The cutoff between "high" and "low" values for Ki-67 varies among laboratories. The 2013 St. Gallen guidelines offered a level of <15 % for the best correlation with the gene expression definition of luminal A tumors. This proposal is based particularly on the results of a single reference laboratory [98]. In the St. Gallen 2015 consensus, the minimum level of Ki-67 for luminal B tumors is generally accepted as 20–29. The value of PR in distinguishing between "luminal A-like" and "luminal B-like" subtypes is derived from the

Table 8.4 St. Gallen recommendations for adjuvant treatment of breast cancer depending on intrinsic subtype and clinicopathological surrogate definitions

Intrinsic subtype	Clinicopathological definition	Treatment	Special considerations
Luminal A	*Luminal A-like*		
	ER (+) and PR (+) and HER2 (−) and Kİ 67 ≤ (14–19 %)[a] and recurrence risk low with multigene tests	Endocrine therapy	Cytotoxics administered when high gene RS (>25), 70-gene high-risk status, grade 3 disease, ≥4 lymph node metastasis, young age (<35 years)[b]
Luminal B	*Luminal B-like (HER2 negative)*		
	ER (+) and HER2 (−) and Ki67≥(20–29 %)[a] or PR low/ negative or recurrence risk high with multigene tests	Endocrine therapy for all, cytotoxics for most	
	Luminal B-like (HER2 positive)		
	HER2 overexpressed or amplified any Ki-67	Cytotoxics and antiHER2 and endocrine therapy	
C-ERB B2 overexpression	*HER2 (+) (nonluminal)*		
	HER2 overexpressed or amplified and ER and PR absent	Cytotoxics and antiHER2	
Basal-like	*Triple negative*		
	ER and PR absent HER2 negative	Cytotoxics	80 % overlap between triple-negative and basal-like subtypes

[a]Panel votes in St. Gallen 2015, the minimum value of Ki67 required for "luminal B-like" is for "14–19 %," 14 %; for "20–29 %," 36 %; and for "30 % or more%," 7 %
[b]The Panel in St. Gallen 2015 was equally divided as to whether young age per se was an indication to add cytotoxics

work of Prat et al. [99], who used a PR cutoff of ≥20 % to best correspond to the luminal A subtype. "Luminal B-like" disease comprises those cases that lack the characteristics noted above for "luminal A-like" disease. Thus, either a high Ki-67 value or a low PR value may be used to distinguish between "luminal A-like" and "luminal B-like (HER2 negative)." According to current guidelines, endocrine therapy is the most critical intervention for the "luminal A-like" subtype and is often used alone. However, the panel suggested the addition of cytotoxics in selected patients. Relative indications for the addition of cytotoxics accepted by the majority included the following: (1) high 21-gene RS (i.e., >25); (2) 70-gene high-risk status, if available; (3) grade 3 disease; and (4) involvement of four or more lymph nodes. A minority require the involvement of only one node as an adequate rationale for the addition of chemotherapy. For "luminal B-like" (HER2-negative) disease, cytotoxic therapy was suggested for most patients. The panel could not conclude whether young age (<35 years) per se was an indication for the addition of cytotoxics. For rare histological subtypes, endocrine therapy alone is recommended for endocrine-responsive subtypes (cribriform, tubular, and mucinous), and cytotoxics are recommended to endocrine nonresponsive subtypes (apocrine, medullary, adenoid cystic, and metaplastic). However, node-negative adenoid cystic carcinoma can be spared from chemotherapy (Table 8.4).

According to NCCN guidelines, patients with lymph node involvement or with tumors greater than 1 cm in diameter are also appropriate candidates for adjuvant systemic therapy [100]. Patients with invasive ductal or lobular tumors of 0.6–1 cm in diameter and no lymph node involvement are classified as low risk of recurrence however those with unfavorable prognostic features may warrant the consideration of adjuvant therapy. Unfavorable prognostic features are defined as intramammary angiolymphatic invasion, high nuclear grade, high histological grade, HER2-positive status, or hormonal receptor-negative status. Adjuvant chemotherapy is not recommended for patients with triple-negative invasive breast cancers less than 0.5 cm (T1aN0M0) in diameter. Patients with T1b and larger tumors should receive adjuvant cytotoxic therapy. An adjuvant chemotherapy regimen for triple-negative tumors should contain anthracyclines and taxanes. Platinum-based chemotherapy regimens are not standard, and data are currently insufficient to recommend these regimens as adjuvant chemotherapy in TNBC patients. The triple-negative phenotype may be an indication for dose-dense chemotherapy with growth factor support.

NCCN member institutions consider performing RT-PCR analysis (e.g., Oncotype DX assay) to further refine risk stratification for adjuvant chemotherapy for patients with node-negative, ER-positive, HER2-negative breast cancers >0.5 cm, whereas others do not. The 21-gene RT-PCR assay is presented as an option when evaluating patients with primary tumors 0.6–1.0 cm in size with unfavorable features or in tumors >1 cm in size and node-negative, hormonal receptor-positive, and HER2-negative disease. The results of the EBCTCG overview have demonstrated convincing reductions in both recurrence and death rates in all age groups with the addition of polychemotherapy and endocrine therapy [9]. Thus, the current guidelines recommend adjuvant chemotherapy regardless of patient age. However, the decision to use adjuvant chemotherapy (CT) in elderly patients is challenging and requires evaluation of both the benefits and risks, including toxicity and comorbidities. The data remain insufficient to recommend adjuvant CT for those >70 years of age.

The Cancer and Leukemia Group B (CALGB) 49907 trial compared standard adjuvant chemotherapy with CMF or doxorubicin plus cyclophosphamide (AC) with capecitabine alone in fit patients over 65 years of age. AC or CMF was superior to capecitabine, and enrollment was discontinued early [101]. However, age is a known risk factor for the development of myelodysplasia and acute myelogenous leukemia after anthracycline-based adjuvant chemotherapy [102]; thus, life expectancy should be taken into consideration when making a decision. In a retrospective review of four randomized CALGB trials, older patients had higher chemotherapy-related mortality (1.5 % of patients aged ≥65 years), and the incidence of treatment-related mortality increased linearly with age [103]. Recently, the phenomenon of "chemobrain" (long-term chemotherapy-induced cognitive impairment) has been described and associated with altered quality of life and functionality [104]. Moreover, adjuvant chemotherapy has been shown to have a progerontogenic effect, estimated as 10.4 years of chronological aging [105].

The French Group of Geriatric Oncology (GERICO) has developed a trial to evaluate the benefit of adjuvant chemotherapy with regard to OS in patients aged over 70 years with pN0 or pN-positive, HR-positive HER2-negative disease and with a high genomic grade index assessed by reverse transcriptase polymerase chain reaction [106]. This study may help resolve uncertainty regarding the benefit of adjuvant CT in elderly patients.

The most recently updated version of the ESMO guidelines does not offer chemotherapy for most luminal A tumors, except those with the highest risk of relapse (extensive nodal involvement) [107]. Luminal B HER2-negative cancers comprise the population of highest uncertainty regarding chemotherapy indications. ESMO guidelines have defined features associated with lower endocrine responsiveness, such as low steroid receptor expression, lack of PR expression, high tumor grade, and high proliferation marker expression. Moreover, two invasion factors, urokinase plasminogen activator (uPA) and plasminogen activator inhibitor 1 (PAI1), also known as tumor markers, have been suggested as prognostic factors and have been utilized to aid treatment decision making in early breast cancer [108].

Treatment of Rare Histological Subtypes

Invasive breast carcinomas comprise several histological subtypes; the most common types (infiltrating ductal, lobular, or mixed) represent approximately 91 % of invasive breast carcinomas, according to Surveillance, Epidemiology, and End Results (SEER) data of the National Cancer Institute from 1992 to 2001 [10]. All other subtypes, including mucinous (colloid), tubular, medullary, papillary, and metaplastic breast cancer, account for fewer than 10 % of cases.

Tubular carcinomas were relatively infrequent in the pre-mammography era, accounting for 2 % or less of all invasive breast cancers. However, in some series of mammographically screened populations, the incidence is higher, accounting for 10–20 % of invasive cancers. These lesions have a relatively better prognosis than infiltrating ductal carcinomas; their natural history is favorable, and metastases are rare. Mucinous carcinoma lesions are another prognostically favorable variant of invasive breast carcinoma [109].

Some guidelines provide systemic treatment recommendations for histologically favorable invasive breast cancers such as tubular and mucinous cancers based on tumor size and ALN status [110]. The treatment options for endocrine therapy and chemotherapy and the sequencing of treatment with other modalities are similar to those for breast cancers with the usual histology. The vast majority of tubular breast cancers are both ER positive and HER2 negative. Thus, the pathological evaluation and accuracy of the ER and/or HER2 determination should be reviewed if a tubular breast cancer is ER negative and/or HER2 positive. If a breast cancer is histologically identified as a tubular or mucinous breast cancer and is confirmed as ER negative, then the tumor should be treated according to the guideline for tumors with the usual histology, ER-negative

breast cancers. Because the prospective data regarding systemic adjuvant therapy of tumors with favorable histology are lacking, decisions regarding treatment should be made on an individual basis.

Medullary carcinomas account for 1–10 % of invasive breast cancers. However, there is considerable interobserver variability in the diagnosis of this type of breast cancer depending in part on the classification system employed. Medullary carcinoma is characterized by high nuclear grade, lymphocytic infiltration, and a pushing tumor border. Despite their aggressive histological appearance, the prognosis of pure medullary carcinomas appears to be more favorable than that of infiltrating ductal carcinomas [111]. However, there is also evidence suggesting that the risk of metastases is equal to that of other high-grade carcinomas, even for cases that meet all of the pathological criteria for typical medullary carcinoma. Moreover, many cases classified as medullary carcinoma do not have all of the pathological features upon subsequent pathological review. Patients may be harmed if a high-grade infiltrating ductal carcinoma is misclassified as a typical medullary carcinoma. Thus, it is often recommended that medullary carcinoma be treated similarly to other infiltrating ductal carcinomas based on tumor size, grade, and lymph node status.

Type, Dosing, and Scheduling of Chemotherapy

Anthracyclines and Other Alkylating Agents

Adjuvant chemotherapy comprising multiple cycles of chemotherapy is a well-established strategy for lowering the risk of recurrence and death due to breast cancer. Initial studies of adjuvant chemotherapy were conducted among patients with higher-risk, lymph node-positive disease. However, subsequent trials with lower-risk groups have extended the benefits of adjuvant chemotherapy.

The Early Breast Cancer Trialists' Collaborative Group (EBCTCG) was first established in 1985 to coordinate individual patient-level meta-analyses of all randomized trials of adjuvant treatments. According to the EBCTCG 1998 meta-analysis, for recurrence, polychemotherapy produced substantial and highly significant proportional reductions among both women aged under 50 at randomization (35 % reduction; $2p < 0.00001$) and women aged 50–69 (20 % reduction; $2p < 0.00001$); few women aged ≥ 70 had been studied. Reductions in mortality were also significant among both women aged under 50 (27 % reduction; $2p < 0.00001$) and women aged 50–69 (11 % reduction; $2p = 0.0001$). The recurrence reductions chiefly emerged during the first 5 years of follow-up, whereas the difference in survival increased throughout the first 10 years [112].

Another report on trials that had begun by 1995 reviewed polychemotherapy vs. no adjuvant chemotherapy and anthracycline-based chemotherapy (with doxorubicin or epirubicin) vs. CMF (cyclophosphamide, methotrexate, fluorouracil) [9]. The analyses of systemic adjuvant treatment for early-stage breast cancer involved a total of nearly 150,000 women in 200 randomized trials, including many with long-term follow-up. For recurrence, several months of polychemotherapy produced, overall, a highly significant 23.5 % reduction in the annual HR ($p < 0.00001$). For mortality, several months of polychemotherapy produced a significant 15.3 % reduction in the annual HR ($p < 0.00001$).

In the 2011 EBCTCG meta-analysis, adjuvant chemotherapy using an anthracycline-based regimen was associated with a significant improvement in the risk of recurrence compared to no treatment (RR 0.73, 95 % CI 0.68–0.79), which translated into an absolute gain of 8.0 % at 10 years, and a significant reduction in overall mortality (RR 0.84, 95 % CI 0.78–0.91), which translated into an absolute gain of 5.0 % [113]. Compared with no treatment, the use of CMF was associated with significant improvement in the risk of recurrence (RR 0.70, 95 % CI 0.63–0.77), which translated into an absolute gain of 10.2 % and a significant reduction in breast cancer mortality (RR 0.76, 95 % CI 0.68–0.84). The reduction in overall mortality, with an absolute

gain of 4.7 %, was also significant (RR 0.84, 95 % CI 0.76–0.93).

The 2005 EBCTCG analysis included an indirect comparison of adjuvant CMF and anthracycline-based chemotherapy [9]. Approximately half of the available evidence was from trials of CMF-based regimens, and approximately a third was from trials of anthracycline-based regimens. For the CMF-based regimens, 84 % of the information was from trials of 6, 9, or 12 months of treatment (with no significant trend toward a greater benefit with longer treatment), and 90 % was from trials that involved no cytotoxic drugs other than CMF (the remainder involved these three drugs and vincristine). In the anthracycline-based trials, the mean duration was 6 months, and the anthracycline used was always doxorubicin (66 %) or epirubicin (34 %). Among both younger and older women, there were no significant differences between the proportional risk reductions (in recurrence or in breast cancer mortality) produced by the CMF-based and anthracycline-based chemotherapy regimens in these particular trials.

Although the indirect comparisons of anthracycline-based and CMF regimens did not suggest any substantial difference in efficacy, the directly randomized comparisons involved smaller standard errors for the comparison between the two treatment effects, particularly at younger ages, favoring anthracyclines [9]. A total of 14,000 women (9000 younger, 5000 older) were included in trials comparing anthracycline-based vs. CMF-based regimens. The anthracyclines tested were doxorubicin (60 %) or epirubicin (40 %), usually administered for approximately 6 months in combination with other cytotoxic drugs (e.g., as FAC or FEC, which were the most widely studied combinations). The CMF-based regimens used in the control groups all involved CMF with no other cytotoxic drugs and were administered for approximately 6 (mean 6.5) months. The overall findings indicated a moderate but highly significant advantage of anthracyclines over CMF (recurrence rate ratio 0.89, $2p = 0.001$; breast cancer death rate ratio 0.84, $2p = 0.00001$). For the probabilities of recurrence, breast cancer mortality, and overall mortality, the absolute difference between anthracycline-based and CMF chemotherapy was approximately 3 % at 5 years and 4 % at 10 years. The proportional risk reductions among older women and those with ER-positive and node-negative disease had relatively wide confidence intervals.

Two randomized prospective trials of CEF (cyclophosphamide, epirubicin, fluorouracil) chemotherapy in ALN-positive breast cancer are available. In one trial, premenopausal women with node-positive breast cancer were randomized to receive classic CMF therapy vs. CEF chemotherapy using high-dose epirubicin. Both 10-year RFS (52 % vs. 45 %; $p = 0.007$) and OS (62 % vs. 58 %; $p = 0.085$) favored the CEF arm of the trial [114]. The second trial compared CEF given intravenously every 3 weeks at two dose levels of epirubicin (50 mg/m^2 vs. 100 mg/m^2) in premenopausal and postmenopausal women with node-positive breast cancer. Five-year DFS (55 % vs. 66 %; $p = 0.03$) and OS (65 % vs. 76 %; $p = 0.007$) both favored the epirubicin 100 mg/m^2 arm [115]. Another trial compared two dose levels of EC chemotherapy with CMF chemotherapy in women with node-positive breast cancer [116]. This study demonstrated that higher-dose EC chemotherapy was equivalent to CMF chemotherapy and superior to moderate-dose EC in event-free survival and OS. Based on the collective experience, multiple cycles of adjuvant chemotherapy, typically including anthracycline-based regimens, are recommended for the majority of patients with node-positive and higher-risk node-negative tumors.

The Story of Taxanes

The introduction of taxanes into early-stage breast cancer treatment was an important development over the historic experience with alkylator and anthracycline-based chemotherapy. The first randomized study of adjuvant taxane therapy was CALGB 9344, which incorporated sequential paclitaxel therapy for women receiving four cycles of cyclophosphamide–doxorubicin (AC) chemotherapy [117]. The study also involved dose escalation for doxorubicin, which did not

reveal a benefit of an increase in dose to 75 or 90 mg/m^2. However, sequential paclitaxel therapy (175 mg/m^2 for four cycles) improved both DFS and OS among women with node-positive breast cancer. At 5 years, DFS was 65 % and 70 %, and OS was 77 % and 80 % after AC alone and AC plus paclitaxel, respectively. Similarly, the NSABP-B28 trial demonstrated that the addition of paclitaxel to AC significantly reduced the HR for DFS events by 17 % (relative risk [RR], 0.83; 95 % CI 0.72–0.95; $p = 0.006$). The 5-year DFS was 76 % for patients randomly assigned to AC followed by paclitaxel compared with 72 % for those randomly assigned to AC [118]. However, the improvement in OS was small and not statistically significant (RR, 0.93; 95 % CI 0.78–1.12; $p = 0.46$). The 5-year OS was 85 % ($\pm$2 %) for both groups. In this trial, an unplanned subset analysis suggested that the addition of paclitaxel was more beneficial in women with tumors that had either a negative or unknown ER status, with a hazard ratio for recurrence of 0.72 (0.59–0.86).

Another adjuvant trial reported on 524 women with T1–3, N0–1 invasive breast cancer who were randomized to four cycles of postoperative paclitaxel followed by four cycles of FAC vs. a control group who received eight cycles of FAC [119]. Therefore, this trial tested the benefit of substituting a single-agent taxane for some cycles of anthracycline-containing chemotherapy while maintaining the overall number of cycles. A total of 174 patients were treated preoperatively (neoadjuvant), and 350 were treated postoperatively (adjuvant); the results were presented together. The hazard ratio was 0.70 (95 % CI 0.47–1.07, $p = 0.09$) for RFS and was not reported for OS. There was a nonsignificant trend suggesting that the addition of paclitaxel was more beneficial in women with tumors that were ER negative.

Similarly, another randomized trial (PACS 01) in women with ALN-positive breast cancer compared six cycles of FEC with three cycles of FEC followed by three cycles of docetaxel [52]. The 5-year DFS (78.4 % vs. 73.2 %; adjusted $p = 0.012$) and OS (90.7 % vs. 86.7 %; $p = 0.017$) of sequential FEC followed by docetaxel were

Table 8.5 Overall and disease-free survival analysis of some of the docetaxel-including trials

Trial	Regimen	Follow-up (years)	DFS (at 5 years)	HR	p	OS (at 5 years)	HR	p
GEICAM 9805 [64]	FAC ×6 vs. TAC ×6	5	90.1 % vs. 85.3 %	0.67	0.03	95.2 % vs. 93.5 %	0.76	0.29
ECOG 2197 [77]	AT ×4 vs. AC ×4	5	85 % vs. 85 %	1.02	0.78	91.2 % vs. 92 %	1.3	0.62
USO 9735 [69]	TC ×4 vs. AC ×4	7	81 % vs. 75 %[a]	0.74	0.033	87 % vs. 82 %[a]	0.69	0.032
UK TACT [61]	FEC ×3-T ×3 vs. FEC ×8 or E ×4 vs. CMF ×4	5	75.6 % vs. 74.3 %	0.95	0.44	82.5 % vs. 83 %	0.99	0.91
BCIRG 001 [58]	TAC ×6 vs. FAC ×6	4.5	75 % vs. 68 %	0.72	0.001	87 % vs. 81 %	0.70	0.008
PACS 01 [53]	FEC ×3-T ×3 vs. FEC ×6	5	73 % vs. 78 %	0.85	0.012	86.7 % vs. 90.7 %	0.73	0.014

DFS disease-free survival, *OS* overall-survival, *A* adriamycin, *C* cyclophosphamide, *E* epirubicin, *F* 5-fluorouracil, *T* docetaxel, *M* methotrexate
[a]DFS and OS rates at 7 years

superior. The GEICAM 9906 study, which compared six cycles of FEC90 with four cycles of FEC90 followed by paclitaxel once a week for 8 weeks, also reported a benefit of paclitaxel for both DFS and OS [120].

The question of the scheduling and dosing of taxanes became more confusing following the results of the Eastern Cooperative Oncology Group (ECOG) E1199 study. The ECOG E1199 study was a four-arm trial that randomized 4950 women to receive AC chemotherapy followed by either paclitaxel or docetaxel given by either an every-3-week schedule or a weekly schedule [121, 122]. At a median of 63.8 months of follow-up, no significant differences in DFS or OS were observed when comparing paclitaxel to docetaxel or weekly vs. every-3-week administration. In a secondary series of comparisons, weekly paclitaxel was superior to every-3-week paclitaxel in DFS (HR 1.27; 95 % CI 1.03–1.57; $p = 0.006$) and OS (HR 1.32; 95 % CI 1.02–1.72; $p = 0.01$), and every-3-week docetaxel was superior to every-3-week paclitaxel in DFS (HR 1.23; 95 % CI 1.00–1.52; $p = 0.02$) but not in OS [123]. Based on these results, as well as on the findings from the CALGB 9741 trial indicating that dose-dense AC followed by paclitaxel every 2 weeks had a

survival benefit compared with the regimen of AC followed by every-3-week paclitaxel, the every-3-week paclitaxel regimen has been removed from the guidelines.

Breast Cancer International Research Group (BCIRG) 001 was an open-label, phase 3, multicenter trial in which 1491 patients aged 18–70 years with node-positive, early-stage breast cancer were randomly assigned to adjuvant treatment with docetaxel, doxorubicin, and cyclophosphamide (TAC) or fluorouracil, doxorubicin, and cyclophosphamide (FAC) every 3 weeks for six cycles [124]. After 55 months of follow-up, the study demonstrated that a regimen incorporating docetaxel reduced the risk of relapse (HR 0.72, 95 % CI 0.59–0.88; $p = 0.001$) and death (HR 0.70, 95 % CI 0.53–0.91; $p = 0.008$) compared with a standard anthracycline-based regimen. The survival advantage for the TAC regimen was maintained at 10-year follow-up. DFS was 62 % (95 % CI 58–65) for patients in the TAC group and 55 % (51–59) for patients in the FAC group (HR 0.80, 95 % CI 0.68–0.93; $p = 0.0043$). Ten-year OS was 76 % (95 % CI 72–79) for patients in the TAC group and 69 % (65–72) for patients in the FAC group (HR 0.74, 0.61–0.90; log-rank $p = 0.0020$) [125]. Some of the adjuvant trials of taxanes are summarized in Tables 8.5 and 8.6.

Table 8.6 Overall and disease-free survival analysis of some of the paclitaxel-including trials

Trials	Regimen	Follow-up (years)	DFS (at 5 years)	HR	p	OS (at 5 years)	HR	p
MDACC 2002 [52]	FAC ×8 vs. P ×4-FAC ×4	5	83 % vs. 86 %	0.83	0.09	NR		
CALGB 9344 [50]	AC ×4 vs. AC ×4-P ×4	5	65 % vs. 70 %	0.83	0.013	77 % vs. 80 %	0.82	0.006
GEICAM/2003-02 [65]	FAC x6 vs. FAC ×3-P (8w)	5	93 % vs. 90.3 %	0.73	0.04	97 % vs. 95 %	0.79	0.34
NSABP B28 [51]	AC ×4 vs. AC ×4-P ×4	5	72 % vs. 76 %	0.83	0.006	85 %vs. 85 %	0.93	0.46
HeCOG 10/97 [76]	E ×4-CMF ×4 vs. E ×3-P ×3-CMF ×3	5	77 % vs. 80 %	1.16	0.31	93 % vs. 90 %	2.42	0.02

DFS disease-free survival, *OS* overall survival, *A* adriamycin, *C* cyclophosphamide

The incorporation of docetaxel with doxorubicin with different schedules has been tested in further trials. At a median follow-up of 73 months, results from the three-arm randomized NSABP B-30 trial comparing TAC vs. AT vs. AC followed by docetaxel (AC→T) demonstrated that AC→T had a significant advantage for DFS (HR:0.83; $p=0.006$) but not OS (HR: 0.86; $p=0.086$) compared with TAC [126]. In addition, both DFS (HR: 0.080; $p=0.001$) and OS (HR:0.83; $p=0.034$) were significantly increased when AC→T was compared with AT, with AT demonstrating non-inferiority compared with TAC.

Not all studies have further supported the use of adjuvant taxanes in early breast cancer. There were no significant differences in DFS in a large ($n=4162$) randomized study (TACT) comparing adjuvant chemotherapy with four cycles of every-3-week FEC followed by four cycles of every-3-week docetaxel with standard anthracycline chemotherapy regimens (e.g., FEC or epirubicin followed by CMF) in women with node-positive or high-risk node-negative operable breast cancer [127]. In addition, the anthracycline–docetaxel sequential schedule was associated with a higher frequency of adverse events and transiently poorer quality of life than the non-taxane control regimen. Generalizations about taxane benefits are difficult to make because individual trials vary in size, are reported at different times since

study initiation, include biologically heterogeneous populations, use one or another taxane with different schedules, and compare different anthracycline control regimens of often unequal duration. Many patients appear to receive benefits of differing magnitude from additional taxanes, particularly in regard to OS. An important role for adjuvant taxanes as a sequential alternative to anthracyclines has been proposed to minimize the overall anthracycline dose and subsequent exposure to associated long-term adverse events (such as the induction of leukemia and cardiotoxicity).

More than a dozen studies have reported improved breast cancer outcomes with the incorporation of the taxanes paclitaxel or docetaxel as substitutes or adjunct treatments to anthracycline-based regimens. A large meta-analysis of 13 studies ($n=22,903$) that incorporated taxanes into anthracycline-based regimens revealed that the pooled HR estimate was 0.83 (95 % CI 0.79–0.87; $p=0.00001$) for DFS and 0.85 (95 % CI 0.79–0.91; $p=0.00001$) for OS. Risk reduction was not influenced by the type of taxane, ER expression, the number of axillary metastases (1–3 lymph nodes vs. ≥4 lymph nodes), patient age/menopausal status, or administration schedule [128]. Taxane incorporation resulted in an absolute 5-year risk reduction of 5 % for DFS and 3 % for OS.

Another meta-analysis of nine trials involving more than 15,000 patients also assessed the impact of paclitaxel or docetaxel on survival [129]. Significant differences in favor of taxanes were observed in DFS in the overall (RR: 0.86; 95 % CI 0.81–0.90; $p=0.00001$) and lymph node-positive populations (RR: 0.84; 95 % CI 0.79–0.89; $p=0.0001$) and in OS in the overall (RR: 0.87; 95 % CI 0.81–0.83; $p=0.0001$) and lymph node-positive populations (RR: 0.84; 95 % CI 0.77–0.92; $p=0.0001$). The absolute benefits in DFS and OS in favor of taxanes ranged from 3.3 % to 4.6 % and from 2.0 % to 2.8 %, respectively.

Collectively, these data suggest that the use of taxanes may contribute to modest improvement in outcomes, particularly among women with node-positive breast cancer. Most taxane trials have included node-positive patients, but the effect of the addition of taxanes to adjuvant chemotherapy for node-negative breast cancer patients has been assessed in a few trials. One pure adjuvant study in node-negative patients was the Spanish Breast Cancer Research Group (GEICAM) 9805 trial [130]. The study assigned 1060 women with axillary node-negative breast cancer and at least one high-risk factor for recurrence to treatment with TAC or FAC every 3 weeks for six cycles after surgery. High-risk factors were defined according to the 1998 St. Gallen criteria: tumor size >2 cm, negative for ER and PR expression, histological tumor grade 2 or 3, and age <35 years. The primary endpoint was DFS after at least 5 years of follow-up. In this study, the combination of docetaxel, doxorubicin, and cyclophosphamide (TAC) significantly reduced the risk of recurrence by 32 % ($p=0.01$) compared with fluorouracil, doxorubicin, and cyclophosphamide (FAC) at the expense of significant toxicity. The benefit of TAC was consistent regardless of hormonal receptor status, menopausal status, or the number of high-risk factors.

Before these results were available, GEICAM/2003-02 began accruing a similar group of high-risk node-negative breast cancer patients to determine the benefits and safety of adding paclitaxel to the standard FAC regimen in this understudied population [131]. Specifically, this trial compared the administration of six cycles of FAC with a regimen of four cycles of FAC followed by eight doses of weekly paclitaxel (FAC-wP). The estimated DFS rates at 5 years were 93 % in the FAC-wP arm and 90.3 % in the FAC arm ($p=0.04$). The difference in DFS between the two arms was mainly due to the greater number of distant breast cancer relapses among those receiving FAC than among those receiving FAC-wP. Subgroup DFS analyses by menopausal status, HR status, tumor grade, and HER2 status suggested that the observed benefit of FAC-wP over FAC in these subpopulations was consistent with that of the overall population. Nonetheless, the 21.4 % reduction in the risk of death in the experimental group failed to reach significance (HR, 0.79; 95 % CI 0.49–1.26, $p=0.31$).

A meta-analysis of 14 studies comparing docetaxel-containing vs. non-taxane-containing regimens revealed that the addition of docetaxel significantly reduced the risk of relapse (16 % relative reduction) and the risk of death (14 % relative reduction) for high-risk early-stage breast cancer [132]. The findings also suggested that the relative benefits for DFS of adding docetaxel were nearly identical in node-negative and node-positive patients [HR 0.86 (0.73–1.00), 4274 patients and HR 0.83 (0.77–0.90), 20,166 patients, respectively]. The authors could not demonstrate a survival advantage with the addition of docetaxel in node-negative patients, but they proposed that this may be due to the lack of statistical power and the short period of follow-up in some of the trials included in the meta-analysis.

Four cycles of AC were demonstrated to be equivalent to 6 months of classic cyclophosphamide, methotrexate, and fluorouracil in two separate National Surgical Adjuvant Breast and Bowel Project (NSABP) studies (NSABP-15 and NSABP-23) [133, 134]. However, whether the benefit of adding a taxane in the adjuvant setting obviates the need for anthracyclines in a subset of patients is not known. While confirmation in larger prospective trials is necessary, one randomized trial supports the use of a non-anthracycline regimen. US Oncology Trial 9735 enrolled 1016 women with stage I to III HER2-negative breast cancer and randomly assigned the women to therapy with AC (doxorubicin and cyclophosphamide) or TC (docetaxel plus cyclophosphamide) [135]. With a median follow-up of 7 years, TC resulted in significantly higher DFS (81 vs. 75 %) and OS (87 vs. 82 %) [136]. Given the scarcity of prospective randomized data addressing this issue, an anthracycline- and taxane-containing regimen is recommended for most women, particularly those with higher-stage tumors and those with triple-negative or HER2-positive cancers. However, for those with contraindications to anthracycline-based therapy, CMF and TC are acceptable alternatives.

Dose-Dense Regimens

Dose escalation studies revealed no benefit, and dose-dense schedules have been evaluated in subsequent trials. Dose density refers to the administration of drugs with a shortened intertreatment interval and is based on the observation that in experimental models, a given dose always kills a certain fraction, rather than a certain number, of exponentially growing cancer cells [137]. Because human cancers in general and breast cancers in particular are believed to grow by non-exponential Gompertzian kinetics, this model has been extended to those situations [138]. The regrowth of cancer cells between cycles of cyto-reduction is more rapid in volume-reduced Gompertzian cancer models than in exponential models. Hence, it has been hypothesized that the more frequent administration of cytotoxic therapy would minimize the residual tumor burden more effectively than dose escalation. The concept of dose density has been strongly influenced by an alternative model developed by Norton and Simon [139], which hypothesizes that logarithmic cell killing is not constant but is proportional to the relative growth rate. Because smaller tumors are growing relatively more rapidly than larger tumors with the same kinetics, chemotherapy induces greater log killing in smaller tumors. However, due to more rapid regrowth, the eventual outcome is the same.

The CALGB 9741 randomized trial evaluated the use of concurrent vs. sequential chemotherapy (doxorubicin followed by paclitaxel followed by cyclophosphamide vs. doxorubicin plus cyclophosphamide followed by paclitaxel) given either every 2 weeks with filgrastim support or every 3 weeks [140]. No significant difference was observed between the two chemotherapy regimens, but a 26 % reduction in the HR of recurrence ($p = 0.01$) and a 31 % reduction in the HR of death ($p = 0.013$) were observed for the dose-dense regimens.

In a different approach, ECOG compared weekly and 3-week interval docetaxel or paclitaxel after four cycles of standard doxorubicin and cyclophosphamide in women with node-positive or high-risk node-negative breast cancer [122]. Neither paclitaxel nor docetaxel emerged as superior with respect to DFS. However, subgroup analyses suggested a potential DFS benefit of dose-dense therapy with paclitaxel (HR: 1.20; $p = 0.06$) but not docetaxel. Those results must be interpreted with caution because the planned dose density and cumulative dose were 37 % higher for weekly paclitaxel compared with 3-weekly therapy, whereas dose-density and cumulative dose were similar for weekly and 3-weekly docetaxel. The schedule for paclitaxel administration was recently analyzed by Budd et al. [141] using a 2×2 factorial design. The study included 3294 high-risk breast cancer patients with stage I–III diseases. High risk was defined as node positive (pN1-N3), any primary tumor ≥ 2 cm, or any primary tumor ≥ 1 cm if it was HR negative or HER2 positive or had a 21-gene RS ≥ 26. Patients were randomized into four arms. Two arms received doxorubicin and cyclophosphamide (AC) every 2 weeks for six cycles, and two arms received AC weekly for 15 cycles. The patients were then randomized to two different paclitaxel regimens. The patients received paclitaxel 175 mg/m^2 every 2 weeks for six cycles or 80 mg/m^2 weekly for 12 cycles. Interim analysis revealed a significant difference in OS but not DFS; all treatments given once every 2 weeks were associated with the highest OS. However, the difference in OS was confined to patients with HR-negative/HER2-negative tumors, although subset analysis by biological type of breast cancer was unplanned. The difference in OS in the absence of a significant difference in DFS is controversial and requires further explanation.

The phase III trial by the European Organization for Research and Treatment of Cancer (EORTC) by Therasse et al. [142] compared six biweekly cycles of epirubicin and cyclophosphamide (EC) with six 4-week-interval cycles of cyclophosphamide, epirubicin, and fluorouracil (CEF) in patients with locally advanced breast cancer. After a median follow-up of 5.5 years, the study failed to show any benefit of dose-dense EC over conventional CEF. Similar efficacy was achieved with both regimens, but duration of treatment was half as long with dose-dense EC without additional significant toxicity.

In contrast to the trials described above, the Hellenic Cooperative Oncology Group (He-COG) trial was the first study to directly compare two different dose-dense sequential regimens for node-positive or high-risk node-negative breast cancer [143]. Patients were randomized to sequential dose-dense epirubicin and paclitaxel or concurrent epirubicin and paclitaxel, both followed by three cycles of intensified combination chemotherapy with CMF. The study failed to show any significant difference in DFS or OS between treatment groups but suggested a potential benefit in ER-negative patients treated with paclitaxel.

Concordantly, the published results of the National Surgical Breast and Bowel Project B-38 (NSABP B-38) trial failed to demonstrate a significant difference between dose-dense regimens and conventional strategies. The trial involved nearly 4900 women (65 % with pathologically involved nodes and 80 % with ER-positive disease) who were randomly assigned to treatment with dose-dense AC-T, dose-dense AC followed by the combination of paclitaxel plus gemcitabine (AC-TG), or TAC [144]. The 5-year DFS rate was similar across treatment groups (82 % with dose-dense AC-T vs. 80 % with both dose-dense AC-TG and TAC). The 5-year OS rate was also similar (89, 90, and 90 %, respectively). However, TAC was associated with significantly more serious (grade 3 or 4) toxicity, including febrile neutropenia (9 % vs. 3 % in both the AC-T and

AC-TG arms) and diarrhea (8 % vs. 2 % with AC-T or AC-TG). However, TAC was associated with significantly less grade 3/4 neurotoxicity (<1 % vs. 7 % and 6 % with AC-T or AC-TG, respectively).

A meta-analysis of dose-dense vs. standard dosing that included data from ten trials and over 11,000 women summarized the findings of the trials described above [145].

1. In three trials that evaluated similar dosing in the treatment arms, dose-dense treatment was associated with an improvement in DFS (hazard ratio [HR] 0.83, 95 % CI 0.73–0.94) and OS (HR 0.84, 95 % CI 0.72–0.98).
2. In seven trials in which modified doses or regimens were evaluated, improvements in DFS (HR 0.81, 95 % CI 0.73–0.88) and OS (HR = 0.85, 95 % CI 0.75–0.96) were also demonstrated.
3. The benefit in DFS was observed in women with ER-negative disease (HR 0.71, 95 % CI 0.56–0.98) but not in women with ER-positive disease (HR 0.92, 95 % CI 0.75–1.12).

Dose-dense strategies have been demonstrated to be feasible and safe with G-CSF support and have a modest impact on disease recurrence and OS of unselected patients with early-stage breast cancer. Emerging data are convincing that the benefits of dose-dense therapy will be greater for specific tumor subtypes such as hormonal receptor-negative, highly proliferative, or HER2-overexpressing tumors [146].

Novel Approaches for Adjuvant Chemotherapy

Adjuvant anthracycline- and taxane-based chemotherapy provides substantial benefits for women diagnosed with node-positive, early-stage breast cancer. However, a significant proportion of women treated with adjuvant chemotherapy still develop disease recurrence, necessitating additional studies to evaluate alternative treatment strategies. However, attempts to improve outcomes with combination regimens by combining additional chemotherapeutic agents with anthracyclines, taxanes, and cyclophosphamide have not yielded promising results.

The randomized, phase III FinXX trial (NCT00114816) investigated whether the integration of capecitabine (X) into a sequential docetaxel (T)→cyclophosphamide+epirubicin+5-FU (CEF) adjuvant regimen might improve clinical outcomes for patients with medium-to-high risk early-stage breast cancer. The primary endpoint of the trial was RFS. The planned interim analysis, after a median follow-up of 3 years, indicated a significant RFS benefit of the X-containing regimen vs. the control (HR: 0.66, 95 % CI 0.47–0.94; $p=0.020$) [147]. However, the final results of the FinXX trial after a median follow-up of 59 months demonstrated that the addition of capecitabine did not provide a significant improvement in RFS compared with docetaxel followed by CEF (HR: 0.79; 95 % CI 0.60–1.04; $p=0.087$) [148]. In exploratory analyses, adding capecitabine appeared to improve BCSS and benefit some women with early-stage breast cancer such as those with triple-negative disease and those with more than three metastatic axillary lymph nodes.

Another trial was performed among 2611 high-risk breast cancer patients who were classified as follows: ≥ 1 positive lymph node, T1–3; node negative with tumors >2 cm; or node negative with tumors >1 cm, both ER and PR negative [149]. The experimental arm comprised four every-3-week cycles of AC (doxorubicin and cyclophosphamide) followed by four cycles of capecitabine and docetaxel (XT) vs. AC followed by every-3-week cycles of docetaxel (T) alone. The primary endpoint of the study was DFS. However, the study failed to meet its primary endpoint of DFS (HR 0.84, 95 % CI: 0.67–1.05; $p=0.125$) after a median follow-up of 5 years, although a statistically significant improvement in OS in patients receiving AC→XT was observed. Similarly, the interim analysis of another open-label study demonstrated an improvement in breast cancer recurrence with a capecitabine-containing chemotherapy regimen [147]. Patients were randomly assigned to either three cycles of capecitabine and docetaxel followed by three cycles of cyclophosphamide, epirubicin, and capecitabine or to three cycles of docetaxel followed by three cycles of cyclophosphamide, epirubicin, and fluorouracil. The primary endpoint was RFS. After a 3-year median follow-up, RFS was higher with the capecitabine regimen compared to the control (93 % vs. 89 %; HR 0.66, 95 % CI 0.47–0.94; $p=0.020$). However, capecitabine administration was frequently discontinued because of adverse effects such as grade 3–4 diarrhea and hand–foot syndrome. The OS data are not yet mature; thus, capecitabine is still not routinely administered in the adjuvant setting.

Attempts to further incorporate different agents into adjuvant protocols have not been limited to capecitabine. The addition of gemcitabine to paclitaxel has yielded improved outcomes in women with metastatic breast cancer. In light of these findings, the tAnGo trial addressed the addition of gemcitabine in adjuvant treatment protocols. The tAnGo trial was a phase III randomized trial of gemcitabine in paclitaxel-containing, epirubicin-based, adjuvant chemotherapy for ER/PR-poor, early-stage breast cancer, which demonstrated that the addition of gemcitabine to sequential epirubicin and cyclophosphamide followed by paclitaxel conferred no therapeutic benefit [150]. Furthermore, the NSABP B-38 study did not indicate a survival advantage for the addition of gemcitabine to a sequential anthracycline- and taxane-based regimen, confirming the results of the tAnGo study [144]. This trial assigned patients with node-positive early-stage breast cancer to dose-dense AC-T, dose-dense AC followed by paclitaxel plus gemcitabine (AC-TG), or TAC. Primary granulocyte colony-stimulating factor support was required; erythropoiesis-stimulating agents (ESAs) were also used at the investigator's discretion. Exploratory analyses of ESAs revealed no association with DFS events. Adding gemcitabine to dose-dense regimens also did not improve outcomes. Whether the combination of these agents with different schemes will produce a significant benefit is a question of debate. However, it appears unlikely that further changes in dosing schedules will result in appreciable gains.

Recommended Adjuvant Chemotherapy Schedules

There is no single standard adjuvant chemotherapy protocol for the treatment of breast cancer.
  Commonly used regimens are described below.

Non-taxane Regimens

1. *AC chemotherapy*
   Doxorubicin 60 mg/m² IV day 1
   Cyclophosphamide 600 mg/m² IV day 1
   (Cycled every 21 days for four cycles)
   (In dose-dense regimen, every 14 days for four cycles with myeloid growth factor support)
2. *EC chemotherapy*
   Epirubicin 100 mg/m² IV day 1
   Cyclophosphamide 830 mg/m² IV day 1
   (Cycled every 21 days for eight cycles)
   (With myeloid growth factor support)
3. *CEF chemotherapy*
   Cyclophosphamide 75 mg/m² PO days 1–14
   Epirubicin 60 mg/m² IV days 1 and 8
   5-Fluorouracil 500 mg/m² IV days 1 and 8
   (With cotrimoxazole support)
   (Cycled every 28 days for six cycles)
4. *FAC chemotherapy*
   5-Fluorouracil 500 mg/m² IV days 1 and 8 or days 1 and 4
   Doxorubicin 50 mg/m2 IV day 1
   (Or by 72-h continuous infusion)
   Cyclophosphamide 500 mg/m² IV day 1
   (Cycled every 21 days for six cycles)
5. *CMF chemotherapy*
   Cyclophosphamide 100 mg/m2 (PO) days 1–14
   Methotrexate 40 mg/m² IV days 1 and 8
   5-Fluorouracil 600 mg/m² IV days 1 and 8
   (Cycled every 28 days for six cycles)
6. *CAF chemotherapy*
   Cyclophosphamide 100 mg/m2 PO days 1–14
   Doxorubicin 30 mg/m2 IV days 1 and 8
   5-Fluorouracil 500 mg/m² IV days 1 and 8
   (Cycled every 28 days for six cycles)
7. *FEC chemotherapy*
   5-Fluorouracil 500 mg/m² IV day 1
   Epirubicin 100 mg/m² IV day 1
   Cyclophosphamide 500 mg/m2 IV day 1

(Cycled every 21 days for three cycles)
(With myeloid growth factor support)

Taxane Regimens

1. *Dose-dense AC followed by paclitaxel chemotherapy*
   Doxorubicin 60 mg/m2 IV day 1
   Cyclophosphamide 600 mg/m2 IV day 1
   (Cycled every 14 days for four cycles)
   Followed by paclitaxel 175 mg/m2 by 3-h IV infusion day 1
   (Cycled every 14 days for four cycles)
   (All cycles with myeloid growth factor support)
2. *Dose-dense AC followed by weekly paclitaxel chemotherapy*
   Doxorubicin 60 mg/m2 IV day 1
   Cyclophosphamide 600 mg/m2 IV day 1
   (Cycled every 14 days for four cycles)
   (All cycles with myeloid growth factor support)
   Followed by paclitaxel 80 mg/m² by 1-h IV infusion weekly for 12 weeks
3. *TAC chemotherapy*
   Docetaxel 75 mg/m2 IV day 1
   Doxorubicin 50 mg/m2 IV day 1
   Cyclophosphamide 500 mg/m2 IV day 1
   (Cycled every 21 days for six cycles)
   (All cycles with myeloid growth factor support)
4. *FEC followed by docetaxel chemotherapy*
   5-Fluorouracil 500 mg/m2 IV day 1
   Epirubicin 100 mg/m2 IV day 1
   Cyclophosphamide 500 mg m2 IV day 1
   (Cycled every 21 days for three cycles)
   Followed by docetaxel 100 mg/m2 IV day 1
   (Cycled every 21 days for three cycles)
   (All cycles with myeloid growth factor support)
5. *FEC followed by weekly paclitaxel*
   5-Fluorouracil 600 mg/m2 IV day 1
   Epirubicin 90 mg/m2 IV day 1
   Cyclophosphamide 600 mg/m2 IV day 1
   (Cycled every 21 days for four cycles)
   (With myeloid growth factor support)
   Followed by paclitaxel 100 mg/m2 IV infusion weekly for 8 weeks
6. *FAC followed by weekly paclitaxel*
   5-Fluorouracil 500 mg/m² IV days 1 and 8 or days 1 and 4

Doxorubicin 50 mg/m2 IV day 1
(Or by 72-h continuous infusion)
Cyclophosphamide 500 mg/m2 IV day 1
(Cycled every 21 days for six cycles)
Followed by paclitaxel 80 mg/m2 by 1-h IV infusion weekly for 12 weeks

7. *AC followed by docetaxel chemotherapy*
Doxorubicin 60 mg/m2 IV on day 1
Cyclophosphamide 600 mg/m2 IV day 1
Cycled every 21 days for four cycles
Followed by docetaxel 100 mg/m2 IV on day 1
(Cycled every 21 days for four cycles)
(All docetaxel cycles with myeloid growth factor support)

8. *TC chemotherapy*
Docetaxel 75 mg/m^2 IV day 1
Cyclophosphamide 600 mg/m^2 IV day 1
(Cycled every 21 days for four cycles)
(All cycles with myeloid growth factor support)

Special Considerations

Adjuvant Chemotherapy for Triple-Negative Disease

TNBC was identified in the early 2000s as a clinically important subgroup of breast cancer characterized by poor prognosis. The risk of distant recurrence was remarkably higher in patients with TNBC than in those with non-TNBC, peaking 3 years after diagnosis. By definition, triple-negative tumors lack expression of ER, PR, and HER2, the established markers used to select patients for adjuvant endocrine therapy or trastuzumab therapy, respectively. Approximately 80 % of TNBCs have a basal-like molecular profile [151]. Beyond the basal-like profile, TNBC encompasses other molecular intrinsic subtypes, particularly normal-like and the recently described claudin-low subtypes. Of basal-like breast cancers, approximately 80 % are TNBC [152]. Most germline mutant BRCA1-associated breast cancers are TNBC, but only a minority of TNBC has a BRCA1 mutation. Somatic TNBCs may have BRCA1 functional loss in the absence of a gene mutation due to downregulated BRCA1 transcription and/or translation and may share phenotypic features with BRCA-mutated tumors [153]. As the overlap between TNBC, basal-like breast cancer, and BRCA1 mutation-associated breast cancer is incomplete, these terms cannot be used synonymously.

Thus far, most clinical trials attempting to define optimal adjuvant regimens have included patients based on clinical stage, irrespective of tumor hormonal receptor or HER2 status. Retrospective subset analyses have attempted to characterize outcomes for patients defined by tumor ER and/or HER2 status. However, such analyses have frequently lacked the power to characterize outcomes in TNBC. Most results suggest high sensitivity to chemotherapy in TNBC. However, due to the lack of randomized phase III trials with a conventional control arm, whether this increased sensitivity is agent specific or reflects general chemosensitivity remains to be determined. Due to the phenotypic similarities between TNBC and BRCA-associated tumors, it is tempting to extend promising therapeutic strategies exploiting defective DNA repair in BRCA-associated tumors to the larger subset of sporadic TN tumors. However, much as the terms for TNBC, basal-like breast cancer and BRCA1-associated breast cancer cannot be used synonymously due to incomplete overlap; extrapolation of treatment results between these groups may be inappropriate. Biological heterogeneity within the TNBC cohort prevents such an assumption. In patients with BRCA mutations, platinum combinations may be an option.

Alkylating Agents

Cyclophosphamide is the most commonly used alkylating agent in breast cancer. Classical CMF (cyclophosphamide, methotrexate, and 5- fluorouracil) is reported to be effective in the treatment of TNBC. The International Breast Cancer Study Group (IBCSG) trials VIII and IX compared three or six courses of CMF (with or without endocrine therapy) with endocrine therapy alone. An analysis of these trials showed a benefit for CMF over endocrine therapy only in the subset of women with TNBC (HR: 0.46; 95 % CI 0.29–0.73; $p = 0.009$) [154].

Anthracyclines

The effectiveness of anthracycline-containing regimens for TNBC has been reported in the neo-adjuvant setting [155]; however, data regarding the benefit of anthracyclines as adjuvant regimens are conflicting. Preclinical evidence also suggests inconsistent results in terms of anthracycline activity in BRCA-deficient breast cancer cells. Cell line studies have revealed differential chemosensitivity based on the BRCA status, with BRCA1/BRCA2 loss associated with increased sensitivity to topoisomerase IIa (topoIIa) inhibitors [156]. In one study, blockade of the topoIIa enzyme prior to exposure to the topoIIa inhibitor markedly reduced cytotoxicity and eliminated any differential BRCA effects, indicating indirect DNA damage via binding of the cytotoxics to the topoIIa protein rather than direct DNA damage [157]. Conversely, other *in vitro* work demonstrated greater sensitivity to doxorubicin in BRCA1 wild type compared with BRCA1-mutant breast cancer cells [158]. Clinical studies have revealed concordant results. For instance, the MA5 adjuvant trial, which compared classical CMF with CEF (cyclophosphamide, epirubicin, and 5-fluorouracil) in premenopausal women with node-positive early-stage breast cancer, determined that classical CMF had similar efficacy as CEF regarding RFS and OS rates (HR: 1.1; 95 % CI 0.6–2.1 for RFS and HR: 1.3; 95 % CI 0.7–2.5 for OS] in a subset of women who had breast cancer of the basal phenotype [22]. However, post hoc analysis of a phase III trial reported that adjuvant CMF was inferior to the combination of epirubicin plus CMF in terms of the 5-year DFS (59 % vs. 85 %, respectively; $p = 0.002$) and overall survival (73 % vs. 91 %, respectively; $p = 0.002$) in TNBC patients [159]. According to the available evidence, anthracyclines should still be considered an important component of chemotherapy for TNBC.

Taxanes

The addition of taxanes to adjuvant anthracycline-based therapy has been evaluated several times in populations unselected for biology in the aforementioned early-stage breast cancer trials. The results specifically in TNBC are limited; however,

a preferential benefit of microtubule-stabilizing agents has not been clearly demonstrated. Subset analyses of several large trials suggest that taxane combinations (with cyclophosphamide and doxorubicin) are also beneficial in the treatment of TNBC and may be more effective in this subset than chemotherapy combinations that do not include a taxane [160]. Moreover, a retrospective analysis of three adjuvant chemotherapy trials coordinated by CALGB and the US Breast Intergroup revealed that women with ER-negative tumors treated with regimens including higher doses, taxanes, and dose-dense scheduling fared better in terms of the risk of recurrence and OS. ER-negative women who received dose-dense doxorubicin and cyclophosphamide followed by paclitaxel (AC→T) compared to low-dose cyclophosphamide, doxorubicin, and 5-fluorouracil (CAF) experienced a 55 % (95 % CI 37–68 %) relative reduction in the risk of recurrence. Unplanned subset analyses of the subgroups demonstrated that women who were both ER and HER2 negative achieved a statistically significant improvement in DFS with the addition of paclitaxel therapy ($p = 0.002$), whereas ER+ HER2(−) individuals did not experience a similar benefit ($p = 0.71$), thereby supporting the inclusion of taxanes in adjuvant therapy for the treatment of patients with TNBC [161].

The Early Breast Cancer Trialists' Collaborative Group has demonstrated that both anthracyclines and taxanes are effective adjuvant chemotherapeutic agents in hormonal receptor-negative breast cancers, with anthracycline-based regimens conferring modest benefits over non-anthracycline, CMF-type regimens, and taxane-based regimens superior to non-taxane alternatives [113]. A meta-analysis of 12 randomized clinical trials demonstrated that adjuvant docetaxel-based chemotherapy is associated with an improvement in DFS and OS in TNBC compared with regimens without taxanes [160]. Similarly, the PACS 01 trial comparing FEC with FEC followed by docetaxel demonstrated significantly better metastasis-free survival and OS for the incorporation of docetaxel among patients with a basal-like profile, as defined by an immunohistochemical panel [162]. Nonsignificant trends in favor of taxanes in TNBC were observed in the GEICAM 9805 trial, which compared docetaxel, doxorubicin, and cyclophosphamide (TAC) with fluorouracil, doxorubicin, and cyclophosphamide (FAC) in node-negative, high-risk breast cancer and in BCIRG 001, which compared TAC with FAC in node-positive disease [130, 163]. In the BCIRG trial, subgroup analyses addressing 3-year DFS revealed a nonsignificant trend ($p = 0.051$) in the TNBC subgroup in favor of TAC over FAC (74 % vs. 60 %, respectively; HR 0.50; 95 % CI 0.29–1.00).

Using immunohistochemical testing for HER2 positivity in tissue blocks from 1322 women, Hayes et al. [161] investigated whether paclitaxel added after adjuvant AC was equally beneficial to all biological subgroups of CALGB9344 participants. Paclitaxel was associated with improved DFS in the subset of women with HER2-negative, ER-negative tumors.

However, an additional benefit from taxanes has not been consistently observed in this subgroup of patients. The TACT trial observed no significant difference between treatment arms in TNBC when FEC followed by docetaxel was compared to a control of FEC or FEC/CMF [127]. Moreover, in the PACS 04 trial, which compared FEC100 with concurrent epirubicin and docetaxel, no differential effect was observed in TNBC [164].

Platinums

A number of recent preclinical studies examining the activity of platinum agents in the treatment of TNBC and BRCA1-associated breast cancers have demonstrated increased sensitivity to these agents. Because BRCA1-associated tumors are deficient in the genes encoding proteins that are critical in DNA integrity, genomic stability, and DNA repair, increased susceptibility to DNA-damaging agents is expected. In preclinical models of BRCA1-deficient breast cancers, increased cytotoxicity of platinum agents through the induction of double-strand breaks has been observed [165, 166]. In addition, the p53 family member p63 has been determined to control a survival pathway that directly mediates cisplatin sensitivity in TNBC. *In vitro*, the co-expression

of p63/p73 in TNBC tumors was identified as a predictor of sensitivity to cisplatin but not to other standard chemotherapy agents in TNBC, warranting further investigation of p63/p73 as biomarkers to predict the response to platinum therapy [167].

Clinical data for carboplatin and cisplatin in TNBC are limited, with data predominantly emerging from small studies and retrospective analyses. In a small study, nine of ten women (90 %) with TNBC and a BRCA1 mutation had a pCR with single-agent cisplatin treatment [168]. A small neoadjuvant study tested 4 cycles of single-agent cisplatin in 28 patients, 2 of whom had a germline BRCA1 mutation and pCR after chemotherapy [169]. The pCR rate was 22 %. A pCR was achieved in 4 of 26 patients with sporadic TNBC (15 %). The only randomized phase II data evaluating the effect of cisplatin in TNBC are from the metastatic setting. A single institution trial included 126 TNBC patients pretreated with anthracycline and taxane therapy and then randomized to metronomic oral cyclophosphamide and methotrexate with or without cisplatin as second-line therapy. The cisplatin arm was associated with improvements in the overall response rate (33 % vs. 63 %), median time to progression (7 months vs. 13 months), and median OS (12 months vs. 16 months).

The issue of cross-sensitivity between carboplatin and cisplatin must also be defined. Currently, there are no randomized phase III data regarding the use of carboplatin instead of cisplatin. Thus, using platinums for the adjuvant treatment of TNBC remains under investigation and is not currently recommended in this setting. Given the small numbers of patients in the above-mentioned trials, it is difficult to draw conclusions regarding reduction in risk of recurrence and survival. However, these data do suggest the activity of platinum agents in the TNBC subgroup and warrant further study.

Capecitabine

Capecitabine has been investigated in the adjuvant setting for the prevention of breast cancer recurrence. CALGB49907, a prospective trial, evaluated the efficacy of the possibly less toxic single-agent capecitabine among elderly breast cancer patients (65 years or older) in the adjuvant setting. In this trial, both the risk of relapse (HR: 2.09; 95 % CI 1.38–3.17; $p < 0.001$) and the risk of death (HR: 1.85; 95 % CI 1.11–3.08; $p = 0.02$) were significantly higher with capecitabine compared with standard chemotherapy [170]. Unplanned subgroup analyses demonstrated that patients with hormonal receptor-negative cancer benefited more from standard therapy than from capecitabine. In the FINXX adjuvant study, three cycles of docetaxel plus capecitabine (TX) followed by three cycles of CEX (cyclophosphamide, epirubicin, and capecitabine) indicated a trend towards improved 5-year recurrence-free survival (RFS) compared with three cycles of docetaxel (T) followed by three cycles of CEF (T-CEF; 87 % vs. 84 %, respectively; HR 0.79; 95 % CI 0.60–1.04; $p = 0.087$) [147]. In an exploratory analysis of the TNBC subgroup comprising 202 patients, TXCEX was associated with longer RFS compared with T-CEF (HR 0.48; 95 % CI 0.26–0.88; $p = 0.018$).

A randomized phase III study of standard adjuvant chemotherapy alone or followed by 1 year of metronomic capecitabine (650 mg/m^2 twice daily) is underway, with DFS as the primary endpoint (NCT01112826). Thus far, capecitabine has not been specifically studied in the triple-negative population. Another multicenter phase III clinical study (NCT01642771) is being conducted among TNBC patients on two adjuvant chemotherapy regimens: sequential docetaxel followed by FEC and sequential docetaxel and capecitabine followed by capecitabine/epirubicin/cyclophosphamide (XEC). The primary outcome measure is 5-year DFS. The results of these trials are awaited to reach further conclusions regarding the efficacy and safety of adjuvant capecitabine among TNBC patients. Other adjuvant trials that are ongoing among TNBC patients are summarized in Table 8.7.

Poly(ADP-Ribose) Polymerase (PARP) Inhibitors

The products of the *BRCA1* and *BRCA2* genes have roles in a highly specialized form of DNA repair, homologous recombination [171, 172]. When the remaining wild-type allele is lost in a tumor precursor cell, this repair mechanism does not function, and the consequent rapid onset of genome instability is sufficient to enable tumor development [173]. Studies of invasive primary breast tumors in individuals with *BRCA1* and *BRCA2* mutations confirm the loss of the remaining wild-type allele [174, 175]. These findings support the clinical usefulness of tumor-specific targeting of the loss of *BRCA1*-associated or *BRCA2*-associated homologous recombination DNA repair in breast cancer patients. Poly(ADP-ribose) polymerase-1 (PARP) is a crucial nuclear enzyme that is involved in the recognition of DNA damage and the facilitation of single-strand DNA repair through the base excision repair (BER) pathway. Following the detection of a DNA strand break, PARP1, as the predominant cellular PARP, catalyzes the synthesis and transfer of ADP-ribose polymers to target proteins to recruit other repair enzymes and facilitate DNA repair and cell survival [176].

The idea of synthetic lethality via the inhibition of PARP has been investigated in preclinical model systems with hereditary mutations in the BRCA1 or BRCA2 genes. The principle hypothesis is based on the assumption that DNA damage by PARP inhibition is irreparable and leads to cell death in homozygote tumor cells but not in normal tissue heterozygote cells, which have one functional BRCA allele [177]. As previously mentioned, preclinical tumor models of BRCA-associated breast cancers have demonstrated increased sensitivity to therapies such as alkylators that induce DNA damage [156, 157]. Farmer et al. [178] demonstrated that BRCA-deficient breast cell lines were highly sensitive to PARP inhibition. Single-agent PARP inhibitors led to impaired single-strand break (SSB) repair, causing double-strand breaks (DSBs) to occur in replicating cells. In BRCA wild-type cells, DSBs are repaired via homologous recombination, but in BRCA-mutant cells, this compensatory repair pathway is impaired, leading to complex rearrangements, repair mechanism loss, and cell death. Concordantly, a phase II study of the PARP inhibitor olaparib verified this strategy in

Table 8.7 Ongoing adjuvant phase III–IV clinical trials involving triple-negative breast cancer patients

NCI ID	Status	Primary location	Stage	Regimen
NCT01112826	Recruiting	Guangzhou, China	T1c-3, N0-2	*Arm A*: standard adjuvant chemotherapy followed by capecitabine 650 mg/m² (1 year)
				Arm B: standard adjuvant chemotherapy
NCT00789581	Active/not recruiting	Nashville, TN	Node-negative T1c-T3 OR node-positive pN1mi -N2b	*Arm A*: doxorubicin and cyclophosphamide D1 ×4 (q21 days) followed by ixabepilone d1 ×4 (q21 days)
				Arm B: doxorubicin and cyclophosphamide D1 ×4 (q21 days) followed by paclitaxel d1 ×12 (q7 days)
NCT01216111	Expanded access	Shanghai, China	Stages I–IIIA	Paclitaxel and cisplatin AUC (2) D1, 8,15 (q28 days)
NCT00630032	Active/not recruiting	Nantes Saint, Herblain/France	Node-positive disease or node-negative and stages II–III or pT>20 mm	*Arm A*: epirubicin and 5-FU and cyclophosphamide D1 ×3 (q21 days) followed by docetaxel ×3 (q21 days)
				Arm B: epirubicin and 5-FU and cyclophosphamide D1 ×3 (q21 days) followed by ixabepilone D1 ×3 (q21 days)
NCT01642771	Recruiting	China	Node positive or node negative and pT>1 cm	*Arm A*: 5-FU and epirubicin and cyclophosphamide D1 ×3 (q21 days) followed by docetaxel ×3 (q21 days)
				Arm B: Docetaxel and capecitabine D1 ×3 (q21 days) followed by docetaxel and capecitabine and epirubicin D1 ×3 (q21 days)
NCT01150513	Recruiting	Beijing, China	Any	*Arm A*: epirubicin and cyclophosphamide D1 ×4 (q21 days)
				Arm B: docetaxel and carboplatin AUC (6) D1 ×6 (q21 days)

patients with advanced or recurrent BRCA1-/BRCA2-mutated breast cancer [179]. The most frequent causally related adverse events in the cohort receiving 400 mg twice daily were fatigue (grade 1 or 2 in 41 %, grade 3 or 4 in 15 %), nausea (grade 1 or 2 in 41 %, grade 3 or 4 in 15 %), vomiting (grade 1 or 2 in 11 %, grade 3 or 4 in 11 %), and anemia (grade 1 or 2 in 4 %, grade 3 or 4 in 11 %). The predominance of grade 1–2 adverse events demonstrated the safety profile of these molecules among patients who were heavily treated with a median of three previous chemotherapy regimens. The results of the trial indicated significant objective response rates of 41 % (95 % CI: 25–59 %) among the cohort receiving 400 mg BID and 22 % (95 % CI 11–41 %) among the cohort receiving 100 mg BID. The median PFS was also significantly prolonged in both cohorts (maximal dose cohort 5.7 months (CI% 4.6–7.4), low-dose cohort 3.8 months (CI% 4.6–7.4), further supporting the efficacy of PARP inhibitors in BRCA-deficient cells. The results are promising but remain inadequate for PARP inhibitors to be considered as part of an adjuvant treatment modality in TNBC patients.

Ixabepilone

Ixabepilone is a member of the epothilone class of macrolide antibiotics, which possess high microtubule-stabilizing activity and low susceptibility to drug resistance mechanisms, including multidrug-resistant protein and P-glycoprotein [180]. In the United States, ixabepilone is approved for use in combination with capecitabine for the treatment of metastatic or locally advanced breast cancer after failure of an anthracycline and a taxane. It is also approved in the United States as a monotherapy in the same setting after failure of an anthracycline, a taxane, and capecitabine.

The utility of ixabepilone among TNBC patients arises from a subgroup analysis of a phase II study in the neoadjuvant setting that demonstrated a pCR rate of 19 % for TNBC [181]. Notably, a retrospective analysis of previous phase II studies (including patients in the neoadjuvant and metastatic setting) showed activity for ixabepilone in TNBC patients, including patients who had previously received or were resistant to anthracyclines, taxanes, and capecitabine [182]. However, a more recent neoadjuvant phase II trial that randomized patients to AC followed by ixabepilone vs. AC followed by paclitaxel did not demonstrate a significant difference in pCR rates between the two regimens, 34 % vs. 41 % [183]. In light of this finding, the two adjuvant phase III trials PACS08 (NCT00630032) and TITAN (NCT00789581)),

which were initiated to compare ixabepilone directly with more commonly used taxanes, have been terminated by Bristol-Myers Squibb. Although it is no longer recruiting patients, the TITAN study remains ongoing. The study randomized early-stage TNBC patients to adjuvant doxorubicin/cyclophosphamide (AC) followed by ixabepilone or AC followed by weekly paclitaxel, and the primary outcome measure was defined as DFS. The findings of this trial should elucidate the efficacy of ixabepilone in the adjuvant setting.

Data from several phase III and phase II studies have indicated a survival benefit for different TNBC subgroups treated with ixabepilone alone or in combination with other agents. In two phase III trials with large TNBC subpopulations, combination therapy with ixabepilone and capecitabine significantly improved the overall response rate (RR) and prolonged PFS compared with single-agent capecitabine in TNBC that had already progressed following treatment with anthracyclines and taxanes. A prospective analysis of the pooled data for TNBC patients from the two studies revealed a median overall RR of 31 % and 15 % for the combination and single-agent capecitabine arms, respectively. The median PFS was 4.2 months in patients receiving combination therapy and 1.7 months in capecitabine monotherapy recipients (HR 0.63; 95 % CI 0.52–0.77) [184]. However, no significant difference in the median OS of the two arms (10.3 months and 9.0 months, respectively, HR: 0.87; 95 % CI 0.71–1.07) was observed.

Targeted Therapies

Bevacizumab

High levels of vascular endothelial growth factor (VEGF) and VEGF-2 in women with TNBC have led to the emergence of agents that target angiogenesis. Thus, VEGF may be a prognostic tool as well as a putative target for therapeutic intervention [185, 186]. Bevacizumab, a humanized monoclonal antibody to VEGF, has been evaluated in large phase III clinical trials in combination with paclitaxel [187]. E2100, an open-label, randomized, phase III trial conducted by

ECOG, demonstrated a significant improvement in PFS and overall response rate (ORR) with paclitaxel plus bevacizumab compared with paclitaxel alone as initial chemotherapy for patients with HER2-negative metastatic breast cancer. The risk of progression was reduced by more than half and the ORR nearly doubled with the addition of bevacizumab to weekly paclitaxel in the analyses, confirming a substantial and robust bevacizumab treatment effect. The PFS was 8.8 months in TNBC patients receiving bevacizumab plus paclitaxel vs. 4.6 months in those receiving paclitaxel alone (HR 0.53; 95 % CI 0.40–0.70). However, OS was not significantly improved in the whole population.

Bevacizumab has been evaluated in further clinical trials in combination with docetaxel or capecitabine as a first-line and second-line treatment for metastatic breast cancer [188–190]. Subgroup analyses of these studies suggested similar PFS benefits for bevacizumab plus a taxane in patients with TNBC and those with non-TNBC [187, 188]. Adjuvant bevacizumab in combination with taxanes was eventually prospectively investigated in TNBC in the BEATRICE trial [191]. The study included T1b–T3 or T1a tumors with ipsilateral axillary node involvement that were centrally confirmed as HER2 negative by FISH or chromogenic in situ hybridization with either negative or low hormone receptor status. A total of 1290 patients were randomized to receive a minimum of four cycles of chemotherapy either alone or with bevacizumab (equivalent of 5 mg/kg every week for 1 year). The primary endpoint was defined as invasive disease-free survival (IDFS). The median follow-up was approximately 32 months for both groups at the time of IDFS analysis. The 3-year IDFS was 82.7 % (95 % CI 80.5–85.0) with chemotherapy alone and 83.7 % (81.4–86.0) with bevacizumab and chemotherapy. There was no difference in OS between the groups (HR 0.84, 95 % CI 0.64–1.12; $p = 0.23$). Nearly half of the study group (49 %) consented to the biomarker study, and 1178 (45 %) were included in the biomarker-assessable population. Analysis of the baseline plasma VEGF-A concentration showed neither prognostic nor predictive value.

By contrast, exploratory biomarker assessment suggested that patients with high pretreatment plasma VEGFR-2 levels might benefit from the addition of bevacizumab (Cox interaction test, $p = 0.029$). However, the use of bevacizumab vs. chemotherapy alone was associated with an increased incidence of adverse events such as grade 3 or worse hypertension (12 % vs. 1 %), severe cardiac events occurring at any point during the 18-month safety reporting period (1 % vs. <0.5 %), and treatment discontinuation. The data are partially immature due to the low rate of events, although the protocol-specified number of events for the primary analysis was reached. The low rate of recurrence was attributed to the high proportion of patients with node-negative disease (63 %) enrolled into BEATRICE; this finding could have important implications for interpretation and follow-up. The investigators concluded that bevacizumab could not be recommended as an adjuvant treatment in otherwise unselected TNBC patients. Final efficacy results with a median follow-up of 56 months also failed to demonstrate a significant difference in OS between the treatment arms. The 5-year OS rates were 88 % (95 % CI 85.7–89.6 %) with CT alone and 88 % (95 % CI 86.0–89.8 %) with chemotherapy plus bevacizumab [192].

Concordantly, another trial investigating the efficacy of adjuvant bevacizumab failed to demonstrate a survival benefit among HER2-expressing high-risk node-negative or node-positive breast cancer patients [193]. The BETH trial included two patient cohorts receiving anthracycline (three cycles of docetaxel+trastuzumab followed by three cycles of FEC followed by 1-year trastuzumab) and non-anthracycline (six cycles of docetaxel+carbo platin+trastuzumab followed by 1-year trastuzumab) regimens. Both of the cohorts were stratified into two arms: bevacizumab combined with chemotherapy and thereafter with trastuzumab and no bevacizumab. High-risk, node-negative early-stage breast cancer was defined as the presence of at least one of the following criteria: age <35 years, ER- and PR-negative disease, pathological tumor size >2 cm, and histological and/or nuclear grade ≥2. The primary objective of the study was comparing invasive disease-free survival (IDFS) for the bevacizumab-included and no bevacizumab arms. The study did not meet its primary endpoint at the median follow-up time of 38 months. The addition of 1-year bevacizumab combined with chemotherapy plus trastuzumab treatment did not prolong IDFS [HR 0.99, 95 % CI 0.79–1.25, $p=0.96$]. In addition, the integration of bevacizumab increased the rate of adverse events such as hypertension (19 % vs. 4 %), congestive heart failure (2.1 % vs. 1 %), and bleeding (2 % vs. 1 %). A similar phase III trial (E5103) comparing doxorubicin and cyclophosphamide followed by paclitaxel with bevacizumab or placebo also failed to demonstrate a survival benefit [194].

EGFR Inhibitors: Cetuximab

EGFR is frequently overexpressed in TNBC (60 %) and is a negative prognostic factor when present [195, 196]. This profile has been suggested as a potential target for EGFR-directed therapies. Clinically, EGFR inhibitors have been studied in the metastatic setting. A randomized, phase II, multicenter trial examined sequential cetuximab followed by carboplatin at the time of progression vs. concurrent cetuximab/carboplatin in pretreated TNBC patients [197]. Due to poor response rates for single-agent cetuximab in the sequential arm, this arm of the trial was closed to accrual early. Most patients rapidly progressed, and the overall median PFS was 2.0 months. Preliminary data from another phase II trial suggested improved response rates in the cetuximab and irinotecan/carboplatin arm (39 % vs. 19 %), thus advocating combination regimens rather than single-agent cetuximab [198]. The triple-therapy regimen achieved a higher overall RR (49 % vs. 30 %) and longer median survival (15.5 months vs. 12.3 months) than chemotherapy alone, although PFS appeared to be shorter (4.7 months vs. 5.1 months). The overall RR with the triple-therapy regimen was higher in TNBC than in the overall study population (49 % vs. 38 %, respectively).

An evaluation of the combination of a standard chemotherapy (FEC100 followed by docetaxel) with panitumumab as neoadjuvant therapy for operable TNBC was recently reported with a pCR rate of 65 % [199]. A neoadjuvant phase II open-label study (NCT 01097642) is currently recruiting T1N1-3M0 or T2-4N0-3M0 patients with TNBC who are candidates for preoperative chemotherapy. Patients are being equally randomized between ixabepilone and ixabepilone plus cetuximab. The primary objective of the study is to determine the pCR rate for the breast and axilla. As a result, cetuximab, used in combination with other agents, may have potential for use in TNBC; however, further studies are warranted to investigate the benefit/risk profile of these combinations.

Adjuvant Chemotherapy for Male Breast Cancer

Male breast carcinoma is a rare condition. Few male breast cancer-specific epidemiological or clinical trial data are available; thus, our understanding of male breast cancer comes from studies of female breast cancer, painting an inaccurate picture of contributing factors. In the United States, approximately 2140 new cases of breast cancer in men are diagnosed annually, and 450 deaths occur; this number represents less than 0.5 % of all cancer deaths in men annually. Approximately 1 % of all breast cancers occur in men, but the male/female ratio is higher among black than among white populations. In areas of Central Africa, breast cancer accounts for up to 6 % of cancers in men, and the male/female ratio is much higher compared with the White population (100:1 vs. 70:1) [200]. African populations also have a poorer prognosis, even after adjustment for clinical, demographic, and treatment factors [201].

There is usually no identifiable risk factor that differs from those for female breast cancer; family history, Jewish ancestry, obesity, low physical activity levels, prior chest wall irradiation, and benign breast disease are all believed to play a role [200]. However, specific to male subjects, gynecomastia, Klinefelter syndrome, a history of testicular or liver pathology, and a history of fracture after age 45 are indicated as having a causal relationship with breast cancer in males [202]. For Klinefelter syndrome, high serum concentrations of gonadotropins in response to low serum testosterone levels result in a high estrogen-to-testosterone ratio [203]. Similarly, testicular injury such as orchitis and cryptorchidism is believed to reduce testosterone levels compared with estrogen levels [204]. Several risk factors involving an imbalance between estrogenic and androgenic influences, as is the case for liver disease, may suppress the protective effect of androgens on breast tissue. However, other conditions associated with an increased estrogen-to-testosterone ratio, such as obesity, thyroid disease, marijuana use, and exogenous estrogen use (e.g., transsexuals, patients undergoing prostate cancer treatment), have a less certain relationship with male breast cancer.

Despite differences in the molecular characteristics of breast cancer associated with both age and ethnicity, the most common subtype of breast cancer in men is hormonal receptor-positive disease, as demonstrated in a registry study of male breast cancer patients in which 82 % comprised the hormonal receptor positive subgroup [205]. Non-Hispanic Black men were more likely to have TNBC than non-Hispanic White or Hispanic men (9 % vs. 3 % and 6 %, respectively). Cancers of the male breast are significantly more likely to express hormonal receptors than cancers of the female breast, even after adjustment for tumor stage, grade, and patient age [206]. As in female breast cancer, the rates of hormonal receptor positivity increase with increasing patient age. By contrast, the HER2-neu proto-oncogene is less likely to be overexpressed in cancers of the male breast [207].

Tumor size and lymph node involvement are two clear prognostic factors for male patients with breast cancer. Men with tumors measuring 2–5 cm have a 40 % higher risk of death than men with tumors with a maximum diameter <2 cm [206]. Similarly, men with lymph node involvement have a 50 % higher risk of death than those without lymph node involvement. In general, the prognosis for male and female patients with breast cancer is similar. Overall survival rates appear to be lower for men; however, this is prob-ably due to older age at diagnosis because the age-adjusted survival rates are comparable between male and female subjects [208].

Local therapy for breast cancer is generally similar in men and women. Most men are treated with modified radical mastectomy with axillary lymph node dissection or sentinel node biopsy. After appropriate surgery, adjuvant systemic therapy is recommended for the majority of men with breast cancer. The same guidelines for adjuvant systemic therapy in women with early-stage breast cancer are generally followed for men with breast cancer [209]. Recommendations for adjuvant chemotherapy are based largely upon the benefits that have been observed in clinical trials performed in women [9]. One prospective study of adjuvant chemotherapy in men was published in 1987 [210]. Twenty-four stage II (node-positive) male breast cancer patients were treated with cyclophosphamide, methotrexate, and 5-fluorouracil (CMF). The 5-year survival rate projected by actuarial means was in excess of 80 % (95 % CI 74–100 %), higher than that for historical controls of similar stage. The authors concluded that the CMF regimen was feasible and was associated with substantial improvement in DFS and OS. Yildirim et al. [211] published follow-up data for 121 male breast cancer patients, 60 % of whom received systemic adjuvant treatment (chemotherapy and hormonal therapy). Adjuvant chemotherapy was associated with a 40 % risk reduction for death. Similarly, publications regarding adjuvant chemotherapy for male breast cancer are mainly retrospective and usually reflect institutional experience [212, 213]. A retrospective study from MD Anderson Cancer Center with a median follow-up of 13 years noted a survival benefit from adjuvant chemotherapy with a 22 % risk reduction among node-positive patients, which was not statistically significant [214]. Chemotherapy was administered to 32 men (84 % as an adjuvant modality); approximately 81 % received anthracycline-based regimens, 9 % received additional taxanes, and 16 % were treated with cyclophosphamide, methotrexate, and 5-fluorouracil (CMF). The 5-year and 10-year OS rates were 86 % and 75 %, respectively, for men with lymph node-negative disease and 70 % and 43 %, respectively, for men with lymph node-positive disease. OS was significantly better for men who received adjuvant hormonal therapy (HR of 0.45; $p = 0.01$).

In view of the findings of a clear benefit for adjuvant chemotherapy in women and the positive trends of adjuvant chemotherapy in small series in men, adjuvant chemotherapy should be considered for men with intermediate- or high-risk primary breast cancer, particularly those with hormonal receptor-negative disease. The role of taxanes or dose-dense chemotherapy in male breast cancer has not been adequately established. Well-powered randomized trials for male breast cancer are unlikely. Therefore, given the established benefit of taxanes in women and the suggestive evidence in men, taxanes may be considered when lymph nodes are involved. Because no specific data are available, adjuvant trastuzumab should be considered according to patient and tumor characteristics following female breast cancer guidelines.

Adjuvant Chemotherapy of Pregnancy-Associated Breast Cancer

Gestational or pregnancy-associated breast cancer is defined as breast cancer that is diagnosed during pregnancy, within the first postpartum year, or during lactation. It is a relatively uncommon event. The incidence of pregnancy-associated breast cancer is approximately 15–35 per 100,000 deliveries, with fewer breast cancer cases diagnosed during pregnancy than during the first postpartum year [215, 216]. With the increasing trend for women to delay childbearing, the co-occurrence of cancer and pregnancy, reported to have an average frequency of 1 in 1000 births, is increasing [217]. Breast cancer during pregnancy requires a multidisciplinary approach because the well-being of both the mother and the fetus must be considered in any treatment planning.

The majority of breast cancers in pregnant women are invasive ductal adenocarcinomas, as in nonpregnant women [217–219]. However, pregnancy-associated breast cancers are predominantly poorly differentiated and diagnosed at an advanced stage, particularly in those diagnosed while lactating [216]. In addition, the incidence of inflammatory breast cancer is higher among pregnancy-associated breast cancer than breast cancer in nonpregnant women, but this trend has not been consistently observed. Despite multiple opportunities for clinical breast examinations arising from the increased frequency of physician visits, breast examination during pregnancy is hampered by hypertrophy, engorgement, and indistinct nodularity of the gland. Moreover, densities and nodularities in the breasts of pregnant women are often overlooked or ascribed to benign proliferative changes. The hyperestrogenic state of pregnancy may also contribute to the development and rapid growth of breast carcinoma in these women. In addition, obstetricians frequently direct their attention to the developing fetus and do not perform a comprehensive physical examination. These factors often cause a delay in diagnosis and advanced disease presentation.

The majority of tumors diagnosed during pregnancy are high-grade tumors [219, 220]. Lymphovascular invasion is a frequent finding and is also a negative prognostic factor [221, 222]. Most series report a lower frequency of ER and PR expression in pregnancy-associated breast cancer compared with breast cancer in nonpregnant patients (approximately 25 % vs. 55–60 %) [221, 223, 224]. This immunohistochemical profile does not appear to differ from age-matched, nonpregnant women [225, 226]. It is believed that the age of the breast carcinoma patient and not the pregnancy itself affects the biological features of the tumor. Therefore, breast carcinomas occurring during pregnancy share many histological and prognostic similarities with breast carcinoma occurring in other young women. Whether there is a higher incidence of HER2 positivity compared with nonpregnant age-matched controls is unclear [227].

The indications for systemic chemotherapy are the same in pregnant patients as in nonpregnant breast cancer patients; however, chemotherapy should not be administered at any point during the first trimester of pregnancy. The most commonly used treatment in pregnancy has been anthracycline and alkylating agent chemotherapy [228, 229]. Anthracyclines are mutagenic and carcinogenic *in vitro* and in animals [230]. Because topoisomerase IIα is overexpressed in rapidly growing tissues, targeting topoisomerase II is a potential source of damage to the embryo or the fetus [231]. By contrast, only low concentrations of anthracyclines have been detected in fetal tissues, and their cytotoxic potential remains unknown. A retrospective analysis of 160 patients with breast cancer during pregnancy revealed that following chemotherapy with an anthracycline-containing regimen, progressive maternal disease was the first cause of fetal death (40 %) [228]. A total of five malformations (3 %) were reported, three in the first trimester (80 %), which is the period of organogenesis, and two following chemotherapy during the second trimester, one of which was a case of Down's syndrome unrelated to chemotherapy and the other a case of eye malformation (congenital adherence of the iris to the cornea, without consequence). In contrast to other anticancer agents, which may rapidly cross the placenta and be completely transferred, anthracyclines cross the placenta incompletely for several reasons. First, drugs with molecular weights greater than 500 Da undergo incomplete transfer across the human placenta; the molecular weights of doxorubicin and daunorubicin are 580 and 564 Da, respectively [232]. Second, anthracyclines are substrates of P-glycoprotein, a placental drug-transporting glycoprotein of great importance *in vivo* in limiting the fetal penetration of potentially harmful compounds [233]. Moreover, the hydrophilic characteristic of doxorubicin likely decelerates its placental transfer [232]. After intravenous injection of anthracyclines, only barely detectable concentrations can be found in the fetus ex vivo. These concentrations are 100- to 1000-fold below those found in adult tissues or in the tumor in similar conditions [234]. Moreover, fetal uptake of anticancer agents can be altered by changes in both uterine and umbilical blood flow [235].

The most commonly used regimens in pregnant women with breast cancer in combination with anthracyclines are cyclophosphamide (AC) or fluorouracil and cyclophosphamide (FAC). Although experience with anthracycline-based regimens in pregnancy suggests their safety and efficacy, there are limited prospective data, particularly on the outcomes of children exposed *in utero*. In a prospective single-arm study, 57 pregnant breast cancer patients were treated with FAC in the adjuvant ($n=32$) or neoadjuvant ($n=25$) setting [236]. Parents/guardians were surveyed by mail or telephone regarding outcomes of children exposed to chemotherapy *in utero*. After a median follow-up of 38.5 months, 40 patients were alive and disease-free, 3 had recurrent breast cancer, and 12 had died from breast cancer. Of the 25 patients who received neoadjuvant FAC, 6 had a pCR, whereas 4 had no tumor response to chemotherapy and eventually died from their disease. All women who delivered had live births. One child had Down's syndrome, and two had congenital anomalies (club foot, congenital bilateral uretcral reflux). The most common neonatal complication was difficulty breathing, with 10 % of the neonates requiring supplemental oxygen (likely due to prematurity). One child who was born vaginally at a gestational age of 38 weeks had a subarachnoid hemorrhage on day 2 postpartum. Although this occurred more than 3 weeks after the mother's last course of chemotherapy and although the mother's complete blood count was normal, the child had both neutropenia and thrombocytopenia. No other etiology for the subarachnoid hemorrhage was found. Other smaller retrospective series regarding the effects of chemotherapy on fetal and maternal health have revealed similar results [237, 238]. The evidence suggests that the incidence of congenital malformations is low (approximately 1.3 %) if chemotherapy is administered to women in the second or third trimester, which is after the major period of organogenesis. The estimated risk of fetal malformation due to first-trimester exposure to chemotherapeutics is 15–20 % [239, 240].

Despite the safety and efficacy of doxorubicin during and after the second trimester, at least four cases of neonatal cardiac effects have been reported after *in utero* exposure to anthracyclines, and several cases of *in utero* fetal death after exposure to idarubicin or epirubicin have also been reported [240–243]. Moreover, chemotherapy in the second or third trimester has been associated with intrauterine growth restriction, lower gestational age at birth (prematurity), and low birth weight in about one-half of exposed infants [240–242]. However, patient fears regarding the side effects of treatment should not cause a delay in the initiation of systemic chemotherapy.

A mathematical model using published data was developed to correlate primary breast tumor size with the percentage of pathologically positive axillary lymph nodes [243]. Using this relationship obtained from pathological data and the accepted relationship of tumor growth and time, an equation estimating the increased risk of axillary metastases due to each day of treatment delay was derived. The model suggests that the daily increased risk of axillary metastases due to treatment delay is 0.028 % for tumors with moderate doubling times of 130 days and 0.057 % for tumors with rapid doubling times of 65 days. Thus, according to the model, for breast cancer with a 65-day doubling time, a 1-month delay increases the risk of axillary metastases by 1.8 %, a 3-month delay by 5.2 %, and a 6-month delay by 10.2 %.

Currently, no data encourage the safety of administering dose-dense AC with or without taxanes; however, G-CSF has been reported to be safe during pregnancy. Moreover, as a general rule, breastfeeding during chemotherapy is contraindicated due to the excretion of cyclophosphamide and doxorubicin into the breast milk [244]. Methotrexate is also avoided during pregnancy due to its abortifacient effect and teratogenic potential [245]. Although no evidence indicates that cisplatin and carboplatin are harmful during pregnancy, higher levels of free drug in the mother and fetus (due to changes in cisplatin protein binding caused by lower albumin levels) may increase the risk of toxicity in both [246].

Data regarding the safety of taxanes during pregnancy are limited. A systematic review of taxane administration during pregnancy identified 23 publications describing a total of 40 women [247]. Twenty-seven patients had breast cancer,

ten had ovarian cancer, and three had non-small-cell lung cancer. Docetaxel was administered in the first trimester in two cases, and the rest received taxanes in the second or third trimester. No spontaneous abortions or intrauterine deaths were reported. In two cases exposed to paclitaxel, neonates born at 30 and 32 weeks developed acute respiratory distress possibly related to prematurity, requiring neonatal intensive care [248, 249]. The only malformation possibly related to taxanes was a case of pyloric stenosis in a neonate whose mother had received multiagent chemotherapy (doxorubicin, cyclophosphamide, paclitaxel, and docetaxel). Because the safety of taxanes is less documented than that of anthracyclines, an additional cycle of anthracycline-based chemotherapy during pregnancy and the completion of taxane-based chemotherapy after delivery can be considered in some situations [250]. According to the limited published data, the major cause of undesirable fetal outcomes appears to be derived from premature delivery rather than from any direct effect of the chemotherapy. Follow-up of children with specialized assessments, including detailed physiological and neurological functions, is necessary.

Treatment of Patients with Cardiac Disease

Adjuvant therapy in early-stage breast cancer typically includes anthracycline-containing chemotherapy, sometimes followed by taxanes, the anti-ERBB2 (-HER2) agent trastuzumab, and radiotherapy; each modality contributes to an increased risk of cardiac disease, including atherosclerotic coronary artery disease and left ventricular (LV) systolic and diastolic dysfunction. Thus, cancer patients who are undergoing chemotherapy have an increased risk of developing cardiovascular complications, and the risk is even greater if there is a known history of heart disease. The most common serious clinical cardiac complications reported are arrhythmias, myocardial necrosis causing dilated cardiomyopathy, and vaso-occlusion or vasospasm resulting in angina or myocardial infarction.

Anthracyclines are believed to cause immediate damage to cardiac myocytes by several mechanisms. Activation of calcium channels triggers intracellular calcium overload, and cardiac contractility may be reduced [251]. The generation of reactive oxygen species, which induce sarcomere degeneration, mitochondrial dysfunction, DNA damage, and gene expression alterations, can cause apoptotic and necrotic cell death [252–254]. The incidence of cardiotoxicity increases with the cumulative dose; however, even low doses of epirubicin in adjuvant chemotherapy for breast cancer have been shown to result in mild left ventricular ejection fraction (LVEF) impairment, an increase in brain natriuretic peptide (a marker of increased cardiac filling pressures and heart failure) levels, and an increased QT interval (QTc), all of which may indicate an increased risk of the development of subsequent heart failure (HF) [254] Reported HF rates associated with epirubicin range from 0.6 % at a cumulative dose of 550 mg/m^2 to 14.5 % at a cumulative dose of 1000 mg/m^2 [255]. A report of 630 patients treated with doxorubicin alone in three controlled trials estimated that as many as 26 % of patients receiving a cumulative doxorubicin dose of 550 mg/m^2 would develop heart failure [256]. Based upon these observations, it has been generally recommended that cumulative doxorubicin doses be limited to 450–500 mg/m^2 and epirubicin doses to 900 mg/m^2 in adults.

Adjuvant radiotherapy causes additional strain on the heart through the development of both ventricular dysfunction and coronary artery disease [257]. Radiation-induced toxicity is typically a late event and comprises diffuse fibrotic and microvascular damage to the myocardium. Radiotherapy can also promote atherosclerosis, resulting in premature coronary artery events [258]. Highly conformal radiotherapy techniques have helped reduce the heart volume at risk, particularly in patients treated for left-sided breast cancer [259]. However, radiation-induced potentially morbid late effects are long-term side effects and add to the adverse effects of other therapeutic modalities such as chemotherapeutics and targeted agents.

Cardiac dysfunction may occur immediately or, more commonly, months or years after finishing chemotherapy. Acute or subacute cardiotoxicity may present as electrocardiographic abnormalities, arrhythmias (both supraventricular and ventricular), heart block (including Mobitz type II second-degree AV block, and complete heart block), ventricular dysfunction, increased plasma brain natriuretic peptide (BNP) levels, or pericarditis–myocarditis syndrome (particularly with mitoxantrone) [260, 261]. Acute–subacute toxicity is a relatively rare event. The most common clinical presentation is chronic cardiotoxicity, which is usually overt within 1 year after the completion of chemotherapy in 1.6–5 % of patients [262]. However, the onset of symptomatic heart failure can occur more than a decade after the last anthracycline dose. Moreover, the risk of breast cancer treatment-induced cardiotoxicity may be increased in patients with coexisting traditional risk factors for cardiovascular disease, such as hypertension and hyperlipidemia [263]. Both the subacute and chronic forms of anthracycline-mediated cardiotoxicity tend not to be reversible.

Risk factors for anthracycline toxicity include the cumulative dose, intravenous bolus administration; higher single doses; a history of prior irradiation; the use of other concomitant agents known to have cardiotoxic effects, including cyclophosphamide, trastuzumab, and paclitaxel; female sex; underlying cardiovascular disease; age (young and elderly); and an increased length of time since the completion of chemotherapy [264, 265].

In addition to anthracyclines, chemotherapeutics included in adjuvant treatment may also cause cardiac side effects. Left ventricular dysfunction has been associated with cyclophosphamide therapy in 7–28 % of patients. Pericardial effusion and myopericarditis have also been reported [266, 267]. The risk of cardiotoxicity appears to be dose related ($\geq$150 mg/kg and 1.5 g/[m^2 days]) and occurs within 1–10 days after administration of the first dose of cyclophosphamide.

According to retrospective analysis, the incidence of HF associated with taxanes is relatively low, ranging from 2.3 % to 8 % for docetaxel [268]. In the BCIRG 001 trial, the

Table 8.8 Cardiac side effects of chemotherapeutic agents commonly utilized for breast cancer treatment

Cardiac toxicity	Chemotherapeutic agent	Incidence (%)
Left ventricular dysfunction	Doxorubicin	3–26
	Epirubicin	0.9–3.3
	Cyclophosphamide	7–28
	Docetaxel	2.3–8
	Bevacizumab	1.7–3.9
	Trastuzumab	2–28
Ischemia	Paclitaxel	<1–5
	Capecitabine	3–9
	Docetaxel	1.7
	5-FU	1–68
QT prolongation	Paclitaxel	0.1–31

overall incidence of congestive HF (including that during follow-up) was 1.6 % among patients treated with docetaxel, doxorubicin, and cyclophosphamide and 0.7 % among patients treated with 5-fluorouracil (5-FU), doxorubicin, and cyclophosphamide ($p=0.09$) [124]. Another study including 46 patients older than 70 years observed five cases of cardiac toxicity related to weekly paclitaxel administration for the treatment of breast cancer [269]. An overview of cardiac toxicity induced by cytotoxic agents utilized in breast cancer treatment is presented in Table 8.8.

Monitoring cardiac function is highly recommended before, during, and after potentially cardiotoxic chemotherapy to detect subclinical cardiac damage, although no clear guidelines are available from any expert group on the frequency or optimal method of LVEF assessment or the best parameters to follow. A baseline cardiovascular examination along with careful cardiovascular management of risk factors such as hypertension or hyperlipidemia is an important and often overlooked component of pretreatment assessment. The most common noninvasive techniques for monitoring LVEF are echocardiography and radionuclide angiography.

Two-dimensional (2D) echocardiography is the most widely available method for monitoring LVEF. Its advantages include portability and the capability of assessing other measures of myocardial dysfunction as well as other cardiac lesions such as valvular disease. The limitations of 2D echocardiography include problems with reproducibility and dependence upon adequate acoustic windows. Thresholds for normal LVEF should be based upon modality- and analysis-specific and population-appropriate normative data. Recent definitions are varied, including a larger change in the LVEF to less than the lower limit of normal or an LVEF less than 50 %. As a result, obtaining a clear understanding of the degree of LV dysfunction with different therapies can be problematic [270]. For a borderline depressed LVEF by echocardiography, further evaluation by radionuclide ventriculography may be necessary. Follow-up assessment of systolic dysfunction is also required throughout the treatment course for the normal initial LVEF. The US FDA-approved labeling for doxorubicin indicates that in adults, a 10 % decrease in the LVEF to below the lower limit of normal, an absolute LVEF of 45 %, or a 20 % decrease in the LVEF at any level is indicative of the deterioration of cardiac function [271].

Dexrazoxane, which is an EDTA-like chelator that may prevent anthracycline damage by binding to iron released secondary to lipid peroxidation, can be used for cardioprotection during chemotherapy with anthracyclines [272]. In some trials conducted among women receiving doxorubicin or epirubicin for breast cancer, concerns have been raised about the possibility that dexrazoxane may interfere with cancer therapy or enhance myelosuppression [273, 274]. However, multiple other randomized trials and two pooled analyses have not confirmed these findings [275–277]. The ASCO guidelines for the use of dexrazoxane in conjunction with doxorubicin include recommendations for cardiac monitoring after a cumulative dose of 400 mg/m² is reached; monitoring should be repeated after a 500 mg/m² cumulative dose is reached and after every 50 mg/m² thereafter [278]. Discontinuing anthracycline and dexrazoxane is recommended in patients who have a decrease in LVEF to below the lower limit of normal or who develop clinical heart failure.

Heart failure is associated with complex neuroendocrine activation, and neuroendocrine blockade with angiotensin-converting enzyme inhibitors (ACEIs), angiotensin receptor blockers (ARBs), and beta-blockers has proven efficient in reducing mortality and morbidity in all stages of HF. Moreover, ACEIs prevent or delay the development of symptomatic HF in patients with asymptomatic LV dysfunction [279, 280]. There is evidence that asymptomatic cardiotoxicity may predispose patients to late-onset cardiac events in the presence of additional factors such as hypertension or ischemia [281]. Thus, early intervention with established HF regimens may prove beneficial. Previous studies indicate that the prophylactic use of established HF therapies in the setting of anthracycline-induced cardiotoxicity may prevent or reduce adverse effects. However, the majority of these studies have been performed in heterogeneous patient groups with different types of cancer and treatment regimens [282–284]. Currently, there are no results from randomized trials concerning the prophylactic effect of beta-blockers, ACEIs, or ARBs in patients receiving standard adjuvant oncological therapy for early-stage breast cancer. The randomized PRADA trial has been designed to evaluate the potential of ARBs, beta-blockers, or both started before chemotherapy to prevent a decline in systolic LV function, as assessed by cardiac magnetic resonance imaging, and diastolic LV function, as assessed by echocardiography [285]. The findings of this trial are expected to contribute to efforts to prevent, detect, and treat the cardiotoxic effects of cancer therapy.

Dose Adjustment for Obese Patients

Obesity is one of the leading environmental causes of cancer in developed countries [286]. A body mass index (BMI) of 30 kg/m² or higher has been used to define obesity in most reports. Although it is not a direct causative factor, obesity results in conditions that can lead to carcinogenesis, such as increases in tumor necrosis alpha and other tumor-promoting factors and increased unopposed estrogen from the aromatase conversion of androstenedione in adipose tissues [287]. Studies have addressed a strong association

between increased adiposity and breast cancer in postmenopausal women. Obesity has also been associated with poorer survival in women diagnosed with breast cancer [288]. The mechanisms underlying the adverse effects of obesity on breast cancer survival are not clearly identified but are probably multifactorial. Obesity is prognostic in part because of its association with less favorable disease features at diagnosis, such as larger tumors and a greater number of involved lymph nodes [289, 290]. Obesity also interferes with the pharmacokinetic behavior of chemotherapeutic agents, possibly due to previously unmeasured factors such as altered metabolic function in the context of fatty liver, inherited hepatic enzyme phenotypes, or changes in the glomerular filtration rate. Impaired clearance and greater body exposure to a variety of adjuvant agents, including doxorubicin, cyclophosphamide, and fluorouracil, have been demonstrated in different trials [291, 292]. Systemic chemotherapy at less than full weight-based dosing and unnecessary dose reductions may in part explain the significantly higher cancer mortality rates observed in overweight and obese individuals.

Previous analyses have indicated that for a clinical trial population of patients with lymph node-negative, ER-positive breast cancer treated with tamoxifen who have a relatively low risk of cancer recurrence, obesity is associated with an increased rate of contralateral breast cancer, second primary cancers, and other noncancer-related deaths [293, 294].

An analysis of three studies involving 6885 women with stage I to III breast cancer evaluated the relationship between BMI and clinical outcomes [295]. The report included patients enrolled in three National Cancer Institute (NCI)-sponsored clinical trials of adjuvant doxorubicin-containing chemotherapy coordinated by ECOG for whom BMI data were available. The findings of this report were consistent with previous studies. Obese patients, defined as having a BMI of 30 kg/m² or higher, exhibited significantly higher risks of recurrence and death. After adjusting for prognostic factors (including age, race, menopausal status, tumor size, number of pathologically involved axillary nodes, and type of surgery), obesity was associated with inferior DFS (HR 1.24, 95 % CI 1.06–1.46) and OS (HR 1.37, 95 % CI 1.13–1.67) among women with hormone receptor-positive breast cancer but not among women with triple-negative or HER2-positive disease. Concordantly, Sestak et al. [296] reported that in postmenopausal women with ER-positive disease enrolled in the ATAC (Arimidex, Tamoxifen, Alone or in Combination) trial, a high baseline BMI was associated with more distant recurrence. Moreover, better outcomes were observed for adjuvant anastrozole compared with tamoxifen, primarily in women who were not obese.

Drug development and clinical trials in oncology are usually conducted irrespective of patient body weight, and obesity is not usually a stratified covariate in data analysis. Therefore, the differing pharmacokinetic parameters of obese patients are frequently overlooked. Consequently, dosing recommendations are limited regarding chemotherapy dosing in obese patients. This has resulted in the inconsistent use of various body weight estimates in chemotherapy dosing and, specifically, the calculation of body surface area (BSA). Most often, oncologists have been conservative by either adjusting body weight for obese patients or by assigning a BSA capped at $2 m^2$ rather than using the actual body weight to calculate the BSA. Although dosing schemas may vary among practices and institutions, many oncologists tend to remain conservative and empirically dose reduce up to 40 % of obese patients, despite data suggesting otherwise. The practice of limiting doses in overweight and obese patients may have unfavorable effects on the quality of care and outcomes at a population level when the increasing frequency of obesity is considered. Although dose capping in obese patients is recommended for other drugs, including low-molecular-weight heparins, some anesthetics, and some antibiotics, it may not be ideal in breast cancer chemotherapy [297].

The major target of dosing in chemotherapy is to achieve the maximum tolerated dose, thereby ensuring efficacy. Toxicity is often dose dependent and is commonly the dose-limiting factor in adjuvant chemotherapy. Chemotherapy has been shown to be more effective at higher doses. Thus, to a certain extent, increasing the dose may lead to greater myelotoxicity and greater efficacy [298, 299]. There are no prospective randomized studies comparing full weight-based chemotherapy dose selection and non-full weight-based dose selection. Obese female patients are at risk of suboptimal treatment due to empiric dose reductions. Concordantly, the previously reported increase in cancer mortality may be partly due to inadequate dosing. A recent review regarding the effect of obesity on the toxicity of chemotherapeutic agents identified ten studies investigating fulfilling the criteria [300]. Seven studies found reduced toxicity in obese compared with non-obese women. Of four studies in which dose capping was precluded or statistically adjusted for, three observed reduced toxicity in obese women. These outcomes included less febrile neutropenia [BMI>23.6; odds ratio (OR) 4.4; 95 % CI 1.65–12.01], fewer hospital admissions (BMI>35; OR 0.61, 95 % CI 0.38–0.97), and fewer neutropenic events (BMI>25; OR 0.49; 95 % CI 0.37–0.66). According to the results of this analysis, obese patients appeared to tolerate chemotherapy better than lean patients. Even after the exclusion of patients with planned dose reductions, a trend toward decreased admission to hospital with febrile neutropenia was observed [301]. Previously, myelosuppression was demonstrated to correlate with the efficacy of treatment and was considered a surrogate [302]. Although the mechanism of low myelosuppression in obese patients has not been elucidated, the tendency to develop less neutropenia suggests a comprised efficacy of chemotherapy. Thus, this tendency is believed to contribute to the poorer prognosis among obese compared to lean patients.

Although not confirmed among breast cancer patients, a study involving lung and colorectal cancer patients has reported equal toxicity rates among lean and obese patients with a higher than traditional BSA cap of 2.2 [303]. Currently there is no evidence for increased short- or long-term toxicity among obese patients receiving full weight-based chemotherapy doses. Most of the data from the aforementioned studies indicate that myelosuppression is the same or is less pronounced among obese compared with non-obese patients when full weight-based doses are administered. According to the most recent ASCO guidelines, the actual body weight should be used when selecting cytotoxic chemotherapy doses, regardless of the obesity status [304]. However, the panel acknowledged that data regarding optimal dose selection among the morbidly obese and other special subgroups are extremely limited. The available evidence indicates that morbidly obese patients treated with curative intent and receiving full weight-based doses are no more likely to experience toxicity than lean patients [305]. Moreover, retrospective analyses and observational studies suggest that dose limits in obese patients may compromise DFS and OS rates [306–308]. An analysis of outcomes among obese patients treated in the CALGB 8541 trial demonstrated that obese patients who received less than 95 % of the expected chemotherapy (based on full weight-based dosing) had worse failure-free survival rates [309]. The panel did not recommend a different management pattern for dosing in the case of high-grade toxicity. The guideline also emphasized the paucity of information on the influence of obesity on the pharmacokinetics of most anticancer drugs from properly powered trials. Overall, there appears to be insufficient pharmacokinetic data to reject the recommendation to use a full weight-based dosing strategy for chemotherapeutic agents in patients with cancer who are obese, regardless of the route of administration and the infusion time.

Conclusion

In breast cancer, the choice of treatment strategy is based on the features and biology of the tumor as well as on the age, general health status, and personal preferences of the patient. The clinical situations in which molecular tests have the greatest relevance for therapeutic decision making are still being established; however, evidence is also increasing as to the types of breast cancer in which good predictions of prognosis can be obtained. One of the current challenges in treatment is the selection of the subset of patients who might preferentially benefit from therapy. Patients with more than three involved lymph nodes, low hormonal receptor positivity, positive HER2 status, triple-negative status, high 21-gene RS, and high-risk 70-gene scores should receive adjuvant chemotherapy. A high Ki67 proliferation index and histological grade 3 tumors are acceptable indications for adjuvant chemotherapy. For women desiring fertility preservation and for patients with certain comorbidities such as cardiovascular disease and diabetic neuropathy, specific chemotherapy regimens may be preferred.

References

1. Landia S, Murray T, Bolden S, Wingo P. Cancer statistics. CA Cancer J Clin. 1999;49:31.
2. Berry D, Cronin KA, Plevritis SK, Fryback DG, Clarke L, Zelen M, et al. Effect of screening and adjuvant therapy on mortality from breast cancer. N Engl J Med. 2005;353:1784–92.
3. Fisher B, Dignam J, Tan-Chiu E, Anderson S, Fisher ER, Wittliff JL, et al. Prognosis and treatment of patients with breast tumors of one centimeter or less and negative axillary lymph nodes. J Natl Cancer Inst. 2001;93:112–20.
4. Clarke M. Meta-analyses of adjuvant therapies for women with early breast cancer: the Early Breast Cancer Trialists' Collaborative Group overview. Ann Oncol. 2006;17 Suppl 10:x59–62.
5. Loprinzi CL, Thome SD. Understanding the utility of adjuvant systemic therapy for primary breast cancer. J Clin Oncol. 2001;19:972–9.
6. Ravdin PM, Siminoff LA, Davis GJ, Mercer MB, Hewlett J, Gerson N, et al. Computer program to assist in making decisions about adjuvant therapy for women with early breast cancer. J Clin Oncol. 2001;19:980–91.
7. Surveillance Research Program, National Cancer Institute SEER*Stat software (seer.cancer.gov/seerstat), released January 2015.
8. van der Hage JA, Mieog JS, van de Velde CJ, Putter H, Bartelink H, van de Vijver MJ. Impact of established prognostic factors and molecular subtype in very young breast cancer patients: pooled analysis of four EORTC randomized controlled trials. Breast Cancer Res. 2011;13:R68.
9. Early Breast Cancer Trialists' Collaborative Group (EBCTCG). Effects of chemotherapy and hormonal therapy for early breast cancer on recurrence and 15-year survival: an overview of the randomised trials. Lancet. 2005;365:1687–717.
10. Li CI, Uribe DJ, Daling JR. Clinical characteristics of different histologic types of breast cancer. Br J Cancer. 2005;93:1046.

11. Prat A, Parker JS, Karginova O, Fan C, Livasy C, Herschkowitz JI, et al. Phenotypic and molecular characterization of the claudin-low intrinsic subtype of breast cancer. Breast Cancer Res. 2010;12:R68.
12. Perou CM, Parker JS, Prat A, Ellis MJ, Bernard PS. Clinical implementation of the intrinsic subtypes of breast cancer. Lancet Oncol. 2010;11:718–9 [author reply 720–711].
13. Perou CM, Sørlie T, Elsen MB, van de Rijn M, Jeffrey SS, Rees CA, et al. Molecular portraits of human breast tumours. Nature. 2000;406:747–52.
14. Sørlie T. Molecular portraits of breast cancer: tumour subtypes as distinct disease entities. Eur J Cancer. 2004;40:2667–75.
15. Loi S, Haibe-Kains B, Desmedt C, Lallemand F, Tutt AM, Gillet C, et al. Definition of clinically distinct molecular subtypes in estrogen receptor-positive breast carcinomas through genomic grade. J Clin Oncol. 2007;25:1239–46.
16. Sorlie T, Tibshirani R, Parker J, Hastie T, Marron JS, Nobel A, et al. Repeated observation of breast tumor subtypes in independent gene expression data sets. Proc Natl Acad Sci U S A. 2003;100(14):8418–23.
17. Cancer Genome Atlas Network. Comprehensive molecular portraits of human breast tumours. Nature. 2012;490:61–70.
18. Russnes HG, Vollan HK, Lingjaerde OC, Krasnitz A, Lundin P, Naume B, et al. Genomic architecture characterizes tumor progression paths and fate in breast cancer patients. Sci Transl Med. 2010;2:38ra47.
19. Sørlie T, Perou CM, Tibshirani R, Aas T, Geisler S, Johnsen H, et al. Gene expression patterns of breast carcinomas distinguish tumor subclasses with clinical implications. Proc Natl Acad Sci U S A. 2001;98:10869–74.
20. Herschkowitz JI, Simin K, Weigman VJ, Mikaelian I, Usary J, Hu Z, et al. Identification of conserved gene expression features between murine mammary carcinoma models and human breast tumors. Genome Biol. 2007;8:R76.
21. Weigelt B, Horlings HM, Kreike B, Hayes MM, Hauptmann M, Wessels LF, et al. Refinement of breast cancer classification by molecular characterization of histological special types. J Pathol. 2008;216:141–50.
22. Cheang MC, Voduc KD, Tu D, Jiang S, Leung S, Chia SK, et al. Responsiveness of intrinsic subtypes to adjuvant anthracycline substitution in the NCIC. CTG MA.5 randomized trial. Clin Cancer Res. 2012;18:2402–12.
23. Parker JS, Mullins M, Cheang MC, Leung S, Voduc D, Vickery T, et al. Supervised risk predictor of breast cancer based on intrinsic subtypes. J Clin Oncol. 2009;27:1160–7.
24. Reis PP, Waldron L, Goswami RS, Xu W, Xuan Y, Perez-Ordonez B, et al. mRNA transcript quantification in archival samples using multiplexed, color-coded probes. BMC Biotechnol. 2011;11:46.
25. Chia SK, Bramwell VH, Tu D, Shepherd LE, Jiang S, Vickery T, et al. A 50-gene intrinsic subtype classifier for prognosis and prediction of benefit from adjuvant tamoxifen. Clin Cancer Res. 2012;18:4465–72.
26. Weigelt B, Mackay A, A'Hern R, Natrajan R, Tan DS, Dowsett M, et al. Breast cancer molecular profiling with single sample predictors: a retrospective analysis. Lancet Oncol. 2010;11:339–49.
27. de Ronde JJ, Hannemann J, Halfwerk H, Mulder L, Straver ME, Vrancken Peeters MJ, et al. Concordance of clinical and molecular breast cancer subtyping in the context of preoperative chemotherapy response. Breast Cancer Res Treat. 2010;119:119–26.
28. Fountzilas G, Valavanis C, Kotoula V, Eleftheraki AG, Kalogeras KT, Tzaida O, et al. HER2 and TOP2A in high-risk early breast cancer patients treated with adjuvant epirubicin-based dose-dense sequential chemotherapy. J Transl Med. 2012;10:10.
29. Foekens JA, Schmitt M, van Putten WL, Peters HA, Bontenbal M, Ja¨nicke F, et al. Prognostic value of urokinase-type plasminogen activator in 671 primary breast cancer patients. Cancer Res. 1992;52:6101–5.
30. Gondi CS, Kandhukuri N, Dinh DH, Gujrati M, Rao JS. Downregulation of uPAR and uPA activates caspase mediated apoptosis, inhibits the PI3k/AKT pathway. Int J Oncol. 2007;31:19–27.
31. Luo J, Sun X, Gao F, Zhao X, Zhong B, Wang H, et al. Effects of ulinastatin and docetaxel on breast cancer invasion and expression of uPA, uPAR and ERK. J Exp Clin Cancer Res. 2011;29:30–71.
32. Look MP, van Putten WL, Duffy MJ, Harbeck N, Christensen IJ, Thomssen C, et al. Pooled analysis of prognostic impact of urokinase-type plasminogen activator and its inhibitor PAI-1 in 8377 breast cancer patients. J Natl Cancer Inst. 2002;94(2):116–28.
33. Duffy MJ. Urokinase plasminogen activator, its inhibitor. PAI-1, as prognostic markers in breast cancer: from pilot to level 1 evidence studies. Clin Chem. 2002;48:1194–7.
34. Ja¨nicke F, Prechtl A, Thomssen C, Harbeck N, Meisner C, Untch M, et al. Randomized adjuvant chemotherapy trial in high-risk, lymph node-negative breast cancer patients identified by urokinase-type plasminogen activator and plasminogen activator inhibitor type 1. J Natl Cancer Inst. 2001;93:913–20.
35. Harbeck N, Kates RE, Gauger K, Willems A, Kiechle M, Magdolen V, et al. Urokinase-type plasminogen activator (uPA) and its inhibitor PAI-I: novel tumor-derived factors with a high prognostic and predictive impact in breast cancer. Thromb Haemost. 2004;91:450–6.
36. Leissner P, Verjat T, Bachelot T, Paye M, Krause A, Puisieux A, et al. Prognostic significance of urokinase plasminogen activator and plasminogen activator inhibitor-1 mRNA expression in lymph node- and hormone receptor-positive breast cancer. BMC Cancer. 2006;31:216.
37. Janicke F, Prechtl A, Thomssen C, Harbeck N, Meisner C, Untch M, et al. Randomized adjuvant chemotherapy trial in high-risk, lymph node-negative

breast cancer patients identified by urokinase-type plasminogen activator and plasminogen activator inhibitor type 1. J Natl Cancer Inst. 2001;93(12): 913–20.

38. Trial ID: NCT0122205. Available at: www.clinical-trials.gov.

39. Harris L, Fritsche H, Mennel R, Norton L, Ravdin P, Taube S, et al. American Society of Clinical Oncology 2007 update of recommendations for the use of tumor markers in breast cancer. J Clin Oncol. 2007;25:5287–312.

40. Cuzick J, Dowsett M, Pineda S, Wale C, Salter J, Quinn E, et al. Prognostic value of a combined estrogen receptor, progesterone receptor, Ki-67, and human epidermal growth factor receptor 2 immunohistochemical score and comparison with the Genomic Health recurrence score in early breast cancer. J Clin Oncol. 2011;29:4273–8.

41. Barton S, Zabaglo L, A'Hern R, Turner N, Ferguson T, O'Neill S, et al. Assessment of the contribution of the IHC4+C score to decision making in clinical practice in early breast cancer. Br J Cancer. 2012;106:1760–5.

42. Stephen J, Murray G, Cameron DA, Thomas J, Kunkler IH, Thomas J, Kunkler IH, Jack W, et al. Time dependence of biomarkers: non-proportional effects of immunohistochemical panels predicting relapse risk in early breast cancer. Br J Cancer. 2014;11:2242–7.

43. Ring BZ, Seitz RS, Beck R, Shasteen WJ, Tarr SM, Cheang MC, et al. Novel prognostic immunohistochemical biomarker panel for estrogen receptorpositive breast cancer. J Clin Oncol. 2006;24:3039–47.

44. Ross DT, Kim CY, Tang G, Bohn OL, Beck RA, Ring BZ, et al. Chemosensitivity and stratification by a five monoclonal antibody immunohistochemistry test in the NSABP B14 and B20 trials. Clin Cancer Res. 2008;14:6602–9.

45. Paik S, Shak S, Tang G, Kim C, Baker J, Cronin M, et al. A multigene assay to predict recurrence of tamoxifen-treated, node-negative breast cancer. N Engl J Med. 2004;35:2817–26.

46. Esteban J, Baker J, Cronin M, Liu M-L, Llamas MG, Walker MG, et al. Tumor gene expression and prognosis in breast cancer: multi-gene RT-PCR assay of paraffin-embedded tissue. Prog Proc Am Soc Clin Oncol. 2003;22:850 abstract.

47. Paik S, Shak S, Tang G, Kim C, Baker J, Cronin M, et al. Multi-gene RT-PCR assay for predicting recurrence in node negative breast cancer patients – NSABP studies B-20 and B-14. Breast Cancer Res Treat. 2003;82:A16 abstract.

48. Paik S, Tang G, Shak S, Kim C, Baker J, Kim W, et al. Gene expression and benefit of chemotherapy in women with node-negative, estrogen receptor-positive breast cancer. J Clin Oncol. 2006;24: 3726–34.

49. Dowsett M, Cuzick J, Wale C, Forbes J, Mallon EA, Salter J, et al. Prediction of risk of distant recurrence using the 21-gene recurrence score in node-negative

and node-positive postmenopausal patients with breast cancer treated with anastrozole or tamoxifen: a TransATAC study. J Clin Oncol. 2010;28:1829–34.

50. Tang G, Cuzick J, Costantino JP, Dowsett M, Forbes JF, Crager M, et al. Risk of recurrence and chemotherapy benefit for patients with node-negative, estrogen receptor-positive breast cancer: recurrence score alone and integrated with pathologic and clinical factors. J Clin Oncol. 2011;29:4365e72.

51. Albain KS, Barlow WE, Shak S, Hortobagyi GN, Livingston RB, Yeh IT, et al. Prognostic and predictive value of the 21-gene recurrence score assay in postmenopausal women with node-positive, oestrogen-receptor-positive breast cancer on chemotherapy: a retrospective analysis of a randomised trial. Lancet Oncol. 2010;11:55–65.

52. Chang JC, Wooten EC, Tsimelzon A, Hilsenbeck SG, Guiterrez MC, Elledge RM, et al. Gene expression profiling predicts therapeutic response to docetaxel (Taxotere(tm)) in breast cancer patients. Lancet. 2003;362:280–7.

53. Ayers M, Symmans WF, Stec J, Damokosh AI, Clark E, Hess K, et al. Gene expression profiles predict complete pathologic response to neoadjuvant paclitaxel and fluorouracil, doxorubicin, and cyclophosphamide chemotherapy in breast cancer. J Clin Oncol. 2004;22:2284–93.

54. Gianni L, Zambetti M, Clark K, Baker J, Cronin M, Wu J, et al. Gene expression profiles in paraffin-embedded core biopsy tissue predict response to chemotherapy in women with locally advanced breast cancer. J Clin Oncol. 2005;23:7265–77.

55. Chang JC, Makris A, Gutierrez MC, Hilsenbeck SG, Hackett JR, Jeong J, et al. Gene expression patterns in formalin-fixed, paraffin embedded core biopsies predict docetaxel chemosensitivity in breast cancer patients. Breast Cancer Res Treat. 2008;108:233–40.

56. Baehner FL, Achacoso N, Maddala T, Shak S, Quesenberry Jr CP, Goldstein LC, Gown AM. Human epidermal growth factor receptor 2 assessment in a case-control study: comparison of fluorescence in situ hybridization and quantitative reverse transcription polymerase chain reaction performed by central laboratories. J Clin Oncol. 2010;28:4300–6.

57. Paik S, Bryant J, Tan-Chiu E, Romond E, Hiller W, Park K, et al. Real-world performance of HER2 testing—National Surgical Adjuvant Breast and Bowel Project experience. J Natl Cancer Inst. 2002;94:852–4.

58. Dabbs DJ, Klein ME, Mohsin SK, Tubbs RR, Shuai Y, Bhargava R. High falsenegative rate of HER2 quantitative reverse transcription polymerase chain reaction of the OncotypeDX test: an independent quality assurance study. J Clin Oncol. 2011;29: 4279–85.

59. Lahr G. RT-PCR from archival single cells is a suitable method to analyze specific gene expression. Lab Invest. 2000;80:1477–9.

60. Schutze K, Lahr G. Identification of expressed genes by laser-mediated manipulation of single cells. Nat Biotechnol. 1998;16:737–42.

61. Cronin M, Pho M, Dutta D, Stephans JC, Shak S, Kiefer MC, et al. Measurement of gene expression in archival paraffin-embedded tissues: development and performance of a 92-gene reverse transcriptase-polymerase chain reaction assay. Am J Pathol. 2004;164(1):35e42.

62. Cobleigh MA, Tabesh B, Bitterman P, Baker J, Cronin M, Liu ML, et al. Tumor gene expression and prognosis in breast cancer patients with 10 or more positive lymph nodes. Clin Cancer Res. 2005;11: 8623e31.

63. Hornberger J, Chien R, Krebs K, Hochheiser L, et al. US insurance program's experience with a multi-gene assay for early-stage breast cancer. J Oncol Pract. 2011;7:e38s–45.

64. Trial ID:NCT00567190. Available at: www.clinical-trials.gov.

65. Tian S, Roepman P, van't Veer LJ, Bernards R, de Snoo F, Glas AM. Biological functions of the genes in the MammaPrint breast cancer profile reflect the hallmarks of cancer. Biomark Insights. 2010;5:129–38.

66. van 't Veer LJ, Dai H, van de Vijver MJ, He YD, Hart AA, Mao M, et al. Gene expression profiling predicts clinical outcome of breast cancer. Nature. 2002;415:530–6.

67. Van de Vijver MJ, He YD, van't Veer LJ, Dai H, Hart AA, Voskuil DW, et al. A gene-expression signature as a predictor of survival in breast cancer. N Engl J Med. 2002;347:1999–2009.

68. Buyse M, Loi S, van't Veer L, Viale G, Delorenzi M, Glas AM, et al. Validation and clinical utility of a 70-gene prognostic signature for women with node-negative breast cancer. J Natl Cancer Inst. 2006;98:1183–92.

69. Bueno-de-Mesquita JM, Linn SC, Keijzer R, Wesseling J, Nuyten DS, van Krimpen C, et al. Validation of 70-gene prognosis signature in node-negative breast cancer. Breast Cancer Res Treat. 2009;117:483–95.

70. Mook S, Schmidt MK, Viale G, Pruneri G, Eekhout I, Floore A, et al. The 70-gene prognosis-signature predicts disease outcome in breast cancer patients with 1–3 positive lymph nodes in an independent validation study. Breast Cancer Res Treat. 2009;116:295e302.

71. Knauer M, Mook S, Rutgers EJ, Bender RA, Hauptmann M, van de Vijver MJ, et al. The predictive value of the 70-gene signature for adjuvant chemotherapy in early breast cancer. Breast Cancer Res Treat. 2010;120:655–61.

72. Drukker CA, Bueno-de-Mesquita JM, Retèl VP, van Harten WH, van Tinteren H, Wesseling J, et al. A prospective evaluation of a breast cancer prognosis signature in the observational RASTER study. Int J Cancer. 2013;133:929–36.

73. Straver ME, Glas AM, Hannemann J, Wesseling J, van de Vijver MJ, Rutgers EJ, et al. The 70-gene signature as a response predictor for neoadjuvant chemotherapy in breast cancer. Breast Cancer Res Treat. 2010;119:551–8.

74. TrialID:NCT00433589. Available at: www.clinical-trials.gov.

75. Rutgers E, Piccart-Gebhart MJ, Bogaerts J, Delaloge S, Veer LV, Rubio IT, et al. The EORTC 10041/BIG 03-04 MINDACT trial is feasible: results of the pilot phase. Eur J Cancer. 2011;47:2742–9.

76. Cardoso F, Piccart-Gebhart M, Van't Veer L, Rutgers E. The MINDACT trial: the first prospective clinical validation of a genomic tool. Mol Oncol. 2007;1: 246–51.

77. Glas AM, Floore A, Delahaye LJ, Witteveen AT, Pover RC, Bakx N, et al. Converting a breast cancer microarray signature into a high-throughput diagnostic test. BMC Genomics. 2006;7:278.

78. Ach RA, Floore A, Curry B, Lazar V, Glas AM, Pover R, et al. Robust interlaboratory reproducibility of a gene expression signature measurement consistent with the needs of a new generation of diagnostic tools. BMC Genomics. 2007;8:148.

79. Perou CM, Jeffrey SS, van de Rijn M, Rees CA, Eisen MB, Ross DT, et al. Distinctive gene expression patterns in human mammary epithelial cells and breast cancers. Proc Natl Acad Sci U S A. 1999;96:9212–7.

80. Sorlie T, Perou CM, Tibshirani R, Aas T, Geisler S, Johnsen H, et al. Gene expression patterns of breast carcinomas distinguish tumor subclasses with clinical implications. Proc Natl Acad Sci U S A. 2001;98:10869–74.

81. Nielsen TO, Parker JS, Leung S, Voduc D, Ebbert M, Vickery T, et al. A comparison of PAM50 intrinsic subtyping with immunohistochemistry and clinical prognostic factors in tamoxifen-treated estrogen receptor-positive breast cancer. Clin Cancer Res. 2010;16:5222–32.

82. Dowsett M, Sestak I, Lopez-Knowles E, Sidhu K, Dunbier AK, Cowens JW, et al. Comparison of PAM50 risk of recurrence score with oncotype DX and IHC4 for predicting risk of distant recurrence after endocrine therapy. J Clin Oncol. 2013;31:2783–90.

83. Sestak I, Cuzick J, Dowsett M, Lopez-Knowles E, Filipits M, Dubsky P, et al. Prediction of late distant recurrence after 5 years of endocrine treatment: a combined analysis of patients from the Austrian breast and colorectal cancer study group 8 and arimidex, tamoxifen alone or in combination randomized trials using the PAM50 risk of recurrence score. J Clin Oncol. 2014;55:6894.

84. Martin M, Prat A, Rodriguez-Lescure A, Caballero R, Ebbert MT, Munarriz B, et al. PAM50 proliferation score as a predictor of weekly paclitaxel benefit in breast cancer. Breast Cancer Res Treat. 2013; 138:457–66.

85. Trial ID NCT01272037. Available at: www.clinical-trials.gov.

86. Sotiriou C, Wirapati P, Loi S, Harris A, Fox S, Smeds J, et al. Gene expression profiling in breast cancer: understanding the molecular basis of histologic grade to improve prognosis. J Natl Cancer Inst. 2006;98:262–72.

87. Desmedt C, Giobbie-Hurder A, Neven P, Paridaens R, Christiaens MR, Smeets A, et al. The Gene expres-

sion Grade Index: a potential predictor of relapse for endocrine-treated breast cancer patients in the BIG 1-98 trial. BMC Med Genomics. 2009;2:40.

88. Toussaint J, Sieuwerts AM, Haibe-Kains B, Desmedt C, Rouas G, Harris AL, et al. Improvement of the clinical applicability of the genomic grade index through a qRT-PCR test performed on frozen and formalin-fixed paraffin embedded tissues. BMC Genomics. 2009;10:424.

89. Ma XJ, Wang Z, Ryan PD, Isakoff SJ, Barmettler A, Fuller A, et al. A two-gene expression ratio predicts clinical outcome in breast cancer patients treated with tamoxifen. Cancer Cell. 2004;5:607–16.

90. Ma XJ, Hilsenbeck SG, Wang W, Ding L, Sgroi DC, Bender RA, et al. The HOXB13: IL17BR expression index is a prognostic factor in early-stage breast cancer. J Clin Oncol. 2006;24:4611–9.

91. Jerevall PL, Brommesson S, Strand C, Gruvberger-Saal S, Malmstrom P, Nordenskjold B, et al. Exploring the two-gene ratio in breast cancer e independent roles for HOXB13 and IL17BR in prediction of clinical outcome. Breast Cancer Res Treat. 2008;107:225–34.

92. Jansen MP, Sieuwerts AM, Look MP, Ritstier K, Meijer-van Gelder ME, van Staveren IL, et al. HOXB13-to-IL17BR expression ratio is related with tumor aggressiveness and response to tamoxifen of recurrent breast cancer: a retrospective study. J Clin Oncol. 2007;25:662–8.

93. Filipits M, Rudas M, Jakesz R, Dubsky P, Fitzal F, Singer CF, et al. A new molecular predictor of distant recurrence in ER-positive, HER2-negative breast cancer adds independent information to conventional clinical risk actors. Clin Cancer Res. 2011;17:6012–20.

94. Dubsky P, Filipits M, Jakesz R, Rudas M, Singer CF, Greil R, et al. EndoPredict improves the prognostic classification derived from common clinical guidelines in ER-positive, HER2-negative early breast cancer. Ann Oncol. 2013;24:640–7.

95. Lohrisch C, Paltiel C, Gelmon K, Speers C, Taylor S, Barnett J, et al. Impact on survival of time from definitive surgery to initiation of adjuvant chemotherapy for early-stage breast cancer. J Clin Oncol. 2006;24:4888–94.

96. Gagliato Dde M, Gonzalez-Angulo AM, Lei X, Theriault RL, Giordano SH, Valero V, et al. Clinical impact of delaying initiation of adjuvant chemotherapy in patients with breast cancer. J Clin Oncol. 2014;32:735–44.

97. Goldhirsch A, Winer EP, Coates AS, Gelber RD, Piccart-Gebhart M, Thürlimann B, et al. Personalizing the treatment of women with early breast cancer: highlights of the St Gallen International Expert Consensus on the Primary Therapy of Early Breast Cancer. Ann Oncol. 2013;24:2206–23.

98. Cheang MCU, Chia SK, Voduc D, Gao D, Leung S, Snider J, et al. Ki67 index, HER2 status, and prognosis of patients with luminal B breast cancer. J Natl Cancer Inst. 2009;101:736–50.

99. Prat A, Cheang MC, Martin M, Parker JS, Carrasco E, Caballero R, et al. Prognostic significance of progesterone receptor positive tumor cells within immunohistochemically defined luminal A breast cancer. J Clin Oncol. 2013;31:203–9.

100. Nccn guidelines version 2.2015. www.nccn.org.

101. Muss HB, Berry DA, Cirrincione CT, Parker JS, Carrasco E, Caballero R, et al. Adjuvant chemotherapy in older women with early-stage breast cancer. N Engl J Med. 2009;360:2055–65.

102. Lyman GH, Dale DC, Wolff DA, Culakova E, Poniewierski MS, Kuderer NM, et al. Acute myeloid leukemia or myelodysplastic syndrome in randomized controlled clinical trials of cancer chemotherapy with granulocyte colony-stimulating factor: a systematic review. J Clin Oncol. 2010;28:2914–24.

103. Muss HB, Berry DA, Cirrincione C, Budman DR, Henderson IC, Citron ML, et al. Toxicity of older and younger patients treated with adjuvant chemotherapy for node-positive breast cancer: the Cancer and Leukemia Group B Experience. J Clin Oncol. 2007;25:3699–704.

104. Tannock IF, Ahles TA, Ganz PA, Van Dam FS. Cognitive impairment associated with chemotherapy for cancer: report of a workshop. J Clin Oncol. 2004;22:2233–9.

105. Sanoff HK, Deal AM, Krishnamurthy J, Torrice C, Dillon P, Sorrentino J, et al. Effect of cytotoxic chemotherapy on markers of molecular age in patients with breast cancer. J Natl Cancer Inst. 2014;106:dju057.

106. Trial ID: NCT01564056. Available at: www.clinicaltrials.gov.

107. Senkus E, Kyriakides S, Penault-Llorca F, Poortmans P, Thompson A, Zackrisson S, on behalf of the ESMO Guidelines Working Group. Primary breast cancer: ESMO Clinical Practice Guidelines for diagnosis, treatment and follow-up. Ann Oncol. 2013;Suppl 6:vi7–23.

108. Harbeck N, Kates RE, Look MP, Meijer-Van Gelder ME, Klijn JG, Krüger A, et al. Enhanced benefit from adjuvant chemotherapy in breast cancer patients classified high-risk according to urokinase-type plasminogen activator (uPA) and plasminogen activator inhibitor type 1 (n=3424). Cancer Res. 2002;62:4617–22.

109. Thurman SA, Schnitt SJ, Connolly JL, Gelman R, Silver B, Harris JR, et al. Outcome after breast-conserving therapy for patients with stage I or II mucinous, medullary, or tubular breast carcinoma. Int J Radiat Oncol Biol Phys. 2004;59:152.

110. Alba E, Calvo L, Albanell J, De la Haba JR, Arcusa Lanza A, Chacon JI, et al. Chemotherapy (CT) and hormonal therapy (HT) as neoadjuvant treatment in luminal breast cancer patients: results from the GEICAM/2006-03, a multicenter, randomized, phase-II study. Ann Oncol. 2012;23:3069–74.

111. Vu-Nishino H, Tavassoli FA, Ahrens WA, Haffty BG. Clinicopathologic features and long-term outcome of patients with medullary breast carcinoma managed with breast-conserving therapy (BCT). Int J Radiat Oncol Biol Phys. 2005;62:1040.

112. Early Breast Cancer Trialists' Collaborative Group. Polychemotherapy for early breast cancer: an overview of the randomised trials. Lancet. 1998;352:930–42.

113. Early Breast Cancer Trialists' Collaborative Group (EBCTCG), Peto R, Davies C, Godwin J, Gray R, Pan HC, et al. Comparisons between different polychemotherapy regimens for early breast cancer: meta-analyses of long-term outcome among 100,000 women in 123 randomised trials. Lancet. 2012;379: 432–44.

114. Levine M, Pritchard K, Bramwell V, Shepherd LE, Tu D, Paul N, et al. Randomized trial comparing cyclophosphamide, epirubicin, and fluorouracil with cyclophosphamide, methotrexate, and fluorouracil in premenopausal women with node-positive breast cancer: update of National Cancer Institute of Canada Clinical Trials Group Trial MA5. J Clin Oncol. 2005;23:5166–70.

115. French Adjuvant Study Group. Benefit of a high-dose epirubicin regimen in adjuvant chemotherapy for node-positive breast cancer patients with poor prognostic factors: 5-year follow-up results of French Adjuvant Study Group 05 Randomized Trial. J Clin Oncol. 2001;19:602–11.

116. Piccart MJ, Di Leo A, Beauduin M, Vindevoghel A, Michel J, Focan C, et al. Phase III trial comparing two dose levels of epirubicin combined with cyclophosphamide with cyclophosphamide, methotrexate, and fluorouracil in node-positive breast cancer. J Clin Oncol. 2001;19:3103–10.

117. Henderson I, Berry D, Demetri G, Cirrincione CT, Goldstein LJ, Martino S, et al. Improved outcomes from adding sequential Paclitaxel but not from escalating Doxorubicin dose in an adjuvant chemotherapy regimen for patients with node-positive primary breast cancer. J Clin Oncol. 2003;21:976–83.

118. Mamounas E, Bryant J, Lembersky B, Fehrenbacher L, Sedlacek SM, Fisher B, et al. Paclitaxel after doxorubicin plus cyclophosphamide as adjuvant chemotherapy for node-positive breast cancer: results from NSABP B-28. J Clin Oncol. 2005;23:3686–96.

119. Buzdar AU, Singletary SE, Valero V, Booser DJ, Ibrahim NK, Rahman Z, et al. Evaluation of paclitaxel in adjuvant chemotherapy for patients with operable breast cancer: preliminary data of a prospective randomized trial. Clin Cancer Res. 2002;8:1073–9.

120. Martin M, Rodriguez-Lescure A, Ruiz A, Alba E, Calvo L, Ruiz-Borrego M, et al. Randomized phase 3 trial of fluorouracil, epirubicin, and cyclophosphamide alone or followed by paclitaxel for early breast cancer. J Natl Cancer Inst. 2008;100:805–14.

121. Sparano JA, Wang M, Martino S, Jones V, Perez E, Saphner T, et al. Phase III study of doxorubicin-cyclophosphamide followed by paclitaxel or docetaxel given every 3 weeks or weekly in patients with axillary node positive or high risk node negative breast cancer [abstract]. San Antonio Breast Cancer Symposium. 2005. Abstract 48.

122. Sparano JA, Wang M, Martino S, Jones V, Perez E, Saphner T, et al. Phase III study of doxorubicin-cyclophosphamide followed by paclitaxel or docetaxel given every 3 weeks or weekly in operable breast cancer: results of Intergroup Trial E1199 [abstract]. J Clin Oncol. 2007;25(Suppl-18):6s Abstract 516.

123. Sparano J, Wang M, Martino S, Jones V, Perez EA, Saphner T, et al. Weekly paclitaxel in the adjuvant treatment of breast cancer. N Engl J Med. 2008; 358:1663–71.

124. Martin M, Pienkowski T, Mackey J, Pawlicki M, Guastalla JP, Weaver C, et al. Adjuvant docetaxel for node-positive breast cancer. N Engl J Med. 2005;352:2302–13.

125. Mackey JR, Martin M, Pienkowski T, Rolski J, Rolski J, Guastalla JP, et al. Adjuvant docetaxel, doxorubicin and cyclophosphamide in node positive breast cancer: 10-year follow-up of the phase 3 randomised BCIRG 001 trial. Lancet Oncol. 2013;14:72–80.

126. Swain SM, Jeong J-H, Geyer CE, Costantino JP, Pajon ER, Fehrenbacher L, et al. NSABP B-30: definitive analysis of patient outcome from a randomized trial evaluating different schedules and combinations of adjuvant therapy containing doxorubicin, docetaxel and cyclophosphamide in women with operable, node-positive breast cancer [abstract]. Cancer Res. 2009;69 (Suppl_1):Abstract 75.

127. Ellis P, Barrett-Lee P, Johnson L, Cameron D, Wardley A, O'Reilly S, et al. Sequential docetaxel as adjuvant chemotherapy for early breast cancer (TACT): an open-label, phase III, randomised controlled trial. Lancet. 2009;373:1681–92.

128. De Laurentiis M, Cancello G, D'Agostino D, Giuliano M, Giordano A, Montagna E, et al. Taxane-based combinations as adjuvant chemotherapy of early breast cancer: a meta-analysis of randomized trials. J Clin Oncol. 2008;26:44–53.

129. Bria E, Nistico C, Cuppone F, Carlini P, Ciccarese M, Milella M, et al. Benefit of taxanes as adjuvant chemotherapy for early breast cancer: pooled analysis of 15,500 patients. Cancer. 2006;106:2337–44.

130. Martín M, Seguí MA, Anto'n A, Ruiz A, Ramos M, Adrover E, et al. Adjuvant docetaxel for high-risk, node-negative breast cancer. N Engl J Med. 2010;363:2200–10.

131. Martín M, Ruiz A, Ruiz Borrego M, Barnadas A, González S, Calvo L, et al. Fluorouracil, doxorubicin, and cyclophosphamide (FAC) versus FAC followed by weekly paclitaxel as adjuvant therapy for high-risk, node-negative breast cancer: results from the GEICAM/2003 02 study. J Clin Oncol. 2013;10(31):2593–9.

132. Epub Jacquin JP, Jones S, Magné N, Chapelle C, Ellis P, et al. Docetaxel containing adjuvant chemotherapy in patients with early stage breast cancer. Consistency of effect independent of nodal and biomarker status: a meta-analysis of 14 randomized clinical trials. Breast Cancer Res Treat. 2012;134:903–13.

133. Fisher B, Brown AM, Dimitrov NV, Poisson R, Redmond C, Margolese RG, et al. Two months of doxorubicin-cyclophosphamide with and without interval reinduction therapy compared with 6 months

of cyclophosphamide, methotrexate, and fluorouracil in positive-node breast cancer patients with tamoxifen-nonresponsive tumors: Results from the National Surgical Adjuvant Breast and Bowel Project B-15. J Clin Oncol. 1990;8:1483–96.

134. Fisher B, Anderson S, Tan-Chiu E, Wolmark N, Wickerham DL, Fisher ER, et al. Tamoxifen and chemotherapy for axillary node negative, estrogen receptor-negative breast cancer: findings from National Surgical Adjuvant Breast and Bowel Project B-23. J Clin Oncol. 2001;19:931–42.

135. Jones SE, Savin MA, Holmes FA, O'Shaughnessy JA, Blum JL, Vukelja S, et al. Phase III trial comparing doxorubicin plus cyclophosphamide with docetaxel plus cyclophosphamide as adjuvant therapy for operable breast cancer. J Clin Oncol. 2006;1(24):5381–7.

136. Jones S, Holmes FA, O'Shaughnessy J, Blum JL, Vukelja SJ, McIntyre KJ, et al. Docetaxel with cyclophosphamide is associated with an overall survival benefit compared with doxorubicin and cyclophosphamide: 7-year follow-up of US Oncology Research Trial 9735. J Clin Oncol. 2009;27:1177–83.

137. Skipper HE. Laboratory models: some historical perspectives. Cancer Treat Rep. 1986;70:3–7.

138. Norton L, Simon R, Brereton JD, Bogden AE. Predicting the course of Gompertzian growth. Nature. 1976;264:542–5.

139. Norton L, Simon R. The Norton–Simon hypothesis revisited. Cancer Treat Res. 1986;70:163–9.

140. Citron ML, Berry DA, Cirrincione C, Hudis C, Winer EP, Gradishar WJ, et al. Randomized trial of dose-dense versus conventionally scheduled and sequential versus concurrent combination chemotherapy as postoperative adjuvant treatment of node-positive primary breast cancer: first report of Intergroup Trial C9741/Cancer and Leukemia Group B Trial 9741. J Clin Oncol. 2003;21:1431–9.

141. Budd GT, Barlow WE, Moore HC, Hobday TJ, Stewart JA, Isaacs C, et al. SWOG S0221: a phase III trial comparing chemotherapy schedules in high-risk early-stage breast cancer. J Clin Oncol. 2015;33:58–64.

142. Therasse P, Mauriac L, Welnicka-Jaskiewicz M, Bruning P, Cufer T, Bonnefoi H, et al. Final results of a randomized phase III trial comparing cyclophosphamide, epirubicin, and fluorouracil with dose-intensified epirubicin and cyclophosphamide plus filgrastim in locally advanced breast cancer. An EORTC-NCIC-SAKK multicenter study. J Clin Oncol. 2003;21:843–50.

143. Fountzilas G, Dafni U, Gogas H, Linardou H, Kalofonos HP, Briasoulis E, et al. Post-operative dose dense sequential chemotherapy with epirubicin, paclitaxel and CMF in patients with high-risk breast cancer: a Hellenic Cooperative Oncology Group Randomized Phase III Trial HE 10/00. Ann Oncol. 2008;19:853–60.

144. Swain SM, Tang G, Geyer Jr CE, Rastogi P, Atkins JN, Donnellan PP, et al. Definitive results of a phase III adjuvant trial comparing three chemotherapy regimens in women with operable, node-positive breast cancer: The NSABP B-38 trial. J Clin Oncol. 2013;31:3197–204.

145. Bonilla L, Ben-Aharon I, Vidal L, Gafter-Gvili A, Leibovici L, Stemmer SM, et al. Dose-dense chemotherapy in nonmetastatic breast cancer: a systematic review and meta-analysis of randomized controlled trials. J Natl Cancer Inst. 2010;102:1845–54.

146. Bayraktar S, Arun B. Dose dense chemotherapy for breast cancer. Breast J. 2012;18:261–6.

147. Joensuu H, Kellokumpu-Lehtinen PL, Huovinen R, Jukkola-Vuorinen A, Tanner M, Asola R, et al. Adjuvant capecitabine in combination with docetaxel and cyclophosphamide plus epirubicin for breast cancer: an open-label, randomised controlled trial. Lancet Oncol. 2009;10:1145–51.

148. Joensuu H, Kellokumpu-Lehtinen PL, Huovinen R, Jukkola-Vuorinen A, Tanner M, Kokko R, et al. Adjuvant capecitabine, docetaxel, cyclophosphamide, and epirubicin for early breast cancer: final analysis of the randomized FinXX trial. J Clin Oncol. 2012;1(30):11–8.

149. O'Shaughnessy J, Paul D, Stokoe C, Pippen JL, Blum JL, Krekow L, et al. First efficacy results of a randomized, open-label, phase II study of adjuvant doxorubicin plus cyclophosphamide, followed by docetaxel with or without capecitabine, in high-risk early breast cancer. 33rd Annual San Antonio Breast Cancer Symposium 2010, San Antonio, 8–12 Dec (abstr S4-2).

150. Wardley AM, Hiller L, Howard HC, Dunn JA, Bowman A, Coleman RE, et al. tAnGo: a randomised phase III trial of gemcitabine in paclitaxel-containing, epirubicin/cyclophosphamide-based, adjuvant chemotherapy for early breast cancer: a prospective pulmonary, cardiac and hepatic function evaluation. Br J Cancer. 2008;99:597–603.

151. Weigelt B, Baehner FL, Reis-Filho JS. The contribution of gene expression profiling to breast cancer classification, prognostication and prediction: a retrospective of the last decade. J Pathol. 2010;220: 263–80.

152. Bertucci F, Finetti P, Cervera N, Esterni B, Hermitte F, Viens P, et al. How basal are triple-negative breast cancers? Int J Cancer. 2008;123:236–40.

153. Turner N, Tutt A, Ashworth A. Hallmarks of 'BRCAness' in sporadic cancers. Nat Rev Cancer. 2004;4:814–9.

154. Colleoni M, Cole BF, Viale G, Regan MM, Price KN, Maiorano E, et al. Classical cyclophosphamide, methotrexate, and fluorouracil chemotherapy is more effective in triple-negative, node-negative breast cancer: results from two randomized trials of adjuvant chemoendocrine therapy for node-negative breast cancer. J Clin Oncol. 2010;28:2966–73.

155. Liedtke C, Mazouni C, Hess KR, André F, Tordai A, Mejia JA, et al. Response to neoadjuvant therapy and long term survival in patients with triple-negative breast cancer. J Clin Oncol. 2008;26:1275–81.

156. Treszezamsky AD, Kachnic LA, Feng Z, Zhang J, Tokadjian C, Powell SN, et al. BRCA1- and BRCA2-deficient cells are sensitive to etoposide-induced DNA double-strand breaks via topoisomerase II. Cancer Res. 2007;67:7078–81.

157. Quinn JE, Kennedy RD, Mullan PB, Gilmore PM, Carty M, Johnston PG, et al. BRCA1 functions as a differential modulator of chemotherapy-induced apoptosis. Cancer Res. 2003;63:6221–8.

158. Tassone P, Tagliaferri P, Perricelli A, Blotta S, Quaresima B, Martelli ML, et al. BRCA1 expression modulates chemosensitivity of BRCA1-defective HCC1937 human breast cancer cells. Br J Cancer. 2003;88:1285–91.

159. Rocca A, Bravaccini S, Scarpi E, Mangia A, Petroni S, Puccetti M, et al. Benefit from anthracyclines in relation to biological profiles in early breast cancer. Breast Cancer Res Treat. 2014;144:307–18.

160. Laporte S, Jones S, Chapelle C, Jacquin J, Martín M. Consistency of effect of docetaxel containing adjuvant chemotherapy in patients with early stage breast cancer independent of nodal status: meta-analysis of 12 randomized clinical trials. Cancer Res. 2009;69 (Suppl 1):Abstr 605.

161. Hayes DF, Thor AD, Dressler LG, Weaver D, Edgerton S, Cowan D, et al. HER2 and response to paclitaxel in node-positive breast cancer. N Engl J Med. 2007;357:1496–506.

162. Jacquemier J, Penault-Llorca F, Mnif H, Charafe-Jauffret E, Marque S, Martin A, et al. Identification of a basal-like subtype and comparative effect of epirubicin-based chemotherapy and sequential epirubicin followed by docetaxel chemotherapy in the PACS 01 breast cancer trial: 33 markers studied on tissue-microarrays (TMA). J Clin Oncol. 2006;24:18s abstract 509.

163. Hugh J, Hanson J, Cheang MC, Nielsen TO, Perou CM, Dumontet C, et al. Breast cancer subtypes and response to docetaxel in node-positive breast cancer: use of an immunohistochemical definition in the BCIRG 001 trial. J Clin Oncol. 2009;27:1168–76.

164. Roche H, Allouache D, Romieu G, Bourgeois H, Canon J, Serin D, et al. Five-year analysis of the FNCLCC-PACS04 Trial: FEC100 vs. ED75 for the adjuvant treatment of node positive breast cancer. Cancer Res. 2010;69:24s abstract 60.

165. Bhattacharyya A, Ear US, Koller BH, Weichselbaum RR, Bishop DK. The breast cancer susceptibility gene BRCA1 is required for subnuclear assembly of Rad51 and survival following treatment with the DNA cross-linking agent cisplatin. J Biol Chem. 2000;275:23899–903.

166. Husain A, He G, Venkatraman ES, Spriggs DR. BRCA1 up-regulation is associated with repair-mediated resistance to cis-diamminedichloroplatinum(II). Cancer Res. 1998;58:1120–3.

167. Leong CO, Vidnovic N, DeYoung MP, Sgroi D, Ellisen LW. The p63/p73 network mediates chemosensitivity to cisplatin in a biologically defined subset of primary breast cancers. J Clin Invest. 2007;117:1370–80.

168. Byrski T, Gronwald J, Huzarski T, Grzybowska E, Budryk M, Stawicka M, et al. Response to neo-adjuvant chemotherapy in women with BRCA1-positive breast cancers. Breast Cancer Res Treat. 2009;115:359–63.

169. Silver DP, Richardson AL, Eklund AC, Wang ZC, Szallasi Z, Li Q, et al. Efficacy of neoadjuvant cisplatin in triple-negative breast cancer. J Clin Oncol. 2010;28:1145–53.

170. Muss HB, Berry DA, Cirrincione CT, Theodoulou M, Mauer AM, Kornblith AB, et al. Adjuvant chemotherapy in older women with early-stage breast cancer. N Engl J Med. 2009;360:2055–65.

171. Moynahan ME, Chiu JW, Koller BH, Jasin M. BRCA1 controls homology-directed DNA repair. Mol Cell. 1999;4:511–8.

172. Moynahan ME, Pierce AJ, Jasin M. BRCA2 is required for homology directed repair of chromosomal breaks. Mol Cell. 2001;7:263–72.

173. Tirkkonen M, Johannsson O, Agnarsson BA, Olsson H, Ingvarsson S, Karhu R, et al. Distinct somatic genetic changes associated with tumor progression in carriers of BRCA1 and BRCA2 germ-line mutations. Cancer Res. 1997;57:1222–7.

174. Collins N, McManus R, Wooster R, Mangion J, Seal S, Lakhani SR, et al. Consistent loss of the wild type allele in breast cancers from a family linked to the BRCA2 gene on chromosome 13q12-13. Oncogene. 1995;10:1673–5.

175. Merajver SD, Frank TS, Xu J, Pham TM, Calzone KA, Bennett-Baker P, et al. Germline BRCA1 mutations and loss of the wild-type allele in tumors from families with early onset breast and ovarian cancer. Clin Cancer Res. 1995;1:539–44.

176. Caldecott W. Mammalian single-strand break repair: mechanisms and links with chromatin. DNA Repair. 2007;6:443–53.

177. Ashworth A. A synthetic lethal therapeutic approach: poly(ADP) ribose polymerase inhibitors for the treatment of cancers deficient in DNA double-strand break repair. J Clin Oncol. 2008;26:3785–90.

178. Farmer H, McCabe H, Lord CJ, Tutt AN, Johnson DA, Richardson TB, et al. Targeting the DNA repair defect in BRCA mutant cells as a therapeutic strategy. Nature. 2005;434:917–21.

179. Tutt A, Robson M, Garber JE, Domchek SM, Audeh MW, Weitzel JN, et al. Oral poly(ADPribose) polymerase inhibitor olaparib in patients with BRCA1 or BRCA2 mutations and advanced breast cancer: a proof-of concept trial. Lancet. 2010;376:235–44.

180. Rivera E, Lee J, Davies A. Clinical development of ixabepilone and other epothilones in patients with advanced solid tumors. Oncologist. 2008;13:1207–23.

181. Baselga J, Zambetti M, Llombart-Cussac A, Manikhas G, Kubista E, Steger GG, et al. Phase II genomics study of ixabepilone as neoadjuvant treatment for breast cancer. J Clin Oncol. 2009;27: 526–34.

182. Fumoleau P, Llombart-Cussac A, Roche H, Pivot X, Martin M, Kubista E, et al. Clinical activity of

ixabepilone, a novel epothilone B analog, across the breast cancer disease continuum. Eur J Cancer. 2007; 5(Suppl): Abstract 2119.

183. Saura C, Tseng LM, Chan S. Phase 2 study of ixabepilone versus paclitaxel as neoadjuvant therapy for early stage breast cancer with comparative biomarker analysis. 33rd Annual San Antonio Breast Cancer Symposium, 2010. San Antonio, Abstract 701.

184. Rugo HS, Roche H, Thomas ES. Ixabepilone plus capecitabine vs capecitabine in patients with triple negative tumors: a pooled analysis of patients from two large phase III clinical studies. Cancer Res. 2009; 69(Suppl 2):Abstract 3057.

185. Linderholm BK, Klintman M, Grabau D. Significantly higher expression of vascular endothelial growth factor (VEGF) and shorter survival after recurrences in premenopausal node negative patients with triple negative breast cancer. Cancer Res. 2009;69(2 Suppl 1):1077 abstract.

186. Ryd´en L, Ferno M, Stal O. Vascular endothelial growth factor receptor 2 is a significant negative prognostic biomarker in triple-negative breast cancer: results from a controlled randomised trial of premenopausal breast cancer. Cancer Res. 2009;69(2 Suppl 1):1087 abstract.

187. Miller K, Wang M, Gralow J, Dickler M, Cobleigh M, Perez EA, et al. Paclitaxel plus bevacizumab versus paclitaxel alone for metastatic breast cancer. N Engl J Med. 2007;357:2666–76.

188. Miles DW, Chan A, Dirix LY, Cortés J, Pivot X, Tomczak P, et al. Phase III study of bevacizumab plus docetaxel compared with placebo plus docetaxel for the first-line treatment of human epidermal growth factor receptor 2-negative metastatic breast cancer. J Clin Oncol. 2010;28:3239–47.

189. Robert NJ, Dieras V, Glaspy J, Brufsky AM, Bondarenko I, Lipatov ON, et al. RIBBON-1: randomized, double-blind, placebo-controlled, phase III trial of chemotherapy with or without bevacizumab for first-line treatment of human epidermal growth factor receptor 2-negative, locally recurrent or metastatic breast cancer. J Clin Oncol. 2011;29:1252–60.

190. Brufsky AM, Hurvitz S, Perez E, Swamy R, Valero V, O'Neill V, et al. RIBBON-2: a randomized, double-blind, placebo-controlled, phase III trial evaluating the efficacy and safety of bevacizumab in combination with chemotherapy for second-line treatment of human epidermal growth factor receptor 2-negative metastatic breast cancer. J Clin Oncol. 2011;29:4286–93.

191. Cameron D, Brown J, Dent R, Jackisch C, Mackey J, Pivot X, et al. Adjuvant bevacizumab-containing therapy in triple-negative breast cancer (BEATRICE): primary results of a randomised, phase 3 trial. Lancet Oncol. 2013;14:933–4.

192. Bell R, Brown J, Parmar M, Toi S ,Suter T, Steger G, et al. Final efficacy and updated safety results of the randomized phase III BEATRICE trial evaluating adjuvant bevacizumab (BEV)-containing therapy for early triple-negative breast cancer (TNBC). San Antonio Breast Cancer Symposium, 2014, San Antonio [PD2-2].

193. Slamon DJ, Swain SM, Buyse M. Primary results from BETH, a phase 3 controlled study of adjuvant chemotherapy and trastuzumab ± bevacizumab in patients with HER2-positive, node-positive or high risk node-negative breast cancer. San Antonio Breast Cancer Symposium, 2013, San Antonio, [S1-03].

194. Miller K, O'Neill AM, Dang CT. Bevacizumab (Bv) in the adjuvant treatment of HER2-negative breast cancer: final results from Eastern Cooperative Oncology Group E5103. J Clin Oncol 32:5s, 2014 (suppl; abstr 500).

195. Siziopikou KP, Ariga R, Proussaloglou KE, Gattuso P, Cobleigh M. The challenging estrogen receptor-negative/ progesterone receptor-negative/HER-2-negative patient: a promising candidate for epidermal growth factor receptor targeted therapy? Breast J. 2006;12:360–2.

196. Corkery B, Crown J, Clynes M, O'Donovan N. Epidermal growth factor receptor as a potential therapeutic target in triple-negative breast cancer. Ann Oncol. 2009;20:862–7.

197. Carey LA, Rugo HS, Marcom PK. TBCRC 001: EGFR inhibition with cetuximab added to carboplatin in metastatic triple-negative (basal-like) breast cancer. J Clin Oncol. 2008;26:1009 abstract.

198. O'Shaughnessy J, Weckstein DJ, Vukelja SJ. Preliminary results of a randomized phase II study of weekly irinotecan/carboplatin with or without cetuximab in patients with metastatic breast cancer. Breast Cancer Res Treat. 2007;106(Suppl -1):S32 abstract 308.

199. Nabholtz J, Weber B, Mouret-Reynier M. Panitumumab in combination with FEC 100 (5-fluorouracil, epidoxorubicin, cyclophosphamide) followed by docetaxel (T) in patients with operable, triple-negative breast cancer (TNBC): preliminary results of a multicenter neoadjuvant pilot phase II study. J Clin Oncol. 2011;29 (suppl):Abstr e11574.

200. Sasco AJ, Lowenfels AB, Pasker-de JP. Review article: epidemiology of male breast cancer. A meta-analysis of published case-control studies and discussion of selected aetiological factors. Int J Cancer. 1993;53:538–49.

201. O'Malley CD, Prehn AW, Shema SJ, Glaser SL. Racial/ethnic differences in survival rates in a population-based series of men with breast carcinoma. Cancer. 2002;94:2836–43.

202. Brinton LA. Breast cancer risk among patients with Klinefelter syndrome. Acta Paediatr. 2011;100: 814–8.

203. Mabuchi K, Bross DS, Kessler II. Risk factors for male breast cancer. J Natl Cancer Inst. 1985;74: 371–5.

204. Thomas DB, Jimenez LM, McTiernan A, Rosenblatt K, Stalsberg H, Stemhagen A, et al. Breast cancer in men: risk factors with hormonal implications. Am J Epidemiol. 1992;135:734–48.

205. Chavez-Macgregor M, Clarke CA, Lichtensztajn D. Male breast cancer according to tumor subtype and

race: a population-based study. Cancer. 2013;119: 1611–7.

206. Giordano SH, Cohen DS, Buzdar AU, Perkins G, Hortobagyi GN. Breast carcinoma in men: a population-based study. Cancer. 2004;101:51–7.

207. Bloom KJ, Govil H, Gattuso P, Reddy V, Francescatti D. Status of HER-2 in male and female breast carcinoma. Am J Surg. 2001;182:389–92.

208. Scott-Conner CE, Jochimsen PR, Menck HR, Winchester DJ. An analysis of male and female breast cancer treatment and survival among demographically identical pairs of patients. Surgery. 1999;126:775–80; discussion 780–781.

209. Giordano SH. A review of the diagnosis and management of male breast cancer. Oncologist. 2005;10: 471–9.

210. Bagley CS, Wesley MN, Young RC, Lippman ME. Adjuvant chemotherapy in males with cancer of the breast. Am J Clin Oncol. 1987;10:55–60.

211. Yildirim E, Berberoğlu U. Male breast cancer: a 22-year experience. Eur J Surg Oncol. 1998;24: 548–52.

212. Patel 2nd HZ, Buzdar AU, Hortobagyi GN. Role of adjuvant chemotherapy in male breast cancer. Cancer. 1989;64:1583–5.

213. Izquierdo MA, Alonso C, De Andres L, Ojeda B. Male breast cancer. Report of a series of 50 cases. Acta Oncol. 1994;33:767–71.

214. Giordano SH, Perkins GH, Broglio K, Garcia SG, Middleton LP, Buzdar AU, Hortobagyi GN. Adjuvant systemic therapy for male breast carcinoma. Cancer. 2005;104:2359–64.

215. Smith LH, Danielsen B, Allen ME, Cress R. Cancer associated with obstetric delivery: results of linkage with the California cancer registry. Am J Obstet Gynecol. 2003;189:1128–35.

216. Stensheim H, Møller B, van Dijk T, Fosså SD. Cause-specific survival for women diagnosed with cancer during pregnancy or lactation: a registry-based cohort study. J Clin Oncol. 2009;27:45–51.

217. Parente JT, Amsel M, Lerner R, Chinea F. Breast cancer associated with pregnancy. Obstet Gynecol. 1998;71:861–4.

218. Tobon H, Horowitz LF. Breast cancer during pregnancy. Breast Dis. 1993;6:127–34.

219. King RM, Welch JS, Martin JK, Coulam CB. Carcinoma of the breast associated with pregnancy. Surg Gynecol Obstet. 1985;160:228–32.

220. Shousha S. Breast carcinoma presenting during or shortly after pregnancy and lactation. Arch Pathol Lab Med. 2000;124:1053–60.

221. Middleton LP, Amin M, Gwyn K, Theriault R, Sahin A. Breast carcinoma in pregnant women: assessment of clinicopathologic and immunohistochemical features. Cancer. 2003;98:1055–60.

222. Ishida T, Yokoe T, Kasumu F, Sakamoto G, Makita M, Tominaga T, et al. Clinicopathologic characteristics and prognosis of breast cancer patients associated with pregnancy and lactation: analysis of case-control study in Japan. Jpn J Cancer Res. 1992;83:1143–9.

223. Reed W, Hannisdal E, Skovlund E, Thoresen S, Lilleng P, Nesland JM. Pregnancy and breast cancer: a population-based study. Virchows Arch. 2003;443:44–50.

224. Bonnier P, Romain S, Dilhuydy JM, Bonichon F, Julien JP, Charpin C, et al. Influence of pregnancy on the outcome of breast cancer: a case-control study. Societe Francaise de Senologie et de Pathologie Mammaire Study Group. Int J Cancer. 1997;72: 720–7.

225. Bertheau P, Steinberg SM, Cowan K, Merino MJ. Breast cancer in young women: clinicopathologic correlation. Semin Diagn Pathol. 1999;16:248–56.

226. Rosen PP, Lesser ML, Kinne DW, Beathie EJ. Breast carcinoma in women 35 years of age or younger. Ann Surg. 1984;199:133–42.

227. Elledge RM, Ciocca DR, Langone G, McGuire WL. Estrogen receptor, progesterone receptor, and HER-2/neu protein in breast cancers from pregnant patients. Cancer. 1993;71:2499–506.

228. Germann N, Goffinet F, Goldwasser F. Anthracyclines during pregnancy: embryo-fetal outcome in 160 patients. Ann Oncol. 2004;15:146–50.

229. Johnson PH, Gwyn K, Gordon N. The treatment of pregnant women with breast cancer and the outcomes of the children exposed to chemotherapy in utero [abstract]. J Clin Oncol. 2005;23(Suppl 16): Abstract 540.

230. Marquardt H, Philips FS, Sternberg SS. Tumorigenicity in vivo and induction of malignant transformation and mutagenesis in cell cultures by Adriamycin and Daunomycin. Cancer Res. 1976;36:2065–9.

231. Pommier Y, Fesen MR, Goldwasser F. Topoisomerase II inhibitors: the epipodophyllotoxins, m-AMSA and the ellipticine derivate. In: Chabner BA, Longo DL, editors. Cancer chemotherapy and biotherapy. 2nd ed. Philadelphia: Lippincott-Raven; 1996. p. 435–61.

232. Pacifici GM, Nottoli R. Placental transfer of drugs administered to the mother. Clin Pharmacokinet. 1995;28:235–69.

233. Smit JW, Huisman MT, Van Tellingen O, Wiltshire HR, Schinkel AH. Absence or pharmacological blocking of placental P-glycoprotein profoundly increases fetal drug exposure. J Clin Invest. 1999;104:1441–7.

234. Stewart DJ, Grewaal D, Green RM, Mikhael N, Goel R, Montpetit VA, et al. Concentrations of doxorubicin and its metabolites in human autopsy heart and other tissues. Anticancer Res. 1993;13:1945–52.

235. He YL, Seno H, Tsujimoto S, Tashiro C. The effects of uterine and umbilical blood flows on the transfer of propofol across the human placenta during in vitro perfusion. Anesth Analg. 2001;93:151–6.

236. Hahn KM, Johnson PH, Gordon N, Kuerer H, Middleton L, Ramirez M, et al. Treatment of pregnant breast cancer patients and outcomes of children exposed to chemotherapy in utero. Cancer. 2006;107: 1219–26.

237. Turchi JJ, Villasis C. Anthracyclines in the treatment of malignancy in pregnancy. Cancer. 1988;61: 435–40.

238. Zemlickis D, Lishner M, Degendorfer P, Panzarella T, Sutcliffe SB, Koren G. Fetal outcome after in utero exposure to cancer chemotherapy. Arch Intern Med. 1992;152:573–6.

239. Ring AE, Smith IE, Jones A, Shannon C, Galani E, Ellis PA. Chemotherapy for breast cancer during pregnancy: an 18-year experience from five London teaching hospitals. J Clin Oncol. 2005;23:4192–7.

240. Giacalone PL, Laffargue F, Bénos P. Chemotherapy for breast carcinoma during pregnancy: a French national survey. Cancer. 1999;86:2266–72.

241. Cardonick E, Iacobucci A. Use of chemotherapy during human pregnancy. Lancet Oncol. 2004;5:283–91.

242. Zemlickis D, Lishner M, Degendorfer P, Panzarella T, Burke B, Sutcliffe SB, et al. Maternal and fetal outcome after breast cancer in pregnancy. Am J Obstet Gynecol. 1992;166:781–7.

243. Nettleton J, Long J, Kuban D, Wu R, Shaefffer J, El-Mahdi A. Breast cancer during pregnancy: quantifying the risk of treatment delay. Obstet Gynecol. 1996;87:414–8.

244. Briggs GG, Freeman RK, Yaffe SJ. Drugs in pregnancy and lactation. 8th ed. Philadelphia: Lippincott Williams & Wilkins; 2008.

245. Doll DC, Ringenberg QS, Yarbro JW. Antineoplastic agents and pregnancy. Semin Oncol. 1989;16:337–46.

246. Zemlickis D, Klein J, Moselhy G, Koren G. Cisplatin protein binding in pregnancy and the neonatal period. Med Pediatr Oncol. 1994;23:476–9.

247. Mir O, Berveiller P, Goffinet F, Treluyer JM, Serreau R, Goldwasser F, et al. Taxanes for breast cancer during pregnancy: a systematic review. Ann Oncol. 2010;21:425–6.

248. Garcia-Gonzalez J, Cueva J, Lamas MJ, Curiel T, Graña B, López-López R. Paclitaxel and cisplatin in the treatment of metastatic non-small-cell lung cancer during pregnancy. Clin Transl Oncol. 2008;10:375–6.

249. Bader AA, Schlembach D, Tamussino KF, Pristauz G, Petru E. Anhydramnios associated with administration of trastuzumab and paclitaxel for metastatic breast cancer during pregnancy. Lancet Oncol. 2007;8:79–81.

250. Amant F, Deckers S, Van Calsteren K, Loibl S, Halaska M, Brepoels L, et al. Breast cancer in pregnancy: recommendations of an international consensus meeting. Eur J Cancer. 2010;46:3158–68.

251. Ferlay J, Héry C, Autier P, Sankaranarayanan R. Global burden of breast cancer. In: Li C, editor. Breast cancer epidemiology. New York: Springer; 2010. p. 1–19.

252. Menna P, Gonzalez Paz O, Chello M, Covino E, Salvatorelli E, Minotti G. Anthracycline cardiotoxicity. Expert Opin Drug Saf. 2012;11:21–36.

253. Roca-Alonso L, Pellegrino L, Castellano L, Stebbing J. Breast cancer treatment and adverse cardiac events: what are the molecular mechanisms? Cardiology. 2012;122:253–9.

254. Meinardi MT, van Veldhuisen DJ, Gietema JA, Dolsma WV, Boomsma F, van den Berg MP, et al. Prospective evaluation of early cardiac damage induced by epirubicin-containing adjuvant chemotherapy and locoregional radiotherapy in breast cancer patients. J Clin Oncol. 2001;19:2746–53.

255. Maxwell CB, Jenkins AT. Drug-induced heart failure. Am J Health Syst Pharm. 2011;68:1791–804.

256. Swain SM, Whaley FS, Ewer MS. Congestive heart failure in patients treated with doxorubicin: a retrospective analysis of three trials. Cancer. 2003;97:2869–79.

257. Darby SC, McGale P, Taylor CW, Peto R. Long-term mortality from heart disease and lung cancer after radiotherapy for early breast cancer: prospective cohort study of about 300,000 women in US SEER cancer registries. Lancet Oncol. 2005;6:557–65.

258. Little MP, Tawn EJ, Tzoulaki I, Wakeford R, Hildebrandt G, Paris F, et al. Review and meta-analysis of epidemiological associations between low/moderate doses of ionizing radiation and circulatory disease risks, and their possible mechanisms. Radiat Environ Biophys. 2010;49:139–53.

259. Schmitz KH, Prosnitz RG, Schwartz AL, Carver JR. Prospective surveillance and management of cardiac toxicity and health in breast cancer survivors. Cancer. 2012;118(Suppl):2270–6.

260. Singal PK, Iliskovic N. Doxorubicin-induced cardiomyopathy. N Engl J Med. 1998;339:900–5.

261. Isncr JM, Ferrans VJ, Cohen SR, Witkind BG, Virmani R, Gottdiener JS, et al. Clinical and morphologic cardiac findings after anthracycline chemotherapy. Analysis of 64 patients studied at necropsy. Am J Cardiol. 1983;51:1167–74.

262. Von Hoff DD, Rozencweig M, Layard M, Slavik M, Muggia FM. Daunomycin-induced cardiotoxicity in children and adults. A review of 110 cases. Am J Med. 1977;62:200–8.

263. Curigliano G, Mayer EL, Burstein HJ, Winer EP, Goldhirsch A. Cardiac toxicity from systemic cancer therapy: a comprehensive review. Prog Cardiovasc Dis. 2010;53:94–104.

264. Gianni L, Baselga J, Eiermann W, Porta VG, Semiglazov V, Lluch A, et al. Phase III trial evaluating the addition of paclitaxel to doxorubicin followed by cyclophosphamide, methotrexate, and fluorouracil, as adjuvant or primary systemic therapy: European Cooperative Trial in Operable Breast Cancer. J Clin Oncol. 2009;27:2474–81.

265. Grenier MA, Lipshultz SE. Epidemiology of anthracycline cardiotoxicity in children and adults. Semin Oncol. 1998;25:72–85.

266. Braverman AC, Antin JH, Plappert MT, Cook EF, Lee RT. Cyclophosphamide cardiotoxicity in bone marrow transplantation: a prospective evaluation of new dosing regimens. J Clin Oncol. 1991;9:1215–23.

267. Goldberg MA, Antin JH, Guinan EC, Rappeport JM. Cyclophosphamide cardiotoxicity: an analysis of dosing as a risk factor. Blood. 1986;68:1114–8.

268. Gharib MI, Burnett AK. Chemotherapy-induced cardiotoxicity: current practice and prospects of prophylaxis. Eur J Heart Fail. 2002;4:235–42.

269. Del Mastro L, Perrone F, Repetto L, Manzione L, Zagonel V, Fratino L, et al. Weekly paclitaxel as firstline chemotherapy in elderly advanced breast cancer patients: a phase II study of the Gruppo Italiano di Oncologia Geriatrica (GIOGer). Ann Oncol. 2005;16:253–8.

270. Bird BR, Swain SM. Cardiac toxicity in breast cancer survivors: review of potential cardiac problems. Clin Cancer Res. 2008;14:14–24.

271. http://dailymed.nlm.nih.gov/dailymed/drugInfo. cfm?id=17003. Accessed on 23 Aug 2010.

272. Smith LA, Cornelius VR, Plummer CJ, Levitt G, Verrill M, Canney P, et al. Cardiotoxicity of anthracycline agents for the treatment of cancer: systematic review and meta-analysis of randomised controlled trials. BMC Cancer. 2010;10:337.

273. Curran CF, Narang PK, Reynolds RD. Toxicity profile of dexrazoxane (Zinecard, ICRF-187, ADR-529, NSC-169780), a modulator of doxorubicin cardiotoxicity. Cancer Treat Rev. 1991;18:241–52.

274. Speyer JL, Green MD, Zeleniuch-Jacquotte A, Wernz JC, Rey M, Sanger J, et al. ICRF-187 permits longer treatment with doxorubicin in women with breast cancer. J Clin Oncol. 1992;10:117–27.

275. Swain SM, Vici P. The current and future role of dexrazoxane as a cardioprotectant in anthracycline treatment: expert panel review. J Cancer Res Clin Oncol. 2004;130:1–7.

276. van Dalen EC, Caron HN, Dickinson HO, Kremer LC. Cardioprotective interventions for cancer patients receiving anthracyclines. Cochrane Database Syst Rev. 2011;(2):CD003917.

277. Seymour L, Bramwell V, Moran LA. Use of dexrazoxane as a cardioprotectant in patients receiving doxorubicin or epirubicin chemotherapy for the treatment of cancer. The Provincial Systemic Treatment Disease Site Group. Cancer Prev Control. 1999;3:145–59.

278. Hensley ML, Hagerty KL, Kewalramani T, Green DM, Meropol NJ, Wasserman TH, et al. American Society of Clinical Oncology 2008 clinical practice guideline update: use of chemotherapy and radiation therapy protectants. J Clin Oncol. 2009;27:127–45.

279. Lee VC, Rhew DC, Dylan M, Badamgarav E, Braunstein GD, Weingarten SR. Meta-analysis: angiotensin-receptor blockers in chronic heart failure and high-risk acute myocardial infarction. Ann Intern Med. 2004;141:693–704.

280. Schocken DD, Benjamin EJ, Fonarow GC, Krumholz HM, Levy D, Mensah GA, et al. Prevention of heart failure. Circulation. 2008;117:2544–65.

281. Minotti G, Salvatorelli E, Menna P. Pharmacological foundations of cardio-oncology. J Pharmacol Exp Ther. 2010;334:2–8.

282. Cardinale D, Colombo A, Sandri MT, Lamantia G, Colombo N, Civelli M, et al. Prevention of high-dose chemotherapy-induced cardiotoxicity in high-risk patients by angiotensin- converting enzyme inhibition. Circulation. 2006;114:2474–81.

283. Cardinale D, Colombo A, Lamantia G, Colombo N, Civelli M, De Giacomi G, et al. Anthracycline-induced cardiomyopathy: clinical relevance and response to pharmacologic therapy. J Am Coll Cardiol. 2010;55:213–20.

284. Kalay N, Basar E, Ozdogru I, Er O, Cetinkaya Y, Dogan A, et al. Protective effects of carvedilol against anthracycline-induced cardiomyopathy. J Am Coll Cardiol. 2006;48:2258–62.

285. Heck SL, Gulati G, Ree AH, Schulz-Menger J, Gravdehaug B, Røsjø H, et al. Rationale and design of the prevention of cardiac dysfunction during an Adjuvant Breast Cancer Therapy (PRADA) Trial. Cardiology. 2012;123:240–7.

286. Danaei G, Vander Hoorn S, Lopez AD, Murray CJL, Ezzati M, Comparative Risk Assessment collaborating group (Cancers). Causes of cancer in the world: comparative risk assessment on nine behavioral and environmental risk factors. Lancet. 2005;366:1784–93.

287. Modesitt SC, Van Nagell JR. The impact of obesity on the incidence and treatment of gynecologic cancers: a review. Obstet Gynecol Surv. 2005;60:683–92.

288. Protani M, Coory M, Martin JH. Effect of obesity on survival of women with breast cancer: systematic review and meta-analysis. Breast Cancer Res Treat. 2010;123:627–35.

289. Zumoff B, Dasgupta I. Relationship between body weight and the incidence of positive nodes at mastectomy in breast cancer. J Surg Oncol. 1983;2:217–20.

290. Verreault R, Brisson J, Deschenes L, Naud F. Body weight and prognostic indicators in breast cancer. Am J Epidemiol. 1989;129:260–8.

291. Barpe DR, Rosa DD, Froehlich PE. Pharmacokinetic evaluation of doxorubicin plasma levels in normal and overweight patients with breast cancer and simulation of dose adjustment by different indexes of body mass. Eur J Pharm Sci. 2010;41:458–63.

292. Gusella M, Toso S, Ferrazzi E, Ferrari M, Padrini R. Relationships between body composition parameters and fluorouracil pharmacokinetics. Br J Clin Pharmacol. 2002;54:131–9.

293. Dignam JJ, Wieand K, Johnson KA, Raich P, Anderson SJ, Somkin C, et al. Effects of obesity and race on prognosis in lymph node-negative, estrogen receptor negative breast cancer. Breast Cancer Res Treat. 2006;97:245–54.

294. Dignam JJ, Wieand K, Johnson KA, Fisher B, Xu L, Mamounas EP. Obesity, tamoxifen use, and outcomes in women with estrogen receptor-positive early-stage breast cancer. J Natl Cancer Inst. 2003; 95:1467–76.

295. Sparano JA, Wang M, Zhao F, Stearns V, Martino S, Ligibel JA, et al. Obesity at diagnosis is associated with inferior outcomes in hormone receptor-positive operable breast cancer. Cancer. 2012;118:5937–46.

296. Sestak I, Distler W, Forbes JF, Dowsett M, Howell A, Cuzick J. Effect of body mass index on recur-

rences in tamoxifen and anastrozole treated women: an exploratory analysis from the ATAC trial. J Clin Oncol. 2010;28:3411–5.

297. Cheymol G. Effects of obesity on pharmacokinetics implications for drug therapy. Clin Pharmacokinet. 2000;39:215–31.

298. Bonadonna G, Valagussa P. Dose-response effect of adjuvant chemotherapy in breast cancer. N Engl J Med. 1981;304:10–5.

299. Wood WC, Budman DR, Korzun AH, Cooper MR, Younger J, Hart RD, et al. Dose and dose intensity of adjuvant chemotherapy for stage-II, node-positive breast-carcinoma. N Engl J Med. 1994;330:1253–9.

300. Carroll J, Protani M, Walpole E, Martin JH. Effect of obesity on toxicity in women treated with adjuvant chemotherapy for early-stage breast cancer: a systematic review. Breast Cancer Res Treat. 2012; 136:323–30.

301. Griggs JJ, Sorbero ME, Lyman GH. Undertreatment of obese women receiving breast cancer chemotherapy. Arch Intern Med. 2005;165:1267–73.

302. Saarto T, Blomqvist C, Rissanen P, Auvinen A, Elomaa I. Haematological toxicity: a marker of adjuvant chemotherapy efficacy in stage II and III breast cancer. Br J Cancer. 1997;75:301–5.

303. Lopes-Serrao MD, Ussery SM, Hall 2nd RG, Shah SR. Evaluation of chemotherapy-induced severe myelosuppression incidence in obese patients with capped dosing. J Oncol Pract. 2011;7:13–7.

304. Griggs JJ, Mangu PB, Anderson H, Balaban EP, Dignam JJ, Hryniuk WM, American Society of Clinical Oncology, et al. Appropriate chemotherapy dosing for obese adult patients with cancer: American Society of Clinical Oncology clinical practice guideline. J Clin Oncol. 2012;30: 1553–61.

305. Smith TJ, Desch CE. Neutropenia-wise and pound-foolish: safe and effective chemotherapy in massively obese patients. South Med J. 1991;84:883–5.

306. Madarnas Y, Sawka CA, Franssen E, Bjarnason GA. Are medical oncologists biased in their treatment of the large woman with breast cancer? Breast Cancer Res Treat. 2001;66:123–33.

307. Wright JD, Tian C, Mutch DG, Herzog TJ, Nagao S, Fujiwara K, et al. Carboplatin dosing in obese women with ovarian cancer: a Gynecologic Oncology Group study. Gynecol Oncol. 2008;109: 353–8.

308. Abdah-Bortnyak R, Tsalic M, Haim N. Actual body weight for determining doses of chemotherapy in obese cancer patients: evaluation of treatment tolerability. Med Oncol. 2003;20:363–8.

309. Rosner GL, Hargis JB, Hollis DR, Budman DR, Weiss RB, Henderson IC, et al. Relationship between toxicity and obesity in women receiving adjuvant chemotherapy for breast cancer: results from Cancer and Leukemia Group B study 8541. J Clin Oncol. 1996;14:3000–8.

Adjuvant Therapy for HER2-Positive Early Breast Cancer

Gul Basaran and Devrim Cabuk

Abstract

The discovery of human epidermal growth factor receptor 2 (HER-2/neu) and its role in the biology of breast cancer is one of the most important success stories in the history of breast cancer. The development of HER-2-targeted therapies has changed the natural history of HER-2-positive breast cancer dramatically in the past two decades. Success in the metastatic setting has been subsequently translated into improved clinical outcomes for women with early-stage HER-2-positive breast cancer. Multiple phase III clinical trials, including HERA, FinHer, Breast Cancer International Research Group (BCIRG) 006, and the National Surgical Adjuvant Breast and Bowel Project (NSABP) B-31, have demonstrated that trastuzumab in combination with or subsequent to chemotherapy was associated with significant improvements in disease-free and overall survival in patients with HER-2-positive early breast cancer. Thus, the monoclonal antibody trastuzumab has been approved as the first and only molecularly targeted agent for the adjuvant treatment of HER-2-positive breast cancer. Despite tremendous progress in the treatment of HER-2-positive breast cancer, many questions regarding the optimal tailoring of anti-HER-2 therapy remain. Current adjuvant anti-HER-2 therapies need to be refined for different patient subsets with HER-2-positive tumors to provide personalized, effective, and minimally toxic treatment. Additional molecular biomarkers beyond HER-2 are necessary for the identification of low-risk patients who could benefit from less intensive or even no chemotherapy in combination with trastuzumab as well as for the identification of patients with resistance to anti-HER-2 therapy.

Keywords

Breast cancer • HER-2/neu • Trastuzumab • Lapatinib • Anti-HER-2 therapy

G. Basaran, MD (✉)
Medical Oncology Department, Medical Faculty,
Acibadem University, Atakent, Istanbul, Turkey
e-mail: gabasaran@gmail.com

D. Cabuk, MD
Department of Medical Oncology,
Kocaeli University Hospital, Kocaeli, Turkey
e-mail: devrimcabuk@yahoo.com

© Springer International Publishing Switzerland 2016
A. Aydiner et al. (eds.), *Breast Disease: Management and Therapies*,
DOI 10.1007/978-3-319-26012-9_9

HER-2/Neu-Positive Early Breast Cancer: From Biology to HER-2-Targeted Therapy

Amplification of the human epidermal growth factor receptor 2 (HER-2/neu) gene was identified as a poor prognostic factor in patients with breast cancer nearly three decades ago, in 1987 [1]. HER-2 gene amplification and/or protein overexpression in breast cancer has subsequently been associated with an aggressive phenotype, increased recurrence, and decreased survival [2]. HER-2 gene amplification and/or protein overexpression has been identified in 10–34 % of invasive breast cancers [3]. Trastuzumab, a monoclonal antibody that binds to the extracellular portion of the HER-2 transmembrane receptor, has been widely studied in metastatic breast cancer. Metastatic trials have demonstrated substantial efficacy of trastuzumab and established criteria to select patients who could benefit from this monoclonal antibody [4]. Soon after US FDA approval of trastuzumab use in metastatic breast cancer, a new molecular classification of breast tumors based on gene expression patterns was developed [5]. This molecular classification identified the HER-2-positive group as one of four molecular subgroups with poor prognosis. Subsequent randomized trials provided clear and consistent evidence that the addition of trastuzumab to adjuvant chemotherapy significantly reduces the likelihood of relapse and death among women with HER-2-positive early breast cancer [6–11].

Metastatic breast cancer trials demonstrated that a high level of HER-2 overexpression is a strong predictor of benefit from trastuzumab [2]. Patients who were likely to respond to trastuzumab therapy were identified either by strong (3+) IHC (immunohistochemistry) for the HER-2 protein or by gene amplification (FISH or CISH). Patients with a 2+ IHC score and gene amplification also received benefit from trastuzumab. Based on the data from the metastatic setting, adjuvant trastuzumab trials have considered breast cancer patients with either 3+ IHC or FISH-positive tumors eligible for enrollment. This algorithm for determining tumor HER-2 status was subsequently outlined as a guideline by a joint consensus of the American Society of Clinical Oncology (ASCO) and the College of American Pathologists (CAP) and was recently updated [12, 13].

Clinical Evidence of Benefit from Adjuvant Trastuzumab

The efficacy and toxicity of trastuzumab in the adjuvant setting have been evaluated by seven large, randomized, multicenter controlled trials that have accrued approximately 17,000 patients [8, 14–24]. These trials had similar eligibility criteria in terms of the assessment of HER-2/neu status (patients with either 3+ IHC or FISH-positive disease were enrolled) but differed in many aspects, including patient population, timing of trastuzumab administration, type of chemotherapy used, duration of trastuzumab use, etc. Table 9.1 provides a summary of pivotal adjuvant trials in HER-2/neu-positive early breast cancer.

The HERA trial, the combined analysis of the NSABP B-31 and NCCTG N9831 trials (joint analysis), and BCIRG 006 trial demonstrated statistically significant improvements in DFS (disease-free survival) as the primary endpoint. The HERA, joint analysis, and BCIRG 006 trials also reported significant improvements in overall survival (OS).

Herceptin Adjuvant (HERA) Trial

HERA was an international, multicenter, randomized, open-label phase III trial comparing trastuzumab for 1 or 2 years with observation in women with centrally confirmed HER-2/neu-positive early breast cancer. All patients completed locoregional therapy and received standard neoadjuvant/adjuvant chemotherapy before randomization. Patients were required to have a left ventricular ejection fraction (LVEF) of 55 % after primary treatment as measured by multigated acquisition (MUGA) scan or echocardiography prior to randomization. After a median follow-up period of

Table 9.1 Overview of adjuvant trastuzumab trials in patients with HER-2-positive early breast cancer

Study	Treatment regimen	Trastuzumab duration (weeks)	Patients (n)	Median follow-up (months)	Disease-free survival			Overall survival		
					HR	95 % CI	P	HR	95 % CI	P
HERA	CT	–	1698	96	0.76	0.66–0.87	<0.0001	0.76	0.65–0.88	0.0005
	CT→T	52	1703							
	CT→T	104	1701		0.99	0.85–1.14	0.86	1.05	0.86–1.28	0.63
Joint analysis				100.8	0.60	0.53–0.68	<0.0001	0.63	0.54–0.73	<0.0001
NSABP B-31	AC→P	–	2018							
NCCTG N9831	AC→PT→T	52	2028							
NCCTG N9831	AC→P	–	1087	72	0.67	0.54–0.81	<0.001	0.88	0.67–1.15	0.343
	AC→P→T	52	1097/954		0.77	0.53–1.11	0.022	0.78	0.58–1.05	0.102
	AC→PT→T	52	949							
BCIRG 006	AC→D	–	1073	65						
	AC→DT→T	52	1074		0.64	0.53–0.78	<0.001	0.63	0.48–0.81	<0.001
	DCarboT→T	52	1075		0.75	0.63–0.90	0.04	0.77	0.60–0.99	0.038
PHARE	CT+T	26	1690	42.5	1.28	1.05–1.56	0.29	1.47	1.07–2.02	NR
	CT+T	52	1690							
FinHer	D/V→FEC	–	116	62	0.65	0.38–1.12	0.12	0.55	0.27–1.11	0.094
	(D/V)T→FEC	9	115							
PACS 04	FEC→ED	–	268	47	0.86	0.61–1.22	0.41	1.27	0.68–2.38	NR
	FEC/ED→T	52	260							

NSABP B-31 the National Surgical Adjuvant Breast and Bowel Project B-31 trial, *NCCTG N9831* the North Central Cancer Treatment Group N9831 trial, *BCIRG 006* the Breast Cancer International Research Group trial, *PHARE* the Protocol for Herceptin as Adjuvant Therapy with Reduced Exposure trial, *FinHer* the Finland Herceptin trial, *PACS 04* the Protocol Adjuvant dans le Cancer du Sein trial, *CT* chemotherapy, *T* trastuzumab, *A* doxorubicin, *C* cyclophosphamide, *P* paclitaxel, *D* docetaxel, *Carbo* carboplatin, *V* vinorelbine, *F* 5-fluorouracil, *E* epirubicin

1 year, the comparison of 1-year treatment versus observation was published in 2005 [6]. There was a statistically significant 36 % reduction in disease recurrence (HR 0.64, 3-year DFS of 81 % versus 74 %) and a significant improvement in overall survival (HR 0.66, 92 % versus 90 % in the trastuzumab and non-trastuzumab groups, respectively). Efficacy outcomes were similar across subgroups as defined by nodal status or hormone receptor expression. Based on these results, trastuzumab became the standard of care in the treatment of HER-2-positive early breast cancer, and there was a protocol amendment allowing the patients in the observation arm who remained event-free to cross over to the trastuzumab arm. The incidence of grade 3 or 4 adverse and serious cardiac toxicity events was higher in the trastuzumab group than in the observation group. Fatal events (six versus three patients), symptomatic congestive heart failure (CHF) (1.7 % versus 0.06 %), and LVEF drops (7.1 % versus 2.2 %) were more frequent in the trastuzumab arm. There was one cardiac death in the observation group, and nine patients (0.54 %) in the treatment group had severe CHF.

With a median follow-up of 23.5 months, the early DFS improvement was confirmed, along with the emergence of a statistically significant OS benefit [14]. There were more grade 3 or 4 adverse events (11 % versus 6 %) and fatal (grade 5) treatment-related toxicities (0.5 % versus 0.2 %) in the trastuzumab arm compared to the control group. The only death due to cardiac causes was in the control arm. Trastuzumab was discontinued by 72 women (4.3 %) because of cardiac problems.

In a subsequent analysis with a median 4-year follow-up, a significant improvement in DFS favoring trastuzumab (4-year DFS 79 versus 72 %, HR 0.76, 95 % CI 0.66–0.87) remained even though 885 of the 1698 controls had crossed over to trastuzumab; however, the survival advantage was no longer statistically significant (HR for death 0.85, 95 % 0.70–1.04) [15]. As reported previously in the 2005 publication, there was one cardiac death in the observation group. More patients on 1-year trastuzumab had symptomatic congestive heart failure and a confirmed

significant LVEF drop than in the observation group. There were fewer cases of symptomatic congestive heart failure and confirmed significant LVEF drops in the selective crossover cohort associated with delayed trastuzumab treatment compared with 1-year trastuzumab.

The results of the 2-year versus 1-year comparison were published at 8 years of median follow-up in 2013 [16]. There was no benefit of 2-year versus 1-year trastuzumab when administered as sequential treatment following chemotherapy. In addition, patients in the 2-year arm experienced more cardiac toxicity with an increase in secondary cardiac adverse events (LVEF <50 % and ≥10 % below baseline confirmed by repeat assessment) (7.2 % versus 4.1 %) and no significant difference in CHF New York Heart Association (NYHA) class III or IV events. HERA results at 8 years of follow-up indicated sustained and statistically significant DFS and OS benefit for 1-year trastuzumab versus observation in intention-to-treat analysis despite the selective crossover rate of 52 %.

Of note, the HERA trial had a different design than North American trials. Patients received adjuvant trastuzumab therapy only after the completion of other local or systemic therapies. The median time from the diagnosis of breast cancer to the initiation of trastuzumab was 8.5 months. This lag time could be particularly important for patients who had a higher risk of relapse. The relapse rates in the observation arms were higher in patients with hormone receptor-negative disease and those with involvement of more than three axillary lymph nodes. Most women did not receive a taxane as a component of their adjuvant chemotherapy; a larger percentage (approximately one-third) had node-negative disease. Trastuzumab was administered on a triweekly schedule (initial loading dose 8 mg/kg and then 6 mg/kg every 3 weeks for 1 year). CNS (central nervous system) metastases were more frequent numerically than those in the observation arm; however, the death rate from CNS metastases was lower in the trastuzumab arm [25]. One year of adjuvant trastuzumab was arbitrarily selected as the study regimen, and HERA is the only adjuvant trial that also tested trastuzumab use for longer than 1 year.

NSABP B-31 and NCCTG N9831 Trials

The two North American cooperative group trials, NCCTG N9831 and NSABP B-31, were both multicenter, randomized, open-label phase III trials with a similar parallel design [7].

The National Surgical Adjuvant Breast and Bowel Project 31 trial (NSABP B-31) randomized 1736 women with HER-2-positive (3+ IHC or FISH-positive), node-positive breast cancer patients either to four cycles of doxorubicin plus cyclophosphamide (AC × 4) followed by four courses of single-agent paclitaxel (175 mg/m^2 over 3 h) (arm 1) or to the same chemotherapy plus weekly trastuzumab (initial loading dose 4 mg/kg and then 2 mg/kg weekly for 1 year) (arm 2), beginning with the first dose of paclitaxel. Weekly paclitaxel was administered after a protocol amendment at 39 months of accrual, and radiation therapy was administered after completion of chemotherapy. Hormonal therapy was initially administered at the start of AC and later following completion of chemotherapy.

In both trials, eligibility required LVEF assessments before entry, after the completion of doxorubicin and cyclophosphamide therapy, and 6, 9, and 18 months after randomization by multigated acquisition scanning or echocardiography. The initiation of trastuzumab required an LVEF that met or exceeded the lower limit of normal and a decrease of less than 16 percentage points from baseline after doxorubicin and cyclophosphamide therapy. Trastuzumab was not permitted in patients with symptomatic left ventricular dysfunction, cardiac ischemia, or arrhythmia while receiving AC. The 6- and 9-month cardiac assessments were used to determine whether trastuzumab should be continued in patients without cardiac symptoms.

The NCCTG N9831 trial randomized 1615 women with HER-2-positive, node-positive, or high-risk node-negative disease (>1 cm ER-negative or >2 cm ER-positive) who received AC × 4 followed by one of three different treatment strategies: weekly paclitaxel (80 mg/m^2) for 12 weeks followed by no further treatment (group A, control arm), the same dose and schedule of paclitaxel followed by sequential trastuzumab for

52 weeks (same schedule and doses as above; group B, sequential arm), or the same dose and schedule of paclitaxel plus concurrent trastuzumab followed by trastuzumab alone for 40 weeks (group C, concurrent arm). Radiation and/or hormonal therapy was administered after the completion of chemotherapy when indicated.

Other than differences in the scheduling of paclitaxel and some aspects of hormonal therapy and radiotherapy, the control groups of the two trials, arm 2 in trial B-31 and the group C concurrent arm in trial N9831, were identical. Therefore, the NCI (National Cancer Institute) and the Food and Drug Administration approved a joint analysis, although this pooled analysis was not part of the original treatment designs. The group B sequential arm of trial N9831 was not included in the combined analysis.

The first joint analysis was published in 2005 and demonstrated a 12 % absolute difference in DFS between the trastuzumab group (3-year DFS 75.4 % in the control group and 87.1 % in the trastuzumab group; HR: 0.48 95 % CI, 0.39–0.59; $P < 0.0001$) and the control group in addition to a 33 % reduction in the risk of death (HR, 0.67; 95 % CI, 0.48–0.93; $P = 0.015$) at a median follow-up of 2.0 years [7]. The 3-year cumulative incidence of class III or IV congestive heart failure or death from cardiac causes in the trastuzumab group was 4.1 % in trial B-31 and 2.9 % in trial N9831.

Efficacy results at 3.9 years of median follow-up were published in 2011 [18] and demonstrated that adjuvant trastuzumab concurrent with paclitaxel resulted in a significant 48 % reduction in recurrence risk (4-year DFS 86 % versus 74 %, HR 0.52) and a 39 % reduction in the risk of death (4-year OS 93 % versus 86 %, HR 0.61).

Updated results from the combined analysis at a median follow-up of 8.4 years were presented at the San Antonio Breast Cancer Symposium in 2012 and were consistent with an 11.5 % gain in DFS and an 8.8 % gain in OS for patients treated with trastuzumab [19]. The relative risk reduction benefit for both DFS and OS was of similar magnitude in virtually all patients, independent of age, nodal status, hormone receptor, tumor size, and histological grade.

After the release of the first joint analysis results at the American Society of Clinical Oncology Annual Meeting in 2005, patients previously randomly assigned to arm A of N9831 and arm 1 of B-31 were allowed to receive trastuzumab based on LVEF measurements. The crossover rate in B-31/N9831 was 20.4 %. Cardiac toxicity was similar to the results in the 7-year follow-up of the B-31 trial; there was a 4.0 % cardiac event rate for patients receiving trastuzumab versus a 1.3 % cardiac event rate in controls [26]. It should be noted that 5 % of patients assigned to the trastuzumab treatment arm never received the antibody due to decreases in LVEF or symptomatic heart disease. A combined review of cardiac toxicity data from the NSABP B-31 and NCCTG N9831 trials has also been published [27].

NCCTG N9831 Trial: Concurrent Versus Sequential Administration of Trastuzumab

N9831 was a three-arm trial that was also designed to compare the sequential and concurrent administration of trastuzumab (arms B and C, respectively). The NCCTG trial was initially designed to allow pairwise comparisons of the treatment strategies with three efficacy interim analyses. The original statistical plan was modified due to the temporary closure of arm C in 2002 because of cardiac safety concerns; this arm was resumed after extensive internal review by an independent cardiac safety monitoring committee.

At the time of the first interim combined analysis of the NSABP B-31 and NCCTG N9831 trials, the data monitoring committee overseeing trial N9831 requested an unplanned comparison of groups B and C. That comparison favored concurrent over sequential taxane treatment (HR for DFS was 0.64, 95 % CI 0.46–0.91; $P=0.00114$), and the HR for OS was 0.74 (95 % CI 0.43–1.26; $P=0.2696$) [28]. Following this preliminary result, the NCCTG independent data monitoring committee (IDMC) recommended the release of all NCCTG N9831 study data from the preplanned second interim analysis, including the comparison of arm A and arm B and the comparison

of arms B and C in 2009, despite low numbers of DFS events. At a 6-year median follow-up, the comparison of arm A and arm B revealed 5-year DFS rates of 71.8 % and 80.1 %, respectively [29]. DFS was significantly increased by the sequential addition of trastuzumab to paclitaxel treatment (log-rank $P=0.001$; HR, 0.69; 95 % CI, 0.57–0.85). Furthermore, there was an increase in DFS with concurrent trastuzumab and paclitaxel relative to sequential administration (arm C/arm B HR, 0.77; 99.9 % CI, 0.53–1.11), but the p value (0.02) did not cross the prespecified O'Brien-Fleming boundary (0.00116) for the interim analysis. The 5-year DFS rates were 80.1 % and 84.4 % in arms B and C, respectively. There was no statistically significant difference in OS. It was recommended that the decision for concurrent administration of trastuzumab with taxanes should be based on the risk-benefit ratio given the trend for superior efficacy profiles at the expense of slightly increased congestive heart failure events and asymptomatic LVEF drops in the concurrent arm C [30].

The BCIRG 006 Trial

The efficacy and safety of combining trastuzumab with a non-anthracycline-containing chemotherapy regimen were evaluated in an international, multicenter open-label phase III trial, the Breast Cancer International Research Group 006 (BCIRG 006) trial. The BCIRG trial enrolled 3222 women with HER-2-positive, node-positive, or high-risk, node-negative disease [8]. Patients with negative lymph nodes (no evidence of involvement in a review of a minimum of six axillary nodes or a negative sentinel node biopsy) were eligible if they had at least one high-risk feature (i.e., age <35 years, tumor >2 cm, ER/PR-negative, or histological and/or nuclear tumor grade 2 or 3). The patients were randomized to four cycles of doxorubicin (60 mg/m²) and cyclophosphamide (600 mg/m²) every 3 weeks followed by four cycles of docetaxel (100 mg/m²) every 3 weeks (ACT, control arm), the same chemotherapy with the concurrent administration of trastuzumab for 1 year beginning with the first dose of docetaxel (weekly during chemotherapy and then every 3 weeks) (ACTH arm) or a non-anthracycline-containing arm with docetaxel (75 mg/m^2) plus carboplatin (dosed at an area under the concentration × time curve [AUC] 6) every 3 weeks for six cycles concurrent with trastuzumab for 1 year (TCH arm). At a median follow-up of 65 months, the DFS rates were 75 % for ACT, 84 % for ACTH, and 81 % for TCH; the OS rates were 87 %, 92 %, and 91 %, respectively [8]. There were significant improvements in estimated DFS and OS at 5 years for both trastuzumab-containing arms (ACTH or TCH) compared to ACT. The BCIRG investigators concluded that the risk-benefit ratio favored the non-anthracycline TCH regimen over ACT plus trastuzumab even though there were no significant differences in DFS and OS between ACTH and TCH, and the study was not powered to detect equivalence between the ACTH and TCH arms. ACTH demonstrated a trend toward improved DFS and OS compared to TCH that did not reach statistical significance as well as small but significantly greater toxicity compared to TCH (the absolute difference in 5-year DFS between ACTH and TCH was 3 %). There were more neutropenia, a significantly lower incidence of congestive heart failure (2 % versus 0.4 % versus 0.7 % in the ACTH, TCH, and ACT arms, respectively), a reduction of mean LVEF (18.6 % versus 9.4 % versus 11.2 % in the ACTH, TCH, and ACT arms, respectively), and less neuropathy, nail changes, and myalgia in the TCH arm compared to ACTH.

The BCIRG 006 study also evaluated topoisomerase II alpha (TOP2A) amplification as a predictor of responsiveness to anthracyclines. The TOP2A gene is amplified in 30–40 % of patient cases of HER-2-positive breast cancer and has been associated with sensitivity to anthracycline-based chemotherapy in some trials [8, 31]. In 35 % of HER-2-positive cancers in which TOP2A was amplified, each of the three treatment arms (ACT, ACTH, and TCH) yielded similar efficacy results, implying no incremental benefit from the addition of trastuzumab to anthracycline-based chemotherapy [32]. Among patients without TOP2A

co-amplification, those treated with trastuzumab received more benefit. A similar analysis from NSABP B-31 determined that adding trastuzumab to anthracycline-based chemotherapy significantly reduced recurrence risk, regardless of TOP2A status [33]. Therefore, based on these mixed results, TOP2A should not presently be used to select the adjuvant chemotherapy regimen or to decide whether to offer trastuzumab.

The data from the BCIRG 0006 study suggest that both ACTH and TCH are superior to non-trastuzumab treatment options. The trade-offs between efficacy and adverse effects are important when selecting adjuvant chemotherapy. There appears to be a slightly higher risk of congestive heart failure (2 % versus 1 %) with ACTH versus TCH. Therefore, TCH represents an effective alternative option for women with contraindications to anthracyclines or patients with lower risk HER-2-positive tumors (small tumors or negative nodes). However, it seems reasonable to use ACTH in women with moderate- to high-risk HER-2-positive tumors without cardiac risk factors.

The FinHer Trial

FinHer was a small sub-study of a national trial conducted in Finland that randomized a total of 1010 women with node-positive and high-risk node-negative disease (defined as tumors greater than 2 cm in diameter and that are progesterone receptor-negative) to three cycles of docetaxel (initially at 100 mg/m^2 but later reduced to 80 mg/m^2 on day 1 every 21 days) or vinorelbine (25 mg/m^2 on days 1, 8, and 15 every 21 days). Both docetaxel and vinorelbine were followed by three cycles of 5-fluorouracil (600 mg/m^2), epirubicin (60 mg/m^2), and cyclophosphamide (600 mg/m^2). FEC is administered on day 1 every 21 days [20]. The primary aim of the trial was to compare docetaxel with vinorelbine. The patients with HER-2-positive tumors ($n = 232$) were further randomized to receive either 9 weeks of docetaxel or vinorelbine with or without trastuzumab given concomitantly followed by three cycles of

FEC. At a median follow-up of 3 years, there was a significant reduction in distant recurrence (HR 0.29; 95 % CI 0.13–0.64; $P = 0.002$), improved 3-year DFS (HR 0.42; 95 % CI 0.21–0.83; $P = 0.01$), and a trend toward improved OS (HR 0.41; 95 % CI 0.16–1.08; $P = 0.07$) favoring patients treated with trastuzumab [20]. This impressive efficacy despite the shorter duration of trastuzumab exposure was attributed to the up-front use of trastuzumab and the use of a synergistic chemotherapy regimen. The results at 62 months of median follow-up were published in 2009 and revealed a trend toward improved 5-year DFS (83 % versus 73 %: HR 0.65, 95 % CI 0.38–1.12) and OS (91 % versus 82 %: HR 0.55, 95 % CI 0.26–1.60) compared to chemotherapy alone that was not statistically significant [21]. Few patients experienced a decline in LVEF compared to those treated with CT alone (6.8 % versus 10.5 %), and there was only one symptomatic congestive heart failure in the trastuzumab group. While the results from this small trial cannot be translated to standard practice until they are compared directly to 1-year therapy in sufficiently powered studies demonstrating non-inferiority, this trial generated intriguing hypotheses for further testing shorter durations of trastuzumab in the adjuvant setting.

The PHARE Trial

Since 2005, 12 months of adjuvant trastuzumab has been the standard treatment for patients with HER-2-positive early-stage breast cancer. However, there has been great interest in shortening the duration of therapy and reducing both the risk of adverse effects and the cost of therapy because trastuzumab is an expensive drug. The PHARE (Protocol for Herceptin as Adjuvant Therapy with Reduced Exposure) trial was designed to address the duration issue in the adjuvant setting. It was a multicenter, phase III French trial randomizing patients with HER-2-positive early breast cancer who had breast-axillary surgery, received at least four cycles of chemotherapy (almost 75 % received an anthracycline-taxane), and previously received up to

6 months of trastuzumab (initial loading dose 8 mg/kg; 6 mg/kg maintenance every 3 weeks). These patients either discontinued trastuzumab at 6 months or continued to receive it for up to 12 months either concomitantly or sequentially to chemotherapy [22, 23]. The primary endpoint was DFS, and the trial was designed to detect a 2 % absolute difference in recurrence and allow a non-inferiority hazard ratio margin of 1.15. After a median follow-up of 42.5 months, 6-month trastuzumab therapy was associated with a hazard ratio of 1.28 versus 12-month therapy (95 % CI 1.05–1.56, $P = 0.29$). Two-year DFS was 93.8 % (95 % CI 92.6–94.9) in the 12-month group and 91.1 % (89.7–92.4) in the 6-month group. Subgroup analysis suggested that the overall results were driven by worse outcomes in patients with estrogen receptor-negative tumors who received sequential systemic therapy (HR 1.57). There was a significant difference in cardiac toxicity in favor of the shorter duration of trastuzumab (5.7 % versus 1.9 % in the 6- versus 12-month trastuzumab arms, respectively; $P < 0.0001$). This trial failed to demonstrate non-inferiority of 6-month trastuzumab compared to 12 months of therapy, and despite the higher rates of cardiac events, 12 months of adjuvant trastuzumab remained the standard of care.

The PACS 04 Trial

The PACS 04 study was a multicenter, randomized phase III French trial initially randomizing women with node-positive early-stage breast cancer to two different chemotherapy regimens (six cycles of epirubicin/docetaxel or FEC) and further randomizing patients with HER-2-positive tumors to either trastuzumab (260 patients) for 1 year after completing chemotherapy or observation (268 patients) [24]. Patients who were randomly assigned to receive trastuzumab had a nonsignificant 14 % reduction in the risk of relapse (HR 0.86; 95 % CI, 0.61–1.22; $P = 0.41$), and this finding questioned the value of the sequential administration of trastuzumab. While these results contradict those reported by the herceptin adjuvant (HERA) trial, which also tested a sequential treatment strategy, it should be noted that the HERA trial randomly assigned significantly larger numbers of patients than the PACS 04 study with a larger statistical power. In PACS 04, random assignment occurred before the completion of chemotherapy in contrast to the random assignment after the completion of neo-adjuvant or adjuvant chemotherapy in the HERA trial. Therefore, patients with early toxicity and/or relapse were not included in the intention-to-treat analysis in the HERA trial. Of note, only 65 % of patients who were randomly assigned to receive trastuzumab fulfilled the cardiac eligibility criteria in the PACS 04 study. In addition, only 75 % of the patients who received trastuzumab were able to complete 1 year of trastuzumab therapy. All these facts need to be considered when interpreting the results from the PACS 04 trial. However, although this study was unable to demonstrate a statistically significant advantage for the trastuzumab-containing arm in terms of its primary endpoint, the HR of 0.86 could still be considered favorable.

Optimal Tailoring of Adjuvant Trastuzumab Therapy

Timing of Trastuzumab in Relation to Radiotherapy

While preclinical studies suggest that concomitant trastuzumab and radiotherapy might be more effective, this issue has not been addressed prospectively in clinical trials [34]. Adjuvant radiotherapy was administered concurrently with trastuzumab in all trials except HERA and FinHer. The incidence of radiotherapy-associated adverse events in the concurrent setting was analyzed in the NCCTG N9831 trial [35]. At a median follow-up of 3.7 years, no significant differences in skin reaction, pneumonitis, dyspnea, cough, esophageal dysphagia, or neutropenia were reported among the treatment arms. A significantly higher incidence of leukopenia was reported in the ACTH arm compared to ACT. Notably, radiotherapy with trastuzumab did

Table 9.2 Adjuvant trastuzumab trials testing duration of therapy

Duration	Trial	Target	Endpoint
1 versus 2 years	HERA	4482	DFS
6 versus 12 months	Persephone	4000	DFS
6 versus 12 months	PHARE	3400	DFS
6 versus 12 months	HORG	478	3 years DFS
9 weeks versus 12 months	Short-HER	2500	DFS, OS
9 weeks versus 12 months	SOLD	3000	DFS

not increase the frequency of cardiac events, although a longer follow-up is needed to evaluate the emergence of delayed toxic effects.

Optimal Duration and Timing of Trastuzumab Administration

The results from large randomized phase III trials of adjuvant trastuzumab currently support 1 year of adjuvant trastuzumab as the standard treatment duration. Although trastuzumab is generally well tolerated, it is a prolonged course of treatment, and a shorter duration would be of great benefit to patients by reducing hospital visits for intravenous administration and side effects. In addition, shorter treatment may also reduce the incidence of the major toxicity of concern, cardiac side effects. The cost of trastuzumab is another issue that healthcare authorities must consider. Following the initial promising results from the FinHer study, the current recommended duration of 1 year was debated, and several trials were launched to test shorter durations of adjuvant trastuzumab. Table 9.2 describes the trials testing adjuvant trastuzumab duration.

Two phase III trials are presently comparing 9-week trastuzumab administration to 1 year of trastuzumab. The Synergism or Long Duration (SOLD) trial compares weekly or triweekly trastuzumab plus three cycles of docetaxel given every 21 days followed by three cycles of FE75C given every 21 days to the same regimen with the addition of trastuzumab to complete 1 year. The primary endpoint is DFS. The Short-HER study is a phase III, randomized non-inferiority trial comparing (arm A, long) four cycles of AC or EC followed by docetaxel or paclitaxel in combination with trastuzumab followed by 14 additional cycles of trastuzumab (total of 18 triweekly administrations) to (arm B, short) three cycles of triweekly docetaxel in combination with weekly trastuzumab (total of nine weekly administrations) followed by three cycles of FEC. The primary objective is DFS for both the SOLD and the multicenter Italian Short-HER trial.

The PHARE trial failed to demonstrate that 6 months of trastuzumab is non-inferior to 12 months [23]. However, the 6-month trastuzumab arm had a more favorable cardiac safety profile. The Hellenic Oncology Research Group trial is a small, multicenter, randomized, phase III, national Greek study comparing 6 versus 12 months of trastuzumab in combination with dose-dense docetaxel following FE75C as adjuvant treatment in women with node-positive disease. The Persephone study is a phase III randomized controlled trial with a non-inferiority design evaluating whether treatment with trastuzumab for 6 months is equivalent to the standard 12-month duration in patients with HER-2-positive early breast cancer. Patients are stratified based on estrogen receptor status, chemotherapy type, chemotherapy timing (adjuvant or neoadjuvant), and trastuzumab timing (concurrent or sequential). Eligible patients are then randomized to receive either 6-month or 12-month trastuzumab administered every 3 weeks. The trial is currently underway in the UK, and the study endpoints are DFS, cardiac safety, and cost-effectiveness. After the completion of the Persephone trial, a meta-analysis combining the results from the PHARE and the Persephone trial is planned.

As mentioned previously, HERA is the only trial that has tested a longer duration of trastuzumab—2 years versus 1 year—and failed to demonstrate the superiority of 2 years of trastuzumab compared to 1 year of trastuzumab [15].

Unfortunately, the results of these ongoing studies will not be available before 2014–2016,

and several ongoing trials testing new anti-HER-2 or dual blockade agents will present their data in the same period. Therefore, the data from these trials testing shorter trastuzumab durations may lose their impact.

Regarding the timing of trastuzumab administration, the data from adjuvant trastuzumab trials have clearly demonstrated a benefit of combining trastuzumab with chemotherapy in the adjuvant setting of HER-2/neu-positive early breast cancer, whether given concomitantly with chemotherapy (joint analysis and BCIRG 006) or sequentially after completing chemotherapy (HERA and arm B of N9831) [6–8]. In addition, the concurrent administration of trastuzumab with an anthracycline-free regimen was also effective in the BCIRG 006 study [8]. Collectively, the magnitude of the benefit was greater in the concurrent regimens than in the sequential ones. Notably, the PACS 04 trial did not demonstrate a statistically significant improvement in DFS or OS, although it was a relatively small trial ($n = 528$) [24]. In the NCCTG N9831 study, the comparison of the sequential versus the concomitant arm tended to favor the latter but did not reach statistical significance [30].

Trastuzumab for Small HER-2-Positive Tumors

Adjuvant trastuzumab is an effective therapy regardless of tumor size and nodal status [9–11]. However, the magnitude of benefit in low-risk tumors, i.e., node-negative small tumors, has been questioned. Data from retrospective studies have revealed that small HER-2-positive tumors (T1 a, b) have significantly higher recurrence rates than HER-2-negative tumors [36]. There was a clear benefit from trastuzumab and chemotherapy in the T1 a, b subgroup of patients in the BCIRG data set [37]. The data from five adjuvant trastuzumab trials, HERA, N9831, NSABP B-31, PACS04, and FinHer, were combined to identify a group of patients who could be excluded from trials evaluating additional therapy to avoid unnecessary side effects. This meta-analysis included patients with tumors up to 2 cm and analyzed hormone receptor-positive and receptor-negative cohorts separately. The primary objectives were DFS and OS. Patients with hormone receptor-positive disease with tumors up to 2 cm and involvement of 0–1 axillary lymph node have a favorable outcome (5-year DFS of 91 % and OS of 97 %) with standard chemotherapy plus trastuzumab therapy. These data suggest that patients with small HER-2-positive tumors with limited nodal involvement and hormone receptor-positive disease could receive less chemotherapy. A recently reported phase II prospective trial investigated the role of weekly paclitaxel given concurrently with weekly trastuzumab for 12 weeks followed by continuation of trastuzumab every 3 weeks for 1 year in 400 patients with node-negative (one lymph node micrometastasis was allowed in the presence of a negative axillary dissection), HER-2-positive tumors less than or equal to 3 cm who had an LVEF $\geq$50 % [38]. The primary endpoint was DFS. With a median follow-up of 3.6 years, 3-year DFS was 98.7 % with few severe events, suggesting that paclitaxel and trastuzumab combination is a reasonable regimen for patients with stage I HER-2-positive breast cancer and that the standard regimens from the pivotal trials could be reserved for patients with high-risk features.

Adjuvant Use of the Tyrosine Kinase Inhibitor Lapatinib

Cost is an important issue for patients with HER-2-positive tumors worldwide, and therefore, adjuvant trastuzumab may not be available to some women. The TEACH (Tykerb Evaluation After Chemotherapy) study is a randomized multicenter phase III trial designed to evaluate the role of lapatinib in women who previously received adjuvant chemotherapy, but not trastuzumab [39]. Patients were assigned (1:1) to receive daily lapatinib (1500 mg) or daily placebo for 12 months and stratified by time since diagnosis, lymph node involvement at diagnosis, and the hormone receptor status of the tumor. The primary endpoint was DFS. After a median follow-up of 4 years, there was no significant difference in DFS between groups in the intention-to-treat analysis. A marginal DFS benefit from adjuvant lapatinib appeared only in the subgroup of patients who had HER-2-positive disease confirmed by central review (79 % of the randomized women). This trial indicated that lapatinib might be an option for women with HER-2-positive breast cancer who did not or could not receive adjuvant trastuzumab. As expected, there was a higher incidence of grade 3–4 diarrhea, rash, and hepatobiliary disorders in the lapatinib arm compared to the placebo arm.

Conclusion and Future Perspective

Trastuzumab is a rationally designed, molecularly targeted therapy for a specific subgroup of breast cancer, the HER-2-positive group. Consistent evidence of clinical benefit of trastuzumab with tolerable toxicity has been obtained in large multicenter randomized phase III trials and meta-analyses [6–11]. Trastuzumab is the first successful example of the translation of an improved understanding of the molecular basis of breast cancer to a rational treatment strategy with greater efficacy and reduced toxicity. Thus, trastuzumab represents a milestone in medical oncology as a practice-changing breast cancer therapy. The adoption of trastuzumab into routine clinical practice in the adjuvant setting began with the announcement of the first results from the adjuvant clinical trials in 2005. Some controversial issues regarding the use of trastuzumab, including the timing of administration, the duration of therapy, and the decision to combine with chemotherapy, have been partly resolved by longer follow-up. However, other questions, such as whether trastuzumab can be used with less toxic chemotherapy regimens or with endocrine therapy in small tumors <1 cm, have not been addressed by large phase III trials thus far. The adjuvant use of trastuzumab has been implemented in well-known international guidelines, and it can be considered globally safe in terms of cardiac toxicity due to its reversible nature, but the cost for 1 year of therapy remains an obstacle.

Advances in molecular biology continue, and the efforts to develop and test new anti-HER-2 strategies complement this progress. The translational/clinical search for biomarkers predicting benefit from trastuzumab has not yet identified any markers other than HER-2 expression/amplification despite numerous publications in the literature. Immune system effectors have recently emerged as a new therapeutic approach in HER-2-positive breast cancer even though breast cancer has not been traditionally considered an immunogenic tumor. Indeed, the presence of tumor-infiltrating lymphocytes in breast cancer samples and their association with prognosis have been reported for many years [40]. The retrospective analysis of several trials suggests that the role of the immune system requires further study in specific subgroups of breast cancer, such as triple-negative and HER-2-positive breast cancer [41]. Each 10 % increase in stromal lymphocytic infiltration was significantly associated with decreased distant recurrence in patients randomized to the trastuzumab arm in the FinHer trial [42]. Thus, patients with HER-2-positive tumors might benefit from a combination of immune modulatory agents and anti-HER-2 treatment strategies in the future.

The standard duration of adjuvant therapy is 1 year with intravenous administration. Efforts to develop a more practical, convenient form of administration to reduce demand on healthcare resources resulted in the development of a subcutaneous form of trastuzumab. The Hannah trial demonstrated that the pharmacokinetic profile and efficacy of subcutaneous trastuzumab were non-inferior to intravenous administration, with a similar safety profile in the locally advanced breast cancer setting [43]. The PrefHer study included women with early-stage HER-2-positive breast cancer and randomized them to receive four cycles of 600 mg fixed-dose subcutaneous adjuvant trastuzumab followed by four cycles of intravenous trastuzumab or these treatments in reverse order [44]. The primary endpoint was the proportion of patients indicating an overall preference for subcutaneous or intravenous trastuzumab as assessed by patient interviews in the evaluable intention-to-treat population. Recently reported results indicated that women with HER-2-positive early breast cancer favored subcutaneous over intravenous administration of trastuzumab.

The direction of adjuvant anti-HER-2 therapy will be further shaped by the results of ongoing trastuzumab trials. The ALTTO (Adjuvant Lapatinib and/or Trastuzumab Treatment Optimisation) study is testing dual blockade with trastuzumab and lapatinib, the APHINITY trial is testing the addition of pertuzumab to trastuzumab, NSABP B-47 is evaluating trastuzumab in patients with low HER-2 expression, NSABP B-43 is exploring the role of trastuzumab in ductal carcinoma in situ, and the KAITLIN study is evaluating the role of TDM-1 plus pertuzumab compared to trastuzumab plus pertuzumab in the adjuvant setting.

It was recently reported that at a median follow-up of 38 months, there was no DFS benefit from the addition of bevacizumab to chemotherapy plus trastuzumab in a large phase III trial, BETH (bevacizumab and trastuzumab adjuvant therapy in HER-2-positive breast cancer), which enrolled 3509 women with HER-2-positive, node-positive, or high-risk node-negative breast cancer [45].

Cost-effectiveness models have justified the use of adjuvant trastuzumab in most countries [46–49]. However, adjuvant trastuzumab therapy remains unaffordable in some countries, and this issue will worsen as the number of other expensive anti-HER-2 therapies increases. This economic dimension will be one of the most important challenges for the future management of HER-2-positive early breast cancer, particularly in developing countries.

The evolution in understanding HER-2-positive breast cancer biology and anti-HER-2 therapies raises future challenges for oncologists. The dissection of heterogeneity within HER-2-positive tumors for developing personalized treatment strategies, the identification of specific biomarkers of resistance to trastuzumab, testing the role of dual blockade in the adjuvant setting, and the identification of clinical and/or biological markers to predict cardiac toxicity are among the clinical issues that must be addressed to improve treatment for patients with HER-2-positive disease in the adjuvant setting.

References

1. Slamon DJ, Clark GM, Wong SG, Levin WJ, Ullrich A, McGuire WL. Human breast cancer: correlation of relapse and survival with amplification of the HER-2/neu oncogene. Science. 1987;235(4785):177–82.
2. Ross JS, Slodkowska EA, Symmans WF, Pusztai L, Ravdin PM, Hortobagyi GN. The HER-2 receptor and breast cancer: ten years of targeted anti-HER-2 therapy and personalized medicine. Oncologist. 2009;14(4):320–68.
3. Schechter AL, Stern DF, Vaidyanathan L, Decker SJ, Drebin JA, Greene MI, et al. The neu oncogene: an erb-B-related gene encoding a 185,000-Mr tumour antigen. Nature. 1984;312:513–6.
4. Verma S, Joy AA, Rayson D, McLeod D, Brezden-Masley C, Boileau JF, et al. HER story: the next chapter in HER-2-directed therapy for advanced breast cancer. Oncologist. 2013;18(11):1153–66.
5. Akslen LA, Fluge O, Pergamenschikov A, Williams C, Zhu SX, Lønning PE, et al. Molecular portraits of human breast tumours. Nature. 2000;406(6797):747–52.
6. Piccart-Gebhart MJ, Procter M, Leyland-Jones B, Goldhirsch A, Untch M, Smith I, et al. Trastuzumab after adjuvant chemotherapy in HER2-positive breast cancer. N Engl J Med. 2005;353(16):1659.
7. Romond EH, Perez EA, Bryant J, Suman VJ, Geyer Jr CE, Davidson NE, et al. Trastuzumab plus adjuvant chemotherapy for operable HER2-positive breast cancer. N Engl J Med. 2005;353(16):1673.
8. Slamon D, Eiermann W, Robert N, Pienkowski T, Martin M, Press M, et al. Adjuvant trastuzumab in HER2-positive breast cancer. N Engl J Med. 2011;365(14):1273–83.
9. Moja L, Tagliabue L, Balduzzi S, Parmelli E, Pistotti V, Guarneri V, et al. Trastuzumab containing regimens for early breast cancer. Cochrane Database Syst Rev. 2012;(4):CD006243.
10. Dahabreh IJ, Linardou H, Siannis F, Fountzilas G, Murray S. Trastuzumab in the adjuvant treatment of early-stage breast cancer: a systematic review and meta-analysis of randomized controlled trials. Oncologist. 2008;13(6):620–30.
11. Viani GA, Afonso SL, Stefano EJ, De Fendi LI, Soares FV. Adjuvant trastuzumab in the treatment of her-2-positive early breast cancer: a meta-analysis of published randomized trails. BMC Cancer. 2007;7:153.
12. Wolff AC, Hammond ME, Schwartz JN, Hagerty KL, Allred DC, Cote RJ, et al. American Society of Clinical Oncology/College of American Pathologists guideline recommendations for human epidermal growth factor receptor 2 testing in breast cancer. J Clin Oncol. 2007;25:118–45.
13. Wolff AC, Hammond ME, Hicks DG, Dowsett M, McShane LM, Allison KH, et al. Recommendations for human epidermal growth factor receptor 2 testing in breast cancer: American Society of Clinical Oncology/College of American Pathologists clinical practice guideline update. J Clin Oncol. 2013;31:3997–4013.
14. Smith I, Procter M, Gelber RD, Guillaume S, Feyereislova A, Dowsett M, et al. 2-year follow-up of trastuzumab after adjuvant chemotherapy in HER-2 positive breast cancer: a randomized controlled trial. Lancet. 2007;369:29–36.
15. Gianni L, Dafni U, Gelber RD, Azambuja E, Muehlbauer S, Goldhirsch A, et al. Treatment with trastuzumab for 1 year after adjuvant chemotherapy in patients with HER2-positive early breast cancer: a 4-year follow-up of a randomised controlled trial. Lancet Oncol. 2011;12:236.
16. Goldhirsch A, Gelber RD, Piccart-Gebhart MJ, de Azambuja E, Procter M, Suter TM, et al. 2 years versus 1 year of adjuvant trastuzumab for HER2-positive breast cancer (HERA): an open-label, randomised controlled trial. Lancet. 2013;382(9897):1021–8.
17. Perez EA, Romond EH, Suman VJ, Jeong J, Davidson NE, Geyer CE, et al. Updated results of the combined analysis of NCCTG N9831 and NSABP B-31 adjuvant chemotherapy with/without trastuzumab in patients with HER2- positive breast cancer. J Clin Oncol. 2007;25(18S, June 20 Suppl):512.
18. Perez EA, Romond EH, Suman VJ, Jeong JH, Davidson NE, Geyer Jr CE, et al. Four-year follow- up of trastuzumab plus adjuvant chemotherapy for operable human epidermal growth factor receptor 2-positive breast cancer: joint analysis of data from NCCTG N9831 and NSABP B-31. J Clin Oncol. 2011;29:3366–73.
19. Perez EA, Romond EH, Suman VJ, Jeong JH, Sledge G, Geyer Jr CE, et al. Trastuzumab plus adjuvant chemotherapy for human epidermal growth factor receptor 2-positive breast cancer: planned joint analysis of overall survival from NSABP B-31 and NCCTG N9831. J Clin Oncol. 2014;32(33):3744–52.
20. Joensuu H, Kellokumpu-Lehtinen PL, Bono P, Alanko T, Kataja V, Asola R, et al. Adjuvant docetaxel or vinorelbine with or without trastuzumab for breast cancer. N Engl J Med. 2006;354(8):809–20.
21. Joensuu H, Bono P, Kataja V, Alanko T, Kokko R, Asola R, et al. Fluorouracil, epirubicin, and cyclophosphamide with either docetaxel or vinorelbine, with or without trastuzumab, as adjuvant treatments of breast cancer: final results of the FinHer trial. J Clin Oncol. 2009;27:5685–92.
22. Pivot X, Romieu G, Bonnefoi H, Pierga J-Y, Kerbrat P, Guastalla J-P, et al. Phare trial results of subset analysis comparing 6 to 12 months of trastuzumab in adjuvant early breast cancer. Cancer Res. 2012;72:S5.
23. Pivot X, Romieu G, Debled M, Pierga JY, Kerbrat P, Bachelot T, et al. 6 months versus 12 months of adjuvant trastuzumab for patients with HER2-positive early breast cancer (PHARE): a randomised phase 3 trial. Lancet Oncol. 2013;14:741–8.
24. Spielmann M, Roché H, Delozier T, Canon JL, Romieu G, Bourgeois H, et al. Trastuzumab for patients with axillary-node-positive breast cancer:

results of the FNCLCC-PACS 04 trial. J Clin Oncol. 2009;27:6129–34.

25. Olson EM, Abdel-Rasoul M, Maly J, Wu CS, Lin NU, Shapiro CL. Incidence and risk of central nervous system metastases as site of first recurrence in patients with HER2-positive breast cancer treated with adjuvant trastuzumab. Ann Oncol. 2013;24(6):1526–33.

26. Romond EH, Jeong JH, Rastogi P, Swain SM, Geyer Jr CE, Ewer MS, et al. Seven-year follow-up assessment of cardiac function in NSABP B-31, a randomized trial comparing doxorubicin and cyclophosphamide followed by paclitaxel (ACP) with ACP plus trastuzumab as adjuvant therapy for patients with node-positive, human epidermal growth factor receptor 2-positive breast cancer. J Clin Oncol. 2012;30:3792–9.

27. Russell SD, Blackwell KL, Lawrence J, Pippen Jr JE, Roe MT, Wood F, et al. Independent adjudication of symptomatic heart failure with the use of doxorubicin and cyclophosphamide followed by trastuzumab adjuvant therapy: a combined review of cardiac data from the National Surgical Adjuvant Breast and Bowel Project B-31 and the North Central Cancer Treatment Group N9831 clinical trials. J Clin Oncol. 2010;28:3416–21.

28. Perez EA, Suman VJ, Davidson N, Martino S, Kaufman P. NCCTG N9831: May 2005 update. Best of ASCO 2005 San Francisco. www.asco.org/ASCO/ Abstracts+%26+Virtual+ Meeting/Virtual+ Meeting.

29. Perez EA, Suman VJ Davidson NE, Gralow J, Kaufman PA, Ingle JN, Dakhil SR, et al. Results of chemotherapy alone, with sequential or concurrent addition of 52 weeks of trastuzumab in the NCCTG N9831 HER2-positive adjuvant breast cancer trial. LBA 80, Program and abstracts of the 32nd Annual San Antonio Breast Cancer Symposium; December 2009; San Antonio, Texas.

30. Perez EA, Suman VJ, Davidson NE, Gralow JR, Kaufman PA, Visscher DW, et al. Sequential versus concurrent trastuzumab in adjuvant chemotherapy for breast cancer. J Clin Oncol. 2011;29:4491–7.

31. Press MF, Sauter G, Buyse M, Bernstein L, Guzman R, Santiago A, et al. Alteration of topoisomerase II-alpha gene in human breast cancer: association with responsiveness to anthracycline-based chemotherapy. J Clin Oncol. 2011;29:859–67.

32. Burstein HJ, Piccart-Gebhart MJ, Perez EA, Hortobagyi GN, Wolmark N, Albain KS, et al. Choosing the best trastuzumab-based adjuvant chemotherapy regimen: should we abandon anthracyclines? J Clin Oncol. 2012;30(18):2179–82.

33. Gianni L, Norton L, Wolmark N, Suter TM, Bonadonna G, Hortobagyi GN. Role of anthracyclines in the treatment of early breast cancer. J Clin Oncol. 2009;27:4798–808.

34. Pietras RJ, Poen JC, Gallardo D, Wongvipat PN, Lee HJ, Slamon DJ. Monoclonal antibody to HER-2/neu receptor modulates repair of radiation-induced DNA damage and enhances radiosensitivity of human breast cancer cells overexpressing this oncogene. Cancer Res. 1999;59(6):1347–55.

35. Halyard MY, Pisansky TM, Dueck AC, Suman V, Pierce L, Solin L, et al. Radiotherapy and adjuvant trastuzumab in operable breast cancer: tolerability and adverse event data from the NCCTG Phase III Trial N9831. J Clin Oncol. 2009;27(16):2638–44.

36. Banerjee S, Smith IE. Management of small HER2-positive breast cancers. Lancet Oncol. 2010;11(12): 1193–9.

37. O'Sullivan CC, Holmes E, Spielmann M, Perez EA, Joensuu H, Costantino JP, et al. The prognosis of small HER2+ breast cancers: a meta-analysis of the randomized trastuzumab trials. Program and abstracts of the 36th Annual San Antonio Breast Cancer Symposium December 10–14, 2013, San Antonio, Texas.

38. Tolaney SM, Barry WT, Dang CT, Yardley DA, Moy B, Marcom PK, et al. A phase II study of adjuvant paclitaxel (T) and trastuzumab (H) (APT trial) for node-negative, HER2-positive breast cancer (BC). Program and abstracts of the 36th Annual San Antonio Breast Cancer Symposium; December 10–14, 2013, San Antonio, Texas.

39. Goss PE, Smith IE, O'Shaughnessy J, Ejlertsen B, Kaufmann M, Boyle F, et al. Adjuvant lapatinib for women with early-stage HER2-positive breast cancer: a randomised, controlled, phase 3 trial. Lancet Oncol. 2013;14(1):88–96.

40. Aaltomaa S, Lipponen P, Eskelinen M, Kosma VM, Marin S, Alhava E, et al. Lymphocyte infiltrates as a prognostic variable in female breast cancer. Eur J Cancer. 1992;28A:859–64.

41. Loi S. Tumor-infiltrating lymphocytes, breast cancer subtypes and therapeutic efficacy. Oncoimmunology. 2013;2(7), e24720.

42. Loi S, Michiels S, Salgado R, Sirtaine N, Jose V, Fumagalli D, et al. Tumor infiltrating lymphocytes are prognostic in triple negative breast cancer and predictive for trastuzumab benefit in early breast cancer: results from the FinHER trial. Ann Oncol. 2014;25(8):1544–50.

43. Ismael G, Hegg R, Muehlbauer S, Heinzmann D, Lum B, Kim SB, et al. Subcutaneous versus intravenous administration of (neo)adjuvant trastuzumab in patients with HER2-positive, clinical stage I–III breast cancer (HannaH study): a phase 3, open-label, multicentre, randomised trial. Lancet Oncol. 2012;13(9):869–7.

44. Pivot X, Gligorov J, Müller V, Barrett-Lee P, Verma S, Knoop A, et al. Preference for subcutaneous or intravenous administration of trastuzumab in patients with HER2-positive early breast cancer (PrefHer): an open-label randomised study. Lancet Oncol. 2013;14:962–70.

45. Slamon DL, Swain SM, Buyse M, Martin M, Geyer CE, Im YH, et al. Primary results from BETH, a phase 3 controlled study of adjuvant chemotherapy and trastuzumab ± bevacizumab in patients with HER2-positive, node-positive, or high-risk node-negative breast cancer. 2013 San Antonio Breast Cancer Symposium. Abstract S1-03.

46. Liberato NL, Marchetti M, Barosi G. Cost effectiveness of adjuvant trastuzumab in human epidermal

growth factor receptor 2-positive breast cancer. J Clin Oncol. 2007;25:625–33.

47. Shiroiwa T, Fukuda T, Shimozuma K, Ohashi Y, Tsutani K. The model-based cost- effectiveness analysis of 1-year adjuvant trastuzumab treatment: based on 2-year follow-up HERA trial data. Breast Cancer Res Treat. 2008;109:559–66.

48. Neyt M, Albrecht J, Cocquyt V. An economic evaluation of Herceptin in adjuvant setting: the Breast Cancer International Research Group 006 trial. Ann Oncol. 2006;17:381–90.

49. Millar JA, Millward MJ. Cost effectiveness of trastuzumab in the adjuvant treatment of early breast cancer: a lifetime model. Pharmacoeconomics. 2007;25:429–42.

Post-mastectomy Adjuvant Radiotherapy (PMRT)

10

İlknur Bilkay Görken

Abstract

Mastectomy can remove any detectable macroscopic disease, but some tumor foci might remain in the locoregional tissue (i.e., chest wall or lymph nodes), that could lead the locoregional recurrence (LRR) of the disease. Post-mastectomy adjuvant radiotherapy (PMRT) has potential to eliminate such microscopic disease. The risk of LRR after mastectomy is 3–46 %, depending on the stage of the disease and prognostic factors. PMRT has been recommended for patients with ≥4 positive axillary lymph nodes but not given for most women with node-negative disease. Patients with one to three positive axillary lymph nodes constitute a gray zone. PMRT indications and side effects will be discussed in this chapter.

Keywords

Mastectomy • Post-mastectomy adjuvant radiotherapy (PMRT)

Introduction

Post-mastectomy adjuvant radiotherapy (PMRT) is the most controversial topic in radiation oncology. The risk of local-regional recurrence (LRR) after mastectomy is 3–46 %, depending on the stage of the disease and prognostic factors [1–7].

İ. B. Görken, MD
Radiation Oncology, Dokuz Eylül University,
Mithatpaşa Cad., İzmir 35340, Turkey
e-mail: Ilknur.gorken@deu.edu.tr;
Ilknur.gorken67@gmail.com

Two different risk groups can be classified according to the radiotherapy (RT) indication:

1. Early-stage breast cancer
2. Locally advanced breast cancer

Early-Stage Breast Cancer

Cases that are assessed as early stage in clinical staging can also be classified into high-risk and low-risk groups depending on the patient and tumor characteristics. We can separate patients into three different groups based on axillary status and the number of involved lymph nodes:

© Springer International Publishing Switzerland 2016
A. Aydiner et al. (eds.), *Breast Disease: Management and Therapies*,
DOI 10.1007/978-3-319-26012-9_10

(a) No axillary lymph nodes, tumor >3 cm (T2–T3N0 (stage IIB))
(b) One to three positive axillary lymph nodes
(c) ≥4 positive axillary lymph nodes (N2 disease)

In cases with ≥4 positive axillary lymph nodes, the LRRs are 24 % and 46 %, respectively [2–4, 7]. In these cases, PMRT decreases the local recurrence risk by 14.8 % [8]. Patients with one to three positive axillary lymph nodes constitute a gray zone.

T2–T3N0 (Stage IIB)

As defined in the American Joint Commission on Cancer (AJCC) Staging Manual, 6th edition, stage IIB breast carcinoma is defined by the following: tumor >5 cm in greatest dimension without direct extension to the chest wall or skin (pT3), no regional lymph node metastasis (N0), and no distant metastasis (M0) [9]. PMRT has been shown to improve locoregional control and survival in T3 and T4 primary breast cancer patients with positive lymph nodes [2–4, 8]. However, axillary-negative patients were not analyzed as a different group in these prospective randomized trials. The British Columbia trial excluded lymph node (LN)-negative patients, and we could not define all node-negative patients in the Danish trials as T3. There was no detailed information regarding the pathological involvement of the pectoralis muscle, fascia, and skin in these trials. Therefore, it is very difficult to extract specific information about T2–T3 patients with negative axilla. The median number of axillary lymph nodes evaluated in these trials was 7, less than the number of lymph nodes reported in most mastectomy series. These trials were criticized for possible under-staging and subtherapeutic surgical staging of the axilla.

Tagihan GA et al. reported results from five National Surgical Adjuvant Breast and Bowel Project (NSABP) randomized trials [10]. Of 8,878 breast cancer patients enrolled in the NSABP B-13, B-14, B-20, and B-23 node-negative trials, 313 patients had tumors 5 cm or larger in their greatest dimension at pathology report and underwent mastectomy. Of the patients, 34.2 % received adjuvant chemotherapy, 21.1 % received tamoxifen, and 19.2 % received adjuvant chemotherapy plus tamoxifen. Another 25.5 % did not receive any systemic therapy. Cumulative incidences for isolated LRR as a first event for patients with tumors of 5 cm or greater than 5 cm were 7.0 % and 7.2 %, respectively (p = 0.2). In patients with stage IIB breast cancer with LN-negative tumors ≥5 cm treated by mastectomy with or without adjuvant systemic therapy and no PMRT, LRR as a first event remained low. The investigator of this trial concluded that PMRT should not be routinely used for these patients.

Using the Surveillance, Epidemiology, and End Results (SEER) database, Yu et al. studied cohorts of pT3N0 tumors treated with mastectomy, of which one-third of patients received PMRT [6]. Women with T3N0 breast disease who met the analysis criteria represented <0.3 % of all breast cancer patients in the SEER database. Of the 1,844 women analyzed for cause-specific survival (CSS), there was no statistically significant difference in CSS between patients who did or did not receive PMRT. Age <50 years and a grade I tumor were statistically significant independent predictors of increased CSS in multivariate analysis. In this trial, PMRT was associated with increased overall survival (OS). For the whole patient population, the actuarial 10-year OS rate was 70.7 % for the PMRT group versus 58.4 % for the group without PMRT (HR, 0.65; 95 % CI, 0.55–0.80; p < 0.001). Age <50 years, grade I tumor, and the number of lymph nodes dissected were associated with increased OS [6]. In a retrospective study of 19,846 nonmetastatic breast cancer patients, Goulart J et al. reported the data for 100 node-negative patients with tumors ≥5 cm (0.5 %) [11]. Of these 100 patients, 44 (44 %) received adjuvant PMRT. The cumulative 10-year LRR was 2.3 % in the PMRT group vs. 8.9 % in the group that did not receive PMRT (p = 0.2). The 10-year breast cancer-specific survival rate was the same between the two groups. In the group that did not receive PMRT, patients with grade 3 histologic features and those who had not received hormonal therapy had the highest LRRs, 17 % (5 of 29) and 15 % (5 of 34), respectively. The investigators of this study recommended that PMRT be considered for grade 3 histological features and for patients not undergoing hormonal therapy.

The South Sweden Breast Cancer Group conducted a randomized trial in which 33 % of the 367 patients were lymph node negative. This three-armed phase III randomized trial compared RT with and without chemotherapy (oral cyclophosphamide for 1 year) and chemotherapy alone. The lymph nodes of the supraclavicular and infraclavicular fossae, the axilla, the chest wall, and the ipsilateral parasternal lymph nodes were included as RT target volumes in this trial. Twenty years of follow-up demonstrated that RT reduced the risk of LRR in chemotherapy-treated patients by 75 % (13.9 % vs. 3.5 %). The risk reduction was highly significant in both N0 and N+ patients. No effect on mortality was observed with 20 years of follow-up [12].

In a combined analysis, Floyd ct al. reported that the 5-year actuarial cumulative rate of LRR in 70 node-negative patients with tumors ≥5 cm was 7.6 %; four of the five failures occurred in the chest wall, and one occurred in the axilla. In a multivariate analysis, lymphatic vessel invasion (LVI) was identified as an independent prognostic factor for LRR, disease-free survival (DFS), and OS [13].

For node-negative patients with tumors ≥5 cm (T3N0), there is no consensus to justify the routine use of PMRT. Unless there is a combination of adverse prognostic factors such as high-grade, young age, positive surgical margin, and infiltration of pectoral fascia, the risk of LRR is low. The Early Breast Cancer Trialists' Collaborative Group (EBCTCG) analysis does not include the T3N0 group in LRR rates with and without radiation [8]. The last meta-analysis of the same group was reported in March 2014. A group of 1,594 women (20 %) with pathologically node-negative disease were included in this analysis. Of the 1,594 women with node-negative disease, 700 (44 %) had axillary dissection. In this group, the locoregional recurrence rate was only 1.4 % for women without RT, suggesting that RT has no effect on locoregional recurrence. However, for the 870 women who had only axillary sampling and node-negative disease, the locoregional recurrence rate was 16.3 % without RT, and RT reduced LRR (2p < 0.00001) and overall recurrence (2p = 0.0003), but had no effect on breast cancer mortality (2p > 0.1) [14]. In the National Comprehensive Cancer Network (NCCN) (2013–2015) and St. Gallen Breast Cancer Conference 2013, panelists strongly recommended PMRT to the chest wall and regional lymphatic area for patients with negative axillary lymph nodes and when the tumor was >5 cm with positive deep and radial margins [15–18]. However, the panelists concluded that PMRT should not be the standard for patients with adverse pathology (such as Her2, grade, LVI), regardless of the presence of nodes. In the NCCN guidelines, PMRT was also recommended for patients with negative axillary nodes, tumors ≤5 cm, and negative margins <1 mm.

One to Three Positive Lymph Nodes (pN1) Breast Cancer

Cuzick et al. published a meta-analysis of the results of the effects of PMRT in 1987 [5]. In this study, the survival rates were lower in the PMRT group than the nonirradiated group. In the PMRT group, non-breast cancer-related death rates were high. However, the studies included in this meta-analysis were older, and most of the patients were treated with Co^{60} and orthovoltage devices. The death rate due to cardiac events was high because of the RT techniques. After this paper was released, the use of PMRT dramatically decreased, and the importance of cardiac doses was emphasized.

In 1997, the Danish 82b (premenopausal) and 82c (postmenopausal) trials were published [2, 3]. In these trials, PMRT not only decreased the LRR but also increased OS significantly in high-risk patients in spite of systemic therapy. This effect was particularly prominent in patients with ≥4 axillary lymph nodes. The Danish Breast Cancer Cooperative Group (DBCG) 82b trial randomized 1,708 premenopausal women with stage II or III breast cancer to mastectomy followed by nine cycles of chemotherapy or to mastectomy, radiation, and eight cycles of chemotherapy [2]. Irradiation was administered as 50 Gy in 25 fractions to the chest wall and peripheral lymphatics, including the internal mammary lymph nodes. The results demonstrated that patients in the radiation arm had lower 10-year LRR (9 % vs. 32 %, $p < 0.001$) and an improved 10-year overall survival rate (54 % vs. 45 %, $p < 0.001$). The British Columbia trial was reported at the same time. In this trial, 318 premenopausal women with high-risk breast cancer were randomized to mastectomy and chemotherapy or chemotherapy plus RT. Patients in the radiation arm exhibited a reduction in 10-year LRR, as in the DBCCG trials. The Danish 82c trial studied the effect of PMRT in high-risk postmenopausal women using a similar design [4]. This trial randomized 1,300 patients to mastectomy and tamoxifen or to mastectomy and tamoxifen plus irradiation. In this study, similar to the premenopausal patient group, despite systemic therapy in the RT arm, a significant reduction in LRR (10-year LRR rates of 8 % vs. 35 %, $p < 0.001$) and an increase in 10-year overall survival (64 % vs. 54 %, $p = 0.07$) were observed.

These three prospective randomized studies reveal that PMRT reduces the LRR significantly, leading to an increase in OS. In these trials, reducing the rate of LRR from 30–35 % to 10 % led to a 10 % increase in survival rates. The irradiation technique in the DBCG trials minimized radiation exposure to the heart. In these trials, the nodal regions were treated with anterior photon fields, except the internal mammary nodes. The internal mammary nodes were treated with an anterior electron field, and custom blocks were used to shield the heart and lungs. At a median 10-year follow-up, similar proportions in each group died of ischemic heart disease (0.8 % in the RT arms vs. 0.9 % in the arm without RT). There was no difference in the rate of ischemic heart disease between left-sided and right-sided RT patients (0.7 % vs. 0.9 %, respectively). Similar rates were observed for death from acute myocardial infarction (MI). When data from patients with local or distant cancer recurrence were censored, deaths from ischemic heart disease were associated with left-sided RT (0.7 % vs. 0.3 %, HR: 2.18) [19]. Decreasing cardiac doses resulted in a decrease in non-breast cancer-related death rates and a significant increase in survival rates.

Since 1995, EBCTCG has gathered all data about breast cancer every 5 years and studied the effect of adjuvant therapies. In the meta-analyses by this group in 2000 and 2005, the effect of RT was studied. In the meta-analysis of 2000, a reduction of approximately two-thirds in local recurrence was observed in all trials during the first decades. The effect was independent of the type of patient or type of RT [20]. Breast cancer mortality was reduced ($2p = 0.0001$), but other mortality, particularly vascular mortality, was increased ($2p = 0.0003$); the overall 20-year survival was 37.1 % with RT versus 35.9 % in the control arm ($2p = 0.06$) [20].

Van de Steene et al. reanalyzed 36 prospective randomized trials that were included in the EBCTCG-1995 meta-analysis according to objective criteria [21]. In their analysis, a significant survival benefit for the RT arm was observed in trials that were recent (designed after 1980) ($2p < 0.05$), large trials (the number of patients accrued in the trial) ($2p < 0.03$), trials that used standard fractionation ($2p < 0.02$), or had favorable crude survival benefit ($2p < 0.0$). Parameter-effect relationships were obtained for these four parameters.

In a meta-analysis by Whelan et al., the effect of PMRT was analyzed in patients who were treated by mastectomy and systemic therapy in 18 randomized trials [22]. In this analysis, an anthracycline-based regimen was used in only nine trials. Radiation was delivered to the chest wall, supraclavicular, axillary, and internal mammary nodal areas. The most common fractionation schedule was 50 Gy in 25 fractions over 5 weeks. Danish trials were not included in this analysis, and radiation therapy was shown to reduce the risk of any recurrence (OR: 0.69, $p = 0.0004$) and LRR with an odds ratio of 0.25 ($p = 0.000001$). A marked difference in LRR resulted in a reduction of BCM with an odds ratio of 0.83 ($p = 0.004$). On multivariate analysis, the timing of radiation therapy ($p = 0.03$) and radiation technique (megavoltage vs. orthovoltage therapy, $p = 0.05$) were independent prognostic factors for a radiation effect.

In the meta-analysis of EBCTCG 2005, treatment data for 42,500 breast cancer patients from 78 randomized trials were studied comparatively. For 23,500 patients (of all 42,500), a comparison of RT vs. non-RT and more surgery vs. less surgery was performed. The patients were grouped according to whether the 5-year LRR exceeded 10 % (<10 % in 17,000 women, >10 % in 25,000 women). These 25,000 women included 8,500 who underwent mastectomy and had axillary clearance and node-positive disease in trials of RT. RT was delivered to the chest wall and regional lymphatics in most of the RT trials. At the 5-year follow-up, LRR was 6 % versus 23 % (absolute reduction 17 %), and 15-year breast cancer mortality (BCM) rate was 54.7 % versus 60.1 % (reduction of 5.4 %, SE 1.3, 2p = 0.0002; overall mortality reduction 4.4 %, SE 1.2, 2p = 0.0009) in the RT group compared to the non-RT group. RT produced similar proportional reductions in local recurrence in all women. This effect was irrespective of age or tumor and radiation therapy treatment characteristics (recent vs. older trials or with vs. without systemic therapy). A 20 % reduction in local recurrence risk resulted in a 5 % reduction in BCM, which implied that for every four local recurrences prevented by RT, one breast cancer death was avoided [23].

The long-term follow-up results of these three prospective randomized trials indicated a clear effect of PMRT on survival because the LRR risk decreased significantly and the survival rates of the RT arm were significantly higher (Table 10.1) [24, 25]. The Danish trials have been criticized by other investigators. One criticism was the inadequacy of axillary surgery because only a median of seven nodes were removed from the axilla. This number is currently defined as inadequate axillary dissection. Most of the patients that had one to three positive nodes in the Overgaard studies would have had ≥4 nodes with a more complete dissection. In response to this issue, Danforth et al. and Saha et al. determined that 64–71 % of patients with one to three positive nodes with limited dissection would remain

Table 10.1 Locoregional control and survival in trials of mastectomy and systemic therapy with or without PMRT

Study	Locoregional recurrence	Overall survival
Danish 82b [2]	@ 10 years	
RT	9 %	45 % $p \leq 0.0001$
No RT	32 %	54 %
Danish 82c [3]	@ 10 years	
RT	8 %	45 % $p \leq 0.003$
No RT	35 %	36 %
Canada [21]	@ 20 years	
RT	7 %	47 % $p \leq 0.003$
No RT	18 %	37 %
Danish 82b and c (1–3 LN +, ≤8 nodes removed) [22]	@ 15 years	
RT	4 %	57 % $p \leq 0.03$
No RT	27 %	48 %

in the same group with more complete dissection [26, 27]. According to DBCG trialists, approximately 50–70 % of the patients in the group with one to three positive nodes would likely remain in the same group with a more complete dissection. The evaluation of 1–3 positive nodes together with ≥4 positive nodes raised another objection to the study. In the re-analysis of the Danish trials after 15-years of follow-up, a subgroup of 1,152 patients with excision of >8 lymph nodes was evaluated. The 15-year OS of the whole subgroup was 39 % for irradiated patients and only 29 % for the no PMRT group ($p = 0.015$). Patients with ≥4 involved axillary nodes experienced an absolute increase in OS of 9 % (21 % vs. 12 %, $p = 0.03$) [25]. The subgroup with one to three positive nodes had an absolute survival gain of 9 % (57 % vs. 48 %, $p = 0.03$). PMRT decreased the 15-year LRR for patients with ≥4 positive nodes by 41 % and for those with 1–3 positive nodes by 25 % (Table 10.2) [25]. The British Columbia trial also evaluated subgroups with ≥4 versus 1–3 positive nodes. In both subgroups, PMRT provided a similar reduction of breast cancer deaths (RR: 0.64, 95 % CI 0.42–0.97 and 0.59, 95 % CI 0.38–0.91, respectively). A similar increase in overall survival was observed. As expected, the impact of PMRT on

LRR was greater for patients with 1–3 positive nodes (RR: 0.46, 95 % CI 0.18–1.13) than for patients with ≥4 positive nodes (RR: 0.30, 95 % CI 0.10–0.85) [24].

In the Danish 82b trial, the 15-year OS rates in patients with ≥4 positive lymph nodes were very low. This is most likely due to the inefficiency of chemotherapy in this trial. Recently, high-risk patients have been treated with anthracycline- or taxane-based chemotherapy regimens. The LRR rates, in studies in which a more efficient systemic treatment was applied and PMRT was not used, were apparently lower than the rates in these prospective studies and meta-analysis.

LRR rates have been published in studies in which systemic therapy was used after mastectomy, and PMRT was not performed. In the MD Anderson Cancer Center (MDACC), the Eastern Cooperative Oncology Group (ECOG), and the National Surgical Adjuvant Breast and Bowel Project (NSABP) studies, the total LRR rates in T1–T2 patients with one to three positive lymph nodes when PMRT was not applied were 14 %, 13 %, and 13 %, respectively [7, 28, 29]. When patients with distant metastasis were excluded, the reported 10-year LRR rates were 11 %, 7–9 %, and 4–7 %, respectively. In these series,

efficient systemic therapy significantly reduced the LRR. When the patients were subdivided into two categories of 1–3 positive nodes and ≥4 positive nodes, the LRR rates were higher in the latter (Table 10.3). The average rate of LRR for patients with one to three positive lymph nodes in these series was approximately 12 %, which is almost three times less than the LRR in the no-radiation arm in the Danish trials. When the LRR is significantly low, the efficiency of RT can also be expected to be low. In these three trials, the LRR rates increased for the following patient or tumor parameters: more involved axillary lymph nodes, less excised axillary lymph nodes, larger tumor, estrogen receptor negativity, presence of extracapsular extension, high-grade tumor, presence of lymphovascular invasion, and younger age. The MDACC trial provided additional information about LRR for patients with one to three positive nodes. An analysis of the data from this subgroup found that the presence of extracapsular extension greater than 2 mm, tumor size over 4 cm, positive or close surgical margins (2 mm), presence of lymphovascular space invasion, resection of less than ten lymph nodes, or invasion of the skin, nipple, or pectoralis muscle were all associated with rates of isolated LRR of ≥25 % [30].

Sharma R et al. reported their series including 1,019 stage II patients who were treated between 1997 and 2002 [31]. With a median follow-up of 7.4 years, the overall 10-year LRR rate was 2.7 % in the whole group. This 10-year LRR rate was similar for patients who had node-negative disease (10-year LRR rates 2.1 %). The only independent factor for LRR was young age ($p = 0.004$).

LRR risks in node-positive patients after mastectomy, and current systemic therapies without RT are no longer as high as those reported by

Table 10.2 Locoregional recurrence and overall survival at 15 years in patients with 1–3 positive versus ≥4 positive lymph nodes

Endpoint at study and subgroup	PMRT (+)	PMRT (−)	p
% LRR @ 15 years			
1–3 LN positive	4	27	0.001
≥4 LN positive	10	51	0.001
% Overall survival @ 15 years			
1–3 LN positive	57	48	0.03
≥4 LN positive	21	12	0.03

Table 10.3 Ten-year LRR rates after mastectomy and systemic therapy in patients with 1–3 positive nodes and ≥4 positive nodes

Study	Number of patients	Systemic therapy	LRR	
			1–3 LN (+)	≥4 LN (+)
MDACC	1,031	Doxorubicin based	10 %	21 %
ECOG	2,016	CMF	13 %	29 %
NSABP	5,758	CMF/AC	8.1 %	15.5 %–18.8 %[*]

*LRR for patients with more than 10 positive axillary lymph nodes

prospective randomized trials and meta-analysis. More complete resection of the axilla combined with more effective systemic therapies such as anthracyclines, taxanes, trastuzumab, and new-generation hormonal therapies with aromatase inhibitors has permitted substantial reductions in LRR rates [32–41].

In the new era, the response to adjuvant therapies will be predicted using biological factors, including genetic alterations and gene expression profiles in the tumor, biological classification, and molecular features of the tumor. Kyndi et al. reanalyzed the molecular features of tumors in a subgroup analysis of the DBCG 82b and c trials [42]. They included 1,000 patients for whom tissue microarray sections were stained for estrogen receptor (ER), progesterone receptor (PgR), and human epidermal growth factor receptor (HER-2) and who were randomly assigned to PMRT. The follow-up time for patients who were alive was 17 years. Significantly improved OS after PMRT was observed among patients who had good prognostic markers, such as hormone receptor-positive and Her-2-negative patients. There was no significant improvement in OS after PMRT among patients with a poor prognosis (particularly hormone receptor-negative and Her-2-positive patients). An obvious lack of improvement in survival was observed for the hormone receptor-negative and Her-2 positive subtype. As an extension of this study, the same investigators divided 1,000 patients with excision of ≥ 8 axillary lymph nodes and for whom paraffin blocks were available into three risk groups. The "good-risk group" was defined by at least four of five favorable criteria (≥ 3 positive nodes, tumor size <2 cm, grade I tumor, ER or PgR positive, Her-2 negative); the "poor-risk group" was defined by at least two of three unfavorable criteria (>3 positive nodes, tumor size >5 cm, grade III tumor); and an intermediate group was defined between these extremes. The lowest LRR at 5 years was observed in patients in the good-risk group. The LRR probability increased from 11 % for the good-risk group to 50 % for the poor-risk group. PMRT reduced 5-year LRR risk significantly for all three subgroups. The largest absolute reduction in LRR probability with PMRT was observed in the poor-risk group [40]. Kyndi et al. also reported increased overall mortality, distant metastasis, and LRR probability in patients with negative bcl2 expression. In contrast to bcl2-positive patients (HR: 0.70 (0.57–0.86), $p = 0.001$), no survival improvement was observed for PMRT in the bcl2-negative subgroup (HR: 0.94 (0.75–1.20), $p = 0.4$) [44]. A significant association was observed between p53 accumulation and other poor prognostic markers, such as grade III malignant tumors, hormone receptor-negative tumors, and Her-2-positive/bcl-2-negative tumors. PMRT improved OS probability for both p53-negative and p53-positive patients. Tourong et al. conducted a retrospective analysis of British Columbia Cancer Agency (BCCA) data for 821 patients with T1–T2 breast cancer and one to three positive lymph nodes who were treated with mastectomy and without adjuvant RT [45]. Adjuvant systemic therapy was used in 94 % of patients, and approximately 66 % of patients received anthracycline-based chemotherapy. The overall 10-year isolated LRR and LRR with or without simultaneous distant recurrence (SDR) rates were 12.7 % and 15.9 %, respectively. A 10-year LRR risk of >20 % was reported in patients with one to three positive nodes plus at least one of the following factors: age <45 years, stage T2, grade III histology, ER-negative disease, medial location of tumor, more than one positive node, or >25 % positive lymph nodes. Multivariate analysis revealed that age <45 years, presence of >25 % positive lymph nodes, medial tumor location, and ER-negative status were statistically significant predictors of isolated LRR and LRR with or without SDR.

RT standards are also important prognostic factors for the survival effect of PMRT. Gebski et al. reanalyzed the results from 36 prospectively randomized trials, 33 of which were included in the EBCTCG meta-analysis [46]. Patients were separated into three different categories according to biologically equivalent dose (BED) and the appropriateness of target volumes: category I, a BED of 40–60 Gy in 2 Gy fractions with an appropriate target volume; category II, an excessive dose of radiation therapy; and category III, an inappropriate target volume. The absolute increase in survival was 2.9 % (OR of death: 0.87, $p = 0.006$) in category I patients with 5-year data and 6.4 % with 10-year data (OR of death: 0.78, $p < 0.001$). No statistically significant change in survival was observed among category II or III patients. Among the 33 EBCTCG trials, the odds of LRR were reduced more among category I trials (80 % lower) than category II (70 % lover) or III (64 % lower) trials. With proper RT techniques, a more precise and effective dose can be delivered to the target volume while preserving normal tissues, i.e., lungs and heart. Demirci et al. analyzed 19 published trials of patients treated between 1968 and 2002 (five randomized controlled trials, five single or multi- institutional trials, and nine national cancer registry database reviews) [47]. All the older trials with a median follow-up time >10 years reported excess cardiac toxicity. By contrast, the majority of RT trials with shorter median follow-up durations (≤10 years) did not report an excess cardiac toxicity risk. For trials that began in or after 1980, the reported relative risk (RR) for cardiac mortality was 0.5–2.1. The recommended optimal follow-up duration for assessing cardiac toxicity is >10–15 years after RT [8, 48, 49]. The follow-up duration in modern studies is shorter than in older RT trials; thus, the long-term safety of modern techniques remains uncertain. However, several trials have reported reduced cardiac risks in patients treated in the modern era (i.e., since 1980) [50–52].

The American Society of Clinical Oncology (ASCO) and the American Society of Therapeutic Radiology and Oncology (ASTRO) recommended PMRT only for patients with ≥4 positive lymph nodes or advanced primary disease, and both statements highlighted the need for additional prospectively randomized data concerning the use of PMRT for patients with T1–T2 and one to three positive lymph nodes [53, 54]. In the last EBCTCG meta-analysis, among the 1,314 women who had one to three axillary positive lymph nodes, RT reduced LRR (2p < 0.00001), overall recurrence (RR 0.68, 2p = 0.00006), and breast cancer mortality (RR 0.80, 2p = 0.01). No significant difference was detected in the proportional reductions in the rates of overall recurrence or breast cancer mortality

with the administration of systemic therapy [14]. Since 2007, the National Comprehensive Cancer Network (NCCN) breast cancer practice guidelines have strongly recommended PMRT in patients with one to three positive lymph nodes [15–17]. In 2009, in the consensus report from St. Gallen, the use of PMRT in patients with one to three lymph nodes positive in the axilla was recommended if the patient was young or had other poor prognostic factors such as high-grade or ER-negative or PgR-negative tumors [55]. The German Cancer Society reported the first guideline in 2004. PMRT was recommended only in patients with microscopic or macroscopic residual disease with ≥4 positive lymph nodes, pT3 tumors >5 cm, and patients with special risk factors. The risk factors were specified in 2005 by the German Society of Radiooncology (Deutsche Gesellschaff für Radiooncologie, DEGRO) [56]: one to three positive lymph nodes plus age <40 years, lymphovascular invasion, tumor >3 cm, grade III histology, multicentric and multifocal tumors, and negative for hormone receptors. Consequently, PMRT should be in used in the one to three lymph node-positive group in the presence of additional adverse prognostic factors. These factors are as follows: age <40 years, grade III histology, ER negative, PgR negative, lymphovascular invasion, tumor >3 cm, c-erb B-2-positive tumor, and high Ki-67 index. Recently, investigators from MDACC reported their series including 1,027 patients with T1–T2 breast cancer and one to three positive lymph nodes who were treated with modern treatment approaches, such as the use of sentinel lymph node surgery and standard systemic therapy (taxanes and aromatase inhibitors). They evaluated the rate of locoregional recurrence for patients treated in two different time periods: the early era (1978–1998) and the later or modern treatment era (2000–2007). They reported that PMRT reduced the locoregional recurrence rate from 14.5 % to 6.1 % in the early era cohort ($p = 0.035$). By contrast, PMRT did not reduce the locoregional recurrence rate in patients who were treated in the modern treatment era cohort; the 5-year LRR rates were 2.8 % without PMRT and 4.2 % with PMRT ($p = 0.48$). It should be kept in mind that this particular trial was a retrospective study and patients treated with PMRT in both eras

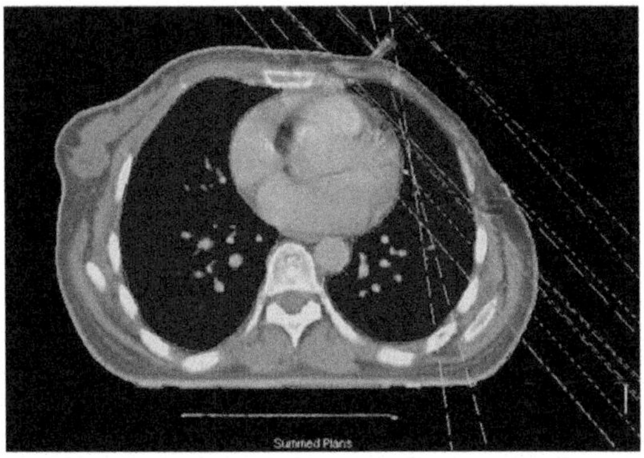

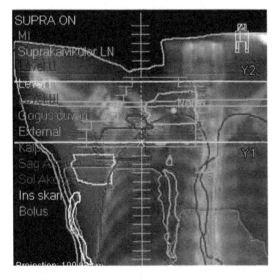

Fig. 10.1 PMRT to chest wall and internal mammary lymph nodes

Fig. 10.2 Supraclavicular field encompasses supraclavicular lymph nodes and level III and half of the level II axillary lymph nodes. Treatment volumes: *light blue*, supracalvicular lymph nodes; *dark blue*, level III axillary lymph nodes; *pink*, level II axillary lymph nodes; *yellow*, level I axillary lymph nodes

had worse prognostic factors than patients treated without PMRT. Patients who were treated with PMRT more commonly are younger, have T2 disease, three positive lymph nodes, and gross extracapsular extension of disease [57].

There is a consensus that the use of PMRT should include the chest wall, the supraclavicular region, and the axillary apex, but not the full axilla for patients treated after a level I–II axillary dissection (Figs. 10.1 and 10.2). The randomized trial supporting the use of PMRT generally treated

internal mammary nodes, which remains controversial [2–4]. A critically important aspect of treatment, particularly for left-sided cancers, is the use of computer-based simulation to ensure that the heart is not included in the treatment field [58, 59].

≥4 Positive Axillary Lymph Nodes (N2 Disease)

Patients with ≥4 positive lymph nodes after mastectomy are defined as having N2 disease pathologically in the AJC manual. As discussed above, the LRR rates are high in these patients, and PMRT is the standard therapy according to all prospective randomized trials, meta-analyses, and guidelines [2–5, 14, 15, 17–19, 21, 39–41, 50–53].

Locally Advanced Breast Cancer

Locally advanced breast cancer (LABC) encompasses breast cancer that is inoperable or operable only by mastectomy at initial diagnosis. LABC includes T3 or T4 tumors and any presence of N2 or N3 disease in the axilla (stage IIB, T3N0 to III A–C, in AJCC 2002 manual) [9]. Because T3N0 cases were discussed in detail previously, only stage III patients will be discussed in this chapter. LABC constitutes 10–20 % of all breast cancer in the United States [60]. Because distant metastases are common, a detailed systemic staging workup is needed. RT plays an important role in the management of LABC. LABC requires multimodal therapy to achieve optimal control of locoregional and distant disease. In the recent past, patients with operable LABC were treated by mastectomy, adjuvant chemotherapy, and PMRT. Currently, neoadjuvant chemotherapy (NAC) has become the preferred treatment method for LABC. The purpose of NAC at LABC is downstaging of the disease and rendering inoperable tumors resectable. After NAC, approximately 80–90 % of patients have changes in the pathological extent of the tumor, and 20 % of patients exhibit eradication of disease within the lymph nodes [61, 62]. In randomized trials, such as the NSABP

B-18, B-27, and the European Organization of Research and Treatment of Cancer (EORTC) 10902 trials, approximately 10 % LRR rates were reported for patients with NAC followed by surgery [63–65].

Trials that study the contribution of PMRT to LABC are usually single-centered nonrandomized studies. Piccart et al. used RT followed by mastectomy in patients treated with doxorubicin, vincristine, and cyclophosphamide and reported an LRR rate of 8 % [66]. According to Bedwinek et al., in LABC patients treated by mastectomy plus PMRT, the LRR rates were 8 %, compared to 61 % when treated by RT alone [67]. These results indicate that all these three treatment modalities should be used effectively. In a trial by the Milan Cancer Institute, a total of 133 LABCs were randomized into two arms after doxorubicin and vincristine neoadjuvant chemotherapy. Sixty-seven patients were treated by RT alone, and 65 patients underwent mastectomy. In the RT arm, LRR was 31 %, whereas in the surgery arm, LRR was 3 % [68]. Kelfström et al. divided patients into three subgroups; LRR was 45 % in the mastectomy and postoperative chemotherapy (vincristine, cyclophosphamide, and doxorubicin) group, 8 % in the mastectomy and PMRT group, and 5 % in the group in which all three treatment modalities were used [69].

A trial from MDACC retrospectively compared 542 patients treated with neoadjuvant chemotherapy, mastectomy, and PMRT with the outcomes of a control group of 134 patients who were treated with neoadjuvant chemotherapy and mastectomy without irradiation. The 10-year LRR rates were significantly lower for irradiated patients, averaging 11 % compared to 22 % [70]. In cases with a pathological complete response to NAC, when PMRT is not used after mastectomy, the LRR is high. In LABC, RT not only increases local control but also has a positive effect on OS. This positive effect is more significant in cases with a pathological complete response to NAC [71]. McGuire et al. also investigated the role of PMRT in patients with LABC who achieved a pCR to NAC. They reported 10-year LRR rates in PMRT and no PMRT groups after pCR to NAC of 5 % and 10 %, respectively [72].

The NCCN guidelines provide recommended indications for RT, and the fields of treatment should be based upon the pretreatment tumor characteristics in patients treated with NAC [15–17]. However, the role of the treatment of the regional lymphatics for patients who were treated with NAC is still unclear. In the MDACC retrospective trial, all patients treated with mastectomy received comprehensive regional nodal irradiation consisting of the supraclavicular and internal mammary chain [70]. Hyun Bae et al. reported that there were no differences in LRR in chest wall-irradiated patients regardless of the inclusion of the supraclavicular region (5 % and 7 %, respectively) [73]. However, this was a retrospective study, and patients in whom the supraclavicular region is treated have higher-risk factors. There has been no prospective randomized trial, and therefore, it is difficult to reach a firm conclusion. It is commonly accepted that RT fields should be chosen according to pre-chemotherapy tumor characteristics.

References

1. Ceiley E, Jagsi R, Goldberg S, Grigon L, Kachnic L, Powell S, et al. Radiotherapy for invasive breast cancer in North America and Europe: results of a survey. Int J Radiat Oncol Biol Phys. 2005;61:365–73.
2. Overgaard M, Hansen PS, Rose C, Andersson M, Kamby C. Postoperative radiotherapy in high risk premenopausal women with breast cancer who receive adjuvant chemotherapy. Danish Breast Cancer Cooperative Group DBCCG 82b trial. N Engl J Med. 1997;337:949–55.
3. Overgaard M, Jensen MB, Overgaard J, Rose C, Andersson M, Bach F, et al. Postoperative radiotherapy in high risk postmenopausal breast cancer patients given adjuvant tamoksifen: Danish Breast Cancer Cooperative Group DBCCG 82c randomised trial. Lancet. 1999;353:1641–8.
4. Ragaz J, Jacson SM, Le N, Plenderleith IH, Spinelli JJ, Bosco VE, et al. Adjuvant radiotherapy and chemotherapy in node positive women with breast cancer. N Engl J Med. 1997;337:956–62.
5. Cuzick J, Stewart H, Peto R, Fisher B, Kaae S, Johansen H, et al. Overview of randomised trials comparing radical mastectomy without radiation therapy against simple mastectomy with radiation therapy in breast cancer. Cancer Treat Rep. 1987;71:7–14.
6. McCammon R, Finlayson C, Schwer A, Rabinovitch R. Impact of postmastectomy radiotherapy in T3N0

invasive carcinoma of the breast: a Surveillance, Epidemiology, and End results database analysis. Cancer. 2008;1113(4):683–9.

7. Recht A, Gray R, Davidson N, Fowble BL, Solin LJ, Cummings FJ, et al. Locoregional failure 10 years after mastectomy and adjuvant chemotherapy with or without tamoxifen without irradiation: experience of the Eastern Cooperative Oncology Group. J Clin Oncol. 1999;17:1689–700.

8. Clarke M, Collins R, Darby S, Davies C, Elphinstone P, Evans E, et al. Effects of radiotherapy and of differences in the extent of surgery for early breast cancer on local recurrence and 15-year survival: an overview of randomised trials. Lancet. 2005;366:2087–106.

9. Gren FL. The American Joint Committee on Cancer: updating the strategies in cancer staging. Bull Am Coll Surg. 2002;87:13–5.

10. Taghian AG, Jeong JH, Mamounas EP, Parda DS, Deutsch M, et al. Low locoregional recurrence rate among node-negative breast cancer patients with tumor 5 cm or larger treated by mastectomy, with or without adjuvant systemic therapy and without radiotherapy: Results from five National Surgical Adjuvant Breast and Bowel Project) randomized clinical trials. J Clin Oncol. 2006;24:3927–32.

11. Goulart J, Truong P, Woods R, Speers CH, Kennecke H, Nichol A, et al. Outcomes of node- negative breast cancer 5 centimeters and larger treated with and without postmastectomy radiotherapy. I J Radiat Oncol Biol Phys. 2011;80:758–64.

12. Killander F, Anderson H, Ryden S, Möller T, Hafström LO, Malmström P, et al. Efficient reduction of loco-regional recurrences but no effect on mortality twenty years after postmastectomy radiation in premenopausal women with stage II breast cancer- a randomized trial from the South Sweden Breast Cancer Group. Breast. 2009;18:309–15.

13. Floyd SR, Bucholz TA, Haffty BG, Goldberg S, Niemierko A, Road RA, et al. Low local recurrence rate without postmastectomy radiation in node- negative breast cancer patients with tumors 5 cm and larger. Int J Radiat Oncol Biol Phys. 2006;66(2): 358–64.

14. Cutter D, Duane F, Ewertz M, Gray G, McGale P, Taylor C, Correa C, EBCTCG (Early Breast Cancer Trialists' Collaborative Group). Effect of radiotherapy after mastectomy and axillary surgery on 10-year recurrence and 20-year breast cancer mortality; meta-analysis of individual patient data for 8135 women in 22 randomised trials. Lancet. 2014;383:2127–35.

15. Theriault RL, Goldstein LJ, Pierce LJ, Carlson RW, Gradishar WJ, Reed EJ, Panel members. National Comprehensive Cancer Network. NCCN breast cancer clinical practice guidelines in oncology. http://www.nccn.org/professionals/physician_gls/PDF/breast.pdf (2.2013). Accessed Jan 2013.

16. Gradishar W, Giordano SH, Pierce LJ, Anderson BO, Goetz M, Reed E, Panel members. National Comprehensive Cancer Network. NCCN breast cancer clinical practice guidelines in oncology. http://

www.nccn.org/professionals/physician_gls/PDF/breast.pdf (2.2014). Accessed 3 2014, 04/01/2014.

17. Gradishar W, Giordano SH, Pierce LJ, Anderson BO, Goetz M, Reed EC, Panel members. National Comprehensive Cancer Network. NCCN breast cancer clinical practice guidelines in oncology. http://www.nccn.org/professionals/physician_gls/PDF/breast.pdf (2.2015). Accessed 3 Nov 2015.

18. www.tukod.org. The Summary of 13th ST. Galen International Breast Cancer Conference 2013.

19. Hojris I, Overgaard M, Christensen JJ, Overgaard J. Morbidity and mortality of ischaemic hard disease in high-risk breast cancer patients after adjuvant postmastectomy systemic treatment with or without radiotherapy: analysis of DBCG 82b and 82c randomised trials. Lancet. 1999;354:1425–30.

20. Early Breast Cancer Trialists Collaborative Group. Favourable and unfavourable effects on long-term survival of radiotherapy for early breast cancer: an overview of the randomised trials. Lancet. 2000;355: 1757–70.

21. Van De Steene J, Soete G, Storme G. Adjuvant radiotherapy for breast cancer significantly improves overall survival: the missing link. Radiother Oncol. 2000;55(3):263–172.

22. Whelan TJ, Julian J, Wright J, Jadad AR, Levine ML. Does locoregional radiation therapy improve survival in breast cancer? A meta-analysis. J Clin Oncol. 2000;18:1220–9.

23. Chung CS, Harris JR. Postmastectomy radiation therapy: translating local benefits into improved survival. Breast. 2007;16:78–83.

24. Ragaz J, Olivotto IA, Spinelli JJ, Phillips N, Jackson SM, Wilson K, et al. Locoregional radiation therapy in patients with high-risk breast cancer receiving adjuvant chemotherapy: 20-year results of the British Columbia randomized trial. J Natl Cancer Inst. 2005;97:116–26.

25. Overgaard M, Nielsen HM, Overgaard J. Is the benefit of postmastectomy irradiation limited to patients with four or more positive nodes, as recommended in international consensus reports? A sub-group analysis of the DBCG 82b&c randomised trials. Radiother Oncol. 2007;82:247–53.

26. Danforth DN, Findlay PA, McDonald HD, Lippman ME, Reichert LM, d'Angelo T, et al. Complete axillary lymph node dissection for stage I–II carcinoma of the breast. J Clin Oncol. 1986;4:655–62.

27. Saha S, Farrar WB, Young DC, Ferrara JJ, Burak Jr WE, et al. Variation in axillary node dissection influences the degree of nodal involvement in breast cancer patients. J Surg Oncol. 2000;73:134–7.

28. Katz A, Strom EA, Buchholz TA, Thames HD, Smith CD, Jhingran A, et al. Locoregional recurrence patterns after mastectomy and doxorubicine-based chemotherapy: implications for postoperative irradiation. J Clin Oncol. 2000;18:2817–27.

29. Taghian AG, Jeong JH, Mamounas E, Anderson S, Bryant J, Deutsch M, et al. Pattern of locoregional and distant failure in patients with breast cancer treated

with mastectomy and chemotherapy with or without tamoxifen without radiation: results from five NSABP randomized trials. J Clin Oncol. 2004;22(21):4247–54. Epub 2004 Sep 27.

30. Katz A, Storm EA, Buchholz TA, Theriault R, Singletary SE, Mc Neese MD, et al. The influence of pathologic tumor characteristics on locoregional recurrence rates following mastectomy. Int J Radiat Oncol Biol Phys. 2001;50:735–42.

31. Sharma R, Bedrosian I, Lucci A, Hwang RF, Rourke LL, Qiao W, et al. Present day locoregional control in patients with T1 or T2 breast cancer with 0 and 1 to 3 positive lymph nodes after mastectomy without radiotherapy. Ann Surg Oncol. 2010;17:2899–908.

32. EBCTCG. Effects of chemotherapy and hormonal therapy for early breast cancer on recurrence and 15 – year survival: an overview of the randomised trials. Lancet. 2005;365:1687–777.

33. Coates AS, Keshaviah A, Thurlimann B, Mouridsen H, Mauriac LL, Forbes JF, et al. Five years of letrozole compared with tamoxifen as initial adjuvant therapy for postmenapausal women with endocrine – responsive early breast cancer: update of study BIG 1-98. J Clin Oncol. 2007;25:486–92.

34. Coombes RC, Kilborn LS, Snowdon CF, Paridaens R, Coleman RE, Jones SE, et al. Survival and safety of exemestane versus tamoxifen after 2–3 years tamoxifen treatment (Intergroup Exemestane Study): a randomized controlled trial. Lancet. 2007;369:359–70.

35. Forbes JF, Cuzick J, Buzdar A, Howell A, Tobias JS, Baum M. Effect of anastrozole and tamoxifen as adjuvant treatment for early stage breast cancer: 100-month analysis of the ATAC trial. Lancet Oncol. 2008;9:45–53.

36. Goss PE, Ingle JN, Martino S, Robert NJ, Muss HB, Piccart MJ, et al. Efficacy of letrozole extended adjuvant therapy according to estrogen receptor and progesterone receptor status of the primary tumor: National Cancer Institute of Canada Clinical Trials Group MA.17. J Clin Oncol. 2007;25:2006–11.

37. Romond EH, Perez EA, Bryant J, Suman VJ, Geyer Jr CE, Davidson NE, et al. Trastuzumab plus adjuvant chemotherapy for operable HER-2 positive breast cancer. N Engl J Med. 2005;353:1673–84.

38. Thürlimann B, Keshaviah A, Coates AS, Mouridsen H, Mauriac L, Forbes JF, et al. A comparison of letrozole and tamoxifen in postmenopausal women with early breast cancer. N Engl J Med. 2005;353: 2747–57.

39. Ward S, Simpson E, Davis S, Hind D, Rees A, Wilinson A, et al. Taxanes fort the adjuvant treatment of early breast cancer: systematic review and economic evaluation. Health Technol Assess. 2007;11: 1–144.

40. Early Breast Cancer Trialists' Colloborative Group (EBCTCG). Comparisons between different polychemotherapy regimens for early breast cancer: meta-analyses of long-term outcome among 100 000 women in 123 randomised trials. Lancet. 2012;379:432–44.

41. Qin YY, Li H, Guo XJ, Yex F, Wei X, Zhou YH, et al. Adjuvant chemotherapy, with or without taxanes, in early or operable breast cancer: a meta-analysis of 19 randomized trials with 30698 patients. PLoS One. 2011;6:1–11.

42. Kyndi M, Sorensen FB, Knudsen H, Overgaard M, Nielsen HM, Overgaard J. Estrogen receptor, progesterone receptor, HER-2, and response to postmastectomy radioteherapy in high risk breast cancer. The Danish Breast Cancer Cooperetive Group. J Clin Oncol. 2008;26:1419–26.

43. Kyndi M, Overgaard M, Nielsen HM, Sorenson FB, Knudsen H, Overgaard J. High local recurrence risk is not associated with large survival reduction after postmastectomy radiotherapy in high risk breast cancer: a subgroup analysis of DBCG 82b&c. Radiother Oncol. 2009;90:74–9.

44. Kyndi M, Sorensen FB, Knudsen H, Overgaard M, Nielsen HM, Anderson J, et al. Impact of BCL2 and p53 on postmastectomy radiotherapy response in high risk breast cancer. A subgroup analysis of DBCG82 b&c. Acta Oncol. 2008;47:608–17.

45. Truong PT, Olivotto IA, Kader HA, Panades M, Speers CH, Berthelet E, et al. Selecting breast cancer patients with T1–T2 tumors and one to three positive axillary nodes at high postmastectomy locoregional recurrence risk for adjuvant radiotherapy. Int J Radiol Oncol Biol Phys. 2005;61(5):1337–47.

46. Gebski V, Lagleva M, Keech A, Sims J, Langlands AO. Survival effects of postmastectomy adjuvant radiation therapy using biologically equivalent doses. J N Cancer Inst. 2006;98:26–38.

47. Demirci S, Nam J, Hubbs J, Thu Nguyen BA, Marks LB. Radiation induced cardiac toxicity after therapy for breast cancer: interaction between treatment era and follow-up duration. Int J Radiat Oncol Biol Phys. 2009;73:980–7.

48. Darby S, McGale P, Peto R, Granath F, Hall P, Ekbom A. Mortality from cardiovascular disease more than 10 years after radiotherapy for breast cancer: nationwide cohort study of 90 000 Swedish women. BMJ. 2003;326:256–7.

49. Harris EE, Correa C, Hwang WT, Liao J, Litt HI, Ferrari VA, et al. Late cardiac mortality and morbidity in early-stage breast cancer patients after breast conservation treatment. J Clin Oncol. 2006;24: 4100–6.

50. Giordano SH, Kuo YF, Freeman JL, Bucholz TA, Hortobagyi GN, Goodwin JS. Risk of cardiac death after adjuvant radiotherapy for breast cancer. J Natl Cancer Inst. 2005;97:419–24.

51. Hooning MJ, Aleman BM, van Rosmalen AJ, Kuenen MA, Klijn JG, van Leeuwen FE. Cause-specific mortality in long-term survivors of breast cancer: a 25-year follow-up study. Int J Radiat Oncol Biol Phys. 2006;64:1081–91.

52. Hooning MJ, Botma A, Aleman BM, Baaijens MH, Bartelink H, Klijn JG, et al. Long-term risk of cardiovascular disease in 10-year survivors of breast cancer. J Natl Cancer Inst. 2007;99:365–75.

53. Recht A, Edge SB, Solin LJ, Robinson DS, Estabrook A, Fine RE, et al. Postmastectomy radiotherapy: clinical practice guidelines of American Society of Clinical Oncology. J Clin Oncol. 2001;19:1539–69.
54. Harris JR, Halpin- Murphy P, McNeese M, Mendenhall NP, Morrow M, Robert NJ. Consensus statement on postmastectomy radiation therapy. Int J Radiat Oncol Biol Phys. 1999;44:989–90.
55. Goldhirsch A, Ingle JN, Gelber RD, Coates AS, Thürlimann B, Senn HJ, Panel Members. Thresholds for therapies: highlights of the St Galen International Expert Consensus on the primary therapy of early breast cancer. 2009. Ann Oncol. 2009;20:1319–29.
56. Sautter-Bihl ML, Souchon R, Budach W, Sedlmayer F, Feyer M, Harm W, Haase W. DEGRO practical guidelines for radiotherapy of breast cancer II. Postmastectomy radiotherapy, irradiation of regional lymphatics, and treatment of locally advanced disease. Strahlenther Onkol. 2008;184:347–53.
57. McBride A, Allen P, Woodward W, Kim M, Kuerer HM, Drinka EK, et al. Locoregional recurrence risk for patients with T1,2 breast cancer with 1–3 lymph nodes treated with mastectomy and systemic treatment. Int J Radiat Oncol Biol Phys. 2014;89:392–8.
58. Stemmer SM, Riel S, Hardon I, Adamo A, Neumann A, Goffman J, et al. The role of irradiation of the internal mammary nodes in high risk stage II to IIIA breast cancer patients after high dose chemotherapy: a prospective sequential non randomized study. J Clin Oncol. 2003;21:2713–8.
59. Obedion E, Haffty BG. Internal mammary nodal irradiation in conservatively managed breast cancer patients: is there a benefit? Int J Radiat Oncol Biol Phys. 1994;44:997–1003.
60. Anderson WF, Chu KC, Chang S. Inflamatory breast carcinoma and non inflamatory locally advanced breast carcinoma: distinct clinicopathologic entities. J Clin Oncol. 2003;21:2254–9.
61. Kuerer HM, Newman LA, Smith TL, Ames FC, Hunt KK, Dhingra K, et al. Clinical course of breast cancer patients with complete pathologic primary tumor and axillary lymph node response to doxorubicin-based neoadjuvant chemotherapy. J Clin Oncol. 1999;17:460–9.
62. Kuerer HM, Sahin AA, Hunt KK, Newman LA, Breslin T, Ames FC, et al. Incidence and impact of documented eradication of breast cancer axillary lymph node metastases before surgery in patients treated with neoadjuvant chemotherapy. Ann Surg. 1999;230:72–8.
63. Fisher B, Brown A, Mamounas E, Wieand S, Robidoux A, Margolese RG, et al. Effect of preoperative chemotherapy on local-regional disease in women with operable breast cancer: findings from National Surgical Adjuvant Breast and Bowel Project B-18. J Clin Oncol. 1997;15:2483–93.
64. Rastgoli P, Anderson SJ, Bear HD, Geyer CE, Kahlenberg MS, Robidoux A, et al. Preoperative chemotherapy: updates of National Surgical Adjuvant Breast and Bowel Project B-18 and B-27. J Clin Oncol. 2008;26:778–85.
65. van der Hage JA, van de Velde CJ, Julien JP, Tubiana-Hulin M, Vandervelden C, Duchateau L, et al. Preoperative chemotherapy in primary operable breast cancer: results from the European Organization for Research and Treatment of Cancer trial 10902. J Clin Oncol. 2001;19:4224–37.
66. Piccart MJ, DE Valeriola D, Paridaens R, Balikdjian D, Mattheiem WH, Loriaux C, et al. Six year results of a multimodality treatment strategy for locally advanced breast cancer. Cancer. 1988;62:2501–6.
67. Bedwinek J, Rao DV, Perez C, Lee J, Fineberg B. Stage II–I and localized stage IV breast cancer: irradiation alone versus irradiation plus surgery. Int J Radiat Oncol Biol Phys. 1982;8:31–6.
68. De Lena M, Varini M, Zucalli R, Rovini D, Viganotti G, Valagussa P, et al. Multimodal treatment for locally advanced breast cancer. Cancer Clin Trials. 1981;4:229–36.
69. Kelfström P, Gröhn P, Heinonen E, Holsti L, Holsti P, et al. Adjuvant postoperative radiotherapy, chemotherapy and immunotherapy in stage III breast cancer. Cancer. 1987;60:936–42.
70. Huang EH, Tucker SL, Strom EA, McNeese MD, Kuerer HM, Buzdar AU, et al. Postmastectomy radiation improves local-regional control and survival for selected patients with locally advanced breast cancer treated with neoadjuvant chemotherapy and mastectomy. J Clin Oncol. 2004;22:4691–9.
71. Bristol IJ, Woodward WA, Strom EA, Cristofanilli M, Domain D, Singletary SE, et al. Locoregional treatment outcomes after multimodality management of inflammatory breast cancer. Int J Radiat Oncol Biol Phys. 2008;72:474–84.
72. McGuire SE, Gonzales-Angulo AM, Huang EH, Tucker SL, Kau SW, Yu TK, et al. Postmastectomy radiation improves the outcome of patients with locally advanced breast cancer who achieve a pathologic complete response to neoadjuvant chemotherapy. Int J Radiat Oncol Biol Phys. 2007;68:1004–9.
73. Bae SH, Park W, Huh SJ, Choi DH, Nam SJ, Im YH, et al. Radiation treatment in pathologic N0–N1 patients treated with neoadjuvant chemotherapy followed by surgery for locally advanced breast cancer. J Breast Can. 2012;15(3):329–36. doi:10.4048/ibc.2012.15.3.329. Epub2012 Sep 28.

Adjuvant Radiation Therapy After Preoperative Chemotherapy

11

Merdan Fayda

Abstract

The decision to treat patients with radiotherapy after preoperative chemotherapy is still largely based on the initial clinical staging of the patients. The use of three-field radiotherapy (RT) including the chest wall/breast and regional lymphatics after surgery in locally advanced, node-positive patients receiving neoadjuvant systemic chemotherapy is well established. Patients with clinically staged T3–T4 tumors, pathological non-complete responders in the axilla, and younger patients (<35) with cT2N1 or worse disease should be treated with RT according to retrospective data. A pooled analysis of the National Surgical Adjuvant Breast and Bowel Project (NSABP) B18 and B27 trials is the only prospective dataset that can assist radiotherapy decisions in the neoadjuvant setting. Although the results of this analysis should be validated with modern studies (i.e., proper anti-Her-2 and hormonal treatment), selected patients (cT1–2, cN1, and >40 years old) with pathological complete response (pCR) (ypT0, ypTis, ypN0) and non-triple-negative histology after neoadjuvant chemotherapy could possibly be followed without postmastectomy radiotherapy (PMRT) and without regional irradiation in a breast-conserving setting. Well-designed randomized, controlled studies are urgently needed in this controversial area.

Keywords

Neoadjuvant chemotherapy • Preoperative chemotherapy • Postmastectomy radiotherapy (PMRT) • Lymphatic radiotherapy • Radiotherapy (RT) • National Surgical Adjuvant Breast and Bowel Project (NSABP) • Lymphovascular space invasion (LVSI) • Extracapsular extension (ECE) • Early Breast Cancer Trialists' Collaborative Group (EBCTCG) • MA-20

M. Fayda, MD
Department of Radiation Oncology, Istanbul
University Institute of Oncology,
Capa, Istanbul, Turkey
e-mail: merdanfayda@yahoo.com

© Springer International Publishing Switzerland 2016
A. Aydiner et al. (eds.), *Breast Disease: Management and Therapies*,
DOI 10.1007/978-3-319-26012-9_11

219

National Cancer Institute of Canada (NCI-C) trial • European Cancer Congress (ECCO) • European Organisation for Research and Treatment of Cancer (EORTC) 22922/10925 trial • Estrogen receptor (ER) • Progesterone receptor (PR) • Human epidermal growth factor receptor 2 neu (HER2) • Magnetic resonance imaging (MRI) • Distant metastasis-free survival (DMFS) • Triple negative (TN) • MD Anderson Cancer Center (MDACC) • NSABP B51 trial • Radiotherapy oncology group (RTOG) 1304 trial • Z1071 study • AMAROS study • Sentinel lymph node biopsy (SLNB) • ALLIANCE (Alliance for Clinical Trials in Oncology) A011202 trial

Introduction

Neoadjuvant systemic chemotherapy has been widely employed for the treatment of locally advanced operable breast cancer, and its use during the early stages of breast cancer has increased [1]. Randomized trials have not observed differences in survival or locoregional control between preoperative and postoperative chemotherapy, with hazard ratios (HRs) of 0.98 (95 % CI, 0.87–1.09; $p=0.67$) and 1.12 (95 % CI, 0.92–1.37; $p=0.25$), respectively [2]. pCR to neoadjuvant chemotherapy is associated with better survival rates compared to non-complete responders [2]. The pathological complete nodal response of the axilla was 41 % (95 % CI, 36.7–45.3 %) in a modern neoadjuvant study [3]. This research also indicates that preoperative treatment supports breast-conserving surgery (BCS) due to tumor shrinkage before surgical intervention (HR 0.82; 95 % CI, 0.76–0.89) [2]. However, many women who receive neoadjuvant chemotherapy still undergo mastectomy, due to either patient preference or a lack of feasibility of BCS [1]. In this chapter, we attempt to determine whether postmastectomy radiotherapy (PMRT) and regional irradiation in the breast-conserving setting are necessary for all patients undergoing systemic neoadjuvant treatment.

PMRT in the Adjuvant Setting

The indication for postmastectomy adjuvant radiotherapy in patients with pT3–pT4 disease and/or four or more positive lymph nodes is well established [4]. Among all node-positive patients with mastectomy and axillary dissection, the absolute

effects of radiotherapy on 5-year local recurrence risk are substantial (6.6 % vs. 21.3 %) [5]. PMRT significantly improves 20-year breast cancer mortality among all node-positive patients (58.3 % vs. 66.4 %, SE, 2.0, $2p$: 0.001) [5]. Although the routine use of PMRT in the subset of patients with small tumor disease (pT1–pT2) and one to three involved lymph nodes is controversial, the recent findings of the Early Breast Cancer Trialists' Collaborative Group (EBCTCG) meta-analysis could affect this practice. Among women with axillary dissection and only one to three positive nodes, PMRT reduced locoregional recurrence (LRR) ($2p<0.00001$), overall recurrence (RR 0.68; 95 % CI 0.57–0.82; $2p=0.00006$), and breast cancer mortality (RR 0.80; 95 % CI 0.67–0.95; $2p=0.01$) [5]. In the absence of these updated results, the selective use of PMRT was generally accepted in the St. Gallen 2013 consensus report for patients with pT1–pT2 and one to three involved nodes [6]. According to National Comprehensive Cancer Network breast guidelines, PMRT should be strongly considered in this patient population [7]. Most of these studies were designed prior to the use of modern systemic agents such as anthracyclines and trastuzumab. Therefore, the results of modern studies, such as SUPREMO, of postmastectomy patients with one to three involved lymph nodes are awaited to reach firm conclusions on this crucial topic.

Regional Radiotherapy in the Adjuvant Setting

The indications for lymphatic radiotherapy are controversial in both postmastectomy and breast-conserving settings. The lymphatic stations of the breast were routinely irradiated in three randomized trials investigating the role of PMRT [8–10]. Thus, regional radiotherapy contributes to the improvement of the overall survival (OS) obtained with PMRT in patients with node-positive disease [5]. The first results of the MA-20 National Cancer Institute of Canada (NCI-C) trial investigating the role of whole lymphatic radiotherapy (supraclavicular and axillary levels and mammaria interna) primarily in one to three node-positive (85 % of patients), breast-conserving patients were reported at the meeting of the American Society of Clinical Oncology (ASCO) in 2011 [11]. Isolated locoregional disease-free survival (DFS) (HR 0.59; 95 % CI 0.37–0.92; $p = 0.02$), distant DFS (HR 0.64; 95 % CI, 0.47–0.85; $p = 0.002$), and a trend toward better OS (HR 0.76; 95 % CI 0.56–1.03; $p = 0.07$) were observed with regional radiotherapy [11]. The European Organisation for Research and Treatment of Cancer (EORTC) 22922/10925 study, presented at the European Cancer Congress (ECCO) in 2013, is also investigating the role of mammaria interna and medial supraclavicular irradiation (IM-MS RT) in patients with medially or centrally located and/or node-positive tumors [12]. At a median follow-up of 10.9 years, IM-MS RT improved the outcome at 10 years: 82.3 vs. 80.7 % OS (HR 0.87; 95 % CI 0.76–1.00; $p = 0.056$), 72.1 vs. 69.1 % DFS (HR 0.89; 95 % CI 0.80–1.00; $p = 0.044$), and 78.0 vs. 75.0 % metastasis-free survival (HR 0.86; 95 % CI 0.76–0.98, $p = 0.020$). Based on these reports, the positive effects of regional radiotherapy on patient outcomes could arguably affect clinical practice. There is no clear consensus on radiotherapy fields and indications for regional irradiation in the adjuvant setting. Longer follow-up and publication of both the NCI-C MA-20 and EORTC 22922/10925 studies are awaited.

Radiotherapy Considerations After Preoperative Chemotherapy

The decision to prescribe radiotherapy after preoperative chemotherapy is still largely based on the initial clinical staging of the patients. Therefore, the initial clinical staging information should be available prior to systemic treatment. History and physical examination, complete blood count, liver function tests, alkaline phosphatase, diagnostic bilateral mammogram (ultrasound as necessary), determination of tumor estrogen (ER)/progesterone receptor (PR), and human epidermal growth factor receptor 2 *neu* (HER2) status should be routinely performed before the start of neoadjuvant chemotherapy in patients at clinical stages IIA–IIB [7]. Chest computed tomography (CT), abdominal CT, and bone scan can be considered for early-stage patients with symptoms (i.e., pulmonary symptoms, abnormal liver function tests, bone pain, or elevated alkaline phosphatase) or clinical stage IIIA or higher disease. Positron emission tomography and magnetic resonance imaging (MRI) of the breast are not considered part of the standard staging procedure. However, MRI could be helpful in patients with mammographically occult tumors [7]. MRI is also more accurate than mammography in detecting residual tumors after neoadjuvant chemotherapy but requires standardization [13]. Before systemic therapy, a pathological confirmation of the axilla via fine needle aspiration biopsy is also strongly suggested [7, 14]. Radiopaque marker insertion may be helpful for clarifying the lumpectomy area after systemic treatment, particularly in patients with a complete tumor response [7, 15].

There is a lack of randomized data to guide decision-making for PMRT after preoperative chemotherapy. Lymphatic irradiation in patients treated with breast-conserving protocols after preoperative chemotherapy and who are staged ypN0 is another area of controversy for which higher-level evidence is urgently needed. Our current source of information in these controversial areas are the retrospective series, the prospective dataset from a pooled analysis of the National Surgical Adjuvant Breast and Bowel Project (NSABP) B18 and B27 trials, and the results of adjuvant randomized trials. A pooled analysis of the NSABP B18 and B27 trials has recently been published. This analysis included cT1–3 cN0–1 patients who underwent preoperative systemic treatment. The median follow-up time was 11.75 years. PMRT and lymphatic irradiation in a breast-conserving setting were not allowed in this trial [16]. Because the NSABP trials form the only prospective dataset, we will compare the retrospective series and NSABP trial data accordingly.

First, we will review the prognostic factors impacting LRR and then focus on LRR rates separately for each stage.

Prognostic Factors for Locoregional Control After Preoperative Neoadjuvant Systemic Treatment

The literature suggests that the most important factors impacting the risk of LRR are the initial clinical stage, the age at the diagnosis, the extent of residual disease after preoperative chemotherapy, and adverse risk factors such as lymphovascular space invasion (LVSI), extracapsular extension (ECE), and a triple-negative (TN) phenotype [17].

Age

In the previous EBCTCG meta-analysis of adjuvant treatments, there was no correlation between age and the 5-year risk of LRR in patients treated with mastectomy, axillary clearance, and node-positive disease. Hence, the absolute effects of adjuvant PMRT on the risk of local recurrence were also approximately independent of age (local recurrence reductions of 17 %, 18 %, and 18 % for women aged <50, 50–59, and 60–69 years, respectively) [37]. Similarly, age was not a significant predictor of LRR in the multivariate Cox proportional hazards model for patients treated with mastectomy and without PMRT in the NSABP B18 and B27 neoadjuvant trials [16]. In a retrospective trial, age <40 was a significant predictor of LRR in patients with stage II disease treated with preoperative chemotherapy and without PMRT [18]. Although age is not a significant predictor of LRR in patients treated with preoperative systemic chemotherapy and mastectomy, younger patients (<35) with stage IIB or worse disease treated with preoperative chemotherapy and mastectomy should also be treated with PMRT, according to the retrospective data [19].

The effect of age on LRR in patients treated with BCS was also studied in the previous EBCTCG

meta-analysis of adjuvant treatments. Most of the local recurrences were in the conserved breast; the 5-year risk of such recurrence in the breast is approximately twofold greater in younger compared to older women. Hence, the absolute effects of post-BCS adjuvant radiotherapy on local recurrence (mainly in the conserved breast) were greater in younger than in older women (5-year risk reductions of 22 %, 16 %, 12 %, and 11 % for those aged ≤50, 50–59, 60–69, and ≥70 years, respectively; test for a trend in absolute benefits $2p = 0.00002$) [37]. Similarly, younger age was a significant predictor of LRR in multivariate analyses of patients treated with preoperative chemotherapy and BCS with whole-breast RT in the NSABP B18–B27 neoadjuvant trial (≥50 vs. <50 years HR 0.71; 95 % CI, 0.53–0.96; $p = 0.025$) [16].

Clinical Tumor Size

In the previous EBCTCG meta-analysis of adjuvant treatments, there was a correlation between T-stage and the 5-year risk of LRR in patients treated with mastectomy, axillary clearance, and node-positive disease. Hence, the absolute effects of adjuvant PMRT on the risk of local recurrence were also dependent on T-stage (local recurrence reductions of 17 %, 24 %, and 28 % for women staged with T1, T2, and T3/T4 disease, respectively) [37]. Similarly, clinical tumor size was an independent predictor of LRR in patients treated with mastectomy and without PMRT in the NSABP B18–B27 neoadjuvant trial (>5 vs. ≤5 cm HR 1.58; 95 % CI, 1.12–2.23; $p = 0.0095$) (Table 11.1) [16].

Conversely, clinical tumor size was not an independent predictor of LRR in multivariate analyses of patients treated with preoperative chemotherapy and BCS with whole-breast RT in the NSABP B18 and B27 neoadjuvant trials [16].

Lymphovascular Space Invasion (LVSI)

Retrospective studies have indicated that the presence of LVSI increases the risk of LRR [17]. LVSI and the risk of LRR were studied in

Table 11.1 Multivariate analysis of independent predictors of 10-year LRR according to type of surgery

Variable	No. of patients	LRR events	HR	95 % CI	p
Patients treated with mastectomy[a]	1,071	131			
Clinical tumor size >5 vs. ≤5 cm[b]			1.58	1.12–2.23	0.0095
Clinical nodal status cN(+) vs. cN(–)[b]			1.53	1.08–2.18	0.017
Nodal/breast pathological status					<0.001
ypN(–)/no breast pCR vs. ypN (–)/breast pCR[b]			2.21	0.77–6.3	
ypN(+) vs. ypN(–)/ breast pCR[b]			4.48	1.64–12.21	
Patients treated with lumpectomy plus breast XRT[a]	1,890	189			
Age ≥50 vs. <50 years[b]			0.71	0.53–0.96	0.025
Clinical nodal status cN(+) vs. cN(–)[b]			1.70	1.26–2.31	<0.001
Nodal/breast pathological status					<0.001
ypN(–)/no breast pCR vs. ypN (–)/breast pCR[b]			1.44	0.9–2.33	
ypN(+) vs. ypN(–)/ breast pCR[b]			2.25	1.41–3.59	

From Mamounas et al. [16], with permission
HR hazard ratio, *LRR* locoregional recurrence, *pCR* pathological complete response, *XRT* external radiation therapy
[a]Includes only patients for whom all covariates are known
[b]Category used as baseline for comparison of risk

a large Canadian cohort. Although LVSI had no impact on LRR in the breast-conserving setting, regional relapses were significantly higher in patients treated with mastectomy (HR 1.73; 1.1–2.7; $p=0.015$) [20]. In a study from MD Anderson Cancer Center (MDACC), the presence of LVSI was associated with worse 5-year LRR (no LVSI 2 % vs. LVSI (+) 15.4 %, $p=0.006$) in patients with cT1–2 N0–1 disease treated with preoperative chemotherapy and mastectomy without PMRT [21]. In another trial, the effects of LVSI on LRR were studied in clinical stage III patients who achieved pCR to neoadjuvant chemotherapy. The presence or absence of LVSI at the time of initial biopsy exhibited a trend toward an association with LRR in univariate analysis that was not statistically significant (45 % ± 24.8 % with and 8.6 % ± 3.6 % without, $p=0.063$) [22].

Extracapsular Extension (ECE)

ECE has not been studied extensively in neoadjuvant studies; however, it is an accepted risk factor for LRR and is widely used to indicate PMRT [17]. In a retrospective study in India, the presence of ECE had no significant effect on LRR in patients with clinical stage II–III disease receiving neoadjuvant chemotherapy, but 5-year distant DFS was 58 % in patients without ECE compared to 10 % in patients with ECE ($p=0.0001$) [23].

Extent of Residual Disease

The presence of residual disease after neoadjuvant chemotherapy was associated with worse outcome in the NSABP B18 and B27 studies for both mastectomy and the breast-conserving setting. Pathological nodal status and pathological breast tumor response (HR, 1.44; 95 % CI, 0.90–2.33 for ypN0/no breast pCR vs. ypN0/ breast pCR and HR, 2.25; 95 % CI, 1.41–3.59 for ypN+ vs. ypN-/breast pCR; $p < 0.001$) were significant independent predictors of LRR in multivariate analyses (Table 11.1) [16].

Receptor Status

In the previous EBCTCG meta-analysis of adjuvant treatments, the 5-year risk of LRR and the contribution of PMRT did not differ according to receptor status in patients treated with mastectomy, axillary clearance, and node-positive disease (ER poor vs. ER positive, 5-year LRR with PMRT 8 vs. 6, and absolute reduction of LRR with PMRT 20 (SE, 2) vs. 18 (SE, 2) [37]. Ten-year local relapse-free survival after mastectomy according to breast cancer subtype was reported in a large Canadian adjuvant trial (10-year LRFS in Luminal A (ER/PR (+), HER2(–), and Ki67≤14 %) vs. TN tumors was 92 % (95 % CI, 89–94) vs. 81 % (95 % CI, 73–87), respectively) [20]. Unfortunately, the status of the receptors (ER, PR, HER-2 status) was unknown in the NSABP B18 and B27 neoadjuvant trials [16]. In a retrospective study by MDACC, ER negativity and not using tamoxifen were significantly and independently associated with increased LRR (HR, 1.69; 95 % CI, 1.04–2.76; $p = 0.033$ and HR, 2.19; 95 % CI 1.19–4.06; $p = 0.012$, respectively) in patients receiving neoadjuvant chemotherapy and mastectomy [24]. Another retrospective neoadjuvant study from Florida demonstrated that TN (negative for ER, PR, and HER2) status had a significantly higher rate of LRR than non-negative status (12.8 % vs. 2.6 %) in stage II–III patients treated with preoperative chemotherapy and mastectomy [25]. In a study from MDACC, patients with TN disease were evaluated. Among the 155 patients treated with neoadjuvant chemotherapy and mastectomy, 27 achieved pCR. All 27 patients had stage I–II disease and were free of LRR. For the entire group of patients treated with neoadjuvant chemotherapy and mastectomy, those who were N0 after

chemotherapy had 99 % 5-year locoregional control (LRC) with or without PMRT. LRC was poor in those patients with 1–3 N+ residual disease (63 %) and was not improved with PMRT ($p = 0.38$). Patients with residual ≥4 N+ also had poor LRC (58 %), although there was a trend toward improved LRC with PMRT (61 % vs. 43 %; $p = 0.07$) [26].

PMRT After Preoperative Systemic Treatment for Initial Clinical Stage I (T1 N0) Disease

There are insufficient data to conclude whether PMRT is necessary for cT1N0 disease treated with neoadjuvant chemotherapy and mastectomy.

PMRT After Preoperative Systemic Treatment for Initial Clinical Stage IIA (T0–1 N1 or T2 N0) Disease

In two retrospective studies, no locoregional failure was observed in cT2N0 patients with complete pathological remission (pCR, no invasive disease in the pathological specimen) [22, 26]. The rates of LRR were 0–7 % in patients with cT1N1 that finally staged ypN0 after neoadjuvant chemotherapy, even with the TN phenotype [17, 18, 27]. In studies from MDACC, the LRR was 4–5 % in older (>35–40) patients with an initial cT1N1 that finally staged ypN(1–3+) after systemic chemotherapy, unless there were adverse risk factors (LVI, ECE, TN) [18, 28]. In another study from MDACC, patients with cT1–2 N0–1 disease were evaluated. In the total cohort of patients who did not receive RT ($n = 181$), those with ypN(≥4+) had the worst 5-year LRR (ypN0 1 %, ypN(1–3+) 5.4 %, yp(≥4+) 20 %, $p = 0.034$). The presence of LVSI was also associated with worse 5-year LRR (no LVSI 2 % vs. LVSI(+) 15.4 %, $p = 0.006$) [28]. The 10-year incidences of LRR were 6.5 %, 11.2 %, and 11.1 % without PMRT in patients with cT1–2 N0 disease that finally staged ypN0, ypN(1–3+), or ypN(≥4+), respectively, in the NSABP trial (Fig. 11.1) [16].

Fig. 11.1 Ten-year cumulative incidence of locoregional recurrence (*LRR*) in patients with (**a**) ≤5-cm tumors treated with mastectomy and (**b**) >5-cm tumors treated with mastectomy. *pCR* pathologic complete response [after neoadjuvant chemotherapy], *ypN* pathologic nodal status [after neoadjuvant chemotherapy] (From Mamounas et al. [16], with permission)

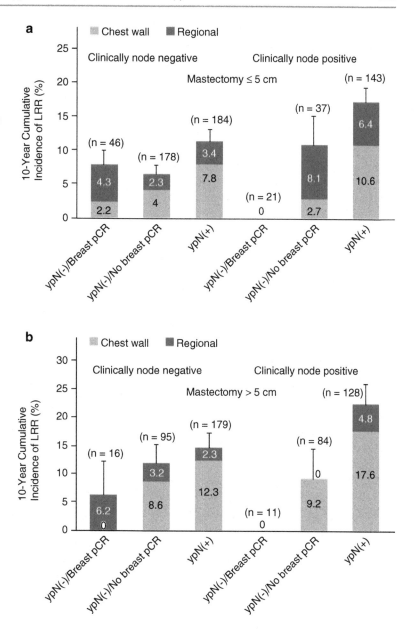

PMRT After Preoperative Systemic Treatment for Initial Clinical Stage IIB (T2 N1 or T3 N0) Disease

Retrospective data from younger patients (<35) with stage IIB or worse disease treated with preoperative chemotherapy and mastectomy indicate that these patients should also be treated with PMRT [19]. In a study from MDACC, 0 %

LRR was observed in patients with cT2N1 disease that finally staged pCR after neoadjuvant chemotherapy [22]. Two retrospective studies have investigated whether PMRT is necessary for patients with clinical stage II–III disease that finally staged ypN0. In a French single-center study, PMRT had no effect on LRR-free survival (HR, 0.37; 95 % CI, 0.09–1.61; $p=0.18$) or OS (HR, 2.06; 95 % CI, 0.71–6; $p=0.18$) for clinical stage II or III disease staged ypN0. A trend was observed toward poorer OS among patients without a pathologically complete in-breast tumor response after neoadjuvant chemotherapy (HR, 6.65; 95 % CI, 0.82–54.12; $p=0.076$) [27]. In a Korean multicenter retrospective study, the addition of PMRT was not correlated with a difference in DFS, LRR-free survival, or OS by multivariate analysis for clinical stage II or III disease that finally staged ypN0. In multivariate analysis, age (≤40 vs. >40 years) and pathological T-stage (0-is vs. 1 vs. 2–4) were significant prognostic factors affecting DFS (HR, 0.35, 95 % CI, 0.135–0.928; $p=0.035$ and HR 2.22, 95 % CI 1.074–4.604; $p=0.031$, respectively) [29]. The 10-year incidences of LRR were 0 %, 10.8 %, 14.4 %, and 19.5 % without PMRT in patients with cT1–2 N1 disease that finally staged pCR, ypN0 (no breast pCR), ypN(1–3+), or ypN(>4+), respectively, in the NSABP trial (Fig. 11.1) [16].

Another study from MDACC evaluated patients with cT3N0 disease treated with neoadjuvant chemotherapy (NAC) and mastectomy. Although all patients were clinically determined to have no nodal disease prior to NAC, 45 % had pathologically confirmed disease in the lymph node. The 5-year LRR rate differed significantly between patients who received PMRT and those who did not: 4 % (95 % CI, 1–9 %) with PMRT vs. 24 % (95 % CI, 10–39 %) without PMRT ($p<0.001$) [31]. Although the LRR rate was 0 % in patients with cT3N0 disease that finally staged pCR after preoperative chemotherapy, MDACC suggests PMRT for all patients with cT3N0 disease [1, 18, 22, 31]. The 10-year incidences of LRR were 6.2 %, 11.8 %, 10.6 %, and 17.6 % without PMRT in patients with cT3N0 disease that finally staged pCR, ypN0 (no breast pCR), ypN(1–3+), or ypN(>4+), respectively, in the NSABP trial (Fig. 11.1) [16].

PMRT After Preoperative Systemic Treatment for Initial Clinical Stage IIIA (T3 N1 or T0–3 N2) Disease

The role of PMRT in cases of pCR in patients with clinical stage III disease was evaluated at MDACC. The 10-year LRR rate for patients with stage III disease was significantly improved with radiation therapy (7.3 % ± 3.5 % with vs. 33.3 % ± 15.7 % without; $p=0.04$). In this cohort, the 10-year distant metastasis-free survival (DMFS) rate was 87.9 % ± 4.6 % for irradiated patients and 40.7 % ± 15.5 % for non-irradiated patients ($p=0.0006$). The 10-year OS rate was 77.3 % ± 6 % for irradiated patients and 33.3 % ± 14 % for non-irradiated patients [22]. The 10-year incidences of LRR were 0 %, 9.2 %, 14.7 %, and 27.2 % without PMRT in patients with cT3N1 disease that finally staged pCR, ypN0 (no breast pCR), ypN(1–3+), or ypN(>4+), respectively, in the NSABP trial (Fig. 11.1) [16]. The indications for PMRT in stage III patients achieving pCR varies between institutions. MDACC suggests PMRT for all clinical stage III patients [22]. If pCR is achieved in patients with cT3N1 disease, aged >40 years, and with no TN histology, PMRT is not necessary, according to NSABP data [16]. Clearly, validation is needed for this controversial topic [17].

PMRT After Preoperative Systemic Treatment for Initial Clinical Stage IIIB (T4 N0–2) Disease

The 5-year LRR risk in clinical stage IIIB patients treated with neoadjuvant chemotherapy and without PMRT was 42 % in a retrospective study from MDACC [31].

Lymphatic Irradiation After Preoperative Systemic Treatment and Breast-Conserving Surgery

The complete nodal pathological response rate in the axilla was 41 % (95%CI, 36.7–45.3) in a modern neoadjuvant study [3]. This encouraging result questions the necessity of axillary lymph node dissection for cN1 patients with good clinical response to neoadjuvant chemotherapy. However, the false-negative rate of sentinel lymph node biopsy after neoadjuvant chemotherapy remains high (12.6 %), and studies are needed to decrease axillary surgical interventions, particularly in patients with cN1 disease and a good clinical response to neoadjuvant chemotherapy [32]. The contribution of lymphatic irradiation to DFS and

Fig. 11.2 Ten-year cumulative incidence of locoregional recurrence (*LRR*) in patients (**a**) age ≥50 years treated with lumpectomy plus breast external radiotherapy (*XRT*) and (**b**) younger than age 50 years treated with lumpectomy plus breast XRT. *IBTR* ipsilateral breast tumor recurrence, *pCR* pathologic complete response [after neoadjuvant chemotherapy], *ypN* pathologic nodal status [after neoadjuvant chemotherapy] (From Mamounas et al. [16], with permission)

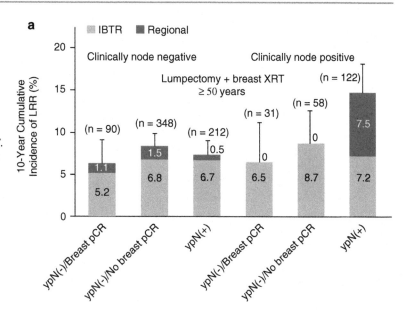

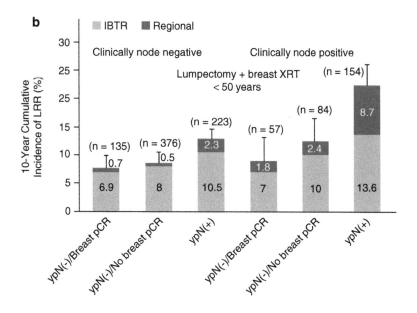

possibly to survival improvement has been demonstrated in modern adjuvant studies such as NCI-C MA20 and EORTC 22922/10925 [11, 12]. How this information will or should be applied in the neoadjuvant setting is not clear. There is no consensus on the optimal management of regional radiotherapy in patients receiving neoadjuvant chemotherapy and axillary dissection.

The role of lymphatic irradiation in clinical stage II–III disease was investigated in a French retrospective study. These researchers compared the outcomes of patients with pN0 status after neoadjuvant chemotherapy and BCS according to whether they received lymphatic irradiation. No improvement in the rates of LRR or survival was observed for nodal irradiation. All patients with initially positive axillary cytology received lymphatic radiotherapy, and 83 % of patients in the no-lymphatic-RT arm had cN0 disease in that study [27]. The risk of regional recurrence was less than 10 % in the NSABP trial after BCS and breast-only RT (Fig. 11.2). Age and the residual disease burden in the axilla had an impact on the 10-year incidence of LRR in the NSABP trial [16].

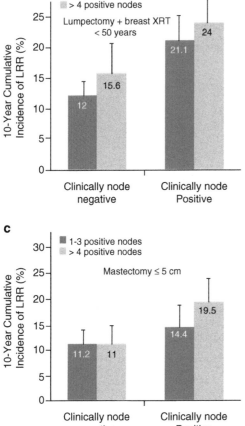

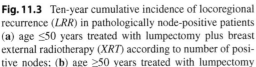

Fig. 11.3 Ten-year cumulative incidence of locoregional recurrence (*LRR*) in pathologically node-positive patients (**a**) age ≤50 years treated with lumpectomy plus breast external radiotherapy (*XRT*) according to number of positive nodes; (**b**) age ≥50 years treated with lumpectomy plus breast XRT according to number of positive nodes; (**c**) with tumors ≤5 cm treated with mastectomy according to number of positive nodes; (**d**) with tumors >5 cm treated with mastectomy according to number of positive nodes (From Mamounas et al. [16], with permission)

The 10-year incidences of LRR (<50 years vs. ≥50 years) were 12 % vs. 5.9 % and 15.6 % vs. 11.3 % with breast-only RT in patients with cN0 disease that finally staged ypN(1–3+) and ypN(>4+), respectively. The 10-year incidences of LRR (<50 years vs. ≥50 years) were 21.1 % vs. 11.4 % and 24 % vs. 19.6 % with breast-only RT in patients with cN+ disease that finally staged ypN(1–3+) and ypN(>4+), respectively (Fig. 11.3) [16].

There are no conclusive data as to whether lymphatic irradiation can be omitted in patients with clinical stage N2 disease that finally staged pCR after neoadjuvant chemotherapy.

Radiotherapy Fields After Preoperative Systemic Chemotherapy

Whole-breast radiotherapy is the standard of practice in patients treated with neoadjuvant chemotherapy and BCS.

If radiotherapy is indicated in the postmastectomy setting, the chest wall should be treated. In most studies from MDACC, full lymphatic irradiation (mammaria interna, supra, level 3, and axillary apex) was also performed [18, 19]. In general, there is no controversy about whether patients with initial clinical stage cN0–1 disease that finally staged ypN(4+) should receive lymphatic radiotherapy including the undissected portion of the axilla (i.e., supraclavicular and level 3). Lymphatic radiotherapy fields may vary between institutions in patients with clinical stage II disease that finally staged ypN(1–3+) [33].

PMRT could be omitted for stage II patients with pCR who are not TN and who are >40 years. All patients with stage II disease but who have had residual disease in the axilla should receive PMRT. One institution is using a supra-level 3 field for stage II patients with no residual axillary cancer but no pCR at the tumor, particularly for younger patients who have no reasonable options for adjuvant systemic therapy (i.e., estrogen receptor (−) and Her-2 Neu(−)). All patients with stage III disease should receive PMRT [33]. The decision to use lymphatic radiotherapy in patients with stage III disease should be based on the pathological status of the axilla, but in a retrospective study from Florida, the omission of the supraclavicular field was significantly associated with LRR by multivariate analysis (HR 3.39; $p = 0.024$) [25]. There are insufficient data examining the omission of radiotherapy in patients with cT4 or cN2 disease. Thus, PMRT with whole lymphatics should be advised for these patients.

Future Directions

Clearly, there is a need for randomized studies to assess the safe omission of PMRT and regional radiotherapy in women with a good response to chemotherapy without compromising breast cancer outcomes. In the NSABP B51/Radiotherapy Oncology Group (RTOG) 1304 study, patients with involved axillary nodes (histologically confirmed) are treated with neoadjuvant chemotherapy. Those who are node negative at subsequent mastectomy are randomly assigned to ± postmastectomy RT (PMRT) to the chest wall and regional nodes. Similarly, patients who undergo subsequent breast conservation surgery and whose nodes have become negative after preoperative chemotherapy will be randomly assigned to breast RT ± regional nodal RT [34].

An analysis of sentinel lymph node biopsy (SLNB) after systemic chemotherapy in patients with cN1 disease has recently been published (Z1071 study) [32]. The false-negative rate after the SLNB procedures was 12.6 % (90 % Bayesian credible interval, 9.85–16.05 %) in the entire group. Both the use of dual-agent mapping (blue dye and radiolabelled colloid) and the recovery of more than 2 SLNs were associated with a lower likelihood of false-negative SLN findings (9.1 % for ≥3 SLNs). According to the recently presented results of the AMAROS trial, both axillary dissection and lymphatic radiotherapy had the same rates of disease control but fewer side effects with RT in patients with positive SLNB cT1–2 N0 disease [35]. For women who receive neoadjuvant chemotherapy and whose lymph nodes remain pathologically positive after surgery, regional radiotherapy is indicated. However, the ALLIANCE (Alliance for Clinical Trials in Oncology) A011202 phase III clinical trial (NCT01901094) has been designed to answer whether axillary node dissection improves the rate of breast cancer recurrence over that observed with SLNB alone when regional radiotherapy is delivered. If SLNB becomes a standard approach in the neoadjuvant setting, some cN1 patients could be treated with SLNB and axillary radiotherapy without axillary dissection. Clearly, more studies are needed in this area [36].

References

1. Hoffman KE, Mittendorf EA, Buchholz TA. Optimizing radiation treatment decisions for patients who receive neoadjuvant chemotherapy and mastectomy. Lancet Oncol. 2012;13(6):e270–6.
2. Mieog JS, van der Hage JA, van de Velde CJ. Preoperative chemotherapy for women with operable breast cancer. Cochrane Database Syst Rev. 2007; 18(2):CD005002.
3. Boughey JC, Suman VJ, Mittendorf EA, Ahrendt GM, Wilke LG, Taback B, et al. Sentinel lymph node surgery after neoadjuvant chemotherapy in patients with node-positive breast cancer: the ACOSOG Z1071 (Alliance) clinical trial. JAMA. 2013;310(14): 1455–61.
4. Eifel P, Axelson JA, Costa J, Crowley J, Curran Jr WJ, Deshler A, et al. National institutes of health consensus development conference statement: adjuvant

therapy for breast cancer. J Natl Cancer Inst. 2001; 93(13):979–89.

5. EBCTCG (Early Breast Cancer Trialists' Collaborative Group), McGale P, Taylor C, Correa C, Darby S, Arriagada R, Clarke M, et al. Effect of radiotherapy after mastectomy and axillary surgery on 10-year recurrence and 20-year breast cancer mortality: meta-analysis of individual patient data for 8135 women in 22 randomized trials. Lancet. 2014; 383(9935):2127–35.

6. Harbeck N, Thomssen C, Gnant M. St. Gallen 2013: brief preliminary summary of the consensus discussion. Breast Care (Basel). 2013;8(2):102–9.

7. National Comprehensive Cancer Network Clinical Practice Guidelines in Oncology. Breast Cancer, Version 1; 2015.

8. Overgaard M, Hansen PS, Overgaard J. Postoperative radiotherapy in high-risk premenopausal women with breast cancer who receive adjuvant chemotherapy. Danish breast cancer cooperative group 82b trial. N Engl J Med. 1997;337(14):949–55.

9. Overgaard M, Jensen MB, Overgaard J, Hansen PS, Rose C, Andersson M, et al. Postoperative radiotherapy in high-risk postmenopausal breast-cancer patients given adjuvant tamoxifen: Danish Breast Cancer Cooperative Group DBCG 82c randomized trial. Lancet. 1999;353(9165):1641–8.

10. Ragaz J, Olivotto IA, Spinelli JJ, Kamby C, Kjaer M, Gadeberg CC, et al. Locoregional radiation therapy in patients with high-risk breast cancer receiving adjuvant chemotherapy: 20-year results of the British Columbia randomized trial. J Natl Cancer Inst. 2005;97(2):116–26.

11. Whelan T, Olivotto IA, Ackerman I. NCICCTG MA.20: an intergroup trial of regional nodal irradiation in early breast cancer. J Clin Oncol. 2011;29:779s. abstr LBA1003.

12. Poortmans PSH, Kirkove C, Budach V, Matuschek C. Irradiation of the internal mammary and medial supraclavicular lymph nodes in stage I to III breast cancer: 10 years results of the EORTC radiation oncology and breast cancer groups phase III trial 2013;22922/10925. EJC 47(Suppl 2).

13. Marinovich ML, Houssami N, Macaskill P, Sardanelli F, Minckwitz G, Mamounas E, et al. Meta-analysis of magnetic resonance imaging in detecting residual breast cancer after neoadjuvant therapy. J Natl Cancer Inst. 2013;105(5):321–33.

14. Park SH, Kim MJ, Park BW, Moon HJ, Kwak JY, Kim EK. Impact of preoperative ultrasonography and fine-needle aspiration of axillary lymph nodes on surgical management of primary breast cancer. Ann Surg Oncol. 2011;18(3):738–44.

15. Oh JL, Nguyen G, Whitman GJ, Hunt KK, Yu TK, Woodward WA, et al. Placement of radiopaque clips for tumor localization in patients undergoing neoadjuvant chemotherapy and breast conservation therapy. Cancer. 2007;110(11):2420–7.

16. Mamounas EP, Anderson SJ, Dignam JJ, James JD, Harry DB, Thomas BJ, et al. Predictors of locoregional recurrence after neoadjuvant chemotherapy: results from combined analysis of national surgical adjuvant breast and bowel project B-18 and B-27. J Clin Oncol. 2012;30:3960–6.

17. Fowble BL, Einck JP, Kim DN, McCloskey S, Mayadev J, Yashar C, et al. Role of postmastectomy radiation after neoadjuvant chemotherapy in stage II–III breast cancer. Int J Radiat Oncol Biol Phys. 2012;83(2):494–503.

18. Garg AK, Strom EA, McNeese MD, Buzdar AU, Hortobagyi GN, Kuerer HM, et al. T3 disease at presentation or pathologic involvement of four or more lymph nodes predict for locoregional recurrence in stage II breast cancer treated with neoadjuvant chemotherapy and mastectomy without radiotherapy. Int J Radiat Oncol Biol Phys. 2004;59(1):138–45.

19. Garg AK, Oh JL, Oswald MJ, Huang E, Strom EA, Perkins GH, et al. Effect of postmastectomy radiotherapy in patients <35 years old with stage II–III breast cancer treated with doxorubicin-based neoadjuvant chemotherapy and mastectomy. Int J Radiat Oncol Biol Phys. 2007;69(5):1478–83.

20. Voduc KD, Cheang MC, Tyldesley, Gelmon K, Nielsen TO, Kennecke H. Breast cancer subtypes and the risk of local and regional relapse. J Clin Oncol. 2010;28(10):1684–91.

21. Yu T, Mittendorf EA, Nagar H, Gomez P, Strom EA, Perkins GH, et al. Local-regional recurrences with and without radiation after neoadjuvant chemotherapy and mastectomy for T1-2/N0-1 breast cancer patients (abstract). Int J Radiat Oncol Biol Phys. 2008; 72:S88–9.

22. McGuire SE, Gonzalez-Angulo AM, Huang EH, Tucker SL, Kau SW, Yu TK, et al. Postmastectomy radiation improves the outcome of patients with locally advanced breast cancer who achieve a pathologic complete response to neoadjuvant chemotherapy. Int J Radiat Oncol Biol Phys. 2007;68:1004–9.

23. Yadav BS, Sharma SC, Singh R, Singh G. Patterns of relapse in locally advanced breast cancer treated with neoadjuvant chemotherapy followed by surgery and radiotherapy. J Can Res Ther. 2007;3:75–80.

24. Huang EH, Tucker SL, Strom EA, McNeese MD, Kuerer HM, Buzdar AU, et al. Postmastectomy radiation improves local-regional control and survival for selected patients with locally advanced breast cancer treated with neoadjuvant chemotherapy and mastectomy. J Clin Oncol. 2004;22(23):4691–9.

25. Wright JL, Takita C, Reis IM, et al. Predictors of locoregional outcome in patients receiving neoadjuvant therapy and postmastectomy radiation. Cancer. 2013;119(1):16–25.

26. Settle S, Gonzalez-Angulo AM, Buchholz TA, Woodward WA, Yu TK, Oh JL, et al. Locoregional outcomes and radiotherapy response in patients with triple negative breast cancer (abstract). Int J Radiat Oncol Biol Phys. 2009;75:S9–10.

27. Le Scodan R, Selz J, Stevens D, Bollet MA, de la Lande B, Daveau C, et al. Radiotherapy for stage II and stage III breast cancer patients with negative

lymph nodes after preoperative chemotherapy and mastectomy. Int J Radiat Oncol Biol Phys. 2012;82(1):e1–7.

28. Buchholz TA, Katz A, Strom EA. Pathologic tumor size and lymph node status predict for different rates of locoregional recurrence after mastectomy for breast cancer patients treated with neoadjuvant versus adjuvant chemotherapy. Int J Radiat Oncol Biol Phys. 2002;53:880–8.

29. Shim SJ, Park W, Huh SJ, Choi SJ, Shin DH, Lee KH, et al. The role of postmastectomy radiation therapy after neoadjuvant chemotherapy in clinical stage II-III breast cancer patients with pN0: a multicenter, retrospective study (KROG 12-05). Int J Radiat Oncol Biol Phys. 2014;88(1):65–72.

30. Nagar H, Mittendorf EA, Strom E, Perkins E, Oh GH, Tereffe JL, et al. Local-regional recurrence with and without radiation after neoadjuvant chemotherapy and mastectomy for clinically staged T3N0 breast cancer patients. Int J Radiat Oncol Biol Phys. 2011; 81:782–7.

31. Buchholz TA, Tucker SL, Masullo L, Kuerer HM, Erwin J, Salas J, et al. Predictors of local-regional recurrence after neoadjuvant chemotherapy and mastectomy without radiation. J Clin Oncol. 2002; 20(1):17–23.

32. Daveau C, Stevens D, Brain E, Berges O, Villette S, Moisson P, et al. Is regional lymph node irradiation necessary in stage II to III breast cancer patients with negative pathologic node status after neoadjuvant chemotherapy? Int J Radiat Oncol Biol Phys. 2010; 78(2):337–42.

33. Bellon JR, Wong JS, Burstein HJ. Should response to preoperative chemotherapy affect radiotherapy recommendations after mastectomy for stage II breast cancer? J Clin Oncol. 2012;30(32):3916–20.

34. White J, Mamounas E. Locoregional radiotherapy in patients with breast cancer responding to neoadjuvant chemotherapy: a paradigm for treatment individualization. J Clin Oncol. 2014;32(6):494–5.

35. Rutgers EJ, Donker M, Straver ME, Meijnen, P Van De Velde CJH, Mansel RE, et al. Radiotherapy or surgery of the axilla after a positive sentinel node in breast cancer patients: final analysis of the EORTC AMAROS trial (10981/22023). J Clin Oncol ASCO Annual Meeting Abstracts. 2013;31(15) suppl: abstract LBA1001.

36. Marks LB, Prosnitz LR. Reducing local therapy in patients responding to preoperative systemic therapy: are we outsmarting ourselves? J Clin Oncol. 2014; 32(6):491–3.

37. Clarke M, Collins R, Darby S. Effects of radiotherapy and of differences in the extent of surgery for early breast cancer on local recurrence and 15-year survival: an overview of the randomised trials. Lancet. 2005;366(9503):2087–106.

Breast-Conserving Therapy: Hypofractionated and Conventional Whole-Breast Irradiation and Accelerated Partial-Breast Irradiation

12

Fusun Tokatlı and Maktav Dincer

Abstract

Breast irradiation after breast-conserving surgery (BCS) is an essential component of breast conservation therapy for maximizing local control and overall survival. The most widely used fractionation regimen is 1.8- to 2-Gy daily fractions for a total of 45–50 Gy to the whole breast over 5 weeks with or without a boost to the surgical bed. However, the optimal dose and fractionation schedule for radiation therapy after BCS has not yet been defined. There is renewed interest in hypofractionation for whole-breast irradiation (WBI), and this approach has important practical advantages and biological implications. The convenience of this method may facilitate patient acceptance and compliance with radiation therapy. Irradiating only the tumor-bearing quadrant of the breast instead of irradiating the whole breast after BCS has also increased in popularity in the last decade.

Keywords

Irradiation • Partial breast • Breast conservation • Accelerated radiotherapy • Radiotherapy complications • Cosmesis • Boost dose • Randomized trials • Breast conserving • Canadian trial • Cosmetic outcome • Fraction size • Hypofractionation • Normal tissue • Local control • Meta-analyses • START-A • START-B • UK FAST • Survival • Whole breast • α/β ratio

F. Tokatlı, MD
Radiation Oncology, Medicana International Hospital, E5 Karayolu, Beylikduzu, Istanbul, Turkey
e-mail: fusun_t@yahoo.com

M. Dincer, MD (✉)
Department of Radiation Oncology, Florence Nightingale Hospital, Gayrettepe, Istanbul 34335, Turkey
e-mail: dincer@superonline.com

Whole-Breast Irradiation

Breast irradiation after breast-conserving surgery (BCS) is an essential component of breast conservation therapy to maximize local control and overall survival. The largest and most recent meta-analysis by the Early Breast Cancer Trialists' Collaborative Group reported the effect of radiotherapy after BCS on 10-year recurrence and 15-year breast cancer death and the absolute magnitudes of these reductions according to various prognostic and other patient characteristics [1]. In this meta-analysis, individual patient data for 10,801 women in 17 randomized trials of radiotherapy versus no radiotherapy after BCS were analyzed to determine if radiotherapy reduces recurrence and breast cancer death more for some subgroups of patients than for others. Overall, radiotherapy reduced the 10-year risk of any (i.e., locoregional or distant) first recurrence from 35.0 % to 19.3 % (absolute reduction 15.7 %, 2p < 0.00001) and reduced the 15-year risk of breast cancer death from 25.2 % to 21.4 % (absolute reduction 3.8 %, 2p = 0.00005). Of the 10,801 patients analyzed, the vast majority (8,337 women) were pathologically confirmed to have node-negative (pN0) cases. In the women with pN0 disease, the absolute reduction in recurrence varied according to age, grade, estrogen receptor status, tamoxifen use, and extent of surgery, and these characteristics were used to predict large (>=20 %), intermediate (10–19 %), or lower (<10%) absolute reductions in the 10-year recurrence risk. The absolute reductions in the 15-year risk of breast cancer death in these three prediction categories were 7.8 %, 1.1 %, and 0.1 %, respectively. In the few women with node-positive disease ($n = 1,050$), radiotherapy reduced the 10-year recurrence risk from 63.7 % to 42.5 % (absolute reduction 21.2 %, 2p < 0.00001) and the 15-year risk of breast cancer death from 51.3 % to 42.8 % (absolute risk reduction 8.5 %, 2p = 0.01). Overall, approximately one breast cancer death was avoided by year 15 for every four recurrences avoided by year 10. In summary, after breast-conserving surgery, breast radiotherapy halved the rate at which the disease recurred and reduced the breast cancer death rate by one-sixth. The most widely used fractionation regimen is 1.8- to 2-Gy daily fractions for a total of 45–50 Gy to the whole breast over 5 weeks with or without a boost to the surgical bed [2, 3]. The National Surgical Adjuvant Breast Project group conducted the NSABP B-06 trial in 1,851 patients with stage I/II breast cancer smaller than 4 cm locally excised with negative margins [2]. The patients were randomized to three arms: total mastectomy versus lumpectomy alone versus lumpectomy plus 50 Gy whole-breast radiotherapy. Node-positive patients received 5-fluorouracil-based adjuvant chemotherapy. At the 20-year follow-up, overall survival (OS), disease-free survival (DFS), and distant metastasis-free survival (DMFS) did not differ significantly among the three arms. The addition of breast radiotherapy to breast-conserving surgery reduced the local recurrence rate from 39 % to 14 %. The Milan group conducted a similar randomized trial in 701 patients with stage I breast cancer [3]. Randomization was to two arms: radical mastectomy versus quadrantectomy plus 60 Gy breast radiotherapy. Node-positive patients received CMF (cyclophosphamide, methotrexate, fluorouracil) combination chemotherapy. At the 20-year follow-up, OS (59 % and 58 %) and cause-specific (76 % and 74 %) survival rates were nearly identical, whereas local recurrence after radical mastectomy was 2.3 % or 8.8 % after BCT. However, an optimal dose and fractionation schedule for radiation therapy (RT) after BCS has not yet been defined. There is renewed interest in hypofractionation for WBI, and this approach has important practical advantages and biological implications. The convenience of this method may facilitate patient acceptance and compliance with radiation therapy [4].

Biological Rationale for Hypofractionation

The rationale for fractionated RT is that reducing the radiation dose per fraction while increasing the number of fractions and the total dose limits damage to normal tissue because an increased dose per fraction is associated with increased normal tissue damage. Interest in hypofractionation has been revived in the last decade as the understanding of the radiobiological parameters that affect fractionation in breast cancer has improved [5]. There are two broad categories of target tissues for radiotherapy: acute and late reacting [6]. The linear-quadratic concept is the most commonly used radiobiological model to predict the differential response of these two types of tissues. The α/β ratio (the dose at which cell killing by the linear (α) and quadratic (β) components is equal) is an essential part of this concept and reflects the inherent radiation sensitivity of the relevant tissue. Acute-reacting tissues, such as skin epidermis and the gastrointestinal tract, develop a reaction to radiation within 1–3 weeks of treatment. These tissues generally have a high α/β ratio (range, 10–30). Although sensitive to the total dose of radiation, they are much less sensitive to the fraction size. By contrast, late-reacting tissues, such as soft tissue and neurological structures, do not display reactions to radiation until several years after beginning treatment. These tissues have a lower α/β ratio in the range of 1–5 and are much more sensitive to dose per fraction. Many tumors (e.g., squamous cancers) have high α/β ratios; however, certain cancers, such as prostate cancer and likely breast cancer, have low α/β ratios and are more sensitive to fraction size [7].

A pilot study was designed in 1986 by Yarnold et al. [8] to test the sensitivity of breast tissue to modest increases in fraction size and estimate the α/β ratio for late effects in the breast. In this randomized study, 1,410 patients with early-stage breast cancer were randomized to three fractionation schedules: 50 Gy in 25 fractions (2 Gy/fraction), 42.9 Gy in 13 fractions (3.3 Gy/fraction), and 39 Gy in 13 fractions (3 Gy/fraction), which were administered over 5 weeks. Patients were followed for a median of 8 years. Based on differences in changes to breast appearance and toxicity over time among the fractionation schedules, α/β ratios were determined. The α/β ratio for late changes in breast appearance was 3.6 Gy (95 % confidence interval (CI), 1.8–5.4), and the α/β ratio for breast induration was 3.1 Gy (95 % CI, 1.8–4.4 Gy). A subsequent analysis estimated the α/β ratio for tumor control to be 4 Gy (95 % CI, 1.0–7.8 Gy) [9]. These data indicate that hypofractionation with a modest increase in fraction size accompanied by a modest decrease in total dose is likely to result in equivalent outcomes compared with standard fractionation with respect to local control and late radiation morbidity.

Trials of Hypofractionation Versus Conventional WBI

Three randomized trials with long-term follow-up and that investigated the effectiveness and safety of hypofractionation compared to conventional fractionation for WBI have been performed in the last decade and published. Additional trials are ongoing.

Canadian Trial (Ontario Clinical Oncology Group)

Between 1993 and 1996, 1,234 women with node-negative breast cancer with clear margins of excision after BCS and axillary dissection were included in the study. Women were randomized to standard WBI of 50 Gy in 25 fractions over 35 days or accelerated hypofractionated WBI of 42.5 Gy in 16 fractions over 22 days. The two groups were similar at baseline: 24.7 % of the women were younger than 50 years of age, 31.3 % had tumors that were 2 cm or larger in diameter, 26.1 % had estrogen-negative disease, and 18.8 % had high-grade disease. All patients had invasive carcinoma of the breast and pT1–T2 pN0. Patients with large breasts (>25 cm width of breast tissue) were excluded. Forty-one percent of the patients received adjuvant tamoxifen, and 11 % received adjuvant chemotherapy, most commonly cyclophosphamide, methotrexate, and fluorouracil (CMF). Radiation therapy was delivered to the whole breast using two opposing tangential fields. Boost irradiation of the tumor bed and regional irradiation were not used. Ninety-eight (7.9 %) patients were lost to follow-up. For the toxicity analysis, 873 patients were evaluated at 5 years, and 455 patients were evaluated at 10 years. The primary outcome was any local recurrence of invasive cancer in the treated breast. Secondary outcomes were distant (including regional) recurrence of breast cancer, second cancers (including contrlateral breast cancer), breast cosmesis, late toxic effects of radiation, and death.

The study was first reported in 2002 [10] and has recently been updated with a median follow-up of 12 years [11]. The cumulative incidence of local recurrence was similar in the two groups. The risk of local recurrence at 10 years was 6.7 %

(42 patients) among the 612 women assigned to standard irradiation, compared with 6.2 % (41 patients) among the 622 women assigned to the hypofractionated regimen (absolute difference, 0.5 %; 95 % CI, −2.5 to 3.5). In addition to the 83 invasive recurrences, there were 13 cases of non-invasive local recurrence (i.e., ductal carcinoma in situ): 6 cases in the control group and 7 in the hypofractionated-radiation group. At 10 years, the cumulative incidence of invasive or noninvasive local recurrence was 7.5 % in the control group and 7.4 % in the hypofractionated-radiation group (absolute difference, 0.1 %; 95 % CI, −3.1 to 3.3). Subgroup analysis demonstrated that the treatment effect was similar regardless of patient age, tumor size, estrogen receptor status, or use or nonuse of systemic therapy. The hypofractionated regimen appeared to be less effective in patients with high-grade tumors; in this subgroup, the cumulative incidence of local recurrence at 10 years was 4.7 % in the control group and 15.6 % in the hypofractionated-radiation group (absolute difference, −10.9 %; 95 % CI, −19.1 to −2.8; test for interaction, $p = 0.01$).

The probability of survival over time was reported to be similar in the two groups ($p = 0.79$). At 10 years, the probability of survival was 84.4 % in the control group and 84.6 % in the hypofractionated-radiation group (absolute difference, −0.2 %; 95 % CI, −4.3 to 4.0). In the control group of 612 patients, 13.4 % of deaths were related to cancer, 1.5 % were related to cardiac disease, and 5.7 % were due to other causes. In the hypofractionated-radiation group of 622 patients, 13.2 % of deaths were related to cancer, 1.9 % were related to cardiac disease, and 4.5 % were due to other causes. No significant differences were observed between groups ($p = 0.56$).

The Canadian trial used the Radiation Therapy Oncology Group/European Organization for Research and Treatment of Cancer (RTOG/EORTC) late scoring schema for skin and subcutaneous tissue toxicity assessment [12]. Moderate and severe toxicity were infrequent and similar between treatment arms at 10 years. Although late toxicity did increase over time, severe toxicity (grade 3) remained less than 4 % at 10 years. However, the progression of these effects was not any worse for hypofractionation compared with conventional fractionation. At 10 years, 71.3 % of women in the control group and 69.8 % of women in the hypofractionated-radiation group had a good or excellent cosmetic outcome (absolute difference, 1.5 %; 95 % CI, −6.9 to 9.8). The repeated-measures logistic regression analysis suggested that the cosmetic outcome was affected by the time from randomization as well as by the patient's age and tumor size, but there was no interaction with treatment.

Rates of pneumonitis, symptomatic lung fibrosis, rib fracture, and ischemic heart disease were also low, and no differences were detected between arms.

START-A Trial

Between 1999 and 2002, 2,236 women with early breast cancer (pT1-3a pN0-1 M0) were randomly assigned after primary surgery to receive 50 Gy in 25 fractions versus 41.6 Gy or 39 Gy in 13 fractions over 5 weeks [13]. Most patients underwent BCS, but in contrast to the Canadian trial, 15 % of patients underwent mastectomy, and there were no exclusions based on breast size. Demographic and clinical characteristics at randomization were well balanced between treatment groups. The mean age was 57 years (range 25–85); 49 % had tumors that were 2 cm or larger in diameter, 29 % had node-positive disease, and 30 % had high-grade disease. No data were available for estrogen receptor status. All patients had invasive carcinoma of the breast. Of the women prescribed chemotherapy (35 % of patients), many (70 %) received an anthracycline-containing regimen, which was similarly balanced between randomized groups. In this study, 79 % of patients received adjuvant tamoxifen. Most patients were treated with 6-MV photons. The planning target volume was the whole breast with a 1-cm margin to palpable breast tissue; where regional radiotherapy was indicated, the planning target volume was supraclavicular nodes with or without axillary nodes with a 1-cm margin. In contrast to the Canadian trial, 14 % of patients received regional radiation therapy, and

61 % received a boost to the tumor bed. Boost irradiation was used according to local indications, and 10 Gy was delivered in five fractions to the tumor bed prescribed at the 100 % isodose using an electron field.

The principal end points specified in the protocol were local-regional relapse and late normal tissue effects. The rates of local-regional relapse at 5 years and 10 years were similar between treatment arms. The rates of relapse at 5 years were 3.6 % (95 % CI 2.2–5.1) after 50 Gy, 3.5 % (95 % CI 2.1–4.3) after 41.6 Gy, and 5.2 % (95 % CI 3.5–6.9) after 39 Gy. The authors recently updated their results [14]. At a median follow-up of 9.3 years (IQR 8.0–10.0, maximum 12.4 years), 139 local-regional relapses had occurred. The 10-year rates of local-regional relapse did not differ significantly between the 41.6 and 50-Gy regimen groups (6.2 %, 95 % CI 4.7–8.5 vs. 7.4 %, 5.5–10.0; hazard ratio (HR) 0.91, 95 % CI 0.59–1.38; $p=0.65$) or the 39-Gy (8.8 %, 95 % CI 6.7–11.4) and 50-Gy regimen groups (HR 1.18, 95 % 0.79–1.76; $p=0.41$). The upper limits of the one-sided 95 % CI for the absolute difference in 10-year local-regional relapse rates indicated an estimated maximum 2.0 % excess risk with 41.6 Gy and 4.5 % with 39 Gy compared with 50 Gy. The estimated α/β value for local-regional relapse in START-A was 4 Gy (95 % CI 0.0–8.9), after adjusting for age, tumor size, primary surgery type, adjuvant chemotherapy use, tamoxifen use, lymphatic radiotherapy, and tumor bed boost radiotherapy.

Rates of distant relapse, disease-free survival, and overall survival were similar among the fractionation schedules, with no evidence of a clinically significant detriment for either of the hypofractionated schedules compared with 50 Gy at 5 and 10 years. At a median follow-up in survivors of 9.3 years, 1,700 of 2,236 patients (76 %) were alive and without relapse, 57 (2.5 %) were alive with local-regional relapse (without distant relapse), 78 (3.5 %) were alive with distant relapse, 392 (17.4 %) had died, and 9 (0.4 %) had been lost to follow-up. In this trial, 273 of 392 deaths (69.6 %) were from breast cancer (92 with 50 Gy, 86 with 41.6 Gy, and 95 with 39 Gy), 26 (6.6 %) were related to cardiac disease only

(7 with 50 Gy, 13 with 41.6 Gy, and 6 with 39 Gy), 34 (8.7 %) were from other cancers (9 with 50 Gy, 10 with 41.6 Gy, and 15 with 39 Gy), 44 (11.2 %) were from other noncancer causes (16 with 50 Gy, 16 with 41.6 Gy, and 12 with 39 Gy), and 15 (3.8 %) were from unknown cause (6 with 50 Gy, 3 with 41.6 Gy, and 6 with 39 Gy). Fifteen (57.7 %) of the 26 deaths from cardiac disease had left-sided primary tumors (4 of 7 with 50 Gy, 10 of 13 with 41.6 Gy, and 1 of 6 with 39 Gy).

Acute toxicity was not reported except for a marked acute reaction observed in the trial, which appeared more common with standard fractionation. Late toxicity was determined from photographs and patient self-assessment questionnaires. Changes in breast appearance and breast hardness were the most common changes. According to patient quality of life self-assessments of five key normal tissue effects on the breast or breast area, rates of moderate or marked breast induration, telangiectasia, and breast edema by 5 years were similar after 41.6 Gy and 50 Gy but generally lower after 39 Gy than after 50 Gy ($p=0.004$). At 10 years, this significant difference between the 39-Gy group and the 50-Gy group continued. α/β estimates for normal tissue end points in this trial (after adjusting for age, breast size, surgical deficit, lymphatic radiotherapy, and tumor bed boost radiotherapy) were reported to be 3.5 Gy (95 % CI 0.7–6.4) for breast shrinkage, 4 Gy (2.3–5.6) for breast induration, 3.8 Gy (1.8–5.7) for telangiectasia, and 4.7 Gy (2.4–7.0) for breast edema. In the 41.6-Gy group, there was one case of brachial plexopathy 2 years after treatment. The incidence of ischemic heart disease, symptomatic rib fracture, and symptomatic lung fibrosis was low during follow-up and balanced among the schedules.

START-B Trial

In the START-B trial, between 1999 and 2001, 2,215 women with node-negative and node-positive breast cancer (pT1-3a pN0-1 M0) were randomized after BCS or mastectomy to standard WBI of 50 Gy in 25 fractions over 5 weeks or accelerated hypofractionated WBI of 40 Gy in 15 fractions over 3 weeks [15]. Most patients (92 %) underwent BCS, but 8 % underwent mastectomy, and there were no exclusions based on breast size. Demographic and clinical characteristics at randomization were well balanced between treatment groups. The mean age was 57 years (range 23–86); 36 % had tumors that were 2 cm or larger in diameter, 23 % had node-positive disease, and 25 % had high-grade disease. No data were available for estrogen receptor status. All patients had invasive carcinoma of the breast. Of the women prescribed chemotherapy (22 % of patients), 59 % received an anthracycline-containing regimen, which was similarly balanced between randomized groups. In this study, 87 % of patients received adjuvant tamoxifen. Most patients were treated with 6-MV photons. The planning target volume was the whole breast with a 1-cm margin to palpable breast tissue; where regional radiotherapy was indicated, the planning target volume was supraclavicular nodes with or without axillary nodes with a 1-cm margin. In contrast to the Canadian trial, 7 % of patients received regional radiation therapy, and 43 % received a boost to the tumor bed. Boost irradiation was used according to local indications, and 10 Gy was delivered in five fractions to the tumor bed prescribed at the 100 % isodose using an electron field.

The principal end points specified in the protocol were local-regional relapse and late normal tissue effects. The rates of local-regional relapse at 6 years and 10 years were similar between treatment arms. The rates of relapse at 6 years were 3.3 % in the 50-Gy group and 2.2 % in the 40-Gy group (estimated absolute difference, 0.7 %; 95 % CI −1.7 to 0.9 %). The authors recently updated their results [14]. At a median follow-up of 9.9 years (IQR 7.5–10.1, maximum 12.5 years), 95 (4.3 %) local-regional relapses had occurred. The 10-year rates of local-regional relapse did not differ significantly between the 40-Gy group (4.3 %, 95 % CI 3.2–5.9) and the 50-Gy regimen group (5.5 %, 95 % CI 4.2–7.2; HR 0.77, 95 % CI 0.51–1.16; $p = 0.21$). The upper limit of the one-sided 95 % CI for the absolute difference in 10-year local-regional relapse rates suggested an estimated 0.4 % excess risk associated with the 15-fraction schedule.

At a median follow-up in survivors of 9.9 years, 1,732 of 2,215 (78.2 %) patients were alive and without relapse, 50 (2.3 %) were alive with local-regional relapse (without distant relapse), 63 (2.8 %) were alive with distant relapse, 351 (15.8 %) had died, and 19 (0.9 %) were lost to follow-up.

In this trial, 236 of 351 deaths (67.2 %) were from breast cancer (130 with 50 Gy and 106 with 40 Gy), 17 (4.8 %) were related to cardiac disease only (12 with 50 Gy and 5 with 40 Gy), 48 (13.7 %) were from other cancers (25 with 50 Gy and 23 with 40 Gy), 40 (11.4 %) were from other noncancer causes (21 with 50 Gy and 19 with 40 Gy), and 10 (2.8 %) were from unknown causes (4 with 50 Gy and 6 with 40 Gy). Eleven (64.7 %) of the 17 deaths from cardiac disease had primary tumors on the left side (8 of 12 with 50 Gy and 3 of 5 with 40 Gy). The 10-year rate of distant relapse was lower in the 40-Gy group (HR 0.74, 95 % CI 0.59–0.94), which contributed to the higher rates of disease-free survival and overall survival compared to the 50-Gy group. The reasons for this difference are unclear. There are many factors that affect relapse and survival, including others that were unknown in the trial, such as HER2 status. The authors could not ascribe the survival difference to any biological or treatment-related factor and only concluded that this difference might be due to chance or an imbalance of unknown prognostic factors and could diminish with further follow-up [4].

Acute toxicity was not reported except for marked acute reactions observed in the trial, which appeared more common with standard fractionation (1.2 % after 50 Gy/25 fractions vs. 0.3 % after 40 Gy/15 fractions). Late toxicity was determined from photographs and patient self-assessment questionnaires. Changes in breast appearance and breast hardness were the most common. An analysis of patient self-assessments of five key normal tissue effects in the breast or breast area revealed that rates of moderate or marked effects within 5 years tended to be lower after 40 Gy than after 50 Gy, with a significantly lower rate of change in skin appearance after radiotherapy at 40 Gy than 50 Gy ($p = 0.02$). At 10 years, this significant difference remained between the 40-Gy group and the 50-Gy group. The various assessments of normal tissue effects were consistently better in the 40-Gy group compared with 50 Gy.

The incidence of ischemic heart disease, symptomatic rib fracture, and symptomatic lung fibrosis was low during follow-up and balanced between the schedules. No cases of brachial plexopathy to the supraclavicular fossa and/or axilla were reported in the 82 women who received 40 Gy in 15 fractions or the 79 women who received 50 Gy in 25 fractions.

The authors performed meta-analyses of START-A, START-B, and the START pilot trial by fitting Cox proportional hazards regression models to all individual patient data from the three trials [9, 13–15]. Post-hoc subgroup analyses of the combined hypofractionated regimens versus the control groups for local-regional relapse in these three trials ($n = 5,861$) indicated that the treatment effect did not differ significantly regardless of age, type of primary surgery, axillary node status, tumor grade, adjuvant chemotherapy use, or the use of tumor bed boost radiotherapy. In a post-hoc analysis, the incidence of any moderate or marked physician-assessed normal tissue effects in the breast (shrinkage, induration, edema, or telangiectasia) for the 4,660 women for whom data were available from these three trials indicated that the treatment effect was similar irrespective of age, breast size, the use of tumor bed boost radiotherapy, adjuvant chemotherapy, or tamoxifen.

UK FAST Trial

The ongoing UK FAST trial is comparing five fractions of 5.7 Gy and 6 Gy at one fraction per week compared with the conventional fractionation of 25 fractions of 2 Gy [16]. Five fractions of 5.7 or 6 Gy are predicted by the linear-quadratic model to be equivalent to 25 fractions of 2.0 Gy, assuming values for α/β of 3.0 and 4.0 Gy, respectively [17]. The aim of this trial was to reduce overall treatment time, not only for patient convenience but also to minimize the potential for rapid tumor growth during radiotherapy. In this trial, women aged ≥50 years with node-negative, early breast cancer were randomly assigned after microscopic complete tumor resection to 50 Gy in 25 fractions versus 28.5 or 30 Gy in 5 once-weekly fractions of 5.7 or 6 Gy, respectively, to the whole breast. Patients with estrogen-positive tumors were eligible for adjuvant endocrine therapy. Exclusion criteria included mastectomy, lymphatic radiotherapy, and tumor bed boost dose as well as neoadjuvant or adjuvant chemotherapy. The primary end point was a 2-year change in photographic breast appearance. In total, 915 women were recruited from 2004 to 2007 (the aim was to recruit 4,000 participants), and 2-year photographic assessments were performed on 729 patients. The risk ratios for mild/marked changes were 1.70 (95 % CI 1.26–2.29, $p < 0.001$) for 30 Gy and 1.15 (95 % CI 0.82–1.60, $p = 0.489$) for 28.5 Gy versus 50 Gy. The 3-year rates of physician-assessed moderate/marked adverse effects in the breast were 17.3 % (95 % CI 13.3–22.3 %, $p < 0.001$) for 30 Gy and 11.1 % (95 % CI 7.9–15.6 %, $p = 0.18$) for 28.5 Gy compared with 9.5 % (95 % CI 6.5–13.7 %) for 50 Gy. The rate was significantly higher in the 30-Gy group than the 50-Gy group (log-rank test $p < 0.001$) or 28.5-Gy group (log-rank test $p < 0.006$), with similar rates in the 28.5- and 50-Gy groups (log-rank test $p = 0.18$).

Thirty-two patients had possible radiotherapy-related adverse effects (10 at 50 Gy, 14 at 30 Gy and 8 at 28.5 Gy), including lymphedema ($n = 25$), rib fracture ($n = 1$), breast pain ($n = 1$), cellulitis ($n = 1$), late-onset asthma ($n = 1$), atrial fibrillation ($n = 1$), irregular heart beat ($n = 1$), and cough ($n = 1$).

At a median of 3 years of follow-up in survivors, there were 2 local relapses (in breast skin or parenchyma), 3 regional relapses (in axilla or supraclavicular fossa), 17 metastases, and 8 patients with a reported second primary cancer. Of 23 patient deaths, 10 were breast cancer related.

In conclusion, the authors suggested that at a median of 3 years of follow-up, 28.5 Gy in five fractions is comparable to 50 Gy in 25 fractions and significantly milder than 30 Gy in 6 fractions in terms of adverse effects in the breast. A five-fraction schedule of WBI delivered in once-weekly fractions has been confirmed to be equivalent to a conventionally fractionated regimen in terms of changes in breast appearance at

2 years and annual clinical assessments of a range of adverse effects in the breast recorded at a median of 3 years. Longer follow-up to a minimum of 5 years is required for reliable estimates of iso-effects.

Use of Hypofractionation in Clinical Practice

The differences in these trials have important implications for the use of hypofractionation in clinical practice. Although most patients had low-risk disease, an important minority had high-risk disease. Subgroup analyses from the Canadian trial did not suggest that hypofractionation was less effective for such patients, except for those with high-grade tumors [4, 11]. The two START trials did not demonstrate any detrimental effect of hypofractionation for high-grade disease [14]. In such instances, additional boost irradiation may be considered, as used in the START trial. However, any biological reasons for a different inherent radiation sensitivity of high-grade tumors or biological subtypes of breast cancer that are associated with high-grade tumors are speculative. The START trials also included patients with tumors 5 cm or larger in diameter and node-positive disease, again suggesting that hypofractionation may be applied to such patients, although for the former category, the numbers would be small.

Although the trials did not include patients with ductal carcinoma in situ (DCIS), the Canadian trial included patients with microinvasive disease and patients with an extensive DCIS component as long as DCIS did not involve the margins of excision [11]. Given the demonstrated effectiveness of hypofractionation for invasive disease, it is likely to be effective for earlier-stage disease that is widely excised [4]. In a retrospective study from Princess Margaret Hospital [18], 104 patients (39 %) were treated with conventional (50 Gy in 25 fractions) and 162 (61 %) with hypofractionated (42.4 Gy in 16 fractions or 40 Gy/16 + 12.5 Gy boost) WBI after BCS. Actuarial risk of recurrence at 4 years was 7 % with hypofractionated WBI and 6 % with

the conventional schedule ($p = 0.9$). In this study, univariate analysis revealed an increased risk of relapse for high nuclear grade tumors (11 % for grade 3 vs. 4 % for grades 1 and 2, $p = 0.029$). Unfortunately, the study had some limitations, including its retrospective nature, short follow-up, and imbalance between groups. However, the results of this trial provide further evidence to guide practice.

The type of systemic treatment might influence local tumor control as well as overall survival and side effects due to normal tissue toxicity. In the Canadian trial, only 10.9 % of patients received adjuvant chemotherapy (mainly CMF), and 41.8 % of patients received adjuvant tamoxifen. Such patients can be at increased risk for an adverse cosmetic outcome with standard radiotherapy, so it is unclear if the outcome of hypofractionation would be worse than that of standard treatment. The Canadian trial reported similar cosmetic appearance after 10 years, which was good or excellent for 69.8 % of women treated with the shorter schedule and 71.3 % of controls [11]. However, a substantial subset of the patients was treated primarily with adjuvant tamoxifen, and only a minority received chemotherapy. Therefore, the results of this trial may not adequately represent the potential long-term complications of WBI in the presence of chemotherapy. Chemotherapy, primarily anthracycline based, was more commonly used in the START trials. Taxane-based chemotherapy was used infrequently in these trials ($n = 28$). Given the application of conventional fractionation after taxane chemotherapy, it seems reasonable to consider hypofractionation as well, provided it is delivered after chemotherapy with at least a 2- to 3-week break [4].

Although most patients in the trials were treated with BCS, an important minority of more than 500 patients were treated after mastectomy, suggesting that hypofractionation is a reasonable choice for the delivery of chest wall irradiation. The Canadian trial excluded women with large breast size, defined as a >25 cm separation at midbreast, because of an increase in adverse cosmesis observed when such patients are treated with standard fractionation [19, 20]. The START trials, which included such patients, did not report increased adverse cosmesis when adjusted for breast size. If such patients are considered for hypofractionation, the variance across the treatment volume should be less than 5 % above the prescribed dose. Boost irradiation was not used in the Canadian trial but was commonly used in the START trials. Despite the use of boost irradiation, no increase in toxicity was observed in patients treated with hypofractionation compared with conventional treatment. In the Canadian trial, the confounding effects of boost irradiation on local recurrence or breast cosmesis have not been examined. Given the acceptable toxicity observed in the START trials, it seems reasonable to consider selective boost irradiation with hypofractionation when delivered as prescribed in these trials.

A major consideration when hypofractionation is used is the treatment of the regional nodes. Previous studies have raised concerns regarding brachial plexopathy in such situations [21–23]. A dose of 40 Gy in 15 fractions at the level of the brachial plexus delivers the equivalent of 46.7 Gy, 47.6 Gy, and 48.9 Gy in 2.0 Gy equivalents, assuming α/β values of 2.0 Gy, 1.5 Gy, and 1.0 Gy, respectively [24]. In other words, 40 Gy in 15 fractions is less damaging to the brachial plexus than 50 Gy in 25 fractions, even under extreme assumptions about the fractionation sensitivity of the nervous system. Regional irradiation was not used in the Canadian study but was used in the 2 START trials. In the START-A trial, one case of brachial plexopathy was observed when 41.6 Gy was used [13]. No cases were observed with 39 Gy or 40 Gy as used in the START-B trial, but a small number of patients were treated ($n=278$). Five-year results suggest that the risk of brachial plexopathy is low (1 % or less with hypofractionation), but radiation oncologists may want more data and longer follow-up before using hypofractionation for regional therapy. In addition, the percentage of lymphedema in START trials did not differ significantly between the treatment groups [14].

Clinically, even more important is the cardiac toxicity after RT. In the Canadian trial, in the conventional schedule group, 9 deaths were related to cardiac disease (1.5 %), compared to 12 deaths (1.9 %) in the hypofractionated group. In the START trials, although follow-up was still short for cardiac events, no major difference was reported between the schedules for the number of cases of heart disease in women with left-sided primary tumors. An increase in long-term risks of cardiac disease (including pericardial, myocardial, cardiovascular disease) related to RT in patients with early-stage breast cancer is detectable at a follow-up of at least 10 years [25, 26]. Unpublished data from the Early Breast Cancer Trialists' Collaborative Group (EBCTCG) revealed an increase in fatal cardiac disease 20 years after RT of approximately 4 %. The heart is sensitive to radiation regardless of the fractionation used, with no lower dose threshold for adverse effects [27]. Thus, the heart should be protected irrespective of the fractionation dose regimen used, and much longer follow-up of the randomized clinical trials investigating hypofractionated RT schedules is needed.

In the long term, radiation therapy may cause skin telangiectasia and fibrosis of subcutaneous tissue, leading to a loss of volume and retraction of the breast, all of which can adversely affect the cosmetic outcome. In the Canadian trial, authors reported a worsening of the cosmetic outcome over time that coincided with the increase in toxic effects of irradiation of the skin and subcutaneous tissue [11]. However, there was no increase in toxic effects in women who received accelerated, hypofractionated-radiation therapy compared with those who received the standard regimen. Although older age and large tumor size were associated with a worse cosmetic outcome, the outcomes of the hypofractionated regimen were similar to those of the standard regimen. However, in the START trials, these outcomes were different [14]. In the START-A trial, moderate or marked breast induration, telangiectasia, and breast edema were significantly less common normal tissue effects in the 39-Gy group than in the 50-Gy group. Normal tissue effects did not differ significantly between the 41.6-Gy and 50-Gy groups. In the START-B trial, breast shrinkage, telangiectasia, and breast edema were significantly less common normal tissue effects in the 40-Gy group than in the 50-Gy group. By applying an α/β value of 3.5 Gy for breast shrinkage and assuming no effect of treatment time on late normal tissue effects, 40 Gy in 15 fractions corresponds to 45 Gy in 2-Gy equivalents. The hypofractionated regimens are less harmful to normal tissues, and there are no suggestions that they are less effective in treating the cancer.

Conclusions

In summary, the results of these studies have confirmed that hypofractionation for WBI is safe and effective. The radiotherapy schedule used in the Canadian trial of 42.5 Gy in 16 fractions over 21 days and two of the schedules used in the START trials, 41.6 Gy in 13 fractions over 25 days and 40 Gy in 15 fractions over 21 days, seem to offer local tumor control and rates of late normal tissue effects at least as good as the accepted international standard of 50 Gy in 25 fractions over 5 weeks. The advantages of hypofractionation include patient convenience, fewer treatment visits, less overall treatment time, and fewer costs to the patient and health-care providers.

Considering the published data hypofractionation most safely could be used in the following patients [28, 29]:

- Age 50 years or older
- pT1-2, pN0 treated with BCS
- No systemic chemotherapy
- No radiation boost to the tumor bed after BCS
- Feasible acceptable dose homogeneity
- Clinically irrelevant long-term risk of cardiac disease

Thus, establishing clinically sufficient selection criteria for patients to identify patients who will benefit from an individualized fractionated WBI remains challenging.

These trials provide results demonstrating that the responsiveness of breast cancer to fraction size is similar to that of the late-responding normal tissues of the breast, as indicated by the α/β estimates. A 13-fraction regimen is unlikely to represent the limits of hypofractionation. This

information can be used to model next approaches to hypofractionation. In the NCCN Guidelines Version 3.2013, a dose of 45–50 Gy in 1.8–2 Gy per fraction or 42.5 Gy at 2.66 Gy per fraction for WBI is now proposed [30]. The real limits of hypofractionation for breast cancer treatment will likely be better determined from the long-term results of the ongoing UK FAST trial. The use of new radiation technologies, such as three-dimensional conformal therapy and intensity-modulated radiation therapy, can also increase the potential application of hypofractionation.

Accelerated Partial-Breast Irradiation

Background

In the last decade, irradiating only the tumor-bearing quadrant of the breast after BCS instead of the whole breast has gained much popularity. This type of breast radiotherapy is termed accelerated partial-breast irradiation (APBI). In this technique, the radiotherapy period is considerably shortened, adjacent normal tissue and organs receive a minimal dose, and parts of the breast distant from the tumor bed receive a minimal dose. One disadvantage of this technique, at least in theory, might be that the parts of the breast distant from the tumor bed that harbor occult tumor foci and that do not receive therapeutic doses of radiotherapy may cause higher rates of in-breast recurrence or new primary tumors with longer follow-up. As a result of increasing interest in this technique, many randomized trials have begun to compare APBI with whole-breast radiotherapy. The results of some of these randomized trials have only recently been published with limited follow-up [31, 32]. A large, multi-institutional trial from the USA has completed accrual, and results are pending [33]. Despite a lack of randomized and solid evidence for the safety and efficacy of APBI, the growing popularity of APBI has driven European and American radiotherapy societies to publish guidelines to guide the selection of patients most suitable for APBI application [34–36]. Researchers, such as

Holland, Vaidya, Faverly, Frazier, and Rosen, have investigated the presence of tumor foci in surgical specimens from the other quadrants of the breast when a tumor mass has been diagnosed in one site [37–41]. In 60 % of the cases, invasive but occult tumor foci were identified in quadrants of the breast other than the quadrant that harbored the index tumor. These findings raised suspicions about the efficacy of APBI. The irradiation period in APBI is shortened to a single fraction to ten fractions in 5 days, which requires very high doses of radiotherapy to be given in very few fractions over a very short time. This type of ultra-hypofractionation raises questions regarding the safety of APBI in terms of late sequelae and cosmesis [42, 43]. In addition, radiobiological considerations regarding the use of a single, very high dose radiation and relating this to the known mathematical models of radiobiological equivalence have raised questions [42]. At this time, according to the guidelines published by larger radiotherapy societies, it is considered safer to use APBI in women who are postmenopausal, have stage I and hormone receptor-positive disease, and have a single tumor focus that has been removed surgically with clear margins [34–36].

Techniques

Interstitial Brachytherapy

The first technique used for APBI was interstitial brachytherapy. In the first results from the Ochsner Clinic, 50 women were treated with multi-plane, multicatheter interstitial brachytherapy applied to the tumor-bearing quadrant between 1992 and 1993; after 6 years of follow-up, only one in-breast recurrence was reported [44]. Vicini et al. reported a larger series of women treated with this technique: 199 cases had implant treatment over 4–5 days using interstitial brachytherapy [45]. After 5 years of follow-up, the in-breast recurrence rate was 1 %, and the excellent-good cosmetic result rate was 99 %. Their technique involved both low-dose rate (LDR) irradiation, in which a 50-Gy prescribed dose was delivered over 4 days, and high-dose

rate (HDR) irradiation, in which 34 Gy in ten fractions was delivered over 5 days with two fractions per day. The implant volume included the lumpectomy cavity plus 1- to 2-cm margins, and multi-planes of implant insertions were performed.

The Radiation Therapy Oncology Group published the results of a phase II trial; in 99 cases treated with interstitial APBI who were followed for 5 years, the rates of in-breast recurrence were 3 % with HDR and 6 % with LDR applications, and major toxicity rates were 3 % (HDR) and 9 % (LDR) [46].

Interstitial APBI using multi-plane insertions was compared to WBI in randomized trials reported from Budapest [47, 48]. After 5 years of follow-up, overall survival, disease-free survival, and breast cancer-specific survival rates were identical, and the cosmetic results were equivalent.

Intracavitary Brachytherapy

A catheter to carry the radioactive source for brachytherapy with a balloon on the tip to fill the lumpectomy cavity that was developed and patented in the USA under the name MammoSite was presented for APBI and rather quickly obtained Food and Drug Administration approval in 2002 for off-protocol use [49].

Cuttino et al. reported a very large series of patients treated with MammoSite [50]. From nine institutions, a total of 483 patients were treated with MammoSite as the sole radiotherapy after BCS. Patients had a single tumor less than 3 cm in diameter that was removed with clear surgical margins and no axillary involvement. By 2-year follow-up, the breast recurrence rate was 1.2 %, and the excellent-good cosmesis rate was 91 %. The American Society of Breast Surgeons conducted a registration trial in patients treated with MammoSite and reported the results in 2009 [51]. Early-stage and good prognosis patients were selected for this treatment. A total of 1,440 patients were registered with a median age of 65 years, a median tumor size of 1 cm, a negative axillary rate of 92 %, and a negative surgical margin rate of 100 %. The prescribed dose was 34 Gy delivered in two fractions per day, with a total of ten fractions in 10 days. In-breast recurrence after 3 years was reported to be 1 %.

Despite these good control rates, publications have reported high rates of infection, symptomatic seroma occurrence, fat necrosis, and difficulties in covering the target volume with this applicator [52]. In recent years, newly designed intracavitary applicators that optimize the dose homogeneity using multiple canals on the tip of the applicator, rather than a single canal as in MammoSite, have been introduced [53].

External Beam Conformal Radiotherapy

Although the first APBI technique was interstitial brachytherapy, this technique has the disadvantages of being invasive, requiring long learning periods before making expert insertions, the limited availability of brachytherapy facilities, and infection and bleeding risks. However, using external beam and three-dimensional conformal techniques for APBI requires a shorter learning period and radiotherapy machines that are readily available in nearly all radiotherapy centers, is noninvasive, and has better options for obtaining dose homogeneity. Selecting the optimal target volume remains controversial [54]. The technique developed by the William Beaumont Hospital is widely used for defining treatment dose, normal tissue tolerance dose, treatment volume, and fractionation [55]. This clinic reported an in-breast recurrence rate of 1 % and a good cosmesis rate of 89 % in 94 patients treated with external APBI and followed for 4 years [56]. Treatment requires 5 days and ten fractions, using two fractions per day to deliver a total prescribed dose of 38.5 Gy. This technique is defined as the external beam APBI technique to be used in the randomized NSABP trial (the largest APBI trial designed, which has been closed to accrual and for which results are pending) [33].

Intraoperative APBI

The intraoperative irradiation of the tumor bed using a single dose with electrons during segmental mastectomy was popularized at the Milan Cancer Institute [57]. After removal of the tumor with clear clinical margins, a special electron generation radiotherapy machine dedicated to the operating theater is used, and the dose is delivered using an appropriately sized conus to the walls of the tumor bed.

A single dose of 21 Gy was tested in a phase II trials. The intraoperative radiotherapy versus external radiotherapy for selected (low-risk) early breast cancer (ELIOT) trial was a randomized, controlled equivalence trial conducted at the European Institute of Oncology, Milan, and the results were published recently [31]. Patients in the intraoperative radiotherapy group received one dose of 21 Gy to the tumor bed during surgery. The patients in the external radiotherapy group received 50 Gy in 25 fractions, followed by a boost of 10 Gy in 5 fractions, with a total treatment time of 6 weeks. In 1,305 patients who were randomized and followed for a median of 5.8 months, ipsilateral breast tumor recurrence was 4.4 % in the intraoperative radiotherapy group and 0.4 % in the external radiotherapy group ($p < 0.0001$). The 5-year overall survival was 96.8 % in the intraoperative radiotherapy group and 96.9 % in the external radiotherapy group. The ipsilateral breast tumor recurrence rate in the intraoperative group was significantly greater than in the external radiotherapy group, and overall survival did not differ between groups. The authors concluded that the improved selection of patients could reduce the rate of ipsilateral breast tumor recurrence with intraoperative radiotherapy with electrons.

One other intraoperative radiotherapy technique involves using a mobile X-ray-generating system adapted for use in the operating theater with various spherical applicators with diameters ranging from 1.5 to 5 cm to match the size of the surgical cavity. A trial of intraoperative radiotherapy using this machine (50 kV generating orthovoltage X-rays) to deliver a single dose of 20 Gy to the surface of the spherical applicator inserted in the tumor bed during BCS has been named "risk-adapted targeted intraoperative radiotherapy versus whole-breast radiotherapy for breast cancer: TARGIT-A randomized trial." Five-year results for this trial have recently been published [32]. In this trial, 1,721 patients were randomized to intraoperative radiotherapy and 1,730 to external beam radiotherapy. The 5-year risk for local recurrence in the conserved breast was 3.3 % for intraoperative radiotherapy versus 1.3 % for external beam breast radiotherapy ($p=0.04$). However, there seemed to be an overall mortality advantage in the intraoperative group. This finding requires some speculative explanation.

Both randomized intraoperative trials summarized above reported less skin complications with intraoperative irradiation and claimed better normal tissue protection. One editorial stated that the new data from TARGIT-A and ELIOT reinforce the notion that intraoperative radiotherapy during BCS is a reliable alternative to conventional postoperative fractionated irradiation, but only in a carefully selected population at low risk for local recurrence [58]. However, concerns regarding the use of a single dose of radiotherapy intraoperatively for breast-conserving treatment have been raised [43, 59, 60]. Concerns have included the delivery by intraoperative radiotherapy of an inadequate dose for the control of microscopic disease; the lack of image verification of target volume coverage or dose to organs at risk; the agnostic nature of the approach to final pathology findings; the use of a linear-quadratic formalism employing an α/β ratio of 10 for tumor control, which is now known to be incorrect, to determine the prescribed dose; and the financial considerations in terms of technical reimbursement for professional fees arising from the use of a single fraction of radiotherapy.

The review article by Njeh et al. provides a further discussion of all available APBI techniques [61]. APBI is a challenging treatment technique with many advantages as well as disadvantages and concerns. APBI may offer acceptable local control in select patients with low-risk breast cancer (possibly in very low-risk patients who actually do not need any radiotherapy after conserving surgery). The optimal patient selection criteria, technique, dose and fractionation, and target definition are active areas of research in APBI, while the results of large phase III trials are pending.

References

1. Early Breast Cancer Trialists' Collaborative Group (EBCTCG). Effects of radiotherapy after breast-conserving surgery on 10-year recurrence and 15-year breast cancer death: meta-analysis of individual patient data for 10801 women in 17 randomized trials. Lancet. 2011;378:1707–16.
2. Fisher B, Anderson S, Bryant J, Margolese RG, Deutsch M, Fisher ER, et al. Twenty-year follow-up of a randomized trial comparing total mastectomy, lumpectomy, and lumpectomy plus irradiation for the treatment of invasive breast cancer. N Engl J Med. 2002;347:1233–41.
3. Veronesi U, Luini A, Del Vecchio M, Greco M, Galimberti V, Merson M, et al. Radiotherapy after breast-preserving surgery in women with localized cancer of the breast. N Engl J Med. 1993;328:1587–91.
4. Theberge V, Whelan T, Shatelman SF, Vicini F. Altered fractionation: rationale and justification for whole and partial breast hypofractionated radiotherapy. Semin Radiat Oncol. 2011;21:55–65.
5. Hall EJ, Giaccia AJ. Radiobiology for the radiologists. Philadelphia: Lippincott Williams & Wilkins; 2006.
6. Thames HD, Bentzen SM, Turesson I, Overgaard M, Van den Bogaert W. Time-dose factors in radiotherapy: a review of the human data. Radiother Oncol. 1990;19:219–35.
7. Williams MV, Denekamp J, Fowler JF. A review of α/β ratios for experimental tumors: implications for clinical studies of altered fractionation. Int J Radiat Oncol Biol Phys. 1985;11:87–96.
8. Yarnold J, Ashton A, Bliss J, Homewood J, Harper C, Hanson J, et al. Fractionation sensitivity and dose response of late adverse effects in the breast after radiotherapy for early breast cancer: long-term results of a randomized trial. Radiother Oncol. 2005;75:9–17.
9. Owen JR, Ashton A, Bliss JM, Homewood J, Harper C, Hanson J, et al. Effect of radiotherapy fraction size on tumor control in patients with early-stage breast cancer after local tumor excision: long-term results of a randomized trial. Lancet Oncol. 2006;7:467–71.
10. Whelan T, MacKenzie R, Julian J, Levine M, Shelley W, Grimard L, et al. Randomized trial of breast irradiation schedules after lumpectomy for women with lymph node-negative breast cancer. J Natl Cancer Inst. 2002;94:1143–50.
11. Whelan T, Pignol J, Levine M, Julian J, Mackenzie R, Parpia S, et al. Long-term results of hypofractionated radiation therapy for breast cancer. N Engl J Med. 2010;362:513–20.
12. Cox JD, Stetz J, Pajak TF. Toxicity criteria of the Radiation Therapy Oncology Group (RTOG) and the European Organization for Research and Treatment of Cancer (EORTC). Int J Radiat Oncol Biol Phys. 1995;31:1341–6.

13. The START Trialists' Group. The UK Standardization of Breast Radiotherapy (START) Trial A of radiotherapy hypofractionation for treatment of early breast cancer: a randomized trial. Lancet Oncol. 2008;9:331–41.
14. Haviland JS, Owen JR, Dewar JA, Agrawal RK, Barrett-Lee PJ, Dobbs HJ, et al. The UK Standardization of Breast Radiotherapy (START) trials of radiotherapy hypofractionation for treatment of early breast cancer: 10-year follow-up results of two randomized controlled trials. Lancet Oncol. 2013;14:1086–94.
15. The START Trialists' Group. The UK Standardization of Breast Radiotherapy (START) trial B of radiotherapy hypofractionation for treatment of early breast cancer: a randomized trial. Lancet. 2008;371:1098–107.
16. The FAST Trialists Group. First results of the randomized UK FAST trial of radiotherapy hypofractionation for treatment of early breast cancer (CRUKE/04/015). Radiother Oncol. 2011;100:93–100.
17. Jones B, Dale RG, Deehan C, Hopkins KI, Morgan DA. The role of biologically effective dose (BED) in clinical oncology. Clin Oncol. 2001;13:71–81.
18. Williamson D, Dinniwell R, Fung S, Pintilie M, Done SJ, Fyles AW. Local control with conventional and hypofractionated adjuvant radiotherapy after breast-conserving surgery for ductal carcinoma in-situ. Radiother Oncol. 2010;95:317–20.
19. Moody AM, Mayles WP, Bliss JM, A'Hern RP, Owen JR, Regan J, et al. The influence of breast size on late radiation effects and association with radiotherapy dose inhomogeneity. Radiother Oncol. 1994;33:106–12.
20. Olivotto IA, Weir LM, Kim-Sing C, Bajdik CD, Trevisan CH, Doll CM, et al. Late cosmetic results of short fractionation for breast conservation. Radiother Oncol. 1996;41:7–13.
21. Galecki F, Hicer-Grzenkowicz J, Grudzien-Kowalska M, Michalska T, Załucki W. Radiation-induced brachial plexopathy and hypofractionated regimens in adjuvant irradiation of patients with breast cancer-a review. Acta Oncol. 2006;45:280–4.
22. Johansson S, Svensson H, Denekamp J. Timescale of evolution of late radiation injury after postoperative radiotherapy of breast cancer patients. Int J Radiat Oncol Biol Phys. 2000;48:745–50.
23. Olsen NK, Pfeiffer P, Johannsen L, Schrøder H, Rose C. Radiation-induced brachial plexopathy: neurological follow-up in 161 recurrence-free breast cancer patients. Int J Radiat Oncol Biol Phys. 1993;26:43–9.
24. Schultheiss TE. The radiation dose-response of the human spinal cord. Int J Radiat Oncol Biol Phys. 2008;71:1455–9.
25. Bartelink H, Arriagada R. Hypofractionation in radiotherapy for breast cancer. Lancet. 2008;371:1050–2.
26. Taylor CW, McGale P, Darby SC. Cardiac risks of breast-cancer radiotherapy: a contemporary view. Clin Oncol (R Coll Radiol). 2006;18:236–46.
27. Darby SC, Ewertz M, McGale P, Bennet AM, Blom-Goldman U, Brønnum D, et al. Risk of ischemic heart disease in women after radiotherapy for breast cancer. N Engl J Med. 2013;368:987–98.
28. Clarke M, Collins R, Darby S, Davies C, Elphinstone P, Evans E, Early Breast Cancer Trialists' Collaborative Group (EBCTCG), et al. Effects of radiotherapy and of differences in the extent of surgery for early breast cancer on local recurrence and 15-year survival: an overview of the randomized trials. Lancet. 2005;366:2087–106.
29. Journal Club. Are three weeks of whole-breast radiotherapy as good as five weeks in early breast cancer? – 10 year follow-up in the Canadian trial of hypofractionated radiation therapy. Breast Care (Basel). 2010;5:272–4.
30. Theriault RL, Carlson RW, Allred C, Anderson BO, Burstein HJ, Edge SB, et al. Breast cancer, version 3. 2013: featured updates to the NCCN guidelines. J Natl Compr Cancer Netw. 2013;11:753–60; Quiz 761.
31. Veronesi U, Orecchia R, Maisonneuve P, Viale G, Rotmensz N, Sangalli C, et al. Intraoperative radiotherapy versus external radiotherapy for early breast cancer (ELIOT): a randomised controlled equivalence trial. Lancet Oncol. 2013;14:1269–77.
32. Vaidya JS, Wenz F, Bulsara M, Saunders C, Alvarado M, Flyger HL, et al. Risk adapted targeted intraoperative radiotherapy versus whole breast radiotherapy for breast cancer: 5-year results for local control and overall survival from TARGIT-a randomised trial. Lancet. 2013;383:1719–20.
33. Barry M, Ho A, Morrow M. The evolving role of partial breast irradiation in early stage breast cancer. Ann Surg Oncol. 2013;20:2534–40.
34. Smith BD, Arthur DW, Buchholz T, Haffty BG, Hahn CA, Hardenbergh PA, et al. Accelerated partial breast irradiation consensus statement from the ASTRO. Int J Radiat Oncol Biol Phys. 2009;74:987–1001.
35. Polgar C, VanLimbergen E, Pötter R, Kovacs G, Polo A, Lyczek J, et al. Patient selection for accelerated partial breast irradiation after breast conserving surgery: recommendations of GEC-ESTRO breast cancer group based on clinical evidence. Radiother Oncol. 2010;94:264–73.
36. Shah C, Vicini F, Wazer DE, Arthur D, Patel RR. The American Brachytherapy Society consensus statement for accelerated partial breast irradiation. Brachytherapy. 2013;12:267–77.
37. Holland R, Veling SHJ, Mravunac M, Hendriks JHCL. Histologic multifocality of Tis, T1-2 breast carcinomas: implications for clinical trials of breast-conserving surgery. Cancer. 1985;56:979–90.
38. Vaidya JS, Vyas JJ, Chinoy RF, Merchant N, Sharma OP, Mittra I. Multicentricity of breast cancer: whole-organ analysis and clinical implications. Br J Cancer. 1996;74:820–4.
39. Faverly DRG, Hendriks JHCL, Holland R. Breast carcinomas of limited extent: frequency, radiologic-pathologic characteristics, and surgical margin requirements. Cancer. 2001;91:647–59.
40. Frazier TG, Wong RWY, Rose D. Implications of accurate pathologic margins in the treatment of primary breast cancer. Arch Surg. 1989;124:37–8.

41. Rosen PP, Fracchia AA, Urban JA. "Residual" mammary carcinoma following simulated partial mastectomy. Cancer. 1975;35:739–47.
42. Khan A, Arthur DW, Dale RG, Haffty BG, Vicini FA. Ultra-short course of adjuvant breast radiotherapy: promised land or primrose path? Int J Radiat Oncol Biol Phys. 2012;82:499–501.
43. Khan AJ, Arthur DW, Vicini FA. On the road to intraoperative radiotherapy: more proceed with caution signs. Oncology. 2013;27(2):1–3.
44. King TA, Bolton JS, Kuske RR, Fuhrman GM, Scroggins TG, Jiang XZ. Long-term results of widefield brachytherapy as the sole method of radiation therapy after segmental mastectomy for T (is, 1,2) breast cancer. Am J Surg. 2000;180:299–304.
45. Vicini FA, Kestin L, Chen P, Benitez P, Goldstein NS, Martinez A. Limited-field radiation therapy in the management of early-stage breast cancer. J Natl Cancer Inst. 2003;95:1205–10.
46. Kuske RR, Winter K, Arthur DW, Bolton J, Rabinowitz R, White J, et al. Phase II trial of brachytherapy alone after lumpectomy for select breast cancer: toxicity analysis of RTOG 2006;95-17. Int J Radiat Oncol Biol Phys. 2006;65:45–51.
47. Polgar C, Sulyok Z, Fodor J, Orosz Z, Major T, Mangel L, et al. Sole brachytherapy of the tumor bed after conservative surgery for T1 breast cancer: five-year results of a phase I–II study and initial findings of a randomized phase III trial. J Surg Oncol. 2002;80:121–8.
48. Polgar C, Fodor J, Major T, Nemeth G, Lövey K, Orosz Z, et al. Breast-conserving treatment with partial or whole breast irradiation for low-risk invasive breast carcinoma: 5 year results of a randomized trial. Int J Radiat Oncol Biol Phys. 2007;69:694–702.
49. Keisch M, Vicini F, Kuske RR, Herbert M, White J, Quiet S, et al. Initial clinical experience with the MammoSite breast brachytherapy applicator in women with early-stage breast cancer treated with breast-conserving therapy. Int J Radiat Oncol Biol Phys. 2003;55:289–93.
50. Cuttino LW, Keisch M, Jenrette JM, Dragun AE, Prestige BR, Quiet CA, et al. Multi-institutional experience using the MammoSite radiation therapy system in the treatment of early-stage breast cancer: 2-year results. Int J Radiat Oncol Biol Phys. 2008;71:107–14.
51. Nelson JC, Beitsch PD, Vicini FA, Quiet CA, Garcia D, Snider HC, et al. Four-year clinical update from the American Society of Breast Surgeons MammoSite brachytherapy trial. Am J Surg. 2009;198:83–91.
52. Biagioli MC, Haris EER. Accelerated partial breast irradiation: potential roles following breast conserving surgery. Cancer Control. 2010;17:191–204.
53. Dickler A, Patel RR, Wazer D. Breast brachytherapy devices. Expert Rev Med Devices. 2009;6:325–33.
54. Kirby AM, Coles CE, Yarnold JR. Target volume definition for external beam partial breast radiotherapy: clinical, pathological and technical studies informing current approaches. Radiother Oncol. 2010;94:255–63.
55. Baglan KL, Sharpe MB, Jaffray D, Frazier RC, Fayad J, Kestin LL, et al. Accelerated partial breast irradiation using 3D conformal radiation therapy (3D-CRT). Int J Radiat Oncol Biol Phys. 2003;55:302–11.
56. Chen PY, Wallace M, Mitchell C. Four-year efficacy, cosmesis, and toxicity using three-dimensional conformal external beam radiation therapy to deliver accelerated partial breast irradiation. Int J Radiat Oncol Biol Phys. 2010;76:991–7.
57. Orecchia R, Veronesi U. Intraoperative electrons. Semin Radiat Oncol. 2005;15:76–83.
58. Azria D, Lemanski C. Intraoperative radiotherapy for breast cancer. Lancet. 2014;383(9917):578–81.
59. Evans SB, Higgins SA. Intraoperative radiotherapy for breast cancer: deceptively simple? Oncology (Williston Park). 2013;27(2):122–4.
60. Ash RB, Williams VL, Wagman LD, Forouzannia A. Intraoperative radiotherapy for breast cancer: its perceived simplicity. Oncology (Williston Park). 2013;27(2):107–13.
61. Njeh CF, Saunders MW, Langton CM. Accelerated partial breast irradiation: a review of available techniques. Radiat Oncol. 2010;5:90–118.

Part II

Preoperative Systemic Therapy

Preoperative Therapy for Operable Breast Cancer

13

Yesim Eralp

Abstract

Preoperative systemic chemotherapy (PSC), also known as "neoadjuvant chemotherapy," is an important therapy option for most patients with breast cancer. PSC has evolved as an integral part of the multidisciplinary treatment approach for breast cancer and has a long history that dates back nearly four decades. Despite previous beliefs that it is more suitable for locally advanced or inflammatory disease, PSC is becoming increasingly popular in the breast oncology community for the treatment of earlier-stage disease. As safe and effective as adjuvant chemotherapy, this approach not only has the advantage of facilitating breast-conserving surgery (BCS) for patients in whom an optimal cosmetic outcome with upfront surgery is not possible but also has the potential to improve drug delivery to the tumor site by retaining intact vasculature before any local intervention is made. Furthermore, PSC provides an ideal setting in which the responsiveness of a given treatment can be observed and provides relevant information on the biology of the tumor by enabling biomarker analysis. Accumulating data on the strong association with survival and pathological complete response (pCR) may lead to a change in the regulatory requirements for drug approval and, consequently, reduce the need for costly and time-consuming large adjuvant trials.

In conclusion, PSC is a valuable research tool for identifying predictive molecular biomarkers and a valid treatment option for patients with early-stage breast cancer. However, the decision to treat a patient with neoadjuvant chemotherapy requires careful clinical judgment and multidisciplinary evaluation by an experienced team.

Y. Eralp, MD
Department of Medical Oncology, Istanbul
University Institute of Oncology, Topkapi,
Istanbul 34390, Turkey
e-mail: yeralp@yahoo.com

© Springer International Publishing Switzerland 2016
A. Aydiner et al. (eds.), *Breast Disease: Management and Therapies*,
DOI 10.1007/978-3-319-26012-9_13

Keywords

Neoadjuvant chemotherapy for breast cancer • Chemotherapy • Biological agents • Pathological complete response • Response-guided treatment

Introduction

A number of large-scale trials have established the role of neoadjuvant chemotherapy in operable and locally advanced breast cancer [1–4]. The common denominator in these studies is the significant association of pathological complete response (pCR) with not only breast conservation but also a prominent improvement in the odds of survival of 50–67 % [5–8]. The current goal of induction treatment is to improve pCR rates using different combinations administered on variable schedules. The incorporation of taxanes has resulted in higher pCR rates of 18–34 %; the range depends on the biology of the tumor. However, we have unfortunately reached a plateau in response rates, despite the utilization of further strategies such as dose-dense regimens or the incorporation of newer agents such as capecitabine, vinorelbine, or gemcitabine in combination, even when used as part of a response-adopted approach [7–9]. Data from these trials and others have suggested that an early clinical response to treatment may also be used to predict a higher probability of pCR at surgery. The main objective of predefining a pCR is to select the best chemotherapy regimen for a given patient. This would also enable treating physicians to switch to better regimens early in the course of treatment and prevent unnecessary toxicity from an ineffective combination. In other words, a "patient-tailored" approach would hypothetically improve the chance of a pCR, which may ultimately lead to an improvement in survival. Some clinicopathological variables, such as a lack of hormone receptors, and high grade, have already been shown to be associated with an improved response to neoadjuvant chemotherapy. Energetic efforts to identify molecular determinants or groups of genetic variables in specific patterns, namely, the "genetic signatures" of response, are in the early stages of development, and there is not yet a reliable predictor of a pCR.

The main advantage of preoperative systemic treatment is the incorporation of genomic analyses into the clinical setting to enable the determination of molecular predictors of response to a given treatment and provide insight into the biology of the tumor. In fact, to carry this approach one step further, recent neoadjuvant trials have focused on investigating the role of various biological agents in the treatment of distinct biological subgroups before confirmation in larger-scale adjuvant trials.

Chemotherapy Regimens

The significant survival advantage achieved by adjuvant chemotherapy led to trials investigating the role of neoadjuvant chemotherapy toward the end of the last century. In fact, the potential benefit of systemic chemotherapy as a primary treatment was initially reported by De Lena et al. [10], who observed a significant improvement in overall survival for administration of a neoadjuvant doxorubicin and vincristine combination before irradiation compared to radiation alone in locally advanced breast cancer. Pivotal trials investigating the role of PSC compared four to eight cycles of anthracycline-based regimens given as a neoadjuvant versus adjuvant treatment in patients with operable clinical T1-3N0-1 disease [1, 2, 4]. None of these trials reported a difference in outcome between either approach as summarized in Table 13.1.

One Step Closer to Improved Response Rates: Integration of Newer-Generation Agents

Taxanes

Encouraged by the favorable results achieved in the adjuvant setting, taxanes were swiftly incorporated into anthracycline-based combinations in the

Table 13.1 Earlier neoadjuvant studies comparing neoadjuvant versus adjuvant anthracycline-based regimens

Trial	n	Disease status	Regimen	pCR	Local recurrence	p	DFS	P	OS	p
NSABP B18 (1)	1,523	T1-3 N0-1	4 AC-surgery	13 %[a]	13 %		58 %		72 %	
			Surgery-4 AC	NA	10 %	NS	55 %[b]	NS	72 %[b]	NS
EORTC (2)	689	T1c-T4b N0-1	4 FEC-surgery	4 %	10 %		65 %		82 %	
			Surgery- 4 FEC	NA	9 %	NS	70 %[c]	NS	84 %[c]	NS
ECTO (4)	1,355	T2-3 N0-1	4 AT-4CMF-surgery	23 %	4.6 %		72 %		84 %	
			Surgery- 4 AT-4CMF	NA	4.1 %	NS	76 %		85 %	
			Surgery- 4 A-4CMF	NA			69 %[d]	NS	82 %[d]	NS

pCR pathological complete response, *DFS* disease-free survival, *OS* overall survival, *NA* not applicable, *NS* not significant, *AC* doxorubicin-cyclophosphamide, *FEC* fluorouracil-epirubicin-cyclophosphamide, *AT* doxorubicin-docetaxel, *CMF* cyclophosphamide-methotrexate-fluorouracil

[a]The ratio of patients with pathologically node-positive disease was significantly lower in the neoadjuvant group (59 % vs. 43 %, $p < 0.001$)
[b]At 8 years
[c]At 4 years
[d]At 7 years

hope of improving response rates in the neoadjuvant setting. As anticipated, taxanes yielded higher pCR rates compared to non-taxane regimens. The largest of these trials was NSABP B-27, which randomized 2,411 patients with operable breast cancer to four cycles of anthracycline (AC) alone, four cycles of AC followed by four cycles of docetaxel before surgery, and four cycles of neoadjuvant AC followed by surgery and four cycles of adjuvant docetaxel [3]. The significantly increased pCR rate (14 % vs. 26 %, $p > 0.001$) compared to the standard referent regimen and the manageable toxicity profile established the AC followed by docetaxel as the state-of-the-art approach in the neoadjuvant setting. However, despite a nearly twofold increase in the pCR rate, the B-27 trial failed to show a significant difference in overall survival, possibly due to the inadequate sample size, which lacked sufficient power to detect the anticipated small improvement of 3–5 % observed in adjuvant taxane trials [5].

The favorable impact of taxanes on response rates is summarized in Table 13.2. Overall, these trials demonstrated that six to eight cycles of anthracycline- and taxane-based combinations, either in sequence or given concomitantly, yield higher pCR rates than non-taxane-based regimens. Furthermore, the response rates attained with dose-dense regimens were not substantially higher than those obtained with the standard dose regimens. Despite the higher pCR rate (21 % vs. 14 %) in the PREPARE trial, which investigated the effect of a dose-dense regimen, disease-free survival (DFS) (3 year 75.8 % vs. 78.8 %) or overall survival (OS) (3 year 88.4 % vs. 91.8 %) did not differ [20]. Although there appears to be an incremental pCR benefit in the hormone receptor-negative subtype, considering the added toxicity, dose-dense regimens incorporating standard 3-weekly doses of paclitaxel or docetaxel should not be used outside of a clinical trial setting.

Capecitabine

Favorable response rates attained by capecitabine in the metastatic setting have led to studies evaluating the role of capecitabine in the neoadjuvant

Table 13.2 Benefit of taxanes with respect to clinical and pathological complete response rates

Trial	Regimen	cRR (%)	pCR (%)
Therasse (2003) [11]	ddEC×6	27	14
	CEF×6	31	10
Romieu (2002) [12]	AP×4	20	17
	AP×6	32	32[a]
Dieras (2004) [13]	AP×4	89	16
	AC×4	70	10
Steger (2004) [14]	ED×3	–	7.7
	ED×6	–	18.6[a]
Han (2009) [15]	ED×6	82	24[a]
	ED×4	72	11
Evans (2005) [16]	AD×6	70	20
	AC×6	61	17
Von Minckwitz (2005) [17]	ddAD×4	75	11
	AC×4-D×4	85	22.3[a]
Bear (2006) [3]	AC×4	85	13
	AC×4-D×4	91	26[a]
Smith (2002) [18]	CVAP×8	64	15
	CVAP×4-D×4	85	31[a]
Von Minckwitz (2008) [19]	TAC×6	48.2	21.0
	TAC×8	52.9	23.5

cRR clinical response rate, *pCR* pathological complete response rate, *dd* dose-dense, *AC* doxorubicin-doxorubicin-cyclophosphamide, *EC* epirubicin-cyclophosphamide, *CEF* fluorouracil-epirubicin-cyclophosphamide, *ED* epirubicin-docetaxel, *AP* doxorubicin-doxorubicin-paclitaxel, *D* docetaxel, *CVAP* cyclophosphamide-vincristine-doxorubicin-doxorubicin-prednisolone, *TAC* docetaxel-doxorubicin-doxorubicin-cyclophosphamide
[a]*p* < 0.05

setting. The GeparQuattro trial, which was the largest in sample size, randomized 1,495 patients with T1-4N0-3M0 to single-agent docetaxel, sequential docetaxel, and capecitabine or concomitant docetaxel and capecitabine following four cycles of epirubicin/cyclophosphamide (EC) [21]. The study failed to demonstrate a significant improvement in pCR rates, and the combination was associated with a higher rate of serious non-hematological toxicity. Similarly, a phase III trial by the Austrian Breast and Colorectal Study Group (ABCSG-24) revealed no difference between a triple combination of epirubicin, docetaxel, and capecitabine and the doublet regimen consisting of docetaxel and capecitabine [22]. Furthermore, in the NSABP B-40 trial, investigators reported a 29.7 % pCR rate

for the combination of docetaxel and capecitabine, somewhat lower than that of single-agent docetaxel (32.7 %) [23].

Despite discouraging data from single studies and a recent meta-analysis of pooled data [24], a meta-analysis including individual patient data from 966 patients from the German neoadjuvant trials suggested a significantly increased rate of pCR with a hazard ratio of 1.62 by multivariate analysis (p: 0.02) [25].

Until further data from ongoing trials including triple-negative patients are reported, there appears to be no role for incorporating capecitabine in standard anthracycline- and taxane-based neoadjuvant chemotherapy regimens.

Gemcitabine

Gemcitabine has established activity when combined with paclitaxel in patients with advanced breast cancer. Preliminary data from the first randomized trial testing the role of this combination in the neoadjuvant setting failed to detect an advantage in terms of pCR compared to single-agent paclitaxel following four cycles of the EC regimen [26]. Likewise, the addition of gemcitabine to docetaxel yielded a lower pCR rate (31.8 %) compared to docetaxel (32.7 %) in the NSABP B-40 trial [23]. In conclusion, there is no evidence supporting a role for adding gemcitabine in the neoadjuvant setting.

Vinorelbine

Limited data exist on the role of vinorelbine in the neoadjuvant setting. In a considerably resistant patient population, a vinorelbine and capecitabine combination yielded a pCR rate of 6 %, which was not different than that of the standard docetaxel-doxorubicin-cyclophosphamide (TAC) combination [19]. In another phase III trial, the epirubicin-vinorelbine combination resulted in similar pCR rates (12 %) and mastectomy rates compared to doxorubicin-cyclophosphamide (AC) [27]. These data do not support a role for vinorelbine in the neoadjuvant setting.

Nanobound Paclitaxel (nab-Pac)

Following approval of this agent for first-line treatment for those progressing within 6 months of adjuvant chemotherapy or second-line treatment of metastatic breast cancer, numerous phase II studies have investigated the role of nab-Pac for earlier disease. However, nearly all of these studies used this agent in combination with carboplatin and bevacizumab, which yielded encouraging response rates ranging between 53 % and 59 %, particularly in the triple-negative subgroup [28–30].

A phase III study that evaluated the role of nab-Pac in the neoadjuvant setting has recently been reported [31]. In the GeparSepto trial, 1,204 patients were randomized to two arms, including standard paclitaxel weekly at 80 mg/m^2 for 12 weeks or nab-Pac weekly at 150 mg/m^2 for 12 weeks followed by four cycles of EC. Patients with HER-2-positive disease received pertuzumab and trastuzumab throughout the treatment period (n: 400). A planned subgroup analysis revealed a significantly improved pCR rate of 48.2 % in the triple-negative subgroup (n: 275 patients), with a hazard ratio of 2.69. Nevertheless, the 25.7 % pCR rate of the standard arm in the triple-negative group was considerably lower than the values of 34.5 % in the GeparSixto trial and 41 % in the CALGB 40603 trials for similar combinations. Therefore, as a subgroup analysis, this result should be regarded with caution, and confirmatory data are required to establish a role of nab-Pac for triple-negative breast cancer.

Biological Agents

HER-2-Targeting Agents

Trastuzumab

Trastuzumab-based combinations have initiated a new era in the treatment of early- and advanced-stage HER-2-positive breast cancer. An early study in the neoadjuvant setting, which was a small randomized pilot trial in operable patients, reported a pCR of 65.2 % [32]. This unprecedented pCR rate has been confirmed by subsequent larger randomized trials that have evaluated the role of trastuzumab as part of standard anthracycline- and taxane-based regimens. One of these, the NOAH trial, had a unique design that permitted the concomitant use of anthracycline

and trastuzumab. In that trial, the combination regimen yielded a pCR rate of 38 % and a 5-year EFS of 71 %, significantly higher than the pCR rate of 19 % (p: 0.001) and EFS rate of 56 % (p: 0.013) in the HER-2-positive patient subset of the control arm. The updated data after a median follow-up period of 5.4 years revealed a significant advantage in terms of overall survival with a hazard ratio of 0.66 (p: 0.05) [33]. In terms of cardiac toxicity, there was no difference with respect to grade 3 and 4 cardiac events; there were only two patients (2 %) that developed transient grade 3 left ventricular dysfunction in the trastuzumab arm. In the GeparQuattro trial, which was originally designed to test the efficacy of capecitabine in the neoadjuvant setting, trastuzumab was allowed as part of the treatment in the HER-2-positive subgroup. The pCR rate including residual DCIS was 48.9 % among 340 HER-2-positive patients. In patients who were unresponsive to four cycles of EC, the pCR rate in the HER-2-positive group was five times that in the HER-2-negative cohort (16.7 % vs. 3.3 %), again confirming the role of trastuzumab even in patients with anthracycline-resistant disease [34].

Lapatinib

Lapatinib, a dual EGFR tyrosine kinase inhibitor, has already been established as an active agent in the metastatic setting. In the GeparQuinto trial, lapatinib (L) was tested head-to-head with trastuzumab (H) as part of a standard regimen consisting of four cycles of EC followed by four cycles of docetaxel (T). Of 620 eligible patients, 30.3 % in the ECH-TH group had a pCR, significantly higher than the rate in the ECL-TL arm (22.7 %) (p: 0.04) [35]. The NeoALTTO trial evaluated the role of lapatinib either as a single agent or in combination with trastuzumab compared to trastuzumab for 6 weeks followed by 12 weeks of paclitaxel added to the three randomized arms before surgery. Despite an amendment for dose reduction in the lapatinib arms due to increased grade 3 and 4 diarrhea and hepatic toxicity, there was a higher pCR rate with the dual blockade (51.3 %) compared to single-agent trastuzumab (29.5 %) or lapatinib (24.7 %) (p: 0.0001) [36]. However, a recently reported subsequent study by the CALGB with a similar design indicated no advantage of dual-targeted therapy in terms of pCR (56 % vs. 46 %) [38]. In the context of these data, there is no evidence supporting a role of lapatinib as a single agent or dual EGFR blockade with lapatinib and trastuzumab at present.

Pertuzumab

Pertuzumab is a monoclonal antibody that inhibits ligand-dependent signaling between HER-2 and HER-3 receptors and is thus complementary with trastuzumab. Based on encouraging data in metastatic patients both as first-line and subsequent treatment options, pertuzumab was also evaluated in the neoadjuvant setting. In the NeoSphere trial, women with operable or locally advanced or inflammatory breast cancer were randomized to receive four cycles every 3 weeks of docetaxel, trastuzumab, or docetaxel, trastuzumab and pertuzumab, or a doublet of the two monoclonal antibodies, or docetaxel and pertuzumab. After surgery, treatment consisted of adjuvant FEC for three cycles and trastuzumab every 3 weeks for one full year for all cases who had already received docetaxel in the neoadjuvant section of the trial, while in patients who received the doublet of antibodies, postsurgical treatment consisted of docetaxel for four cycles and FEC for three cycles with trastuzumab. The in-breast pCR rate when pertuzumab was added to the conventional trastuzumab and docetaxel combination was 46.8 %, significantly higher than the 24 % pCR rate for the pertuzumab and docetaxel doublet and 29 % pCR rate for the trastuzumab and docetaxel combination. Furthermore, there was a small subset of patients (16.8 %) who had a pCR with the doublet antibody regimen, suggesting the possibility that there may be a group of patients who do not require any chemotherapy [38]. There was some concern regarding toxicity because the triplet combination resulted in more neutropenia and febrile neutropenia, and there was one treatment-related death with fulminant hepatitis. In light of the accumulating evidence, further studies are needed to identify predictive markers that would facilitate the accurate identification of patients who would derive benefit from combined treatment strategies.

Antiangiogenic Agents

Bevacizumab

Bevacizumab, a monoclonal antibody targeting VEGF, has unfortunately been withdrawn by the FDA for its indication as a treatment option for metastatic breast cancer patients in light of recent data that failed to show a significant overall survival advantage despite favorable DFS rates. In the neoadjuvant setting, two trials evaluated the role of this antibody in combination with various cytotoxic regimens. In a subset of the GeparQuinto trial, HER-2-negative patients were randomized to four cycles of EC with bevacizumab and continued to four cycles of docetaxel plus bevacizumab if responsive to EC or to chemotherapy only. This trial failed to show a benefit in terms of pCR for the addition of bevacizumab in the general population (17.5 % vs. 15 %) with a subgroup benefit in the receptor-negative subset [39]. A subsequent study by the NSABP Group (NSABP B-40) randomized 1,206 patients to evaluate the role of capecitabine and gemcitabine with docetaxel followed by four cycles of AC and a second randomization with or without bevacizumab. In this trial, the addition of bevacizumab significantly increased the pCR rate, which was the primary endpoint, from 28.2 % to 34.5 % (p: 0.02), with greater benefit observed in the hormone receptor-positive subset [23]. Recently, an overall survival advantage was reported that was most evident in this subgroup as well [40]. However, it is not clear if the benefit observed in this trial is due to a compensatory effect due to the lower dose of docetaxel in the two-third of patients who received the antimetabolites. In conclusion, considering the conflicting evidence regarding the efficacy of bevacizumab within distinct molecular subgroups and the lack of a valid predictive marker, bevacizumab cannot be considered standard in the neoadjuvant setting at this time.

M-TOR Inhibitors

Everolimus

The mammalian target rapamycin (m-TOR) is a valid target that is frequently disrupted in breast cancer pathogenesis. The accumulation of favorable data in combination with hormonal and cytotoxic agents led to the randomized GeparQuinto trial to evaluate the role of everolimus in combination with paclitaxel as a second randomization in patients who were resistant to neoadjuvant EC with or without bevacizumab. The trial was stopped prematurely after 395 patients were randomized due to completion of the main trial. In terms of pCR, there was no difference between study arms (3.6 % vs. 5.6 %). Almost half of the patient group had to stop the treatment due to side effects in the combination arm, and there were concerns about whether everolimus attenuated the cytotoxic effects of paclitaxel on inhibition of cell-cycle progression. In addition, there was no indication that any subgroup may have benefited from the addition of everolimus to paclitaxel in this resistant group of patients [41].

Pathological Complete Response

Substantial evidence from randomized trials has consistently demonstrated a positive correlation between pCR and outcome, as summarized in Table 13.3. Therefore, pCR has been universally accepted as the primary endpoint in nearly all neoadjuvant trials. However, the definition of pCR remains controversial, and the substantial heterogeneity of this definition across different trials complicates the comparison of outcomes. As summarized in Table 13.4, definitions range from no invasive disease in the breast only to no invasive or noninvasive tumor deposits in the breast and lymph nodes (ypT0N0), most of which exhibit a significant association with DFS or OS. A meta-analysis of seven neoadjuvant German trials including data from 6,377 patients demonstrated that no invasive or noninvasive residual in both the breast and lymph nodes was the most sensitive definition of pCR predicting a better outcome in terms of OS and DFS [25]. These data contradict the most recent meta-analysis reporting individual patient data from 12 large randomized trials, which demonstrated that the presence of in situ carcinoma in the breast does not influence the favorable effect of pCR on OS (HR ypT0ypN0 vs. ypT0/isypN0 vs. ypT0/is:

Table 13.3 Pathological complete response classification systems and correlations with outcome

Author/group	pCR definition	Outcome correlation
Fisher/NSABP [8]	Breast: no invasive tumor	OS; DFS
Kuerer/MD Anderson CC [7]	Breast and lymph nodes: no invasive tumor	OS; DFS
Pierga/Institut Curie [43]	Breast and lymph nodes: no invasive tumor	OS; DFS
Van der Hage/EORTC [2]	Breast and lymph nodes: no malignant cells	OS
Ogston/Aberdeen [44]	Breast: no invasive tumor	OS; DFS
Von Minckwitz/ GBCSG [45]	Breast and lymph nodes: no invasive or noninvasive tumor	OS; DFS

pCR pathological complete response, *OS* overall survival, *DFS* disease-free survival

0.36, 0.36 vs. 0.51, respectively). According to this meta-analysis, the definition of pCR should be an absence of invasive tumor in the breast and lymph nodes (ypT0/is ypN0) [49].

Predictive Biomarkers

With the evolution of molecular and genetic testing in modern oncology, numerous multigene signatures with potential predictive and prognostic roles have been identified. However, correlative validation studies have demonstrated that these classifiers are not only associated with substantially different outcomes but also display a wide variation in response to standard chemotherapy regimens. However, trials evaluating the role of biomarkers have consistently concluded that tumors with a high proliferative capacity, as assessed by a high Ki-67 level or grade, hormone receptor negativity, or HER-2 positivity, display a high probability of response and a higher chance of survival in those patients with a pCR. Although

Table 13.4 Survival outcome of neoadjuvant chemotherapy and pathological complete response rates

Author	Regimen	pCR (%)	pCR site	P	DFS, EFS (%)	P	OS (%)	p
Aberdeen [18]	CVAP	16	b		77		84	
	CVAP-D	34		0.034	90 (3-year DFS)	0.03	97 (3-year OS)	0.05
AGO [46]	EP	10	bl		50		77	
	E-P	18		0.008	70 (5-year DFS)	0.011	83 (5-year OS)	0.04
SICOG [47]	EP q3 week	6	bl		55		69	
	EPC is q week	16		0.02	73 (5-year DMFS)	0.04	82 (5-year OS)	0.07
NOAH [33]	AP-P-CMF	19	bl		56		79	
	AP-P-CMF + Trastz	38		0.001	71 (3-year EFS)	0.013	87 (3-year OS)	NS
NSABP B-27 [5]	AC–surgery	13	bl		59		74	
	AC–surgery-D	14.5			62		75	
	AC–D–surgery	26		<0.001	62 (8-year DFS)	NS	75 (8-year OS)	NS
ACCOG [16]	AC	16	bl		NA		NA	
	AD	12		NS		NS		NS
MDA [48]	CAF	8	bl		89		NA	
	P	17		NS	94 (2-year DFS)	NS		NS
Baldini [47]	CED	2.6	bl		48		52	
	dd CEF	4.1		NS	60 (5-year DFS)	NS	54 (5-year OS)	NS
TOPIC [49]	AC	25	bl		63		74	
	ECisF	24		NS	62 (5-year RFS)	NS	82 (5-year OS)	NS
TOPIC 2 [27]	AC	12	bl					
	VE	12		NS	HR: 1.18 (2-year DFS)	NS	HR: 1.41 (2-year OS)	NS

pCR pathological response rate, *dd* dose-dense, *EFS* event-free survival, *Cis* cisplatin, *AC* doxorubicin-cyclophosphamide, *D* docetaxel, *EC* epirubicin-cyclophosphamide, *CEF* fluorouracil-epirubicin-cyclophosphamide, *ED* epirubicin-docetaxel, *CED* fluorouracil-epirubicin-docetaxel, *AP* doxorubicin-paclitaxel, *D* docetaxel, *CVAP* cyclophosphamide-vincristine-doxorubicin-prednisolone, *VE* vincristine-epirubicin, *wk* week, *b* breast, *bl* breast and lymph nodes, *yr* year, *OS* overall survival, *DFS* disease-free survival, *RFS* relapse-free survival, *DMFS* distant metastasis-free survival
p<0.05

molecular tests specifically developed to predict pCR have not demonstrated any predictive superiority over the combination of standard clinicopathological parameters (ER status, grade, and age), there are emerging data that some of those molecular tests that have been compared with a survival endpoint may have a role in identifying patients who may or may not benefit from chemotherapy. A retrospective evaluation of gene expression profiling data from eight studies including 996 patients revealed that an immunogenic genomic module added to clinical characteristics significantly increased the accuracy of predicting a pCR in the HER-2 subgroup [6]. In the remaining intrinsic subgroups as assessed by the PAM50 assay, there were no specific genomic signatures that would identify patients who would benefit from standard neoadjuvant chemotherapy. I-SPY, a recently reported multicenter trial, prospectively evaluated the role of multigene classifiers as well as standard pathological biomarkers in 237 patients treated with neoadjuvant anthracycline- and taxane-based chemotherapy [50]. This trial confirmed the general consensus that highly proliferative tumors respond better to chemotherapy because pCR rates ranged from approximately 5–9 % for luminal A tumors and those with a low Ki-67 level or low-risk genomic profiles (ROR-S, wound healing signature, PAM-50, 70-gene classifier) to 35 % and 54 % for high-risk and HER-2-positive tumors, respectively [50, 51]. In terms of outcome, patients with luminal or low-risk tumors had longer survival rates despite lower pCR rates, consistent with a meta-analysis of individual patient data across 12 large randomized neoadjuvant trials and the GeparTrio trial reported recently [49, 52]. As expected, in higher-risk patients, a pCR improved the likelihood of a better outcome. Multivariate analysis demonstrated that most molecular signatures and clinical stage improved the ability to predict RFS, suggesting that molecular classifiers can identify patients with a favorable prognostic profile among the non-pCR hormone receptor-positive subtypes. The wound healing signature was the most accurate classifier for identifying lower-risk patients, consistent with previous studies suggesting that

the tumor microenvironment and the inflammatory response may have relevant roles in the pathogenesis of breast cancer.

Response-Guided Treatment

Accurate early-response assessment during chemotherapy is an important component of the neoadjuvant treatment strategy to identify patients who are unlikely to benefit from the given regimen. There are substantial data from randomized trials indicating a strong correlation between achieving a pCR and favorable long-term survival, as summarized previously in this chapter. As expected, a poor or minimal response usually suggests a poorer outcome. Numerous neoadjuvant trials have evaluated the role of an early response to standard chemotherapy regimens in the selection of subsequent non-cross-resistant agents. An earlier study by the MD Anderson group randomized patients with a larger than 1-cm^2 residual tumor burden following five cycles of an anthracycline-based combination to either five additional cycles of the same regimen or five cycles of a different combination including vinblastine, methotrexate, and fluorouracil [53]. Despite the limited sample size, there was a trend for survival advantage for patients treated with the alternative regimen (p: 0.08). Contradicting this data, the TAX 301 Aberdeen Trial showed no advantage in switching to docetaxel in patients who were unresponsive to four cycles of an anthracycline-based combination [18]. However, there was a significant increase in the pCR rate (31 % vs. 15 %) when responding patients received four additional cycles of docetaxel, which translated to a survival advantage. The recently reported GeparTrio trial included 2,090 patients who initially received two cycles of the TAC regimen and randomized nonresponding patients to six more cycles of the same regimen or to two cycles of TAC followed by four cycles of a vinorelbine and capecitabine combination [19]. Although an earlier report failed to show an advantage in terms of pCR in the experimental group, an update analysis suggested a significant survival advantage favoring response-guided treatment that was limited to patients in the luminal A and luminal B subgroups [19, 52]. The results of this study indicated that pCR may not be a good surrogate endpoint for survival in patients with hormone receptor-positive tumors. Despite accumulating data suggesting that neoadjuvant chemotherapy may be tailored according to response early during the course of treatment, further study is needed before neoadjuvant chemotherapy can be adopted as a standard approach.

Conclusion

Neoadjuvant chemotherapy offers an ideal setting to identify regimens or agents for prioritization for adjuvant confirmatory trials and to identify biomarkers or genomic signatures to predict response or resistance to a given regimen. Numerous trials over the last three or four decades have provided valuable information on the biology of breast cancer, as well as efficacy data that have improved treatment strategies in earlier stages. Substantial evidence from meta-analyses suggests that pCR is an important surrogate endpoint for outcome in most subgroups, arguing that costly, time-consuming large trials may be spared for agents exhibiting a high pCR rate with survival advantage in the neoadjuvant setting. With the advent of molecular diagnostic techniques and translational medicine, the last decade has proved to be an exciting era for oncology research. However, the more we examine the basic mechanisms of oncogenesis, the deeper we find ourselves in the abyss of the cancer enigma.

Even more remains to be accomplished than has been thus far to develop better treatment options for patients with breast cancer.

References

1. Wolmark N, Wang J, Mamounas E, Bryant J, Fisher B. Preoperative chemotherapy in patients with operable breast cancer: nine-year results from National Surgical Adjuvant Breast and Bowel Project B-18. J Natl Cancer Inst Monogr. 2001;30:96–102.

2. van der Hage JA, van de Velde CJ, Julien JP, Tubiana-Hulin M, Vandervelden C, Duchateau L. Preoperative chemotherapy in primary operable breast cancer: results from the European Organization for Research and Treatment of Cancer trial 10902. J Clin Oncol. 2001;19:4224–37.

3. Bear HD, Anderson S, Smith RE, Geyer Jr CE, Mamounas EP, Fisher B, et al. Sequential preoperative or postoperative docetaxel added to preoperative doxorubicin plus cyclophosphamide for operable breast cancer National Surgical Adjuvant Breast and Bowel Project Protocol B-27. J Clin Oncol. 2006; 24:2019–27.

4. Gianni L, Baselga J, Eiermann W, Porta VG, Semiglazov V, Lluch A, et al. Phase III trial evaluating the addition of paclitaxel to doxorubicin followed by cyclophosphamide, methotrexate, and fluorouracil, as adjuvant or primary systemic therapy: European Cooperative Trial in Operable Breast Cancer. J Clin Oncol. 2009;27:2474–81.

5. Rastogi P, Anderson SJ, Bear HD, Geyer CE, Kahlenberg MS, Robidoux A, et al. Preoperative chemotherapy: updates of National Surgical Adjuvant Breast and Bowel Project Protocols B-18 and B-27. J Clin Oncol. 2008;26:778–85.

6. Untch M, Mobus V, Kuhn W, Muck BR, Thomssen C, Bauerfeind I, et al. Intensive dose-dense compared with conventionally scheduled preoperative chemotherapy for high-risk primary breast cancer. J Clin Oncol. 2009;27:2938–45.

7. Kuerer HM, Newman LA, Smith TL, Ames FC, Hunt KK, Dhingra K, et al. Clinical course of breast cancer patients with complete pathologic primary tumor and axillary lymph node response to doxorubicin-based neoadjuvant chemotherapy. J Clin Oncol. 1999; 17:460–9.

8. Fisher B, Bryant J, Wolmark N, Mamounas E, Brown A, Fisher ER, et al. Effect of preoperative chemotherapy on the outcome of women with operable breast cancer. J Clin Oncol. 1998;16:2672–85.

9. Ring AE, Smith IE, Ashley S, Fulford LG, Lakhani SR. Oestrogen receptor status, pathological complete response and prognosis in patients receiving neoadjuvant chemotherapy for early breast cancer. Br J Cancer. 2004;91(12):2012–7.

10. De Lena M, Zucali R, Viganotti G, Valagussa P, Bonadonna G. Combined chemotherapy-radiotherapy approach in locally advanced (T3b–T4) breast cancer. Cancer Chemother Pharmacol. 1978;1:53–9.

11. Therasse P, Mauriac L, Welnicka-Jaskiewicz M, Bruning P, Cufer T, Bonnefoi H, EORTC, et al. Final results of a randomized phase III trial comparing cyclophosphamide, epirubicin, and fluorouracil with a dose-intensified epirubicin and cyclophosphamide + filgrastim as neoadjuvant treatment in locally advanced breast cancer: an EORTC-NCIC-SAKK multicenter study. J Clin Oncol. 2003;21(5):843–50.

12. Romieu G, Tubiana-Hulin M, Fumoleau P, Dieras V, Namer M, Mauriac L, et al. A multicenter randomized phase II study of 4 or 6 cycles of adriamycin/Taxol

(paclitaxel) (AT) as neoadjuvant treatment of breast cancer (BC). Ann Oncol. 2002;13 Suppl 5:33–9.

13. Diéras V, Fumoleau P, Romieu G, Tubiana-Hulin M, Namer M, Mauriac L, et al. Randomized parallel study of doxorubicin plus paclitaxel and doxorubicin plus cyclophosphamide as neoadjuvant treatment of patients with breast cancer. J Clin Oncol. 2004;22(24):4958–65.

14. Steger GG, Kubista E, Hausmaninger H, Gnant M, Tausch C, Lang A et al. 6 vs. 3 cycles of epirubicin/docetaxel + G-CSF in operable breast cancer: results of ABCSG-14 [abstract]. 2004;22 (Jul 15 Suppl 14S):A553.

15. Han S, Kim J, Lee J, Chang E, Gwak G, Cho H, et al. Comparison of 6 cycles versus 4 cycles of neoadjuvant epirubicin plus docetaxel chemotherapy in stages II and III breast cancer. Eur J Surg Oncol. 2009; 35(6):583–7.

16. Evans TR, Yellowlees A, Foster E, et al. Phase III randomized trial of doxorubicin and docetaxel versus doxorubicin and cyclophosphamide as primary medical therapy in women with breast cancer: an anglo-celtic cooperative oncology group study. J Clin Oncol. 2005;23(13):2988–95.

17. von Minckwitz G, Raab G, Caputo A, Earl H, Cameron DA, Hutcheon AW, et al. Doxorubicin with cyclophosphamide followed by docetaxel every 21 days compared with doxorubicin and docetaxel every 14 days as preoperative treatment in operable breast cancer: the GEPARDUO study of the German Breast Group. J Clin Oncol. 2005;23:2676–85.

18. Smith IC, Heys SD, Hutcheon AW, Miller ID, Payne S, Gilbert FJ, et al. Neoadjuvant chemotherapy in breast cancer: significantly enhanced response with docetaxel. J Clin Oncol. 2002;20(6):1456–66.

19. von Minckwitz G, Kümmel S, Vogel P, Hanusch C, Eidtmann H, Hilfrich J, German Breast Group, et al. Neoadjuvant vinorelbine-capecitabine versus docetaxel-doxorubicin-cyclophosphamide in early nonresponsive breast cancer: phase III randomized GeparTrio trial. J Natl Cancer Inst. 2008;100(8): 542–51.

20. Untch M, von Minckwitz G, Konecny GE, Conrad U, Fett W, Kurzeder C, on behalf of; Arbeitsgemeinschaft Gynäkologische Onkologie PREPARE investigators, et al. PREPARE trial: a randomized phase III trial comparing preoperative, dose-dense, dose-intensified chemotherapy with epirubicin, paclitaxel, and CMF versus a standard-dosed epirubicin-cyclophosphamide followed by paclitaxel with or without darbepoetin alfa in primary breast cancer – outcome on prognosis. Ann Oncol. 2011;22(9):1999–2006.

21. von Minckwitz G, Rezai M, Loibl S, Fasching PA, Huober J, Tesch H, et al. Capecitabine in addition to anthracycline- and taxane-based neoadjuvant treatment in patients with primary breast cancer: phase III GeparQuattro study. J Clin Oncol. 2010;28(12):2015–23.

22. Steger GG, Greil R, Jakesz R, Lang A, Mlineritsch B, Melbinger-Zeinitzer E, et al. Final results of ABCSG-24, a randomized phase III study comparing

epirubicin, docetaxel, and capecitabine (EDC) to epirubicin and docetaxel (ED) as neoadjuvant treatment for early breast cancer and comparing ED/EDC + trastuzumab (T) to ED/EDC as neoadjuvant treatment for early HER-2 positive breast cancer. Cancer Res. 2009;69(24 Suppl):564s (abstract 1081).

23. Bear HD, Tang G, Rastogi P, Geyer Jr CE, Robidoux A, Atkins JN, et al. Bevacizumab added to neoadjuvant chemotherapy for breast cancer. N Engl J Med. 2012;366(4):310–20.

24. Li Q, Jiang Y, Wei W, Yang H, Liu J. Clinical efficacy of including capecitabine in neoadjuvant chemotherapy for breast cancer: a systematic review and meta-analysis of randomized controlled trials. PLoS One. 2013;8(1):e53403. doi:10.1371/journal.pone.0053403.

25. von Minckwitz G, Untch M, Nüesch E, Loibl S, Kaufmann M, Kümmel S, et al. Impact of treatment characteristics on response of different breast cancer phenotypes: pooled analysis of the German neoadjuvant chemotherapy trials. Breast Cancer Res Treat. 2011;125(1):145–56.

26. Earl HM, Vallier A, Hiller L, Fenwick N, Iddawela M, Hughes-Davies L, et al. Neo-tAnGo: a neoadjuvant randomized phase III trial of epirubicin/cyclophosphamide and paclitaxel± gemcitabine in the treatment of women with high-risk early breast cancer (EBC): first report of the primary endpoint, pathological complete response (pCR). J Clin Oncol. 2009;27:15s (abstract 522).

27. Chua S, Smith IE, A'Hern RP, Coombes GA, Hickish TF, Robinson AC, et al. Neoadjuvant vinorelbine/epirubicin (VE) versus standard adriamycin/cyclophosphamide (AC) in operable breast cancer: analysis of response and tolerability in a randomised phase III trial (TOPIC 2). Ann Oncol. 2005;16:1435–41.

28. Snider JN, Sanchev JC, Allen JW, Schwartzberg LS, Young RR, Javed AY et al. Pathologic complete response with weekly nanoparticle albumin bound paclitaxel plus carboplatin followed by doxorubicin plus cyclophosphamide with concurrent bevacizumab for triple negative breast cancer. J Clin Oncol (meeting abstracts). 2013;31 (Suppl) (abstract 1068).

29. Mrozek E, Lustber MB, Knopp MV, Spigos DG, Yang X, Houton LA et al. Phase II trial of neoadjuvant chemotherapy with weekly nanoparticle albumin bound paclitaxel, carboplatin and bevacizumab in women with clinical stages II–III breast cancer: pathologic response prediction by changes in angiogenic volüme by dynamic contrast enhanced magnetic resonance imaging. J Clin Oncol (meeting abstracts). 2010;28(Suppl) (abstract 604).

30. Sinclair NF, Abu-Khalaf MM, Rizack T, Rosati K, Chung G, Legare RD et al. Neoadjuvant weekly nanoparticle albumin bound paclitaxel, carboplatin plus bevacizumab with or without dose-dense doxorubicin-cyclophosphamide plus B in ER+/Her-2 negative and triple negative breast cancer: a BrUOG study. J Clin Oncol (meeting abstracts). 2012; 30(Suppl) (abstract 1045).

31. Untch M, Jackisch C, Schneeweiß A, Conrad B, Aktas B, Denkert C, et al. A randomized phase III trial comparing neoadjuvant chemotherapy with weekly nanoparticle-based paclitaxel with solvent-based paclitaxel followed by anthracyline/cyclophosphamide for patients with early breast cancer (GeparSepto); GBG 69. 37th San Antonio Breast Cancer Conference 9–13 Dec 2014, San Antonio; Meeting Abstract (S2–07).

32. Buzdar AU, Ibrahim NK, Francis D, Booser DJ, Thomas ES, Theriault RL, et al. Significantly higher pathologic complete remission rate after neoadjuvant therapy with trastuzumab, paclitaxel, and epirubicin chemotherapy: results of a randomized trial in human epidermal growth factor receptor 2-positive operable breast cancer. J Clin Oncol. 2005;23:3676–85.

33. Gianni L, Eiermann W, Semiglazov V, Manikhas A, Lluch A, Tjulandin S, et al. Neoadjuvant chemotherapy with trastuzumab followed by adjuvant trastuzumab versus neoadjuvant chemotherapy alone, in patients with HER2-positive locally advanced breast cancer (the NOAH trial): a randomised controlled superiority trial with a parallel HER2-negative cohort. Lancet. 2010;375(9712):377–84.

34. Untch M, Rezai M, Loibl S, Fasching PA, Huober J, Tesch H, et al. Neoadjuvant treatment with trastuzumab in HER2-positive breast cancer: results from the GeparQuattro study. J Clin Oncol. 2010;28(12): 2024–31.

35. Untch M, Loibl S, Bischoff J, Eidtmann H, Kaufmann M, Blohmer JU, Arbeitsgemeinschaft Gynäkologische Onkologie-Breast (AGO-B) Study Group, et al. Lapatinib versus trastuzumab in combination with neoadjuvant anthracycline-taxane-based chemotherapy (GeparQuinto, GBG 44): a randomised phase 3 trial. Lancet Oncol. 2012;13(2):135–44.

36. Baselga J, Bradbury I, Eidtmann H, Di Cosimo S, de Azambuja E, Aura C et al. NeoALTTO Study Team. Lapatinib with trastuzumab for HER2-positive early breast cancer (NeoALTTO): a randomised, open-label, multicentre, phase 3 trial. Lancet. 2012;379:(9816):633–40. Carey LA, Berry DA, Ollila D, Harris L, Krop IE, Weckstein D et al. Clinical and translational results of CALGB 40601. Proc ASCO 49th Annual Meeting. 2013. 31 May–3 June 2013;15 S (Abstract 500).

37. Carey LA, Berry DA, Ollila D, et al. (2013) Clinical and translational results of CALGB 40601. Proc ASCO 49th Annual Meeting. May 31-June 3, 2013; 15 S (Abstract 500).

38. Gianni L, Pienkowski T, Im YH, Roman L, Tseng LM, Liu MC, et al. Efficacy and safety of neoadjuvant pertuzumab and trastuzumab in women with locally advanced, inflammatory, or early HER2-positive breast cancer (NeoSphere): a randomised multicentre, open-label, phase 2 trial. Lancet Oncol. 2012;13(1):25–32.

39. von Minckwitz G, Eidtmann H, Rezai M, Fasching PA, Tesch H, Eggemann H, German Breast Group; Arbeitsgemeinschaft Gynäkologische Onkologie–Breast Study Groups, et al. Neoadjuvant chemotherapy and bevacizumab for HER2-negative breast cancer. N Engl J Med. 2012;366(4):299–309.

40. Bear HD, Tang G, Rastogi P, Geyer CE Jr., Robidoux A, Atkins JN, et al. The effect on overall and disease-free survival (OS & DFS) by adding bevacizumab and/or antimetabolites to standard neoadjuvant chemotherapy: NSABP Protocol B-4037 the San Antonio Breast Cancer Conference 9–13 Dec 2014, San Antonio; Meeting Abstract (PD2-1).

41. Huober J, Fasching PA, Hanusch C, Rezai M, Eidtmann H, Kittel K, et al. Neoadjuvant chemotherapy with paclitaxel and everolimus in breast cancer patients with non-responsive tumours to epirubicin/cyclophosphamide (EC) ± bevacizumab – results of the randomised GeparQuinto study (GBG 44). Eur J Cancer. 2013;49(10):2284–93.

42. Pierga JY, Mouret E, Diéras V, Laurence V, Beuzeboc P, Dorval T, et al. Prognostic value of persistent node involvement after neoadjuvant chemotherapy in patients with operable breast cancer. Br J Cancer. 2000;83(11):1480–7.

43. Ogston KN, Miller ID, Payne S, Hutcheon AW, Sarkar TK, Smith I, Schofield A, Heys SD. A new histological grading system to assess response of breast cancers to primary chemotherapy: prognostic significance and survival. Breast. 2003;12(5):320–7.

44. von Minckwitz G, Untch M, Blohmer JU, Costa SD, Eidtmann H, Fasching PA, et al. Definition and impact of pathologic complete response on prognosis after neoadjuvant chemotherapy in various intrinsic breast cancer subtypes. J Clin Oncol. 2012;30(15):1796–804.

45. Frasci G, D'Aiuto G, Comella P, D'Aiuto M, Di Bonito M, Ruffolo P, et al. Preoperative weekly cisplatin, epirubicin, and paclitaxel (PET) improves prognosis in locally advanced breast cancer patients: an update of the Southern Italy Cooperative Oncology Group (SICOG) randomised trial 9908. Ann Oncol. 2010;21:707–16.

46. Buzdar AU, Singletary SE, Theriault RL, Booser DJ, Valero V, Ibrahim N, et al. Prospective evaluation of paclitaxel versus combination chemotherapy with fluorouracil, doxorubicin, and cyclophosphamide as neoadjuvant therapy in patients with operable breast cancer. J Clin Oncol. 1999;17:3412–7.

47. Baldini E, Gardin G, Giannessi PG, Evangelista G, Roncella M, Prochilo T, et al. Accelerated versus standard cyclophosphamide, epirubicin and 5-fluorouracil or cyclophosphamide, methotrexate and 5-fluorouracil: a randomized phase III trial in locally advanced breast cancer. Ann Oncol. 2003;14:227–32.

48. Smith IE, A'Hern RP, Coombes GA, Howell A, Ebbs SR, Hickish TF, TOPIC Trial Group, et al. A novel continuous infusional 5-fluorouracil-based chemotherapy regimen compared with conventional chemotherapy in the neoadjuvant treatment of early breast cancer: 5 year results of the TOPIC trial. Ann Oncol. 2004;15:751–8.

49. Cortazar P, Zhang L, Untch M, Mehta K, Costantino JP, Wolmark N, et al. Pathological complete response and long-term clinical benefit in breast cancer: the

CTNeoBC pooled analysis. Lancet. 2014;384(9938): 164–72.

50. Esserman LJ, Berry DA, Cheang MC, Yau C, Perou CM, Carey L, I-SPY 1 TRIAL Investigators, et al. Chemotherapy response and recurrence-free survival in neoadjuvant breast cancer depends on biomarker profiles: results from the I-SPY 1 TRIAL (CALGB 150007/150012; ACRIN 6657). Breast Cancer Res Treat. 2012;132(3):1049–62.

51. Esserman LJ, Berry DA, DeMichele A, Carey L, Davis SE, Buxton M, et al. Pathologic complete response predicts recurrence-free survival more effectively by cancer subset: results from the I-SPY 1 TRIAL – CALGB 150007/150012, ACRIN 6657. J Clin Oncol. 2012;30(26):3242–9.

52. von Minckwitz G, Blohmer JU, Untch M, Costa SD, Eidtmann H, Fasching PA et al. Neoadjuvant chemotherapy adapted by interim response improves overall survival of primary breast cancer patients – results of the GeparTrio Trial. Proc SABCS 34th Annual San Antonio Breast Cancer Symposium 15 Dec 2011. Cancer Res 71. 2011:24(S 3):S3–2.

53. Thomas E, Holmes FA, Smith TL, Buzdar AU, Frye DK, Fraschini G, et al. The use of alternate, non-cross-resistant adjuvant chemotherapy on the basis of pathologic response to a neoadjuvant doxorubicin-based regimen in women with operable breast cancer: long-term results from a prospective randomized trial. J Clin Oncol. 2004;22(12): 2294–302.

Neoadjuvant Hormonal Therapy in Breast Cancer

14

Nil Molinas Mandel and Fatih Selcukbiricik

Abstract

The various types of ER-positive and HER-2-negative breast cancers have different treatment modalities. There are two options for the treatment of locally advanced breast cancer: chemotherapy or hormonal therapy. Chemotherapy can be particularly toxic for elderly postmenopausal patients, and neoadjuvant hormonal therapy (NHT) is an alternative for patients with hormone receptor-positive, locally advanced, postmenopausal breast cancer. This treatment is also highly beneficial for patients with comorbidities and can comprise tamoxifen and steroidal or nonsteroidal aromatase inhibitors (AIs). The best activities in clinical trials are observed with AIs. NHT produces good response rates (RRs) as well as adequate downstaging of tumor size such that breast-conserving surgery (BCS) may become an option. The optimal duration of such treatments should not be less than 4 months and may be continued for as long as 8 months.

There are no studies showing benefits of neoadjuvant endocrine therapy in premenopausal patients.

Keywords

Hormonotherapy • Neoadjuvant hormonal therapy (NHT) • Letrozole • Anastrozole • Exemestane • Tamoxifen • Aromatase inhibitors (AIs) • IMPACT study • PROACT study • Postmenopausal • Premenopausal • Breast-conserving surgery (BCS) • Luteinizing hormone-releasing hormone agonist (LHRH)

N. Molinas Mandel, MD (✉)
Department of Medical Oncology, Koc University
Medical Faculty, Topkapi/İstanbul, Turkey

Department of Medical Oncology, VKV American
Hospital, Güzelbahce Sokak, Nısantas, SISLI,
Istanbul, Turkey
e-mail: nmmandel@gmail.com

F. Selcukbiricik, MD
Department of Medical Oncology,
Koc University Medical Faculty,
Topkapi/İstanbul, Turkey

© Springer International Publishing Switzerland 2016
A. Aydiner et al. (eds.), *Breast Disease: Management and Therapies*,
DOI 10.1007/978-3-319-26012-9_14

Introduction

Until recently, conventional treatment of estrogen receptor (ER)-/progesterone receptor (PgR)-positive breast cancer patients, particularly in postmenopausal women, consisted of surgery, adjuvant endocrine therapy, radiation therapy, and/or chemotherapy depending on the tumor stage [1]. However, in practice, chemotherapy can lead to additional toxicity in postmenopausal elderly patients. Consequently, different treatment modalities have been developed [2]. One of these is neoadjuvant hormonal therapy (NHT) or neoadjuvant chemotherapy. Neoadjuvant therapy is administered prior to surgery to reduce the size of the tumor and to make an inoperable tumor operable or to allow breast-conserving surgery (BCS) [3]. Tamoxifen, which is a selective estrogen-receptor modulator, has been used as an adjuvant therapy for early breast cancer as well as metastatic disease. Recent studies have demonstrated that tamoxifen can also be used for neoadjuvant purposes [3, 4]. Aromatase inhibitors (AIs) have become the main focus for NHT in postmenopausal patients [5].

Neoadjuvant treatment approaches continue to be applied in the treatment of breast cancer. The use of neoadjuvant hormonal therapy (NHT) was widely accepted at the 13th St Gallen International Breast Cancer Conference [6]. The general purposes of neoadjuvant treatments in breast cancer include making inoperable large tumors operable, increasing the probability of breast-conserving surgery (BCS), obtaining high antitumoral efficiency benefits, and prolonging general survival and the time until progression. While neoadjuvant treatment may be performed with classical chemotherapy agents, it may also be performed with hormonal therapy in hormone receptor-positive patients. The efficiency of NHT continues to be investigated [7]. The aims of neoadjuvant hormonal therapy include reducing the size of breast tumors, maintaining efficient control through early-onset systematic treatment, enabling resection, and increasing the responsiveness of tumor cells to the administered systematic treatment. However, NHT may induce the development of resistance to systematic treatments at an early stage. In addition, the administration of NHT delays surgery, and the condition of the axilla may be obscure unless tissue biopsy is available. NHT is administered as tamoxifen, letrozole, anastrozole, exemestane, and other hormonal treatments.

Various assessments of NHT have been conducted, including 13 single-arm studies [8], four studies involving aromatase inhibitors (AIs) versus tamoxifen [3], five studies comparing AIs [3], and four studies of NHT and neoadjuvant chemotherapy (NCT) [8]. In addition, a comprehensive systematic review of NHT has just been published [8]. In these studies, the clinical response rate (RR) was 13.5–110 %, and the duration of treatment was 3–24 months. NHT studies began in the 1990s with the administration of tamoxifen. However, preliminary studies demonstrated that tamoxifen could not sufficiently control the tumors [9]. A subsequent study demonstrated that neoadjuvant tamoxifen treatment reduced the need for surgery [10]. In addition, in an attempt to assess responsiveness, studies were conducted with tamoxifen+AIs in addition to studies with tamoxifen treatment alone. Patient responsiveness was assessed by breast ultrasonography, mammography, and breast examination.

A total of 171 postmenopausal hormone receptor-positive patients were included in the Edinburgh study. The study was designed to include extended resection ($n=35$), tamoxifen ($n=65$), letrozole ($n=36$), anastrozole ($n=23$), and exemestane ($n=12$) [11]. The study revealed that the RR of patients who received AIs was high. Instead of radical mastectomy, patients underwent BCS (Table 14.1). In this study, they received treatment with 2.5 and 10 mg of letrozole and 1 and 10 mg of anastrozole. No improvement in RR was observed for the 10-mg dose in patients who received AIs. In addition, patients who received AIs exhibited a better RR than patients who received 20 mg of tamoxifen. RRs were 81 % with letrozole, 87 % with anastrozole, and 48 % with tamoxifen.

The Bergonie study also examined NHT. In this study, postmenopausal patients 50–70 years of age were evaluated, and neoadjuvant tamoxifen treatment was assessed. Of the 199 patients who

Table 14.1 Neoadjuvant hormonal therapy (Edinburgh study) [11]

Drug	Number of patients	Mastectomy at onset	Surgery after neoadjuvant	Rate of breast conservation (%)
Tamoxifen	65	41	15	63
Letrozole	36	24	2	93
Anastrozole	24	19	2	89
Exemestane	12	10	2	80

received neoadjuvant tamoxifen, 97 had operable tumors (T2–T3, N0/1), and 102 patients had T4 tumors. During follow-up for a median treatment duration of 5.3 months, 92 % of T2-T3 (89 patients) and 91 % of T4 (93 patients) patients underwent surgery. The BCS rates in the T2–T3 and T4 groups were 53.6 %, and 44 %, respectively. General survival was assessed in the 83rd month. The results of this study indicated that NHT is administrable [12].

NHT was examined in the French Exemestane Study. In this phase II study, postmenopausal patients with hormone receptor-positive and T2–T4 tumors (locally advanced) were administered 25 mg/day exemestane as a neoadjuvant for 16 weeks. For patients who received neoadjuvant exemestane, the RR was 73.3 %, while the BCS rate was 57.1 %. In this study, exemestane reduced Ki-67 expression and PgR expression. The significant decrease in PgR expression was correlated with the clinical response. No relationship between the generated response and aromatase mRNA or ER-beta expression was observed. These results indicated that exemestane features efficiency and safety profiles as a neoadjuvant therapy [13]. The first phase III clinical study of NHT is that conducted by Eiermann et al. In the PO-24 letrozole efficiency study, letrozole and tamoxifen were compared as NHTs [14]. In this study, the clinical response rate was significant in the letrozole arm based on the palpation ($p < 0.001$), ultrasonography ($p < 0.042$), and mammography ($p < 0.001$). The letrozole arm was significant in the ER-positive and HER-2-positive arms. In the IMPACT (Immediate Preoperative Arimidex Compared with Tamoxifen) study, anastrozole+tamoxifen was compared with anastrozole or tamoxifen alone [15]. A total of 337 patients were enrolled in the study. The drugs were used as a preoperative treatment for 12 weeks.

In this study, although the RRs were the same in all groups, BCS was more performable in the anastrozole group. Again in this study, the RR for anastrozole was significant in the HER-2-positive patients. This study concluded that anastrozole is applicable as an NHT.

This trial did not observe a superior effect of the combination treatment. The RR and BCS rates were 37 % and 44 %, respectively, in the anastrozole arm, but 36 % and 21 %, respectively, in the tamoxifen arm. The differences between the two arms were not significant. In addition, there was no difference according to HER-2 status.

In the PROACT (Preoperative Arimidex Compared to Tamoxifen) study, anastrozole was compared with tamoxifen, and the efficiency of anastrozole was assessed by ultrasonography [16]. A summary of phase III studies assessing NHT is presented in Table 14.2.

In the PROACT study, 451 postmenopausal locally advanced breast cancer patients were enrolled. The patients were randomized to anastrozole and tamoxifen arms for 3 months. The RRs and BCS rates were 39.5 % and 38 %, respectively, in the anastrozole arm, but 35.4 % and 29.9 %, respectively, in the tamoxifen arm. The differences between the two arms were not significant.

While there are no data from the Edinburgh Study related to the assessment of local relapse after NHT, in another study, 112 patients were administered BCS after NHT. The median follow-up was 62 months, and during the relapse assessment in the fifth year of follow-up, no difference was observed between tamoxifen and AIs [5]. In another study, preoperational and postoperational NHT was assessed, and no significant difference was observed between anastrozole and letrozole [17].

In postmenopausal cases, the optimal NHT duration is >3–4 months [5]. In the St Gallen

Table 14.2 Summary of phase III studies assessing neoadjuvant hormonal therapy

	Letrozole 024 [14]	IMPACT [15]	PROACT [16]
Number (*n*)	337	330	451
Patient characteristic	BCS not appropriate (14 % inoperable)	96 appropriate BCS	Inoperable
Duration	4 months	12 weeks	3 months
Response oRR	55 % L vs. 35 % T (*p*<0.001)	37 % A vs. 24 % AT vs. 31 % T *p*>0.05	43 % A vs. 30.8 % T *p*>0.05
BCS	45 % L vs. 35 % T (*p*<0.022)	%44 A vs. %24 AT vs. %31 T *p*>0.05	43 % A vs. 30.8 % T *p*>0.05

BCS breast-conserving surgery

Consensus Panel, for postmenopausal patients with strong hormone-receptor positivity and low-proliferating disease, the authors advised hormonal therapy alone as a neoadjuvant treatment. Moreover, the general consensus was that this treatment should be continued until the maximal response was achieved [6].

Response assessments at 0–3 months, 3–6 months, and 6–12 months for cases in which the patients received postmenopausal NHT revealed that the size of the tumor was reduced in each stage. In a phase II study [13], the objective median response was determined to be 3.9 months, and the maximum RR was determined to be 4.2 months. In these studies, the histological subtype was generally reported to be invasive ductal and lobular breast cancer [18–20].

Studies involving NHT have also been conducted in premenopausal patients [21]. Thirteen estrogen receptor-positive premenopausal patients were administered NHT and goserelin, and a response was obtained in seven of these cases. Thirty-two patients were included in another premenopausal NHT study. Patients were administered LHRH analogs and letrozole treatment. While pathological complete response was obtained in one patient, clinical partial response was observed in 15 cases. As a result, this treatment modality may be administered in select clinical cases; however, comprehensive clinical studies are required [22]. In a study by Masuda et al., premenopausal patients were administered ovarian ablation with goserelin and received anastrozole or tamoxifen. A significant clinical response was obtained in patients who received anastrozole [23].

In another study, researchers used exemestane, anastrozole, and letrozole in NHT [24]. In this study, the RR was 74.8 % in the letrozole arm, but 62.9 % and 69.1 % in the exemestane and anastrozole arms, respectively. There was no significant difference in BCS rates among these three groups.

A comprehensive study comparing NHT and NCT [25] demonstrated that NHT provides effective RRs at least as often as NCT. Moreover, the administration rate of BCS in the arm that received NHT was higher. In another study of 95 patients, NHT provided a better RR compared to NCT (*p*=0.075) [26].

In the ACOSOG Z1031 study, 377 patients were enrolled with clinical stage II/III and strongly ER-positive (Allred score 6–8) disease. The patients were randomized into three arms, letrozole, anastrozole, and exemestane. The RRs were 70.9 %, 66.7 %, and 60.5 %, respectively. There were no differences between the arms. Marker panel studies were also performed in this study.

A randomized study compared NHT to neoadjuvant chemotherapy in postmenopausal hormone receptor-positive breast cancer patients. In the study, preoperative four-cycle chemotherapy and 12 weeks of anastrozole and exemestane were compared [25]. The RRs were 63.4 % and 64.5 %, respectively. The BCS rates were 24 % and 33 %, respectively. There was no difference between the arms. By contrast, the toxicity of neoadjuvant chemotherapy was greater than that of NHT [26].

Finally, the first report of a clinicopathological analysis of a neoadjuvant treatment phase in NEOS was also noted in a report presented at the 2014 San Antonia Breast Cancer annual meeting as the New primary Endocrine-therapy Origination Study (NEOS: N-SAS BC06 study: UMIN 000001090). The trial was conducted in a randomized controlled manner to verify the necessity of adjuvant chemotherapy in node-negative, *ER+*, and *HER2−* postmenopausal breast cancer patients who responded to neoadjuvant endocrine therapy. The trial has demonstrated that neoadjuvant letrozole therapy improves breast-conserving surgery rates. MRI was useful for predicting the residual pathological invasive tumor size. PgR positivity and small tumor size at baseline were significant independent predictors of clinical response.

There are two ongoing clinical trials: the Alliance A011106, ALTernate approaches for clinical stage II or III Estrogen Receptor positive breast cancer NeoAdjuvant TrEatment (*ALTERNATE*) in postmenopausal women: A phase III study; and a prospective multicenter study evaluating the effect of impaired tamoxifen metabolism on efficacy in breast cancer patients receiving tamoxifen in the neoadjuvant or metastatic setting – The *CYPTAM-BRUT 2* trial. These studies will soon open up new horizons in neoadjuvant endocrine treatment for breast cancer.

Neoadjuvant endocrine therapy is not recommended in premenopausal patients. There have been no studies of the administration of NHT to premenopausal patients, except case reports [27].

As a result, NHT is safe, and BCS does not increase local relapse. Particularly in elderly patients, NHT is a good alternative that may provide high response and BCS rates. A better response has been observed with AIs. According to the St Gallen recommendations [1], NHT may be administered in postmenopausal patients if ER is *>50 %*, and treatment with AIs may be continued until the maximal response is obtained.

References

1. Fisher B, Redmond C, Fisher ER, Bauer M, Wolmark N, Wickerham DL, et al. Ten-year results of a randomized clinical trial comparing radical mastectomy and total mastectomy with or without radiation. N Engl J Med. 1985;312:674–81.

2. Silliman RA. What constitutes optimal care for older women with breast cancer? J Clin Oncol. 2003; 21:3554–6.

3. Krainick-Strobel UE, Lichtenegger W, Wallwiener D, Tulusan AH, Jänicke F, Bastert G, et al. Neoadjuvant letrozole in postmenopausal estrogen and/or progesterone receptor positive breast cancer: a phase IIb/III trial to investigate optimal duration of preoperative endocrine therapy. BMC Cancer. 2008;26(8):62.

4. Mustacchi G, Milani S, Pluchinotta A, De Matteis A, Rubagotti A, Perrota A, et al. Tamoxifen or surgery plus tamoxifen as primary treatment for elderly patients with operable breast cancer: the G.R.E.T.A. Trial. Group for research on endocrine therapy in the elderly. Anticancer Res. 1994;14:2197–200.

5. Buzdar A, Howell A. Advances in aromatase inhibition: clinical efficacy and tolerability in the treatment of breast cancer. Clin Cancer Res. 2001;7:2620–35.

6. Goldhirsh A, Winer EP, Coates AS, Gelber RD, Piccart-Gebhart M, Thürlimann B, et al. Personalizing the treatment of women with early breast cancer: highlights of the St Gallen International Expert Consensus on the Primary Therapy of Early Breast Cancer. Ann Oncol. 2013;24(9):2206–23.

7. Powles TJ, Hickish TF, Makris A, Ashley SE, O'Brien ME, Tidy VA, et al. Randomized trial of chemoendocrine therapy started before or after surgery for treatment of primary breast cancer. J Clin Oncol. 1995;13(3):547–52.

8. Charehbili A, Fontein DB, Kroep JR, Liefers GJ, Mieog JS, Nortier JW, et al. Neoadjuvant hormonal therapy for endocrine sensitive breast cancer: a systematic review. Cancer Treat Rev. 2014;40(1):86–92.

9. Horobin JM, Preece PE, Dewar JA, Wood RA, Cuschieri A. Long-term follow-up of elderly patients with locoregional breast cancer treated with tamoxifen only. Br J Surg. 1991;78(2):213–7.

10. Dixon JM, Love CD, Bellamy CO, Cameron DA, Leonard RC, Smith H, et al. Letrozole as primary medical therapy for locally advanced and large operable breast cancer. Breast Cancer Res Treat. 2001;66(3):191–9.

11. Dixon JM, Anderson TJ, Miller WR. Neoadjuvant endocrine therapy of breast cancer: a surgical perspective. Eur J Cancer. 2002;38(17):2214–21.

12. Mauriac L, Debled M, Durand M, Floquet A, Boulanger V, Dagada C, et al. Neoadjuvant tamoxifen for hormone-sensitive non-metastatic breast carcinomas in early postmenopausal women. Ann Oncol. 2002;13(2):293–8.

13. Tubiana-Hulin M, Becette V, Bieche I, Mauriac L, Romieu G, Bibeau F, et al. Exemestane as neoadjuvant hormonotherapy for locally advanced breast cancer: results of a phase II trial. Anticancer Res. 2007;27(4C):2689–96.

14. Eiermann W, Paepke S, Appfelstaedt J, Llombart-Cussac A, Eremin J, Vinholes J, et al. Preoperative treatment of postmenopausal breast cancer patients with letrozole: a randomized double blind multicenter study. Ann Oncol. 2001;2(11):1527–32.

15. Smith IE, Dowsett M, Ebbs SR, Dixon JM, Skene A, Blohmer JU, et al. Neoadjuvant treatment of postmenopausal breast cancer with anastrozole, tamoxifen, or both in combination: the immediate preoperative anastrozole, tamoxifen, or combined with tamoxifen (IMPACT) multicenter double-blind randomized trial. J Clin Oncol. 2005;23(22): 5108–16.

16. Cataliotti L, Buzdar AU, Noguchi S, Bines J, Takatsuka Y, Petrakova K, et al. Comparison of anastrozole versus tamoxifen as preoperative therapy in postmenopausal women with hormone receptor-positive breast cancer: the pre-operative "Arimidex" Compared to Tamoxifen (PROACT) trial. Cancer. 2006;106(10):2095–103.

17. Murray J, Young OE, Renshaw L, White S, Williams L, Evans DB, et al. A randomised study of the effects of letrozole and anastrozole on oestrogen receptor positive breast cancers in postmenopausal women. Breast Cancer Res Treat. 2009;114(3):495–501.

18. Hille U, Soergel P, Langer F, Schippert C, Makowski L, Hillemanns P. Aromatase inhibitors as solely treatment in postmenopausal breast cancer patients. Breast J. 2012;18(2):145–50.

19. Dixon JM, Renshaw L, Dixon J, Thomas J. Invasive lobular carcinoma: response to neoadjuvant letrozole therapy. Breast Cancer Res Treat. 2011;130(3):871–7.

20. Olson Jr JA, Budd GT, Carey LA, Harris LA, Esserman LJ, Fleming GF, et al. Improved surgical outcomes for breast cancer patients receiving neoadjuvant aromatase inhibitor therapy: results from a multicenter phase II trial. J Am Coll Surg. 2009;208(5):906–14.

21. Gazet JC, Ford HT, Gray R, McConkey C, Sutcliffe R, Quilliam J, Makinde V, et al. Estrogen-receptor-directed neoadjuvant therapy for breast cancer: results of a randomised trial using formestane and methotrexate, mitozantrone and mitomycin C (MMM) chemotherapy. Ann Oncol. 2001;12(5):685–91.

22. Torrisi R, Bagnardi V, Pruneri G, Ghisini R, Bottiglieri L, Magni E, et al. Antitumour and biological effects of letrozole and GnRH analogue as primary therapy in premenopausal women with ER and PgR positive locally advanced operable breast cancer. Br J Cancer. 2007;97(6):802–8.

23. Masuda N, Sagara Y, Kinoshita T, Iwata H, Nakamura S, Yanagita Y, et al. Neoadjuvant anastrozole versus tamoxifen in patients receiving goserelin for premenopausal breast cancer (STAGE): a double-blind, randomised phase 3 trial. Lancet Oncol. 2012;13(4): 345–52.

24. Ellis MJ, Suman VJ, Hoog J, Lin L, Snider J, Prat A, et al. Randomized phase II neoadjuvant comparison between letrozole, anastrozole, and exemestane for postmenopausal women with estrogen receptor-rich stage 2–3 breast cancer: clinical and biomarker outcomes and predictive value of the baseline PAM50-based intrinsic subtype – ACOSOG Z1031. J Clin Oncol. 2011;29(17):2342–9.

25. Semiglazov VF, Semiglazov VV, Dashyan GA, Ziltsova EK, Ivanov VG, Bozhok AA, et al. Phase 2 randomized trial of primary endocrine therapy versus chemotherapy in postmenopausal patients with estrogen receptor-positive breast cancer. Cancer. 2007;110(2):244–54.

26. Alba E, Calvo L, Albanell J, De la Haba JR, Arcusa Lanza A, Chacon JI, et al. Chemotherapy (CT) and hormonotherapy (HT) as neoadjuvant treatment in luminal breast cancer patients: results from the GEICAM/2006-03, a multicenter, randomized, phase-II study. Ann Oncol. 2012;23(12):3069–74.

27. Colleoni M, Montagna E. Neoadjuvant therapy for ER-positive breast cancers. Ann Oncol. 2012;23 Suppl 10:x243–8.

Systemic Therapy for Locally Advanced Breast Cancer

15

Serkan Keskin and Adnan Aydiner

Abstract

Neoadjuvant therapy refers to the systemic treatment of breast cancer prior to definitive surgical therapy. Neoadjuvant therapy is administered with the objective of improving surgical outcomes in patients with breast cancer for whom a primary surgical approach is technically not feasible and for patients with operable breast cancer who desire breast conservation but for whom either a mastectomy is required or a partial mastectomy would result in a poor cosmetic outcome. In addition, neoadjuvant chemotherapy is appropriate for patients with HER2-positive or triple-negative breast cancer who are most likely to have a good locoregional response to treatment, regardless of the size of their breast cancer at presentation.

Keywords

Neoadjuvant chemotherapy • Locally advanced • Breast cancer

Introduction

Neoadjuvant therapy refers to the systemic treatment of breast cancer prior to definitive surgical therapy (i.e., preoperative therapy). Locally advanced breast cancer (LABC) has always

S. Keskin, MD
Department of Medical Oncology, Memorial Hospital, Istanbul, Turkey

A. Aydiner, MD (✉)
Department of Medical Oncology, Istanbul University Istanbul Medical Faculty, Institute of Oncology, Istanbul, Turkey
e-mail: adnanaydiner@superonline.com

included a heterogeneous group of presentations. According to the American Joint Committee on Cancer (AJCC) staging system, LABC technically can include a patient with a clinically apparent internal mammary or paraclavicular node as well as the more commonly accepted presentations, which include a primary breast cancer larger than 5 cm, disease fixed to the chest wall or involving the skin, or bulky palpable disease in the axilla. Inflammatory breast cancer can also be called LABC. The approach to LABC has evolved considerably over the years. Surgery and radiation therapy were once the only available treatments, but multimodal approaches that emphasize *systemic therapy* have become the standard of treatment [1–3].

© Springer International Publishing Switzerland 2016
A. Aydiner et al. (eds.), *Breast Disease: Management and Therapies*,
DOI 10.1007/978-3-319-26012-9_15

Conversely, neoadjuvant therapy should be considered for women with large clinical stage IIA, stage IIB, and T3N1M0 tumors who meet the criteria for breast-conserving therapy except tumor size and wish to undergo breast-conserving therapy. Preoperative chemotherapy is not indicated unless invasive breast cancer is confirmed. In the available data from clinical trials of preoperative systemic therapy, pretreatment biopsies have been limited to core-needle biopsy or fine-needle aspiration (FNA) cytology. Therefore, in patients anticipated to receive preoperative systemic therapy, core biopsy of the breast tumor and placement of image-detectable marker(s) should be considered to demarcate the tumor bed for any future (post-chemotherapy) surgical management. Clinically positive axillary lymph nodes should be sampled by FNA or core biopsy, and positive nodes must be removed following preoperative systemic therapy at the time of definitive surgery. Patients with clinically negative axillary lymph nodes should have axillary ultrasound prior to neoadjuvant treatment. For those with clinically suspicious axillary lymph nodes, positive nodes indicated by core biopsy should be removed following neoadjuvant therapy at the time of definitive surgery [4, 5].

The primary objective of neoadjuvant therapy is to improve surgical outcomes in patients for whom a primary surgical approach is technically not feasible and in patients with operable breast cancer who desire breast conservation but for whom either a mastectomy is required or a partial mastectomy would result in a poor cosmetic outcome [6–8].

Neoadjuvant chemotherapy includes the delivery of systemic therapy early in treatment to attempt to reduce subclinical micrometastatic disease and an evaluation of chemotherapy response, reducing local and regional tumor bulk and increasing the likelihood of successful surgical resection. In addition, the appropriateness of the systemic agents chosen can be assessed by following the patient's locoregional clinical response. Neoadjuvant therapy also enables early evaluation of the effectiveness of systemic therapy.

In addition to these clinical objectives, neoadjuvant therapy gives researchers the opportunity to obtain tumor specimens (both fresh and formalin fixed) and blood samples prior to and during preoperative treatment. This enables research aimed at identifying tumor- or patient-specific biomarkers [9].

Although it was hypothesized that overall survival would be improved with earlier initiation of systemic therapy in patients at risk of distant recurrence, clinical studies have not yet demonstrated a mortality benefit for pre- versus postoperative delivery of systemic therapy.

Neoadjuvant therapy is most appropriate for patients likely to have a good locoregional response, regardless of tumor size at presentation, including those with HER2-positive or triple-negative breast cancers (TNBC) [10, 11]. By contrast, patients with HER2-negative, ER-positive breast cancers are *less likely* to have a clinical or pathological complete response (pCR) to neoadjuvant therapy [12].

Patients with HER2-positive cancers have a relatively high rate of pCR to neoadjuvant therapy, particularly if treatment includes a HER2-directed agent. This result has been observed in several clinical trials. For patients with HER2-positive disease who receive trastuzumab as part of their neoadjuvant therapy, pCR is associated with improvements in disease-free and overall survival [13, 14]. For this reason, we recommend the addition of targeted treatment against HER2 to neoadjuvant therapy in these patients.

Rates of pCR to neoadjuvant therapy among TNBC patients range from 27 % to 45 %, while the pCR rate for HER2-negative, hormone receptor-positive patients is generally less than 10 %. However, while TNBC patients who achieve a pCR appear to have a prognosis similar to that of patients with other breast cancer subtypes who achieve a pCR, TNBC patients with more than minimal residual disease at surgery have a much higher risk of early distant disease recurrence [15].

Pretreatment Evaluation

As with all patients presenting with a new diagnosis of breast cancer, histopathological confirmation and an evaluation of receptor status

(ER, PR, and HER2) must be obtained before initiating treatment. Patients should undergo an appropriate initial staging workup prior to neoadjuvant systemic therapy. This workup may include imaging studies to rule out detectable metastatic disease depending upon clinical stage and other characteristics. The detection of metastatic disease would likely alter the overall treatment goals and plan.

Tumor Evaluation

In some patients, preoperative systemic therapy results in a sufficient tumor response that enables breast-conserving therapy. Prior to the start of neoadjuvant therapy, radiopaque clips can be placed in the tumor at the time of diagnostic biopsy or at some other time prior to the initiation of neoadjuvant therapy. Because the aim of neoadjuvant therapy is to shrink the primary tumor, the clip facilitates the planning of locoregional treatment (surgery and radiation therapy) and subsequent pathological assessment of the surgical specimen. In addition to the placement of a clip in the tumor bed, the tumor size should be documented prior to treatment. In most cases, an ultrasound of the breast is sufficient to document tumor size. However, breast MRI is often helpful to evaluate disease extent, including assessing the presence of multicentric disease or invasion of the underlying chest wall [16].

The results of the NSABP B-18 trial demonstrate that breast conservation rates are higher after preoperative systemic therapy [17]. However, preoperative systemic therapy has no demonstrated disease-specific survival advantage over postoperative adjuvant chemotherapy in patients with stage II tumors. NSABP B-27 is a three-arm, randomized, phase III trial of women with invasive breast cancer treated with preoperative systemic therapy with AC (doxorubicin/cyclophosphamide) for four cycles followed by local therapy alone, preoperative AC followed by preoperative docetaxel for four cycles followed by local therapy, or AC followed by local therapy followed by four cycles

of postoperative docetaxel [18]. Results from this study, which involved 2,411 women, documented a higher rate of pCR at the time of local therapy in patients treated preoperatively with four cycles of AC followed by four cycles of docetaxel versus four cycles of preoperative AC. There were no differences in DFS and OS between the preoperative and postoperative groups.

Node Evaluation

For patients with palpable axillary adenopathy, physicians can perform ultrasound-guided FNA and/or core needle biopsy of one or more suspicious nodes prior to neoadjuvant treatment to determine whether the axillary nodes are pathologically involved. If FNA is negative, we suggest a sentinel lymph node biopsy to stage the axilla *prior* to treatment. If FNA is positive, no further evaluation is required. For patients with a clinically negative axillary exam, a sentinel lymph node biopsy can be performed prior to the initiation of neoadjuvant therapy. The results of this procedure may more accurately reflect the status of the axillary nodes if performed before the initiation of neoadjuvant therapy rather than following completion of treatment, although the status of the lymph nodes after neoadjuvant therapy may have greater prognostic significance. If the sentinel lymph node biopsy is negative, no further evaluation is necessary. If the sentinel lymph node biopsy is positive, further treatment will depend on the outcome following neoadjuvant therapy. At some centers, an axillary ultrasound with FNA of any enlarged or otherwise suspicious lymph node(s) is the initial diagnostic exam of choice, even in patients with a clinically negative axillary exam. This is a reasonable alternative.

According to our view, axillary staging after preoperative systemic therapy may include sentinel node biopsy or level I/II dissection. Level I/II dissection should be performed when patients are confirmed as node positive prior to neoadjuvant therapy. False-negative sentinel lymph node biopsy either pre- or post-pCR following chemotherapy may occur in lymph node metastases previously undetected by clinical exam. A sentinel lymph node excision can be considered before administering preoperative systemic therapy because it provides additional information to guide local and systemic treatment decisions. When sentinel lymph node resection is performed after the administration of preoperative systemic therapy, both the pre-chemotherapy clinical and the post-chemotherapy pathological nodal stages must be used to determine the risk of local recurrence. Close communication between members of the multidisciplinary team, including the pathologist, is particularly important when any treatment strategy involving preoperative systemic therapy is planned.

Treatment Options

The options for neoadjuvant treatment include chemotherapy, endocrine therapy, and the incorporation of biological therapy in appropriate patients. Much of the information regarding neoadjuvant therapy comes from trials utilizing chemotherapy, with recent studies assessing the role of biologics. There are limited data regarding the use of neoadjuvant endocrine therapy, and clinical studies have predominantly evaluated only postmenopausal women.

A treatment plan is as follows:

Patients with TNBC should be offered neoadjuvant therapy. These patients have an excellent chance of achieving a clinical and pathological complete response to treatment.

For women with HER2-negative, estrogen-receptor (ER)- and/or progesterone-receptor (PR)-positive breast cancers who are not candidates for initial resection, we suggest neoadjuvant chemotherapy rather than endocrine therapy [19, 20]. While few of these patients will achieve a clinical or pathological complete response, tumor shrinkage may enable surgery for some unresectable patients and breast conservation for some borderline patients. However, those who are medically

unfit for or refuse chemotherapy may be treated with neoadjuvant endocrine therapy.

Patients with HER2-positive breast cancer should be offered neoadjuvant therapy. We recommend the addition of HER2-tatrgeted agents (trastuzumab plus pertuzumab) to neoadjuvant therapy.

Chemotherapy

Several chemotherapy regimens have been studied as preoperative systemic therapy. We believe that the regimens recommended in the adjuvant setting are appropriate for consideration in the preoperative systemic therapy setting [21].

For patients with locally advanced breast cancer, neoadjuvant therapy is associated with high rates of clinical response and a higher likelihood of allowing cosmetically acceptable surgery. However, neoadjuvant therapy does not improve overall survival compared to adjuvant chemotherapy.

The outcomes of neoadjuvant therapy were demonstrated in a 2007 meta-analysis that included data for 5,500 women participating in 1 of 14 trials reported between 1991 and 2001. Compared to adjuvant chemotherapy, neoadjuvant therapy resulted in the following:

- Equivalent overall survival (hazard ratio [HR] 0.98; 95 % CI, 0.87–1.09) and disease-free survival (HR 0.97; 95 % CI, 0.89–1.07)
- A reduction in the likelihood of modified radical mastectomy (HR 0.71; 95 % CI, 0.67–0.75)

Those patients with a documented pCR at surgery had significant improvements in survival compared to patients with residual invasive disease.

The choice of specific chemotherapy drugs and regimens should be based on tumor biology and intrinsic subsets (i.e., triple-negative, estrogen receptor-positive, HER2-positive) [22–24]. There is no reason to assume that regimens administered in the adjuvant setting would be less active when used prior to surgery.

Commonly used regimens for patients with HER2-negative disease include the following:

- AC—neoadjuvant doxorubicin (60 mg/m^2) and cyclophosphamide (600 mg/m^2) (AC) every two (dose-dense) or 3 weeks for four cycles
- AC/taxane—AC followed by docetaxel (100 mg/m^2) every 3 weeks for four cycles
- AC/weekly T—AC followed by weekly paclitaxel (80 mg/m^2) for 12 weeks
- FEC—fluorouracil (600 mg/m^2), epirubicin (100 mg/m^2), and cyclophosphamide (600 mg/m^2) (FEC) every 3 weeks for four cycles
- FAC—fluorouracil (600 mg/m^2), doxorubicin (60 mg/m^2), and cyclophosphamide (600 mg/m^2) (FAC) every 3 weeks for four cycles
- TAC—docetaxel (75 mg/m^2), doxorubicin (50 mg/m^2), and cyclophosphamide (500 mg/m^2) for six cycles

Because a reduction in tumor size to permit surgery is the primary objective of neoadjuvant therapy, all planned treatment should be administered *prior* to definitive surgery, provided there is no evidence of disease progression during treatment.

Anthracycline-Taxane-Based Regimens

Multiple studies have demonstrated that anthracycline-based regimens incorporating a taxane (either concurrently or in sequence with anthracycline-based regimens) are associated with increased response rates in the neoadjuvant setting compared to the use of non-taxane-containing regimens [25]. As an example, in the NSABP B-27 trial, 2,411 patients received four cycles of neoadjuvant AC, after which they were randomly assigned to one of three groups: one group received no further chemotherapy, another group was treated with four cycles of neoadjuvant docetaxel (100 mg/m^2) every 3 weeks, and the third group underwent surgery followed by four cycles of adjuvant docetaxel. Compared to AC alone, the incorporation of docetaxel prior to surgery resulted in the following [18]:

- A higher overall clinical response rate (CRR, 91 % versus 86 %)
- A higher pCR rate (26 % versus 13 %)
- No difference in overall survival (74 % with neoadjuvant AC only and 75 % in the arms containing docetaxel) or disease-free survival at 8 years (disease-free survival, 59 % and 62 %)

Alternative Regimens

Ongoing clinical research is examining whether the addition of non-cross-resistant agents with demonstrated activity in metastatic breast cancer might improve the clinical and pathologic response rates observed with the use of an anthracycline and/or a taxane. However, there is no evidence that this approach improves survival outcomes or response rates. Thus, we suggest not administering additional agents with standard anthracycline- and taxane-based neoadjuvant therapy.

Response-Adjusted Sequential Therapy

Response-adjusted sequential therapy refers to the use of one chemotherapy regimen for a set number of cycles, followed by a clinical assessment of the response and subsequent administration of either the same or a non-cross-resistant chemotherapy regimen based on the observed response to the first regimen. This design allows for an independent evaluation of different drug regimens and the potential to individualize therapy based on the response of a patient's tumor. This approach has been evaluated in a limited number of studies in the neoadjuvant setting and is not recommended outside of a clinical trial.

Endocrine Therapy

At the present time, we restrict the administration of neoadjuvant endocrine therapy to postmenopausal patients who are medically unfit to receive or refuse chemotherapy. However, there is growing interest in studying neoadjuvant endocrine therapy in a broader cohort of postmenopausal patients. However, few studies have evaluated neoadjuvant endocrine therapy in premenopausal women, and none have been performed in the context of a randomized trial. Therefore, a neoadjuvant endocrine therapy approach should be considered investigational as a treatment option for premenopausal women. If a premenopausal woman refuses neoadjuvant therapy, we suggest definitive surgical treatment. Premenopausal women who refuse surgery can also be offered neoadjuvant endocrine therapy, but they should be aware that there is no data regarding the risks and benefits of this approach in this population [26].

Several randomized trials have assessed the value of neoadjuvant endocrine therapy in postmenopausal women with ER-positive breast cancer. These studies have generally compared the rates of objective response and the rates of breast-conserving surgery among treatment with tamoxifen, anastrozole, anastrozole plus tamoxifen, or letrozole. These studies have consistently demonstrated that the use of either anastrozole or letrozole alone provides superior rates of breast-conserving surgery. Preoperative endocrine therapy is usually utilized; an aromatase inhibitor is preferred for the treatment of postmenopausal women with hormone receptor-positive disease [2, 27–30].

Endocrine Therapy Versus Chemotherapy

There is a small body of evidence suggesting that the use of endocrine therapy may be equivalent to chemotherapy in postmenopausal women. However, until more data are available, we recommend chemotherapy for most patients in the neoadjuvant setting.

In a phase II trial, 239 postmenopausal women with hormone receptor-positive stage II–III breast cancer were randomly assigned to neoadjuvant treatment with an aromatase inhibitor (AI) (either exemestane or anastrozole) for 3 months or chemotherapy (four cycles of doxorubicin and paclitaxel every 21 days). There were no differences in overall response rates between exemestane, anastrozole, and chemotherapy (67 %, 62 %, and 63 %, respectively). Compared to chemotherapy, neoadjuvant AI resulted in a similar median time to clinical response (57 versus 51 days) and a similar rate of pCR (3 % versus

6 %). Breast-conserving surgery was performed in 33 % of the patients assigned to an AI compared to 24 % of the patients assigned to chemotherapy.

Duration of Endocrine Therapy

For patients undergoing neoadjuvant endocrine therapy, we continue treatment for at least 3–4 months. If the tumor is amenable to surgery after 3–4 months, we recommend proceeding with definitive surgical treatment. However, if the tumor responds to endocrine therapy, extending treatment to 6 months or longer with clinical monitoring of the response may permit a higher percentage of patients to undergo breast-conserving surgery. If at any time there is evidence of progression or non-response, we recommend surgery. A response to endocrine therapy may not be evident for at least 3–4 months, and a maximal response may not be achieved until much later. Thus, the duration of endocrine treatment prior to surgery must be individualized based on the patient's clinical status and the clinical response.

HER2-Directed Therapy

The benefit of adding trastuzumab to chemotherapy was demonstrated in a pooled analysis of two randomized studies that evaluated neoadjuvant therapy with or without trastuzumab [31]. The addition of trastuzumab to chemotherapy resulted in the following:

- An improvement in the rate of pCR (43 % versus 20 %; relative risk for achieving pCR [RR] 2.07; 95 % CI, 1.41–3.03)
- A reduction in the relapse rate (26 % versus 39 %; RR for relapse 0.67; 95 % CI, 0.48–0.94)
- A trend toward a lower mortality rate (13 % versus 20 %; RR for mortality 0.67; 95 % CI, 0.39–1.15) that did not reach statistical significance

The GeparQuinto phase III trial led by the German Breast Group studied 620 women who were randomized to receive four cycles of epirubicin/cyclophosphamide followed by docetaxel administered concurrently with either trastuzumab or lapatinib [32]. The primary endpoint, pCR, was achieved in 30.3 % of patients who received trastuzumab plus chemotherapy compared with 22.7 % of patients who received lapatinib plus chemotherapy [33, 34].

The NeoALTTO trial randomized 455 patients with HER2-positive primary breast cancer to receive lapatinib plus paclitaxel, trastuzumab plus paclitaxel, or a combination of lapatinib and trastuzumab plus paclitaxel [35]. The pCR rate was 51.3 % (95 % CI, 43.1–59.5) in the lapatinib plus trastuzumab combination arm, 24.7 % (CI, 18.1–32.3) in the lapatinib arm, and 29.5 % (CI, 22.4–37.5) in the trastuzumab arm. The difference in pCR rates between the lapatinib plus trastuzumab arm and the trastuzumab arm was statistically significant (difference 21.1 %, 9.1–34.2, $p = 0.0001$). The difference in pCR rates between the lapatinib and trastuzumab arms was not statistically significant (difference −4.8 %, −17.6–8.2; $p = 0.34$). Grade 3/4 liver enzyme abnormalities occurred more frequently with trastuzumab plus lapatinib or lapatinib alone compared to trastuzumab alone.

These studies thus confirm that the use of HER2-targeted therapy is important in the preoperative treatment of HER2-positive primary breast cancer. There remains significant uncertainty regarding the optimal regimen of HER2 targeting. The results of the NeoALTTO study confirm the potential of dual HER2-targeted therapy in the neoadjuvant setting.

For patients with HER2-positive breast cancer who are candidates for neoadjuvant therapy, we do not recommend administering lapatinib in place of trastuzumab. Multiple randomized studies have reported similar or inferior pCR rates when lapatinib is substituted for trastuzumab.

Pertuzumab is a recombinant, humanized, monoclonal antibody that inhibits the ligand-dependent dimerization of HER2 and its downstream signaling. Pertuzumab and trastuzumab bind to different epitopes of the HER2 receptor and have complementary mechanisms of action. When administered together in HER2-positive tumor models and in humans, pertuzumab and trastuzumab provide a greater overall antitumor effect than either alone. Because the combination of pertuzumab and trastuzumab exhibited a significant overall survival benefit in a metastatic setting, it has also been examined in the neoadjuvant setting.

The combination of trastuzumab plus pertuzumab was evaluated in the neoadjuvant setting with responses noted even without the use of chemotherapy. These results are fascinating not only because of the higher pCR rate associated with chemotherapy plus trastuzumab and pertuzumab but also because of the frequency of pCR associated with dual HER2-targeted therapy alone, particularly in patients with ER-negative disease.

The FDA recently granted accelerated approval for pertuzumab in combination with trastuzumab and docetaxel as a neoadjuvant treatment for patients with HER2-positive, early-stage breast cancer, including patients with tumors greater than 2 cm in diameter (≥T2) or who are node positive (≥N1). The accelerated approval was based on the results of two phase II trials, the NeoSphere trial and the TRYPHAENA study, that observed significant improvements in pCR in patients receiving pertuzumab, trastuzumab, and docetaxel [36, 37].

In the NeoSphere trial, 417 patients were randomized 1:1:1:1 to receive trastuzumab plus docetaxel, pertuzumab and trastuzumab plus docetaxel, pertuzumab and trastuzumab, or pertuzumab plus docetaxel [36]. Of the patients who received pertuzumab plus trastuzumab and docetaxel, 45.8 % [95 % CI, 36.1–55.7] achieved pCR, compared with only 29 % [CI, 20.6–38.5] of patients who received the trastuzumab plus docetaxel regimen ($p = 0.0063$).

TRYPHAENA was a phase II, randomized, multicenter trial designed to evaluate the safety and tolerability of trastuzumab and pertuzumab in combination with anthracycline- or carboplatin-based neoadjuvant chemotherapy [37]. A total of 225 patients with HER2-positive, locally advanced (T2-3, N2-3, M0; T4a-c, any N, M0), inflammatory (T4d, any N, M0), or early-stage breast cancer (tumors >2 cm) were enrolled and randomized 1:1:1 to receive six cycles of neoadjuvant therapy with FEC plus trastuzumab and pertuzumab followed by docetaxel, trastuzumab, and pertuzumab; FEC followed by docetaxel, trastuzumab, and pertuzumab; or docetaxel, carboplatin, and trastuzumab along with pertuzumab. Based on pCR assessment, all three regimens appear to be active. The reported pCR ranged from 57.3 % to 66.2 %. The highest pCR, 66.2 %, was observed in patients who received pertuzumab, trastuzumab, docetaxel, and carboplatin chemotherapy.

Treatment Evaluation

Patients receiving neoadjuvant systemic therapy should be followed by clinical exam at regular intervals during treatment to ensure that the disease is not progressing. At the end of treatment, an assessment of tumor response is important to help guide the surgical approach.

Clinical Response Assessment During Treatment

Patients undergoing neoadjuvant systemic therapy for breast cancer should undergo periodic clinical evaluations during treatment to assess response and ensure that their tumor is not progressing.

There are no formal guidelines regarding the ideal assessment strategy during neoadjuvant treatment. Our approach is as follows:

• For patients on neoadjuvant therapy, we perform a clinical examination every 2–4 weeks (i.e., prior to each cycle of treatment). This should include evaluation of the affected breast and ipsilateral axilla.
• For patients undergoing neoadjuvant endocrine therapy, we perform clinical evaluations every 4–8 weeks. The response to treatment is expected to take a longer time to become evident.
• Imaging studies (ultrasound [US] or magnetic resonance imaging [MRI]) should only be performed if disease progression is suspected based on clinical exam.

• Limited data suggest that fluoro-2-deoxyglucose positron emission tomography (FDG-PET) may have a sensitivity and specificity as high as 80 %, but there are insufficient prospective data to evaluate the ability of FDG-PET to accurately predict the response to neoadjuvant therapy.
• There is no role for repeat biopsy of the index tumor during neoadjuvant treatment unless performed as part of a clinical trial. Although repeat measurement of biological factors (such as Ki-67) may identify patients who are unlikely to respond to neoadjuvant endocrine therapy, validation of such tests is needed before repeat pathological assessment during treatment is incorporated into clinical practice.

Clinical Response Assessment After Treatment

Once a patient has completed neoadjuvant therapy (typically six to eight cycles of chemotherapy or 3–4 months of endocrine therapy), an assessment of tumor response helps guide the surgical approach. Tumor size is typically assessed using World Health Organization-International Union against Cancer (WHO-UICC) or Response Evaluation Criteria in Solid Tumors (RECIST) criteria. However, the correlation between tumor measurements by physical examination, imaging (mammography, US, or MRI), and tumor size on final pathological analysis is modest at best, as illustrated in the following examples:

• A 2010 meta-analysis of 25 studies involving a total of 1,212 patients receiving neoadjuvant therapy concluded that while contrast-enhanced MRI has high specificity (91 %), its sensitivity to predict pCR is low (63 %) [38].
• In another study involving 189 patients, the reported accuracy (defined as the ability to predict the greatest tumor dimension within 1 cm) of clinical exam, US, and mammography were 66 %, 75 %, and 70 %, respectively, compared with findings at final pathological analysis [39].

The lack of concordance between the clinical and pathologic assessments of response may be due to the variable patterns of tumor response to neoadjuvant treatment, which range from symmetric shrinkage around a central core (that may contain residual cancer or fibrotic tissue) to the complete resolution of a discrete mass despite the persistence of microscopic foci of residual invasive cancer.

Local therapy following a complete or partial response to preoperative systemic therapy is usually a lumpectomy if possible along with surgical axillary staging. If a lumpectomy is not possible or progressive disease is confirmed, mastectomy is performed along with surgical axillary staging with or without breast reconstruction. Surgical axillary staging may include sentinel lymph node biopsy or level I/II dissection. If a sentinel lymph node biopsy is performed before administering preoperative systemic therapy and the findings are negative, then further axillary lymph node staging is not necessary. If a sentinel lymph node procedure is performed before administering preoperative systemic therapy and the findings are positive, then a level I/II axillary lymph nodes dissection should be performed.

If an inoperable tumor fails to respond, if the response is minimal after several cycles of preoperative systemic therapy, or if the disease progresses at any point, an alternative chemotherapy regimen and/or preoperative radiation therapy should be considered followed by local therapy, usually a mastectomy plus axillary dissection, with or without breast reconstruction.

Postsurgical adjuvant treatment for these patients consists of the completion of planned chemotherapy if not completed preoperatively followed by endocrine therapy in women with ER- and/or PR-positive tumors. Up to 1 year of trastuzumab therapy should be completed if the tumor is HER2-positive.

chemotherapy in patients receiving neoadjuvant treatment can increase pCR rates, it is not clear which patients are most likely to benefit from this approach [40]. Given that the benefits are unclear but the risks can be quite serious, bevacizumab should not be used as part of neoadjuvant therapy outside of a well-designed clinical trial.

The evidence to support this conclusion comes from four trials.

In one German trial (GeparQuinto), the pCR rate with the addition of bevacizumab was significantly higher only in patients with hormone receptor-negative disease [41]. However, in an American trial (NSABP B-40), hormone receptor-positive patients had a significant improvement in pCR with incorporation of bevacizumab [42].

In the TNBC study conducted by CALGB (CALGB 40603), a significant increase in the pCR rate within the breast was observed in women who received bevacizumab; however, if the pCR definition included the axilla, the improvement in the pCR rate was not statistically significant [43].

In all of these studies, bevacizumab resulted in higher rates of serious (grade 3/4) toxicities, including febrile neutropenia, hypertension, and mucositis. Higher rates of bleeding, thromboembolic events, and postsurgical complications (early and late) were also observed with bevacizumab therapy and are all known complications of the drug.

Finally, none of these studies reported whether the pCR rate with bevacizumab improves survival outcomes. Taken together, these data illustrate that the benefits of adding bevacizumab to neoadjuvant therapy are unclear at best and do not justify the risks of toxicity. We therefore do not administer bevacizumab as part of neoadjuvant therapy unless it is within a well-designed clinical trial.

Novel Approaches

Incorporation of Angiogenesis Inhibitors

Although studies suggest that the addition of the angiogenesis inhibitor bevacizumab to

Incorporation of a PARP Inhibitor

Mutations that result in dysfunction of either the BRCA1 or BRCA2 gene predispose patients to the development of breast cancers with deficiencies in DNA repair. This appears to confer sensitivity to chemotherapeutic agents that damage DNA, such as platinum analogs, and to agents that affect alternative mechanisms of DNA repair, such as poly ADP ribose polymerase (PARP) inhibitors. Similarities in tumor characteristics and gene expression patterns between BRCA-associated and sporadic TNBC led to speculation that the addition of these same agents might improve responses in TNBC, including in the neoadjuvant setting.

In the Investigation of Serial Studies to Predict Your Therapeutic Response with Imaging and Molecular Analysis 2 (I-SPY 2) trial, one arm evaluated standard chemotherapy (dose-dense AC/weekly T) with or without the oral PARP inhibitor veliparib. As presented at the 2013 San Antonio Breast Cancer Symposium, patients with TNBC who received carboplatin and veliparib as part of their treatment achieved a higher pCR rate (52 % versus 26 % in those who did not receive veliparib) [44]. However, whether the improvement in pCR was due to carboplatin, veliparib, or the combination cannot be determined. Thus, we do not administer this agent or other PARP inhibitors in the neoadjuvant setting outside of a clinical trial. Data from studies investigating the addition of carboplatin to neoadjuvant therapy for TNBC are discussed above.

Prognosis

The prognosis of patients with breast cancer who undergo neoadjuvant therapy correlates with the pathological response observed at the time of surgery but is also influenced by presenting clinical stage and tumor characteristics (particularly hormone receptor and HER2 status). As described above, clinical response is not an accurate predictor of pathological response, and achieving a pCR in the breast and axilla is a better predictor of survival than a clinical complete response.

The prognostic significance of pCR on survival endpoints has been evaluated in several meta-analyses [45, 46]. The largest of these was conducted by the Collaborative Trials in Neoadjuvant Breast Cancer (CTNeoBC) working group and included 12 randomized trials and nearly 12,000 patients [45]. Their major findings were as follows:

- Patients who achieved pCR had significant improvements in event-free survival (hazard ratio [HR] 0.48, $p < 0.001$) and overall survival ([OS] HR 0.36, $p < 0.001$) compared to patients who did not achieve pCR.
- The inclusion of patients with residual ductal carcinoma in situ (DCIS) only (ypT0/is, ypN0) did not diminish the benefit of achieving pCR for event-free survival and overall survival. However, the inclusion of patients with residual axillary nodal involvement in the definition of pCR reduced its prognostic value for both event-free survival and overall survival.

pCR rates and improvement in event-free survival for patients who achieved pCR varied by breast cancer subtype:

- Hormone receptor (HR)-positive, HER2-negative, grade 1–2: 8 % (HR for event-free survival 0.63, $p = 0.07$)
- HR-positive, HER2-negative, grade 3: 16 % (HR 0.27, $p < 0.001$)
- HR-positive, HER2-positive (treated with a trastuzumab-containing regimen): 31 % (HR 0.58, $p = 0.001$)
- HR-negative, HER2-negative (triple-negative): 34 % (HR 0.24, $p < 0.001$)
- HR-negative, HER2-positive (treated with a trastuzumab-containing regimen): 50 % (HR 0.25, $p < 0.001$)

Despite these results, the threshold of benefit (defined by an increase in the pCR rate) associated with an improvement in event-free survival and/or overall survival is not clear. The investigators hypothesized that the lack of an association may have been due to the heterogeneous patient populations in many of the studies, the relatively low pCR rates (even in the "superior" treatment arm), and/or the lack of effective targeted agents for many of the patient populations studied.

Several models are being developed to better define the prognosis of patients treated with neoadjuvant therapy. Examples of these include calculation of the residual cancer burden (RCB) score, the breast cancer index (BCI), and, for patients treated specifically with neoadjuvant endocrine therapy, the preoperative endocrine prognostic index (PEPI) score [47, 48].

The RCB takes into account residual tumor size, the percentage of the residual tumor composed of invasive cancer cells (as opposed to fibrosis or in situ disease), the number of positive axillary nodes, and the largest nodal metastatic deposit. In the original analysis, the RCB score correlated with prognosis in patients who received anthracycline- and taxane-containing neoadjuvant therapy regimens.

The measurement of the RCB requires the collection of pathological variables, which are not routinely recorded. In addition, the validation of this prognostic index is limited. Therefore, a further evaluation of the RCB is required before it becomes part of routine practice.

References

1. Hortobagyi GN, Ames FC, Buzdar AU, Kau SW, McNeese MD, Paulus D, et al. Management of stage III primary breast cancer with primary chemotherapy, surgery, and radiation therapy. Cancer. 1988;62: 2507–16.
2. Eiermann W, Paepke S, Appfelstaedt J, Llombart-Cussac A, Eremin J, Vinholes J, et al. Preoperative treatment of postmenopausal breast cancer patients with letrozole: a randomized double-blind multicenter study. Ann Oncol. 2001;12:1527–32.
3. Schwartz GF, Hortobagyi GN. Proceedings of the consensus conference on neoadjuvant chemotherapy in carcinoma of the breast, April 26–28, 2003, Philadelphia, Pennsylvania. Cancer. 2004;100: 2512–32.
4. Lyman GH, Giuliano AE, Somerfield MR, Benson 3rd AB, Bodurka DC, Burstein HJ, et al. American Society of Clinical Oncology guideline recommendations for sentinel lymph node biopsy in early-stage breast cancer. J Clin Oncol. 2005;23:7703–20.
5. Citron ML, Berry DA, Cirrincione C, Hudis C, Winer EP, Gradishar WJ, et al. Randomized trial of dose-dense versus conventionally scheduled and sequential versus concurrent combination chemotherapy as postoperative adjuvant treatment of node-positive primary breast cancer: first report of Intergroup Trial C9741/

Cancer and Leukemia Group B Trial 9741. J Clin Oncol. 2003;21:1431–9.
6. Van der Hage JA, Van de Velde CJ, Julien JP, Tubiana-Hulin M, Vandervelden C, Duchateau L. Preoperative chemotherapy in primary operable breast cancer: results from the European Organization for Research and Treatment of Cancer trial 10902. J Clin Oncol. 2001;19:4224–37.
7. Gralow JR, Burstein HJ, Wood W, Hortobagyi GN, Gianni L, von Minckwitz G, et al. Preoperative therapy in invasive breast cancer: pathologic assessment and systemic therapy issues in operable disease. J Clin Oncol. 2008;26:814–9.
8. Davidson NE, Morrow M. Sometimes a great notion – an assessment of neoadjuvant systemic therapy for breast cancer. J Natl Cancer Inst. 2005;97:159–61.
9. Hayes DF. Targeting adjuvant chemotherapy: a good idea that needs to be proven! J Clin Oncol. 2012;30:1264–7.
10. Coates AS, Colleoni M, Goldhirsch A. Is adjuvant chemotherapy useful for women with luminal a breast cancer? J Clin Oncol. 2012;30:1260–3.
11. Shannon C, Smith I. Is there still a role for neoadjuvant therapy in breast cancer? Crit Rev Oncol Hematol. 2003;45:77–90.
12. Untch M, Fasching PA, Konecny GE, Hasmuller S, Lebeau A, Kreienberg R, et al. Pathologic complete response after neoadjuvant chemotherapy plus trastuzumab predicts favorable survival in human epidermal growth factor receptor 2-overexpressing breast cancer: results from the TECHNO trial of the AGO and GBG study groups. J Clin Oncol. 2011;29:3351–7.
13. Von Minckwitz G, Untch M, Blohmer JU, Costa SD, Eidtmann H, Fasching PA, et al. Definition and impact of pathologic complete response on prognosis after neoadjuvant chemotherapy in various intrinsic breast cancer subtypes. J Clin Oncol. 2012;30:1796–804.
14. Kaufmann M, Hortobagyi GN, Goldhirsch A, Scholl S, Makris A, Valagussa P, et al. Recommendations from an international expert panel on the use of neoadjuvant (primary) systemic treatment of operable breast cancer: an update. J Clin Oncol. 2006;24:1940–9.
15. Carey LA, Dees EC, Sawyer L, Gatti L, Moore DT, Collichio F, et al. The triple negative paradox: primary tumor chemosensitivity of breast cancer subtypes. Clin Cancer Res. 2007;13:2329–34.
16. Jones S, Holmes FA, O'Shaughnessy J, Blum JL, Vukelja SJ, McIntyre KJ, et al. Docetaxel with cyclophosphamide is associated with an overall survival benefit compared with doxorubicin and cyclophosphamide: 7-year follow-up of US Oncology Research Trial 9735. J Clin Oncol. 2009;27:1177–83.
17. Wolmark N, Wang J, Mamounas E, Bryant J, Fisher B. Preoperative chemotherapy in patients with operable breast cancer: nine-year results from National Surgical Adjuvant Breast and Bowel Project B-18. J Natl Cancer Inst Monogr. 2001;30:96–102.
18. Bear HD, Anderson S, Smith RE, Geyer Jr CE, Mamounas EP, Fisher B, et al. Sequential preoperative or postoperative docetaxel added to preoperative

doxorubicin plus cyclophosphamide for operable breast cancer: National Surgical Adjuvant Breast and Bowel Project Protocol B-27. J Clin Oncol. 2006;24:2019–27.

19. Berry DA, Cirrincione C, Henderson IC, Citron ML, Budman DR, Goldstein LJ, et al. Estrogen-receptor status and outcomes of modern chemotherapy for patients with node-positive breast cancer. JAMA. 2006;295:1658–67.

20. Schneeweiss A, Huober J, Sinn HP, von Fournier D, Rudlowski C, Beldermann F, et al. Gemcitabine, epirubicin and docetaxel as primary systemic therapy in patients with early breast cancer: results of a multicentre phase I/II study. Eur J Cancer. 2004;40: 2432–8.

21. Schott AF, Hayes DF. Defining the benefits of neoadjuvant chemotherapy for breast cancer. J Clin Oncol. 2012;30:1747–9.

22. Untch M, Mobus V, Kuhn W, Muck BR, Thomssen C, Bauerfeind I, et al. Intensive dose-dense compared with conventionally scheduled preoperative chemotherapy for high-risk primary breast cancer. J Clin Oncol. 2009;27:2938–45.

23. Smith IC, Heys SD, Hutcheon AW, Miller ID, Payne S, Gilbert FJ, et al. Neoadjuvant chemotherapy in breast cancer: significantly enhanced response with docetaxel. J Clin Oncol. 2002;20:1456–66.

24. Von Minckwitz G, Kummel S, Vogel P, Hanusch C, Eidtmann H, Hilfrich J, et al. Neoadjuvant vinorelbine-capecitabine versus docetaxel-doxorubicin-cyclophosphamide in early nonresponsive breast cancer: phase III randomized GeparTrio trial. J Natl Cancer Inst. 2008;100:542–51.

25. Von Minckwitz G, Rezai M, Loibl S, Fasching PA, Huober J, Tesch H, et al. Capecitabine in addition to anthracycline- and taxane-based neoadjuvant treatment in patients with primary breast cancer: phase III GeparQuattro study. J Clin Oncol. 2010;28:2015–23.

26. Torrisi R, Bagnardi V, Pruneri G, Ghisini R, Bottiglieri L, Magni E, et al. Antitumour and biological effects of letrozole and GnRH analogue as primary therapy in premenopausal women with ER and PgR positive locally advanced operable breast cancer. Br J Cancer. 2007;97:802–8.

27. Alba E, Calvo L, Albanell J, De la Haba JR, Arcusa Lanza A, Chacon JI, et al. Chemotherapy (CT) and hormonotherapy (HT) as neoadjuvant treatment in luminal breast cancer patients: results from the GEICAM/2006-03, a multicenter, randomized, phase-II study. Ann Oncol. 2012;23:3069–74.

28. Cataliotti L, Buzdar AU, Noguchi S, Bines J, Takatsuka Y, Petrakova K, et al. Comparison of anastrozole versus tamoxifen as preoperative therapy in postmenopausal women with hormone receptor-positive breast cancer: the Pre-Operative "Arimidex" Compared to Tamoxifen (PROACT) trial. Cancer. 2006;106:2095–103.

29. Smith IE, Dowsett M, Ebbs SR, Dixon JM, Skene A, Blohmer JU, et al. Neoadjuvant treatment of postmenopausal breast cancer with anastrozole, tamoxifen, or both in combination: the Immediate Preoperative Anastrozole, Tamoxifen, or Combined with Tamoxifen (IMPACT) multicenter double-blind randomized trial. J Clin Oncol. 2005;23:5108–16.

30. Ellis MJ, Suman VJ, Hoog J, Lin L, Snider J, Prat A, et al. Randomized phase II neoadjuvant comparison between letrozole, anastrozole, and exemestane for postmenopausal women with estrogen receptor-rich stage 2 to 3 breast cancer: clinical and biomarker outcomes and predictive value of the baseline PAM50-based intrinsic subtype – ACOSOG Z1031. J Clin Oncol. 2011;29:2342–9.

31. Petrelli F, Borgonovo K, Cabiddu M, Ghilardi M, Barni S. Neoadjuvant chemotherapy and concomitant trastuzumab in breast cancer: a pooled analysis of two randomized trials. Anticancer Drugs. 2011;22:128–35.

32. Untch M, Loibl S, Bischoff J, Eidtmann H, Kaufmann M, Blohmer JU, et al. Lapatinib versus trastuzumab in combination with neoadjuvant anthracycline-taxane-based chemotherapy (GeparQuinto, GBG 44): a randomised phase 3 trial. Lancet Oncol. 2012;13: 135–44.

33. Untch M, Rezai M, Loibl S, Fasching PA, Huober J, Tesch H, et al. Neoadjuvant treatment with trastuzumab in HER2-positive breast cancer: results from the GeparQuattro study. J Clin Oncol. 2010;28: 2024–31.

34. Dieras V, Fumoleau P, Romieu G, Tubiana-Hulin M, Namer M, Mauriac L, et al. Randomized parallel study of doxorubicin plus paclitaxel and doxorubicin plus cyclophosphamide as neoadjuvant treatment of patients with breast cancer. J Clin Oncol. 2004; 22:4958–65.

35. De Azambuja E, Holmes AP, Piccart-Gebhart M, Holmes E, Di Cosimo S, Swaby RF, et al. Lapatinib with trastuzumab for HER2-positive early breast cancer (NeoALTTO): survival outcomes of a randomised, open-label, multicentre, phase 3 trial and their association with pathological complete response. Lancet Oncol. 2014;15:1137–46.

36. Gianni L, Pienkowski T, Im YH, Roman L, Tseng LM, Liu MC, et al. Efficacy and safety of neoadjuvant pertuzumab and trastuzumab in women with locally advanced, inflammatory, or early HER2-positive breast cancer (NeoSphere): a randomised multicentre, open-label, phase 2 trial. Lancet Oncol. 2012;13: 25–32.

37. Schneeweiss A, Chia S, Hickish T, Harvey V, Eniu A, Hegg R, et al. Pertuzumab plus trastuzumab in combination with standard neoadjuvant anthracycline-containing and anthracycline-free chemotherapy regimens in patients with HER2-positive early breast cancer: a randomized phase II cardiac safety study (TRYPHAENA). Ann Oncol. 2013;24:2278–84.

38. Yuan Y, Chen XS, Liu SY, Shen KW. Accuracy of MRI in prediction of pathologic complete remission in breast cancer after preoperative therapy: a meta-analysis. AJR Am J Roentgenol. 2010;195:260–8.

39. Chagpar AB, Middleton LP, Sahin AA, Dempsey P, Buzdar AU, Mirza AN, et al. Accuracy of physical

examination, ultrasonography, and mammography in predicting residual pathologic tumor size in patients treated with neoadjuvant chemotherapy. Ann Surg. 2006;243:257–64.

40. von Minckwitz G, Eidtmann H, Rezai M, Fasching PA, Tesch H, Eggemann H, et al. Neoadjuvant chemotherapy and bevacizumab for HER2-negative breast cancer. N Engl J Med. 2012;366:299–309.

41. Gerber B, von Minckwitz G, Eidtmann H, Rezai M, Fasching P, Tesch H, et al. Surgical outcome after neoadjuvant chemotherapy and bevacizumab: results from the GeparQuinto study (GBG 44). Ann Surg Oncol. 2014;21:2517–24.

42. Bear HD, Tang G, Rastogi P, Geyer CE Jr, Liu Q, Robidoux A, et al. Neoadjuvant plus adjuvant bevacizumab in early breast cancer (NSABP B-40 [NRG Oncology]): secondary outcomes of a phase 3, randomised controlled trial. Lancet Oncol. 2015;16: 1037–48.

43. Sikov WM, Berry DA, Perou CM, Singh B, Cirrincione CT, Tolaney SM, et al. Impact of the addition of carboplatin and/or bevacizumab to neoadjuvant once-per-week paclitaxel followed by dose-dense doxorubicin and cyclophosphamide on pathologic complete response rates in stage II to III triple-negative breast cancer: CALGB 40603 (Alliance). J Clin Oncol. 2015;33:13–21.

44. Rugo HS, Olopade O, DeMichele A, van't Veer L, Buxton M, Hylton N, et al. Veliparib/carboplatin plus standard neoadjuvant therapy for high-risk breast cancer: first efficacy results from the I-SPY 2 TRIAL. The San Antonio Breast Cancer Symposium 2013. Abstr S5-02.

45. Cortazar P, Zhang L, Untch M, Mehta K, Costantino JP, Wolmark N, et al. Pathological complete response and long-term clinical benefit in breast cancer: the CTNeoBC pooled analysis. Lancet. 2014;384: 164–72.

46. Kong X, Moran MS, Zhang N, Haffty B, Yang Q. Meta-analysis confirms achieving pathological complete response after neoadjuvant chemotherapy predicts favourable prognosis for breast cancer patients. Eur J Cancer. 2011;47:2084–90.

47. Symmans WF, Peintinger F, Hatzis C, Rajan R, Kuerer H, Valero V, et al. Measurement of residual breast cancer burden to predict survival after neoadjuvant chemotherapy. J Clin Oncol. 2007;25: 4414–22.

48. Mathieu MC, Mazouni C, Kesty NC, Zhang Y, Scott V, Passeron J, et al. Breast Cancer Index predicts pathological complete response and eligibility for breast conserving surgery in breast cancer patients treated with neoadjuvant chemotherapy. Ann Oncol. 2012; 23:2046–52.

Systemic Therapy for Inflammatory Breast Cancer

16

Nilüfer Güler

Abstract

Inflammatory breast carcinoma (IBC) is the most aggressive, lethal, and rare form of breast cancer. IBC is characterized by the rapid development of erythema, edema, and peau d'orange over a third or more of the skin of the breast due to the occlusion of dermal mammary lymphatics by tumor emboli. IBC is associated with rapid progression, with a high risk of axillary lymph node involvement and distant metastases at initial diagnosis. The most striking progress in the management of IBC has been the sequential incorporation of preoperative systemic chemotherapy [an induction regimen containing an anthracycline and a taxane (plus trastuzumab in *HER2*-positive patients)], followed by surgery and radiation therapy. This multidisciplinary approach has essentially transformed IBC from a uniformly fatal disease with 5-year overall survival rates of less than 5 % to one in which 5-year overall survival rates range from 46 % to 61 % and 15-year survival rates vary between 20 % and 30 %. The response to primary chemotherapy is a strong indicator of survival. The 15-year survival rate is 44 % in patients who achieve a pathological complete response after primary chemotherapy. In this chapter, preoperative systemic therapy for the disease is discussed after a brief outline of inflammatory breast carcinoma.

Keywords

Inflammatory breast cancer • Epidemiology • Etiology • Risk factors • Diagnosis • Pathology • Imaging studies • Preoperative systemic therapy • Preoperative systemic chemotherapy • Neoadjuvant chemotherapy • Dose-dense chemotherapy • High-dose chemotherapy • Preoperative-targeted therapies • Anti-HER2 agents • Antiangiogenic agents • Endocrine therapy • Statins • Monitoring response • Follow-up

N. Güler, MD
Retared Member of Department of Medical
Oncology, Hacettepe University Cancer Institute,
Sıhhiye, Ankara, Turkey
e-mail: nguler@hacettepe.edu.tr

© Springer International Publishing Switzerland 2016
A. Aydiner et al. (eds.), *Breast Disease: Management and Therapies*,
DOI 10.1007/978-3-319-26012-9_16

Introduction

Inflammatory breast carcinoma (IBC) is a rare and aggressive subtype of breast carcinoma that is diagnosed clinically [1–5] and was first identified by Lee and Tannenbaum in 1924 [6]. IBC is characterized by skin changes that are suggestive of infection and inflammation, usually with fairly abrupt onset and rapid progression. The duration of symptoms before diagnosis is usually less than 3 months [1–5]. The most common symptoms are a feeling of warmth and heaviness, itching, nipple retraction, and pain in the affected breast. IBC is frequently misdiagnosed as cellulitis or acute mastitis. Acute-phase radiation dermatitis, sarcoma or lymphoma of the breast, inflammatory metastatic melanoma, and Paget's disease of the nipple can also mimic IBC.

The minimum diagnostic criteria for the diagnosis of IBC are the following [7–9]:

- Rapid onset of breast erythema (with a palpable border), edema and/or dermal edema (peau d'orange), and/or warm breast, with or without an underlying palpable mass
- A duration of symptom history of no more than 6 months
- Erythema occupying at least one-third of the breast
- Pathological   confirmation   of   invasive   carcinoma

Primary IBC is classified as T4d according to the American Joint Commission for Cancer (AJCC) staging system and is staged as IIIB, IIIC, or IV according to nodal involvement and distant metastases [8, 9]. IBC is not an entity of locally advanced breast carcinoma (LABC) but is completely separate according to epidemiological and molecular evidence. The outcomes of these two diseases are quite different: younger age at diagnosis, higher tumor grade, and the absence of the estrogen receptor (*ER*) in the tumor are more suggestive of primary IBC than LABC [1, 2, 4]. According to the National Cancer Institute (NCI) Surveillance, Epidemiology, and End Results (SEER) program records for 828 IBC and 3,476 non-IBC LABC patients, 2-year

breast cancer-specific survival (BCSS) was 84 % in patients with IBC (95 % CI: 80–87 %) compared to 91 % (95 % CI: 90–91 %) in patients with non-IBC LABC after a median follow-up of 19 months [10]. In a multivariate model, the mortality risk in patients with IBC is 43 % higher than that in non-IBC LABC patients (hazard ratio 1.43, 95 % CI: 1.10–1.86, $p = 0.008$) In addition, a distinction must also be made between primary and secondary IBC [2]. In primary IBC, skin alterations and carcinoma develop concurrently from the previously healthy breast, whereas in secondary IBC, inflammatory skin alterations appear subsequent to malignancy development [1, 2, 4, 5].

Epidemiology, Etiology, and Risk Factors

The reported incidence of IBC varies due to a lack of consensus regarding the case definition for the disease [11]. In the United States, the incidence of IBC ranges from 1 % up to 6 % [12–14]. Data from the SEER program have demonstrated that the age-adjusted incidence rates for IBC increased significantly between 1988–1990 and 1997–1999 (from 2.0 to 2.5 cases/100,000 woman-years; $p < 0.001$) [15]. The incidence of IBC is significantly higher in African-American women than that in Caucasian women (3.1/100,000 woman-years vs. 2.2/100,000 woman-years, respectively) [15]. The incidence is lowest among Asian Pacific Islander women (0.7 cases/100,000 woman-years) [16]. In Morocco, Egypt, Algeria, and Tunisia, the reported incidence rates are very high, and nearly 10–15 % of all breast cancers are stated to present as IBC [17–20]. According to data from two single institutions in Turkey and Spain, however, the incidence of IBC is 5 % and 2.9 %, respectively [21, 22].

IBC generally has an early onset. Maximal peak age at diagnosis is approximately 50 years. However, maximal peak age at diagnosis is 69 years for non-T4 tumors and 74 years for LABC. According to the SEER database, the median age at diagnosis is lower in patients with IBC (58.8 years) than patients with non-T4 breast cancer (61.7 years, $p < 0.0001$) and LABC (66.2 years, $p < 0.0001$) [15]. In addition, race seems to be an important risk factor, as African-American women are at higher risk for developing the disease. The age of onset also varies according to race and ethnicity [16]. Compared to Caucasians, African-Americans present at a younger age of onset (median age 55.2 versus 58.1 years) with inferior prognosis. However, Hispanic women present with the youngest average age (median 50.5 years) at the initial diagnosis of IBC. In one study, the epidemiology, biology, and prognosis of IBC in Japanese and US populations were compared [23]. No differences were observed between the two populations regarding age at diagnosis, hormone receptor (HR) status, human epidermal growth factor receptor-2 (*HER2*) overexpression, or overall survival (OS). However, body-mass index (BMI) and nuclear grade were lower in Japanese patients than US patients. For OS, *ER* status and race were prognostic when the two populations were combined.

Possible risk factors for IBC are young age at first birth (<20 years), pregnancy (21–26 % of IBC cases develop during or after pregnancy), lactation (longer cumulative duration of breastfeeding history), increased BMI (>26.65; the odds ratio for IBC vs. other types of BC is 2.45), blood group A, and rural residency [1–4, 14, 24–27]. However, it should be recognized that these risk factors are currently based on smaller studies and have not been well established.

Immunological factors have been examined in Tunisian studies. Immunodeficiency was not observed studies, but the results suggested that a hyperimmune response may be the cause of this rapidly progressing breast cancer [28, 29].

Because of the rapid onset and clinical characteristics of IBC, the involvement of viral infection was suggested by Pogo et al. [30]. They detected *human mammary tumor virus (HMTV)*, a provirus structure with 96 % homology with *Mouse Mammary Tumor virus (MMTV)*, in 71 % of IBC cases compared to 40 % of non-IBC cases in American patients [30]. *HMTV*-positive IBC was significantly higher in breast cancer patients in Tunisia (74 %) compared with those in the

United States (36 %), Italy (38 %), Argentina (31 %), and Vietnam (0.8 %) [31]. Another study from Egypt demonstrated that *human cytomegalovirus (HCMV)* infection enhances the expression and activation of transcription factor *NF-κB (nuclear factor-κB/p65*, which controls different cytokines) signaling in IBC patients [32]. *HCMV* infection may be associated with the etiology and progression of IBC versus non-IBC. The relationship between viral etiology and IBC is under investigation in the United States [2].

Although the median age of IBC is younger than that of non-IBC, *BRCA1*, *BRCA2*, and *PTEN* do not play a strong role in IBC. *BRCA* testing is not routinely recommended, except in cases with a strong family history [9]. In one retrospective study, there was no statistically significant difference ($p = 0.169$) in the rate of *BRCA1* and *BRCA2* mutations between IBC (35.9 %; total 39 patients) and non-IBC (26.1 %; total 992 patients) [33]. In another study, the percentage of patients with a positive family history was 13 % in IBC cases and 8 % in non-IBC [24]. This difference was not statistically significant. Family history was significantly more common in IBC cases than in non-IBC cases (20 % versus 5 %, respectively) in one Pakistani study [34].

Imaging Studies

Among various diagnostic imaging modalities, mammography is the least sensitive and effective method for the diagnosis of IBC and detects only 43 % of breast parenchymal lesions [35]. Therefore, IBC is usually not detected by mammographic scanning. The most common signs of IBC by mammography are skin thickening and trabecular distortion; a mass is often visible by ultrasonography (USG) [5, 7, 21, 36]. Both the mammary tissue and local lymph nodes should be evaluated by USG. Axillary lymph node metastases are detected in 90 % of all patients. Parenchymal lesions in the breasts can be identified in nearly 95 % of IBC patients by USG, which is also a useful method for obtaining biopsies from lesions. Recently, magnetic resonance imaging (MRI) has become a popular method for visualizing the breast. The reported success rates of MRI, USG, and mammography in detecting parenchymal lesions in patients with proven IBC are 100 %, 95 % and 80 %, respectively [36]. Although MRI appears to be the best method, it is not recommended for routine diagnostic imaging because it is expensive and time consuming and breast coils are available in only one size. Therefore, MRI is advised only under two conditions [7]: when parenchymal lesions cannot be detected with mammography or USG and when patients are recruited for research studies that evaluate the use of MRI of the breast in the diagnosis of IBC.

Local-regional disease is present in all patients diagnosed with IBC; however, approximately 30 % of patients have metastatic disease at the time of diagnosis. Therefore, a systemic staging workup [computed tomography, bone scintigraphy, ^{18}F FDG PET/CT (fluorodeoxyglucose positron emission tomography/computed tomography), etc.] should be performed in every patient [1–5, 7, 9]. In addition, cross-sectional imaging of the neck and an evaluation of infra- and supraclavicular lymph nodes during radiological imaging and planning of radiotherapy are equally important [7].

Tissue Sampling and Pathology

Preoperative systemic chemotherapy (PSC) is the standard therapy for IBC treatment [1–5]. Sufficient tissue sampling from the parenchymal lesion in the affected breast during the pretreatment period is essential for both future treatment planning and subsequent research studies because no cancerous tissue will be available following treatment in patients with pathological complete response (pCR) [1–4, 7]. The presence of an invasive cancer, the identification of the histological type and grade of the tumor, and the expression of the *ER*, progesterone receptor (*PR*), and *HER2* should be clarified with utmost care. If there is doubt about metastasis in the axillary and/or supraclavicular lymph nodes, image-guided core biopsies and analysis of prognostic and predictive markers are suggested [7]. For patients who meet the diagnostic criteria for IBC, obtaining at least two skin punch biopsies to determine dermal lymphatic invasion (DLI) is recommended. Apart from their significance in indicating the presence of DLI, these biopsies are also important for the diagnosis of invasive cancer in patients with no detectable intraparenchymal breast lesions or regional metastases. The best site for sampling is believed to be the region with the most significant color alteration on the breast skin [7]. A 2- to 8-mm biopsy specimen taken from that region is sufficient to demonstrate the presence of DLI. However, although DLI is responsible for the clinically observed inflammatory alterations in IBC, it is not necessary for diagnosis [7, 9, 37].

All pathological subtypes of invasive adenocarcinoma can be associated with IBC [4, 37, 38]. IBC is also rarely seen in male patients [39]. IBC is often in the form of ductal carcinoma. It is a highly angiogenic and invasive type of cancer characterized by high histological grade and *HER2* positivity with a high rate of *ER* negativity. *p53* mutations are common (70 % in IBC and 48 % in non-IBC, $p = 0.0238$) [34].

There are three subtypes of IBC: clinicopathologically apparent IBC, clinically apparent IBC, and pathological (occult) IBC [2]. Two population-based studies used this classification for IBC to demonstrate that patients with occult IBC have better disease-free survival (DFS) (5-year DFS 51.6 % vs. 25.6 %, respectively) and OS than patients with clinically apparent IBC (5-year OS 40 % vs. 28.6 %, respectively) [22, 40].

The molecular subtypes of IBC are the same as those of non-IBC (luminal, triple negative, and *HER2* positive). Twenty to 40 % of all IBC cases are triple negative (TN), whereas 15–20 % of non-IBC cases display this molecular subtype [41]. The distribution of the seven subtypes of triple-negative breast cancers (TNBC) (basal-like 1, basal-like 2, immunomodulatory, mesenchymal, mesenchymal stem cell-like, luminal androgen receptor, unstable) in patients with TN IBC and TN non-IBC has been by investigating microRNA gene expression profiles [42]. The distribution of molecular subtypes did not differ significantly between the two patient groups.

Moreover, no associations between IBC characteristics and TNBC subtype were observed. Similarly, the influence of the expression of various target genes on prognosis, response to therapy, and classification has been evaluated [43–45]. In one study, the expression of approximately 8,000 genes was analyzed in tumor samples from 81 patients with breast carcinoma (37 IBC and 44 non-IBC), and 109 genes were identified as beneficial for the differentiation of IBC and non-IBC [43]. In addition, a set of 85 genes (associated with signal transduction, cell motility, adhesion, and angiogenesis) selected to determine the aggressiveness of IBC were significantly useful in distinguishing two different patient groups with distinct pCR rates (70 % vs. 0 % pCR) [43]. In another study, gene expression analysis and comparative genomic hybridization were performed in IBC samples using a microdissection technique [44]. No IBC-specific gene signature that distinguishes IBC from non-IBC was identified using this technique. However, these studies must be validated, and further research studies are required [45].

Preoperative Systemic Therapy (PST)

Historically, radical mastectomy was the primary modality for the treatment of IBC. Surgery alone resulted in a very poor prognosis and a 5-year survival of less than 5 %, with a median survival of 12–32 months [46, 47]. During the past 30 years, the treatment of IBC has significantly evolved. Because of the systemic nature of the disease, adding radiotherapy (RT) after surgery increased only locoregional control without increasing OS [48–50]. The addition of PSC (also referred to as neoadjuvant, preoperative, or induction) before surgery and RT has been associated with significantly increased survival rates of 30–50 % for 5-year survival and 24 % for 15-year survival [51–56]. SEER data from 7,679 stage/grade III IBC patients from 1990 to 2010 were analyzed according to survival [57]. The diagnosed patients were classified over four time periods (1990–1995, 1996–2000, 2001–2005,

2006–2010), and BCSS during these periods was calculated. Two-year BCSS was 62 %, 67 %, 72 % and 76 %, respectively ($p < 0.0001$). Multivariate analysis revealed that mortality risks decreased with increasing diagnosis year (HR, 0.98; 95 % CI 0.97–0.99; $p < 0.0001$).

Historically, PST included only chemotherapy (CT). However, in recent years, some targeted therapies have been used together with CT based on tumor characteristics. Survival was analyzed in IBC cases who were treated before and after October 2006 at MD Anderson Cancer Center (MDACC) [58]. The date October 2006 was chosen because this date was the beginning of anti-*HER2* usage in standard neoadjuvant chemotherapies (NACT) and the opening of a multidisciplinary IBC clinic. Before this date, 3-year OS was 63 %; after this date, the ratio increased to 82 % ($p = 0.02$). Multivariate analysis demonstrated that anti-*HER2* therapies (HR = 0.38; 95 % CI 0.17–0.84; $p = 0.02$) and *ER* positivity (HR = 0.032; CI 0.14–0.74, $p = 0.01$) are important factors for survival.

Breast-conserving surgery is not suggested for IBC because it is a disease that often has a diffuse character [1–4]. When first diagnosed, mastectomy is not suggested; after NACT application, mastectomy can be performed. Mastectomy and axillary lymph node dissection are the optimal surgical procedure. Axillary lymph node metastasis is noted in 55–85 % of IBC cases at first diagnosis. A clinical response evaluation by physical examination and imaging techniques may underestimate the extent of residual disease [1–5, 9, 54, 55]. The removal of all gross disease is important because skin lymphatic involvement may extend beyond the area of visible skin changes. After mastectomy, postmastectomy RT to the chest wall and axillary, infraclavicular, and supraclavicular, and internal mammary lymph nodes (if involved; consider internal mammary nodes if not clinically involved) is part of standard multimodality treatment [1–4, 9, 56].

Randomized clinical trials assessing therapy have not been performed because of the rare occurrence of the disease. Many of the cases are evaluated in protocols in the same way as the LABC study. Data are gathered from one-armed studies and retrospective case series [51–56]. Collaborations between the surgeon, medical oncologist, and radiation oncologist are important in IBC application for optimal therapy [7, 9]. An analysis of 10,197 nonmetastatic IBC patients from the National Cancer Database who underwent surgery and were observed between 1998 and 2010 [59] revealed that trimodality therapy (NACT + surgery + RT) was less common in patients who were old, low paid, and far from health centers and who received therapy during the early period of the study, had other serious health problems, and had insufficient health insurance ($p < 0.05$). The 5- and 10-year survival rates of patients who received all three therapies (55.4 % and 37.3 %, respectively) were higher than those of the surgery + RT group (40.7 % and 23.5 %, respectively), the surgery + chemotherapy group (42.9 % and 28.5 %, respectively), and the surgery-only group (10-year survival 16.5 %).

The treatment should begin with NACT. There is no standard primary CT regimen or combination. However, anthracyclines and taxanes are constant members of primary chemotherapy regimens currently. The optimal sequence, dose, duration, and intensity of the CT regimen remain to be defined, and the optimal sequence and type of locoregional therapy have not yet been resolved.

Preoperative Systemic Chemotherapy (PSC)

In pre-1970 clinical trials, IBC cases were excluded because of the rarity and poor overall prognosis. Most IBC cases were treated with the same regimens used for the treatment of non-IBC cases. In recent years, specifically designed CT trials for patients with IBC have increased. The response to PSC has prognostic significance. Patients with pCR (complete clearance of the tumor in the breast and axilla) have a significantly increased DFS rate. Here, I would like to discuss PSC chronologically.

MDACC is the most experienced center for IBC. Since 1974, MDACC has been planning prospective studies on only IBC patients. As of 2010, 242 IBC patients had been enrolled in clinical trials. These studies demonstrated that PSC is necessary for this group of patients. The response to NACT is a surrogate marker for long-term survival. The survival of patients without a response to NACT is shorter than those with a response. In one study, NACT was applied to 175 IBC patients [60]. After NACT and surgery, 61 of 175 patients had residual disease in the breast and axillary lymph nodes. Five-year relapse-free survival (RFS) was 82.5 % and OS was 78.6 % in patients with pCR after NACT, but in the group with residual disease after NACT, RFS was 37.1 % and OS was 25.4 %.

First CMF (cyclophosphamide, methotrexate, 5-fluorouracil) and similar regimens, then anthracycline-containing CT regimens, and finally taxanes have been used for NACT in IBC. A total of 527 stage III IBC patients who were observed between January 1989 and January 2011 were retrospectively analyzed in a study at MDACC [61]. The pCR ratio was 15.2 % in all groups. The pCR ratio was lowest in the *HR*-positive/*HER2*-negative group (7.5 %) and highest in the *HR*-negative/*HER2*-positive group (30.6 %). The survival of TN-IBC patients was lowest. DFS and OS were related to pCR achievement after therapy, the absence of vascular invasion, non-TNBC type, adjuvant hormonal therapy, and radiotherapy. This study indicated that the predictive and prognostic roles of both *HR* and *HER2* status are limited and that prognosis is poor in all groups. It is valuable to use new subtype-specific therapies.

Anthracyclines

Active chemotherapy applications for IBC began in 1970. Anthracycline-containing NACT studies involving 15–192 patients have reported improvements in response rates from 20 % to 93 % and in complete response (CR) rates from 4 % to 55 % [49]. pCR ratios improved from 3 % to 16 % [53].

The use of CMF±VP (vincristine-prednisone) and FAC (fluorouracil-doxorubicin-cyclophosphamide) combinations for NACT in 38 IBC cases was reviewed retrospectively [62]

Table 16.1 Important neoadjuvant chemotherapy trials in patients with stage III inflammatory breast cancer [51, 54, 55, 63–67]

Study group	Chemotherapy protocol	n	ORR % (complete+partial)	Median survival (months)	DFS %	OS %
MDACC Protocol A	FAC-RT-FAC FAC-RT-CMF	40	80	38	–	–
MDACC Protocol B	FAC-surgery FAC-RT	23	57	38	–	–
MDACC Protocol C	FACVP-surgery FACVP-CMF-RT	43	76	64	–	–
MDACC Protocol D	FACVP-surgery-FACVP or FACVP ± MV or MV according to the response to induction CT	72	77	34+	–	–
MDACC-Ueno-whole group [64]	FAC ± VP	178	72	37	32 (5-year) 28 (10-year) 28 (15-year)	40 (5-year) 35 (10-year)
Bauer et al. [62]	CMF ± VP	38	57	18	–	–
	FAC		100	30		
Harris et al. [54]	CMF or CAF	54	54		–	56 (5-year)
Low et al. [55]	CAFM	46	46	–	–	27 (10-year) 20 (15-year)
Cristofanilli et al. [65]	FAC-3 weekly P-surgery-FAC-weekly P-RT	44	77	46	–	74 (2-year OS)
Cristofanilli et al. [66]	FAC	178	72	–	39 (3-year PFS)	53 (3-year)
	FAC-P (weekly or 3-weekly)	62	79		46 (3-year PFS)	71 (3-year)

CAF cyclophosphamide-doxorubicin-fluorouracil, *CMF* cyclophosphamide-methotrexate-fluorouracil, *CMF±VP* CMF plus/minus vincristine-prednisone, *DFS* disease-free survival, *FAC* fluorouracil-doxorubicin-cyclophosphamide, *FACVP* FAC plus vincristine-prednisone, *FACVP-MV* FACVP plus methotrexate and vinblastine, *MDACC* MD Anderson Cancer Center, *ORR* overall response rate, *OS* overall survival, *P* paclitaxel, *PFS* progression-free survival, *RT* radiotherapy

(Table 16.1). The overall response rate (ORR) was 57 % in the CMF ± VP group and 100 % in the FAC group; the median OS was 18 months in the CMF ± VP group and 30 months in the FAC group. Harris et al. evaluated the long-term follow-up of combined modality therapy in 54 IBC patients [54] (Table 16.1). CMF or CAF (cyclophosphamide-doxorubicin-fluorouracil) was applied as PSC. The clinical CR rate was 52 % in patients treated with PSC with or without preoperative radiotherapy. pCR was achieved in 37 % (13 patients) of the PSC and RT group and 12 % (2 patients) of the PSC-only group. Ten-year overall survival was 46 % in patients who achieved pCR and 31 % in patients with residual disease in the breast and axilla ($p = 0.09$).

A total of 107 stage III breast cancer patients were included in one prospective, randomized NCI study [55] (Table 16.1). Forty-six of the patients had IBC. CAF and methotrexate were applied as NACT until the maximal response was achieved. The median follow-up time was 16.8 years. ORR was 57 % within IBC patients.

Two hundred forty-two IBC patients who were enrolled between 1974 and 2001 were examined in five study protocols by MDACC [51, 63–67]. A total of 178 patients received neoadjuvant therapy with four different chemotherapy regimens containing anthracycline [63, 64, 67] (Table 16.1).

1. Protocol A (First Protocol): Patients received FAC neoadjuvant therapy first and then received radiotherapy, followed by FAC or CMF therapies.
2. Protocol B (Second Protocol): Patients received FAC neoadjuvant therapy first and then surgery, followed by adjuvant FAC and radiotherapy.
3. Protocol C (Third Protocol): Patients received FACVP (fluorouracil-doxorubicin-cyclophosphamide-vincristine prednisone) as induction therapy first and then surgery, followed by FACVP and CMF radiotherapy.
4. Protocol D (Fourth Protocol): Patients received FACVP as induction therapy and then surgery. After surgery, patients with complete responses received adjuvant FACVP. Patients with partial responses (tumors that become decreased in diameter by more than half) received FACVP with MV (methotrexate-vincristine). Patients received MV therapy only when tumors became smaller in diameter by approximately 25–50 %.

The response rate for all studies was 72 %, and the clinical CR rate was 12 % [52, 64, 67] (Table 16.1). There were no differences within the four studies in terms of DFS and OS. The median survival was 37 months. DFS for 5, 10, and 15 years was 32 %, 28 % and 28 %, respectively. The 15-year DFS for patients with complete or partial responses who received induction chemotherapy was 44 % and 31 %, respectively, and the 15-year OS was 51 % and 31 %, respectively. The 15-year DFS and OS of patients whose responses were less than partial with induction chemotherapy decreased to 7 %. These results indicate the importance of the response to induction chemotherapy for prognosis.

VP or MV therapy combinations in the third and fourth study protocols had no effect on DFS and OS. Surgery after a poor response to NACT did not alter local relapse risk. Surgery and RT application instead of RT-only as a local therapy did not effect DFS and OS. At the 20-year follow-up, the local relapse rate was 20 % [64]. Distant metastasis was observed in 39 % of patients, and central nervous system (CNS) metastasis was observed in 9 % of patients.

Taxanes

The effect of taxane use in NACT for IBC cases was investigated in 1994 and included 44 patients in a MDACC study (Protocol E) [65] (Table 16.1). FAC chemotherapy was used as NACT and adjuvant therapy in all patients. Paclitaxel (P) was added to the therapy regimen of patients with stable disease or who had a minor response to NACT during the preoperative period, and P was added as an adjuvant therapy in all patients. NACT and then surgery, followed by adjuvant chemotherapy and then radiotherapy, were applied. The objective/clinical response rate was 77 % (vs. 72 % in regimens containing only anthracycline), and the median survival time was 46 months (vs. 37 months in regimens containing only anthracycline). The results were not statistically significant.

In another study, anthracycline-based and taxane-based NACT protocols were compared in patients with IBC. Group 1 included 178 patients who received anthracycline-containing induction chemotherapy, and group 2 included 62 patients who received taxane-containing chemotherapy (Tables 16.1 and 16.2) [65, 66]. The median follow-up period was 148 months (range: 85–283 months) for group 1 and 45 months (range: 21–99 months) for group 2. The 3-year OS was 71 % in group 2 and 53 % in group 1. In conclusion, P is an important agent in IBC therapy. The 3-year OS for patients with *ER*-negative tumors in groups 1 and 2 was 43 % and 71 %, respectively (32 months and 54 months, respectively ($p = 0.03$)); progression-free survivals (PFS) was 31 % and 39 %, respectively (18 months and 27 months, respectively; $p = 0.04$). Taxanes are clearly more effective, particularly in *ER*-negative tumors. The pCR ratio was 10 % in the FAC-only group and 25 % in the anthracycline-P group; this difference was statistically significant ($p = 0.012$).

Table 16.2 MDACC comparison of neoadjuvant-only anthracycline and anthracycline-taxane containing chemotherapy protocols in patients with inflammatory breast cancer [64, 66]

Parameter	Group 1	Group 2
n	178 patients	62 patients
Follow-up years	1973–1993	1994–2000
Median follow-up (months)	148 (85–283)	45 (21–99)
Chemotherapy protocol	FAC-based regimens	FAC followed by 3 weekly P or weekly high-dose P
ORR	72 %	79 %
3-year PFS	39 %	46 % $p=0.19$
3-year OS	53 %	71 % $p=0.12$
pCR rate	10 %	25 %
ER-negative tumors	33 %	65 %
Median PFS (*ER*-negative group)	18 months	27 months $p=0.042$
Median OS (*ER*-negative group)	32 months	54 months $p=0.035$
3-year PFS (*ER*-negative group)	31 %	39 %
3-year OS (*ER*-negative group)	43 %	71 %

ER estrogen receptor, *FAC* fluorouracil-doxorubicin-cyclophosphamide, *MDACC* MD Anderson Cancer Center, *ORR* overall response rate (complete+partial response), *OS* overall survival, *P* paclitaxel, *pCR* pathological complete response, *PFS* progression-free survival

A retrospective analysis substantiated these findings using data from 308 IBC patients who were observed between 1980 and 2000 in a study performed in England [68]. Taxane-containing chemotherapy regimens (AP, cisplatin, P) were better than anthracycline-containing chemotherapy regimens in the 1990s for 10-year BCSS (43.7 % and 23.6 %, respectively, $p=0.03$).

In the GeparTrio trial, an anthracycline and taxane combination (docetaxel/doxorubicin/cyclophosphamide (TAC)) was used as NACT [69]. Participants were stratified by stage (93 IBC, 194 LABC, and 1,777 operable breast cancers) and randomized to arms with six or eight cycles of TAC or two cycles of TAC followed by four cycles of vinorelbine/capecitabine chemotherapy. pCR rates and ORRs were not significantly different between IBC and LABC patients (8.6 % vs. 11.3 % for pCR, respectively; 71 % vs. 69.6 % for ORR, respectively) but were significantly lower compared with operable breast cancer (17.7 % and 83.4 %, respectively; $p=0.002$ and $p<0.001$, respectively). In IBC patients, there was a nonsignificant trend toward higher pCR rates with a response at midcourse in patients who received eight cycles of TAC compared with those patients who received only six cycles (17.2 % vs. 3.3 %; $p=0.103$).

These studies demonstrate that anthracyclines and taxanes are important and are necessary for primary chemotherapies for IBC. pCR rates are higher with the use of weekly paclitaxel regimens [70, 71]. The optimal dosage and sequence for anthracycline-taxane remain under investigation (taxane first followed anthracycline, anthracycline first followed by taxane, or an anthracycline-taxane combination).

Other Chemotherapies

Dose-dense chemotherapy and high-dose chemotherapy with stem cell support may be effective for some selected patient groups. Survival advantages were observed in small, phase II studies (3–4 year DFS of 45–65 % and OS of 52–89 %), but because there have been no prospective, randomized studies of these protocols, they are not standard and are not suggested except in clinical research trials [1, 2, 53, 72–78].

High-risk primary breast cancer patients were included in one prospective study at MDACC [77]. Eighteen patients in the study had IBC. High-dose weekly paclitaxel chemotherapy was applied following FAC therapy as NACT. After surgery, cyclophosphamide, etoposide, and cisplatin (CVP) combined therapy was applied, followed by bone marrow mobilization and high-dose cyclophosphamide, carmustine, and thiotepa CT with stem cell support. The clinical CR ratio was 31 %, and the mastectomy ratio was 72 %. The 5-year OS rate was 36 %, and the DFS rate was 28 %. The therapy was more effective in young patients and patients with less lymph node metastasis.

The PEGASE 02 study included 95 nonmetastatic IBC patients [75]. After high-dose FAC therapy, blood stem cell support was applied. Mastectomies were performed in 86 patients following PSC. Radiotherapy was performed. The clinical response rate (RR) was 90 %, and the pCR rate in the breast was 32 %. The 3-year RFS was 44 % (95 % CI, 33–54 %), and the estimated 3-year survival was 70 % (95 % CI, 60–79 %).

One retrospective study from Somlo et al. included 120 IBC patients who received dose-intense CT as NACT [76]. Patients received conventional-dose chemotherapy and surgery and sequentially developed single- or tandem-cycle dose-intense CT. The median observation time was 61 months, the 5-year RFS rate was 44 %, and the OS was 64 %. Multivariate analysis demonstrated that *ER/PR* positivity and <4 positive axillary lymph node metastasis were the best predictors of which patients would benefit from tandem, dose-intense chemotherapy.

The GETIS 02 trial was conducted by the French Adjuvant Study Group [79]. In that study, the efficacy of primary chemotherapy with four cycles of high-dose FEC (fluorouracil-epirubicin-cyclophosphamide) with or without lenograstim in 120 nonmetastatic IBC patients was evaluated. After preoperative CT, surgery and RT were administered as locoregional therapy, and then maintenance CT with four cycles of FEC-75 was applied. The median DFS was 39 months. After a median of 10 years of follow-up, the DFS and OS rates were 36 % and 41 %, respectively.

An international expert panel on IBC recommended a minimum of six cycles of PSC be administered over a course of 4–6 months before surgery [7]. If the response is insufficient, different CT regimens or RT can be applied [7, 9]. RT is applied after surgery, and if the CT program is not completed before surgery, it should be completed during the postoperative period.

Targeted Therapies

Anti-HER2 Therapies

The *HER2* positivity ratio in IBC is very high and varies between 42 % and 57 % [1–4, 37, 38]. *HER2* positivity is important for the prognosis of non-IBC, but its importance for IBC is not known. A retrospective study that included 179 stage III IBC patients [80] determined that *HER2* positivity or negativity is not related to RFS. Another study of more than 2,000 patients conducted in California demonstrated improved BCSS in *HER2*-positive patients compared to *HER2*-negative patients (HR, 0.82; 95 % CI 0.68–0.99) [81].

Although the prognostic importance of *HER2* for IBC is not known, *HER2* positivity is important for predicting the response to anti-*HER2* therapies in *HER2*-positive patients. Trastuzumab (Tr) is a monoclonal antibody against HER2 and the first of the anti-HER2 agents. The addition of Tr to anthracycline- and taxane-containing PSC regimens yielded a significantly increased response and improved survival compared to non-Tr PSC regimens [5, 78, 81–86]. The increase in the pCR rate from 17 % to 62.5 % was also statistically significant. Unfortunately, the studies included many LABC and fewer IBC cases. Studies including only IBC cases are very rare.

Dawood et al. reported that the pCR rate was 62.5 % in *HER2*+ IBC cases receiving NACT combined with Tr therapy, and the 2-year PFS was 59.4 % [86]. In that study, 3 of 16 IBC patients had metastatic disease at the beginning of treatment. Forty-eight *HER2*+ LABC (IBC-containing) patients were enrolled in a study by Hurley et al. [87]. Docetaxel-cisplatin-Tr was applied as induction therapy. After chemotherapy, surgery, adjuvant chemotherapy and radiotherapy were perform consecutively. The OS was 100 % in patients with pCR. In patients with residual disease after NACT, the OS ratio ranged from 76 % to 83 %.

In another study including 9 IBC and 22 LABC patients, docetaxel and Tr were applied as the primary chemotherapy, and the CR rate was 40 % [88].

The NOAH (neoadjuvant Herceptin) trial was a prospective, open-label, phase 3, multicenter, randomized study [89]. *HER2*-positive, locally advanced ($n = 174$) or IBC ($n = 61$) cases were enrolled in the study. The patients received anthracycline-based and taxane-based NACT alone or with 1 year of Tr (concurrently with NACT and continued after surgery). A parallel group with *HER2*-negative disease was included and received NACT alone. Relapse, progression, and mortality risks were statistically significantly decreased in the Tr group compared with the CT-only group. The pCR ratio was twofold higher in the Tr group than in CT-only group (38 % and 19 %, respectively). After a median follow-up of 5.4 years, the event-free survival (EFS) benefit of the addition of Tr was maintained in patients with *HER2*-positive disease [90]. The 5-year EFS was 58 % in the Tr group and 43 % in the CT group (HR, 0.64; 95 % CI 0.44–0.93; $p = 0.016$). Similarly, during that time period, EFS was strongly associated with pCR in patients who received Tr. In that study, 27 % of *HER2*(+) patients had IBC. The 3-year EFS was 70.1 % in the Tr group and 53.3 % in the CT-only group ($p = 0.0007$). The pCR (complete disappearance of the tumors from both the breast and lymph nodes) rate was 48 % in the Tr group and only 13 % in the CT-only group ($p = 0.002$) [91].

Tr should be started in the induction chemotherapy period for the treatment of *HER2*-positive LABC or IBC patients. Although there has been no prospective randomized study, Tr therapy should be extended to 1 year. An anthracycline-Tr combination is not suggested because of enhanced cardiotoxicity [5, 7, 9].

Lapatinib is another anti-*HER2* (reversible dual inhibitor of both *HER1* and *HER2*) targeted drug, and studies with lapatinib or lapatinib with paclitaxel are ongoing [92–94]. The clinical RR was 80 % for 21 IBC patients who received a lapatinib-paclitaxel combination [93]. In one multicenter, open-label, phase II study with 49 IBC patients, a lapatinib-paclitaxel combination was used as NACT [94]. Patients were divided into two groups: cohort A was positive for *HER2* 2+ or 3+ by immunohistochemical (IHC) methods or FISH (fluorescence in situ hybridization) ± epidermal growth factor receptor (*EGFR*) expression; cohort B was *HER2* negative/*EGFR* positive. *HER2* 3+ or FISH-positive patients were analyzed separately. First, patients received lapatinib only for 14 days, followed by 12 weeks of lapatinib and paclitaxel weekly. Cohort B was stopped because of slow enrollment and a lack of efficacy in IBC patients with *HER2*-negative/*EGFR*-positive tumors enrolled in a parallel study, EGF103009. Thirty-five patients completed the study and underwent surgery. The pCR rate of cohort A was 18.2 %, and the clinical RR was 78.6 % for all groups and 78.1 % in the *HER2* 3+ group. The clinical RR was 31 % in the *HER2*-positive group receiving only lapatinib, and the pCR rate was 17.6 % in all patients who underwent surgery after therapy. The most common side effects of lapatinib were diarrhea and skin eruptions. Lapatinib is currently suggested only for clinical research studies and not for routine clinical applications and should only be administered to patients who have *HER2*-positive BC.

In one German randomized, phase III trial (GeparQuinto, GBG 44 trial), lapatinib versus trastuzumab in combination with neoadjuvant anthracycline-taxane-based chemotherapy was compared in the neoadjuvant setting [95]. IBC cases were also included in the study (83 patients had T4d disease). A total of 620 patients were randomly assigned in a 1/1 ratio to receive neoadjuvant therapy with four cycles of EC (epirubicin+cyclophosphamide) every 3 weeks and four cycles of docetaxel (D) with either Tr (every 3 weeks for eight cycles) or lapatinib (L: 1,000–1,250 mg/day throughout all cycles) before surgery. Of 620 patients, 309 received ECTr-DTr, and 311 received ECL-DL. The pCR rate was 30.3 % in the ECTr-DTr group and 22.7 % in the ECL-DL group. The difference was statistically significant ($p = 0.04$). This study demonstrated that the pCR rate was significantly lower in the lapatinib+CT group compared to the Tr+CT group. The investigators concluded that unless long-term outcome data showed different results, lapatinib should not be used outside of clinical trials as a single anti-*HER2* treatment in combination with NACT.

Table 16.3 Pathological complete response and survival rates according to neoadjuvant chemotherapy protocol in inflammatory breast cancer

Trial	Type of study	*n*	pCR rate	Survival
	NACT protocol			
Ueno et al. [64]	Retrospective	178	10 %	15-year DFS 28 %
	Anthracycline-containing regimens			10-year OS 35 %
Cristofanilli et al. [66]	Retrospective	62	25 %	3-year PFS 46 %
	Anthracycline+paclitaxel			3-year OS 71 %
Dawood et al. [86]	Retrospective	16 (3 patients with stage 4 disease)	62.5 %	2-year PFS 59.4 %
	Anthracycline+paclitaxel+trastuzumab in HER2-positive patients			
Baselga et al. [91]	Prospective randomized study	61		3-year EFS
	(NOAH trial)		48 % (+Tr) vs. 13 % (−Tr)	70.1 % (+Tr) vs. 53.3 % (−Tr)
	Anthracycline+taxane±trastuzumab in HER2-positive patients			

DFS disease-free survival, *EFS* event-free survival, *NACT* neoadjuvant chemotherapy, *NOAH* neoadjuvant Herceptin trial, *pCR* pathological complete response, *PFS* progression-free survival, *OS* overall survival, *Tr* trastuzumab

In one prospective randomized study, a lapatinib plus Tr combination was compared to Tr and lapatinib (NeoALTTO trial) [96]. Only early breast cancer patients were enrolled in this study. The NeoALTTO trial demonstrated that dual anti-HER2 inhibition with Tr+lapatinib combined with weekly P significantly increased the proportion of patients achieving pCR (51.3 %; 95 % CI 43.1–59.5) in the combination group compared with Tr alone (29.5 %; 95 % CI 22.4–37.5) and lapatinib alone (24.7 %; 95 % CI 18.1–32.3). The difference was statistically significant ($p=0.0001$). The EFS and OS did not differ between treatment groups. However, the 3-year EFS and 3-year OS were significantly improved in women who achieved pCR (HR 0.38, $p=0.0003$, and HR 0.35, $p=0.005$, respectively) [97]. Findings from this study confirmed that pCR after neoadjuvant anti-*HER2* therapy is an important prognostic factor for survival.

The NeoSphere study was a multicenter, open-label, phase II randomized trial. IBC cases (29 of 417 patients) were also enrolled in this study. Tr and another anti-*HER2* targeted agent, pertuzumab, were used during the preoperative CT period [98]. The pCR ratio was higher in the pertuzumab+Tr+docetaxel combination arm then in the Tr+docetaxel combination arm (39.3 %

vs. 21.5 %; $p=0.0063$). The TRYPHANEA study, a phase II cardiac safety study, was a randomized, three-arm study [99]. A total of 225 *HER2*-positive LABC, IBC and operable breast cancer patients were enrolled in the study. In the first arm, NACT+Tr+pertuzumab was followed by Tr+pertuzumab+docetaxel. In the second arm, NACT only was followed by docetaxel+Tr+pertuzumab. In the third arm, docetaxel+carboplatin+Tr+pertuzumab combination was administered. The pCR ratio was the same in all treatment groups but was highest in the third arm (66.2 %). After these two studies, the Food and Drug Administration (FDA) approved the use of Tr+pertuzumab+docetaxel combination as NACT for *HER2*-positive LABC, IBC, and early breast cancer (>2 cm tumor or axillary lymph node positive) [100].

The pCR rates and survival after anthracycline, anthracycline+taxane, and CT+trastuzumab-containing NACT regimens for the treatment of IBC are outlined in Table 16.3.

In another study, a new anti-*HER2* agent, afatinib (an oral tyrosine kinase inhibitor and irreversible binder of *HER1*, *HER2*, and *HER3*), was compared to Tr and lapatinib in a neoadjuvant setting in patients with *HER2*-positive stage IIIA, B, C, and IBC [101]. A total of 29 patients were randomized to afatinib ($n=10$), lapatinib ($n=8$), or trastuzumab ($n=11$). These drugs were administered for a duration of 6 weeks until the patients underwent surgery. The ORR was determined for eight afatinib-, six lapatinib-, and four trastuzumab-treated patients. Drug-related adverse events were recorded in all afatinib-treated patients and commonly included diarrhea, acneiform dermatitis, and paronychia. Diarrhea and rash were documented in six of eight lapatinib-treated patients. The authors concluded that afatinib demonstrated more favorable clinical activity than lapatinib and trastuzumab for neoadjuvant treatment of *HER2*-positive LABC and IBC.

Antiangiogenic Therapies

Vascular endothelial growth factor (*VEGF*) expression is increased in IBC. Therefore, antiangiogenic drugs have been suggested as therapy targets. The antiangiogenic drug bevacizumab has been used together with chemotherapy in induction therapy but did not meet the expectations [1–4, 56, 83, 102, 103]. NCI-0173 was a small, phase II study that included 21 patients and assessed the efficacy of doxorubicin and docetaxel combined with bevacizumab in the preoperative treatment of LABC/IBC cases [104]. The clinical RR was 67 %, and the pCR rate was 5 %. The BEVERLY-2 study was a multicenter, one-armed, open-label, phase II study performed in France with *HER2*-positive nonmetastatic IBC patients [105]. First, four cycles of a FEC-bevacizumab combination were applied, followed by four cycles of docetaxel-bevacizumab-Tr combination every 21 days. Forty-two (8 %) of 52 patients completed eight cycles of therapy, and 49 patients (94 %) underwent surgery. The pCR rate was 63.5 %. The 3-year DFS rate was 68 %, and the OS was 90 %; the 3-year DFS rate for patients who achieved pCR was 80 %. Astheny and vomiting were reported as the most common side effects. In the other part of this study, the numbers of circulating tumor cells (CTCs) and circulating endothelial cells (CECs) were counted before the study

began, at the fifth cycle, before surgery, during the postoperative period, and during the first year [106]. The 3-year DFS was 95 % in patients with pCR, and these patients were CTC-free after treatment. For baseline (before treatment) patient CTC numbers of <1 and ≥1, the 3-year survival was 81 % and 43 %, respectively; this difference was statistically significant ($p=0.01$). Prognostic importance was not detected for CEC. This study is important in terms of demonstrating the prognostic effect of CTC. In another study, CTCs were determined to be a strong predictor of worse prognosis in patients with newly diagnosed IBC [107].

Semaxanib (*SU5416*) is an organic small receptor tyrosine kinase inhibitor that inhibits *VEGF*-mediated signaling through *VEGFR2*. The effectiveness of a doxorubicin and semaxanib combination was investigated in 18 stage IIIB and IBC patients in a phase IB study [108]. The median survival has not yet been provided. After treatment, the density of microvessels and blood flow through the tumor decreased. Neutropenia was reported as a factor in dose-limiting toxicity. Congestive heart failure was monitored in four patients (22 %).

Antiangiogenic drug studies continue with pazopanib, a new multi-targeted tyrosine kinase inhibitor.

New Targets

There are many ongoing targeted therapy drug studies (*p53* gene therapy, *p53* stabilizer agents, proteasome inhibitors, *Tie-2* kinase inhibitors, *E-cadherin* inhibitors, phosphatidyl-inositol-3-kinase inhibitors, farnesyltransferase inhibitors, etc.) [1–4, 52, 56, 83, 102, 103]. *p53* mutations are associated with decreased responses to CT and decreased survival outcomes.

EGFR overexpression occurs in 30 % of IBC cases. Mortality risk is increased with increased expression of *EGFR* and chemokine receptors (*CXCR4* and *CCR7*) in IBC [109]. The 5-year OS was 24.8 % in an IHC analysis of *CXCR4*-positive patients and 42.3 % in the negative group. The 5-year OS was 20 % in an IHC analysis of

CCR7-positive patients and 41.9 % in the negative group. These genes have been announced as new targets for therapy. The effectiveness of the human-*EGFR* antibody panitumumab and chemotherapy (nanoparticle paclitaxel and carboplatin) combination will be investigated in *HER2*-negative IBC cases during the preoperative period.

A deficiency in the Ras signaling pathway member low-affinity insulin-like growth binding protein (*LIBC/WINT1*) and overexpression of Ras homolog gene family member C (*RhoC*) guanosine triphosphatase (*GTPase*) have been established in IBC [110]. In situ hybridization analysis of paraffin blocks demonstrated that LIBC deficiency was 80 % in IBC cases and 21 % in non-IBC cases ($p = 0.0013$). The *RhoC GTPase* overexpression ratio was 90 % in IBC cases and 38 % in non-IBC cases ($p = 0.0095$). These genes may be a target for the treatment of IBC. Farnesyltransferase inhibitors (*FTIs*) inhibit RhoC and angiogenesis. *FTIs* have been investigated for IBC. The FTI tipifarnib (T) enhances the antitumor effects of chemotherapy in vitro, has activity in metastatic breast cancer, and enhances the pCR rate of neoadjuvant AC chemotherapy. In one phase I–II trial, T plus weekly P and 2-week AC CT were tested as a neoadjuvant treatment for *HER2*-negative *ER* and/or *PR*-positive LABC (stratum A: 33 patients) and IBC (stratum B: 22 patients) irrespective of *ER/PR* expression [111]. The breast pCR rate was 18 % in stratum A and 4 % in stratum B. These results are not sufficient to indicate the use of *FTIs* for the neoadjuvant treatment of IBC.

Anaplastic lymphoma kinase (*ALK*) gene amplification or overexpression may occur in IBC [112, 113]. IBC patients are currently being evaluated for the presence of *ALK* genetic abnormalities and, when eligible, enrolled into clinical trials evaluating *ALK*-targeted therapies (the small-molecule dual tyrosine kinase *cMET/ALK* inhibitor crizotinib).

Endocrine Therapies

ER and *PR* negativity is higher in IBC than in other types of breast cancer [1–4, 37, 38]. Some studies have reported that up to 83 % of IBC tumors are *ER* negative [114, 115]. HR negativity is associated with more aggressive clinical course, shorter survival, and poor prognosis. The median survival for HR-positive IBC is superior to that of HR-negative IBC according to SEER data (4 vs. 2 year; $p = 0.0001$) [15].

There are no studies of neoadjuvant hormonal therapy in primary IBC. Antiestrogen therapy should be applied after induction therapy and adjuvant chemotherapy are completed for HR-positive patients [7, 10]. Antiestrogen therapy should include either tamoxifen or an aromatase inhibitor depending on the patient's menopausal status. The minimum period for use is 5 years.

The anti-inflammatory and cholesterol-lowering effects of statins suggest they may have antitumor effects as well. The effect of statins on IBC was determined in a cohort study conducted by MDACC [116]. PFS was improved in patients who received hydrophobic statins (atorvastatin, pravastatin, rosuvastatin) (HR, 0.49; 95 % CI 0.28–0.84; $p < 0.01$). No significant response was observed in patients who received lipophilic statins (fluvastatin, lovastatin, simvastatin). The mechanism of this effect is not known. Double-blind, prospective randomized studies are needed to explain this effect.

Monitoring the Response to Treatment

The international IBC consensus panel recommends that monitoring of the response to PSC entails a combination of physical examination and imaging techniques [7]. Physical examination of the breast and regional lymph nodes for response may be conducted every 6–9 weeks [117]. The breasts are usually photographed during the examination because the response to treatment can be monitored by the reduction in erythema and edema [118]. After therapy is complete, radiological evaluation should be performed and compared with the initial examination data. If necessary, radiological evaluation can be performed in the middle of the treatment course to confirm or refute the clinical findings.

Mammography and USG are recommended for radiological evaluation. MRI may be a better option to evaluate the response to therapy if it is available and affordable [5, 7]. In one trial, FDG-PET/CT was used to evaluate the response to NACT [119]. Thirty-two patients were included in the study. In patients with CR according to the PET/CT imaging, only 26 % had pCR. In conclusion, more research is needed to use PET/CT to evaluate the response to therapy.

Follow-Up After Therapy

After the completion of treatment, regular history, physical examination, and mammography are recommended for follow-up by the American Society of Clinical Oncology (ASCO) and the European Society of Medical Oncology (ESMO) [120, 121]. Physical examinations should be performed at 3- to 6-month intervals for the first 3 years, every 6–12 months for years 4 and 5, and annually thereafter. Yearly mammography of the other breast is suggested by ASCO [120]. The examination of local lymph nodes with yearly USG has been suggested, although data are insufficient [7]. Genetic consultations are particularly important for patients with a family history of breast and ovarian cancer [9]. Prophylactic contralateral mastectomy should not be performed unless there are risk factors that make this obligatory. Routine performance of other radiological examinations, blood tests, and tumor markers are not suggested in asymptomatic patients. Distant metastases are common during the follow-up period of the disease. Metastasis was observed in 203 of 478 stage III IBC patients at a median observation time of 29 months [122]. The most common metastasis locations were the bone (28 %), lung (21 %), liver (21 %), and CNS (21 %). CNS metastasis was most frequent in *HER2*-positive and triple-negative subtypes, as with non-IBC subtypes ($p = 0.001$).

Conclusion

Multimodal therapy (PST, surgery, and radiotherapy) is the main treatment method for IBC [1–5, 7, 9, 123] (Fig. 16.1). Underuse of trimodal therapy is associated with decreased survival [59]. Currently, anthracycline- and taxane-containing chemotherapy protocols as PSC are preferred (with the addition of trastuzumab in *HER2*+ patients). Following PSC, surgical assessment is suggested. A modified radical mastectomy can be performed in patients with recovered skin eruption. Next, adjuvant RT is applied. In patients with no response to PSC, additional systemic CT and/or preoperative RT is planned. Trastuzumab therapy should be started during the NACT period with taxanes and extended to 1 year for *HER2*-positive patients. Antiestrogen therapy is suggested for at least 5 years for HR-positive patients. New combined CT regimens and new targeted therapies are being investigated to increase the pCR ratio and survival times.

In recent years, an international congress devoted to IBC has been planned [124]. Opening specific IBC clinics similar to that established by MDACC will improve outcomes and promote well-designed research trials.

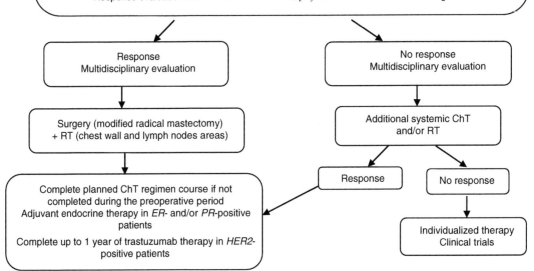

Fig. 16.1 Flowchart for diagnosis, follow-up, and treatment of inflammatory breast cancer [1–4, 7–9, 52, 118]. *Abbreviations*: *ChT* chemotherapy, *CT* computed tomography, *ER* estrogen receptor, *FDG-PET/CT* fluorodeoxyglucose positron emission tomography/computed tomography, *HER2* human epidermal growth factor receptor 2, *PR* progesterone receptor, *PSC* primary systemic chemotherapy, *RT* radiotherapy

References

1. Barsky SH, Mrozek E, Love R. Inflammatory breast cancer. In: Bland KI, Copeland III EM, editors. The breast comprehensive management of benign and malignant diseases. 4th ed. Philadelphia: Saunders; 2009. p. 1393–402.
2. Dean-Colomb WM, Cristofanilli M. Inflammatory breast cancer. In: Kantarjian HM, Wolff RA, Koller CA, editors. The MD Anderson manual of medical oncology. 2nd ed. China: Mc Graw-Hill; 2011. p. 712–29.
3. Woodward WE, Cristofanilli M. Inflammatory breast cancer. Semin Radiat Oncol. 2009;19:256–65.
4. Overmoyer B, Pierce LJ. Inflammatory breast cancer. In: Harris JR, Morrow M, Osborne JK, editors. Disease of the breast. 5th ed. Philadelphia: Wolters Kluwer; 2015. p. 800–15.
5. Yamauchı H, Woodward WA, Valero V, Alvarez RH, Lucci A, Buchholz TA, et al. Inflammatory breast cancer: what we know and what we need to learn. Oncologist. 2012;17:891–9.
6. Lee BJ, Tannenbaum NE. Inflammatory carcinoma of the breast; report of twenty-eight cases from the breast clinic of Memorial Hospital. Surg Gynecol Obstet. 1924;39:580–95.
7. Dawood S, Merajver SD, Viens P, Vermeulen PB, Swain SM, Buchholz TA, et al. International expert panel on inflammatory breast cancer: consensus statement for standardized diagnosis and treatment. Ann Oncol. 2011;22:515–23.
8. Rabban J. Breast. In: Edge SB, Byrd DB, Compton CC, Fritz AG, Grene FI, Trotti A, editors. AJCC cancer staging manual. 7th ed. Chicago: Springer; 2010; p. 345–77.
9. National Comprehensive Cancer Network (NCCN). NCCN clinical practice guideline in oncology. Breast Cancer v.3 2014. www.nccn.org
10. Dawood S, Ueno NT, Valero V, Woodward WA, Buchholz TA, Hortobagyi GN, et al. Differences in survival among women with stage III inflammatory and noninflammatory locally advanced breast cancer appear early. Cancer. 2011;117:1819–26.
11. Hirko KA, Soliman AS, Banerjee M, Ruterbusch J, Harford JB, Merajver SD, et al. A comparison of criteria to identify inflammatory breast cancer cases from medical records and the surveillance, epidemiology and end results data base. 2007–2009. Breast J. 2014;20:185–91.
12. Levine PH, Venerosa C. The epidemiology of inflammatory breast cancer. Semin Oncol. 2008;35:11–6.
13. Dawood S, Cristofanilli M. What progress have we made in managing inflammatory breast cancer? Oncology (Willingston Park). 2007;21:673–9.
14. Anderson WF, Schairer C, Chen BE, Hance KW, Levine PH. Epidemiology of inflammatory breast cancer (IBC). Breast Dis. 2005;22:9–23.
15. Hance KW, Anderson WF, Devesa SS, Young HA, Levine PH. Trends in inflammatory breast carcinoma incidence and survival: the surveillance, epidemiology, and end results program at the National Cancer Institute. J Natl Cancer Inst. 2005;97:966–75.
16. Wingo PA, Jamison PM, Young JL, Gargiullo P. Population- based statistics for women diagnosed with inflammatory breast cancer. Cancer Causes Control. 2004;15:321–8.
17. Corbex M, Bouzbid S, Boffetta P. Features of breast cancer in developing countries, examples from North-Africa. Eur J Cancer. 2014;50:1808–18.
18. Slaoui M, Razine R, İbrahimi A, Attaleb M, Mzibri ME, Amrani M. Breast cancer in Morocco: a literature review. Asian Pac J Cancer. 2014;15:1067–74.
19. Chiedozi LC. Rapidly progressing breast cancer in Nigeria. Eur J Surg Oncol. 1987;13:505–9.
20. Maalej M, Frikha H, Ben Salem, Daoud J, Bouaouina N, Ben Abdallah M, et al. Breast cancer in Tunisia: clinical and epidemiological study. Bull Cancer. 1999;86:302–6.
21. Gunhan BI, Üstün EE, Memiş A. Inflammatory breast carcinoma: mammographic, ultrasonographic, clinical and pathologic findings in 142 cases. Radiology. 2002;223:929–38.
22. Amparo RS, Angel CD, Ana LH, Antonio LC, Vicente MS, Carlos FM, et al. Inflammatory breast carcinoma: pathological or clinical entity? Breast Cancer Res Treat. 2000;64:269–73.
23. Natori A, Hayashi N, Soejima K, Deshpande GA, Takahashi O, Cristofanilli M, et al. A comparison of epidemiology, biology, and prognosis of inflammatory breast cancer in Japanese and US populations. Clin Breast Cancer. 2013;13:460–4.
24. Chang S, Buzdar AU, Hursting SD. Inflammatory breast cancer and body-mass index. J Clin Oncol. 1998;16:3731–5.
25. Chang S, Alderfer JR, Asmar L, Buzdar AU. Inflammatory breast cancer survival: the role of obesity and menopausal status at diagnosis. Breast Cancer Res Treat. 2000;64:157–63.
26. Schairer C, Li Y, Frawley P, Graubard BI, Wellman RD, Buist DS, et al. Risk factors for inflammatory breast cancer and other invasive breast cancer. J Natl Cancer Inst. 2013;105:1373–84.
27. Mohamed MM, Al-raawi D, Sabet SF, El-Shinawi M. Inflammatory breast cancer: new factors contribute to disease etiology: review. J Adv Res. 2013;6:526–35.
28. Levine PH, Mourali N, Tabbane F, Loon J, Terasaki P, Tsang P, et al. Studies on the role of cellular immunity and genetics in the etiology of rapidly progressing breast cancer in Tunisia. Int J Cancer. 1981;27:611–5.
29. Mourali N, Levine PH, Tabanne F, Belhassen S, Bahi J, Bennaceur M, et al. Rapidly progressing breast cancer (poussee evolutive) in Tunisia: studies on delayed hypersensitivity. Int J Cancer. 1978; 22:1–3.
30. Pogo BG, Holland JF, Levine PH. Human mammary tumor virus in inflammatory breast cancer. Cancer. 2010;116(11 suppl):2741–4.

31. Levine PH, Pogo BG, Klouj A, Coronel S, Woodson K, Melana SM, et al. Increasing evidence for a human breast carcinoma virus with geographic differences. Cancer. 2004;101:721–6.

32. El-Shinawi M, Mohamed HT, El-Ghonaimy EA, Tantawy M, Younis A, Schneider RJ, et al. Human cytomegalovirus infection enhances NF/kB/p65 signaling in inflammatory breast cancer patients. PLoS One. 2013;8:1–10.

33. Gutierrez-Barrera AM, Turco DL, Alvarez RH, Litton JK, Valero V, Hortobagyi GN, et al. BRCA mutations in women with inflammatory breast cancer. J Clin Oncol. 2010; (ASCO breast cancer symposium abstracts) 28: Abstract 192.

34. Aziz SA, Pervez S, Khan S, Kayani N, Azam SI, Rahbar MH. Case control study of prognostic markers and disease outcome in inflammatory carcinoma breast: a unique clinical experience. Breast J. 2001;7:398–404.

35. Chow CK. Imaging in inflammatory breast carcinoma. Breast Dis. 2005;22:45–54.

36. Yang WT, Le-Petross HT, Macapinlac H, Carkaci S, Gonzalez-Angulo AM, Dawood S, et al. Inflammatory breast cancer: PET/CT, MRI, mammography and ultrasonography findings. Breast Cancer Res Treat. 2008;109:417–26.

37. Morgensztern D. Breast pathology. In: Silva OE, Zurrida S, editors. Breast cancer, a practical guide. 3rd ed. Edinburgh: Elsevier; 2005. p. 84–94.

38. Stamatakos MD. Invasive breast cancer. In: Jacops L, Finlayson CA, editors. Early diagnosis and treatment of cancer: breast cancer. Philadelphia: Saunders-Elsevier; 2011. p. 21–54.

39. Abner A, Kaufman M, Pories S, Gauvin G. Unusual presentations of malignancy. Case 1. Male inflammatory (?) breast cancer. J Clin Oncol. 2001;19:3288–9.

40. Lucas FV, Perez-Mesa C. Inflammatory carcinoma of the breast. Cancer. 1978;41:1595–605.

41. Li J, Gonzalez-Angulo AM, Allen PK, Yu TK, Woodward WA, Ueno NT, et al. Triple-negative subtype predicts poor overall survival and high locoregional relapse in inflammatory breast cancer. Oncologist. 2011;16:1675–83.

42. Masuda H, Baggerly KA, Wang Y, Iwamoto T, Brewer T, Pusztai L, et al. Comparison of molecular subtype distribution in triple-negative inflammatory and non-inflammatory breast cancer. Breast Cancer Res. 2013;15:R112 (1–9).

43. Bertucci F, Finetti P, Rougemont J, Charafe-Jauffret E, Nasser V, Loriod B, et al. Gene expression profiling for molecular characterization of inflammatory breast cancer and prediction of response to chemotherapy. Cancer Res. 2004;64:8558–65.

44. Woodward WA, Krishnamurthy S, Yamauchi H, El-Zein R, Ogura D, Kitadai E, et al. Genomic and expression analysis of microdissected inflammatory breast cancer. Breast Cancer Res Treat. 2013;138:761–72.

45. Bertucci F, Finetti P, Birnbaum D, Viens P. Gene expression profiling of inflammatory breast cancer. Cancer. 2010;116(11 suppl):2783–93.

46. Taylor G, Meltzer A. Inflammatory carcinoma of the breast. Am J Cancer. 1938;33:33–49.

47. Kell MR, Morrow M. Surgical aspects of inflammatory breast cancer. Breast Dis. 2005;22:67–73.

48. Bruckman JE, Harris JR, Levene MB, Chaffey JT, Hellman S. Results of treating stage III carcinoma of the breast by primary radiation therapy. Cancer. 1979;43:985–93.

49. Perez CA, Fields JN. Role of radiation therapy for locally advanced and inflammatory carcinoma of the breast. Oncology (Huntingt). 1979;1:81–94.

50. Barker JL, Nelson AJ, Montague ED. Inflammatory carcinoma of the breast. Radiology. 1976;121:173–6.

51. Singletary SE, Ames FC, Buzdar AU. Management of inflammatory breast cancer. World J Surg. 1994;18:87–92.

52. Cristofanilli M, Buzdar AU, Hortobagyi GN. Update on the management of inflammatory breast cancer. Oncologist. 2003;8:141–8.

53. Giordano SH. Update on locally advanced breast cancer. Oncologist. 2003;8:521–30.

54. Harris EE, Schultz D, Bertsch H, Fox K, Glick J, Solin LJ. Ten-year outcome after combined modality therapy for inflammatory breast cancer. Int J Radiat Oncol Biol Phys. 2003;55:1200–8.

55. Low JA, Berman AW, Steinberg SM, Danforth DN, Lippman ME, Swain SM. Long-term follow-up for locally advanced and inflammatory breast cancer patients treated with multimodality therapy. J Clin Oncol. 2004;22:4067–74.

56. Sinclair S, Swain SM. Primary systemic chemotherapy for inflammatory breast cancer. Cancer. 2010;116(11 suppl):2821–8.

57. Dawood S, Lei X, Dent R, Gupta S, Sirohi B, Cortes J, et al. Survival of women with inflammatory breast cancer : a large population-based study. Ann Oncol. 2014;25:1143–51.

58. Tsai CJ, Li J, Gonzales-Angulo AM, Allen PK, Woodward WA, Ueno NT, et al. Outcomes after multidisciplinary treatment of inflammatory breast cancer in the era of neoadjuvant HER-2 directed therapy. Am J Clin Oncol. 2015;38(3):242–7.

59. Rueth NM, Lin HY, Bedrosian I, Shaitelman SF, Ueno NT, Shen Y, et al. Underuse of trimodality treatment affects survival for patients with inflammatory breast cancer: an analysis of treatment and survival trends from National Cancer Database. J Clin Oncol. 2014;32:2018–24.

60. Hennessy BT, Gonzales-Angulo AM, Hortobagyi GN, Cristofanilli M, Kau SW, Broglio K, et al. Disease-free and overall survival after pathologic complete disease remission of cytologically proven inflammatory breast carcinoma axillary lymph node metastases after primary systemic chemotherapy. Cancer. 2006;106:1000–6.

61. Masuda H, Brewer TM, Liu DD, Iwamoto T, Shen Y, Hsu L, et al. Long-term treatment efficacy in primary inflammatory breast cancer by hormonal receptor and HER2 defined subtypes. Ann Oncol. 2014;25:384–91.

62. Bouer RL, Busch E, Levine F, Edge SB. Therapy for inflammatory breast cancer: impact of doxorubicin based therapy. Ann Surg Oncol. 1995;2:288–94.

63. Koh EH, Buzdar AU, Ames FC, Koh EH, Buzdar AU, Ames FC, et al. Inflammatory carcinoma of the breast: results of a combined modality approach – M.D. Anderson Cancer Center Experience. Cancer Chemother Pharmacol. 1990;27:94–100.

64. Ueno NT, Buzdar AU, Singletary SE, Ames FC, McNeese MD, Holmes FA, et al. Combined modality treatment of inflammatory breast cancer. Twenty years experience at M.D. Anderson Cancer Center. Cancer Chemother Pharmacol. 1997;40:321–9.

65. Cristofanilli M, Buzdar AU, Sneige N, Smith T, Wasaff B, Ibrahim N, et al. Paclitaxel in the multi-modality treatment for inflammatory breast carcinoma. Cancer. 2001;92:1775–82.

66. Cristofanilli M, Gonzalez-Angulo AM, Buzdar AU, Kau SW, Frye DK, Hortobagyi GN. Paclitaxel significantly improves the prognosis in ER negative inflammatory breast cancer. The M.D. Anderson Cancer Center Experience (1974–2000). Breast Cancer Res Treat. 2002;76 suppl 1:S158a.

67. Buzdar AU, Singletary SE, Booser DJ, Frye DK, Wasaff B, Hortobagyi GN. Combined modality treatment of stage III and inflammatory breast cancer. M.D. Anderson Cancer Center Experience. Surg Oncol Clin N Am. 1995;4:715–34.

68. Panades M, Olivotto IA, Speers CH, Shenkier T, Olivotto TA, Weir L, et al. Evolving treatment strategies for inflammatory breast cancer: a population based survival analysis. J Clin Oncol. 2005;23:1941–50.

69. Costa SD, Loibl S, Kaufmann M, Zahm DM, Hilfrich J, Huober J, et al. Neoadjuvant chemotherapy shows similar response in patients with inflammatory or locally advanced breast cancer when compared with operable breast cancer: a secondary analysis of the GeparTrio trial data. J Clin Oncol. 2010;28:83–91.

70. Cristofanilli M, Fratarcangeli T, Esteva F, Rosales M, Booser D, Ibrahim M, et al. Weekly high dose paclitaxel has significant antitumor activity in inflammatory breast cancer (IBC). Proceeding of the ECCO 11. Eur J Cancer. 2001;37:S173.

71. Green MC, Buzdar AU, Smith T, et al. Weekly (wkly) paclitaxel (P) followed by FAC as primary systemic chemotherapy (PSC) of operable breast cancer improves pathologic complete remission (pCR) rates when compared to every 3-week (Q3 wk) P therapy (tx) followed by FAC- final results of a prospective phase III randomized trial. Proc Am Soc Clin Oncol. 2002;21:35a.

72. Chevallier B, Roche H, Olivier JP, Chollet P, Hurteloup P. Inflammatory breast cancer: pilot study of intensive induction chemotherapy (FEC-HD) results in a high histologic response rate. Am J Clin Oncol. 1993;16:223–8.

73. Cagnoni PJ, Nieto Y, Shpall EJ, Bearman SI, Barón AE, Ross M, et al. High-dose chemotherapy with autologous hematopoietic progenitor-cell support as part of combined modality therapy in patients with inflammatory breast cancer. J Clin Oncol. 1998;16:1661–8.

74. Dazzi C, Cariello A, Rosti G, Tienghi A, Molino A, Sabbatini R, et al. Neoadjuvant high dose chemotherapy plus peripheral blood progenitor cells in inflammatory breast cancer: a multicenter phase II pilot study. Haematologica. 2001;86:523–9.

75. Viens P, Palangie T, Janvier M, Fabbro M, Roché H, Delozier T. First-line high-dose sequential chemotherapy with r-GCSF and repeated blood stem cell transplantation in untreated inflammatory breast cancer: toxicity and response (PEGASE 02 Trial). Br J Cancer. 1999;81:449–56.

76. Somlo G, Frankel P, Chow W, Leong L, Margolin K, Morgan Jr R. Prognostic indicators and survival in patients with stage IIIB inflammatory breast carcinoma after dose-intense chemotherapy. J Clin Oncol. 2004;10:1839–48.

77. Cheng YC, Rondon G, Yang Y, Smith TL, Gajewski JL, Donato ML. The use of high dose cyclophosphamide, carmustine, and thitepa plus autologous hematopoietic stem cell transplantation as consolidation therapy for high risk primary breast cancer after primary surgery or neoadjuvant chemotherapy. Biol Blood Marrow Transpl. 2004;10:794–804.

78. Viens P, Tarpin C, Roche H, Bertucci F. Systemic therapy of inflammatory breast cancer from high-dose chemotherapy to targeted therapies: the French experience. Cancer. 2010;116(11 suppl):2829–36.

79. Veyret C, Levy C, Chollet P, Merrouche Y, Roche H, Kerbrat P. Inflammatory breast cancer outcome with epirubicin based induction and maintenance chemotherapy: ten-year results from the French Adjuvant Study Group GETIS 02 Trial. Cancer. 2006;107:2535–44.

80. Dawood S, Broglio K, Gong Y, Yang WT, Cristofanilli M, Kau SW. Prognostic significance of HER2 status in women with inflammatory breast cancer. Cancer. 2008;112:97–103.

81. Zell JA, Tsang WY, Taylor TH, Mehta RS, Anton-Culver H. Prognostic impact of human epidermal growth factor like receptor 2 and hormone receptor status in inflammatory breast cancer (IBC): analysis of 2.014 IBC cases from the California Cancer Registry. Breast Cancer Res. 2009;11:R9.

82. Buzdar AU, Valero V, Ibrahim NK, Francis D, Broglio KR, Theriault RL, et al. Neoadjuvant therapy with paclitaxel followed by 5 fluorouracil, epirubicin and cyclophosphamide chemotherapy and concurrent trastuzumab in HER2 positive operable breast cancer: an update of the initial randomized study population and data of additional patients treated with the same regimen. Clin Cancer Res. 2007;13:228–33.

83. Cristofanilli M. Novel targeted therapies in inflammatory breast cancer. Cancer. 2010;116(11 suppl):2837–9.

84. Dawood S, Gonzales Angulo AM, Peintinger F, Broglio K, Symmans WF, Kau SW, et al. Efficacy

and safety of neoadjuvant trastuzumab combined with paclitaxel and epirubicin: a retrospective review of the MD Anderson experience. Cancer. 2007;110:1195–200.

85. Chang HR. Trastuzumab-based neoadjuvant therapy in patients with *HER2*-positive breast cancer. Cancer. 2010;116:2856–67.

86. Dawood S, Gong Y, Broglio K, Buchholz TA, Woodward W, Lucci A, et al. Trastuzumab in primary inflammatory breast cancer, high pathologic response rates and improved outcome. Breast J. 2010;16:529–32.

87. Hurley J, Doliny P, Reis I, Silva O, Gomez-Fernandez C, Velez P, et al. Docetaxel, cisplatin, and trastuzumab as primary systemic therapy for human epidermal growth factor receptor 2-positive locally advanced breast cancer. J Clin Oncol. 2006;24:1831–8.

88. Van Pelt AE, Mohsin S, Elledge RM, Hilsenbeck SG, Gutierrez MC, Lucci Jr A, et al. Neoadjuvant trastuzumab and docetaxel in breast cancer: preliminary results. Clin Breast Cancer. 2003;4:348–53.

89. Gianni L, Eiermann W, Semiglazov V, Manikhas A, Lluch A, Tjulandin S, et al. Neoadjuvant chemotherapy with trastuzumab followed by adjuvant trastuzumab versus neoadjuvant chemotherapy alone, in patients with HER-2-positive locally advanced breast cancer (the NOAH trial): a randomised controlled superiority trial with a parallel *HER2*-negative cohort. Lancet. 2010;375:377–84.

90. Gianni L, Eiermann W, Semiglazov V, Lluch A, Tjulandin S, Zambetti M, et al. Neoadjuvant and adjuvant trastuzumab in patients with HER-2-positive locally advanced breast cancer (the NOAH trial): follow-up of a randomised controlled superiority trial with a parallel *HER2*-negative cohort. Lancet Oncol. 2014;15:640–7.

91. Baselga J, Semiglazov V, Manikhas GM, et al. Efficacy of neoadjuvan trastuzumab in patients with inflammatory breast cancer: data from the NOAH (neoadjuvant herceptin) phase III trial (abstract 2030)(ECCO meeting 2007). Eur J Cancer. 2007;5:193.

92. Hall PS, Hanby A, Cameron DA. Lapatinib for inflammatory breast cancer. Lancet Oncol. 2009;10:538–9.

93. Cristofanelli M, Boussen J, Baselga J, et al. Phase II combination study of lapatinib and paclitaxel as neoadjuvant therapy in patients with newly diagnosed inflammatory breast cancer. Breast Cancer Res Treat. 2006;100:1A. Abstract.

94. Boussen H, Cristofanilli M, Zaks T, DeSilvio M, Salazar V, Spector N. Phase II study to evaluate the efficacy and safety of neoadjuvant lapatinib plus paclitaxel in patients with inflammatory breast cancer. J Clin Oncol. 2010;28:3248–55.

95. Untch M, Loibl S, Bischoff J, Eidtmann H, Kaufmann M, Blohmer JU, et al. Lapatinib versus trastuzumab in combination with neoadjuvant anthracycline-taxane-based chemotherapy

(GeparQuinto, GBG44): a randomised phase III trial. Lancet Oncol. 2012;13:135–44.

96. Baselga J, Bradbury I, Eidtmann H, Di Cosimo S, de Azambuja E, Aura C, et al. Lapatinib with trastuzumab for *HER2* positive early breast cancer (NeoALTTO). A randomized, open label, multicentre phase III trial. Lancet. 2012;379:633–40.

97. Azambuja E, Holmes AP, Piccart M, Holmes E, Di Cosimo S, Swaby F, et al. Lapatinib with trastuzumab for *HER2* positive early breast cancer (NeoALTTO): survival outcomes of a randomised, open-label, multicentre, phase 3 trial and their association with pathological complete response. Lancet Oncol. 2014;15:1137–46.

98. Gianni L, Pienkowski T, Im YH, Roman L, Tseng LM, Liu MC, et al. Efficacy and safety of neoadjuvant pertuzumab and trastuzumab in women with locally advanced, inflammatory, or early HER2-positive breast cancer (NeoSphere): a randomized multicentre, open label phase 2 trial. Lancet Oncol. 2012;13:25–32.

99. Schneeweiss A, Chia S, Hickish T, Harvey V, Eniu A, Hegg R, et al. Pertuzumab plus trastuzumab in combination with standard neoadjuvant anthracycline-containing and anthracycline-free chemotherapy regimens in patients with *HER2*-positive early breast cancer: a randomised phase II cardiac safety study (TRYPHAENA). Ann Oncol. 2013;24:2278–84.

100. Amiri-Kordestani L, Wedam S, Zhang L, Tang S, Tilley A, Ibrahim A, et al. First FDA approval of neoadjuvant therapy for breast cancer: pertuzumab for the treatment of patients with *HER2*-positive breast cancer. Clin Cancer Res. 2014;20:5359–64.

101. Riawi MF, Aleixo SB, Rozas AA, Nunes de Matos Neto J, Caleffi M, Figueira AC, et al. A neoadjuvant, randomized, open-label phase II trial of afatinib versus trastuzumab versus lapatinib in patients with locally advanced HER2-positive breast cancer. Clin Breast Cancer. 2015;15(2):101–9.

102. Yamauchi H, Cristofanilli M, Nakamura S, Hortobaghy GN, Ueno NT. Molecular targets for treatment of inflammatory breast cancer. Nat Rev Clin Oncol. 2009;6:387–94.

103. Monneur A, Bertucci F, Viens P, Gonçalves A. Systemic treatment of inflammatory breast cancer: an overview. Bull Cancer. 2014;101:1080–8.

104. Wedam SB, Low JA, Yang SX, Chow CK, Choyke P, Danforth D, et al. Antiangiogenic and antitumor effects of bevacizumab in patients with inflammatory and locally advanced breast cancer. J Clin Oncol. 2006;24:769–77.

105. Pierga JY, Petit T, Delozier T, Ferrero JM, Campone M, Gligorov J, et al. Neoadjuvant bevacizumab, trastuzumab, and chemotherapy for primary inflammatory *HER2* positive breast cancer (BEVERLY-2): an open-label, single-arm phase II study. Lancet Oncol. 2012;13:375–84.

106. Pierga JY, Petit T, Levy C, Ferrero JM, Campone M, Gligorov J, et al. Pathological response and circulating tumor cell count identifies treated *HER2*+

inflammatory breast cancer patients with excellent prognosis: BEVERLY-2 survival data. Clin Cancer Res. 2015;21(6):1298–304.

107. Mego M, Giordano A, De Giorgi U, Masuda H, Hsu L, Giuliano M, et al. Circulating tumor cells in newly diagnosed inflammatory breast cancer. Breast Cancer Res. 2015;17:2.

108. Overmoyer B, Fu P, Hoppel C, Radivoyevitch T, Shenk R, Persons M, et al. Inflammatory breast cancer as a model disease to study tumor angiogenesis: results of a phase IB trial of combination *SU5416* and doxorubicin. Clin Cancer Res. 2007;13:5862–8.

109. Cabioglu N, Gong Y, Islam R, Broglio KR, Sneige N, Sahin A, et al. Expression of growth factor and chemokine receptors: new insights in the biology of inflammatory breast cancer. Ann Oncol. 2007;18:1021–9.

110. van Golen KL, Wu ZF, Qiao XT, Bao LW, Merajver SD. RhoC GTPase, a novel transforming oncogene for human mammary epithelial cells that partially recapitulates the inflammatory breast cancer phenotype. Cancer Res. 2000;60:5832–8.

111. Andreopoulou E, Vigoda IS, Hershman DL, Hershman DL, Raptis G, Vahdat LT, et al. Phase I-II study of farnesyl transferase inhibitor tipifarnib plus sequential weekly paclitaxel and doxorubicin-cyclophosphamide in *HER2*/neu-negative inflammatory carcinoma and non-inflammatory estrogen-receptor positive breast carcinoma. Breast Cancer Res. 2013;141:429–35.

112. Krisnamurthy S, Woodward W, Yang W, Reuben JM, Tepperberg J, Ogura D, et al. Status of the anaplastic lymphoma kinase (*ALK*) gene in inflammatory breast carcinoma. SpringerPlus. 2013;2:409.

113. Robertson FM, Petricoin III EF, Van Laere SJ, Bertucci F, Chu K, Fernandez SV, et al. Presence of anaplastic lymphoma kinase in inflammatory breast cancer. SpringerPlus. 2013;2:497.

114. Harvey HA, Lipton A, Lawrence BV, White DS, Wells SA, Blumenschein G, et al. Estrogen receptor status in inflammatory breast carcinoma. J Surg Oncol. 1982;21:42–4.

115. Nguyen DM, Sam K, Tsimelzon A, Li X, Wong H, Mohsin S, et al. Molecular heterogeneity of inflammatory breast cancer: a hyperproliferative phenotype. Clin Cancer Res. 2006;12:5047–54.

116. Brewer TM, Masuda H, Liu DD, Shen Y, Liu P, Iwamoto T, et al. Statin use in primary inflammatory breast cancer: a cohort study. BJC. 2013;109:318–24.

117. Kaufmann M, von Minckwitz G, Bear HD, Buzdar A, McGale P, Bonnefoi H, et al. Recommendations from an international expert panel on the use of neoadjuvant (primary) systemic treatment of operable breast cancer: new perspectives 2006. Ann Oncol. 2007;18:1927–34.

118. Dushkin H, Cristofanilli M. Inflammatory breast cancer. J Natl Compr Cancer Netw. 2011;9(2):233–40; quiz 241.

119. Woodward WA, Buchholz TA. Unpublished observations from Yamauchi H, Woodward WA, Valero V, et al. Inflammatory breast cancer: what we know and what we need to learn. Oncologist. 2012;17:891–9.

120. Khatcheressian JL, Hurley P, Bantug E, Esserman LJ, Grunfeld E, Halberg F, et al. Breast cancer follow-up and management after primary treatment: American Society of Clinical Oncology clinical practice guideline update. J Clin Oncol. 2013;3:961–5.

121. Senkus E, Kyriakides S, Penault-Llorca P, Poortmans P, Thompson A, Zackrisson S, et al. Primary breast cancer: ESMO clinical practice guidelines for diagnosis, treatment and follow-up. Ann Oncol. 2013;24(supplement 6):vi7–23.

122. Matro JM, Cristofanilli M, Hughes ME, Hughes ME, Ottesen RA, Weeks JC, et al. Inflammatory breast cancer management in the National Comprehensive Cancer Network: the disease, recurrence pattern, and outcome. Clin Breast Cancer. 2015;15:1–7.

123. Guler N, Karabulut B, Koçdor MA, et al. Locally advanced breast cancer-2010 Istanbul Breast Cancer Consensus Meeting. J Breast Health. 2011;7:68–89.

124. van Golen KL, Cristofanilli M. The third international inflammatory breast cancer conference. Breast Cancer Res. 2013;15:318.

Part III

Surgical Management of Patient with Preoperative Systemic Therapy

Surgical Management of Operable Breast Cancer After Neoadjuvant Systemic Therapy

17

Atilla Soran, Ebru Menekse,
and Kandace P. McGuire

Abstract

The primary goal of neoadjuvant chemotherapy (NCT) in operable breast cancer is tumor down-sizing to facilitate breast-conserving surgery (BCS). The use of NCT in early-stage breast cancer in carefully selected patients is increasing. Despite a shift in the treated patient population to patients with earlier-stage tumors, the principles of surgery after NCT remain the same. Monitoring response to therapy is important for surgical planning and prognostic information. Preoperative marking of the tumor is essential for guiding BCS after NCT and should be performed in all patients. Axillary staging can be performed prior to or after NCT, and both methods are associated with specific risks and benefits. Early literature supported the use of pre-NCT sentinel lymph node biopsy (SLNB), but current literature suggests increased accuracy and decreased use of axillary dissection in patients who undergo SLNB after NCT. A multidisciplinary approach to breast cancer care is essential during NCT for improved outcomes and decreased morbidity.

A. Soran, MD, MPH, FACS (✉)
Department of Surgery, Division of Surgical
Oncology, Magee-Women's Hospital,
University of Pittsburgh Medical Center,
Pittsburgh, PA, USA
e-mail: asoran@upmc.edu, asoran65@gmail.com

E. Menekse, MD
Department of Surgery, Division of Surgical
Oncology, University of Pittsburgh School
of Medicine, Magee-Women's Hospital, University
of Pittsburgh Medical Center, 300 Halket St,
Suite 2601, Pittsburgh, PA, USA

Surgical Oncology Department, Breast Surgery Unit,
Magee-Women's Hospital, University of Pittsburgh
School of Medicine, Pittsburgh, PA, USA
e-mail: drebrumenekse@gmail.com

K.P. McGuire, MD
Department of Surgery, Division of Surgical
Oncology, University of North Carolina School
Lineberger Comprehensive Cancer Center,
170 Manning Dr., CB# 7203, Chapel Hill, NC, USA

Department of Surgery, University of North Carolina,
Lineberger Comphrensive Cancer Center,
Chapel Hill, NC, USA
e-mail: kandace_mcguire@med.unc.edu

© Springer International Publishing Switzerland 2016
A. Aydiner et al. (eds.), *Breast Disease: Management and Therapies*,
DOI 10.1007/978-3-319-26012-9_17

Keywords

Breast cancer • Chemotherapy • Neoadjuvant treatment • Surgery • Surgical procedure

Introduction

Although routinely used for locally advanced and inflammatory breast cancer, neoadjuvant chemotherapy for early-stage breast cancer (defined as stages I and II) should also be considered for appropriate patients [1–3]. As surgery for breast cancer has become less invasive, gradually progressing from Halsted's radical mastectomy in 1894 and toward modern techniques of breast-conserving surgery (BCS) and skin- and nipple-sparing mastectomy, the need to decrease tumor size prior to surgery has increased. Even in the setting of early-stage breast cancer, neoadjuvant chemotherapy (NCT) can decrease tumor size and improve cosmetic results [4]. Randomized trials in early breast cancer demonstrate that neoadjuvant chemotherapy can increase the use of breast conservation by decreasing tumor size. Approximately 25 % of patients exhibit a pathological complete response (pCR) and greater than 80 % exhibit a partial response [5]. Some physicians suggest that decreasing micrometastatic disease and altering tumor kinetics in early breast cancer contributes to improved overall survival [4]. Various trials indicate that neoadjuvant therapy is superior to adjuvant therapy in preventing the spread of micrometastatic disease [4]. However, NCT has not improved overall survival in any large randomized controlled trial [6].

The National Surgical Adjuvant Breast and Bowel Project B-18 (NSABP B-18) randomized patients with operable breast cancer to preoperative versus postoperative administration of adjuvant chemotherapy. Patients in the neoadjuvant group demonstrated a statistically significant increase in the use of breast-conservation surgery compared with mastectomy ($p=0.001$). However, the difference in disease-free survival (DFS) and overall survival was not statistically significant [7, 8].

The primary benefit of neoadjuvant chemotherapy for early breast cancer is tumor downstaging, which improves the opportunity for breast-conservation surgery. In addition, neoadjuvant chemotherapy provides other advantages, such as nodal downstaging, which can reduce the extent of axillary surgery, in vivo evaluation of tumor resistance or sensitivity, prognostic information based on tumor response, and the ability to assess the efficacy of new chemotherapeutic agents in clinical trials. However, potential disadvantages of NCT exist. Tumor downstaging can be inadequate to achieve the preferred surgical therapy. Chemotherapy-resistant tumors can progress, rendering patients inoperable. Knowledge regarding initial lymph node status can be lost, and patients with favorable tumor phenotypes (luminal tumors) could be potentially overtreated [4].

Initial Evaluation, Staging, and Diagnosis

The first step in the management of any breast cancer is the establishment of a diagnosis of cancer. Next, prognostic tumor markers (estrogen/progesterone/HER2 receptor positivity and, when possible, Ki-67 %) should be evaluated and staging of the primary tumor performed. A pathological diagnosis is determined by core biopsy in patients receiving neoadjuvant therapy. A post-biopsy localization clip that will be detectable post chemotherapy should be deployed, and its location should be confirmed prior to initiation of therapy based on NCCN 2014 guidelines [3]. If appropriate (particularly for patients with stage IIB and greater tumors), staging for distant metastasis should be performed prior to the initiation of NCT. Several imaging modalities are available for staging both local and metastatic disease, including diagnostic mammography and tomosynthesis, breast and axillary ultrasound, MRI, molecular breast imaging for local disease,

CT, bone scan, and PET/CT [3]. The relative benefits of these modalities are beyond the scope of this chapter.

When planning surgical management, the surgeon and the patient must decide between BCS and mastectomy. If a patient does not have contraindications to BCS (multicentric disease, prior history of radiation or other contraindications to radiation, BRCA mutation, or simply a desire to undergo mastectomy) but has a tumor to breast size ratio that is unfavorable for BCS, NCT can be offered [3, 9].

Once the decision for NCT is made, both medical oncology and surgery personnel will develop a care plan, including pre-NCT tumor assessment, frequency of tumor response assessment, and final clinical, staging plans. Patients should be prepared that a change in NCT course can be made based on response to therapy. As mentioned previously, initial tumor staging can be performed using a variety of imaging modalities. Consistent imaging modalities are important to accurately assess the response to therapy. Many authors recommend MRI in initial and post-therapy evaluation given its increased sensitivity compared with traditional imaging [10–12]. However, the use of MRI is also associated with increased mastectomy rates. Ongoing tumor assessment during therapy can be performed via physical exam and ultrasound and mammogram or MRI should progression be a concern.

Evaluation of Response to Neoadjuvant Therapy

The evaluation of response to neoadjuvant chemotherapy includes clinical and pathological assessment. The clinical response should be determined with physical exam and imaging. Physical exam alone is inaccurate. Mammogram, ultrasound, and MRI are used as adjuncts to increase accuracy. Some clinicians hypothesize that MRI is advantageous for evaluating response to NCT given its ability to detect angiogenic changes, which can be observed before the tumor size is reduced [12]. Multiple studies have reported that MRI is a good predictor of response in all tumor types, particularly triple-negative and HER2+ patients, for which its ability to predict pCR was statistically superior compared to luminal tumors ($p < 0.005$) [13, 14]. A clinical complete response is defined as complete resolution of all detectable palpation and imaging disease findings. Clinical partial response is defined as a greater than 50 % decrease in tumor size. Clinical progressive disease is defined as a greater than 50 % increase in tumor mass [7]. Pathological response is determined via surgical pathology. Responses can be measured using a variety of methods, including the Response Evaluation Criteria in Solid Tumors (RECIST) criteria. pCR is defined by different organizations in various manners. The strictest definition is that of the German Breast Group (GBG) and requires the complete absence of invasive or noninvasive disease in breast or axillary lymph nodes. The Austrian Breast and Colorectal Cancer Study Group, Neo-Breast International Group, and MD Anderson define complete response as the lack of invasive tumor in the breast or lymph nodes, whereas residual in situ disease is allowed. The NSABP defines pCR as no residual invasive disease in the breast; however, this criterion allows in situ disease and does not measure residual nodal disease. Using the Sataloff index, various groups actually allow for the persistence of focal invasive tumors [15].

A discrepancy often exists between clinical and pathologic tumor responses. Tumor responses to NCT were categorized as a clinical complete response in 36 % patients. However, pCR was observed only in 26 % of these patients [8]. This discordance between pathological and radiological responses is attributed to the fact that breast tumors responses exhibit two response patterns to NCT: concentric decrease and patchy regression [4]. These multiple microscopic residual areas cannot be observed via imaging assessments. This discrepancy is also due to intraductal tumors that do not respond to chemotherapy [5].

The NSABP trials B-18 and B-27 established the efficacy of NCT and also evaluated response to therapy as a prognostic indicator. B-18 compared pre- and postoperative treatment with doxorubicin and cyclophosphamide in patients with T1-3, N0-1 operable breast cancer. The trial indicated that the degree of response (complete, partial, or none) was strongly related to overall survival, DFS, and recurrence-free survival (0.0008, 0.005, and 0.002, respectively). The risk of death decreased 50 % in patients with pCR. However, the death rate increased 28 % in patients with a partial response and 45 % in nonresponders [16]. In the study, the incidence of pathologically negative axillary lymph nodes was increased in the preoperative group compared with the postoperative group (48 % and 42 %, respectively; $p < 0.0001$) [5]. However, as a prognostic factor, primary tumor response is more valuable than pathological lymph node status [16].

NSABP B-27 compared three different neoadjuvant/adjuvant regimens: doxorubicin and cyclophosphamide followed by surgery, doxorubicin and cyclophosphamide followed by surgery and then paclitaxel and doxorubicin, and cyclophosphamide and paclitaxel followed by surgery [5, 7]. The clinical response in the preoperative doxorubicin, cyclophosphamide, and paclitaxel group was increased compared with the other two groups (91 % and 86 %, respectively; $p < 0.001$). The clinical complete response and pCR rates for the group receiving preoperative taxane were 40 % and 26 %, respectively, superior to the other groups ($p < 0.001$). pCR was a significant predictor of DFS and overall survival ($p < 0.001$). Post-neoadjuvant nodal status was also a highly significant predictor of DFS and overall survival ($p < 0.001$) [7].

An early response of the primary tumor after two or three cycles of chemotherapy is a predictor of pCR [4]. Factors including age <40, tumor size <2 cm, ductal pathology, high nuclear grade, high rate of cellular proliferation (association with Ki-67), estrogen receptor-negative status, triple-negative status, and human epidermal growth factor receptor 2 (HER2)-positive status are directly proportional with increased frequency of pCR [6]. Similar to the NSABP trials, a number of contemporary studies have demonstrated that pCR after neoadjuvant chemotherapy is strongly associated with prolonged DFS and overall survival [17, 18]. Primary tumor response and axillary lymph node response to neoadjuvant chemotherapy are separate prognostic factors [4]. pCR after neoadjuvant chemotherapy can improve the prognosis for patients with ER-negative and triple-negative disease. Unfortunately, pCR is obtained in only 20–25 % of breast cancer patients following neoadjuvant chemotherapy. Failure to achieve pCR can lead to delays in surgery and/or hormonal therapy and is potentially detrimental in terms of overall outcome [7, 15].

Surgical Management

Surgical Management of the Breast After Neoadjuvant Chemotherapy

Once the response to neoadjuvant chemotherapy has been assessed, a surgical plan can be made by the surgeon and the patient. Generally, surgery is performed approximately 4 weeks after neoadjuvant chemotherapy due to the myelosuppressive toxicity of chemotherapeutic agents [19]. If neoadjuvant chemotherapy was administered for the purpose of downstaging the tumor to facilitate BCS, then imaging will guide the decision for BCS post NCT. Acceptable BCS responses vary from patient to patient and depend on a number of factors, including original tumor size and location as well as the patient's breast size. Several algorithms are available to aid decision making. Some algorithms include the option to continue with additional NCT if the response is inadequate and second-line therapy may prove effective [3] (Fig. 17.1).

According to NSABP B18, 68 % of patients in the NCT group underwent breast-conserving surgery compared with 60 % of patients in the adjuvant chemotherapy group ($p = 0.0001$) [7]. However, despite modern chemotherapy regimens and targeted therapies that increase the pCR rate, BCS rates after neoadjuvant chemotherapy remain stable since NSABP B18. In fact, estrogen receptor-positive tumors, which exhibit the lowest pCRs, are associated with the highest rates of BCS after neoadjuvant chemotherapy [20]. Many researchers have correlated the difficulty in determining post-NCT tumor size clinically with the lack of improvement in BCS rates [1, 5].

Due to the limitations of modern imaging, a discrepancy remains between imaging complete response and pCR. Thus, regardless of clinical

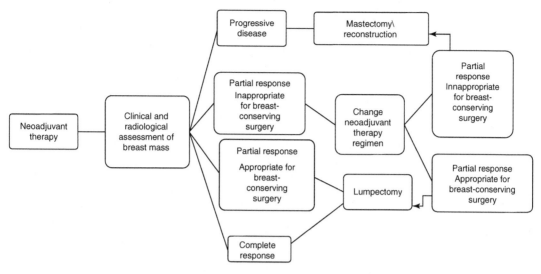

Fig. 17.1 Algorithm for the management of the primary tumor after neoadjuvant therapy (Modified NCCN guidelines)

response, the biopsy clip should be targeted for surgical removal after NCT. If post-treatment imaging suggests residual disease, the surgeon should attempt to remove the area of residual tumor as suggested radiographically [13, 19, 21]. However, removal of the entire tumor bed as it existed prior to neoadjuvant treatment is not necessary. It is important to note that the tumor may respond to neoadjuvant treatment as scattered microscopic islands. In this case, negative margins may be difficult to achieve despite response to chemotherapy. Many of these patients will require re-excision or completion mastectomy [19].

In the GEPARDUO trial, a more recent prospective, multicenter study, BCS rates after NCT for operable breast cancer were measured. After neoadjuvant therapy, breast-conserving surgery was attempted in approximately 82 % of patients. Re-excision was performed in 12.4 % patients. Completion mastectomy was performed in 8.7 % of patients. According to the GEPARDUO trial, tumor size ≤40 mm pre-chemotherapy, tumor size ≤20 mm post-chemotherapy, treatment with doxorubicin/cyclophosphamide/taxane vs. doxorubicin/taxane, clinical response, and treatment at a high-volume (>10 enrolled patients) center were correlated with successful breast-conserving surgery after NCT. In addition, non-lobular histopathology and intraoperative evaluation of margins with frozen section analysis decreased the re-excision rate ($p=0.015$) [22].

Response is often inadequate; no second-line therapy is recommended, and mastectomy is necessary. By contrast, a patient initially motivated for BCS may opt for mastectomy during treatment. If this is the case and the patient desires reconstruction, decisions must be made regarding the potential for postmastectomy radiotherapy and the ability to perform immediate reconstruction. Traditional guidelines for postmastectomy radiotherapy include treatment of positive margins, a tumor that is >5 cm at time of resection or lymph node positivity before or after chemotherapy. However, recent trials suggest that a patient who is clinically node positive prior to chemotherapy but is rendered N0 with NCT does not significantly benefit from postmastectomy radiation [23, 24]. Patients with a low likelihood of radiation should be referred for immediate reconstruction barring other contraindications to reconstruction. Patients who absolutely require radiation should be reconstructed in a delayed fashion or in an immediate fashion with caution. In patients for whom the decision for postmastectomy radiotherapy is uncertain, the "delayed-immediate" form of reconstruction can be employed [25, 26].

Table 17.1 Comparison of SLND before and after neoadjuvant treatment

SLND before neoadjuvant treatment		SLND after neoadjuvant treatment	
Advantage	Disadvantage	Advantage	Disadvantage
Higher detection rate	Increased ALND rate and increased morbidity	Lower ALND rate and reduced morbidity	Lower detection rate
Lower FNR	Lack of information regarding response	Proven to predict differences in DFS/OS	Higher FNR
Guides decision regarding type of NCT	Makes subsequent SLNB attempts less successful	Decreases the time between diagnosis and systemic therapy	Questionable alteration of lymphatic drainage
	Increases # of surgical procedures	Decreases # of surgical procedures	

SLNB sentinel lymph node biopsy, *ALND* axillary lymph node dissection, *FNR* false-negative rate, *DFS* disease-free survival, *OS* overall survival, *NCT* neoadjuvant chemotherapy

Surgical Management of the Axilla After Neoadjuvant Chemotherapy

Numerous completed and ongoing studies have examined optimal management of the axilla either before or after NCT [27]. Therefore, no standard axillary approach for breast cancer patients who are undergoing neoadjuvant therapy is available.

Sentinel lymph node biopsy (SLNB) is widely accepted in the setting of primary surgery for breast cancer. Landmark trials, such as NSABP B-32 and ACOSOG Z0010, have demonstrated sentinel node detection rates of 95–99 % and a false-negative rate (FNR) of 9.8 % [28, 29].

However, the management of the axilla and the timing of SLNB in relation to NCT are controversial. Varying reports have described SLNB in the clinically node-negative patient both before and/or after NCT, and each option possesses inherent advantages and disadvantages [19, 30–32] (Table 17.1).

Proponents of pre-NCT SLNB note that valuable staging information is lost if nodal staging is performed after chemotherapy and that SLNB has a higher detection rate and lower FNR if performed prior to NCT. In addition, for borderline candidates, axillary status may aid the decision for preoperative systemic therapy. Concerns also exist regarding whether chemotherapy may cause scarring that could affect lymphatic drainage, thus making SN identification more difficult and/or less accurate. Single institution studies typically describe identification rates of approximately 96 % for pre-NCT SLNB and 90 % after NCT. FNRs are approximately 7 % pre-NCT and 12 % after NCT [33]. Large multicenter trials, such as NSABP B18 and B27, have demonstrated slightly reduced FNRs of 11 % [34]. Despite these arguments, outcomes for patients undergoing SLN either before or after NCT do not vary significantly.

We can predict greater success in post-NCT SLNB in specific subsets of patients. Pecha et al. have demonstrated that the success of finding SLNs increased in breast cancer patients administered NCT and <50 years of age, clinically lymph node negative at the time of diagnosis, harbored ER (+) primary tumors, exhibited a KI 67 proliferation index of ≤15 %,, and without lymphatic and/or vascular space invasion. The absence of lymphovascular space invasion was also predictive of a lower FNR in this study [35].

There is also a strong argument for performing SLNB after NCT. NCT can convert 30–40 % of patients from node positive to node negative. This efficacy enables a single surgery and decreases the morbidity of patients undergoing axillary dissection for what has been rendered a negative axilla. Additionally, post-NCT axillary assessment provides the care team with important prognostic information. In B18 and B27 protocols, patients who presented with clinically

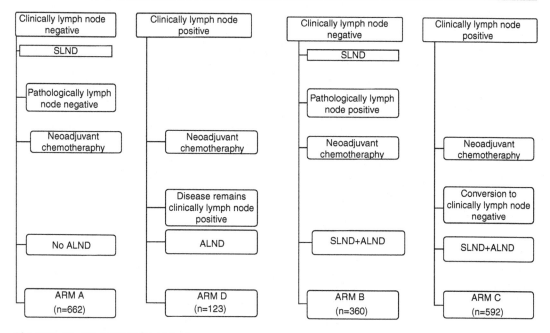

Fig. 17.2 Modified SENTINA trial schema

node-positive disease and were node negative by SLNB after chemotherapy exhibited improved DFS and overall survival.

Two recent prospective trials have examined the issue of SLNB either before or after NCT, particularly in patients who were clinically node positive at presentation. SENTINA (SENTinel Neo Adjuvant) divided 1,737 patients undergoing NCT into two groups based on clinical nodal status at presentation. The clinically node-negative patients underwent SLNB prior to NCT. If these patients were confirmed as SLN−, no further axillary staging was performed. If the patients were SLN+, they underwent SLNB followed by ALND post-NCT. Clinically node-positive patients were randomized to SLNB followed by ALND after NCT or ALND only after NCT (Fig. 17.2). The trial compared the detection rate of SLNB before and/or after NCT. Patients who underwent SLNB before NCT exhibited a detection rate of 99 % compared with 87.8 % after NCT (Arm C). Those undergoing repeat SLNB after NCT exhibited the lowest detection rate (61 %), and their FNR values were greater than 50 %. SLNB after NCT in patients

who were clinically node-positive at presentation was associated with an FNR of 14.2 %. However, the FNR was <10 % in the subset of patients who had two or more SLNs removed. Furthermore, if combined mapping (blue dye and radiotracer) was used, the FNR was 8.6 % [36].

The second recent trial, ACOSOG Z1071, identified 641 patients who were clinically staged as N1–2 at presentation either by clinical exam or axillary ultrasound/biopsy. All patients underwent SLNB followed by ALND after NCT with removal of two or more SLNs (if possible). At least one SLN was identified in 92.7 % of the patients in this study. The overall FNR was 12.6 %, higher than the predetermined threshold of 10 %. However, when a dual tracer was used, the FNR was reduced to 10.8 %. Moreover, the FNR was 9.1 % when >3 SLNs were removed [32]. Unpublished data presented at the San Antonio Breast Cancer Symposium in 2012 also noted that if a pre-therapy positive lymph node was biopsied and clipped and its removal was confirmed at the time of SLNB, the FNR was 7.4 % [37]. The findings of both studies have resulted in changes in practice patterns (Fig. 17.3) [3, 34].

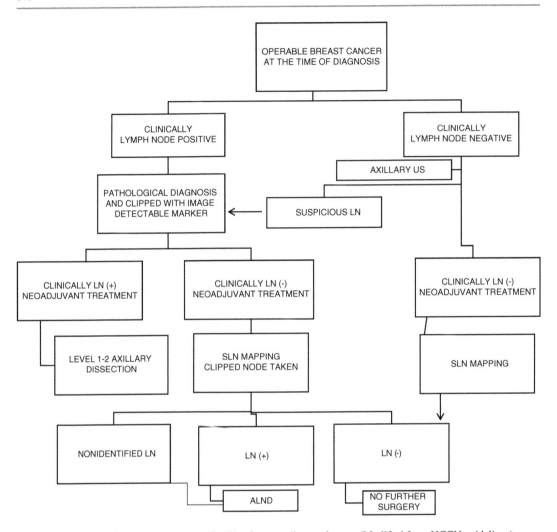

Fig. 17.3 Algorithm for the management of axilla after neoadjuvant therapy (Modified from NCCN guidelines)

Adjuvant therapy in patients who present with clinically positive axilla is another fertile area of debate and study. Two current trials are examining the role of radiotherapy in the management of these patients. NSABP B51 randomizes patients with positive axilla at presentation (cT1-3, N1) who converted to node negative on SLNB to axillary radiation versus no axillary radiation. Alliance A011202 randomizes patients with persistently positive axillary nodes to axillary dissection plus comprehensive breast/chest wall/regional nodal irradiation or axillary radiation plus comprehensive breast/chest wall/regional nodal irradiation. The primary endpoint for both of these studies is recurrence-free survival [38, 39].

Surgical Management After Neoadjuvant Hormonal Therapy

Neoadjuvant hormonal therapy can be considered to decrease tumor size to facilitate breast-conserving surgery in postmenopausal women with hormone receptor-positive breast cancer. Studies comparing neoadjuvant hormonal therapy and neoadjuvant chemotherapy in patients with HR-positive disease indicate that neoadjuvant hormonal therapy is as effective as NCT in downstaging tumors and promoting breast-conserving surgery in postmenopausal women [40–42]. In studies comparing neoadjuvant hormonal therapy regimens, aromatase inhibitors are superior to tamoxifen in regard to tumor response and breast-conserving surgery rates [43]. ACOSOG Z1031 revealed that in patients with a tumor-to-breast size ratio considered marginal for breast conservation, exemestane, letrozole, and anastrozole made breast-conserving surgery possible in 45.2 %, 40.0 %, and 48.7 % of patients, respectively, with an overall breast-conserving surgery rate of 83.1 % for the study. Moreover, this study revealed that for patients who were candidates for mastectomy only, breast-conserving surgery could be performed following neoadjuvant hormonal therapy with exemestane, letrozole, and anastrozole in 21.7 %, 20.0 %, and 27.4 % of patients, respectively. However, clinical response and breast-conserving surgery rates did not significantly differ for exemestane, anastrozole and letrozole [44]. Length of treatment is an important question addressed in many studies. Patients who receive neoadjuvant hormonal therapy with letrozole and anastrozole for longer than 4 months exhibited clinical response rates of 55.2–98.7 % and breast-conserving surgery rates of 43–86 % [45–50].

Locoregional Recurrence

NSABP B-18 and NSABP B-27 described locoregional recurrence rates (LRRs) in early breast cancer patients who underwent NCT. Patients undergoing NCT exhibited higher overall recurrence rates compared with those who underwent adjuvant therapy. Mamounas et al. reported LRR of 12.3 % (8.9 % local; 3.4 % regional) for patients who underwent mastectomy and 10.3 % for patients (8.1 % local; 2.2 % regional) treated with breast-conserving surgery followed by radiotherapy after NCT at a median follow-up of 10 years. Table 17.2 presents independent predictors for LRRs based on NSABP B-18 and NSABP B-27. LRRs were higher in patients who did not achieve pCR in both the breast and axilla. This effect was particularly pronounced in young patients [51]. Similar findings were described by von Minckwitz et al. These researchers evaluated tumor response at surgery and its association with long-term outcomes in 6,377 patients with primary breast cancer receiving NCT in seven randomized trials.

Table 17.2 Independent predictors of locoregional recurrence rate according to type of surgery in patients receiving neoadjuvant chemotherapy

Patients undergoing mastectomy	Patients undergoing breast-conserving surgery
Clinical tumor size >5 cm	Age <50 years
Clinically lymph node + disease	Clinically lymph node + disease
Pathologically lymph node + disease	Pathologically lymph node + disease
	M.D. Anderson Prognostic Index
	1. Clinically N2,3 lymph node
	2. pT >2 cm
	3. Multifocal tumor pattern
	4. Lymphovascular invasion

DFS was significantly superior in patients with no invasive and no in situ residuals in the breast or nodes [15].

According to the studies noted above, LRR differs significantly based on intrinsic tumor subtype (luminal, HER2, and triple negative). In the seven German Breast Group trials, pCR was associated with improved DFS in luminal B/HER2- ($p=0.005$), HER2+ ($p<0.001$), and triple-negative ($p<0.001$) tumors but not in luminal A ($p=0.39$) or luminal B/HER2+ ($p=0.45$) tumors. pCR in HER2-positive (nonluminal) and triple-negative tumors was associated with excellent prognosis [15].

In the NSABP B18 and NSABP B27 trials, patients who received systemic therapy before and after surgery were compared. No differences between groups were noted for cancer-related death, disease progression, or distant recurrence [52]. A significant relationship between treatment age and overall survival ($p=0.01$) was observed. In patients younger than 50 years, overall survival and DFS rates were 55 % and 38 %, respectively, in the adjuvant chemotherapy group compared with 61 % and 44 %, respectively, in the neoadjuvant group ($p=0.06$ and 0.09, respectively) [7].

MD Anderson has developed a prognostic index that stratifies risk of LRR in patients who undergo breast-conserving surgery following NCT. This index includes four predictors of an increased risk of locoregional recurrence: clinical

N2–3 disease, residual pathologic tumor size >2 cm, multifocal pattern of residual disease, and lymphovascular space (Table 17.2) [53].

Postoperative Complications

One of the concerns regarding NCT is the rate of surgical complications after therapy. However, these concerns are not supported by the literature. Numerous studies have reported postoperative complication rates in this situation, and the rates are statistically equivalent. Broadwater et al. compared patients undergoing mastectomy after NCT and patients undergoing mastectomy followed by adjuvant chemotherapy. No differences were noted between the two groups regarding wound infection and wound necrosis rates. Interestingly, seroma formation was significantly decreased in the preoperative chemotherapy group compared with the postoperative chemotherapy group ($p = 0.04$) [54]. A more recent study by Unalp and Onal found no correlation between seroma formation and the use of NCT [55].

Several studies have described outcomes in mastectomy and immediate reconstruction after NCT. Recent studies have evaluated outcomes after both autologous tissue reconstruction and tissue expander/implant-based reconstruction following NCT. Both studies reported no difference in overall complication rates in patients who received preoperative chemotherapy [56, 57]. The only statistically significant difference observed was the rate of skin necrosis in patients receiving tissue expander or implant-based reconstruction. However, this difference did not result in an increased rate of implant loss [57].

Certainly, one of the greatest concerns after surgery of the breast and axilla is lymphedema. A commonly stated reason for NCT is the opportunity to downstage the axilla and reduce the extent of axillary surgery. The major advantage of SLNB compared with ALND is reduced lymphedema rates. NASBP B32 reported lymphedema rates of 12.5 % in patients after ALND, whereas the rate was 0 % in patients who had SLNB only. Z0010 and Z0011 reported lymphedema in 7 % of patients at 6 months [58]. SLNB may be particularly important in this population as recent data suggests that patients who receive ALND after NCT exhibit significantly higher rates of lymphedema at 5 years compared with those receiving adjuvant therapy (41.6 % vs. 21.7 %, respectively) ($p < 0.001$) [59]. Studies such as NSABP B51 and A011202 will provide an opportunity to study the long-term rates of lymphedema after SLNB in the setting of NCT as the data mature.

References

1. Kummel S, Holtschmidt J, Loibl S. Surgical treatment of primary breast cancer in the neoadjuvant setting. Br J Surg. 2014;101(8):912–24.
2. Edge SB, Byrd DR, Compton CC, Fritz AG, Greene FL, Trotti A. AJCC cancer staging manual. 7th ed. Chicago: Springer; 2010. p. 345–76.
3. Breast Cancer. NCCN clinical practice guidelines in oncology 2014. 3.2014. http://www.nccn.org/professionals/physician_gls/pdf/breast.pdf. Accessed 31 July 2014.
4. Mieog JS, van de Velde CJ. Neoadjuvant chemotherapy for early breast cancer. Expert Opin Pharmacother. 2009;10(9):1423–34.
5. Redden MH, Fuhrman GM. Neoadjuvant chemotherapy in the treatment of breast cancer. Surg Clin North Am. 2013;93(2):493–9.
6. Teshome M, Hunt KK. Neoadjuvant therapy in the treatment of breast cancer. Surg Oncol Clin N Am. 2014;23(3):505–23.
7. Rastogi P, Anderson SJ, Bear HD, Geyer CE, Kahlenberg MS, Robidoux A, et al. Preoperative chemotherapy: updates of National Surgical Adjuvant Breast and Bowel Project Protocols B-18 and B-27. J Clin Oncol. 2008;26(5):778–85.
8. Fisher B, Brown A, Mamounas E, Wieand S, Robidoux A, Margolese RG, et al. Effect of preoperative chemotherapy on local-regional disease in women with operable breast cancer: findings from National Surgical Adjuvant Breast and Bowel Project B-18. J Clin Oncol. 1997;15(7):2483–93.
9. Rapoport BL, Demetriou GS, Moodley SD, Benn CA. When and how do I use neoadjuvant chemotherapy for breast cancer? Curr Treat Options Oncol. 2014;15(1):86–98.
10. Warren RM, Bobrow LG, Earl HM, Britton PD, Gopalan D, Purushotham AD, et al. Can breast MRI help in the management of women with breast cancer treated by neoadjuvant chemotherapy? Br J Cancer. 2004;90(7):1349–60.
11. Rosen EL, Blackwell KL, Baker JA, Soo MS, Bentley RC, Yu D, Samulski TV, et al. Accuracy of MRI in the detection of residual breast cancer after neoadjuvant chemotherapy. Am J Roentgenol. 2003;181(5):1275–82.
12. Marinovich ML, Sardanelli F, Ciatto S, Mamounas E, Brennan M, Macaskill P, et al. Early prediction of

pathologic response to neoadjuvant therapy in breast cancer: systematic review of the accuracy of MRI. Breast. 2012;21(5):669–77.

13. McGuire KP, Toro-Burguete J, Dang H, Young J, Soran A, Zuley M, et al. MRI staging after neoadjuvant chemotherapy for breast cancer: does tumor biology affect accuracy? Ann Surg Oncol. 2011;18(11): 3149–54.

14. De Los Santos JF, Cantor A, Amos KD, Forero A, Golshan M, Horton JK, et al. Magnetic resonance imaging as a predictor of pathologic response in patients treated with neoadjuvant systemic treatment for operable breast cancer: Translational Breast Cancer Research Consortium trial 017. Cancer. 2013;119(10):1776–83.

15. von Minckwitz G, Untch M, Blohmer JU, Costa SD, Eidtmann H, Fasching PA, et al. Definition and impact of pathologic complete response on prognosis after neoadjuvant chemotherapy in various intrinsic breast cancer subtypes. J Clin Oncol. 2012;30(15): 1796–804.

16. Wolmark N, Wang J, Mamounas E, Bryant J, Fisher B. Preoperative chemotherapy in patients with operable breast cancer: nine-year results from National Surgical Adjuvant Breast and Bowel Project B-18. J Natl Cancer Inst Monogr. 2001;30(30):96–102.

17. Chollet P, Amat S, Cure H, de Latour M, Le Bouedec G, Mouret-Reynier MA, et al. Prognostic significance of a complete pathological response after induction chemotherapy in operable breast cancer. Br J Cancer. 2002;86(7):1041–6.

18. Mieog JS, van der Hage JA, van de Velde CJ. Neoadjuvant chemotherapy for operable breast cancer. Br J Surg. 2007;94(10):1189–200.

19. Veronesi U, Bonadonna G, Zurrida S, Galimberti V, Greco M, Brambilla C, et al. Conservation surgery after primary chemotherapy in large carcinomas of the breast. Ann Surg. 1995;222(5):612–8.

20. Straver ME, Rutgers EJ, Rodenhuis S, Linn SC, Loo CE, Wesseling J, et al. The relevance of breast cancer subtypes in the outcome of neoadjuvant chemotherapy. Ann Surg Oncol. 2010;17(9):2411–8.

21. Buchholz TA, Lehman CD, Harris JR, Pockaj BA, Khouri N, Hylton NF, et al. Statement of the science concerning locoregional treatments after preoperative chemotherapy for breast cancer: a National Cancer Institute conference. J Clin Oncol. 2008;26(5): 791–7.

22. Loibl S, von Minckwitz G, Raab G, Blohmer JU, Dan Costa S, Gerber B, et al. Surgical procedures after neoadjuvant chemotherapy in operable breast cancer: results of the GEPARDUO trial. Ann Surg Oncol. 2006;13(11):1434–42.

23. Hoffman KE, Mittendorf EA, Buchholz TA. Optimising radiation treatment decisions for patients who receive neoadjuvant chemotherapy and mastectomy. Lancet Oncol. 2012;13(6):e270–6.

24. Shim SJ, Park W, Huh SJ, Choi DH, Shin KH, Lee NK, et al. The role of postmastectomy radiation therapy after neoadjuvant chemotherapy in clinical stage II-III breast cancer patients with pN0: a multicenter,

retrospective study (KROG 12-05). Int J Radiat Oncol Biol Phys. 2014;88(1):65–72.

25. Kronowitz SJ, Robb GL. Radiation therapy and breast reconstruction: a critical review of the literature. Plast Reconstr Surg. 2009;124(2):395–408.

26. Berbers J, van Baardwijk A, Houben R, et al. 'Reconstruction: before or after postmastectomy radiotherapy?' A systematic review of the literature. Eur J Cancer. 2014;50(16):2752–62.

27. Lyman GH, Temin S, Edge SB, Newman LA, Turner RR, Weaver DL, et al. Sentinel lymph node biopsy for patients with early-stage breast cancer: American Society of Clinical Oncology clinical practice guideline update. J Clin Oncol. 2014;32(13):1365–83.

28. Krag DN, Anderson SJ, Julian TB, Brown AM, Harlow SP, Costantino JP, et al. Sentinel-lymph-node resection compared with conventional axillary-lymph-node dissection in clinically node-negative patients with breast cancer: overall survival findings from the NSABP B-32 randomised phase 3 trial. Lancet Oncol. 2010;11(10):927–33.

29. Posther KE, McCall LM, Blumencranz PW, Burak Jr WE, Beitsch PD, Hansen NM, et al. Sentinel node skills verification and surgeon performance: data from a multicenter clinical trial for early-stage breast cancer. Ann Surg. 2005;242(4):593–9; discussion 599–602.

30. Mamounas EP. Timing of determining axillary lymph node status when neoadjuvant chemotherapy is used. Curr Oncol Rep. 2014;16(2):364.

31. Shimazu K, Noguchi S. Sentinel lymph node biopsy before versus after neoadjuvant chemotherapy for breast cancer. Surg Today. 2011;41(3):311–6.

32. Boughey JC, Suman VJ, Mittendorf EA, Ahrendt GM, Wilke LG, Taback B, et al. Sentinel lymph node surgery after neoadjuvant chemotherapy in patients with node-positive breast cancer: the ACOSOG Z1071 (Alliance) clinical trial. JAMA. 2013;310(14):1455–61.

33. Iwase H, Yamamoto Y, Kawasoe T, Ibusuki M. Advantage of sentinel lymph node biopsy before neoadjuvant chemotherapy in breast cancer treatment. Surg Today. 2009;39(5):374–80.

34. Mittendorf EA, Caudle AS, Yang W, Krishnamurthy S, Shaitelman S, Chavez-MacGregor M, et al. Implementation of the american college of surgeons oncology group z1071 trial data in clinical practice: is there a way forward for sentinel lymph node dissection in clinically node-positive breast cancer patients treated with neoadjuvant chemotherapy? Ann Surg Oncol. 2014;21(8):2468–73.

35. Pecha V, Kolarik D, Kozevnikova R, Hovorkova K, Hrabetova P, Halaska M, et al. Sentinel lymph node biopsy in breast cancer patients treated with neoadjuvant chemotherapy. Cancer. 2011;117(20):4606–16.

36. Kuehn T, Bauerfeind I, Fehm T, Fleige B, Hausschild M, Helms G, et al. Sentinel-lymph-node biopsy in patients with breast cancer before and after neoadjuvant chemotherapy (SENTINA): a prospective, multicentre cohort study. Lancet Oncol. 2013;14(7):609–18.

37. Boughey JC. Role of sentinel node surgery explored in node-positive breast cancer. Paper presented at: San Antonio Breast Cancer Symposium; San Antonio; 2012.

38. Mamounas E. NSABP B-51/RTOG 1304: Randomized phase III clinical trial evaluating the role of postmastectomy chest wall and regional nodal XRT (CWRNRT) and post-lumpectomy RNRT in patients (pts) with documented positive axillary (Ax) nodes before neoadjuvant chemotherapy (NC) who convert to pathologically negative Ax nodes after NC. Paper presented at: ASCO annual meeting; Chicago; 2014.

39. Smith BD. Using chemotherapy response to personalize choices regarding locoregional therapy: a new era in breast cancer treatment? J Clin Oncol. 2012;30(32):3913–5.

40. Alba E, Chacon JI, Lluch A, Anton A, Estevez L, Cirauqui B, et al. A randomized phase II trial of platinum salts in basal-like breast cancer patients in the neoadjuvant setting. Results from the GEICAM/2006-03, multicenter study. Breast Cancer Res Treat. 2012;136(2):487–93.

41. Generali D, Buffa FM, Berruti A, Brizzi MP, Campo L, Bonardi S, et al. Phosphorylated ERalpha, HIF-1alpha, and MAPK signaling as predictors of primary endocrine treatment response and resistance in patients with breast cancer. J Clin Oncol. 2009;27(2): 227–34.

42. Semiglazov VF, Semiglazov VV, Dashyan GA, Ziltsova EK, Ivanov VG, Bozhok AA, et al. Phase 2 randomized trial of primary endocrine therapy versus chemotherapy in postmenopausal patients with estrogen receptor-positive breast cancer. Cancer. 2007; 110(2):244–54.

43. Eiermann W, Paepke S, Appfelstaedt J, Llombart-Cussac A, Eremin J, Vinholes J, et al. Preoperative treatment of postmenopausal breast cancer patients with letrozole: a randomized double-blind multicenter study. Ann Oncol. 2001;12(11):1527–32.

44. Ellis MJ, Suman VJ, Hoog J, Lin L, Snider J, Prat A, et al. Randomized phase II neoadjuvant comparison between letrozole, anastrozole, and exemestane for postmenopausal women with estrogen receptor-rich stage 2 to 3 breast cancer: clinical and biomarker outcomes and predictive value of the baseline PAM50-based intrinsic subtype – ACOSOG Z1031. J Clin Oncol. 2011;29(17):2342–9.

45. Dixon JM, Renshaw L, Macaskill EJ, Young O, Murray J, Cameron D, et al. Increase in response rate by prolonged treatment with neoadjuvant letrozole. Breast Cancer Res Treat. 2009;113(1):145–51.

46. Dixon JM, Renshaw L, Dixon J, Thomas J. Invasive lobular carcinoma: response to neoadjuvant letrozole therapy. Breast Cancer Res Treat. 2011;130(3):871–7.

47. Olson Jr JA, Budd GT, Carey LA, Harris LA, Esserman LJ, Fleming GF, et al. Improved surgical outcomes for breast cancer patients receiving neoadjuvant aromatase inhibitor therapy: results from a multicenter phase II trial. J Am Coll Surg. 2009;208(5):906–14.

48. Llombart-Cussac A, Guerrero Á, Galán A, Carañana V, Buch E, Rodríguez-Lescure Á, et al. Phase II trial with letrozole to maximum response as primary systemic therapy in postmenopausal patients with ER/PgR[+] operable breast cancer. Clin Transl Oncol. 2012;14(2):125–31.

49. Krainick-Strobel UE, Lichtenegger W, Wallwiener D, Tulusan AH, Jänicke F, Bastert G, et al. Neoadjuvant letrozole in postmenopausal estrogen and/or progesterone receptor positive breast cancer: a phase IIb/III trial to investigate optimal duration of preoperative endocrine therapy. BMC Cancer. 2008;8:62.

50. Salmon RJ, Alran S, Malka I, Rosty C, Languille O, Campana F, et al. Estrogen receptors evolution in neoadjuvant aromatase inhibitor (AI) therapy for breast cancer in elderly women: stability of hormonal receptor expression during treatment. Am J Clin Oncol. 2006;29(4):385–8.

51. Mamounas EP, Anderson SJ, Dignam JJ, Bear HD, Julian TB, Geyer Jr CE, et al. Predictors of locoregional recurrence after neoadjuvant chemotherapy: results from combined analysis of National Surgical Adjuvant Breast and Bowel Project B-18 and B-27. J Clin Oncol. 2012;30(32):3960–6.

52. Mauri D, Pavlidis N, Ioannidis JP. Neoadjuvant versus adjuvant systemic treatment in breast cancer: a meta-analysis. J Natl Cancer Inst. 2005;97(3):188–94.

53. Huang EH, Strom EA, Perkins GH, Oh JL, Chen AM, Meric-Bernstam F, et al. Comparison of risk of local-regional recurrence after mastectomy or breast conservation therapy for patients treated with neoadjuvant chemotherapy and radiation stratified according to a prognostic index score. Int J Radiat Oncol Biol Phys. 2006;66(2):352–7.

54. Broadwater JR, Edwards MJ, Kuglen C, Hortobagyi GN, Ames FC, Balch CM. Mastectomy following preoperative chemotherapy. Strict operative criteria control operative morbidity. Ann Surg. 1991;213(2): 126–9.

55. Unalp HR, Onal MA. Analysis of risk factors affecting the development of seromas following breast cancer surgeries: seromas following breast cancer surgeries. Breast J. 2007;13(6):588–92.

56. Narui K, Ishikawa T, Satake T, Adachi S, Yamada A, Shimada K, et al. Outcomes of immediate perforator flap reconstruction after skin-sparing mastectomy following neoadjuvant chemotherapy. Eur J Surg Oncol. 2014;41(1):94–9.

57. Donker M, Hage JJ, Woerdeman LA, Rutgers EJ, Sonke GS, Vrancken Peeters MJ. Surgical complications of skin sparing mastectomy and immediate prosthetic reconstruction after neoadjuvant chemotherapy for invasive breast cancer. Eur J Surg Oncol. 2012;38(1):25–30.

58. Wilke LG, Ballman KV, McCall LM, Giuliano AE, Whitworth PW, Blumencranz PW, et al. Adherence to the National Quality Forum (NQF) breast cancer measures within cancer clinical trials: a review from ACOSOG Z0010. Ann Surg Oncol. 2010;17(8):1989–94.

59. Jung SY, Shin KH, Kim M, Chung SH, Lee S, Kang HS, et al. Treatment factors affecting breast cancer-related lymphedema after systemic chemotherapy and radiotherapy in stage II/III breast cancer patients. Breast Cancer Res Treat. 2014;148(1):91–8.

Surgical Management of Locally Advanced Breast Cancer

18

Abdullah İğci and Enver Özkurt

Abstract

Patients with locally advanced breast cancer (LABC) have historically been considered inoperable cases. However, in light of recent research and studies, even metastatic breast cancers have been down-staged to operable cases using new treatment modalities. The incidence of LABC is less than 5 % [1–3]. Annually, 300,000–450,000 new cases of LABC are diagnosed worldwide.

According to the American Joint Committee on Cancer (AJCC) staging system, LABC is classified as follows: T3, large tumors; T4, tumors with skin or chest wall involvement; N2, nodal disease with fixed or matted axillary lymph nodes; and N3, nodal disease with involvement of the ipsilateral subclavicular and supraclavicular lymph nodes [4]. However, tumors that do not clinically match the criteria for LABC according to the AJCC staging system, such as tumors 3–5 cm in size located in a low-volume breast, behave similarly to LABC; thus, these tumors are optimally treated with combined modality approaches.

The administration of preoperative systemic therapy (PST) as the first modality of treatment is favored by most expert groups for the management

A. İğci, MD, FACS (✉)
Breast Unit, Department of General Surgery,
Istanbul University, Istanbul Medical Faculty,
Istanbul, Turkey
e-mail: aigci@istanbul.edu.tr

E. Özkurt, MD
Department of General Surgery, Istanbul Medical
Faculty, Istanbul University, Istanbul, Turkey
e-mail: doctorenver@gmail.com

© Springer International Publishing Switzerland 2016
A. Aydiner et al. (eds.), *Breast Disease: Management and Therapies*,
DOI 10.1007/978-3-319-26012-9_18

of stage III and most large stage II breast cancers [5–11]. This treatment may enable down-staging in approximately 70–95 % of patients [5, 10–13]. Several studies have compared preoperative systemic therapy with postoperative (adjuvant) systemic therapy and demonstrated that these new treatment modalities prolong disease-free and overall survival [14–16].

Patients treated with PST were significantly more likely to undergo breast-conserving surgery (BCS) without a significant increase in local recurrence (LR) compared with patients treated with surgery first [14–16]. In addition, PST results in down-staging the axillary lymph nodes in up to 40 % of patients [14, 15, 17, 18]. Down-staging the axilla can reduce morbidity due to decreased rates of axillary dissection. Several randomized and non-randomized studies have demonstrated a significant achievement of pathologic complete response (pCR) in the breast and axillary nodes and improved outcome. According to these studies, clinical and pathologic response to PST can be used as an intermediate marker of chemotherapy efficacy, thus prompting the decision as to which chemotherapy regimen should be used following surgery. Furthermore, the efficacy of chemotherapy is slightly enhanced prior to surgery based on robust vascular and lymphatic drainage of the breast and the tumor itself. Based on the findings above, multidisciplinary collective and coordinated work between surgical and oncological teams as well as other clinicians is crucial when evaluating patients with LABC.

Keywords

Locally advanced breast cancer • Neoadjuvant chemotherapy • Sentinel lymph node biopsy • Breast-conserving surgery

Introduction

Patients with locally advanced breast cancer (LABC) have been historically considered inoperable cases. However, in the light of recent research and studies, even metastatic breast cancers have been down-staged to operable cases using new treatment modalities. The incidence of LABC is less than 5 % [1–3]. Annually, 300,000–450,000 new cases of LABC are diagnosed worldwide.

According to the American Joint Committee on Cancer (AJCC) staging system, LABC is classified as follows: T3, large tumors; T4, tumors with skin or chest wall involvement; N2, nodal disease with fixed or matted axillary lymph nodes; and N3, nodal disease with involvement of the ipsilateral subclavicular and supraclavicular lymph nodes [4]. However, tumors that do not clinically match the criteria for LABC according to the AJCC staging system, such as tumors 3–5 cm in size located in a low-volume breast, behave similarly to LABC; thus, these tumors are optimally treated with combined modality approaches.

The administration of preoperative systemic therapy (PST) as the first modality of treatment is favored by most expert groups for the management of stage III and most large stage II breast cancers [5–11]. This treatment may result in down-staging for approximately 70–95 % of patients [5, 10–13]. Several studies have compared preoperative systemic therapy with postoperative (adjuvant) systemic therapy and demonstrated that these new treatment modalities prolong disease-free and overall survival [14–16].

Patients treated with PST were significantly more likely to undergo breast-conserving surgery (BCS) without significant increase in local recurrence (LR) compared with patients treated with surgery first [14–16]. In addition, PST enabled down-staging of the axillary lymph nodes in up to 40 % of patients [14, 15, 17, 18]. Down-staging the axilla can reduce morbidity due to decreased rates of axillary dissection. Several randomized and non-randomized studies have demonstrated a significant achievement of pathologic complete response (pCR) in the breast and axillary nodes and improved outcome. According to these studies, clinical and pathological response to PST can be used as an intermediate marker of chemotherapy efficacy, thus enabling a decision as to which chemotherapy regimen should be used following surgery. Furthermore, the efficacy of chemotherapy is slightly enhanced prior to surgery based on robust vascular and lymphatic drainage of the breast and the tumor itself. Based on the findings above, multidisciplinary collective and coordinated work between surgical and oncological teams as well as other clinicians is crucial when evaluating patients with LABC.

Evaluation of Primary Tumor Between Diagnosis and Surgery in Patients Who Will Receive Preoperative Systemic Therapy

Patients who are candidates for PST should be assessed before, during, and after chemotherapy. One of the most important benefits of PST is the potential for converting patients who require mastectomy to patients who can undergo BCS. Therefore, assessment of patients before, during, and after chemotherapy clinically via physical examination and radiologically is crucial before deciding on a surgical strategy.

Chagpar et al. reported that physical examination appears to be at least as accurate as mammography or ultrasound in estimating residual tumor size [19]. However, the false-negative rate (FNR) is approximately 60 %; thus, many small tumors may be missed with this approach.

Before starting the treatment, a pathologic assessment of the tumor is needed via fine-needle aspiration (FNA) or core biopsy (CB). Additionally, defining prognostic and predictive factors, such as estrogen/progesterone receptors (ER/PR) and human epidermal growth factor receptor 2 (HER2), before chemotherapy is particularly important in cases of pCR in the breast and axillary nodes. In addition, in patients who plan to undergo BCS, the tumor bed should be marked during CB. Thus, if pCR is determined at the end of PST, the surgeon can resect exact tumor location.

Although the rate of a false-positive FNA is very low in patients with newly diagnosed breast cancer [20], this technique cannot readily differentiate invasive from noninvasive carcinoma. By contrast, CB results in minimal tumor perturbation while providing important diagnostic information, including the identification of tumors that are predominantly or completely in situ [21]. Furthermore, CB can provide sufficient material to evaluate prognostic and predictive tumor biomarkers, such as ER/PR, HER2, Ki-67, etc. [22, 23].

Clinical and Radiological Assessment

Mammography
When estimating the extent of the primary tumor and to eliminate the presence of diffuse malignant microcalcifications potentially indicative of an extensive intraductal component, careful physical examination and a pre-chemotherapy mammogram are important [24]. The extent of the mass and the presence of microcalcifications in the breasts must be determined before and after PST, particularly in patients who are candidates for BCS (Fig. 18.1).

Ultrasound and Elastography (Sonoelastography)
Although primary tumor assessments are potentially laborious in patients with dense breasts, ultrasound can be useful to determine the extent of the tumor and monitor the tumor during PST [25] (Fig. 18.2). Ultrasound elastography (sonoelastography or elastography) is a novel ultrasound method that provides a representation of tissues and organs and evaluation of their

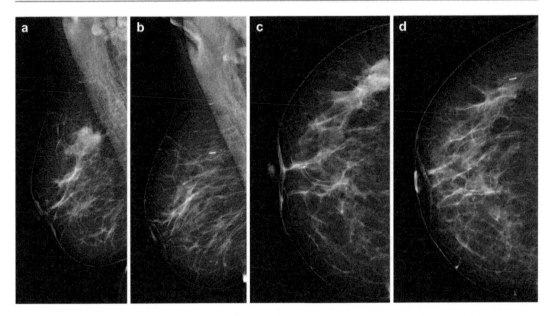

Fig. 18.1 Mammography imaging of the patient before (**a**, **c**) and after (**b**, **d**) PST with complete pathological response. Titanium clip for tumor bed localization is also seen in mammograms

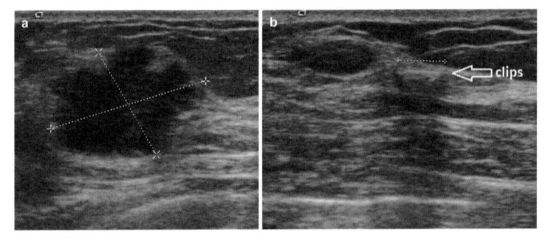

Fig. 18.2 Ultrasonographic imaging of the patient before (**a**) and after (**b**) PST with complete pathological response. Titanium clip for tumor bed localization is also seen in ultrasound

elasticity and stiffness. In this procedure, slight repeated pressure is placed on the examined organ with the ultrasound transducer. Elasticity and deformations are processed and presented in real time as color-coded maps called elastograms. Masses are typically coded from blue to red (blue for rigid masses and red for soft masses) (Fig. 18.3). This method is based on the fact that pathological changes in tissues generally also affect their stiffness [26–29].

Ianculescu et al. reported Virtual Touch IQ shear wave elastography results for 110 breast lesions [30]. Of these lesions, 48 were benign, and 62 were malignant. Breast Imaging-Reporting and Data System (BIRADS)-based B-mode evaluation of the 48 benign and 62 malignant lesions achieved 92 % sensitivity and 62.5 % specificity. Elastography was performed using visual interpretation of the color overlay displaying relative shear wave velocities with

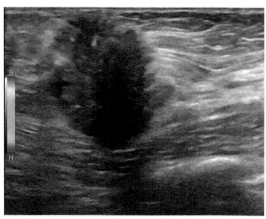
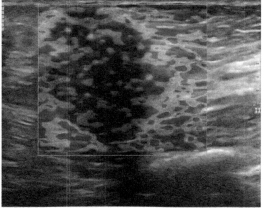

Fig. 18.3 A malignant characterized mass in the left upper quadrant with irregular margins. The mass is showing a rigid color (*blue*) in elastography (This image is used by the permission of Dr. Ravza Yilmaz from Istanbul University Istanbul School of Medicine, Department of Radiology)

similar stand-alone diagnostic performance with 92 % sensitivity and 64.6 % specificity. Lesion and surrounding tissue shear wave speed values were calculated, and a significant difference was observed between the benign and malignant populations (Mann-Whitney U test, $p < 0.0001$). Using a lesion cutoff value of 3.31 m/s, 80.4 % sensitivity and 73 % specificity were achieved. Exclusively applying this threshold to BIRADS 4a masses, overall levels of 92 % sensitivity and 72.9 % specificity were achieved. VTIQ qualitative and quantitative elastography has the potential to further characterize B-mode-detected breast lesions, increasing specificity and reducing the number of unnecessary biopsies.

Although recent studies suggest that elastography reduces unnecessary biopsy numbers [30–32], additional prospective randomized trials with a large number of patients are required to evaluate the clinical use of this novel technique.

Magnetic Resonance Imaging

Magnetic resonance imaging (MRI) has emerged as a very useful tool for defining the extent and patterns of primary breast tumor growth [33], particularly in high-risk patients [34, 35] and patients with increased mammographic density [36]. MRI is also valuable in assessing tumor response to PST [37, 38] and demonstrates superior accuracy compared with mammography [33]. MRI also provides valuable information regarding the extent of surgical margins in patient who are candidates for BCS as well as the response of the axillary lymph nodes to PST (Figs. 18.4 and 18.5). MRI before and after PST can identify distinct patterns of tumor growth and shrinkage (concentric versus dendritic) [39] and thus can be useful in identifying appropriate candidates for BCS after PST [40]. Although MRI is less predictive of the true residual tumor size when a substantial clinical response is noted [41, 42], the residual tumor size based on MRI correlates well with microscopic findings on pathologic examination [43, 44]. However, the use of MRI has raised concerns regarding the potential of decreasing the pool of BCS candidates regardless of whether patients receive PST or not [45]. Thus, for patients who are not good candidates for BCS based on the presence of multicentric lesions on the original or post-chemotherapy MRI, consideration should be given to obtaining histological confirmation of these additional MRI abnormalities before the decision to proceed with mastectomy [45].

In a meta-analysis of MRI detection of residual breast cancer after neoadjuvant therapy, 44 studies including 2,050 patients were reviewed [46]. MRI exhibited increased accuracy compared with mammography ($p = 0.02$); the evidence only weakly indicated that MRI exhibited increased accuracy compared with clinical examination ($p = 0.10$). No difference in MRI and ultrasound accuracy was observed ($p = 0.15$).

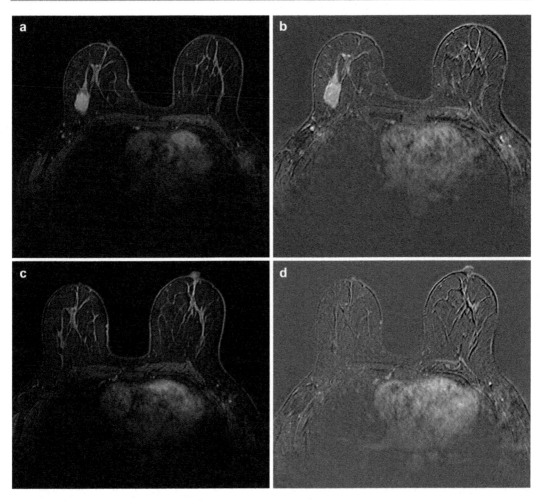

Fig. 18.4 Magnetic resonance imaging of the patient with a mass in her right breast. (**a, b**) Before PST. (**c, d**) After PST with complete pathological response

Contrast-Enhanced Computed Tomography

When determining tumor extent in the breast and identifying appropriate candidates for BCS, contrast-enhanced computed tomography (CE-CT) also exhibits increased sensitivity and specificity before and after PST [47]. Similar to MRI, CE-CT classifies breast tumors into localized and diffuse patterns of growth [48]. Tumors exhibiting a diffuse growth type shrink in a mosaic pattern, exhibit reduced rates of pCR, and are not generally suitable for BCS. By contrast, tumors exhibiting a localized growth pattern generally shrink concentrically, exhibit increased rates of pCR, and are often appropriate candidates for BCS [48]. CE-CT can be a less expensive and readily attainable alternative to MRI, but studies comparing these two imaging modalities are needed.

Positron Emission Tomography

Recent studies of technetium-99 sestamibi scintimammography and 18-fluoro-deoxy-glucose positron emission tomography (^{18}FDG-PET) indicate that these imaging modalities are useful when assessing patients undergoing PST before, during, and after chemotherapy. Alterations in ^{18}FDG uptake exhibit a strong correlation with clinical response [48–51] (Fig. 18.6). However, the value of this technique in identifying pathologic complete responders among clinical complete responders is variable [48, 50]. Intraductal cancer is typically not affected by cytotoxic

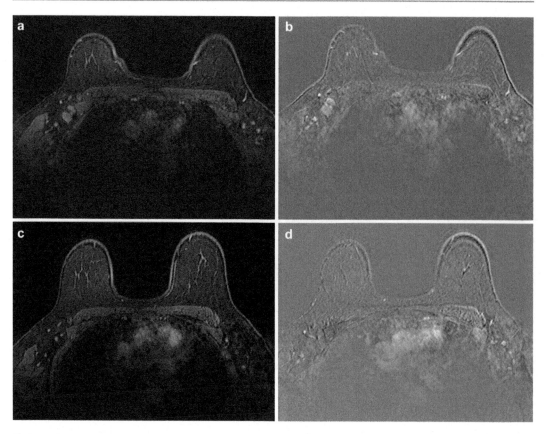

Fig. 18.5 Magnetic resonance imaging of positive lymph nodes before (**a**, **b**) and after (**c**, **d**) PST with complete pathological response

chemotherapy and will persist during treatment [52]. Thus, the discrepancy between a radiographic and pathologic response can be attributed to the persistence of intraductal cancer.

Mghanga et al. reviewed 15 FDG-PET studies with 745 patients who underwent PST with the diagnosis of breast cancer [53]. In their meta-analysis, the pooled sensitivity and specificity of FDG-PET or PET/CT were 80.5 % (95 % CI, 75.9–84.5 %) and 78.8 % (95 % CI, 74.1–83.0 %), respectively; the positive predictive and negative predictive values were 79.8 % and 79.5 %, respectively. After one and two courses of chemotherapy, the pooled sensitivity and false-positive rate were 78.2 % (95 % CI, 73.8–82.5 %) and 11.2 % and 82.4 % (95 % CI, 77.4–86.1 %) and 19.3 %, respectively. Analysis of the findings suggests that FDG-PET exhibits moderately increased sensitivity and specificity in the early detection of responders compared with nonresponders. In addition, this technique can be applied in the evaluation of breast cancer response to neoadjuvant chemotherapy in breast cancer patients.

In another meta-analysis of 17 studies and a total of 781 patients, FDG-PET/FDG-CT and PET exhibited reasonable sensitivity in evaluating the response to neoadjuvant chemotherapy in breast cancer; however, the specificity was relatively low. The authors of this analysis recommended combining other imaging methods with FDG-PET/FDG-CT or PET [54].

Determining the Tumor Bed Location in Patients with Clinical or Pathological Complete Response

Determining the exact tumor bed location in patients, especially those with clinical complete response or pCR who receive PST, is crucial before

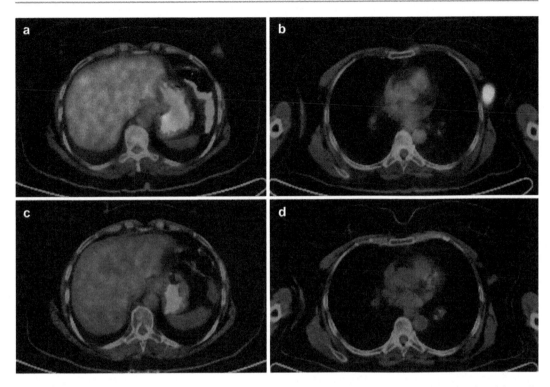

Fig. 18.6 Positron emission tomography imaging of the invasive ductal carcinoma in the left breast and positive axillary lymph nodes before (**a**, **b**) and after (**c**, **d**) PST

and during chemotherapy. When complete response is assessed, there is no evidence of the tumor after PST using imaging modalities. Thus, care should be taken, and all patients who undergo PST should be assessed promptly [55, 56]. Approximately 30 % of these patients (and up to 60 % of those treated with trastuzumab) will achieve a clinical complete response, making it difficult to locate the tumor site during surgery [57].

The exact tumor location must be marked with a radiopaque marker (embolization coils, titanium clips, and metallic harpoon) under mammographic or sonographic guidance before administering chemotherapy or early during chemotherapy when there is evidence of response [55, 56]. Studies have indicated that the identification of the tumor site is difficult or impossible in as many as half of patients receiving NACT without the placement of such a marker [58, 59]. Marker placement is crucial for both the surgeon and pathologist before and after surgery. The surgeon will decide where to operate and how much volume to remove in patients who are candidates for BCS, and the pathologist will focus on that particular area in

search of a residual tumor [55, 56]. Nearly two-thirds of patients with a clinical complete response will have residual tumor on final pathology, and thus it is critically important to precisely localize and remove the original tumor site and ensure that the surgical specimen has clean margins [57].

Determining the Axillary Nodal Status Before Preoperative Systemic Therapy

Radiological Assessment

Although considerable advances in imaging modalities, such as CE-CT, MRI, and PET-CT, have been made, none of these techniques are as accurate as FNA of the axillary lymph nodes. The sensitivity of these imaging modalities ranges from 70 % to 90 % [47, 49, 60]. However, in the presence of micrometastases or small macrometastases, the sensitivity is considerably reduced [49]. Consequently, the recent approach to identify pathologically enlarged lymph nodes in the axillary region involves the use of ultrasound and subsequent biopsy of these lymph nodes by FNA [61, 62]. This method can also provide important information for decision-making before starting PST. Common causes of decreased sensitivity of this approach include failure to visualize all lymph nodes by ultrasound and small size of axillary metastases in some patients [62]. In addition, the radiologist may occasionally sample from a nonmetastatic portion of the lymph node, and the biopsy result will therefore mislead the clinician.

Sentinel Node Biopsy

Sentinel node biopsy (SNB) can also be used to assess axillary nodal status before PST [63–65]. SNB may provide valuable information regarding the nodal status of the axilla, allowing the clinician to choose an appropriate regimen and estimate the effects of PST. The feasibility and accuracy of SNB in patients who are the typical candidates for PST has been demonstrated in several studies [63–67]. Moreover, patients with large operable breast cancer have been included in several multicenter and randomized trials. None of these trials has demonstrated reduced feasibility or accuracy of SNB according to tumor size [68–71].

A considerable number of studies have suggested that SNB can be performed either before or after PST [72–75]. The appropriate timing of SNB is an important and controversial locoregional therapy issue for patients who are candidates for neoadjuvant chemotherapy. However, the current trend is SNB after PST [72, 75]. A detailed review of this topic is presented in the section on the surgical management of the axilla.

Surgical Management of the Primary Breast Tumor After Preoperative Systemic Therapy

The most important advantage of PST in women with large primary tumors or those with moderate size tumors but large tumor size to breast size ratio is the potential for tumor shrinkage to facilitate breast-conserving surgery [76–78].

Vlastos et al. [78] reported that at MD Anderson Cancer Center, 129 patients treated with preoperative chemotherapy (either paclitaxel or FAC [fluorouracil, doxorubicin, and cyclophosphamide]) exhibited significant tumor downsizing. Although the number of patients eligible for breast conservation was not defined preoperatively, 26 % of tumors initially categorized as T2 were down-staged to less than 1.0 cm, and 11 % of patients experienced pCR in the breast. In addition, of those tumors clinically larger than 5 cm, 29 % decreased to less than 1.0 cm, and 9 % exhibited no residual disease at surgery [78].

Bonadonna et al. [77] reported the 8-year results of two prospective trials from the Milan Cancer Institute in women with primary tumors larger than 2.5 cm. Following a variety of preoperative chemotherapy regimens, 85 % of the patients were able to undergo breast-conserving surgery. In addition, breast conservation was possible in 62 % of patients who presented with primary tumors larger than 5.0 cm [77]. Overall, 34 % underwent breast-conserving surgery. By contrast, in the National Surgical Adjuvant Breast and Bowel Project (NSABP) B-18 trial [79], in which patients were randomized to preoperative versus adjuvant chemotherapy and surgeons were required to state beforehand whether a patient was a candidate for breast conservation, breast conservation rates were significantly improved but only increased from 60 % to 67 %. Similarly, in the Royal Marsden randomized trial of preoperative plus adjuvant chemotherapy (mitoxantrone/methotrexate with or without mitomycin) versus the same chemotherapy administered in the adjuvant setting, breast conservation was increased from 13 % to 28 % [80]. In addition, 23 % of patients in the European Organization for Research and Treatment of Cancer (EORTC) randomized trial of preoperative fluorouracil, epirubicin, and cyclophosphamide (FEC) underwent breast conservation instead of planned mastectomy [15].

Another important issue is the quantity of breast tissue removed from patients who are candidates for BCS. This issue is particularly important for patients with pCR. The surgeon should consider the original tumor configuration, the pattern of tumor shrinkage, and the presence or absence of suspicious microcalcifications. Accordingly, the surgeon must identify the extent of the tumor before and after chemotherapy via clinical and imaging assessments. The surgeon must consider additional removal of tissue instead of removing the center of tumor bed if the lumpectomy margins are found to be compromised on pathologic evaluation or if there is evidence of "honeycomb" tumor regression.

Invasive lobular carcinoma is often multicentric, can extensively involve the breast without significant clinical or imaging findings of a defined mass [45, 81, 82], and is associated with reduced clinical response rates compared with invasive ductal carcinoma [83, 84]. Thus, particular attention is needed when planning the extent of lumpectomy in patients who present with invasive lobular carcinoma. Among patients with lobular invasive histology, the rate of pCR is low [84–86]. In one series, lobular histology was identified as one of the independent predictors of ineligibility for BCS after preoperative chemotherapy [87]. Thus, it is unlikely that preoperative chemotherapy will convert patients who present with extensive lobular invasive carcinoma requiring mastectomy to lumpectomy candidates.

Breast-Conserving Surgery After Preoperative Systemic Therapy

For selected patients (i.e., complete resolution of skin edema [*peau d'orange*], adequate reduction in tumor size, no extensive intramammary lymphatic invasion, absence of extensive suspicious microcalcifications, and no evidence of multicentricity), BCS can be an appropriate local treatment option. In patients meeting these criteria, the LR rate and 10-year overall survival after BCS are equivalent to those observed in early-stage breast cancer patients [88].

Second-generation randomized phase III trials incorporating paclitaxel and docetaxel into neoadjuvant regimens as well as those evaluating preoperative targeted therapies, such as trastuzumab, continue to demonstrate improved BCS rates and, importantly, increased pCR rates: 10–28 % for trials incorporating paclitaxel and docetaxel and

36–78 % for trials incorporating trastuzumab [89]. Achievement of pCR is associated with improved overall survival and disease-free survival. At this point, a question emerges. What will be the margins of resection and the extent of the lumpectomy? Surgical excision does not attempt to remove the pre-chemotherapy volume of tumor. The goal is to remove any residual lesion with 1 cm of clear margins. Alternatively, if no detectable residual lesion is evident, a 2-cm specimen with the metal coil in the center is removed. While the patient is still in surgery, the specimen is then sectioned by a pathologist. If there is any indication of positive margin, the surgeon must remove additional tissue from the positive site to obtain a negative margin.

Radiation therapy plays a crucial role in successful BCS and reduces LR risk by approximately 50 % [90]. The 5-year LR risk is significantly reduced from 26 % after lumpectomy alone to 7 % after lumpectomy with radiation therapy, with an absolute reduction of 19 % [90].

Ipsilateral Breast Tumor Recurrence Following Preoperative Systemic Therapy and Lumpectomy

LR after BCS can be described as follows:

1. True recurrence, one within the primary tumor bed
2. Marginal miss, one within the same quadrant just outside of the tumor bed
3. Recurrence elsewhere, one in a separate quadrant of the breast

The Early Breast Cancer Trialists' Collaborative Group (EBCTCG) demonstrated that greater than 75 % of all recurrences occur within 5 years [90].

Studies in patients with operable breast cancer and in those with locally advanced disease have demonstrated that BCT can be safely performed in patients who respond to preoperative chemotherapy without compromising local control [14, 15, 18, 91]. The evidence is stronger in patients with operable breast cancer, for whom large randomized trials have demonstrated no statistically significant increase in LR between the preoperative and adjuvant chemotherapy arms of the trials [14, 15, 18]. In the European Organization for Research and Treatment of Cancer (EORTC) trial, which compared preoperative versus postoperative 5-fluorouracil, epirubicin, and cyclophosphamide chemotherapy in 689 patients, no significant difference in locoregional recurrence (LRR) was observed [15]. Similarly, in the NSABP B-18 trial, in which 1,523 women were randomized to preoperative versus postoperative doxorubicin and cyclophosphamide chemotherapy, a small difference in LRR favoring the adjuvant chemotherapy arm was observed but was not statistically significant.

Kümmel S. et al. reported LR rates in a recently published review [92]. Long-term follow-up results of the NSABP B-18 and B-27 trials have recently been published [93]. These two studies included a total of 3,088 patients undergoing PST or adjuvant chemotherapy. All underwent surgery in the course of treatment. RT was limited to whole-breast irradiation following BCS. The 10-year cumulative LRR rate after NACT was 12.3 % for patients who underwent mastectomy and 10.3 % for those treated with BCS and consecutive whole-breast irradiation. Clinical tumor sizes larger than 5 cm in patients who underwent mastectomy and age <50 years in the BCS group had a significant impact on the risk of LR by 10 years. Clinically node-positive (cN+) disease before PST and pathological nodal involvement after PST were independent predictors of LR, regardless of the type of surgical therapy. Patients who failed to achieve down-staging of the axilla (cN+ to ypN0) and breast pCR were at higher risk of LR. In addition, data concerning hormone receptor and HER2 status were not available; thus, it could not be determined whether certain subgroups may benefit more or may be at increased risk of LR after PST. Moreover, a direct comparison of LR rates between the two groups in NSABP B-18 that received the same type of chemotherapy (one group before and one after surgery) was not reported.

LR may occur in both mastectomy and BCS patients. The slightly increased rates of LR in patients with BCS are due to regression of tumors in a "honeycomb" pattern rather than a "concentric" pattern after PST.

Breast Reconstruction After Preoperative Chemotherapy and Mastectomy

Several studies have demonstrated that immediate breast reconstruction with autologous tissue is safe [94–96], does not delay further adjuvant therapy [94, 97], and is not associated with an increase in LR [94, 98] or a delay in detecting such a recurrence in patients who have received prior PST [99]. However, evidence suggests that immediate reconstruction can compromise the quality of RT, which can lead to more radiation to the heart and lung [100]. The optimal type of reconstruction remains the subject of debate because the effect of RT on breast implants or autologous tissue is unpredictable and may lead to increases in capsular contraction or flap contraction, respectively [96, 98, 101]. Given this concern, some investigators have recently adopted the so-called immediate-delayed or delayed-delayed reconstruction approach in patients who are likely to require postmastectomy RT [102]. With reference to this approach, a submuscular expander is placed and partially inflated during the skin-sparing mastectomy procedure. After the final pathology report, if RT is not required, expansion continues until sufficient space is obtained for the replacement of the expander by the permanent implant. However, if adjuvant RT is required, the expander is deflated for adequate skin or chest wall and ipsilateral regional lymph node irradiation. After completion of radiotherapy, reconstruction is performed at the appropriate time.

Surgical Complications After Preoperative Systemic Therapy

The effect of preoperative systemic therapy on surgical complications has not been investigated widely. The influence of new agents on postoperative wound healing, wound infection, and other complications regarding the need for reoperation remains unknown. In a current retrospective analysis [103], data were collected from 44,533 patients after breast surgery. To identify predictors of postoperative wound complications, a multivariable regression analysis was performed; 2,006 patients received PST prior to surgery. Wound complication rates were generally low and comparable in the neoadjuvant treatment and primary surgery groups (3.4 % versus 3.1 %). In the study, PST did not influence postoperative wound healing, although a trend toward a higher rate of wound complications (4.0 %) was noted among patients who underwent mastectomy and immediate reconstruction after PST. Postoperative complication rates were higher for mastectomies with immediate or delayed reconstruction compared with BCS [104]. In smaller series [105–107] of immediate breast reconstruction following PST, complication rates after mastectomy and immediate autologous or expander/implant reconstruction with or without preceding PST were similar. In light of this information, PST does not appear to affect postoperative complication rates.

Surgical Management of the Axillary Nodes After Preoperative Systemic Therapy

SNB for detecting axillary nodal status is crucial for breast cancer patients regardless of whether they receive PST or undergo surgery. As previously mentioned, the nodal status of the patient at the time of admission guides the clinician in the selection of the treatment modality. The use of PST for LABC patients has increased continuously since its introduction in clinical practice. Preoperative chemotherapy downstages axillary lymph nodes in a considerable proportion of patients (up to 40 % with anthracycline- and taxane-containing regimens). Thus, if SNB is accurate following preoperative chemotherapy, patients who present with involved axillary nodes at the time of diagnosis may potentially be spared from axillary dissection if the sentinel node is found to be negative following preoperative chemotherapy. At this point, relevant questions include whether axillary dissection is feasible, the false-negative and false-positive rates of SNB, the potential for PST to affect the results of SNB and mislead the surgeon, and the LR rate after SNB without axillary dissection.

Newman et al. [108] reported 54 consecutive breast cancer patients with biopsy-proven axillary nodal metastases at initial diagnosis who underwent SNB and axillary lymph node dissection after receiving PST. The sentinel node identification rate was 98 %, and the FNR was consistent with the literature. Based on their results, the authors concluded that SNB after PST in patients with documented nodal disease at presentation accurately identified cases that were down-staged and commented that this approach can potentially spare this subset of patients (32 %) from the morbidity of an axillary dissection.

Lee et al. [109] reported on 238 patients with positive axillary nodes at presentation and underwent SNB and axillary dissection following PST. The identification rate was 77.6 % in patients who received PST, and the FNR was 5.6 %. Based on these results, the authors concluded that for patients who present with involved axillary nodes and who achieve complete clinical axillary response with PST, SNB could replace axillary node dissection.

Shen et al. [110] reported on 69 patients with clinical T1-4, N1-3 disease in whom axillary metastases were identified by ultrasound-guided FNA and who then underwent SNB following PST using prospective, institutional protocols. The sentinel node identification rate was 92.8 %, and the FNR was 25 %. Based on these results, the authors concluded that SNB is feasible after PST.

Larger single-institution studies have been reported, including various studies in which the axillary nodes were documented to be involved prior to PST [108–113]. When these studies are examined collectively [114, 115] or when larger, multicenter data sets are analyzed [116, 117], the performance characteristics of SNB after PST appear to be similar to those of SNB prior to systemic therapy [68, 69, 71, 117, 118].

The largest report to date comes from the NSABP B-27 trial [116], in which 428 of the 2,411 patients treated with PST underwent lymphatic mapping and attempted SNB prior to the required axillary node dissection. The identification rate was 85 %, which was significantly increased when radiocolloid (with or without Lymphazurin (isosulfan blue: Tyco Healthcare Group, North Haven, Connecticut)) was used for lymphatic mapping (88–89 %) compared with Lymphazurin alone (78 %). The FNR was 11 %, and this result was also lower when radiocolloid (with or without Lymphazurin) was used for lymphatic mapping (8 %) compared with Lymphazurin alone (14 %). By contrast, no significant differences in the FNRs were observed for patients who presented with clinically negative versus clinically positive axillary nodes (12.4 % versus 7.0 %, respectively; $p = 0.51$).

Xing et al. [114] published a meta-analysis of 21 studies of SNB after PST. Studies were eligible for inclusion if they evaluated patients with operable breast cancer who underwent SNB after PST followed by axillary dissection. A total of 1,273 patients were included in the 21 studies. The reported identification rates ranged from 72 % to 100 % with a pooled estimate of 90 %. The sensitivity of SNB ranged from 67 % to 100 % with a pooled estimate of 88 % (95 % CI, 85–90 %). Thus the FNR ranged from 0 % to 33 % with a pooled estimate of 12 %. Based on their results, the authors concluded that SNB is a reliable tool for planning treatment after PST.

The identification rates are slightly lower for SNB after PST in multicenter studies and in the meta-analysis compared with those from other multicenter and randomized trials of SNB before systemic therapy, but the FNRs are similar [68, 69, 71, 118].

In the NSABP B-27 [17] as well as other large PST trials [18, 79, 119], patients achieving pCR in the breast had the lowest rate of involved axillary nodes (13–15 %). However, in the NSABP B-27 SNB, no significant differences were noted in the sentinel node FNRs according to clinical or pathological breast tumor response. Thus, as expected, in the NSABP B-27 trial, the rate of remaining positive non-sentinel nodes was the lowest among patients with pCR (1.7 %) compared with those with clinical complete response but residual invasive cancer in the breast (4.0 %) and those with any other type of clinical response (5.5 %). However, these differences did not reach statistical significance.

The accuracy and utility of SLNB in patients who present with axillary node involvement and undergo PST remain controversial. Two prospective clinical trials regarding the characteristics of SLNB after PST in patients with documented axillary nodal involvement were recently published [120, 121]. The German SENTINA (SENTInel NeoAdjuvant) trial [120, 122] is a four-arm prospective multicenter cohort study designed to (1) evaluate a specific algorithm for the timing of SLNB in patients who undergo PST and (2) provide reliable data regarding the detection rate and FNR in different settings. Patients were categorized into four treatment arms according to the clinical axillary staging before and after PST. Patients with cN0 status underwent SLNB prior to PST (arms A and B). If the SLN was histologically negative, no further axillary surgery was performed after PST (arm A). However, if the SLN was positive, a second SLNB and axillary dissection were performed after PST (arm B). Patients with cN1 status before PST did not undergo axillary surgery prior to PST and were stratified as arms C and D. If patients converted to cN0 after PST, SLNB plus axillary dissection were performed (arm C), but patients who remained cN1 after PST underwent axillary dissection (arm D). A total of 1,737 eligible patients were accrued. The detection rate for SLN was 99.1 % before PST (arms A and B), 80.1 % in arm C (after PST), and 60.8 % in arm D (after PST and prior SLNB) ($p < 0.001$). In arm C, the FNR was 14.2 %. However, in the multivariate regression analysis, the number of removed SLNs was a significant predictor of the FNR (OR for >1 SLN versus 1 SLN removed $= 0.505$, $p = 0.008$). Thus, the FNR was 24.3 % when one SLN was removed, 18.5 % when two SLNs were removed, and only 5 % when more than two SLNs were removed. The SLNB FNR was 51.6 % in arm B, indicating that SLNB prior to PST significantly impairs the detection rate and accuracy of SLNB after PST. Based on these findings, the authors concluded that the SLNB detection rate is significantly reduced compared with primary SLNB in patients who convert from a positive to a negative clinical nodal stage during PST. The FNR was less favorable after PST compared with primary SLNB, but the FNR improved with removal of more than one SLN in this setting.

The second recently reported prospective trial is the ACOSOG Z0171 [121] trial, a single-arm prospective trial of women with clinical T0-4/N1-2/M0 breast cancer receiving PST. At the time of surgery, all patients underwent SLNB followed by axillary lymph node dissection. The primary endpoint was FNR in women with cN1 disease with two or more SLNs reviewed. The protocol encouraged use of the dual-tracer technique. A total of 756 patients were enrolled from July 2009 to July 2011. In patients with SLNB and ALND, the SLN identification rate was 92.5 % (92.7 % in cN1, 90 % in cN2). For patients with cN1 disease and >2 SLNs identified, the FNR was 12.8 %. In patients subjected to the dual-tracer technique, the FNR was 11.1 %. Based on these results, the authors concluded that SLN surgery after NAC in node-positive breast cancer patients correctly identified nodal status in 84 % of all patients and was associated with a FNR of 12.8 %. This FNR was higher than the prespecified study endpoint of 10 %; thus, the authors suggested that further analysis of factors associated with FNR should be performed prior to the widespread use of SLN in these patients. Studies regarding the timing of SLN status in the presence of PST were also mentioned in a review by Mamounas [73] and Fontein et al. [75].

Ultimately, the surgeon must decide whether to perform an axillary dissection. Preoperative imaging studies as well as traditional frozen section can be used for preoperative and intraoperative assessment of pCR in the breast, respectively. Touch imprint cytology is reliable for intraoperative detection of nodal metastases after PST [123]. Patients achieving a clinical complete response or, more importantly, pCR are the best candidates for preserving the axilla and reducing morbidity due to axillary dissection if the sentinel node is negative.

References

1. Seidman H, Gelb SK, Silverberg E, LaVerda N, Lubera JA. Survival experience in the Breast Cancer Detection Demonstration Project. CA Cancer J Clin. 1987;37:258–90.
2. Zeichner GI, Mohar BA, Ramirez UMT. Epidemiologia del Cancer de Mama en el Institute Nacional de Cancerologia (1989–1990). Cancerologia. 1993;39:1825–30.
3. Moisa FC, Lopez J, Raymundo C. Epidemiologia del carcinoma del seno mamario en Latino America. Cancerologia. 1989;35:810–4.
4. Anonymous. Part VII. Breast. In: Green FL, Page DL, Fleming ID, et al., editors. AJCC cancer staging handbook. 6th ed. New York: Springer; 2002. p. 255–81.
5. Jacquillat C, Baillet F, Weil M, Auclerc G, Housset M, Auclerc M, et al. Results of a conservative treatment combining induction (neoadjuvant) and consolidation chemotherapy, hormonotherapy, and external and interstitial irradiation in 98 patients with locally advanced breast cancer (IIIA–IIIB). Cancer. 1988;61:1977–82.
6. DeLena M, Varini M, Zucali R, Rovini D, Viganotti G, Valagussa P, et al. Multimodal treatment for locally advanced breast cancer: results of chemotherapy-radiotherapy versus chemotherapy-surgery. Cancer Clin Trials. 1981;4:229–36.
7. Cocconi G, di Blasio B, Bisagni G, Alberti G, Botti E, Anghinoni E. Neoadjuvant chemotherapy or chemotherapy and endocrine therapy in locally advanced breast carcinoma. Am J Clin Oncol. 1990;13:226–32.
8. Touboul E, Lefranc JP, Blondon J, Ozsahin M, Mauban S, Schwartz LH, et al. Multidisciplinary treatment approach to locally advanced noninflammatory breast cancer using chemotherapy and radiotherapy with or without surgery. Radiother Oncol. 1992;25:167–75.
9. Lippman ME, Sorace RA, Bagley CS, Danforth Jr DW, Lichter A, Wesley MN. Treatment of locally advanced breast cancer using primary induction chemotherapy with hormonal synchronization followed by radiation therapy with or without debulking surgery. NCI Monogr. 1986;1:153–9.
10. Schwartz GF, Cantor RI, Biermann WA. Neoadjuvant chemotherapy before definitive treatment for stage III carcinoma of the breast. Arch Surg. 1987;122:1430–4.
11. Bonadonna G, Veronesi U, Brambilla C, Ferrari L, Luini A, Greco M, et al. Primary chemotherapy to avoid mastectomy in tumors with diameters of three

centimeters or more. J Natl Cancer Inst. 1990;82:1539–45.

12. Hortobagyi GN, Buzdar AU. Locally advanced breast cancer: a review including the M.D. Anderson experience. In: Ragaz J, Ariel IM, editors. High-risk breast cancer. Berlin: Springer; 1991. p. 382–415.

13. Hortobagyi GN, Ames FC, Buzdar AU, Kau SW, McNeese MD, Paulus D, et al. Management of stage III primary breast cancer with primary chemotherapy, surgery, and radiation therapy. Cancer. 1988;62:2507–16.

14. Wolmark N, Wang J, Mamounas E, Bryant J, Fisher B. Preoperative chemotherapy in patients with operable breast cancer: nine-year results from National Surgical Adjuvant Breast and Bowel Project B-18. J Natl Cancer Inst Monogr. 2001;30:96–102.

15. van der Hage JA, van de Velde CJ, Julien JP, Tubiana-Hulin M, Vandervelden C, Duchateau L. Preoperative chemotherapy in primary operable breast cancer: results from the European Organization for Research and Treatment of Cancer trial 10902. J Clin Oncol. 2001;19:4224–37.

16. Gianni L, Baselga J, Eirmann W, Guillem Porta V, Semiglazov V, Lluch A, et al. European cooperative trial in operable breast cancer (ECTO): improved freedom from progression (FFP) from adding paclitaxel (T) to doxorubicin (a) followed by cyclophosphamide methotrexate and fluorouracil (CMF). J Clin Oncol. 2005;23:7S. abst 513.

17. Bear HD, Anderson S, Brown A, Smith R, Mamounas EP, Fisher B, et al. The effect on tumor response of adding sequential preoperative docetaxel to preoperative doxorubicin and cyclophosphamide: preliminary results from National Surgical Adjuvant Breast and Bowel Project Protocol B-27. J Clin Oncol. 2003;21:4165–74.

18. Gianni L, Baselga J, Eiermann W, et al. First report of the European cooperative trial in operable breast cancer (ECTO): effect of primary systemic therapy. Proc Am Soc Clin Oncol. 2002;21:34A. abst 132.

19. Sperber F, Weinstein Y, Sarid D, Ben Yosef R, Shalmon A, Yaal-Hahoshen N. Preoperative clinical, mammographic and sonographic assessment of neoadjuvant chemotherapy response in breast cancer. Israel Med Assoc J. 2006;8:342–6.

20. Chaiwun B, Settakorn J, Ya-In C, Wisedmongkol W, Rangdaeng S, Thorner P. Effectiveness of fine-needle aspiration cytology of breast: analysis of 2,375 cases from Northern Thailand. Diagn Cytopathol. 2002;26:201–5.

21. El-Tamer M, Axiotis C, Kim E, Kim J, Wait R, Homel P, et al. Accurate prediction of the amount of in situ tumor in palpable breast cancers by core needle biopsy: implications for neoadjuvant therapy. Ann Surg Oncol. 1999;6:461–6.

22. Kaneko S, Gerasimova T, Butler WM, Cupples TE, Guerry PL, Greene GR, et al. The use of FISH on breast core needle samples for the presurgical assessment of HER-2 oncogene status. Exp Mol Pathol. 2002;73:61–6.

23. Taucher S, Rudas M, Gnant M, Thomanek K, Dubsky P, Roka S, et al. Sequential steroid hormone receptor measurements in primary breast cancer with and without intervening primary chemotherapy. Endocr Relat Cancer. 2003;10:91–8.

24. Herrada J, Iyer RB, Atkinson EN, Sneige N, Buzdar AU, Hortobagyi GN. Relative value of physical examination, mammography, and breast sonography in evaluating the size of the primary adjuvant tumor and regional lymph node metastases in women receiving neoadjuvant chemotherapy for locally advanced breast carcinoma. Clin Cancer Res. 1997;3:1565–9.

25. Kuerer HM, Singletary SE, Buzdar AU, Ames FC, Valero V, Buchholz TA, et al. Surgical conservation planning after neoadjuvant chemotherapy for stage II and operable stage III breast carcinoma. Am J Surg. 2001;182:601–8.

26. Parker KJ, Taylor LS, Gracewski S, Rubens DJ. A unified view of imaging the elastic properties of tissue. J Acoust Soc Am. 2005;117:2705.

27. Bamber J. EFSUMB guidelines and recommendations on the clinical use of ultrasound elastography. Part 1: basic principles and technology. Ultraschall Med. 2013;34:169–84.

28. Cosgrove D. EFSUMB guidelines and recommendations on the clinical use of ultrasound elastography. Part 2: clinical applications. Ultraschall Med. 2013;34:238–53.

29. Itoh A, Ueno E, Tohno E, Kamma H, Takahashi H, Shiina T, et al. Clinical application of US elastography for diagnosis. Radiology. 2006;239:341–50.

30. Ianculescu V, Ciolovan LM, Dunant A, Vielh P, Mazouni C, Delaloge S, et al. Added value of virtual touch IQ shear wave elastography in the ultrasound assessment of breast lesions. Eur J Radiol. 2014;83(5):773–7.

31. Zaleska-Dorobisz U, Kaczorowski K, Pawluś A, Puchalska A, Inglot M. Ultrasound elastography – review of techniques and its clinical applications. Adv Clin Exp Med. 2014;23(4):645–55.

32. Zhang X, Xiao Y, Zeng J, Qiu W, Qian M, Wang C, et al. Computer-assisted assessment of ultrasound real-time elastography: initial experience in 145 breast lesions. Eur J Radiol. 2014;83(1):e1–7.

33. Esserman L, Hylton N, Yassa L, Barclay J, Frankel S, Sickles E. Utility of magnetic resonance imaging in the management of breast cancer: evidence for improved preoperative staging. J Clin Oncol. 1999;17(1):110–9.

34. Stoutjesdijk MJ, Boetes C, Jager GJ, Beex L, Bult P, Hendriks JH, et al. Magnetic resonance imaging and mammography in women with a hereditary risk of breast cancer. J Natl Cancer Inst. 2001;93(14):1095–102.

35. Kriege M, Brekelmans CT, Boetes C, Besnard PE, Zonderland HM, Obdeijn IM, et al. Efficacy of MRI and mammography for breast-cancer screening in women with a familial or genetic predisposition. N Engl J Med. 2004;351:427–37.

36. Esserman L, Kaplan E, Partridge S, Tripathy D, Rugo H, Park J, et al. MRI phenotype is associated with response to doxorubicin and cyclophosphamide neoadjuvant chemotherapy in stage III breast cancer. Ann Surg Oncol. 2001;8:549–59.

37. Drew PJ, Kerin MJ, Mahapatra T, Malone C, Monson JR, Turnbull LW, et al. Evaluation of response to neoadjuvant chemoradiotherapy for locally advanced breast cancer with dynamic contrast-enhanced MRI of the breast. Eur J Surg Oncol. 2001;27:617–20.

38. Balu-Maestro C, Chapellier C, Bleuse A, Chanalet I, Chauvel C, Largillier R. Imaging in evaluation of response to neoadjuvant breast cancer treatment benefits of MRI. Breast Cancer Res Treat. 2002; 72:145–52.

39. Nakamura S, Kenjo H, Nishio T, Kazama T, Doi O, Suzuki K. Efficacy of 3D-MR mammography for 62 breast conserving surgery after neoadjuvant chemotherapy. Breast Cancer. 2002;9:15–9.

40. Nakamura S, Kenjo H, Nishio T, Kazama T, Do O, Suzuki K. 3D-MR mammography-guided breast conserving surgery after neoadjuvant chemotherapy: clinical results and future perspectives with reference to FDG-PET. Breast Cancer. 2001;8:351–4.

41. Wasser K, Sinn HP, Fink C, Fink C, Klein SK, Junkermann H, et al. Accuracy of tumor size measurement in breast cancer using MRI is influenced by histological regression induced by neoadjuvant chemotherapy. Eur Radiol. 2003;13:1213–23.

42. Rosen EL, Blackwell KL, Baker JA, Soo MS, Bentley RC, Yu D, et al. Accuracy of MRI in the detection of residual breast cancer after neoadjuvant chemotherapy. AJR Am J Roentgenol. 2003;181:1275–82.

43. Cheung YC, Chen SC, Su MY, See LC, Hsueh S, Chang HK, et al. Monitoring the size and response of locally advanced breast cancers to neoadjuvant chemotherapy (weekly paclitaxel and epirubicin) with serial enhanced MRI. Breast Cancer Res Treat. 2003;78:51–8.

44. Partridge SC, Gibbs JE, Lu Y, Esserman LJ, Sudilovsky D, Hylton NM. Accuracy of MR imaging for revealing residual breast cancer in patients who have undergone neoadjuvant chemotherapy. AJR Am J Roentgenol. 2002;179:1193–9. 59.

45. Morris EA. Review of breast MRI: indications and limitations. Semin Roentgenol. 2001;36:226–37.

46. Marinovich ML, Houssami N, Macaskill P, Sardanelli F, Irwig L, Mamounas EP, et al. Meta-analysis of magnetic resonance imaging in detecting residual breast cancer after neoadjuvant therapy. J Natl Cancer Inst. 2013;105(5):321–33.

47. Akashi-Tanaka S, Fukutomi T, Sato N, Miyakawa K. The role of computed tomography in the selection of breast cancer treatment. Breast Cancer. 2003; 10:198–203.

48. Akashi-Tanaka S, Fukutomi T, Sato N, Iwamoto E, Watanabe T, Katsumata N, et al. The use of contrast-enhanced computed tomography before neoadjuvant

49. Danforth Jr DN, Aloj L, Carrasquillo JA, Bacharach SL, Chow C, Zujewski J, et al. The role of 18F-FDG-PET in the local/regional evaluation of women with breast cancer. Breast Cancer Res Treat. 2002; 75:135–46.

chemotherapy to identify patients likely to be treated safely. Ann Surg. 2004;239(2):238–43.

50. Burcombe RJ, Makris A, Pittam M, Lowe J, Emmott J, Wong WL. Evaluation of good clinical response to neoadjuvant chemotherapy in primary breast cancer using [18F]-fluorodeoxyglucose positron emission tomography. Eur J Cancer. 2002;38:375–9.

51. Mankoff DA, Dunnwald LK, Gralow JR, Ellis GK, Schubert EK, Tseng J, et al. Changes in blood flow and metabolism in locally advanced breast cancer treated with neoadjuvant chemotherapy. J Nucl Med. 2003;44:1806–14.

52. Mazouni F, Peintinger S, Wan-Kau S, Andre F, Gonzalez-Angulo AM, Symmans WF, et al. Effect on patient outcome of residual DCIS in patients with complete eradication of invasive breast cancer after neoadjuvant chemotherapy. J Clin Oncol. 2007;25 Suppl 18:530.

53. Mghanga FP, Lan X, Bakari KH, Li C, Zhang Y. Fluorine-18 fluorodeoxyglucose positron emission tomography-computed tomography in monitoring the response of breast cancer to neoadjuvant chemotherapy: a meta-analysis. Clin Breast Cancer. 2013;13(4):271–9.

54. Cheng X, Li Y, Liu B, Xu Z, Bao L, Wang J. 18F-FDG PET/CT and PET for evaluation of pathological response to neoadjuvant chemotherapy in breast cancer: a meta-analysis. Acta Radiol. 2012;53(6):615–27.

55. Baron LF, Baron PL, Ackerman SJ, Durden DD, Pope Jr TL. Sonographically guided clip placement facilitates localization of breast cancer after neoadjuvant chemotherapy. AJR Am J Roentgenol. 2000;174:539–40.

56. Alonso-Bartolome P, Ortega Garcia E, Garijo Ayensa F, de Juan Ferre A, Vega Bolivar A. Utility of the tumor bed marker in patients with breast cancer receiving induction chemotherapy. Acta Radiol. 2002;43:29–33.

57. Nadeem R, Chagla LS, Harris O, Desmond S, Thind R, Flavin A, et al. Tumor localization with a metal coil before the administration of neo-adjuvant chemotherapy. Breast. 2005;14:403–7.

58. Shen J, Valero V, Buchholz TA, Singletary SE, Ames FC, Ross MI, et al. Effective local control and long-term survival in patients with T4 locally advanced breast cancer treated with breast conservation therapy. Ann Surg Oncol. 2004;11:854–60.

59. Guth U, Wight E, Schotzau A, Langer I, Dieterich H, Rochlitz C, et al. Breast carcinoma with noninflammatory skin involvement (T4b). Cancer. 2005;104: 1862–70.

60. Mankoff DA, Dunnwald LK, Gralow JR, Ellis GK, Drucker MJ, Livingston RB. Monitoring the response of patients with locally advanced breast

carcinoma to neoadjuvant chemotherapy using technetium 99m3-sestamibi scintimammography. Cancer. 1999;85:2410–23.

61. Oruwari JU, Chung MA, Koelliker S, Steinhoff MM, Cady B. Axillary staging using ultrasound-guided fine needle aspiration biopsy in locally advanced breast cancer. Am J Surg. 2002;184:307–9.

62. Krishnamurthy S, Sneige N, Bedi DG, Edieken BS, Fornage BD, Kuerer HM, et al. Role of ultrasound-guided fine-needle aspiration of indeterminate and suspicious axillary lymph nodes in the initial staging of breast carcinoma. Cancer. 2002;95:982–8.

63. Bedrosian I, Reynolds C, Mick R, Callans LS, Grant CS, Donohue JH, et al. Accuracy of sentinel lymph node biopsy in patients with large primary breast tumors. Cancer. 2000;88:2540–5.

64. Schrenk P, Hochreiner G, Fridrik M, Wayand W. Sentinel node biopsy performed before preoperative chemotherapy for axillary lymph node staging in breast cancer. Breast J. 2003;9:282–7.

65. Sabel MS, Schott AF, Kleer CG, Merajver S, Cimmino VM, Diehl KM, et al. Sentinel node biopsy prior to neoadjuvant chemotherapy. Am J Surg. 2003;186:102–5.

66. Ollila DW, Neuman HB, Sartor C, Carey LA, Klauber-Demore N. Lymphatic mapping and sentinel lymphadenectomy prior to neoadjuvant chemotherapy in patients with large breast cancers. Am J Surg. 2005;190:371–5.

67. Chung MH, Ye W, Giuliano AE. Role for sentinel lymph node dissection in the management of large (> or = 5 cm) invasive breast cancer. Ann Surg Oncol. 2001;8:688–92.

68. Krag DN, Anderson SJ, Julian TB, Brown AM, Harlow SP, Ashikaga T, et al. Technical outcomes of sentinel-lymph-node resection and conventional axillary-lymph-node dissection in patients with clinically node-negative breast cancer: results from the NSABP -32 randomised phase III trial. Lancet Oncol. 2007;8:881–8.

69. Veronesi U, Paganelli G, Viale G, Luini A, Zurrida S, Galimberti V, et al. A randomized comparison of sentinel-node biopsy with routine axillary dissection in breast cancer. N Engl J Med. 2003;349:546–53.

70. Tafra L, Lannin DR, Swanson MS, Van Eyk JJ, Verbanac KM, Chua AN, et al. Multicenter trial of sentinel node biopsy for breast cancer using both technetium sulfur colloid and isosulfan blue dye. Ann Surg. 2001;233:51–9.

71. McMasters KM, Tuttle TM, Carlson DJ, Brown CM, Noyes RD, Glaser RL, et al. Sentinel lymph node biopsy for breast cancer: a suitable alternative to routine axillary dissection in multi-institutional practice when optimal technique is used. J Clin Oncol. 2000;18:2560–6.

72. Boughey JC, Suman VJ, Mittendorf EA, Ahrendt GM, Wilke LG, Taback B, et al. Sentinel lymph node surgery after neoadjuvant chemotherapy in patients with node-positive breast cancer: the ACOSOG Z1071 (Alliance) clinical trial. Alliance for Clinical Trials in Oncology. JAMA. 2013;310(14):1455–61.

73. Mamounas EP. Timing of determining axillary lymph node status when neoadjuvant chemotherapy is used. Curr Oncol Rep. 2014;16(2):364.

74. Elliott RM, Shenk RR, Thompson CL, Gilmore HL. Touch preparations for the intraoperative evaluation of sentinel lymph nodes after neoadjuvant therapy have high false-negative rates in patients with breast cancer. Arch Pathol Lab Med. 2014;138(6):814–8.

75. Fontein DB, van de Water W, Mieog JS, Liefers GJ, van de Velde CJ. Timing of the sentinel lymph node biopsy in breast cancer patients receiving neoadjuvant therapy – recommendations for clinical guidance. Eur J Surg Oncol. 2013;39(5):417–24.

76. Mauriac L, MacGrogan G, Avril A, Durand M, Floquet A, Debled M, et al. Neoadjuvant chemotherapy for operable breast carcinoma larger than 3 cm: a unicentre randomized trial with a 124 – month median follow-up. Institut Bergonie Bordeaux Groupe Sein (IBBGS). Ann Oncol. 1999;10:47–52.

77. Bonadonna G, Valagussa P, Brambilla C, Ferrari L, Moliterni A, Terenziani M, et al. Primary chemotherapy in operable breast cancer: eight-year experience at the Milan Cancer Institute. J Clin Oncol. 1998;16:93–100.

78. Vlastos G, Mirza NQ, Lenert JT, Hunt KK, Ames FC, Feig BW, et al. The feasibility of minimally invasive surgery for stage IIA, IIB, and IIIA breast carcinoma patients after tumor downstaging with induction chemotherapy. Cancer. 2000;88:1417–24.

79. Fisher B, Brown A, Mamounas E, Wieand S, Robidoux A, Margolese RG, et al. Effect of preoperative chemotherapy on local-regional disease in women with operable breast cancer: findings from National Surgical Adjuvant Breast and Bowel Project B-18. J Clin Oncol. 1997;15:2483–93.

80. Powles TJ, Hickish TF, Makris A, Ashley SE, O'Brien ME, Tidy VA, et al. Randomized trial of chemoendocrine therapy started before or after surgery for treatment of primary breast cancer. J Clin Oncol. 1995;13:547–52.

81. Bazzocchi M, Facecchia I, Luiani C, Puglisi F, Di Loreto C, Smania S. Diagnostic imaging of lobular carcinoma of the breast: mammographic, ultrasonographic and MR findings. Radiol Med. 2000;100:436–43.

82. Lesser ML, Rosen PP, Kinne DW. Multicentricity and bilaterality in invasive breast carcinoma. Surgery. 1982;91:234–40.

83. Sinn HP, Schmid H, Junkermann H, Huober J, Leppien G, Kaufmann M, et al. Histologic regression of breast cancer after primary (neoadjuvant) chemotherapy. Geburtshilfe Frauenheilkd. 1994;54:552–8.

84. Cocquyt VF, Blondeel PN, Depypere HT, Praet MM, Schelfhout VR, Silva OE, et al. Different responses to preoperative chemotherapy for invasive lobular and invasive ductal breast carcinoma. Eur J Surg Oncol. 2003;29:361–7.

85. Cristofanilli M, Gonzalez-Angulo A, Sneige N, Kau SW, Broglio K, Theriault RL, et al. Invasive lobular

carcinoma classic type: response to primary chemotherapy and survival outcomes. J Clin Oncol. 2005;23:41–8.

86. Julian TB, Anderson S, Fourchotte V, Haile SR, Fisher ER, Mamounas EP, et al. Is invasive lobular breast cancer a prognostic factor for neoadjuvant chemotherapy response and long term outcomes? Breast Cancer Res Treat. 2006;100:S146. abst 3065.

87. Newman LA, Buzdar AU, Singletary SE, Kuerer HM, Buchholz T, Ames FC, et al. A prospective trial of preoperative chemotherapy in resectable breast cancer: predictors of breast-conservation therapy feasibility. Ann Surg Oncol. 2002;9:228–34.

88. Chen AM, Meric-Bemstam F, Hunt KK, Chen AM, Meric-Bemstam F, Hunt KK, et al. Breast conservation after neoadjuvant chemotherapy. Cancer. 2005;103:4689–95.

89. Mieog JS, van der Hage JA, van de Velde CJ. Preoperative chemotherapy for women with operable breast cancer. Cochrane Database Syst Rev. 2007;94(10):1189–200.

90. Clarke M, Collins R, Darby S, Davies C, Elphinstone P, Evans E, et al. Effects of radiotherapy and of differences in the extent of surgery for early breast cancer on local recurrence and 15-year survival: an overview of the randomized trials. Lancet. 2005;366(9503):2087–106.

91. Kuerer HM, Hunt KK, Newman LA, Ross MI, Ames FC, Singletary SE. Neoadjuvant chemotherapy in women with invasive breast carcinoma: conceptual basis and fundamental surgical issues. J Am Coll Surg. 2002;190:350–63.

92. Kümmel S, Holtschmidt J, Loibl S. Surgical treatment of primary breast cancer in the neoadjuvant setting. Br J Surg. 2014;101(8):912–24.

93. Mamounas EP, Anderson SJ, Dignam JJ, Bear HD, Julian TB, Geyer Jr CE, et al. Predictors of locoregional recurrence after neoadjuvant chemotherapy: results from combined analysis of National Surgical Adjuvant Breast and Bowel Project B-18 and B-27. J Clin Oncol. 2012;30:3960–6.

94. Styblo TM, Lewis MM, Carlson GW, Murray DR, Wood WC, Lawson D, et al. Immediate breast reconstruction for stage III breast cancer using transverse rectus abdominis musculocutaneous (TRAM) flap. Ann Surg Oncol. 1996;3:375–80.

95. Deutsch MF, Smith M, Wang B, Ainsle N, Schusterman MA. Immediate breast reconstruction with the TRAM flap after neoadjuvant therapy. Ann Plast Surg. 1999;42:240–4.

96. Newman LA, Kuerer HM, Hunt KK, Ames FC, Ross MI, Theriault R, et al. Feasibility of immediate breast reconstruction for locally advanced breast cancer. Ann Surg Oncol. 1999;6:671–5.

97. Sultan MR, Smith ML, Estahrook A, Schnabel F, Singh D. Immediate breast reconstruction in patients with locally advanced disease. Ann Plast Surg. 1997;38:345–51.

98. Hunt KK, Baldwin BJ, Strom EA, Ames FC, McNeese MD, Kroll SS, et al. Feasibility of postmastectomy radiation therapy after TRAM flap breast reconstruction. Ann Surg Oncol. 1997; 4:377–84.

99. Slavin SA, Love SM, Goldwyn RM. Recurrent breast cancer following immediate reconstruction with myocutaneous flaps. Plast Reconstr Surg. 1994;93:1191–207.

100. Motwani SB, Strom EA, Schechter NR, Butler CE, Lee GK, Langstein HN, et al. The impact of immediate breast reconstruction on the technical delivery of postmastectomy radiotherapy. Int J Radiat Oncol Biol Phys. 2006;66:76–82.

101. McKeown DJ, Hogg FJ, Brown IM, Walker MJ, Scott JR, Weiler-Mithoff EM. The timing of autologous latissimus dorsi breast reconstruction and effect of radiotherapy on outcome. J Plast Reconstr Aesthet Surg. 2009;62(4):488–93.

102. Kronowitz SJ. Immediate versus delayed reconstruction. Clin Plast Surg. 2007;34:39–50. abst 6.

103. Decker MR, Greenblatt DY, Havlena J, Wilke LG, Greenberg CC, Neuman HB. Impact of neoadjuvant chemotherapy on wound complications after breast surgery. Surgery. 2012;152:382–8.

104. Garvey EM, Gray RJ, Wasif N, Casey WJ, Rebecca AM, Kreymerman P, et al. Neoadjuvant therapy and breast cancer surgery: a closer look at postoperative complications. Am J Surg. 2013;206:894–8.

105. Schaverien MV, Munnoch DA. Effect of neoadjuvant chemotherapy on outcomes of immediate free autologous breast reconstruction. Eur J Surg Oncol. 2013;39:430–6.

106. Warren Peled A, Itakura K, Foster RD, Hamolsky D, Tanaka J, Ewing C, et al. Impact of chemotherapy on postoperative complications after mastectomy and immediate breast reconstruction. Arch Surg. 2010;145:880–5.

107. Zweifel-Schlatter M, Darhouse N, Roblin P, Ross D, Zweifel M, Farhadi J. Immediate microvascular breast reconstruction after neoadjuvant chemotherapy: complication rates and effect on start of adjuvant treatment. Ann Surg Oncol. 2010;17:2945–50.

108. Newman EA, Sabel MS, Nees AV, Schott A, Diehl KM, Cimmino VM, et al. Sentinel lymph node biopsy performed after neoadjuvant chemotherapy is accurate in patients with documented node positive breast cancer at presentation. Ann Surg Oncol. 2007;14(10):2946–52.

109. Lee S, Kim EY, Kang SH, Kim SW, Kim SK, Kang KW, et al. Sentinel node identification rate, but not accuracy, is significantly decreased after preoperative chemotherapy in axillary node-positive breast cancer patients. Breast Cancer Res Treat. 2007;102:283–8.

110. Shen J, Gilcrease MZ, Babiera GV, Ross MI, Meric-Bernstam F, Feig BW, et al. Feasibility and accuracy of sentinel lymph node biopsy after preoperative chemotherapy in breast cancer patients with documented axillary metastases. Cancer. 2007;109:1255–63.

111. Tanaka Y, Maeda H, Ogawa Y, Nishioka A, Itoh S, Kubota K, et al. Sentinel node biopsy in breast

cancer patients treated with neoadjuvant chemotherapy. Oncol Rep. 2006;15:927–31.

112. Yu JC, Hsu GC, Hsieh CB, Yu CP, Chao TY. Role of sentinel lymphadenectomy combined with intraoperative ultrasound in the assessment of locally advanced breast cancer after neoadjuvant chemotherapy. Ann Surg Oncol. 2007;14:174–80.

113. Kinoshita T. Sentinel lymph node biopsy is feasible for breast cancer patients after neoadjuvant chemotherapy. Breast Cancer. 2007;14:10–5.

114. Xing Y, Foy M, Cox DD, Kuerer HM, Hunt KK, Cormier JN. Meta-analysis of sentinel lymph node biopsy after preoperative chemotherapy in patients with breast cancer. Br J Surg. 2006;93:539–46.

115. Mamounas EP. Sentinel lymph node biopsy after neoadjuvant systemic therapy. Surg Clin North Am. 2003;83:931–42.

116. Mamounas EP, Brown A, Anderson S, Smith R, Julian T, Miller B, et al. Sentinel node biopsy after neoadjuvant chemotherapy in breast cancer: results from National Surgical Adjuvant Breast and Bowel Project Protocol B-27. J Clin Oncol. 2005;23:2694–702.

117. Tafra L, Verbanac KM, Lannin DR. Preoperative chemotherapy and sentinel lymphadenectomy for breast cancer. Am J Surg. 2001;182:312–5.

118. Krag D, Weaver D, Ashikaga T, Moffat F, Klimberg VS, Shriver C, et al. The sentinel node in breast cancer: a multicenter validation study. N Engl J Med. 1998;339:941–6.

119. Kuerer HM, Newman LA, Buzdar AU, Dhingra K, Hunt KK, Buchholz TA, et al. Pathologic tumor response in the breast following neoadjuvant chemotherapy predicts axillary lymph node status. Cancer J Sci Am. 1998;4:230–6.

120. Kuehn T, Bauerfeind I, Fehm T, Fleige B, Hausschild M, Helms G, et al. Sentinel lymph node biopsy before or after neoadjuvant chemotherapy – final results from the prospective German, multi-institutional SENTINA-Trial. Cancer Res. 2012;72(24 Suppl):95S. Abstract S2-2.

121. Boughey JC, Suman VJ, Mittendorf EA, Ahrendt GM, Wilke LG, Taback B, et al. The role of sentinel lymph node surgery in patients presenting with node positive breast cancer (T0-T4, N1-2) who receive neoadjuvant chemotherapy – results from the ACOSOG Z1071 trial. Cancer Res. 2012;72(24 Suppl):94S. Abstract S2-1.

122. Kuehn T, Bauerfeind I, Fehm T, Fleige B, Hausschild M, Helms G, et al. Sentinel lymph node biopsy in patients with breast cancer before and after neoadjuvant chemotherapy (SENTINA): a prospective, multicentre cohort study. Lancet Oncol. 2013;14:609–18.

123. Jain P, Kumar R, Anand M, Asthana S, Deo SV, Gupta R, et al. Touch imprint cytology of axillary lymph nodes after neoadjuvant chemotherapy in patients with breast carcinoma. Cancer. 2003;99:346–51.

Surgical Management of Inflammatory Breast Cancer

19

Atilla Soran, Bulent Unal, and Tara Grahovac

Abstract

Inflammatory breast cancer (IBC) is a rare clinicopathological entity but remains one of the most aggressive types of breast cancer. The acute edematous infiltration of the skin and breast is met with occasionally, and it is without doubt the most acute and fatal form of cancer found in the breast. Such cases as these have been mistaken for inflammation, but knowledge of the probability of this affection being cancerous should prevent such a mistake from being made. Here, we review the current epidemiology, clinical characteristics, diagnostic modalities, and treatment of IBC.

Keywords

IBC • Mastitis • Mammography • HER2 • Modified radical mastectomy

A. Soran, MD, MPH, FACS (✉) • T. Grahovac, MD
Department of Surgery, Division of Surgical
Oncology, Magee-Womens Hospital, University of
Pittsburgh Medical Center, Pittsburgh, PA, USA
e-mail: asoran@upmc.edu, asoran65@gmail.com,
tara.l.grahovac@gmail.com

B. Unal, MD
Department of Surgery, Turgut Ozal Medical
Center, Inonu University Faculty of Medicine,
Malatya, Turkey
e-mail: bulentunal2005@yahoo.com.tr

Introduction

Inflammatory breast cancer (IBC) has been characterized by rapid progression and poor outcome since its first description by Sir Charles Bell in 1814. Patients present with the clinical signs of edema (peau d'orange) and erythema of the skin overlying the breasts. Upon histopathological examination, plugging of the dermal lymphatics of the breast is noted, but this finding is not mandatory for diagnosis. Bryant first noted this "lymphatic absorption" of cancer cells, which leads to edema, in 1887. He also acknowledged how easily IBC could be confused with a benign etiology, given that IBC is often not associated with a palpable mass, as well as the magnitude of this misdiagnosis. The diagnosis of IBC equates to a T4d classification according to the American Joint Committee

© Springer International Publishing Switzerland 2016
A. Aydiner et al. (eds.), *Breast Disease: Management and Therapies*,
DOI 10.1007/978-3-319-26012-9_19

on Cancer (AJCC) staging system and has significant prognostic implications. Early distant metastasis is present in approximately 30 % of patients at diagnosis, and disease-related death occurs twice as often compared with noninflammatory breast cancers [1–5]. Recognizing IBC as a distinct entity, an international expert panel gathered in 2008 to develop guidelines for diagnosis and management. In addition, international IBC registries have been developed, and several clinical trials have been initiated in the last decade to address the unmet need for therapeutic advancements specific to this deadly form of breast cancer.

Epidemiology and Risk Factors

According to the National Cancer Institute's Surveillance, Epidemiology, and End Results (SEER) Program registry database, diagnosis of IBC represents 1 and 0.59 % of all newly diagnosed breast cancer cases among women and men, respectively [8, 9]. IBC remains a rare disease, but the incidence is increasing worldwide [3, 4]. The true incidence is difficult to determine due to regional differences in diagnostic criteria as well as a lack of attention to clinical symptoms. The percentage of IBC among breast cancers varies geographically, with lower proportions in the United States (1–2 %) than other parts of the world (i.e., Turkey, Morocco, Tunisia, Egypt, Nigeria, 10–17 %) [6, 7]. The results of large population-based studies indicate that the incidence of IBC is higher in black women (3.1/100,000) than white women (2.2/100,000). IBC is also diagnosed at earlier ages than non-IBC (median age 57 vs. 62 years, respectively). Patients with IBC are more likely to have had their first pregnancy at younger ages compared with non-IBC patients. Other reproductive parameters, such as menarche at an early age, premenopausal status, and older age at first live birth, are not associated with IBC. Some authors report that higher BMI and a family history of IBC are associated with IBC in both premenopausal and postmenopausal women [2, 9, 10].

IBC was defined to be lethal before 1974 with a median survival time period of 1.2 years and a five year survival rate of 5% [10, 33]. The SEER program noted an overall increase in survival for IBC patients throughout the 1990s; however, survival remains poor compared with non-IBC patients. Among microscopically confirmed malignancies of the breast diagnosed in the SEER 9 Registries database between 1988 and 2000, median survival times differed significantly among women with non-T4 breast cancer, non-IBC T4 breast cancer, and IBC (10 vs. 6.4 vs. 2.9 years, respectively) [1].

Diagnosis

Clinical Characteristics

The American Joint Committee on Cancer (AJCC) defines IBC as "a clinicopathologic entity characterized by diffuse erythema and edema (peau d'orange) of the breast, often without an underlying palpable mass." These clinical findings should involve the majority of the skin of the breast (Figs. 19.1 and 19.2) [4, 12, 13]. Less than 50 % of IBC patients present with a discretely palpable mass. Peau d'orange refers to the unique appearance of the breast skin, which may have ridges or pits resembling the surface of an orange. Other symptoms of inflammatory breast cancer include a rapid increase in breast size, sensations of heaviness, burning or tenderness in the breast, or a retracted nipple [11]. Metastatic axillary lymph nodes are present at diagnosis in over half of IBC patients. Distant metastases are also noted

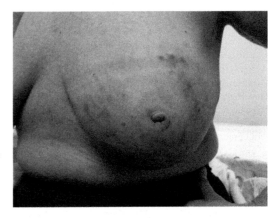

Fig. 19.1 Clinical findings in patients with IBC

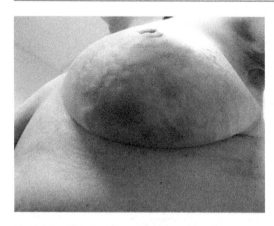

Fig. 19.2 Clinical findings in patients with IBC

in approximately 30 % of IBC patients at diagnosis [14]. The term "primary IBC" or "de novo IBC" is defined as the new development of IBC in a previously normal breast, whereas the term "secondary IBC" describes the inflammatory recurrence of non-IBC breast cancer [10]. "Occult IBC" has also been described and refers to cases in which dermal lymphatic invasion is present in the absence of clinical criteria.

The differential diagnosis for IBC primarily includes mastitis and locally advanced breast cancer. The distinction among these entities is important because the treatment algorithm and prognostic information differ drastically. Recognizing the nonspecificity of the traditionally used diagnostic criteria, the expert panel of the First International Conference on Inflammatory Breast Cancer developed the following guidelines for a more standardized diagnosis of IBC [15].

The following minimum clinical diagnostic criteria are required for the diagnosis of IBC:

- Rapid onset of breast erythema, edema and/or peau d'orange, and/or warm breast with or without an underlying palpable mass.
- History of flattening, crusting, or retraction of the nipple may be present.
- Patients may have a history of being diagnosed with mastitis not responding to at least 1 week of antibiotic administration.
- Duration of no longer than 6 months.
- Clinical examination revealing erythema occupying at least one-third of the breast.

- Clinical examination may reveal underlying palpable mass with or without palpable locoregional lymph nodes with or without nipple abnormalities.
- Pathological confirmation of invasive carcinoma from a core biopsy of the breast.
- Recommendation to obtain adequate skin punch biopsy to possibly document dermal lymphovascular tumor emboli.

Pathological and Molecular Criteria

No pathological diagnostic criteria are available for IBC, although dermal lymphatic involvement is pathognomonic. Patients with IBC typically have ductal tumors with high histological grades. Skin punch biopsies should be a standard requirement in the diagnostic work-up of all clinically suspected cases of IBC [15, 16]. Histopathologically, IBC is characterized by the presence of cancer cells involving and plugging dermal lymphatic vessels of the involved skin, but dermal lymphatic involvement is not a prerequisite for diagnosis (Fig. 19.3). Dermal lymphatic invasion is evident in up to 75 % of IBC patients. There is no correlation between the extent of this invasion and the severity and distribution of the cutaneous manifestations of the disease [10, 17].

No established molecular criteria are available for distinguishing IBC from non-IBC. Molecular subtypes of IBC are similar to molecular subtypes of non-IBC. Compared to other forms of breast cancer; IBC typically exhibits negative ER and PR status and is associated with poor prognosis. Moreover, IBC exhibits increased HER2 overexpression compared with non-IBC cases. Molecular studies demonstrate increased angiogenesis and lymphangiogenesis in IBC based on endothelial cell proliferation fraction assessment. Several markers have been studied, but limited evidence is available regarding the prognostic or predictive role of these markers in IBC. However, p53 mutations and elevated CXCR4/CCR7 receptor expression have been demonstrated in IBC and may reduce the chemotherapeutic response and patient survival [15, 17]. Notch-1, E-cadherin, MUC1, RhoC guanosine triphosphatase (GTPase), and

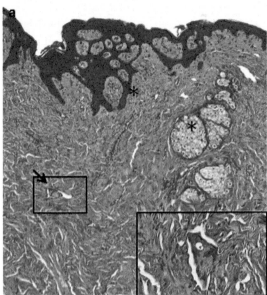
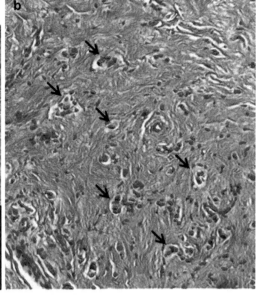

Fig. 19.3 Inflammatory mammary carcinoma, involving dermal lymphatics. (**a**) H&E, 4×: skin surface and adnexa (*epidermis, rete, sebaceous glands) with a tumor embolus within superficial dermal lymphatics (*arrow* and *box/ inset*, H&E 20×). (**b**) H&E, 10×: numerous tumor emboli were present within lymphatics of deep dermis

vascular endothelial growth factor (e.g., VEGF-C, VEGF-D, VEGFR-3, Prox-1, and lymphatic vessel endothelial receptor1) expressions are also increased in IBC tumors compared with non-IBC tumors and have been associated with high histological grade, advanced stage, and poor prognostic outcome [15, 18–22].

Imaging Modalities

Use of suitable imaging methods is important in IBC for the following reasons [10]:

- Identifying a primary breast tumor and facilitating image-guided diagnostic biopsy to enable optimal biomarker evaluation.
- Staging locoregional disease (most authors recommend the use of the AJCC tumor-node-metastasis (TNM) system for staging; IBC is defined as T4d according the TNM system).
- Diagnosing distant metastases and recurrent diseases.
- Evaluating tumor response to neoadjuvant therapy.

Standard breast-imaging techniques, such as mammography and ultrasound, are still frequently used for diagnosis, clinical staging, and therapeutic monitoring of breast cancer. In recent years, magnetic resonance imaging (MRI) and positron emission tomography-computed tomography (PET/CT) have also been used frequently. No specific radiological diagnostic criteria are available.

Mammographic breast abnormalities associated with IBC include masses, global skin thickening, and trabecular distortion [23]. Both skin thickening and trabecular distortion are observed in 80 % of IBC patients. These abnormalities are also associated with mastitis or locally advanced breast cancer. Calcification and focal mass lesions are less commonly observed in IBC compared with non-IBC. Calcification rates vary from 41 to 47 % in different series [23–25].

Ultrasonography is a practical and useful imaging modality in IBC patients. Ultrasound imaging is an important localizing tool for biopsy of underlying masses and nodal involvement. Some authors argue that breast ultrasound imaging is useful in determining the presence of breast

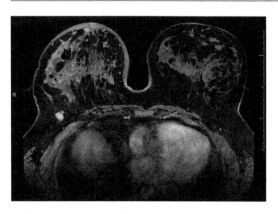

Fig. 19.4 Breast MRI of a patient with right inflammatory breast cancer. Note the large mass-like enhancement and skin thickening on right compared to left. This patient had no palpable breast mass. *Arrow* denotes an abnormal axillary lymph node

parenchymal lesions, which are detected in approximately 95 % of breasts affected with IBC [26]. Common sonographic findings include a singular mass or masses (50 % of patients with a clinical diagnosis of IBC), skin thickening, heterogeneous infiltration of the breast parenchyma, lymphatic dilatation, lymphadenopathy, architectural distortions, and skin and subcutaneous edema [27]. In addition, ultrasonography may affect locoregional therapeutic planning based on initial disease involvement and is useful for evaluating responses to induction chemotherapy.

More advanced imaging techniques, such as MRI and PET/CT, have an evolving role in IBC. MRI T2-weighted images are particularly promising; this technique is more reliable and accurate in distinguishing between IBC, non-IBC, and acute mastitis [28]. In a study of IBC patients at the University of Texas MD Anderson Cancer Center, breast MRI detected 100 % of breast parenchymal lesions, whereas mammography and ultrasound exhibited detection rates of 80 % and 95 %, respectively [23]. MRI is currently recommended for patients with suspected IBC when a breast parenchymal lesion is not identified on mammography or ultrasonography (Fig. 19.4).

All IBC patients should be staged at the time of diagnosis because early distant metastasis is detected in approximately 30 % of patients at

diagnosis. CT of the chest, abdomen, and pelvis along with a bone scan is standard. F18-FDG PET is used as an alternative staging imaging modality in women with locally advanced breast cancer and can be considered in IBC as well [29, 30]. However, the role of PET/CT in IBC diagnoses remains underinvestigated and does not have a defined role [31].

In summary, most authors recommend diagnostic mammogram accompanying ultrasound of the breast and regional lymph nodes as the initial imaging steps for patients with suspected IBC. All patients should be imaged to evaluate distant metastases. MRI and PET/CT have evolving roles in mapping locoregional diseases and documenting distant metastases, but routine use of diagnostic MRI and PET is not recommended [4].

Management of IBC

The management of IBC has changed significantly in recent years, and no standard regimen has been defined for IBC. However, IBC treatment should be multimodal, including systemic therapy, surgery, and radiation. ER/PR status is commonly negative in IBC, and chemotherapy is considered the mainstay systemic treatment [32]. Algorithms for IBC management are summarized in Fig. 19.5.

Primary Systemic Treatment

The widely accepted consensus for the treatment of IBC patients without evidence of distant metastases at the time of diagnosis is systemic chemotherapy followed by surgery and subsequent radiation. An early report from MD Anderson investigators indicated that taxane-based combination chemotherapy was effective as neoadjuvant therapy for IBC [7, 34]. The same group of researchers studied the beneficial effects of adding paclitaxel to fluorouracil, doxorubicin, and cyclophosphamide in a group of 178 IBC patients. The benefits were more obvious in patients with ER-negative disease. Following the combination of these components, taxane-based neoadjuvant

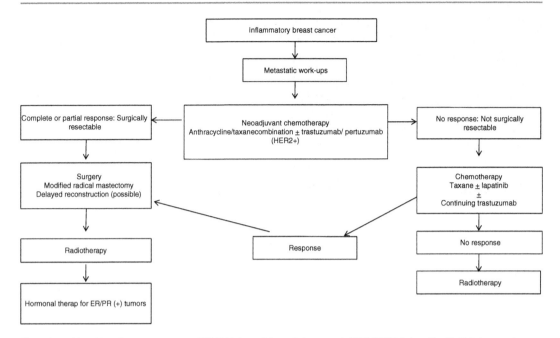

Fig. 19.5 Algorithm for management of IBC (Adapted from Iniesta et al. [32]. If ER (+) and/or PgR (+) tumor)

chemotherapy has improved the prognosis for IBC when combined with an anthracycline. Twenty years of experience (1974–1993) with anthracycline-based chemotherapy in patients with IBC at MD Anderson resulted in an increase in overall survival rates at 5 years to %40 and at ten years to %33. The researchers of this extended study reported the effect of four different multimodal anthracycline-containing protocols for the prognosis of and survival in IBC. Overall clinical response and complete response rates were 72 % and 12 %, respectively. For patients on all four protocols, the median survival was 37 months [35–37]. Two prospective randomized trials involving IBC patients treated with three cycles of either cyclophosphamide, doxorubicin, and 5-fluorouracil or cyclophosphamide, epirubicin, and 5-fluorouracil followed by surgical operation, adjuvant therapy, and radiation therapy reported overall survival rates of 44 % at 5 years and 32 % at 10 years [38].

Several studies have reported a higher incidence of epidermal growth factor receptor 2 (HER2) overexpression in patients with IBC. For patients with HER2-positive disease, trastuzumab and lapatinib therapy (an antibody targeting HER2) may be an option. Anti-HER2 therapy can be administered as a part of neoadjuvant therapy and adjuvant therapy. Women with IBC who receive trastuzumab in addition to chemotherapy exhibit better responses to treatment and survival rates. Several anthracycline-based, anthracycline+taxane-based, trastuzumab-based, lapatinib, and high-dose regimens are preoperatively used in IBC, and their effects on survival are reported in the literature [39–45]. Other targeted therapies, such as those targeting vasculolymphatic pathways (angiogenesis, lymphangiogenesis, and vasculogenesis), RhoC GTPase overexpression, or loss of WISP3, as well as high-dose chemotherapy may be considered for the treatment of IBC in the near future. In the case of hormone receptor-positive patients, tamoxifen or aromatase inhibitor therapy should be started as components of a long-term therapeutic regimen [10, 46].

Locoregional Therapy

Following neoadjuvant chemotherapy (NAC), modified radical mastectomy (MRM) and subsequent radiotherapy are the widely accepted approaches to achieve maximum local control in patients with IBC [47, 48]. A systematic review of studies prior to 1980 of mastectomy alone revealed dismal survival rates of 12 % at 5 years, with a mean survival of 19.8 months and local recurrence rates of approximately 50 % [49]. A review of more recent studies utilizing multimodality therapy indicated improved locoregional recurrence rates of 20 % on average. Other studies of the role of chemotherapy and radiation without mastectomy have reported similar outcomes [35]. However, these studies are small and challenged by other retrospective studies that demonstrate a benefit to adding MRM. The MD Anderson group reported OS and LRR rates of 48 % and 41 %, respectively, for complete multimodal treatment compared with 37 % and 35 %, respectively, for chemotherapy/RT without mastectomy [36]. In the absence of prospective, randomized data, multimodal treatment including MRM should be considered the standard of care. Combined RT and surgery can also provide information regarding the pathological response to NAC. This combination has prognostic significance for both IBC and non-IBC [39]. The aim of the surgery should be to achieve complete resection of residual gross disease with negative margins. The degree of the clinical response of the skin to NAC often underestimates the amount of pathological residual disease, and skin-sparing mastectomy is contraindicated [15]. Axillary lymph node involvement rates are 55–85 % in patients with IBC at the time of presentation [5]. Therefore, complete axillary lymph node dissection is a standard approach for IBC patients. Historically there have been concerns for the accuracy of sentinel lymph node biopsy (SLNB) following neoadjuvant chemotherapy. Although recent data suggests that NAC is not a contraindication to SLNB, this has not been evaluated specifically in IBC patients. In fact, the small numbers of IBC cases included in these studies appear to have higher false-negative rates and higher rates of failed SLNB [49]. SLNB should remain contraindicated in IBC

patients. The timing of reconstruction is controversial. Therefore, delayed breast reconstruction is preferred for IBC patients who request reconstructive surgery.

RT is a crucial component of multimodal therapy approaches. All IBC patients undergoing MRM are recommended for postmastectomy RT. RT fields are planned to target the chest wall and possible undissected axillary lymphatics, including supraclavicular-infraclavicular regions and internal mammary lymph nodes. Different approaches for preoperative and postoperative and/or radical RT series in IBC are presented in the literature [35, 36, 39, 48, 50–56]. Pretreatment imaging, including PET/CT, is extremely useful for correlated pretreatment-posttreatment status. Postmastectomy radiation therapy should be provided to all IBC patients, but questions concerning accelerated hyperfractionated radiation therapy, the role of preoperative radiation therapy, and the effect of concurrent chemoradiation remain to be answered.

Metastatic IBC

Up to 30 % of women with newly diagnosed IBC have metastatic disease at diagnosis compared with 4 % of women with newly diagnosed non-IBC. Metastatic IBC currently follows the same treatment as metastatic non-IBC. At this point, clinical trials should be considered, including phase I trials, if appropriate. Currently, no standard systemic treatment is available for metastatic IBC. No standard approaches are available for locoregional therapy in metastatic IBC patients. Locoregional treatment is challenging, and its effect is limited. It is generally suggested that patients with metastatic IBC should first undergo systemic CT followed by radiation and/or surgery for palliation. No prospective randomized studies have assessed the biological behavior of metastatic IBC. Moreover, the differences in the characteristics of metastatic non-IBC and metastatic IBC are unknown [10, 15].

Follow-Up and Outcome

Following multimodal treatment, physical examinations should be conducted every 3–6 months in combination with yearly mammograms of the contralateral breast. Despite the limited data offered by this procedure, ultrasound of the locoregional lymph nodes may also be considered. However, additional imaging methods and laboratory examinations are not recommended [57].

Again, despite trimodal therapy, IBC remains a fatal and aggressive disease. The expected median survival time for patients with IBC is less than 15 months, with a local recurrence rate of approximately 50 % with surgery and/or RT before the introduction of comprehensive multimodality treatment for IBC. In cases of recurrence, suggested management algorithms for these patient scan can be considered for more RT and CT. Currently, overall survival among women with IBC is less than 48 months [40]. Survival analyses of patients with IBC have yielded conflicting results depending on subtypes, such as "clinical-only," "pathological only," or clinical-pathological IBC. Localization, disease stage, patient age, and response to therapy may influence prognosis. IBC survival is 48.5 % for ER-positive cases and 25.3 % for ER-negative cases according to SEER's comprehensive data from 1988 to 2002 [5]. Given appropriate treatment, disease-free survival in IBC patients ranges from 24 to 49 % at 5 years [1, 8].

References

1. Hance KW, Anderson WF, Devesa SS, Young HA, Levine PH. Trends in inflammatory breast carcinoma incidence and survival: the surveillance, epidemiology, and end results program at the National Cancer Institute. J Natl Cancer Inst. 2005;97:966–75.
2. Taylor GW, Meltzer A. Inflammatory carcinoma of the breast. Am J Cancer. 1938;33:33–49.
3. Bonnier P, Charpin C, Lejeune C, Romain S, Tubiana N, Beedassy B, et al. Inflammatory carcinomas of the breast: a clinical, pathological, or a clinical and pathological definition? Int J Cancer. 1995;62:382–5.
4. Yamauchi H, Woodward WA, Valero V, Alvarez RH, Lucci A, Buchholz TA, et al. Inflammatory breast cancer: what we know and what we need to learn. Oncologist. 2012;17:891–9.
5. Anderson WF, Schairer C, Chen BE, Hance KW, Levine PH. Epidemiology of inflammatory breast cancer (IBC). Breast Dis. 2006;22(1):9–23.
6. Jaiyesimi IA, Buzdar AU, Hortobagyi G. Inflammatory breast cancer: a review. J Clin Oncol. 1992;10:1014–24.
7. Woodward, Wendy A, Cristofanilli M. Inflammatory breast cancer. Semin Radiat Oncol. 2009;19:4. WB Saunders.
8. Chang S, Parker SL, Pham T, Buzdar AU, Hursting SD. Inflammatory breast carcinoma incidence and survival. Cancer. 1998;82(12):2366–72.
9. Wingo PA, Jamison PM, Young JL, Gargiullo P. Population-based statistics for women diagnosed with inflammatory breast cancer (United States). Cancer Causes Control. 2004;15(3):321–8.
10. Robertson FM, Bondy M, Yang W, Yamauchi H, Wiggins S, Kamrudin S, et al. Inflammatory breast cancer: the disease, the biology, the treatment. CA Cancer J Clin. 2010;60(6):351–75.
11. Schairer C, Soliman AS, Omar S, Khaled H, Eissa S, Ayed FB, et al. Assessment of diagnosis of inflammatory breast cancer cases at two cancer centers in Egypt and Tunisia. Cancer Med. 2013;2(2):178–84.
12. Haagensen CD. Diseases of the breast. Philadelphia: WB Saunders; 1971. p. 576–84.
13. Grren F, Page D, Flemming I, Fritz AG, Balch CM, Haller DG, et al. AJCC cancer staging manual, 6th Edition. 2002:221–40.
14. Shenkier T, Weir L, Levine M, Olivotto I, Whelan T, Reyno L, et al. Clinical practice guidelines for the care and treatment of breast cancer. CMJA. 2004;170:983–94.
15. Dawood S, Merajver S D, Viens P, Vermeulen P B, Swain SM, Buchholz T A, et al. International expert panel on inflammatory breast cancer: consensus statement for standardized diagnosis and treatment. Annals Oncol. 2011;22:511–23.
16. Ellis DL, Teitelbaum SL. Inflammatory carcinoma of the breast. A pathologic definition. Cancer. 1974;33(4):1045–7.
17. Boussen H, Bouzaiene H, Ben Hassouna J, Dhiab T, Khomsi F, Benna F, et al. Inflammatory breast cancer in Tunisia. Cancer. 2010;116:2730–5.
18. Overmoyer BA. Inflammatory breast cancer: novel preoperative therapies. Clin Breast Cancer. 2010;10(1):27–32.
19. Dawood S, Broglio K, Gong Y, Yang WT, Cristofanilli M, Kau SW, et al. Prognostic significance of HER-2 status in women with inflammatory breast cancer. Cancer. 2008;112(9):1905–11.
20. Gonzalez Angulo AM, Sneige N, Buzdar AU, Valero V, Kau SW, Broglio K, et al. p53 expression as a prognostic marker in inflammatory breast cancer. Clin Cancer Res. 2004;10(18):6215–21.
21. Gong Y, González Angulo AM, Broglio K, Huo L, Sneige N, Cen P, et al. Expression of Notch-1 and beta-catenin: defining the molecular portrait of inflammatory breast cancer. Breast Cancer Res Treat. 2006;100:299.

22. Kleer CG, Griffith KA, Sabel MS, Gallagher G, van Golen KL, Wu ZF, et al. RhoC-GTPase is a novel tissue biomarker associated with biologically aggressive carcinomas of the breast. Breast Cancer Res Treat. 2005;93(2):101–10.

23. Yang WT, Le-Petross HT, Macapinlac H, Carkaci S, Gonzalez Angulo AM, Dawood S, et al. Inflammatory breast cancer: PET/CT, MRI, mammography, and sonography findings. Breast Cancer Res Treat. 2008; 109(3):417–26.

24. Chow CK. Imaging in inflammatory breast carcinoma. Breast Dis. 2006;22(1):45–54.

25. Gunhan Bilgen I, Ustun EE, Memis A. Inflammatory breast carcinoma: mammographic, ultrasonographic, clinical, and pathologic findings in 142 cases 1. Radiology. 2001;223(3):829–38.

26. Vetto JT. Breast diseases in males. In: Management of breast diseases. Springer: Berlin Heidelberg; 2010; 471–96.

27. Le Petross H, Uppendahl L, Stafford J. Sonographic features of inflammatory breast cancer. Semin Roentgenol. 2011;46:275–9. WB Saunders.

28. Uematsu T. MRI findings of inflammatory breast cancer, locally advanced breast cancer, and acute mastitis: T2-weighted images can increase the specificity of inflammatory breast cancer. Breast Cancer. 2012;19(4):289–94.

29. Danforth Jr DN, Aloj L, Carrasquillo JA, Bacharach SL, Chow C, Zujewski J, et al. The role of 18F-FDG-PET in the local/regional evaluation of women with breast cancer. Breast Cancer Res Treat. 2002;75(2): 135–46.

30. Eubank WB, Mankoff DA. Evolving role of positron emission tomography in breast cancer imaging. Semin Nucl Med. 2005;35:84–99. WB Saunders.

31. Eubank WB, Mankoff DA, Takasugi J, Vesselle H, Eary JF, Shanley TJ, et al. 18fluorodeoxyglucose positron emission tomography to detect mediastinal or internal mammary metastases in breast cancer. J Clin Oncol. 2001;19(15):3516–23.

32. Iniesta MD, Mooney CJ, Merajver SD. Inflammatory breast cancer: what are the treatment options? Expert Opin Pharmacother. 2009;10(18):2987–97.

33. Scotti V, Desideri I, Meattini I, Cataldo VD, Cecchini S, Petrucci A, et al. Management of inflammatory breast cancer: focus on radiotherapy with an evidence-based approach. Cancer Treat Rev. 2013;39(2): 119–24.

34. Cristofanilli M, Buzdar AU, Sneige N, Smith T, Wasaff B, Ibrahim N, et al. Paclitaxel in the multimodality treatment for inflammatory breast carcinoma. Cancer. 2001;92(7):1775–82.

35. Ueno NT, Buzdar AU, Singletary SE, Ames FC, McNeese MD, Holmes FA, et al. Combined-modality treatment of inflammatory breast carcinoma: twenty years of experience at MD Anderson Cancer Center. Cancer Chemother Pharmacol. 1997;40(4):321–9.

36. Koh EH, Buzdar AU, Ames FC, Singletary SE, McNeese MD, Frye D, et al. Inflammatory carcinoma of the breast: results of a combined-modality approach—MD Anderson Cancer Center experience. Cancer Chemother Pharmacol. 1990;27(2):94–100.

37. Buzdar AU, Singletary SE, Booser DJ, Frye DK, Wasaff B, Hortobagyi GN. Combined modality treatment of stage III and inflammatory breast cancer. MD Anderson Cancer Center experience. Surg Oncol Clin N Am. 1995;4(4):715–34.

38. Baldini E, Gardin G, Evangelista G, Prochilo T, Collecchi P, Lionetto R. Long-term results of combined-modality therapy for inflammatory breast carcinoma. Clin Breast Cancer. 2004;5(5):358–63.

39. Harris EE, Schultz D, Bertsch H, Fox K, Glick J, Solin LJ. Ten-year outcome after combined modality therapy for inflammatory breast cancer. Int J Radiat Oncol Biol Phys. 2003;55(5):1200–8.

40. Low JA, Berman AW, Steinberg SM, Danforth DN, Lippman ME, Swain SM. Long-term follow-up for locally advanced and inflammatory breast cancer patients treated with multimodality therapy. J Clin Oncol. 2004;22(20):4067–74.

41. Van Pelt AE, Mohsin S, Elledge RM, Hilsenbeck SG, Gutierrez M, Lucci Jr A, et al. Neoadjuvant trastuzumab and docetaxel in patients with breast cancer: preliminary results. Clin Breast Cancer. 2003;4(5):348–53.

42. Burstein HJ, Harris LN, Gelman R, Lester SC, Nunes RA, Kaelin CM, et al. Preoperative therapy with trastuzumab and paclitaxel followed hy sequential adjuvant doxorubicin/cyclophosphamide for HER2 overexpressing stage II or III breast cancer: a pilot study. J Clin Oncol. 2003;21(1):46–53.

43. Gianni L, Eiermann W, Semiglazov V, Manikhas A, Lluch A, Tjulandin S, et al. Neoadjuvant chemotherapy with trastuzumab followed by adjuvant trastuzumab versus neoadjuvant chemotherapy alone, in patients with HER2-positive locally advanced breast cancer (the NOAH trial): a randomised controlled superiority trial with a parallel HER2-negative cohort. Lancet. 2010;375:377–84.

44. Conti F, Carpano S, Sergi D, Di Lauro L, Amodio A, Vici P, et al. High-dose CEF (cyclophosphamide, epirubicin, fluorouracil) as primary chemotherapy in locally advanced breast cancer: long-term results. La Clinicaterapeutica. 2006;158(4):331–41.

45. Viens P, Palangie T, Janvier M, Fabbro M, Roche H, Delozier T, et al. First-line high-dose sequential chemotherapy with rG-CSF and repeated blood stem cell transplantation in untreated inflammatory breast cancer: toxicity and response (PEGASE 02 trial). Br J Cancer. 1999;81(3):449.

46. Specht J, Gralow JR. Neoadjuvant chemotherapy for locally advanced breast cancer. Semin Radiat Oncol. 2009;19:222–8. WB Saunders.

47. Perez CA, Graham ML, Taylor ME, Levy JF, Mortimer JE, Philpott GW, et al. Management of locally advanced carcinoma of the breast I. Noninflammatory. Cancer. 1994;74:453–65.

48. Panades M, Olivotto IA, Speers CH, Shenkier T, Olivotto TA, Weir L, et al. Evolving treatment strategies for inflammatory breast cancer: a population-based survival analysis. J Clin Oncol. 2005;23(9):1941–50.

49. Kell R, Morrow M. Surgical aspects of inflammatory breast cancer. Breast Dis. 2005;22:67–73.

50. Stearns V, Ewing CA, Slack R, Penannen MF, Hayes DF, Tsangaris TN. Sentinel lymphadenectomy after neoadjuvant chemotherapy for breast cancer may reliably represent the axilla except for inflammatory breast cancer. Ann Surg Oncol. 2002;9(3):235–42.

51. Pisansky TM, Schaid DJ, Loprinzi CL, Donohue JH, Schray MF, Schomberg PJ. Inflammatory breast cancer: integration of irradiation, surgery, and chemotherapy. Am J Clin Oncol. 1992;15(5):376–98.

52. Thomas F, Arriagada R, Spielmann M, Mouriesse H, Chevalier TL, Fontaine F, Tursz T. Pattern of failure in patients with inflammatory breast cancer treated by alternating radiotherapy and chemotherapy. Cancer. 1995;76(11):2286–90.

53. Fleming RD, Asmar L, Buzdar AU, McNeese MD, Ames FC, Ross MI, et al. Effectiveness of mastectomy by response to induction chemotherapy for control in inflammatory breast carcinoma. Ann Surg Oncol. 1997;4(6):452–61.

54. Abrous Anane S, Savignoni A, Daveau C, Pierga JY, Gautier C, Reyal F, et al. Management of inflammatory breast cancer after neoadjuvant chemotherapy. Int J Radiat Oncol Biol Phys. 2011;79(4):1055–63.

55. Bristol IJ, Woodward WA, Strom EA, Cristofanilli M, Domain D, Singletary SE, et al. Locoregional treatment outcomes after multimodality management of inflammatory breast cancer. Int J Radiat Oncol Biol Phys. 2008;72(2):474–84.

56. Damast S, Ho AY, Montgomery L, Fornier MN, Ishill N, Elkin E, et al. Locoregional outcomes of inflammatory breast cancer patients treated with standard fractionation radiation and daily skin bolus in the taxane era. Int J Radiat Oncol Biol Phys. 2010;77(4): 1105–12.

57. Khatcheressian JL, Wolff AC, Smith TJ, Grunfeld E, Muss HB, Vogel VG, et al. American Society of Clinical Oncology 2006 update of the breast cancer follow-up and management guidelines in the adjuvant setting. J Clin Oncol. 2006;24(31):5091–7.

Part IV

Special Therapeutic Problems

Occult Primary Breast Cancer with Axillary Metastases

20

Lejla Hadzikadic Gusic and Ronald Johnson

Abstract

Occult primary cancer is defined as the presence of metastatic cancer with an undetectable primary at the time of presentation. Occult breast cancer remains controversial. The low incidence of this cancer precludes prospective trials, and thus evidence-based conclusions must be based on retrospective data.

Keywords

Occult primary cancer • DCIS • Sentinel lymph node • SLN

Introduction

In 2011, an estimated 31,000 cases of occult primary tumors were diagnosed in the United States, comprising 2 % of all cancers diagnosed in the United States. Deaths from cancer of unknown primary were estimated to be 45,900 in 2012. Occult primary cancer is defined as the presence of metastatic cancer with an undetectable primary at the time of presentation. This chapter focuses specifically on occult primary breast cancer presenting with axillary metastases, a rare form of breast cancer with an incidence of 0.3–1 % across the literature [1–8]. A positive family history has been observed in 20–30 % of patients with an axillary presentation of occult breast cancer [2, 9]. First described by Halsted in 1907, this disease process continues to be described in the literature [2, 9]. In 1909, Cameron recommended ipsilateral mastectomy for occult breast carcinoma presenting with axillary metastases, and this remained the standard of care for some time [2, 10]. However, treatment has changed drastically over time in parallel with

L.H. Gusic, MD, MSc (✉)
Division of Surgical Oncology, Department of Surgery, Levine Cancer Institute, Carolinas Medical Center, Charlotte, NC, USA

Department of Surgery, Carolinas Medical Center, Charlotte, NC, USA

Magee-Womens Hospital, UPMC, Pittsburgh, PA, USA
e-mail: hoyalh@gmail.com

R. Johnson, MD, FACS
Division of Surgical Oncology, Department of Surgery, Magee-Womens Hospital, UPMC, Pittsburgh, PA, USA
e-mail: rjohnson@upmc.edu

© Springer International Publishing Switzerland 2016
A. Aydiner et al. (eds.), *Breast Disease: Management and Therapies*,
DOI 10.1007/978-3-319-26012-9_20

advancements in the management of primary breast cancer. This chapter examines the clinical presentation, evaluation, and management of occult primary breast cancer with axillary metastases.

Clinical Presentation

The peak incidence of occult breast cancer is in postmenopausal females (age 50–55), as observed in multiple retrospective studies [1–16]. A patient will typically present to a primary care physician with isolated axillary lymphadenopathy without other physical complaints. Although cancer is in the differential diagnosis, all sources of possible axillary lymphadenopathy must be considered. The differential diagnosis includes disease processes of benign and malignant etiology, including inflammatory processes, hidradenitis, lymphoma, metastatic melanoma, or metastases from the thyroid, pancreas, stomach, colon/rectum, and lung (all references). Another source to consider in the axilla is cancer in the axillary tail or in ectopic breast tissue within a lymph node [2]. An astute primary care physician is critical in the diagnosis of this disease. If the initial workup is not complete, the diagnosis can easily be missed, thus allowing the disease process to continue silently until a more classic or ominous presentation presents, with a timeline from months to years.

Many breast surgeons contribute to the education of their local communities about breast cancer by providing various presentations to both the medical community and the general public. Particularly in presentations to the medical community, it is important to include the rare presentation of occult breast cancer presenting as axillary metastases and to thoroughly review the workup required to ensure that this diagnosis has been considered and investigated.

Initial Evaluation

When a patient presents with isolated axillary lymphadenopathy, a complete history should be obtained that includes a thorough review of risk factors for breast cancer by inquiring about the patient's history of childbearing, start and end of menses, and any past use of hormone therapy. Past breast biopsies should be reviewed, as should any pathology, inquiries about any nipple discharge or eversion, or masses palpated by the patient. Perhaps most importantly, a thorough family history of cancer should be evaluated, focusing on breast and gynecological malignancies. It is important to ask if there is a paucity of women in the family on either the maternal or paternal side, as this may complicate the discernment of a familial pattern and should not be overlooked. Once the history has been completed, a complete physical exam should be performed, focusing on a thorough breast exam with the patient in sitting and supine positions and with arms placed at the side as well as overhead. The head and neck nodes and both axillae should be carefully examined. Once a complete history and physical exam have been conducted, a search for the primary disease should begin after a differential diagnosis has been formulated. Once other disease processes have been ruled out and breast cancer has become a concern, the search for a breast primary cancer must proceed in a logical manner. NCCN guidelines suggest starting with a mammogram and/or breast ultrasound for women and/or a CT of the neck, chest, abdomen, and pelvis for either men or women. Mammograms can detect a primary lesion in 7–29 % of clinically false-negative cases [9, 14]. If these examinations are negative, proceeding with an MRI is the next step in the current NCCN guidelines. If presented with imaging from an outside institution, the physician and the physician's radiology department should thoroughly review the images to confirm the findings and determine if the imaging is adequate in quality and extent. Pathology from an outside institution should also be reviewed thoroughly. When available, fine needle aspiration (FNA) or core needle biopsy (CNBx) of the isolated axillary lymph node must be reviewed to confirm the diagnosis. Specifically, the sampled material should be evaluated for cytokeratins, specifically CK7+20− (90 % of breast cancers have this cytokeratin/keratin distribution) and immunohistochemical markers such as GCDFP-15 and mammaglobin, ER/PR, and MABm4G3 [11]. However, only 50–60 % of breast cancers are ER/PR positive; thus, a negative result does not rule out breast cancer [3, 9, 15]. Generic assessments such as CBC, liver function tests, and alkaline phosphatase, with inclusion of cancer markers such as CEA, should also be performed [11]. A proposed pathway for workup is presented in Fig. 20.1.

Imaging

As stated above, diagnostic mammography should be the first attempt to identify the location of a primary breast tumor. There can be significant variation between the quality of mammography and additional views; thus, the clinician must ensure that high-quality diagnostic mammography is performed. Ultrasound should be used as an adjunct to mammography to search for masses. If these modalities fail to find a primary lesion, the NCCN guidelines suggest that a bilateral MRI be performed. MRI is able to identify the primary tumor in 75–86 % of mammographically negative patients [7, 8, 14, 15]. MRI has a reported sensitivity of 88–100 % for detecting breast masses. The specificity, however, is much lower, with some reports indicating values as low as 35 % [14]. In one study, among patients with a negative MRI, tumors were identified in pathology specimens from mastectomy in two of eight patients (25 %) [15]. Additional studies are indicated only if signs or symptoms suggest additional disease. For example, a bone scan is indicated if a patient describes localized bone pain or if alkaline phosphatase levels are elevated. Abdominal and pelvic CT scans are indicated if there are elevated liver function test values, if the patient exhibits abdominal symptoms, or if the physical exam of the abdomen or pelvis is abnormal. Chest CT is indicated if the patient presents with pulmonary symptoms. PET has been used experimentally to detect breast disease but has not yet been endorsed for routine use in this scenario [2, 11].

NCCN Guidelines for the Treatment of Occult Primary Breast Cancer

Due to the low incidence of this disease presentation, only a few small retrospective studies are available for review. Regardless of when these studies were conducted, they present a similar picture of how a patient may present and how the management has changed over time. There are no prospective trials on this topic, and a prospective

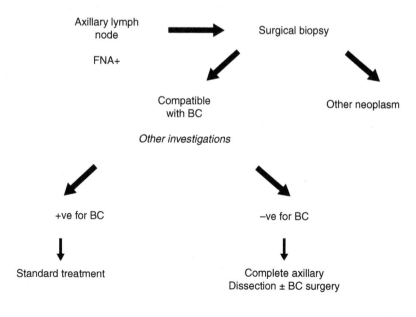

Fig. 20.1 Proposed guidelines for the workup of patients presenting with axillary disease (Galimberti et al. [2])

trial will likely never be conducted given the low incidence of occult primary breast cancer. We thus rely on these retrospective studies, which were taken into account when establishing the NCCN guidelines, to provide options for the treatment of this disease.

According to the NCCN guidelines, after a comprehensive workup has been performed and a primary breast cancer has been identified, treatment should be performed according to the clinical stage of the breast cancer. However, if the workup determines no primary breast cancer, there are specific guidelines for men and for women. A patient without an identified primary breast cancer but with an isolated axillary lymph node proven to be of breast origin is designated as T0N1M0-T0N2M0 or stage II/III [13]. Therefore, the NCCN guidelines for stage II/III breast cancer are followed for locoregional treatment. For men, the guidelines state that an axillary lymph node dissection (ALND) should be performed; following this, radiotherapy and chemotherapy should be administered if clinically indicated. For women, the guidelines state that for those with MRI-negative disease, treatment should be based on nodal status. For patients with T0N1M0 disease, the options include traditional mastectomy and ALND with or without postmastectomy radiation or axillary nodal dissection followed by whole-breast irradiation with or without nodal irradiation. Systemic chemotherapy, endocrine therapy, or anti-HER2 therapy should be administered according to the pathological status of the disease. Patients who present with T0N2M0-T0N3M0 disease should be considered for neoadjuvant chemotherapy and/or neoadjuvant anti-HER2 therapy and endocrine therapy, followed by axillary nodal dissection and mastectomy [11].

Literature Review

As mentioned above, the standard treatment of occult breast disease presenting as axillary metastases has historically been total mastectomy and ALND. This technique has traditionally yielded occult cancer in approximately two-thirds of

patients. However, pathological evaluation of the removed breast fails to show carcinoma in one-third of these patients, suggesting that the surgery was unnecessary [9]. If locoregional treatment of the axilla and breast are separated, several options exist. Here, we examine select retrospective studies to review the data. For the axilla, we can consider radiation vs. ALND, although most retrospective series included ALND unless the patients refused surgical treatment [1, 2, 7–10, 12–16].

For locoregional treatment of the breast, we consider mastectomy vs. whole-breast radiotherapy vs. segmental mastectomy vs. observation. The Memorial Sloan-Kettering Cancer Center series demonstrated that 45 % of the identified occult cancers were multifocal, suggesting that partial mastectomy of suspicious areas on mammogram or MRI might miss additional disease [9]. When the ipsilateral breast is left untreated in occult breast cancer following ALND, clinical disease in the ipsilateral breast develops in approximately 40 % of patients [12]. Therefore, it is prudent to consider some form of treatment to the ipsilateral breast, despite the absence of a definite primary. Baron et al. observed no 5-year survival benefit of mastectomy vs. breast preservation. They suggested that omitting mastectomy in the treatment of occult breast cancer is a valid option and that salvage mastectomy should be reserved for recurrences if the breast received prior whole-breast radiation [9]. To evaluate the role of ipsilateral breast radiotherapy, Barton et al. and Masinghe et al. compared outcome data for patients with occult primary breast cancer presenting with axillary metastases treated with breast preservation and radiotherapy vs. observation. Patients who had radiotherapy to the preserved breast exhibited superior 5-year local recurrence-free survival (84 % vs. 34 %, $p < 0.001$) and relapse-free survival (64 % vs. 34 %, $p = 0.05$). Barton et al. also observed no difference in overall survival (Figs. 20.2 and 20.3) [12]. Barton et al. did not observe a difference in 5-year local recurrence-free survival between the traditional dose of 50 Gy in 25 fractions and doses >60 Gy, suggesting that additional doses are not necessary (Fig. 20.4) [12].

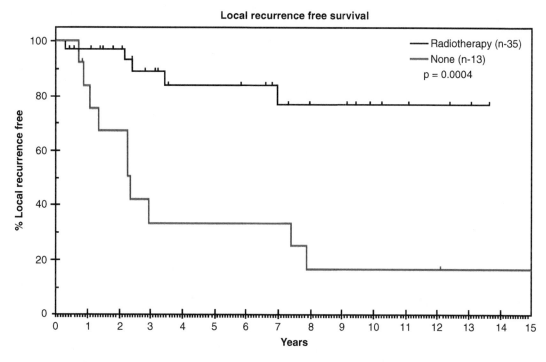

Fig. 20.2 Local recurrence-free survival according to whether the patient was treated with ipsilateral breast radiotherapy (IBR) (Barton et al. [12])

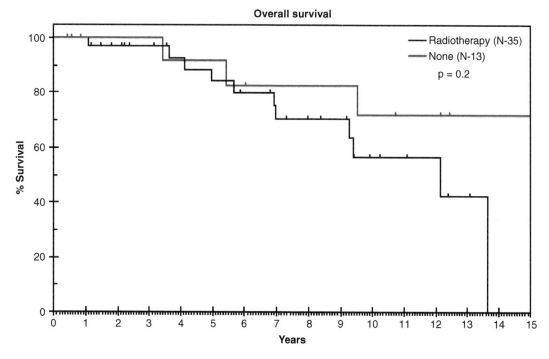

Fig. 20.3 Overall survival according to whether the patient was treated with ipsilateral breast radiotherapy (IBR) (Barton et al. [12])

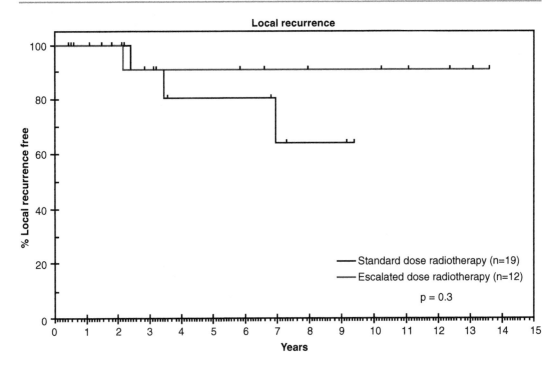

Fig. 20.4 Local recurrence-free survival according to whether the patient was treated with escalated/high-dose radiotherapy to the ipsilateral breast (60/30 or 50/25 with boost) or with a standard dose (50/25 or 40/15) (Barton et al. [12])

In a series at MD Anderson, no difference in survival was observed between patients whose breast was preserved compared to those who underwent mastectomy, indicating that local therapy to the breast in occult breast cancer need not necessarily include removal of the breast [1]. This sentiment was echoed by Galimberti et al. [2]. Merson et al. actually observed no difference in survival between whole-breast radiation or breast surgery compared to observation only and agree that less treatment to the breast is better than more [4]. They also noted that the primary tumor distribution observed no pathological sectioning and was no different from the distribution in common cases of primary breast cancer (Table 20.1), with ductal invasive histology as the predominant type.

Wang et al. demonstrated that patients who underwent mastectomy had better disease-free survival and overall survival compared with those who had no local therapy to the breast. Their series, however, did not include a group with other local therapies to the breast [16].

Table 20.1 Histological review: the distribution of cancers according to the site within the breast (among 37 patients in whom a tumor was identified)

Site	Number of patients
Upper outer quadrant	20
Lower outer quadrant	3
Upper inner quadrant	2
Lower inner quadrant	3
Central quadrant	2
Multicentricity	4
Total	34[a]

Merson et al. [4]

[a]Three cases: no information on the exact site

Another MD Anderson series used SEER data from 1983 to 2006 to perform a population-based analysis of T0N1M0 breast cancer. This study included four groups: observation (i.e., no treatment), ALND only, TM + ALND plus or minus postmastectomy radiotherapy (PMRT), and breast conservation therapy with ALND and XRT. Patients who underwent definitive locoregional treatment with either mastectomy or breast conservation therapy with ALND and XRT to the breast had significantly increased 10-year overall survival compared with patients who underwent ALND only or observation (65 % compared with 59 % and 48 %, respectively). There was no difference in the 10-year cause-specific survival for breast conservation therapy with ALND and XRT compared to mastectomy (Figs. 20.5 and 20.6). Multivariate analysis revealed that ER-negative tumors, >10 positive lymph nodes, and <10 resected lymph nodes were correlated with an unfavorable outcome. This population-based SEER analysis included 750 patients, making it the largest study to date, and supports the conclusions of smaller retrospective studies that locoregional treatment of occult breast disease does not necessarily include mastectomy. This series, published in 2010, also confirmed that in recent years the trend for treatment has favored whole-breast radiation without mastectomy [15].

Khandelwal and Garguilo conducted a survey of the American Society of Breast Surgeons (ASBS) of surgeons' preferences for management of the breast in occult primary breast cancer presenting with axillary metastasis. With a response rate of 42 %, they observed that despite recent literature supporting the use of whole-breast radiation, 43 % of responders preferred mastectomy, whereas 37 % opted for whole-breast radiation [14]. This suggests that the correct treatment of this rare form of breast cancer remains controversial in the surgical community.

Even more disputed is modern breast conservation therapy, i.e., partial mastectomy or quadrantectomy, in the setting of occult primary breast cancer, suggesting that resection may be performed based on an abnormality deemed suspicious on imaging despite negative pathological analysis by biopsy. Several of these retrospective studies have included patients who received a partial mastectomy or quadrantectomy as their surgical treatment, although these patients and those who received mastectomy were not compared directly [2, 4, 9].

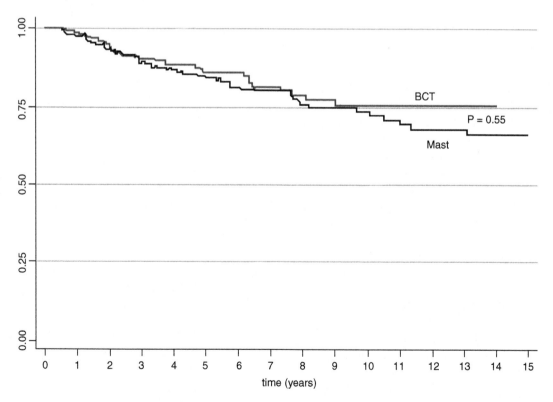

Fig. 20.5 Kaplan-Meier curve for cause-specific survival for patients who underwent breast-conserving therapy (BCT; *red line*) and patients who underwent mastectomy (Mast; *blue line*) (Walker et al. [15])

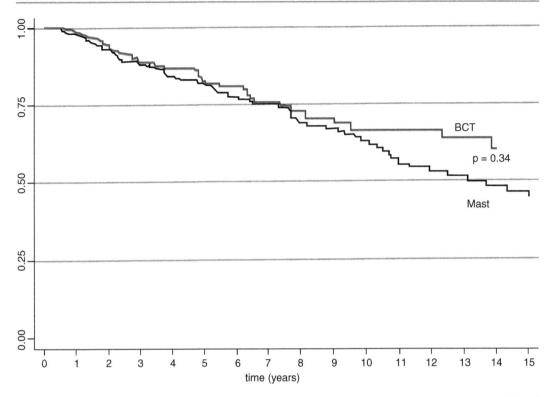

Fig. 20.6 Kaplan-Meier curve for overall survival for patients who underwent breast-conserving therapy (BCT; *red line*) and patients who underwent mastectomy (Mast; *blue line*) (Walker et al. [15])

Although mostly comprised of small retrospective studies, the data available to us suggest no survival benefit or locoregional control benefit of mastectomy compared to whole-breast irradiation with breast preservation. Due to the low incidence of this disease, there will not likely be any future prospective study on this topic; thus, we are left to interpret the currently available data. Given this information and the cosmetic advantage of breast preservation, whole-breast irradiation has become the treatment of choice [9, 12, 14].

Adjuvant Systemic Therapy

In their series, Baron et al. demonstrated that there was no statistically significant survival benefit for those patients who received adjuvant chemotherapy compared to those who did not, with 5-year survival rates of 79 % vs. 77 % (Fig. 20.7). They note, however, that this result suggests a benefit of adjuvant therapy because patients with positive nodes should have had decreased survival [9]. Ellerbroek et al. also reported no survival benefit of chemotherapy but did note a trend in favor of chemotherapy, concluding that all patients should be treated according to the same guidelines matched stage for stage as patients with a known breast primary [1]. Most other studies, as well as NCCN guidelines, recommend adjuvant chemotherapy and hormone therapy when appropriate, similar to the guidelines for staged disease of a known primary breast cancer. The current NCCN guidelines also endorse neoadjuvant chemotherapy for N2 disease [11].

Survival Data and Prognosis

As noted in the above series, no difference in survival has been demonstrated for mastectomy vs. whole-breast radiotherapy for definitive

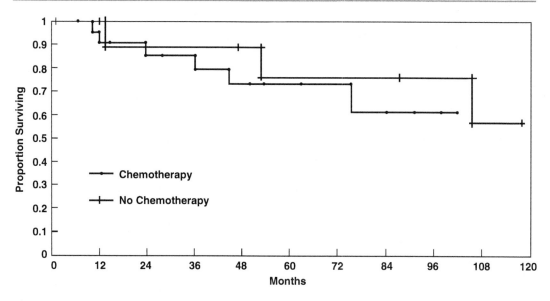

Fig. 20.7 Overall survival based on whether adjuvant systemic therapy was administered (Baron et al. [9])

locoregional treatment of the breast in occult primary breast cancer. Less radical treatment appears to correlate well with the reported better prognosis of this presentation of breast cancer compared to matched stage II/III cancer with a breast primary [2, 4]. Some studies have also reported worse and equivalent survival among matched groups, but the overall trend is toward an improved prognosis. However, there has been some evidence of improved disease-free and overall survival in certain circumstances and treatment options. This section examines these data.

Baron et al. reported that patients who underwent an ALND following a positive lymph node biopsy had the same 5- and 10-year survival rates, both 80 %, if all subsequent nodes were negative, compared with rates of 72 % and 43 %, respectively, if at least one other node was positive on the final pathological examination [9]. Ellerbroek et al. also noted that local control and survival were improved at 5 years for N1 compared with N2 disease [1, 4, 5, 14, 16]. Baron et al. also noted that 5- and 10-year survival did not significantly differ for patients in whom the primary breast cancer was found on final pathological examination compared to those in whom it was not discovered. They also demonstrated decreased 5- and 10-year

survival for patients who were ER negative compared with those who were ER positive [9].

Montagna et al. specifically compared 80 patients with occult primary breast cancer to 80 patients with early-stage breast cancer. The groups were matched for age, nodal status, and biological features, and immunohistochemical differences, and outcomes were compared. No significant differences in disease-free survival (DFS: 66 vs. 68 %) and overall survival (OS: 80 and 86 %) were observed between the two groups; however, the findings did add to the existing literature indicating a worse prognosis for occult breast cancer with more than four involved lymph nodes and triple-negative tumors [5].

Ductal Carcinoma In Situ (DCIS)

Interestingly, the reported rate of axillary lymph node metastases among patients with DCIS is 1–2 % in the literature. By definition, DCIS is an in situ disease and cannot metastasize, but there have been reports of its metastasis in the literature [2, 16]. The significance of these findings remains unclear; however, this phenomenon is another indication that we do not yet fully understand the mechanism of this disease and the tumor/host relationship.

Looking Forward: What Does the Future Hold?

This rare occurrence of breast cancer remains controversial. The low incidence of this cancer precludes prospective trials; thus, we must rely on retrospective data to make evidence-based conclusions.

The treatment of occult breast cancer with axillary presentation is a particularly interesting topic in light of the recent trend of less invasive axillary treatment. The recent findings of ACOSOG Z11, which suggested that complete axillary dissection is not necessary in postmenopausal women with hormone receptor-positive disease treated with breast conservation therapy, including lumpectomy and whole-breast irradiation, with findings of limited disease in the axilla after a sentinel lymph node biopsy [17]. In the specific population of women studied, who had limited nodal disease and were treated with breast conservation therapy, a completion axillary nodal dissection did not improve survival. With careful patient selection, this has greatly affected current therapy and will likely continue to do so.

Similarly, the findings of ACOSOG Z1071 suggest that in women with biopsy-proven node-positive disease, a negative sentinel lymph node biopsy may be sufficient axillary treatment after neoadjuvant chemotherapy [18]. The examination of two or more sentinel nodes had a false-negative rate of 12.6 % among women with residual N1 nodal disease, based on the completion of ALND. The false-negative rate decreased to 9.0 % when at least three sentinel lymph nodes were removed, which has significant implications for women presenting with nodal disease who will undergo neoadjuvant therapy. The literature suggests that 34–40 % of node-positive women convert to node-negative status following systemic therapy. Recent data suggest that in this cohort of women, ALND is not indicated, which would prevent a significant number of women from experiencing complications such as lymphedema.

As treatments for the staging and treatment of the axilla in breast cancer develop, it will be interesting to observe how these developments affect the treatment of occult primary breast cancer presenting with axillary metastases.

References

1. Ellerbroek N, Holmes F, Singletary E, Evans H, Oswald M, McNeese M. Treatment of patients with isolated axillary nodal metastases from an occult primary carcinoma consistent with breast origin. Cancer. 1990;66:1461–7.
2. Galimberti V, Bassani G, Monti S, Simsek S, Villa G, Renne G, Luini A. Clinical experience with axillary presentation breast cancer. Breast Cancer Res Treat. 2004;88:43–7.
3. Masinghe SP, Faluyi OO, Kerr GR, Kunkler IH. Breast radiotherapy for occult breast cancer with axillary nodal metastases-does it reduce the local recurrence rate and increase overall survival? Clin Oncol. 2011;23:95–100.
4. Merson M, Andreola S, Galimberti V, Bufalino R, Marchini S, Veronesi U. Breast carcinoma presenting as axillary metastases without evidence of a primary tumor. Cancer. 1992;70(2):504–8.
5. Montagna E, Bagnardi V, Rotmensz N, Viale G, Cancello G, Mazza M, et al. Immunohistochemically defined subtypes and outcome in Occult Breast Carcinoma with axillary presentation. Breast Cancer Res Treat. 2011;129:867–75.
6. Surveillance Epidemiology and End Results (SEER) Database. Available at http://seer.cancer.gov/statistics/.
7. Siegel R, Naishadham D, Jemal A. Cancer statistics. Cancer J Clin. 2012;62:10–29.
8. Varadarajan R, Edge SB, Yu J, et al. Prognosis of occult breast carcinoma presenting as isolated axillary nodal metastasis. Oncology. 2006;71:456–9.
9. Baron PL, Moore MP, Kinne DW, Candela FC, Osborne MP, Petrek JA. Occult breast cancer presenting with axillary metastases. Arch Surg. 1990;125:210–4.
10. Cameron HC. Some clinical facts regarding mammary cancer. B Med J. 1909;I:577–82.
11. National Comprehensive Cancer Network (NCCN). NCCN Clinical Practice Guidelines in Oncology. Breast Cancer. v2.2015. Available at http://www.nccn.org.
12. Barton SR, Smith IE, Kirby AM, Ashley S, Walsh G, Parton M. The role of ipsilateral breast radiotherapy in management of occult primary breast cancer presenting as axillary lymphadenopathy. Eur J Cancer. 2011;47:2099–106.

13. Green FL, Page DL, Fleming ID, Fritz A, Balch CM, Haller DG, et al. American joint committee on cancer: cancer staging handbook. 6th ed. New York: Springer; 2002. p. 255–81.

14. Khandelwal AK, Garguilo GA. Therapeutic options for occult breast cancer: a survey of the American Society of Breast Surgeons and Review of the Literature. Am J Surg. 2005;190:609–13.

15. Walker GV, Smith GL, Perkins GH, Oh JL, Woodward W, Yu TK, et al. Population-based analysis of occult primary breast cancer with axillary lymph node metastasis. Cancer. 2010;116:4000–6.

16. Wang X, Zhao Y, Cao X. Clinical benefits of mastectomy on treatment of occult breast carcinoma presenting axillary metastases. Breast J. 2010;16(1):32–7.

17. Giuliano AE, McCall L, Beitsch P, Whitworth PW, Blumencranz P, Leitch AM, et al. Locoregional recurrence after sentinel lymph node dissection with or without axillary dissection in patients with sentinel lymph node metastases: the American College of Surgeons Oncology Group Z0011 randomized trial. Ann Surg. 2010;252(3):426–32.

18. Boughey JC, Suman VJ, Mittendorf EA, Ahrendt GM, Wilke LG, Taback B, et al. Alliance for Clinical Trials in Oncology. Sentinel lymph node surgery after neoadjuvant chemotherapy in patients with node-positive breast cancer: the ACOSOG Z1071 (Alliance) clinical trial. JAMA. 2013;310(14):1455–61.

Breast Cancer in Older Women

Denise Monahan and Nora Hansen

Abstract

Breast cancer risk increases with age and as life expectancy continues to increase; therefore, breast cancer in older women has become a significant public health concern. The basic principles of imaging, diagnosis, and treatment remain standard for all women with breast cancer. However, in the elderly population, comorbid conditions, life expectancy, and quality of life take on particular importance for the clinician to consider and balance with treatment decisions. Historically, older women have been poorly represented in breast cancer trials, and their surgical and adjuvant treatment often differs from that of younger women. More information is needed regarding the impact of breast cancer and its treatment on the growing population of older women with breast cancer. In this chapter, the role of screening, diagnosis, and treatment of breast cancer in older women and some of the special considerations relevant to this population of patients will be reviewed.

Keywords

Older women • Screening mammography • Diagnosis • Treatment • Endocrine therapy

Introduction

Worldwide, breast cancer is the most frequently diagnosed cancer. According to data from GLOBOCAN, breast cancer is the leading cause of cancer death in women in less developed countries and is the second leading cause of cancer death in more developed countries [1]. In 2001–2012, breast cancer accounted for 25 % (1.67 million) of all new cancer cases and

D. Monahan, MD (✉)
Department of Surgery, John H. Stroger, Jr. Hospital of Cook County and Rush University Medical Center, Chicago, IL, USA
e-mail: dmona12@gmail.com

N. Hansen, MD
Department of Surgery, Feinberg School of Medicine, Northwestern University, Chicago, IL, USA
e-mail: nhansen@nm.org

© Springer International Publishing Switzerland 2016
A. Aydiner et al. (eds.), *Breast Disease: Management and Therapies*,
DOI 10.1007/978-3-319-26012-9_21

14 % (458,400) of all cancer deaths [1, 2]. Data from 18 countries for 1993–1997 were evaluated, revealing that the United States, Switzerland, Israel, Denmark, and Australia had the highest incidence of age-adjusted breast cancer and that Asian countries had the lowest incidence [3].

The probability of developing breast cancer is positively correlated with increasing age. Greenlee et al. reported that in the United States, the probability of developing invasive breast cancer is 0.43 % (1 in 235) in women younger than 39 years, 4.06 % (1 in 25) in women aged 40–59 years, and 6.88 % (1 in 15) in women aged 60–79 years. The overall lifetime risk was calculated to be 12.56 % (1 in 8) [4].

Based on the Surveillance Epidemiology and End Results (SEER) data, it is estimated that 232,340 new breast cancer cases were diagnosed in the United States in 2013 and that 39,620 deaths occurred due to breast cancer. Using the SEER data for 2005–2009, the median age of women diagnosed with breast cancer is 61 years, and 41 % of women with breast cancer are diagnosed after the age of 65 (Fig. 21.1). Specifically, 21 % are between the ages of 65 and 74, 15 % are between the ages of 75 and 84, and 6 % are 85 or older [5]. Thus, approximately 100,000 women aged 65 or older will be diagnosed with breast cancer each year in the United States alone.

Screening

Several randomized trials have demonstrated mortality reduction from regular screening mammograms [6–11]. Only some of these studies included older women, and the available information that includes women aged 70 or older is therefore limited [12]. The Swedish Two-County Trial included women aged 40–74 and revealed a significant reduction in breast cancer mortality in women who underwent screening mammography [13]. The Malmo trial included women aged 45–69 years at the start of the trial and concluded that women older than 55 had a 20 % reduction in mortality from breast cancer [10].

Countries around the world have developed guidelines regarding the age at which to start mammographic screening and the frequency of screening. For instance, the American Cancer Society Guidelines for the Early Detection of Cancer recommends an annual screening mammogram for women at average risk beginning at the age of 40, with annual screening continuing as long as a woman is in good health [14]. According to the Canadian Task Force on Preventive Healthcare, women aged 40–49 at average risk are not recommended to undergo routine screening, and those aged 50–74 are recommended to undergo routine screening every 2–3 years [15].

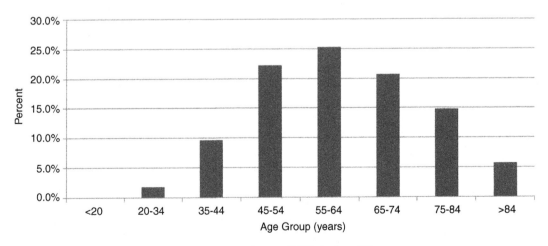

Fig. 21.1 Percent of new breast cancer cases by age (Source: SEER database [5])

Knowing that breast cancer risk increases with age, it is sensible to screen older women; however, it remains unknown at what age screening with mammography may lose its benefit. Moreover, given that some breast cancers prevented by screening may not become clinically relevant for approximately 10 years, accurately estimating an older woman's life expectancy may be relevant.

One study reported by Van Dijck et al. evaluated breast cancer mortality in women aged 68–83 years. The control group included women from the same birth cohort in a neighboring city without a screening program. The women were enrolled from 1977 to 1978 and were followed until 1990. The cumulative mortality rate ratio was 0.80 (95 % CI = 0.53–1.22). The cumulative mortality rate ratio decreased to 0.53 % (95 % CI = 0.27–1.04) 9–13 years after screening. With the follow-up data, the authors concluded that mammographic screening in women over 65 years old yielded a 40 % reduction in breast cancer mortality after 10 years [16].

One study reported that 36 % of American women older than 75 and with a life expectancy of less than 5 years received a screening mammogram [17]. Given the anxiety, false positives, additional tests, and procedures that may result from a mammogram, screening in this group may not always be beneficial. However, it has been demonstrated that the false-positive rate decreases slightly with older age [18].

Another study reported that mammographic detection of breast cancer was associated with a decreased risk of death for women older than 65, even those with mild to moderate comorbidities, but was not associated with improved overall survival in older women with severe or multiple comorbidities [19]. A study by Mandelblatt et al. utilized a decision analysis model to determine whether screening extends life for women over age 65 with and without comorbidities. Comorbidities included mild hypertension and symptomatic congestive heart failure. The authors reported that for women who had breast cancer, screening extended life by 617 days for average-health women aged 65–69 years and by 311 days for women in the same age group but with congestive heart failure.

This result compares to 178 days for women aged 85 years and over and 126 days for women in the same age group with congestive heart failure. Therefore, the authors concluded that older women continue to benefit from screening, with the potential exception of those older than 85 years, in whom anxiety and discomfort may outweigh the benefit. However, no inherent reason has been found to oblige an upper age limit on screening mammography [20].

The utilization of prognostic tools to estimate life expectancy may aid decision-making. Cruz et al. used data from the Health and Retirement Study, a cohort of community-dwelling adults aged 50 years and older to estimate 10-year mortality. The prediction model included the following indices: age, sex, body mass index, diabetes, tobacco use, noncutaneous cancer, chronic lung disease, and heart failure, as well as difficulty bathing, managing finances, walking several blocks, and pushing large objects. Based on these indices, subjects were stratified into groups with varying 10-year mortality [21].

Currently, women who are in good or moderately good health with a reasonable life expectancy are considered appropriate for screening mammograms. The patient and the clinician should each consider the potential benefit and harm of the test as well as whether the patient would be amenable to undergoing diagnostic tests and therapeutic treatment should an abnormal finding be discovered. Specifically, is the woman able and willing to undergo biopsy and possibly surgery? The ultimate decision should be made after a thorough conversation between the patient and her primary care physician.

Diagnosis

For older women undergoing screening mammography during which an abnormality is seen, the diagnostic workup proceeds in the standard fashion. The workup begins with additional spot compression mammographic views and targeted ultrasound. Either ultrasound or mammography-guided core needle biopsy can provide tissue for histologic diagnosis and tumor markers. Some elderly women may have physical limitations that preclude their ability to lie prone for a stereotactic biopsy. If a patient is not able to lie prone for biopsy and the lesion is occult on ultrasound, then stereotactic needle localization can be performed with the woman in a seated position and followed by a wire-localized excisional biopsy. Ultrasound-guided biopsies are performed with the woman lying supine; however, significant respiratory disease may require the procedure to be performed with the head and torso of the patient elevated to offload the thoracic cavity. It is important to keep these possible limitations in mind.

Clinicians must be cognizant of the prevalence of anticoagulation and antiplatelet medications taken by some older women and should manage this appropriately during any invasive procedure. Ideally, these medications are withheld prior to invasive procedures, but one must consider the underlying medical condition that is being treated to determine the safety of that approach.

The use of breast magnetic resonance imaging (MRI) in newly diagnosed breast cancer patients has become increasingly common. More data are needed regarding the effects of information obtained from MRI on therapy and outcome.

Tumor Characteristics

Older women with breast cancer tend to have tumors with more favorable biology. A review of the San Antonio breast cancer and SEER databases found that older women had more lobular and mucinous carcinomas [22]. Although tumors in older women tend to be larger at presentation, tumor biological characteristics are more favorable than in younger women. Specifically, tumors tend to be hormone receptor positive and exhibit lower proliferation rates, normal p53, and the absence of epidermal growth factor receptor and c-erbB2 expression [22, 23].

Treatment

The treatment of breast cancer has become more tailored to the patient and tumor biology than ever before. This is especially important when treating elderly women. The tumor biology and disease burden should be balanced with the patient's general health status.

Several studies have examined the undertreatment of elderly women with breast cancer and its impact on outcomes. By conventional criteria, many older women are treated less aggressively than younger women who present with breast cancer. Reports from single-surgeon databases demonstrate that older women are treated with less aggressive surgery, less chemotherapy, less radiotherapy, and more endocrine therapy. Regardless of these differences in treatment, the reported rates of local recurrence and distant metastasis are similar in the younger and older patient populations [24, 25]. Data from the San Antonio breast cancer and SEER databases confirm the findings of less chemotherapy and less radiotherapy and reported equal endocrine therapy in older women [22]. A report from the Netherlands examined age-related differences in treatment and found that there was no effect on survival [26].

However, some reports do identify differences in the outcomes of elderly women who are treated with less aggressive therapy. One analysis from the Rhode Island state tumor registry found that survival was impaired in patients older than 65 years who underwent lumpectomy alone relative to those who had lumpectomy, axillary dissection and radiation, or mastectomy [27]. Another analysis from the Geneva Cancer Registry reports that age was independently associated with less cancer treatment and that less cancer treatment was associated with an increased risk of dying as a result from breast cancer [28].

Clearly, more data are needed regarding how age influences treatment strategies and whether less treatment portends a worse outcome for elderly women.

Preoperative Clinical Evaluation

All patients should be assessed for risk factors for perioperative morbidity. In general, this assessment includes taking a history that focuses on prior cardiac disorders, including coronary artery disease, congestive heart failure, arrhythmias, and the presence of a pacemaker or cardiac defibrillator. Patients should also be asked about any history of renal disease, diabetes, pulmonary disease, peripheral vascular disease, or functional status. An electrocardiogram (EKG) is obtained, and if significant risk factors or abnormalities are noted on EKG, further cardiac assessment may be warranted.

Surgery

The surgical treatment of breast cancer centers on achieving local control by removing the primary tumor with negative margins, as is the central tenet of the field of surgical oncology as a whole. However, modern breast surgery has become quite tailored. Local control can be gained by mastectomy, breast conservation consisting of excision and radiation, or excision alone. The axilla will be addressed below. The type of surgical treatment, whether breast conservation or mastectomy, is often made by the patient after a thoughtful discussion with her physician, who explains the pros and cons of each. The surgeon should also keep in mind that if a patient is unlikely to be a good candidate for radiation therapy, then mastectomy might offer better local control. Sometimes women may opt for mastectomy to decrease the need for future mammograms, possible biopsies, and anxiety of a second breast cancer. If the cancer is multicentric, occupying two or more quadrants of the breast, then mastectomy remains the standard procedure.

The Primary Tumor

The primary tumor should be excised with negative margins by either excision (lumpectomy) or mastectomy. The width of the negative margin

remains highly debated but can be defined as no tumor cells at the inked margin. When choosing excision versus mastectomy in a patient with significant comorbidities, the surgeon must keep in mind that excision can be easily performed with sedation and local anesthesia, whereas mastectomy is usually performed under general anesthesia. The ability to avoid general anesthesia may lead some surgeons to recommend excision to some patients, especially those with significant pulmonary or cardiovascular disease.

The Axilla

Clinically involved axillary lymph nodes should be resected when the primary tumor is removed. Sentinel lymph node biopsy can be used to evaluate the axilla in patients who have a negative axillary lymph node exam. If a patient with a clinically negative axilla has significant comorbidities that would preclude her from receiving chemotherapy, a sentinel lymph node biopsy may not provide any useful information, and some surgeons chose to eliminate this procedure. If sentinel lymph node biopsy is positive for metastatic involvement by frozen pathology at the time of mastectomy, it is currently standard to perform an axillary dissection. While performing a lumpectomy, the sentinel lymph node can be submitted for permanent pathology. If the sentinel lymph node biopsy reveals metastatic carcinoma in one or two lymph nodes after lumpectomy, the Z0011 protocol can be followed with no further surgery in the axilla, and the patient can proceed to treatment with radiotherapy. If three or more lymph nodes have metastatic involvement, the patient no longer meets the Z0011 criteria, and an axillary dissection should be performed [29].

Reconstruction

Research has shown that postmastectomy reconstruction is associated with improved patient quality of life. In 1998, President Bill

Clinton signed the Women's Health and Cancer Rights Act of 1998, requiring healthcare insurance companies to cover breast reconstruction after mastectomy. However, overall reconstruction rates continue to be low in the United States and decrease with increasing patient age [30, 31]. Some women may chose not to undergo reconstruction as a personal preference; however, whether reconstruction is performed has also been shown to be influenced by the institution at which patients received care [31]. Patient preference and medical comorbidities may influence the decision to forgo reconstruction, which often requires longer surgeries and additional procedures; however, the surgeon should address this issue with each patient and provide access to reconstruction for those women who are good candidates.

Adjuvant Therapy

As stated previously, some studies have reported that older women with breast cancer receive less chemotherapy and radiotherapy than younger women. When making decisions regarding adjuvant therapy, the clinician must consider the functional status, life expectancy, and comorbidities of the patient. Because most breast cancer in the elderly is hormone receptor-positive and patients can receive endocrine therapy, researchers have asked how much benefit is provided by the addition of chemotherapy. The data demonstrating improved survival from combined chemotherapy and endocrine therapy in women with hormone receptor-positive early-stage breast cancer do not include a large population of women older than 70 [32]. In fact, patients aged 65 years and older are significantly underrepresented in clinical trials of cancer treatment [33]. Gene-based assays can provide more information regarding tumor biology and the likelihood of recurrence, and this information in turn can help guide decisions regarding adjuvant therapy.

Another study from the United States randomly assigned women aged 70 or older with stage I estrogen receptor-positive breast cancer to lumpectomy and tamoxifen with or without radiation. There was a significant difference in the rate of local or regional recurrence at 5 years (1 % in those treated with lumpectomy, radiation, and tamoxifen versus 4 % in those treated with lumpectomy and tamoxifen), and there was no difference reported in distant metastases or 5-year overall survival [34].

Currently, the most common radiotherapy regimen in the United States takes approximately 6 weeks to complete. However, shorter regimens of higher doses over fewer weeks (resulting in lower total doses) are an alternative. Data from Canada and the United Kingdom report that hypofractionated radiation regimens are just as effective in terms of local and regional recurrence [35, 36].

Whelan et al. studied women with invasive cancer who had undergone lumpectomy with negative lymph nodes and were randomized to 50 Gy in 25 fractions over 35 days or 42.5 Gy in 16 fractions over 22 days. The risks of local recurrence were 6.7 % and 6.2 % (95 % CI = −2.5 to 3.5), respectively [35].

Haviland et al. recently reported 10-year follow-up data from the UK Standardisation of Breast Radiotherapy trial (START), which demonstrated that hypofractionated radiotherapy is safe and effective. The START-A trial compared 50 Gy in 25 fractions over 5 weeks to 41.6 Gy or 39 Gy in 13 fractions over 5 weeks, and no difference in local-regional recurrence was detected between the 41.6 Gy (6.3 %, 95 % CI = 4.7–8.5) and either the 50 Gy (7.4 % CI = 5.5–10.0) or the 39 Gy regimen (8.8 %, 95 % CI = 6.7–11.4). The START-B trial compared 50 Gy in 25 fractions over 5 weeks to 40 Gy in 15 fractions over 3 weeks and also demonstrated no significant difference in local-regional recurrence in the two groups (4.3 %, 95 % CI = 3.2–5.9 and 5.5 %, 95 % CI = 4.2–7.2) [36].

Another development in the quest to shorten the duration of radiotherapy after lumpectomy is intraoperative radiation (TARGIT). The 5-year risk of local recurrence was reported to be 3.3 % (95 % CI=2.1–5.1) for women in the TARGIT group compared with 1.3 % (95 % CI=0.7–2.5) for external beam radiation. Notably, there were also fewer non-breast cancer deaths in the TARGIT group [37].

Shorter radiation regimens and intraoperative radiation provide alternatives to the widespread use of longer duration radiotherapy. There are also some data indicating that it may be safe to omit radiation therapy in women over 70 years old. Hughes et al. reported data from the CALGB 9343 study in which women with estrogen receptor-positive stage I breast cancer treated with lumpectomy were randomized to tamoxifen plus radiation or tamoxifen alone. In this study, there were no significant differences in time to consequent mastectomy, time to distant metastasis, breast cancer-specific survival, or overall survival [38]. The National Comprehensive Cancer Network Guidelines allow for lumpectomy with negative margins plus endocrine therapy in women aged 70 years or older with T1, node-negative, ER-positive breast cancer to omit breast radiation [39].

Endocrine Therapy

Several studies have examined endocrine therapy as a primary treatment in elderly breast cancer patients. One study from the United Kingdom compared primary tamoxifen treatment to mastectomy with tamoxifen in women aged 70 or older with estrogen receptor-positive, node-negative breast cancer. Both groups exhibited similar regional recurrence, metastasis, breast cancer-specific survival, and overall survival, but the local control was better after mastectomy and tamoxifen [40]. Another study from the Netherlands noted an increasing trend in primary endocrine therapy; however, the study reported compromised survival (from all causes) in those who received primary endocrine treatment [40]. It is important to note that this was not a randomized study and that the patients treated with primary endocrine therapy were older and exhibited more comorbidities at baseline [41].

Other Treatments

Clinicians and researchers are exploring other modalities to treat breast cancer. For instance, ultrasound-guided percutaneous radiofrequency ablation with endocrine therapy in a small group of patients has been reported as well tolerated but is not recommended for lobular carcinoma [42]. Other studies have investigated cryotherapy for breast cancer treatment and report minimal patient discomfort with no short-term recurrences detected [43]. Further research regarding recurrence and disease-free survival relative to conventional treatment is needed.

Special Considerations

There are many special considerations inherent to caring for an elderly patient. Some important issues to highlight are difficulties with transportation and social support. The elderly patient may have difficulty arranging transportation to appointments for imaging, biopsies, consultations, surgery, chemotherapy, and radiotherapy. Standard breast radiation in the United States entails 33 treatments given 5 days a week over a 6.5-week period. During this time, the patient needs daily transportation to and from the radiation facility, and alternative radiation regimens may eliminate this problem. As always, it is important to involve family in the care of the patient. Providing social support either through family involvement or through various cancer organizations can have a meaningful impact on the patient's experience.

References

1. Ferlay J, Soerjomataram I, Ervik M, Dikshit R, Eser S, Mathers C, et al. GLOBOCAN 2012 v 1.0, cancer incidence and mortality worldwide: IARC CancerBase No. 11 [internet]. Lyon: International Agency for Research on Cancer; 2013. Available from: http://globocan.iarc.fr, accessed on 3/11/2015.
2. Jemal A, Bray F, Center MM, Ferlay J, Ward E, Forman D. Global cancer statistics. CA Cancer J Clin. 2011;61:69–90.
3. Althuis MD, Dozier JM, Anderson WF, Devesa SS, Brinton LA. Global trends in breast cancer incidence and mortality 1973–1997. Int J Epidemiol. 2005;34:405–12.
4. Greenlee RT, Murray T, Bolden S, Wingo P. Cancer, statistics, 2000. CA Cancer J Clin. 2000;50:7–33.
5. Surveillance, Epidemiology, and End Results (SEER) Program (www.seer.cancer.gov) SEER*Stat Database: SEER 18 2006–2010.
6. Alexander FE, Anderson TJ, Brown HK, Forrest AP, Hepburn W, Kirkpatrick AE, et al. 14 years of follow-up from the Edinburgh randomized trial of breast-cancer screening. Lancet. 1999;353:1903–8.
7. Bjurstam N, Bjorneld L, Duffy SW, Smith TC, Cahlin E, Eriksson O, et al. The Gothenburg breast screening trial: first results on mortality, incidence, and mode of detection for women ages 39–49 years at randomization. Cancer. 1997;80:2091–9.
8. Frisell J, Lidbrink E, Hellstrom L, Rutqvist LE. Follow-up after 11 years: update of mortality results in the Stockholm mammographic screening trial. Breast Cancer Res Treat. 1997;45:263–70.
9. Tabár L, Fagerberg CJ, Gad A, Baldetorp L, Holmberg LH, Gröntoft O, et al. Reduction in mortality from breast cancer after mass screening with mammography: randomised trial from the Breast Cancer Screening Working Group of the Swedish National Board of Health and Welfare. Lancet. 1985;1:829–32.
10. Andersson I, Aspergren K, Janzon L, Landberg T, Lindholm K, Linell F, et al. Mammographic screening and mortality from breast cancer: the Malmo mammographic screening trial. BMJ. 1988;297:943–8.
11. Shapiro S. Periodic screening for breast cancer: the HIP randomized controlled trial. Health insurance plan. J Natl Cancer Inst Monogr. 1997;22:27–30.
12. Fletcher SW, Black W, Harris R, Rimer BK, Shapiro S. Report of the international workshop on screening for breast cancer. J Natl Cancer Inst. 1993;85:1644–56.
13. Tabár L, Vita B, Chen TH, Yen AM, Cohen A, Tot T, et al. Swedish two-county trial: impact of mammographic screening on breast cancer mortality during 3 decades. Radiology. 2011;260:658–63.

14. American Cancer Society Guidelines for the Early Detection of Cancer http://www.cancer.org/healthy/findcancerearly/cancerscreeningguidelines/american-cancer-society-guidelines-for-the-early-detection-of-cancer. Accessed 28 Mar 2013.
15. Canadian Task Force on Preventive Health Care. http://canadiantaskforce.ca/guidelines/2011-breast-cancer/. Accessed 28 Mar 2013.
16. Van Dijck JA, Verbeek AL, Beex LV, Hendriks JH, Holland R, Mravunac M, et al. Breast-cancer mortality in a non-randomized trial on mammographic screening in women over age 65. Int J Cancer. 1997;70:164–8.
17. Schonberg MA, Breslau ES, McCarthy EP. Targeting of mammography screening according to life expectancy in women aged 75 and older. J Am Geriatr Soc. 2013;61:388–95.
18. Hubbard RA, Kerlikowske K, Flower CI, Yankaskas BC, Zhu W, Miglioretti DL. Cumulative probability of false-positive recall or biopsy recommendation after 10 years of screening mammography: a cohort study. Ann Intern Med. 2011;155:481–92.
19. McPherson CP, Swenson KK, Lee MW. The effects of mammographic detection and comorbidity on the survival of older women with breast cancer. JAGS. 2002;50:1061–8.
20. Mandelblatt JS, Wheat ME, Monane M, Moshief RD, Hollenberg JP, Tang J. Breast cancer screening for elderly women with and without comorbid conditions: a decision analysis model. Ann Intern Med. 1992;116:722–30.
21. Cruz M, Covinsky K, Wildera EW, Stijacic-CenzerI I, Lee SJ. Predicting 10-year mortality for older adults. JAMA. 2013;309:874–6.
22. Diab S, Elledge R, Clark G. Tumor characteristics and clinical outcome of elderly women with breast cancer. J Natl Cancer Inst. 2000;92:550–6.
23. Clark GM. The biology of breast cancer in older women. J Gerontol. 1992;47:19–23.
24. Malik MK, Tartter PI, Belfer R. Undertreated breast cancer in the elderly. J Cancer Epidemiol. 2013;2013:893104. doi:10.1155/2013/893104.
25. Gajdos C, Tartter PI, Bleiweiss IJ. The consequence of undertreating breast cancer in the elderly. J Am Coll Surg. 2001;192:698–707.
26. Bergman L, Kluck HM, van Leeuwen FE, Crommelin MA, Dekker G, Hart AA, et al. The influence of age on treatment choice and survival of elderly breast cancer patients in south-eastern Netherlands: a population-based study. Eur J Cancer. 1992;28A:1475–80.
27. Wanebo H, Cole B, Chung M, Vezeridis M, Schepps B, Fulton J, et al. Is surgical management compromised in elderly patients with breast cancer? Ann Surg. 1997;225:579–86.

28. Bouchardy C, Rapiti E, Fioretta G, Laissue P, Neyroud-Casper I, et al. Undertreatment strongly decreases prognosis of breast cancer in elderly women. J Clin Oncol. 2003;21:3580–7.

29. Giuliano AE, Hunt KK, Ballman KV, Beitsch PD, Whitworth PW, Blumencranz PW, et al. Axillary dissection vs no axillary dissection in women with invasive breast cancer and sentinel node metastasis: a randomized clinical trial. JAMA. 2011;305:569–75.

30. Wilkins ED, Alderman AK. Breast reconstruction practices in North America: current trends and future priorities. Semin Plast Surg. 2004;18:149–55.

31. In H, Jiang W, Lipsitz SR, Neville BA, Weeks JC, Greenberg CC. Variation in the utilization of reconstruction following mastectomy in elderly women. Ann Surg Oncol. 2012;20:1872–9.

32. Jones EL, Leak A, Muss HB. Adjuvant therapy of breast cancer in women 70 years of age and older: tough decision, high stakes. Oncology. 2012;26:793–801.

33. Hutchins LF, Unger JM, Crowley JJ, Coltman Jr CA, Albain KS. Underrepresentation of patients 65 years of age or older in cancer-treatment trials. N Engl J Med. 1999;341:2061–7.

34. Hughes KS, Schnaper LA, Berry D, Cirrincione C, McCormick B, Shank B, et al. Lumpectomy plus Tamoxifen with or without irradiation in women 70 years of age or older with early breast cancer. N Engl J Med. 2004;351:971–7.

35. Whelan TJ, Pignol JP, Levine MN, Julian JA, MacKenzie R, Parpia S, et al. Long-term results of hypofractionated radiation therapy for breast cancer. N Engl J Med. 2010;362:513–20.

36. Haviland JS, Owen JR, Dewar JA, Agrawal RK, Barrett J, Barrett-Lee PJ, et al. The UK Standardisation of Breast Radiotherapy (START) trials of radiotherapy hypofractionation for treatment of early breast cancer: 10 year follow-up results of two randomized controlled trials. Lancet Oncol. 2013;14:1086–94.

37. Vaidya JS, Wenz F, Bulsara M, Tobias JS, Joseph DJ, Keshtgar M, et al. Risk-adapted targeted intraoperative radiotherapy versus whole-breast radiotherapy for breast cancer: 5-year results for local control and overall survival from the TARGIT-A randomised trial. Lancet. 2014;383(9917):603–13.

38. Hughes KS, Schnaper LA, Bellon JR, Cirrincione CT, Berry DA, McCormick B, et al. Lumpectomy plus tamoxifen with or without irradiation in women age 70 years or older with early breast cancer: long-term follow-up of CALGB 9343. J Clin Oncol. 2013;31:2382–7.

39. National Comprehensive Cancer Network. Breast cancer version 2.2015 clinical practice guidelines in oncology.

40. Johnston SJ, Kenny FS, Syed BM, Robertson JF, Pinder SE, Winterbottom L, et al. A randomized trial of primary tamoxifen versus mastectomy plus adjuvant tamoxifen in fit elderly women with invasive breast carcinoma of high oestrogen receptor content: long-term results at 20 years of follow-up. Ann Oncol. 2012;23:2296–300.

41. Wink CJ, Woensdregt K, Nieuwenhuijzen GA, van der Sangen MJ, Hutschemaekers S, Roukema JA, et al. Hormone treatment without surgery for patients aged 75 years or older with operable breast cancer. Ann Surg Oncol. 2012;19:1185–91.

42. Palussiere J, Henriques C, Mauriac L, Asad-Syed M, Valentin F, Brouste V, et al. Radiofrequency ablation as a substitute for surgery in elderly patients with non-resected breast cancer: pilot study with long-term outcomes. Radiology. 2012;264:597–605.

43. Littrup PJ, Jallad BJ, Chandiwala-Mody P, D'Agostini M, Adam BA, Bouwman D. Cryotherapy for breast cancer: a feasibility study without excision. J Vasc Interv Radiol. 2009;20:1329–41.

Breast Cancer in Young Women (Premenopausal Breast Cancer)

Kandace P. McGuire

Abstract

Breast cancer in women of childbearing age (premenopausal breast cancer) accounts for almost one-quarter of all breast cancer diagnoses in the United States. Advances in diagnosis and treatment have led to improved outcomes in this population that echo those in the postmenopausal population. Despite these advances, premenopausal women with breast cancer still show a significantly worse prognosis than their postmenopausal counterparts. Differences in presentation, tumor phenotype, and options for therapy may explain some of the difference in outcome. However, research is underway to identify the inherent differences that lead to differential outcomes.

Keywords

Breast cancer • Premenopausal • Young • MRI • Tomosynthesis • Mastectomy • BRCA • Chemotherapy • Endocrine therapy • Prognosis

Introduction

In 2013, over 230,000 new cases of breast cancers will be diagnosed in the United States, and almost 40,000 women will die from breast cancer [1]. Almost one-quarter of new breast cancer cases occur in premenopausal women [2], and substantial improvements in breast cancer outcomes have been achieved over time in younger women [3]. Despite these advances, premenopausal women with breast cancer still exhibit a significantly worse prognosis than their postmenopausal counterparts (Table 22.1) [4].

Prognosis/Clinical Features

Whether younger patients exhibit poorer outcomes due to age alone or because they present with more advanced tumors remains an ongoing research question. Compared with patients older than age 50, younger patients (<35) tend to present

K.P. McGuire, MD, FACS
Department of Surgery, Division of Surgical Oncology, University of North Carolina,
170 Manning Dr., CB#7203, Chapel Hill, NC 27599, USA
e-mail: kandace.mcguire@med.unc.edu

© Springer International Publishing Switzerland 2016
A. Aydiner et al. (eds.), *Breast Disease: Management and Therapies*,
DOI 10.1007/978-3-319-26012-9_22

Table 22.1 Five-year overall survival by age at diagnosis

	Total	Five-year survival				Crude		Adjusted[a]	
Age	No.	Expected	Observed	RSR	95 % CI	RER	95 % CI	RER	95 % CI
20–34	471	99.8	74.7	74.8	70.1–78.9	2.84	2.31–3.49	1.63	1.32–2.01
35–39	858	99.7	83.8	84.1	81.2–86.6	7.16	1.45–2.14	1.08	0.89–1.32
40–49	4,789	99.1	88.3	89.0	88.0–90.0	1.17	1.04–1.31	0.84	0.75–0.94
50–69	15,899	96.8	87.8	90.7	90.1–91.2	1.00	(Ref.)	1.00	(Ref.)

Courtesy of Fredholm et al. [4]

RSR relative survival ratio, *RER* relative excess risks of mortality

[a]Adjusted for year and stage

with significantly larger, multifocal primary tumors with a greater percentage of lymph node positivity. Younger patients also tend to present with tumors that are more commonly estrogen receptor (ER) and progesterone receptor (PR) negative and higher grade, with more lymphovascular invasion (LVI) and greater degrees of tumor necrosis [4–8]. However, in most cases, age remains a significant predictor of poor outcomes even after accounting for these factors [4, 6–8].

Detection

Detection of breast cancer in the premenopausal population can be difficult for numerous reasons. In most countries, women at average risk for breast cancer do not receive screening until age 40. There is little data to suggest any benefit in screening earlier than age 40. Even in patients age 40–49, only statistically nonsignificant improvements in overall survival have been demonstrated [9, 10]. The risk-benefit ratio with respect to true-positive results versus false-positive results and consequent unnecessary biopsy prompted the US Preventative Services Task Force to recommend only biannual screening prior to age 50, if screening is provided at all [11].

With few exceptions, there is an inverse relationship between age and mammographic density. In a study by Checka et al., 74 % of patients between 40 and 49 years old exhibited dense breasts in mammography. This percentage decreased to 57 % of women in their 50s [12]. Increased mammographic density has been associated with difficulty in identifying early breast

cancers and has also been described as an independent risk factor for breast cancer [12–14].

Patients at high risk of developing cancer due to genetic mutations, strong family history or personal history of atypia, or Mantle radiation are recommended to undergo earlier screening with alternative methods [15]. The most commonly recommended adjuvant screening test is magnetic resonance imaging (MRI). MRI is far more sensitive in detecting earlier breast cancers, especially in dense breasts. MRI, however, remains inadequate to detect the presence of calcifications and other anatomic variations. Furthermore, its low sensitivity can lead to false-positive screening results and numerous unnecessary biopsies [16–26].

Other alternative screening methods include screening ultrasound and tomosynthesis (also known as "3-D mammography"). Early studies into these imaging modalities as screening methods have met with mixed results [22, 25–29]. Thus far, neither of these methods is considered a primary screening method. The methods are, instead, considered adjuncts to screening [30, 31]. Molecular breast imaging (MBI) or beta-specific gamma imaging (BSGI) has also emerged as a useful screen in the detection of breast cancer. The use of MBI as a screening modality has not been widely studied. However, early trials suggest a benefit from using this technology in combination with mammography [32].

Locoregional Therapy

For most patients with premenopausal breast cancer, effective locoregional therapy does not differ significantly from that provided to postmenopausal patients. It is generally believed that both breast conservation therapy (BCT) and mastectomy are safe and efficacious in younger patients. However, with decreasing age, the chance of local recurrence increases after BCT [5, 33, 34]. Several studies have found age to be an independent risk factor on multivariate analysis for local recurrence. Despite the increase in local recurrence, whether overall survival is significantly different after recurrence in younger, premenopausal patients remains controversial [33, 35].

Perhaps due to the higher likelihood of local recurrence after breast conservation in the young, the rates of mastectomy are higher in younger patients [36–39]. Tumor size at presentation is also larger in the premenopausal population, which may necessitate mastectomy in some patients. Increased T stage is likely a result of a lack of effective screening in these patients and the biologic aggressiveness of tumors in this population. In addition, decreasing age is an independent predictor for contralateral prophylactic mastectomy (CPM) [36, 40–44]. Although there is currently no evidence that CPM in this population improves overall survival, contralateral disease occurrence is certainly reduced. The surgery is also highly cost-effective when performed in patients age 45–54 [45].

In the event of a BRCA mutation, the benefit of mastectomy and CPM changes. The rate of recurrent or contralateral breast cancer approaches 2–3 %/year for patients with BRCA mutations, compared with 0.5 %/year for the average breast cancer survivor. BRCA patients, especially those with BRCA1 mutations, are more likely to present at younger ages [46]. It has been suggested that patients with breast cancer and a BRCA mutation derive a survival benefit from CPM, although larger-scale studies are needed to confirm these findings [47].

Beyond the debate surrounding surgical therapy of the breast and the contralateral breast, there exists a debate regarding surgical therapy of the axilla in young patients. Traditional staging of the axilla includes a full axillary dissection. Such dissection historically consisted of axilla levels I, II, and III during the radical mastectomy era, followed by the elimination of level III upon the advent of modified

radical mastectomy. Oncologists continued to employ axillary dissection after the introduction of breast-conserving therapy. Unfortunately, even with modern axillary dissection, lymphedema rates can range anywhere from 15 % to 30 %.

The 1990s brought the widespread use of the sentinel node biopsy for staging in melanoma. This concept was adopted for use in breast surgery and is now considered the standard of care for axillary staging in the clinically node-negative axilla. Numerous large-scale studies, most notably ACOSOG Z0010 and NSABP B-32, established the equivalence in locoregional recurrence rates between sentinel node and axillary dissection [48–50]. More recently, it has been suggested that for patients undergoing breast conservation and whole-breast irradiation, axillary dissection offers no advantage in terms of locoregional recurrence over sentinel node biopsy in patients who are clinically node negative by physical exam but have one to two sentinel lymph nodes (SLNs) harboring metastatic disease [51, 52].

The application of these changes in patient management has been slow to extend into the premenopausal population, largely due to the low numbers of young women in the large studies that have established equivalent outcomes. However, most large governing bodies, such as the European Society of Breast Cancer Specialists, endorse the limited use of axillary dissection for staging in patients of all ages, including young patients [53].

With respect to adjuvant radiotherapy, there is little difference in the application of this therapy for the young. The risk-benefit ratio appears to remain the same regardless of age. When used in combination with breast conservation or lumpectomy, radiation decreases the risk of recurrence by more than half. However, in the case of postmastectomy radiotherapy (PMRT), the benefit does appear to be greater in young patients, who are thus more likely to receive PMRT for lower stage disease. In the sentinel studies regarding PMRT by the Danish Breast Trialists' Cooperative Group, postmastectomy radiotherapy exhibited a benefit in premenopausal patients with one to two positive lymph nodes, whereas the benefit of PMRT was demonstrated in postmenopausal patients with >3 positive lymph nodes [54, 55].

Adjuvant Systemic Therapy

Cytotoxic Chemotherapy

The efficacy of adjuvant systemic therapy in improving distant disease-free and overall survival has long been established in both pre- and postmenopausal patients. Such therapy will be discussed elsewhere in this book, and we will therefore concentrate on the implications of systemic cytotoxic chemotherapy on premenopausal patients. Several issues surround the use of chemotherapy in young patients, including premature amenorrhea and its consequences (namely, infertility, osteoporosis, and sexual dysfunction), as well as the use of preoperative (neoadjuvant) chemotherapy in the young.

One of the important issues that surround the treatment of young women with breast cancer is the issue of fertility. Many women delay childbearing until after schooling and beginning careers. In fact, the average age at first birth has risen in most developed countries over the last decade (Fig. 22.1) [56]. Many women who develop premenopausal breast cancer, therefore, have not completed their families and wish to preserve fertility. Unfortunately, many standard chemotherapeutic agents can cause amenorrhea during treatment, which can lead to infertility (Table 22.2) [57]. Even those patients who resume normal menstrual cycles can experience infertility after treatment, mostly due to the cytotoxicity of traditional chemotherapeutic agents towards the declining oocyte pool (Fig. 22.2) [58].

Several approaches can be used to preserve fertility in young cancer patients. The most important component of fertility preservation is to begin frank and open discussion with the patient *before* beginning any systemic therapy. Consideration must be given to the risks and benefits of therapy, such as delay in systemic therapy, the likelihood of infertility after therapy, and the likelihood of success in achieving pregnancy with the current techniques available.

The most traditional form of fertility preservation is embryo cryopreservation, which is endorsed by several organizations, including the European Society of Medical Oncology (ESMO) and the American Society of Clinical Oncology (ASCO) in their recent consensus statements [59, 60]. This method provides the best chance of achieving pregnancy after chemotherapy. However, it requires that the patient have a partner with whom she would like to produce children or that she use donor sperm. A newer alternative used with increasing success is oocyte cryopreservation [61]. Both methods require ovarian stimulation, which can be achieved with a number of agents, including letrozole and GnRH agonists [62]. Hormonal stimulation with traditional ovarian stimulators is avoided, as there is limited data on the use of these agents in breast cancer patients. One to two cycles is recommended to improve the likelihood of successful future implantation, and this can delay therapy by as much as 4–6 weeks [63].

An alternative to both of these methods is ovarian tissue harvesting and cryopreservation. This approach is an emerging technology, and extremely limited data/success rates have been reported. At the time of this report, ovarian tissue harvesting and cryopreservation is considered an experimental technique [64, 65].

Another option to be discussed is the use of GnRH agonists during chemotherapy for the protection of ovarian function. Due to the low risk, the practice is largely being used in the premenopausal population, although the data regarding success in preventing infertility and amenorrhea/menopause is variable [66–69].

Randomized trials have demonstrated that ovarian suppression with GnRH agonist therapy administered during adjuvant chemotherapy in premenopausal women with ER-negative tumors may preserve ovarian function and diminish the likelihood of chemotherapy-induced amenorrhea. In patients with ER-positive disease, conflicting results have been reported with respect to the protective effect of GnRH agonist therapy on fertility.

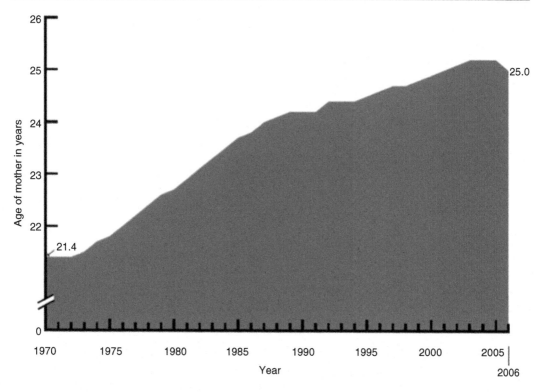

Fig. 22.1 Average age of mother at first birth, United States 1970–2006 (Courtesy of the Centers for Disease Control, CDC/NCHS, National Vital Statistics System)

Table 22.2 Incidence of amenorrhea with chemotherapy

Adjuvant chemotherapy	Incidence of amenorrhea
CMF	61 % (<40 year)
	95 % (≥40 year)
AC	34 %
FAC	32.8 %
TAC	51.4 %
Doxorubicin based	59 %
CEF	51 %

Courtesy of Minton and Munster [57]
CMF cyclophosphamide, methotrexate, 5FU; AC doxorubicin, cyclophosphamide; FAC 5FU, doxorubicin, cyclophosphamide; TAC docetaxel, doxorubicin, cyclophosphamide; *CEF* cyclophosphamide, epirubicin, 5FU

In addition to infertility, premature menopause associated with chemotherapy can cause a host of other problems, including sexual dysfunction and osteoporosis. Sexual dysfunction can be a problem after diagnosis as well as during and after therapy and can affect both pre- and postmenopausal women. Recent evidence suggests that younger women and their partners can have greater problems with intimacy [70]. In a study performed by Alder et al., it was noted that while the only predictor for desire was the quality of the relationship, chemotherapy was predictive for problems with arousal, lubrication, orgasm, and sexual pain [71]. Treatment is typically targeted at symptom management for physical dysfunction with lubrication, for which it includes local estrogen therapy, especially in patients with a history of hormone receptor-negative disease, and it is targeted at psychological/family therapy for intimacy issues [72–74].

Osteopenia/osteoporosis can be induced by premature menopause due to the acute and premature withdrawal of estrogen, which supports bone mineral density [75, 76]. The use of tamoxifen can increase bone density in postmenopausal women, but tamoxifen decreases bone density in premenopausal women, so it is quite difficult to assess its true impact on patients with chemotherapy-induced menopause

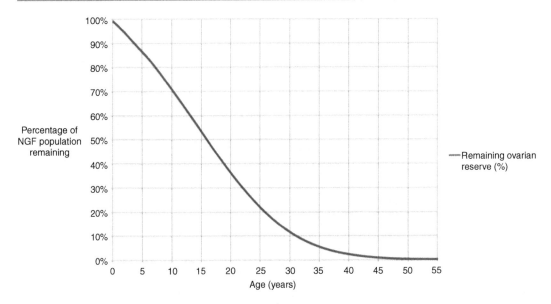

Fig. 22.2 Human female oocyte reserve by age (years) (Courtesy of Wallace and Kelsey [58])

[77]. Supplementation with calcium and vitamin D is recommended, as well as maintaining moderate physical activity with weight-bearing exercise, just as is recommended for those at risk for standard postmenopausal bone loss.

Bisphosphonates have also been used for the last decade to treat osteoporosis, and their effect on chemotherapy-related bone loss is now being widely studied. Studies involving large cohorts of women both in North America and Asia have reported that zoledronic acid can ameliorate bone loss in premenopausal patients undergoing cytotoxic chemotherapy, with its effects lasting at least 1 year [78–81].

Neoadjuvant Chemotherapy

The concept of preoperative or neoadjuvant chemotherapy for the treatment of locally advanced breast cancer is well studied. There are several known indications for neoadjuvant chemotherapy, including converting an inoperable tumor to an operable one and converting a mastectomy candidate into a breast conservation candidate.

For various reasons, neoadjuvant chemotherapy is often used in the treatment of premenopausal

women with breast cancer. Typically, as noted previously, younger women present with more advanced disease, which may benefit from downstaging. These women also typically exhibit a greater preponderance of hormone receptor-negative and/or HER2-positive disease, both of which would otherwise require adjuvant chemotherapy and are more likely to respond to neoadjuvant chemotherapy [82, 83] (Fig. 22.3). Additionally, even within specific tumor subtypes, premenopausal women are more likely to demonstrate a pathologic complete response to therapy than their postmenopausal counterparts [84].

Endocrine Therapy

Despite the extensive research noted previously, the optimal systemic therapy for premenopausal women remains elusive. Questions remain regarding the type and duration of endocrine therapy. Moreover, information about the value of ovarian suppression/ovarian ablation (OS/OA) continues to emerge, but it remains unclear whether the addition of such strategies to tamoxifen and chemotherapy is necessary.

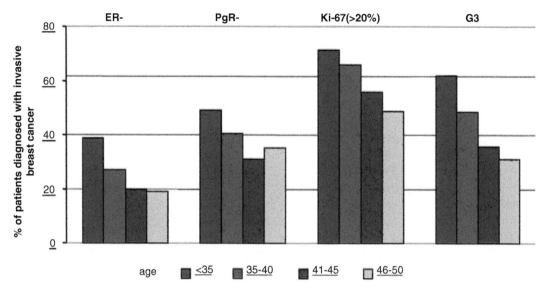

Fig. 22.3 Variation in immunohistochemical subtype by age [83]

Ovarian Ablation or Ovarian Suppression

Both OA and OS have been shown to improve survival in patients with early-stage breast cancer. The Early Breast Cancer Trialists' Collaborative Group (EBCTCG) overview, also known as the Oxford Overview, represents a meta-analysis of the existing trial data of adjuvant therapy with tamoxifen, chemotherapy, and OA/OS. The most recent overview on ovarian ablation for breast cancer contained data from almost 8,000 women ≤50 years of age with either ER-positive or ER-unknown disease who were randomized into trials of OA [85]. OA and OS both reduced recurrence and breast cancer mortality, but this occurred only in the absence of other systemic treatments.

Opinions regarding the efficacy of the combined use of OS/OA alone or in combination with endocrine therapy and chemotherapy in premenopausal patients have varied over the last several years, with much conflicting data. As recently as 2011, the American Society of Clinical Oncology (ASCO) endorsed the Cancer Care Ontario practice guidelines on adjuvant OS/OA in the treatment of premenopausal women with early-stage breast cancer [86]. The opinion of both groups, based on the preponderance of available data, was as follows: "OA should not be routinely added to systemic therapy with chemotherapy, tamoxifen, or the combination of tamoxifen and chemotherapy." The guidelines also recommended against using OA as an alternative to other systemic therapy, providing that the patient was a candidate for other systemic therapy.

More recently, analysis of the Austrian Breast and Colorectal Cancer Study Group trial-12 (ABCSG-12) at the 62-month follow-up reported outcomes in premenopausal, early-stage patients receiving goserelin who were randomized to anastrozole or tamoxifen with or without zoledronic acid. Investigators observed improved disease-free survival (DFS) in patients taking zoledronic acid with anastrozole or tamoxifen [87], but the difference lost statistical significance when measuring the anastrozole arms separately. Overall, the outcomes of the ABCSG-12 trial are excellent, with >96 % of patients alive at the 62-month follow-up, despite the facts that 31 % of the patients were node-positive and that only 5.4 % of patients received chemotherapy.

As evidenced above, much has been written about combined pharmacologic ovarian OA/OS and endocrine therapy in the premenopausal population, but few recent studies have addressed surgical ovarian ablation and endocrine therapy. Ovarian ablation by oophorectomy can be a cost-effective alternative to pharmacologic ovarian suppression, especially in economically disadvantaged areas of the world. In combination with tamoxifen, ovarian ablation by oophorectomy provides equivalent DFS and overall survival for a fraction of the cost [88]. Previous reports have suggested that variations in the hormonal milieu related to the menstrual cycle may affect the short-term DFS and overall survival (3.6-year median) associated with oophorectomy and tamoxifen [88, 89].

Neoadjuvant Endocrine Therapy

Despite the wide acceptance of neoadjuvant endocrine therapy in the postmenopausal population [90], neoadjuvant endocrine therapy in the premenopausal population with or without ovarian suppression remains controversial [91]. Early studies reported the use of tamoxifen, buserelin, or both in premenopausal women with metastatic or locally advanced breast cancer [92, 93].

The only prospective randomized trial of neoadjuvant endocrine therapy in premenopausal women, the Study of Tamoxifen or Arimidex plus Goserelin Acetate to Compare Efficacy and Safety (STAGE), evaluated goserelin plus either anastrozole or tamoxifen for 24 weeks prior to surgery [94]. This Japanese study found that the likelihood of a complete or partial response was significantly higher in the anastrozole group. These results appear to be in direct opposition to those from ABCSG-12, in which tamoxifen plus goserelin led to better overall survival. However, the authors of this study noted that this effect in ABCSG-12 was only observed in a subset of patients with body mass index (BMI) higher than 25 kg/m². The percentage of patients with a BMI ≥25 in the ABCSG-12 study was nearly twice that of the STAGE trial (33.0 % vs. 17.3 %). This discrepancy may explain the improved efficacy of anastrozole in comparison with tamoxifen in the STAGE trial but may also raise questions as to whether these results can be extrapolated to Western populations, where BMI is typically higher (as seen in ABCSG-12).

Duration of Adjuvant Endocrine Therapy in Premenopausal Women

The question of the duration of adjuvant endocrine therapy in premenopausal women is highly important. The NSABP B14 extension study randomized over 1,100 premenopausal patients to either placebo or tamoxifen after completing 5 years of adjuvant tamoxifen therapy. Seven years of follow-up showed a slight advantage in patients who discontinued tamoxifen relative to those who continued to receive it [95, 96]. These findings, along with concern for cumulative toxicity with ongoing tamoxifen, previously established 5 years of adjuvant tamoxifen therapy as the standard of care for premenopausal women.

However, recently, an analysis of the Adjuvant Tamoxifen: Longer Against Shorter (ATLAS) trial, which included almost 13,000 women with early breast cancer who had completed 5 years of treatment with tamoxifen and then were randomly allocated to continue tamoxifen for 10 years or to stop at 5 years, reported improved recurrence and mortality rates with continuation of tamoxifen [97]. The mortality reduction was only significant after year 10.

ATLAS and other studies have reported mild to serious side effects with endocrine therapy, including hot flashes, night sweats, irritability, insomnia, and weight gain, as well as other more serious issues of uterine cancer and complications from hypercoagulability. Extended treatment with 10 years of tamoxifen can yield a significantly increased risk of uterine and pulmonary embolus, but there appears to be no increase in stroke, and ischemic heart disease can be decreased.

The challenge, however, lies in the determination of appropriate timing for switching premenopausal women who become postmenopausal during their first 10 years on tamoxifen to an aromatase inhibitor. The MA17 study demonstrated that extended adjuvant therapy with 5 years of letrozole after 5 years of tamoxifen improved relapse rates and survival [98]. Because there are no comparisons between such sequencing strategies and 10 years of tamoxifen treatment, it remains unknown whether switching to an AI after 2–3 years of tamoxifen (or vice versa) or switching to an AI after 5 years of tamoxifen would be superior to 10 years of tamoxifen alone.

Conclusion

Breast cancer is a common disease among women, and it is complex and can be difficult to treat. Premenopausal breast cancer presents a special challenge; the disease can be difficult to detect and can require alterations in therapy due to more aggressive disease, risks of therapy, and the effect on the young patient's life. Much is known about local and systemic therapy in this population, but research to define the special needs of premenopausal breast cancer patients is ongoing.

References

1. Singletary SE, Allred C, Ashley P, Bassett LW, Berry D, Bland KI, et al. Revision of the American Joint Committee on Cancer staging system for breast cancer. J Clin Oncol. 2002;20(17):3628–36.
2. Leal CB, Schmitt FC, Bento MJ, Maia NC, Lopes CS. Ductal carcinoma in situ of the breast. Histologic categorization and its relationship to ploidy and immunohistochemical expression of hormone receptors, p53, and c-<I>erb</I>B-2 protein. Cancer. 1995;75(8):2123–31.
3. Smith BD, Jiang J, McLaughlin SS, Hurria A, Smith GL, Giordano SH, et al. Improvement in breast cancer outcomes over time: are older women missing out? J Clin Oncol. 2011;29(35):4647–53.
4. Fredholm H, Eaker S, Frisell J, Holmberg L, Fredriksson I, Lindman H. Breast cancer in young women: poor survival despite intensive treatment. PLoS One. 2009;4(11):e7695.
5. Crowe Jr JP, Gordon NH, Shenk RR, Zollinger Jr RM, Brumberg DJ, Shuck JM. Age does not predict breast cancer outcome. Arch Surg. 1994;129(5):483–7; discussion 7–8.
6. Nixon AJ, Neuberg D, Hayes DF, Gelman R, Connolly JL, Schnitt S, et al. Relationship of patient age to pathologic features of the tumor and prognosis for patients with stage I or II breast cancer. J Clin Oncol. 1994;12(5):888–94.
7. de la Rochefordiere A, Asselain B. Age as prognostic factor in premenopausal breast carcinoma. Lancet. 1993;341(8852):1039.
8. Yıldırım E, Dalgıç T, Berberoğlu U. Prognostic significance of young age in breast cancer. J Surg Oncol. 2000;74(4):267–72.
9. Miller AB, To T, Baines CJ, Wall C. The Canadian National Breast Screening Study-1: breast cancer mortality after 11 to 16 years of follow-up: a randomized screening trial of mammography in women age 40 to 49 years. Ann Intern Med. 2002;137(5_Part_1):305–12.
10. Moss SM, Cuckle H, Evans A, Johns L, Waller M, Bobrow L. Effect of mammographic screening from age 40 years on breast cancer mortality at 10 years' follow-up: a randomised controlled trial. Lancet. 2006;368(9552):2053–60.
11. Calonge NPD, DeWitt TG, Dietrich AJ, Gregory KD, Grossman D, Isham G, et al. Screening for breast cancer: U.S. Preventive Services Task Force recommendation statement. Ann Intern Med. 2009;151(10):716–26.
12. Checka CM, Chun JE, Schnabel FR, Lee JToth H. The relationship of mammographic density and age: implications for breast cancer screening. Am J Roentgenol. 2012;198(3):W292–5.
13. Boyd N, Martin L, Chavez S, Gunasekara A, Salleh A, Melnichouk O, et al. Breast-tissue composition and other risk factors for breast cancer in young women: a cross-sectional study. Lancet Oncol. 2009;10(6):569–80.
14. McCormack VA, dos Santos Silva I. Breast density and parenchymal patterns as markers of breast cancer risk: a meta-analysis. Cancer Epidemiol Biomarkers Prev. 2006;15(6):1159–69.
15. Breast Cancer Screening and Diagnosis 2013 (cited 9 Apr 2013). Available from: http://www.nccn.org/professionals/physician_gls/pdf/breast-screening.pdf.
16. Feig S. Cost-effectiveness of mammography, MRI, and ultrasonography for breast cancer screening. Radiol Clin North Am. 2010;48(5):879–91.
17. Le-Petross HT, Whitman GJ, Atchley DP, Yuan Y, Gutierrez-Barrera A, Hortobagyi GN, et al. Effectiveness of alternating mammography and magnetic resonance imaging for screening women with deleterious BRCA mutations at high risk of breast cancer. Cancer. 2011;117(17):3900–7.
18. Lowry KP, Lee JM, Kong CY, McMahon PM, Gilmore ME, Cott Chubiz JE, et al. Annual screening strategies in BRCA1 and BRCA2 gene mutation carriers: a comparative effectiveness analysis. Cancer. 2012;118(8):2021–30.
19. Passaperuma K, Warner E, Causer PA, Hill KA, Messner S, Wong JW, et al. Long-term results of screening with magnetic resonance imaging in women with BRCA mutations. Br J Cancer. 2012;107(1):24–30.
20. Pavic D, Koomen MA, Kuzmiak CM, Lee YH, Pisano ED. The role of magnetic resonance imaging in diagnosis and management of breast cancer. Technol Cancer Res Treat. 2004;3(6):527–41.

21. Plevritis SK, Kurian AW, Sigal BM, Daniel BL, Ikeda DM, Stockdale FE, et al. Cost-effectiveness of screening BRCA1/2 mutation carriers with breast magnetic resonance imaging. JAMA. 2006;295(20):2374–84.

22. Podo F, Sardanelli F, Canese R, D'Agnolo G, Natali PG, Crecco M, et al. The Italian multi-centre project on evaluation of MRI and other imaging modalities in early detection of breast cancer in subjects at high genetic risk. J Exp Clin Cancer Res. 2002;21(3 Suppl):115–24.

23. Sardanelli F, Podo F, Santoro F, Manoukian S, Bergonzi S, Trecate G, et al. Multicenter surveillance of women at high genetic breast cancer risk using mammography, ultrasonography, and contrast-enhanced magnetic resonance imaging (the high breast cancer risk italian 1 study): final results. Invest Radiol. 2011;46(2):94–105.

24. Warner E. Impact of MRI surveillance and breast cancer detection in young women with BRCA mutations. Ann Oncol. 2011;22 Suppl 1:i44–9.

25. Warner E, Plewes DB, Shumak RS, Catzavelos GC, Di Prospero LS, Yaffe MJ, et al. Comparison of breast magnetic resonance imaging, mammography, and ultrasound for surveillance of women at high risk for hereditary breast cancer. J Clin Oncol. 2001;19(15):3524–31.

26. Warner E, Plewes DB, Hill KA, Causer PA, Zubovits JT, Jong RA, et al. Surveillance of brca1 and brca2 mutation carriers with magnetic resonance imaging, ultrasound, mammography, and clinical breast examination. JAMA. 2004;292(11):1317–25.

27. Berg W, Zhang Z, Lehrer D, Jong RA, Pisano ED, Barr RG, et al. Detection of breast cancer with addition of annual screening ultrasound or a single screening mri to mammography in women with elevated breast cancer risk. JAMA. 2012;307(13):1394–404.

28. Kuhl C, Weigel S, Schrading S, Arand B, Bieling H, König R, et al. Prospective multicenter cohort study to refine management recommendations for women at elevated familial risk of breast cancer: the EVA trial. J Clin Oncol. 2010;28(9):1450–7.

29. Kuhl CK, Kuhn W, Schild H. Management of women at high risk for breast cancer: new imaging beyond mammography. Breast. 2005;14(6):480–6.

30. Brandt KR, Craig D, Hoskins TL, Henrichsen TL, Bendel EC, Brandt SR, Mandrekar J. Can digital breast tomosynthesis replace conventional diagnostic mammography views for screening recalls without calcifications? A comparison study in a simulated clinical setting. Am J Roentgenol. 2013;200(2):291–8.

31. Skaane P, Bandos AI, Gullien R, Eben EB, Ekseth U, Haakenaasen U, et al. Comparison of digital mammography alone and digital mammography plus tomosynthesis in a population-based screening program. Radiology. 2013;267(1):47–56.

32. Sun Y, Wei W, Yang H-W, Liu J-L. Clinical usefulness of breast-specific gamma imaging as an adjunct modality to mammography for diagnosis of breast cancer: a systemic review and meta-analysis. Eur J Nucl Med Mol Imaging. 2013;40(3):450–63.

33. Miles RC, Gullerud RE, Lohse CM, Jakub JW, Degnim AC, Boughey JC. Local recurrence after breast-conserving surgery: multivariable analysis of risk factors and the impact of young age. Ann Surg Oncol. 2012;19(4):1153–9.

34. Elkhuizen PH, van de Vijver MJ, Hermans J, Zonderland HM, van de Velde CJ, Leer JW. Local recurrence after breast-conserving therapy for invasive breast cancer: high incidence in young patients and association with poor survival. Int J Radiat Oncol Biol Phys. 1998;40(4):859–67.

35. Clarke M, Collins R, Darby S, Davies C, Elphinstone P, Evans E, Early Breast Cancer Trialists' Collaborative Group (EBCTCG), et al. Effects of radiotherapy and of differences in the extent of surgery for early breast cancer on local recurrence and 15-year survival: an overview of the randomised trials. Lancet. 2005;366(9503):2087–106.

36. Dragun AE, Pan J, Riley EC, Kruse B, Wilson MR, Rai S, et al. Increasing use of elective mastectomy and contralateral prophylactic surgery among breast conservation candidates: a 14-year report from a comprehensive cancer center. Am J Clin Oncol. 2013;36(4):375–80.

37. Lee MC, Rogers K, Griffith K, Diehl KA, Breslin TM, Cimmino VM, et al. Determinants of breast conservation rates: reasons for mastectomy at a comprehensive cancer center. Breast J. 2009;15(1):34–40.

38. McGuire KP, Santillan AA, Kaur P, Meade T, Parbhoo J, Mathias M, et al. Are mastectomies on the rise? A 13-year trend analysis of the selection of mastectomy versus breast conservation therapy in 5865 patients. Ann Surg Oncol. 2009;16(10):2682–90.

39. Feigelson HS, James TA, Single RM, Onitilo AA, Aiello Bowles EJ, Barney T, et al. Factors associated with the frequency of initial total mastectomy: results of a multi-institutional study. J Am Coll Surg. 2013;216(5):966–75.

40. Bedrosian I, Hu C-Y, Chang GJ. Population-based study of contralateral prophylactic mastectomy and survival outcomes of breast cancer patients. J Natl Cancer Inst. 2010;102(6):401–9.

41. Graves K, Peshkin B, Halbert C, DeMarco T, Isaacs C, Schwartz M. Predictors and outcomes of contralateral prophylactic mastectomy among breast cancer survivors. Breast Cancer Res Treat. 2007;104(3):321–9.

42. Howard-McNatt M, Schroll RW, Hurt GJ, Levine EA. Contralateral prophylactic mastectomy in breast cancer patients who test negative for BRCA mutations. Am J Surg. 2011;202(3):298–302.

43. Stucky CC, Gray RJ, Wasif N, Dueck AC, Pockaj BA. Increase in contralateral prophylactic mastectomy: echoes of a bygone era? Surgical trends for unilateral breast cancer. Ann Surg Oncol. 2010;17 Suppl 3:330–7.

44. Tuttle TM, Habermann EB, Grund EH, Morris TJ, Virnig BA. Increasing use of contralateral prophylactic mastectomy for breast cancer patients: a trend toward more aggressive surgical treatment. J Clin Oncol. 2007;25(33):5203–9.

45. Zendejas B, Moriarty JP, O'Byrne J, Degnim AC, Farley DR, Boughey JC. Cost-effectiveness of contra-

lateral prophylactic mastectomy versus routine surveillance in patients with unilateral breast cancer. J Clin Oncol. 2011;29(22):2993–3000.

46. Robson ME, Chappuis PO, Satagopan J, Wong N, Boyd J, Goffin JR, et al. A combined analysis of outcome following breast cancer: differences in survival based on BRCA1/BRCA2 mutation status and administration of adjuvant treatment. Breast Cancer Res. 2004;6(1):R8–17.

47. Evans DG, Ingham S, Baildam A, Ross G, Lalloo F, Buchan I, et al. Contralateral mastectomy improves survival in women with BRCA1/2-associated breast cancer. Breast Cancer Res Treat. 2013;140(1): 135–42.

48. Giuliano AE, Chung AP. Long-term follow-up confirms the oncologic safety of sentinel node biopsy without axillary dissection in node-negative breast cancer patients. Ann Surg. 2010;251(4):601–3.

49. Giuliano AE, Dale PS, Turner RR, Morton DL, Evans SW, Krasne DL. Improved axillary staging of breast cancer with sentinel lymphadenectomy. Ann Surg. 1995;222(3):394–9; discussion 9-401.

50. Krag DN, Anderson SJ, Julian TB, Brown AM, Harlow SP, Ashikaga T, et al. Technical outcomes of sentinel-lymph-node resection and conventional axillary-lymph-node dissection in patients with clinically node-negative breast cancer: results from the NSABP B-32 randomised phase III trial. Lancet Oncol. 2007;8(10):881–8.

51. Giuliano AE, Hunt KK, Ballman KV, Beitsch PD, Whitworth PW, Blumencranz PW, et al. Axillary dissection vs no axillary dissection in women with invasive breast cancer and sentinel node metastasis: a randomized clinical trial. JAMA. 2011;305(6):569–75.

52. Giuliano AE, McCall L, Beitsch P, Whitworth PW, Blumencranz P, Leitch AM, et al. Locoregional recurrence after sentinel lymph node dissection with or without axillary dissection in patients with sentinel lymph node metastases: the American College of Surgeons Oncology Group Z0011 randomized trial. Ann Surg. 2010;252(3):426–32; discussion 32–3.

53. Cardoso F, Loibl S, Pagani O, Graziottin A, Panizza P, Martincich L, et al. The European Society of Breast Cancer Specialists recommendations for the management of young women with breast cancer. Eur J Cancer. 2012;48(18):3355–77.

54. Overgaard M, Hansen PS, Overgaard J, Rose C, Andersson M, Bach F, et al. Postoperative radiotherapy in high-risk premenopausal women with breast cancer who receive adjuvant chemotherapy. Danish Breast Cancer Cooperative Group 82b Trial. N Engl J Med. 1997;337(14):949–55.

55. Overgaard M, Jensen MB, Overgaard J, Hansen PS, Rose C, Andersson M, et al. Postoperative radiotherapy in high-risk postmenopausal breast-cancer patients given adjuvant tamoxifen: Danish Breast Cancer Cooperative Group DBCG 82c randomised trial. Lancet. 1999;353(9165):1641–8.

56. Mathews T, Hamiltom BE. Delayed childbearing: more women are having their first child later in life, NCHS data brief, no 21. Hyattsville: National Center for Health Statistics; 2009.

57. Minton SE, Munster PN. Chemotherapy-induced amenorrhea and fertility in women undergoing adjuvant treatment for breast cancer. Cancer Control. 2002;9(6):466–72.

58. Wallace WH, Kelsey TW. Human ovarian reserve from conception to the menopause. PLoS One. 2010;5(1):e8772.

59. Pentheroudakis G, Pavlidis N, Castiglione M. Cancer, fertility and pregnancy: ESMO clinical recommendations for diagnosis, treatment and follow-up. Ann Oncol. 2009;20 Suppl 4:178–81.

60. Loren AW, Mangu PB, Beck LN, Brennan L, Magdalinski AJ, Partridge AH, et al. Fertility preservation for patients with cancer: American Society of Clinical Oncology clinical practice guideline update. J Clin Oncol. 2013;31(19):2500–10.

61. Combelles CM, Chateau G. The use of immature oocytes in the fertility preservation of cancer patients: current promises and challenges. Int J Dev Biol. 2012;56(10–12):919–29.

62. Azim AA, Costantini-Ferrando M, Oktay K. Safety of fertility preservation by ovarian stimulation with letrozole and gonadotropins in patients with breast cancer: a prospcctive controlled study. J Clin Oncol. 2008;26(16):2630–5.

63. Rodriguez-Wallberg KA, Oktay K. Fertility preservation in women with breast cancer. Clin Obstet Gynecol. 2010;53(4):753–62.

64. Chung K, Donnez J, Ginsburg E, Meirow D. Emergency IVF versus ovarian tissue cryopreservation: decision making in fertility preservation for female cancer patients. Fertil Steril. 2013;99(6):1534–42.

65. Donnez J, Dolmans MM, Pellicer A, Diaz-Garcia C, Sanchez Serrano M, Schmidt KT, et al. Restoration of ovarian activity and pregnancy after transplantation of cryopreserved ovarian tissue: a review of 60 cases of reimplantation. Fertil Steril. 2013;99(6):1503–13.

66. Bouchlariotou S, Tsikouras P, Benjamin R, Neulen J. Fertility sparing in cancer patients. Minim Invasive Ther Allied Technol. 2012;21(4):282–92.

67. Del Mastro L. Temporary ovarian suppression with goserelin and ovarian function protection in patients with breast cancer undergoing chemotherapy. J Clin Oncol. 2011;29(24):3339–40; author reply 41–2.

68. Kim SS, Lee JR, Jee BC, Suh CS, Kim SH, Ting A, et al. Use of hormonal protection for chemotherapy-induced gonadotoxicity. Clin Obstet Gynecol. 2010;53(4):740–52.

69. Lee MC, Gray J, Han HS, Plosker S. Fertility and reproductive considerations in premenopausal patients with breast cancer. Cancer Control. 2010;17(3):162–72.

70. Northouse LL. Breast cancer in younger women: effects on interpersonal and family relations. J Natl Cancer Inst Monogr. 1994;16:183–90.

71. Alder J, Zanetti R, Wight E, Urech C, Fink N, Bitzer J. Sexual dysfunction after premenopausal stage I and II breast cancer: do androgens play a role? J Sex Med. 2008;5(8):1898–906.

72. Al-Baghdadi O, Ewies AA. Topical estrogen therapy in the management of postmenopausal vaginal atrophy: an up-to-date overview. Climacteric. 2009;12(2):91–105.

73. Melisko ME, Goldman M, Rugo HS. Amelioration of sexual adverse effects in the early breast cancer patient. J Cancer Surviv. 2010;4(3):247–55.

74. Sinha A, Ewies AA. Non-hormonal topical treatment of vulvovaginal atrophy: an up-to-date overview. Climacteric. 2013;16(3):305–12.

75. Lindsay R, Hart DM, Aitken JM, MacDonald EB, Anderson JB, Clarke AC. Long-term prevention of postmenopausal osteoporosis by oestrogen. Evidence for an increased bone mass after delayed onset of oestrogen treatment. Lancet. 1976;1(7968):1038–41.

76. Abdalla HI, Hart DM, Lindsay R, Leggate I, Hooke A. Prevention of bone mineral loss in postmenopausal women by norethisterone. Obstet Gynecol. 1985;66(6):789–92.

77. Powles TJ, Hickish T, Kanis JA, Tidy A, Ashley S. Effect of tamoxifen on bone mineral density measured by dual-energy x-ray absorptiometry in healthy premenopausal and postmenopausal women. J Clin Oncol. 1996;14(1):78–84.

78. Shapiro C, Halabi S, Gibson G, et al. CALGB 78909: phase III trial of intravenous zoledronic acid in the prevention of bone loss in localized breast cancer patients with chemotherapy-induced ovarian failure. Clin Adv Hematol Oncol. 2005;3(2):105–6.

79. Kim JE, Ahn JH, Jung KH, Kim SB, Kim HJ, Lee KS, et al. Zoledronic acid prevents bone loss in premenopausal women with early breast cancer undergoing adjuvant chemotherapy: a phase III trial of the Korean Cancer Study Group (KCSG-BR06-01). Breast Cancer Res Treat. 2011;125(1):99–106.

80. Hershman DL, McMahon DJ, Crew KD, Cremers S, Irani D, Cucchiara G, et al. Zoledronic acid prevents bone loss in premenopausal women undergoing adjuvant chemotherapy for early-stage breast cancer. J Clin Oncol. 2008;26(29):4739–45.

81. Hershman DL, McMahon DJ, Crew KD, Shao T, Cremers S, Brafman L, et al. Prevention of bone loss by zoledronic acid in premenopausal women undergoing adjuvant chemotherapy persist up to one year following discontinuing treatment. J Clin Endocrinol Metab. 2010;95(2):559–66.

82. Houssami N, Macaskill P, von Minckwitz G, Marinovich ML, Mamounas E. Meta-analysis of the association of breast cancer subtype and pathologic complete response to neoadjuvant chemotherapy. Eur J Cancer. 2012;48(18):3342–54.

83. Colleoni M, Rotmensz N, Robertson C, Orlando L, Viale G, Renne G, et al. Very young women (<35 years) with operable breast cancer: features of disease at presentation. Ann Oncol. 2002;13(2):273–9.

84. Huober J, von Minckwitz G, Denkert C, Tesch H, Weiss E, Zahm DM, et al. Effect of neoadjuvant anthracycline-taxane-based chemotherapy in different biological breast cancer phenotypes: overall results from the GeparTrio study. Breast Cancer Res Treat. 2010;124(1):133–40.

85. Early Breast Cancer Trialists' Collaborative Group (EBCTCG). Effects of chemotherapy and hormonal therapy for early breast cancer on recurrence and 15-year survival: an overview of the randomised trials. Lancet. 2005;365(9472):1687–717.

86. Griggs JJ, Somerfield MR, Anderson H, Henry NL, Hudis CA, Khatcheressian JL, et al. American Society of Clinical Oncology endorsement of the cancer care Ontario practice guideline on adjuvant ovarian ablation in the treatment of premenopausal women with early-stage invasive breast cancer. J Clin Oncol. 2011;29(29):3939–42.

87. Gnant M, Mlineritsch B, Stoeger H, Luschin-Ebengreuth G, Heck D, Menzel C, et al. Adjuvant endocrine therapy plus zoledronic acid in premenopausal women with early-stage breast cancer: 62-month follow-up from the ABCSG-12 randomised trial. Lancet Oncol. 2011;12(7):631–41.

88. Love RR, Duc NB, Allred DC, Binh NC, Dinh NV, Kha NN, et al. Oophorectomy and tamoxifen adjuvant therapy in premenopausal Vietnamese and Chinese women with operable breast cancer. J Clin Oncol. 2002;20(10):2559–66.

89. Love RR, Duc NB, Dinh NV, Shen TZ, Havighurst TC, Allred DC, et al. Mastectomy and oophorectomy by menstrual cycle phase in women with operable breast cancer. J Natl Cancer Inst. 2002;94(9):662–9.

90. Ellis MJ, Suman VJ, Hoog J, Lin L, Snider J, Prat A, et al. Randomized phase II neoadjuvant comparison between letrozole, anastrozole, and exemestane for postmenopausal women with estrogen receptor-rich stage 2 to 3 breast cancer: clinical and biomarker outcomes and predictive value of the baseline PAM50-based intrinsic subtype – ACOSOG Z1031. J Clin Oncol. 2011;29(17):2342–9.

91. Takei H, Kurosumi M, Yoshida T, Hayashi Y, Higuchi T, Uchida S, et al. Neoadjuvant endocrine therapy of breast cancer: which patients would benefit and what are the advantages? Breast Cancer. 2011;18(2):85–91.

92. Klijn JG, Beex LV, Mauriac L, van Zijl JA, Veyret C, Wildiers J, et al. Combined treatment with buserelin and tamoxifen in premenopausal metastatic breast cancer: a randomized study. J Natl Cancer Inst. 2000;92(11):903–11.

93. Torrisi R, Bagnardi V, Pruneri G, Ghisini R, Bottiglieri L, Magni E, et al. Antitumour and biological effects of letrozole and GnRH analogue as primary therapy in premenopausal women with ER and PgR positive locally advanced operable breast cancer. Br J Cancer. 2007;97(6):802–8.

94. Masuda N, Sagara Y, Kinoshita T, Iwata H, Nakamura S, Yanagita Y, et al. Neoadjuvant anastrozole versus tamoxifen in patients receiving goserelin for

premenopausal breast cancer (STAGE): a double-blind, randomised phase 3 trial. Lancet Oncol. 2012;13(4):345–52.

95. Fisher B, Dignam J, Bryant J, Wolmark N. Five versus more than five years of tamoxifen for lymph node-negative breast cancer: updated findings from the National Surgical Adjuvant Breast and Bowel Project B-14 randomized trial. J Natl Cancer Inst. 2001;93(9):684–90.

96. Fisher B, Dignam J, Bryant J, DeCillis A, Wickerham DL, Wolmark N, et al. Five versus more than five years of tamoxifen therapy for breast cancer patients with negative lymph nodes and estrogen receptor-positive tumors. J Natl Cancer Inst. 1996;88(21):1529–42.

97. Davies C, Pan H, Godwin J, Gray R, Arriagada R, Raina V, et al. Long-term effects of continuing adjuvant tamoxifen to 10 years versus stopping at 5 years after diagnosis of oestrogen receptor-positive breast cancer: ATLAS, a randomised trial. Lancet. 2013;381(9869):805–16.

98. Goss PE, Ingle JN, Martino S, Robert NJ, Muss HB, Piccart MJ, et al. Efficacy of letrozole extended adjuvant therapy according to estrogen receptor and progesterone receptor status of the primary tumor: National Cancer Institute of Canada Clinical Trials Group MA.17. J Clin Oncol. 2007;25(15):2006–11.

Abdullah İğci, Mustafa Tükenmez,
and Enver Özkurt

Abstract

Breast cancer is observed in men 100-fold less often than in women. The risk of breast cancer in men is approximately 1 in 1,000 throughout life. The American Association of Cancer predicted that 2,360 men would be diagnosed with breast cancer in 2014 and that 430 male patients with breast cancer would die. Anderson et al. reported on male breast cancer (MBC) from the Surveillance, Epidemiology, and End Result (SEER) database during the period of 1973–2005 and found an annual increase in incidence of 1.19 %, with a peak in 2000 of 1.24 cases per 100,000 men. The frequency is 0.1 deaths per 100,000 cases at 35 years of age and reaches up to 11.1 deaths per 100,000 cases after 85 years of age. The mean age of diagnosis of MBC is 67.68, which is 5–10 years older than for female breast cancer (FBC) patients in the USA, but in other parts of the world, such as the Middle East and South Asia, the age gap is smaller.

In a study based on an international population, the world-standardized incidence rates of breast cancer were 66.7 per 105 person-years in women and 0.40 per 105 person-years in men.

Previous studies have shown that MBC cases are significantly different from female cases, whereas new studies have reported that breast cancer has similar characteristics at the same stages in both genders.

Keywords

Male breast cancer • Sentinel lymph node • Mastectomy • Axillary dissection • Adjuvant therapy

A. İğci, MD, FACS (✉)
Breast Unit, Department of General Surgery,
Istanbul University, Istanbul Medical Faculty,
Istanbul, Turkey
e-mail: aigci@istanbul.edu.tr

M. Tükenmez, MD • E. Özkurt, MD
Department of General Surgery, Istanbul Medical
Faculty, Istanbul University, Istanbul, Turkey
e-mail: mdmustafatukenmez@gmail.com;
doctorenver@gmail.com

© Springer International Publishing Switzerland 2016
A. Aydiner et al. (eds.), *Breast Disease: Management and Therapies*,
DOI 10.1007/978-3-319-26012-9_23

Introduction

Breast cancer is observed in men 100-fold less often than in women [1, 2]. The risk of breast cancer for men is approximately 1 in 1,000 throughout life. The American Association of Cancer predicts that 2,360 men will be diagnosed with breast cancer in 2014 and 430 male patients with breast cancer will die [3, 4]. Breast cancer is responsible for 0.1 % of cancer-dependent deaths in men [5, 6]. Similar to women, breast cancer is observed more frequently in the left breast in men [7]. The bilateral case rate is 1.4 % [8]. The incidence is lower in Japan, Colombia, Singapore, Finland, and Hungary, whereas the incidence is higher in North America and England and very high in some African countries [9, 10].

Anderson et al. reported on male breast cancer (MBC) from the Surveillance, Epidemiology, and End Result (SEER) database during the period of 1973–2005 and found an annual increase in incidence of 1.19 %, with a peak in 2000 of 1.24 cases per 100,000 men [11].

There is no difference in the frequency of death from MBC between Europe and the USA [3]. The frequency is 0.1 deaths per 100,000 cases at 35 years of age and reaches up to 11.1 deaths per 100,000 cases after 85 years. One percent of MBC is observed in males younger than 30, and 6 % of cases are detected below the age of 40 [12]. The mean age of diagnosis of MBC is 67.68, which is 5–10 years older than for female breast cancer (FBC) patients in the USA, but in other parts of the world, such as the Middle East and South Asia, the age gap is smaller [3, 13–16].

In a study based on an international population [17], the world-standardized incidence rates of breast cancer were 66.7 per 105 person-years in women and 0.40 per 105 person-years in men. Women were diagnosed at a younger median age (61.7 years) than men (69.6 years).

Previous studies have shown that MBC cases are significantly different from female cases, but new studies have reported that breast cancer has similar characteristics at the same stages in both genders [12].

Epidemiology and Risk Factors

The majority of cases are sporadic. Only 5–10 % of all male breast cancer cases are considered to be related to a genetic predisposition [18–21]. In a study investigating the familial characteristics of men with breast cancer, FBC or ovarian cancer cases were reported by 30 % of the families that included men with breast cancer [22, 23]. The risk of breast cancer in the sister or daughter of a patient with breast cancer is increased by two to threefold [10]. Breast cancer was reported in two brothers, one of whom also had prostate cancer [24]. BRCA1 is a suppressor gene that has been isolated and located on chromosome 17q. The risk of breast cancer increases in the presence of this germline mutation, and the disease appears at early ages in patients with mutations in BRCA1. BRCA2, which has been localized to chromosome 13, has been reported to be responsible for 70 % of hereditary breast cancer cases [25]. The genetic presence of the BRCA2 germline mutation is a risk factor for early-age MBC. A mutation in BRCA2 is not likely to exist in MBC cases without a family history of breast cancer [16, 22, 26]. BRCA2 and BRCA1 were detected by 77 % and 19 % of cases with familial MBC, respectively [27]. Breast cancer eventually develops in 5–10 % of men with BRCA2 mutations (and in a smaller proportion of those with BRCA1 mutations) [28].

In a study conducted in Iceland, mutations in BRCA2 were found at rates of 0.6 % in the community, 7.7 % in patients with FBC, and 40 % in the patients with MBC [20]. Breast cancer cases with the BRCA2 mutation generally have similar prognostic characteristics as the cases without the mutation; however, the nuclear grade tends to be higher in those with the mutation, and the frequency of p53 mutation is increased [22]. In another collaborative multicenter study from Italy [29], BRCA2 mutations were associated with a family history of breast/ovarian cancer ($p=0.0001$), a personal history of other cancers ($p=0.044$), and contralateral breast cancer (BC) ($p=0.001$). BRCA2-associated MBCs presented with high tumor grade ($p=0.001$), PR- ($p=0.026$), and HER2+ ($p=0.001$) status. Ding et al. reported from the USA that the difference in BRCA2 mutation frequencies between cases with and without a family history of breast cancer was not statistically significant ($p=0.145$), suggesting that in males, family history is not a strong predictor of carrying a mutation [30]. They observed that carrying a pathogenic BRCA2 mutation showed a highly significant association with a high tumor grade ($p=0.001$) and a weak association with positive lymph nodes ($p=0.02$). Of the 97 BRCA2-negative MBC cases, they identified one PALB2 mutation with confirmed pathogenicity and one mutation predicted to be pathogenic, corresponding to a prevalence of pathogenic PALB2 mutations of 1–2 %. Based on their results and previous studies, they recommend genetic testing for BRCA2 for any diagnosed MBC case, regardless of the family history of breast cancer.

Data are mixed regarding the relevance of other germline mutations such as those in PALB2, the androgen receptor (AR), CYP17, and CHEK2 [31–34]. Other mutations that increase the risk of FBC (e.g., BRIP1 and RAD51C) have not been found to increase the risk of MBC [35, 36], and one study reports that polymorphisms in the vitamin D receptor do not appear to be associated with risk [37]. Lists of main risk factors for male breast cancer are listed in Table 23.1.

In the studies conducted on the BRCA1 and BRCA2 genes, MBC was shown to have a greater association with the BRCA2 gene [18]. BRCA2 is considered a useful marker for identifying men with higher risk of breast cancer [18].

Mutations in p53, a tumor suppressor gene, result in Li-Fraumeni syndrome. It is reported that the incidence of breast cancer and many other tumor types increases when suppression disappears upon p53 mutation [15]. There is no convincing evidence for the association of MBC with gynecomastia, which is considered to be related to common hormonal risk factors [38].

Klinefelter's syndrome (genotype XXY) is a syndrome including characteristics such as less developed sex organs, gynecomastia, small testicles, aspermatogenesis, and increased FSH. It is the strongest risk factor for MBC, and the risk increases by 50-fold compared to a male with a

Table 23.1 Main risk factors for male breast cancer

Genetics	Endocrine
Klinefelter's syndrome	Liver disease
Family history of breast cancer	Exogenous estrogens
BRCA2 mutations	Androgen deficiency (prolactinoma)
BRCA1 mutations	
Ashkenazi Jewish men	
Cowden syndrome	

Environmental, occupational, and other factors
Chest wall radiation
Testicular disorders
Undescended testes, congenital
Inguinal hernia, orchiectomy
Orchitis, infertility
Lifestyle
Obesity, alcohol, diet
Occupational and environmental exposures
Occupational exposure to heat
High ambient temperature
Exhaust emissions
Electromagnetic field radiation

normal genotype [39–43]. Hypertrophy in the breasts of such men is secondary to gynecomastia and the development of acini and lobules [44]. Patients with Klinefelter's syndrome have significant hyperestrogenemia in their blood, and the incidence of breast cancer in such male patients reaches 6 % [25]. Whether causes of gynecomastia other than Klinefelter's syndrome increase, the risk for MBC remains unknown. However, when slides from Klinefelter's syndrome patients with MBC are examined histologically, microscopic findings of gynecomastia are observed in 40 % of cases [45]. The most common side effect of finasteride, which is used for the treatment of prostate hyperplasia, is gynecomastia; additionally, breast cancer was reported in three patients who used finasteride [46].

In the MBC pooling project [47] involving a consortium of 11 case-control and 10 cohort investigations involving 2,405 case patients ($n=1,190$ from case-control and $n=1,215$ from cohort studies) and 52,013 control subjects, individual participant data were harmonized and pooled. Risk of MBC was significantly associated with weight (highest/lowest tertile: OR=1.36; 95 % CI=1.18–1.57), height (OR=1.18; 95 % CI=1.01–1.38), and body mass index (BMI; OR=1.30; 95 % CI=1.12–1.51), with evidence that recent rather than distant BMI was the strongest predictor. Klinefelter's syndrome (OR=24.7; 95 % CI=8.94–68.4) and gynecomastia (OR=9.78; 95 % CI=7.52–12.7) were also significantly associated with the risk, independent of BMI, and diabetes emerged as another independent risk factor (OR=1.19; 95 % CI=1.04–1.37). Additionally, there were trends indicating relationships with cryptorchidism (OR=2.18; 95 % CI=0.96–4.94) and orchitis (OR=1.43; 95 % CI=1.02–1.99). Although age at the onset of puberty and histories of infertility were unrelated to risk, never having had children was statistically significantly related (OR=1.29; 95 % CI=1.01–1.66). Among individuals diagnosed at older ages, a history of fractures was statistically significantly related (OR=1.41; 95 % CI=1.07–1.86).

In men, obesity is associated with high levels of estrogen and low levels of testosterone and sex-hormone-binding globulin [48], leading to greater estrogen bioavailability. Thyroid diseases, marijuana use, and external estrogen cause gynecomastia, but their associations with MBC are much weaker. Only 2 of more than 17,000 patients who were treated with estrogen because of prostate cancer developed breast cancer [20]. Increases in estrogen circulation and hepatic metabolism may explain the increased incidence for MBC as follows: hepatic dysfunction because of cirrhosis and chronic malnutrition is common in some territories of Africa and is connected with increased rates of MBC [49]. The incidence of MBC is increased in regions where schistosomiasis is common. This parasitic infestation causes hepatic failure and hyperestrogenemia. In Egypt, where schistosomiasis is endemic, MBC was reported more frequently than prostate cancer [25].

Chronic liver diseases with other etiologies have also theoretically increased the risk for the development of MBC; however, severe hepatic dysfunction has a high mortality rate; thus, the increased risk may become significant [38]. MBC accompanying liver disease is observed in younger ages (40–50) and more frequently (15 %) in Zambia [10].

In testicular abnormalities that cause androgen deficiency, an increase in the incidence of MBC was reported in men with orchitis, undescended testicles, and testicle injuries [50, 51]. Radiation is also a risk factor for men and women. Cancer develops 12–36 years after contact with radiation [52]. Exposure to radiation of over 50–100 cGy during childhood or adolescence increases the risk of cancer similarly in both sexes [44, 49]. Unlike in women, white race does not appear to be a risk factor in men [53].

Work and environmental factors may also play an increasing role in MBC. Based on a multicenter case-control study that was conducted in eight European countries and included 104 cases and 1,901 controls, it was concluded that some environmental chemicals are possible mammary carcinogens [54]. Petrol, organic petroleum solvents, or polycyclic aromatic hydrocarbons are suspect because of the consistent elevated risk of MBC observed in motor vehicle mechanics. Endocrine disruptors such as alkylphenolic compounds may play a role in breast cancer. The prevalence is increased in those who work in high temperature ovens and steel factories because of cancer potentialization; in other words, testicular failure appeared as a result of heat [12, 18]. Vapors of gasoline and other flammable substances were shown to play a role in the appearance of breast cancer in men [54, 55].

Long-term therapy with the drugs which are commonly used today and cause hyperestrogenemia such as digital agents, cimetidine, methyldopa, and spironolactone has higher risk of breast cancer [56]. Obesity of which the frequency gradually increases in economically developed countries has become a social problem. Especially, obesity under age of 30 is a risk factor for breast cancer in women as well as men. The suggested mechanism of appearance is the increase in conversion of androgens into estrogen in increased fat tissue. Other risk factors include being unmarried, being Jewish, the presence of previous benign breast disease history, late puberty, and hypercholesterolemia [56].

Clinical Progress

Patients with MBC generally refer with a hard and painless mass located centrally under the nipple. The mass secondly settles in the upper-outer quadrant [57]. Nipple ulceration is commonly observed, but first referral with an efflux from the nipple is rare [25]. However, if serous-hemorrhagic efflux comes out of the nipple, the underlying disease is cancer in general (75 %). If metastasis exists, patients may complain about cough and bone pain [10]. It is more common in the left breast [58]. Bilateral masses are very rare (0–1.9 %). The period between onset of the disease and diagnosis is 18 weeks to 6 months [10]. Moreover, easy invasion of the dermal tissue in MBC because its superficial and central location causes to diagnose the disease during advanced stages [59].

Diagnosis

Breast cancer biology is distinct in men, but diagnostic approaches and treatments for men are generally extrapolated from those in women due to inadequate research in men [60]. Perhaps due to poor awareness of the disease and diagnostic delays, most (but not all) studies suggest that men are diagnosed with higher stage tumors and have a poorer prognosis overall [61, 62]. It often presents as a painless subareolar lump [63].

MBC is diagnosed with biopsy. Fine-needle aspiration biopsy (FNAB) may be performed in medical centers where experienced cytopathologists are employed. If FNAB is not appropriate, tru-cut biopsy should be performed. Removal of sufficient tissue is important both for diagnosis and determination of hormone receptors [12, 49]. Two studies that compared FNA with core and/or excision biopsies demonstrated that the former had sensitivity and specificity that approached 100 % [64]. Chest X-ray, bone scintigraphy, and liver enzymes should be assessed to determine invasion of the disease before the treatment [41]. Clinical examination is invaluable, although it must be noted that concurrent gynecomastia, the most common breast-related diagnosis in men, may mask an underlying tumor [65].

Gynecomastia which is generally confused with MBC in mammography is observed as a nodular lesion with three edges and small extensions in subareolar area. Edges are irregular in general. It should be noted that cancers may be hidden well in such benign density increases and nodularities. Although microcalcifications are not cancer specific, they are the most important traces for malignancy in mammography. Evaluation with mammography only is difficult for men [16, 65] (Fig. 23.1). Calcifications are not in spot or stick form like observed in women; they are generally wider and round. The mass is solid, spiculated, and located eccentrically associated with the nipple (Fig. 23.2) in general [65]. The mass in gynecomastia is symmetrically associated with the nipple. Breast skin retraction may exist in malignancies. Enlargements on axillary lymph nodes may be observed via mammography [66, 67]. Male patients with cancer on one breast may be followed by mammography to search a secondary tumor on the other breast. Cases with non-palpable breast cancer were reported by mammography in the normal breast which seems clinically normal.

Subareolar triangular, anechoic, and hyperechoic fibroglandular appearances exist in gynecomastia by ultrasound. Ultrasonographic microcalcifications in MBC are not detected in the ultrasound. Structural distortion, asymmetric

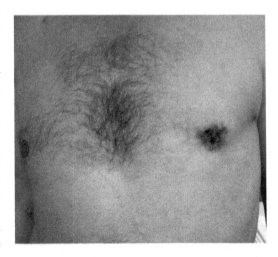

Fig. 23.1 Physical examination finding of a 45-year-old male showing ulceration around his nipple

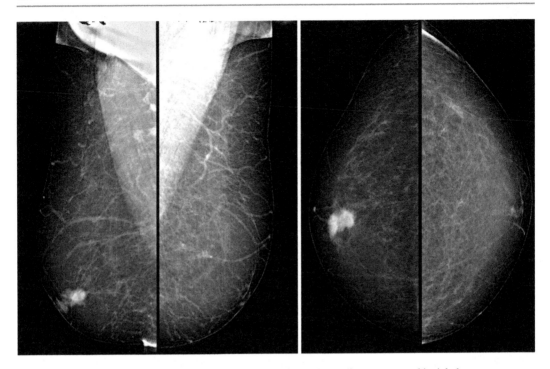

Fig. 23.2 Mammography imaging of a 65-year-old male patient with a malignant mass on his right breast

appearance in nipple shadows, and shadowing around the nipple may be detected by the ultrasound (Fig. 23.3). Ultrasonography generally visualizes a mass with hypoechogenicity and indistinct or irregular margins [65]. The use of ultrasound alone is deemed insufficient for male breast growths. However, much attention should be paid during diagnosis when suspicious changes are found by either ultrasound or mammography. In some cases, the combination of both techniques may be required for the final diagnosis [66, 67]. Clinical examination, ultrasound, and mammography may reduce the need for biopsy in patients who are considered to have a benign disease [68].

Smear examination is required for patients with nipple efflux. When a mass is detected on the breast of a man, a procedure should be run for histological diagnosis to definitively differentiate between benign and malign disease. This may be performed by fine needle aspiration, core needle biopsy, or open biopsy. A cytological examination performed by fine needle aspiration biopsy depends on the experience of the clinician and cytopathologist. In fact, the use of such a technique is safer with increased experience; however, fine needle aspiration biopsy is not

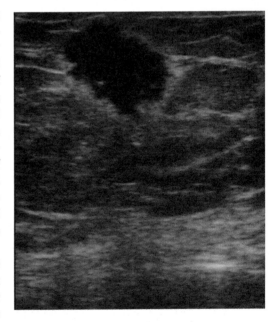

Fig. 23.3 Ultrasonographic imaging of a 65-year-old male patient with a malignant mass on his right breast

commonly used for differentiation of the lesion on the male breast. The gold standard is open biopsy [49]. Cellularity, dyshesion, and morphism are important criteria for the diagnosis of cancer, which is also assisted by nuclear changes.

A mild cellularity or cellular failure exists in gynecomastia. Although anisonucleosis may exist in gynecomastia, a smooth surface of the membrane indicates a benign case. Honeycomb pattern, macronucleus, and mixed cell groups support malignancy [69].

Differential Diagnosis

The differential diagnosis should be made between gynecomastia and cancer for male breast masses. The most common unilateral or bilateral benign mass is gynecomastia [70]. It is generally detected by physical examination. Gynecomastia is characteristically a symmetrical, bilateral discoid under the nipple and areola. Carcinomas have an eccentric settlement and a hard mass; no sensitivity exists. Breast skin adjacencies may be observed both in gynecomastia and carcinoma. However, adjacency to the pectoral fascia, nipple efflux, nipple inversion, and ulceration are only detected in breast cancer. These characteristics are difficult to determine in adults, and a biopsy should be performed in any suspicious case [12]. Benign neoplasms are extremely rare in a male breast. Cystosarcoma phyllodes, phylloid papillomatosis, ductal papillomas, lipomas, and other tumor types that are not associated with the breast may be detected on the breast [49].

Pathology

The distribution of breast cancer in male and female patients differs because of the lack of lobule development in the male breast. Because a normal male breast does not contain any lobular elements, the most frequent cancer type detected in men is invasive ductal carcinoma (85–90 %) [71]. Invasive lobular cancer or lobular carcinoma in situ has been reported in several cases with a normal genetic profile and without any history of hormone use [8]. All histological types of the breast cancer observed in women (ductal carcinoma in situ, medullary, papillary, and colloid) can also be observed in men (Table 23.2). Inflammatory breast cancer and Paget disease were also reported in men. Granular cell tumor, adenoid cystic carcinoma, myofibroblastoma,

Table 23.2 Frequency of histological types observed

Histology	Incidence (%)
Invasive ductal carcinoma	90
Ductal carcinoma in situ	10
Invasive papillary carcinoma	2
Medullary carcinoma	2
Mucinous carcinoma	1
Paget disease	1
Lobular carcinoma	1

carcinoid tumor, and metastatic tumors (generally originating from the lungs and prostate) are other possible tumor types [38].

The vast majority of MBCs are hormone sensitive [72, 73]. MBC shows higher estrogen (75–94 %) and progesterone (67–96 %) hormone receptor positivity than does breast cancer in women. In the National Cancer Institute's Surveillance, Epidemiology, and End Result (SEER) database between 1973 and 2005, 92 % of the 5,494 MBCs but only 78 % of the 838,805 FBCs were estrogen receptor (ER) positive [53]. Receptor positivity was not reported to be associated with age, histological grade, stage, and axillary lymph node involvement [8].

Information with other molecular and genetic markers is limited for MBC [74]. The Mayo Clinic assessed 111 cases and reported positive estrogen receptors in 91 % of cases; positive progesterone receptors in 96 % of cases; positive androgen receptors in 95 % of cases; the expression of bcl-2, which is a determinant for apoptosis, in 94 % of cases; p53, which is one of the proto-oncogenes, in 21 % of cases; HER-2 in 29 % of cases; and cyclin D1, which is one of the cell cycle regulatory proteins, in 58 % of cases [75]. The overexpression of cyclin D1 and c-myc may correlate with better outcomes [76]. In addition, studies have reported higher rates of HER-2 in 40 % of cases and p52 in 54 % of cases [10, 72, 77, 78].

Treatment

Treatment for Early-Stage Male Breast Cancer

Treatment in early-stage MBC patients is surgical followed by adjuvant endocrine, chemotherapy, or radiotherapy according to the prognostic factors. A large population-based study conducted in Europe and Asia demonstrated that males with BC were significantly less likely to receive surgery and radiation therapy (RT) than females with BC. However, the rates of the use of chemotherapy and hormonal therapy were similar [17].

Surgical Treatment

Surgical options for men with early-stage breast cancer include breast-conserving therapy and mastectomy [79]. Standard treatment is mastectomy and sentinel node biopsy or axillary lymph node dissection [23, 80]. Radical mastectomy has been performed throughout the history of MBC. Today, this method is applied for wide chest wall invasions only. Currently, most patients undergo modified radical mastectomy [79]. The rarity of breast-protective therapy may be because men have less breast tissue than women and have tumors located more centrally; in addition, male patients do not request breast-protective therapy [18].

In a study from the USA, the Surveillance, Epidemiology, and End Result (SEER) database was used to identify all MBC patients who underwent either mastectomy or less than mastectomy between 1983 and 2009 [81]. A total of 4,707 (86.8 %) men underwent mastectomy and 718 (13.2 %) underwent lumpectomy. They mentioned that lumpectomy was performed in a small but growing proportion of MBC patients. These patients were not only older and more likely to have advanced disease at the time of diagnosis but were also less likely to receive standard therapies such as lymph node sampling and adjuvant radiotherapy. Despite those observations, breast cancer-specific survival was unaffected by the type of surgery. A recent report found a considerable desire by men to preserve their breast to maintain a positive self-image [82].

A retrospective analysis of MBC identified a total of 42 patients to undergo localized treatment [83]. Musculoskeletal functionality (tissue fibrosis, arm edema, and range of motion) and treatment outcome (local-regional control, disease-free survival, and overall survival) were evaluated. The actuarial overall 1-year fair-poor documented tissue fibrosis, arm edema, and

decreased range of motion rates were 13 %, 23 %, and 27 % for patients receiving MRM; 25 %, 0 %, and 50 % for patients who underwent total simple mastectomy (TSM); and 13 %, 0 %, and 0 % for those undergoing BCS, respectively. The overall survival and disease-free survival were not significantly different between the groups. These data suggest that breast conservation therapy may be considered a reasonable local treatment option for male patients presenting with breast cancer because it may offer functional advantages over mastectomy with comparable rates of local control and disease-free survival and overall survival.

In the guidelines of the American Society for Clinical Oncology, sentinel lymph node biopsy is reported as acceptable in MBC [16, 84]. More radical surgical procedures do not improve survival. Preoperative chemotherapy may be useful for cases with a critical tumor load. Simple mastectomy or localized tumor excision can be performed for patients who have a metastatic disease or non-suitable overall status; this may be combined with postoperative radiotherapy [9].

Adjuvant Chemotherapy

The benefit of systemic adjuvant treatment for MBC was not assessed in randomized clinical surveys; however, progress and response to the therapy in patients with metastatic MBC is similar to that in female patients. Therefore, patients with early-stage MBC are considered to benefit from adjuvant therapy [4]. There is not yet sufficient information about various prognostic factors for selecting specific adjuvant chemotherapy. Generally, the prognostic factors used for women are also valid for men. Deciding on the treatment is difficult, particularly for lymph node-negative cases or cases with one to three positive lymph nodes and strongly positive for estrogen receptor. Chemotherapy is applied to lymph node-negative patients according to the indications in FBC. There is an indication for chemotherapy in those with positive lymph nodes [85]. The same chemotherapeutic drugs are used both for male and female patients. The agents generally used are CMF (cyclophosphamide, methotrexate, 5-fluorouracil) and FAC

(5-fluorouracil, doxorubicin, cyclophospha-mide) regimes. However, treatment regimens including doxorubicin are superior to classical CMF [9]. Bagley [86] and Patel [87] reported in two small-scaled retrospective studies that survival was increased by adjuvant systemic therapy. Bagley reported a 5-year survey in which patients with stage II MBC who received 12 courses of CMF therapy showed a survival rate of 80 % and a mean overall survival of 98 months; he also suggested adjuvant therapy for its benefits. The precision of such data should be supported by prospective studies; however, because MBC is rare, it is difficult to perform large randomized studies.

Adjuvant Endocrine Therapy

Based on the positive clinical study results of adjuvant endocrine therapy solely or in combination with chemotherapy in female patients with early-stage breast cancer, adjuvant endocrine therapy is also recommended for male patients [88]. Likewise, in a Chinese retrospective single-institution study of 72 male patients over 40 years old, a multivariate regression found that the receipt of endocrine therapy was associated with better survival [89]. Tamoxifen or another hormone treatment is recommended for male patients with estrogen receptor-positive cancer, based on the prognostic factors for female patients [85]. Adjuvant therapy combined with radiotherapy was applied after surgery in 39 patients with Stage II and Stage III MBC with positive axillary nodes; the 5-year disease-free survival rate was reported as 55 % and the overall survival as 61 %. For former patients who were not treated systemically, the 5-year disease-free survival and overall survival were reported as 28 % and 44 %, respectively. Based on these indirect comparisons, tamoxifen increases both 5-year disease-free survival and overall survival. The long-term use of tamoxifen is suggested because it does not cause severe bone marrow toxicity or drug-induced death. However, tamoxifen may not be tolerated well in male patients. Men often experience bothersome symptoms from endocrine therapy, and approximately one in four discontinue treatment early because of hot flashes or sexual dysfunction [90, 91].

A limiting factor in the duration of tamoxifen therapy in men is the high incidence of adverse effects, with 20 % of participants in one study discontinuing therapy as a result. Common adverse effects include weight gain, sexual dysfunction, hot flashes, neurocognitive deficits, and thromboembolic events [91]. One study reported few adverse effects of tamoxifen [15]. However, further studies reported high rates of treatment-limiting side effects upon tamoxifen treatment in male patients, including a decrease in libido (29.2 %), weight gain (25 %), hot flashes (20.8 %), mental disorders (20.8 %), depression (16.6 %), sleeping disorders (12.5 %), and deep vein thrombosis (4.1 %). The rate of those who discontinued the treatment because of side effects was reported to be as high as 20.8 % within 1 year, compared with approximately 4 % for women who received tamoxifen [92]. Eggeman et al. [93] studied adjuvant therapy with tamoxifen compared to aromatase inhibitors for 257 hormone receptor-positive MBC patients. They found that the overall survival with MBC was significantly better after adjuvant treatment with tamoxifen compared to adjuvant treatment with an aromatase inhibitor. In conclusion, tamoxifen should be considered the treatment of choice for hormone receptor-positive MBC.

Adjuvant Radiotherapy

Postsurgical radiation criteria are generally extrapolated from data in women [94]. There are no prospective randomized studies evaluating the clinical effects of postoperative adjuvant radiotherapy in MBC. A case series of 75 men treated with curative intent in Ontario found significantly improved local recurrence-free survival in the 46 patients who received postmastectomy radiation, but their overall survival was not different [95].

Such studies have different technical characteristics, making clinical assessments difficult. Radiotherapy decreases local and regional relapse after mastectomy; however, it is not significantly effective for survival [41]. Radiotherapy should be considered based on similar criteria as for female cancer patients, and the indications are related to local findings. Tumors invading the skin and the chest wall require radiotherapy. Skin and nipple invasion occurs more frequently in men than in women. This may be associated with breast size and the distance of the tumor to these formations. Radiotherapy is imperative for patients who choose breast-protective surgery [10]. Consistent with the results of two studies on the benefits of radiotherapy after mastectomy on overall survival for patients with FBC, radiotherapy was considered a requirement after mastectomy for male patients with positive axillary lymph nodes [96]. Raguse et al. [97] showed that radiotherapy reduced the first 2-year local relapse (from 60 % to 20 %) for the patients with positive nodes. However, a decrease in local relapse does not reflect overall survival. Postoperative radiotherapy is a basic component of the treatment plan for localized advanced tumors [9, 98].

Treatment in Advanced-Stage Male Breast Cancer

Metastasis and the relapse pattern in MBC are similar to that in women. Metastasis is detected in 4–17 % of patients during diagnosis. Metastasis will develop in 18–54 % of the patients who do not have metastasis at the beginning. Distant metastases are commonly observed on the bones, lungs, and brain [87]. Isolated metastases are best treated by excision or radiotherapy. Systemic treatment options include ablative hormone treatment, additive hormone treatment, and chemotherapy; however, ablative hormone treatment is no longer commonly used. Ablative hormonal treatments include orchiectomy, adrenalectomy, and hypophysectomy. In 1942, bilateral orchiectomy was shown to be effective as hormone therapy in the treatment of patients with metastatic MBC [86]. Orchiectomy has a low morbidity rate. The remission rate was reported as 55 % in a study including 271 cases between 1959 and 1987 [12]. Some researchers have reported a remission rate of 60–83 % by this treatment [99]. The basis for performing adrenalectomy was not clearly explained. The treatment response in an adrenalectomy series including 38 patients was shown to be 7.4 % [12]. In another study, the effect of adrenalectomy followed by orchiectomy

was reported as 80 % [99]; however, when chemotherapy and hormone treatment options are available, adrenalectomy followed by orchiectomy is not preferred because of the low achievement rate and the presence of morbidity.

Tamoxifen and other antiestrogen substances used as additive hormonal treatments, such as clomiphene and nafoxidine, bind to estrogen receptors and reduce the hormone intake of the target tissue. Tamoxifen has fewer side effects and is more commonly used for FBC than are other drugs. A response rate of 48 % was obtained in 73 male patients with metastatic breast cancer who received tamoxifen treatment. All the patients responded to tamoxifen treatment, regardless of whether they responded to orchiectomy. Tamoxifen and orchiectomy are two individual treatment methods that do not show cross resistance [12, 41, 100]. Second-generation hormone therapy is currently used for FBC by inhibiting estrogen production through aromatase inhibitors, and good outcomes have been obtained. The role of aromatase inhibitors in male patients is limited. A case series including five patients who were treated with aromatase inhibitors was published [101]: three of the five patients had a stable period; however, those patients showed slow disease progress before adding aromatase inhibitors, and no objective response could be obtained from the patients. In another study, anastrozole was tested on healthy male volunteers [102]. Unlike in women, men treated with anastrozole did not show complete estrogen suppression; instead, a decrease of 50 % was observed in the estradiol concentration. Furthermore, testosterone levels were increased by 58 %. Two case studies reported responses to letrozole [103, 104]. Additional studies are required for evaluating both the adjuvant and metastatic efficiency of aromatase inhibitors on MBC. Luteinizing hormone-releasing hormone (LH-RH) agonists were reported as effective for the treatment of MBC with or without antiandrogens [105–107]. An LH-RH analogue drug called buserelin was introduced for use in advanced MBC. This drug first causes stimulation and then causes a paradoxical decrease in LH and FSH release; it presents an effect that can be called medical orchiectomy. Partial remission was obtained for 12 months in one of five patients who were treated with buserelin only. This period was extended to 24 months by the addition of flutamide, which is a nonsteroidal antiandrogenic agent. A partial response for 15 months was observed in four of five patients who were treated with a combination of buserelin and flutamide [12]. Treatments including progesterone (megestrol acetate and medroxyprogesterone acetate) may be used for metastatic MBC; however, these studies included fewer patients. A 7-month partial remission was observed in five of six patients treated with a high dose of medroxyprogesterone acetate [12, 41, 100].

Prognosis

Men with breast cancer reportedly have poorer outcomes than matched women patients, even at the same disease stages, which might be because of variations in tumor biology between male and female patients [108]. Mortality in MBC has continued to improve over the past 30 years, despite its late presentation [12, 23]. The most important prognostic factor in MBC, similar to FBC, is positive axillary lymph nodes [45, 57, 72, 89, 98, 109]. The poorer progress in male patients was explained by the anatomic location of the tumor. It has been reported that nipple invasion occurs very early because of such placement, and increased lymphovascular invasion and higher axillary lymph node invasion were observed compared to FBC, despite the small tumor size; those characteristics and the referral of the patient at advanced stages result in poor prognosis [110, 111]. When matched by stage and age, men appear to have a similar or better prognosis compared to women [17, 112].

In an international population-based study including 459,846 women and 2,665 men diagnosed with breast cancer in Denmark, Finland, Geneva, Norway, Singapore, and Sweden over the last 40 years, male patients had a poorer 5-year relative survival ratio than women (0.72 [95 % CI, 0.70–0.75] vs. 0.78 [95 % CI, 0.78–0.78], respectively), corresponding to a relative

excess risk (RER) of 1.27 (95 % CI, 1.13–1.42). However, after adjustment for age and the year of diagnosis, stage, and treatment, male patients had a significantly better relative survival from breast cancer than female patients (RER, 0.78; 95 % CI, 0.62–0.97) [13].

In a multivariate analysis of the prognostic factors performed on patients with MBC, tumor size and nodal invasion were presented as significant prognostic factors [72]. Published data also indicate that advanced age is a predictor of lower overall survival [113]. Guinee et al. [114] showed that both axillary lymph node involvement and clinical tumor size play important roles in prognosis in 335 patients. Patients with palpable axillary lymph nodes have a twofold greater risk for disease-related death, and a tumor diameter larger than 3 cm increases the risk of treatment failure. Fixation of the tumor to the skin or chest wall and tumor ulceration was reported more often in men than in women, but these factors were not shown to affect prognosis in multivariate analyses [49].

In a retrospective analysis of Egyptian patients, the collective 5-year survival in this cohort was 46.4 % [115]. Kiluk et al. reported that the 5-year survival estimates for node-positive and node-negative diseases were 68.5 % and 87.5 %, respectively, (p = 0.3) [80]. Ethnic differences might also affect the prognosis of MBC [116]. In a Turkish cohort of 86 male patients treated over 37 years, Selcukbiricik and his coworkers reported a 65.8 % 5-year overall survival rate [117]. Similar in an Iranian cohort of 64 patients, the 5-year overall survival rate was 66 % [13].

The most significant protective factor is ER and PR receptor positivity. The significance of HER2 status in MBC remains unclear because there are few studies that have assessed its significance in terms of treatment options and prognosis [23]. There is no demonstrable correlation between Ki-67 expression and MBC prognosis [118]. To identify risk factors, the period between the appearance of the symptoms and diagnosis and less differentiated tumor must indicate a bad prognosis [12]. The prognosis of ductal-type carcinoma is worse than that of the medullary, colloidal, and papillary types [41]. In another study, no connection could be found between C-erbB2 and c-myc oncogenes, p53 suppressor genes, and survival [119]. The overexpression of cyclin D1 and c-myc may correlate with better outcomes [76]. One recent study identified more high-grade, progesterone-receptor negative, HER2-positive disease male patients who carried BRCA2 mutations [29], and earlier research found a poorer prognosis in men with BRCA2-associated tumors.

Survivorship issues in men may include sexual and hormonal side effects of endocrine therapies and unique psychosocial effects of the disease [60]. In a quality of life and symptom survey over MBC survivors, patients experience substantial sexual and hormonal symptoms [120].

References

1. Siegel R, Naishadham D, Jemal A. Cancer statistics. CA Cancer J Clin. 2013;63(1):11–30.
2. Siegel R, DeSantis C, Virgo K, Stein K, Mariotto A, Smith T, et al. Cancer treatment and survivorship statistics. CA Cancer J Clin. 2012;62(4):220–41.
3. American Cancer Society. Cancer facts and figures. Atlanta: American Cancer Society; 2014.
4. DeSantis C, Siegel R, Bandi P, Jemal A. Breast cancer statistics. CA Cancer J Clin. 2011;61(6):409–18.
5. Siegel R, Ma J, Zou Z, Jemal A. Cancer statistics. CA Cancer J Clin. 2014;64(1):9–29.
6. Giordano SH, Cohen DS, Buzdar AU, Perkins G, Hortobagyi GN. Breast carcinoma in men: a population-based study. Cancer. 2004;101:51–7.
7. Nirmul D, Pegoraro RJ, Jialal I, Naidoo C, Joubert SM. The sex hormone profile of male patient with breast cancer. Br J Cancer. 1983;48(3):423–7.
8. Sanchez AG, Villanueva AG, Redondo C. Lobular carcinoma of the breast in a patient with Klinefelter's syndrome. A case with bilateral, synchronous, histologically different breast tumors. Cancer. 1986;57(6):1181–3.
9. Schuchardt U, Seegenschmiedt MH, Kirschner MJ, Renner H, Sauer R. Adjuvant radiotherapy for breast carcinoma in men: a 20-year clinical experience. Am J Clin Oncol. 1996;19(4):330–6.
10. Gradishar WJ. Male breast cancer. In: Harris JR, Lippman ME, Morrow M, Osborn CK, editors. Disease of the breast. Philadelphia: Lippincott Williams and Wilkins; 2000. p. 661–7.
11. Anderson WF, Jatoi I, Tse J, Rosenberg PS. Male breast cancer: a population-based comparison with female breast cancer. J Clin Oncol. 2010;28(2):232–9.
12. Crichlow RW, Galt SW. Male breast cancer. Surg Clin N Am. 1990;70(5):1165–77.
13. Salehi A, Zeraati H, Mohammad K, Mahmoudi M, Talei AR, Ghaderi A, et al. Survival of male breast cancer in Fars, South of Iran. Iran Red Crescent Med J. 2011;13(2):99–105.
14. Tawil AN, Boulos FI, Chakhachiro ZI, Otrock ZK, Kandaharian L, El Saghir NS, et al. Clinicopathologic and immunohistochemical characteristics of male breast cancer: a single center experience. Breast J. 2012;18(1):65–8.
15. Ribeiro G, Swindell R. Adjuvant tamoxifen for male breast cancer (MBC). Breast J Cancer. 1992;65:252–4.
16. Johansen Taber KA, Morisy LR, Osbahr 3rd AJ, Dickinson BD. Male breast cancer: risk factors, diagnosis, and management (review). Oncol Rep. 2010;24(5):1115–20. Review.
17. Miao H, Verkooijen HM, Chia KS, Bouchardy C, Pukkala E, Larønningen S, et al. Incidence and outcome of male breast cancer: an international population-based study. J Clin Oncol. 2011;29(33):4381–6.
18. Gómez-Raposo C, Zambrana Tévar F, Sereno Moyano M, López Gómez M, Casado E. Male breast cancer. Cancer Treat Rev. 2010;36(6):451–7.
19. Volpe CM, Raffetto JD, Collure DW, Hoover EL, Doerr RJ. Unilateral male breast masses: cancer risk and their evaluation and management. Am Surg. 1999;65(3):250–3.
20. Thorlacius S, Struewing JP, Hartge P, Olafsdottir GH, Sigvaldason H, Tryggvadottir L, et al. Population-based study of risk of breast cancer in carriers of BRCA-2 mutation. Lancet. 1998;352(9137):1337–9.
21. Satram-Hoang S, Moran EM, Anton-Culver H, Burras RW, Heimann TM, Boggio I, et al. A pilot study of male breast cancer in the Veterans Affairs healthcare system. J Environ Pathol Toxicol Oncol. 2010;29(3):235–44.
22. Winer EP, Morrow M, Osborne CK, Harris JR. Malignant tumors of the breast. In: Devita VT, Hellman S, Rosenberg SA, editors. Cancer principles and practice of oncology. 6th ed. Philadelphia: Lippincott Williams and Wilkins pub; 2001. p. 1651–717.
23. Korde LA, Zujewski JA, Kamin L, Giordano S, Domchek S, Anderson WF, et al. Multidisciplinary meeting on male breast cancer: summary and research recommendations. J Clin Oncol. 2010;28(12):2114–22.
24. Marger D, Urdaneta N, Fischer JJ. Breast cancer in brothers: case reports and review of 30 cases of male breast cancer. Cancer. 1975;36(2):458–61.
25. Basham VM, et al. BRCA1 and BRCA2 mutations in a populationbased study of male breast cancer. Breast Cancer Res BCR. 2002;4(1):R2.
26. Gilbert SF, Soliman AS, Karkouri M, Quinlan-Davidson M, Strahley A, Eissa M, et al. Clinical profile, BRCA2 expression, and the androgen receptor CAG repeat region in Egyptian and Moroccan male breast cancer patients. Breast Dis. 2011;33(1):17–26.
27. Bishop DT. BRCA1 and BRCA2 and breast cancer incidence: a review. Ann Oncol. 1999;10 Suppl 6:113–9.

28. Evans DG, Susnerwala I, Dawson J, Woodward E, Maher ER, Lalloo F. Risk of breast cancer in male BRCA2 carriers. J Med Genet. 2010;47(10):710–1.

29. Ottini L, Silvestri V, Rizzolo P, Falchetti M, Zanna I, Saieva C, Masala G, Bianchi S, et al. Clinical and pathologic characteristics of BRCA-positive and BRCA-negative male breast cancer patients: results from a collaborative multicenter study in Italy. Breast Cancer Res Treat. 2012;134(1):411–8.

30. Ding YC, Steele L, Kuan CJ, Greilac S, Neuhausen SL. Mutations in BRCA2 and PALB2 in male breast cancer cases from the United States. Breast Cancer Res Treat. 2011;126(3):771–8.

31. Blanco A, de la Hoya M, Balmana J, Ramón y Cajal T, Teulé A, Miramar MD, et al. Detection of a large rearrangement in PALB2 in Spanish breast cancer families with male breast cancer. Breast Cancer Res Treat. 2012;132(1):307–15.

32. Gilbert SF, Soliman AS, Iniesta M, Eissa M, Hablas A, Seifeldin IA, et al. Androgen receptor polyglutamine tract length in Egyptian male breast cancer patients. Breast Cancer Res Treat. 2011;129(2):575–81.

33. Silvestri V, Rizzolo P, Zanna I, Falchetti M, Masala G, Bianchi S, et al. PALB2 mutations in male breast cancer: a population-based study in Central Italy. Breast Cancer Res Treat. 2010;122(1): 299–301.

34. Sauty de Chalon A, Teo Z, Park DJ, Odefrey FA, kConFab, Hopper JL, Southey MC. Are PALB2 mutations associated with increased risk of male breast cancer? Breast Cancer Res Treat. 2010;121(1):253–5.

35. Silvestri V, Rizzolo P, Falchetti M, Zanna I, Masala G, Bianchi S, et al. Mutation analysis of BRIP1 in male breast cancer cases: a population-based study in Central Italy. Breast Cancer Res Treat. 2011;126(2):539–43.

36. Silvestri V, Rizzolo P, Falchetti M, Zanna I, Masala G, Palli D, et al. Mutation screening of RAD51C in male breast cancer patients. Breast Cancer Res. 2011;13(1):404.

37. Kizildag S, Gulsu E, Bagci O, Yuksel E, Canda T. Vitamin D receptor gene polymorphisms and male breast cancer risk in Turkish population. J BUON. 2011;16(4):640–5.

38. Fentiman IS, Fourguet A, Hortobagyi GN. Male breast cancer. Lancet. 2006;367:595–604.

39. Giordano SH. A review of the diagnosis and management of male breast cancer. Oncologist. 2005;10(7):471–9.

40. Ottini L, Masala G, D'Amico C, Mancini B, Saieva C, Aceto G, et al. BRCA1 and BRCA2 mutation status and tumor characteristics in male breast cancer: a population-based study in Italy. Cancer Res. 2003;63:342–7.

41. Donegan WL, Redlich PN. Breast cancer in men. Surg Clin N Am. 1996;76(2):343–63.

42. Brinton LA. Breast cancer risk among patients with Klinefelter syndrome. Acta Paediatr. 2011;100(6):814–8.

43. Ottini L, Palli D, Rizzo S, Federico M, Bazan V, Russo A. Male breast cancer. Crit Rev Oncol Hematol. 2010;73:141–55.

44. Evans DB, Crichlow RW. Carcinoma of the male breast and Klinefelter's syndrome: is there an association? CA Cancer J Clin. 1987;37(4):246–51.

45. Heller K, Rosen P, Schottenfeld D. Male breast cancer: a clinicopathologic study of 97 cases. Ann Surg. 1978;188:60–5.

46. Green L, Wysowski DK, Fourcroy JL. Gynecomastia and breast cancer during finasteride therapy. N Eng J Med. 1996;335(11):823.

47. Brinton LA, Cook MB, McCormack V, Johnson KC, Olsson H, Casagrande JT, et al. Anthropometric and hormonal risk factors for male breast cancer: male breast cancer pooling project results. J Natl Cancer Inst. 2014;106(3):djt465.

48. Rohrmann S, Shiels MS, Lopez DS, Rifai N, Nelson WG, Kanarek N, et al. Body fatness and sex steroid hormone concentrations in US men: results from NHANES III. Cancer Causes Control. 2011;22(8): 1141–51.

49. Moore MP, Harris RH, Lippman ME, Morrow M, Hellman S. Male Breast Cancer. Diseases of the Breast. First Edition. Philadelphia: Lippincott-Raven; 1996:859–63.

50. Sasco AJ, Lowenfels AB, Pasker-de Jong P. Epidemiology of male breast cancer: a meta analysis published case-control studies and discussion of selected a etiological factors. Int J Cancer. 1993;53(4):538–49.

51. Brinton LA, Carreon JD, Gierach GL, McGlynn KA, Gridley G. Etiologic factors for male breast cancer in the U.S. Veterans Affairs medical care system database. Breast Cancer Res Treat. 2010;119(1):185–92.

52. Eldar S, Nash E, Abrahanson J. Radiation carcinogenesis in the male breast. Eur J Surg Oncol. 1989;15(3):274–8.

53. Anderson WF, Jatoi I, Tse j, Rosenberg PS. Male breast cancer: a population-based comparison with female breast cancer. J Clin Oncol. 2010;28(2):232–9.

54. Villeneuve S, Cyr D, Lynge E, Orsi L, Sabroe S, Merletti F, et al. Occupation and occupational exposure to endocrine disrupting chemicals in male breast cancer: a case-control study in Europe. Occup Environ Med. 2010;67(12):837–44.

55. Hansen J. Elevated risk for male breast cancer after occupational exposure to gasoline and vehicular combustion products. Am J Ind Med. 2000;37(4):349–52.

56. Ewertz M, Holmberg L, Tretli S, Pedersen BV, Kristensen A. Risk factors for male breast cancer a case-control study from Scandinavia. Acta Oncol. 2001;40(4):467–71.

57. Borgen PI, Wong GY, Vlamis V, Potter C, Hoffmann B, Kinne DW, et al. Current management of male breast cancer: a review of 104 cases. Ann Surg. 1992;215(5):451–7.

58. Donegan WL, Redlich PN, Lang PJ, Gall MT. Carcinoma of the breast in males. A multi institutional survey. Cancer. 1998;83(3):498–509.

59. Bezwoda WR, Hesdorffer C, Dansey R, de Moor N, Derman DP, Browde S, et al. Breast cancer in men: clinical features, hormone receptor status, and response to therapy. Cancer. 1987;60(6):1337–40.

60. Ruddy KJ, Winer EP. Male breast cancer: risk factors, biology, diagnosis, treatment, and survivorship. Ann Oncol. 2013;24(6):1434–43.

61. Xia LP, Zhou FF, Guo GF, Wang F, Wang X, Yuan ZY, et al. Chinese female breast cancer patients show a better overall survival than their male counterparts. Chin Med J. 2010;123(17):2347–52.

62. Gnerlich JL, Deshpande AD, Jeffe DB, Seelam S, Kimbuende E, Margenthaler JA. Poorer survival outcomes for male breast cancer compared with female breast cancer may be attributable to instage migration. Ann Surg Oncol. 2011;18(7):1837–44.

63. Bourhafour M, Belbaraka R, Souadka A, M'rabti H, Tijami F, Errihani H. Male breast cancer: a report of 127 cases at a Moroccan institution. BMC Res Notes. 2011;4:219.

64. Wauters CAP, Kooistra BW, de Kievit-van der Heijden IM, Strobbe LJ. Is cytology useful in the diagnostic workup of male breast lesions? A retrospective study over a 16-year period and review of the recent literature. Acta Cytol. 2010;54: 259–64.

65. Doyle S, Steel J, Porter G. Imaging male breast cancer. Clin Radiol. 2011;66:1079–85.

66. Jackson VP, Gilmor RL. Male breast carcinoma and gynecomastia: comparison of mammography with sonography. Radiology. 1983;149(2):533–6.

67. Kapdi CC, Parekh NJ. The male breast. Radiol Clin N Am. 1983;21(1):137–48.

68. Evans GF, Anthony T, Turnage RH. The diagnostic accuracy of mammography in the evaluation of male breast disease. Am J Surg. 2001;181(2):96–100.

69. Bhagat P, Kline TS. The male breast and malignant neoplasms. Diagnosis by aspiration biopsy cytology. Cancer. 1990;65(10):2338–41.

70. Gill MS, Kayani N, Khan MN, Hasan SH. Breast diseases in males a morphological review of 150 cases. J Pak Med Assoc. 2000;50(6):177–9.

71. Tahmasebi S, Akrami M, Omidvari S, Salehi A, Talei A. Male breast cancer; analysis of 58 cases in Shiraz, South of Iran. Breast Dis. 2010;31(1):29–32.

72. Arslan UY, Oksuzoglu B, Ozdemir N, Aksoy S, Alkış N, Gök A, et al. Outcome of non-metastatic male breast cancer: 118 patients. Med Oncol. 2012;29(2):554–60.

73. Liukkonen S, Saarto T, Maenpaa H, Sjöström-Mattson J. Male breast cancer: a survey at the Helsinki University Central Hospital during 1981–2006. Acta Oncol. 2010;49(3):322–7.

74. Rizzolo P, Silvestri V, Tommasi S, Pinto R, Danza K, Falchetti M, et al. Male breast cancer: genetics, epigenetics, and ethical aspects. Ann Oncol. 2013;24 Suppl 8:viii75–82.

75. Rayson D, Erlichman C, Suman VJ, Roche PC, Wold LE, Ingle JN, Donohue JH. Molecular markers in male breast carcinoma. Cancer. 1998;83(9):1947–55.

76. Kanthan R, Fried I, Rueckl T, Senger JL, Kanthan SC. Expression of cell cycle proteins in male breast carcinoma. World J Surg Oncol. 2010;8:10.

77. Kornegoor R, Verschuur-Maes AH, Buerger H, Hogenes MC, de Bruin PC, Oudejans JJ, et al. Molecular subtyping of male breast cancer by immunohistochemistry. Mod Pathol. 2012;25(3):398–404.

78. Shaaban AM, Ball GR, Brannan RA, Cserni G, Di Benedetto A, Dent J, et al. A comparative biomarker study of 514 matched cases of male and female breast cancer reveals gender-specific biological differences. Breast Cancer Res Treat. 2012;133(3):949–58.

79. Zhou FF, Xia LP, Guo GF, Wang X, Yuan ZY, Zhang B, et al. Changes in therapeutic strategies in Chinese male patients with breast cancer: 40 years of experience in a single institute. Breast. 2010;19(6):450–5.

80. Kiluk JV, Lee MC, Park CK, Meade T, Minton S, Harris E, et al. Male breast cancer: management and follow-up recommendations. Breast J. 2011;17(5):503–9.

81. Cloyd JM, Hernandez-Boussard T, Wapnir IL. Outcomes of partial mastectomy in male breast cancer patients: analysis of SEER, 1983–2009. Ann Surg Oncol. 2013;20(5):1545–50.

82. Nguyen T, Cowher M. Demand for breast-conserving surgery among male breast cancer patients. Presented at: 13th annual meeting of American Society of Breast Surgeons, Phoenix. 2012.

83. Fogh S, Kachnic LA, Goldberg SI, Taghian AG, Powell SN, Hirsch AE. Localized therapy for male breast cancer: functional advantages with comparable outcomes using breast conservation. Clin Breast Cancer. 2013;13(5):344–9.

84. Lyman GH, Giuliano AE, Somerfield MR, Benson 3rd AB, Bodurka DC, Burstein HJ, et al. American society of clinical oncology guideline recommendations for sentinel lymph node biopsy in early stage breast cancer. J Clin Oncol. 2005;23:7703.

85. Jaiyesimi IA, Buzdar AU, Sahin AA, Ross MA. Carcinoma of the male breast. Ann Intern Med. 1992;117(9):771–7.

86. Bagley CS, Wesley MN, Young RC, Lippman ME. Adjuvant chemotherapy in males with cancer of the breast. Am J Clin Oncol. 1987;10(1):55–60.

87. Patel 2nd HZ, Buzdar AU, Hortobagyi GN. Role of adjuvant chemotherapy in male breast cancer. Cancer. 1989;64(8):1583–5.

88. Fogh S, Hirsch AE, Langmead JP, Goldberg SI, Rosenberg CL, Taghian AG, et al. Use of tamoxifen with postsurgical irradiation may improve survival in estrogen and progesterone receptor-positive male breast cancer. Clin Breast Cancer. 2011;11(1):39–45.

89. Zhou FF, Xia LP, Wang X, Guo GF, Rong YM, Qiu HJ, et al. Analysis of prognostic factors in male breast cancer: a report of 72 cases from a single institution. Chin J Cancer. 2010;29(2):184–8.

90. Visram H, Kanji F, Dent SF. Endocrine therapy for male breast cancer: rates of toxicity and adherence. Curr Oncol. 2010;17(5):17–21.

91. Pemmaraju N, Munsell MF, Hortobagyi GN, Giordano SH. Retrospective review of male breast cancer patients: analysis of tamoxifen-related side-effects. Ann Oncol. 2012;23(6):1471–4.

92. Anelli TF, Anelli A, Tran KN, Lebwohl DE, Borgen PI. Tamoxifen administration is associated with a high rate of treatment-limiting symptoms in male breast cancer patients. Cancer. 1994;74(1):74–7.

93. Eggemann H, Ignatov A, Smith BJ, Altmann U, von Minckwitz G, Röhl FW, et al. Adjuvant therapy with tamoxifen compared to aromatase inhibitors for 257 male breast cancer patients. Breast Cancer Res Treat. 2013;137(2):465–70.

94. Bratman SV, Kapp DS, Horst KC. Evolving trends in the initial locoregional management of male breast cancer. Breast. 2012;21(3):296–302.

95. Yu E, Suzuki H, Younus J, Elfiki T, Stitt L, Yau G, et al. The impact of post-mastectomy radiation therapy on male breast cancer patients—a case series. Int J Radiat Oncol Biol Phys. 2012;82(2):696–700.

96. Overgaard M, Hansen PS, Overgaard J, Rose C, Andersson M, Bach F, et al. Postoperative radiotherapy in high risk premenopausal women with breast cancer who receive adjuvant chemotherapy. Danish Breast cancer Cooperative Group 82b Trial. N Engl J Med. 1997;337(14):949–55.

97. Ragaz J, Jackson SM, Le N, Plenderleith IH, Spinelli JJ, Basco VE, et al. Adjuvant radiotherapy and chemotherapy in node positive premenopausal women with breast cancer. N Engl J Med. 1997;337(14):956–62.

98. Erlichman C, Murphy KC, Elhakim T. Male breast cancer: a 13-year review of 89 patients. J Clin Oncol. 1984;2(8):903–9.

99. Patel JK, Nemoto T, Dao TL. Metastatic breast cancer in males. Assessment of endocrine therapy. Cancer. 1984;53(6):1344–6.

100. Donegan WL. Cancer of the male breast. In: Donegan WL, Spratt JS, editors. Cancer of the breast. Philadelphia: WB Saunders; 1995. p. 774–5.

101. Giordano SH, Valero V, Buzdar AU, Hortobagyi GN. Efficacy of anastrozole in male breast cancer. Am J Clin Oncol. 2002;25(3):235–7.

102. Mauras N, O'Brien KO, Klein KO, Hayes V. Estrogen suppression in males: metabolic effects. J Clin Endocrinol Metab. 2000;85(7):2370–7.

103. Zabolotny BP, Zalai CV, Meterissian SH. Successful use of letrozole in male breast cancer: a case report and review of hormonal therapy for male breast cancer. J Surg Oncol. 2005;90(1):26–30.

104. Italiano A, Largillier R, Marcy PY, Foa C, Ferrero JM, Hartmann MT, et al. Complete remission obtained with letrozole in a man with metastatic breast cancer. Rev Med Interne. 2004;25(4):323–4.

105. Labrie F, Dupont A, Belanger A, Lacourcière Y, Béland L, Cusan L, et al. Complete response to combination therapy with an LHRH agonist and flutamide in metastatic male breast cancer: a case report. Clin Invest Med. 1990;13(5):275–8.

106. Lopez M, Natali M, Di Lauro L, Vici P, Pignatti F, Carpano S. Combined treatment with buserelin an cyproterone acetate in metastatic male breast cancer. Cancer. 1993;72(2):502–5.

107. Doberauer C, Niederle N, Schmidt CG. Advanced male breast cancer treatment with the LH-RH analogue buserelin alone or in combination with the antiandrogen flutamide. Cancer. 1988;62(3):474–8.

108. Chen X, Liu X, Zhang L, Li S, Shi Y, Tong Z. Poorer survival of male breast cancer compared with female breast cancer patients may be due to biological differences. Jpn J Clin Oncol. 2013;43(10):954–63.

109. Cutuli B, Le-Nir CC, Serin D, Kirova Y, Gaci Z, Lemanski C, et al. Male breast cancer. Evolution of treatment and prognostic factors. Analysis of 489 cases. Crit Rev Oncol Hematol. 2010;73(3):246–54.

110. Joshi MG, Lee AK, Loda M, Camus MG, Pedersen C, Heatley GJ, et al. Male breast carcinoma: an evaluation of prognostic factors contributing to a poorer outcome. Cancer. 1996;77(3):490–8.

111. Donegan WL. Cancer of the male breast. J Gend Specif Med. 2000;3(4):55–8.

112. Foerster R, Foerster FG, Wulff V, Schubotz B, Baaske D, Wolfgarten M, et al. Matched-pair analysis of patients with female and male breast cancer: a comparative analysis. BMC Cancer. 2011;11:335.

113. Tural D, Selcukbiricik F, Aydogan F, Beşc N, Yetmen O, Ilvan Ş, et al. Male breast cancers behave differently in elderly patients. Jpn J Clin Oncol. 2013;43(1):22–7.

114. Guinee VF, Olsson H, Moller T, Shallenberger RC, van den Blink JW, Peter Z, et al. The prognosis of breast cancer in males: a report of 335 cases. Cancer. 1993;71(1):154–61.

115. Soliman AA, Denewer AT, El-Sadda W, Abdel-Aty AH, Refky B. A retrospective analysis of survival and prognostic factors of male breast cancer from a single center. BMC Cancer. 2014;14:227.

116. O'Malley CD, Prehn AW, Shema SJ, Glaser SL. Racial/ethnic differences in survival rates in a population-based series of men with breast carcinoma. Cancer. 2002;94(11):2836–43.

117. Selcukbiricik F, Tural D, Aydogan F, Beşe N, Büyükünal E, Serdengeçti S, et al. Male breast cancer: 37-year data study at a single experience center in Turkey. J Breast Cancer. 2013;16(1):60–5.

118. Xia Q, Shi YX, Liu DG, Jiang WQ. Clinicopathological characteristics of male breast cancer: analysis of 25 cases at a single institution [in Chinese with English abstract]. Nan Fang Yi Ke Da Xue Xue Bao. 2011;31:1469–73.

119. Andre S, Fonseca I, Pinto AE, Cardoso P, Pereira T, Soares J, et al. Male breast cancer-a reappraisal of clinical and biologic indicators of prognosis. Acta Oncol. 2001;40(4):472–8.

120. Ruddy KJ, Giobbie-Harder A, Giordano SH, Goldfarb S, Kereakoglow S, Winer EP, et al. Quality of life and symptoms in male breast cancer survivors. Breast. 2013;22(2):197–9.

Breast Cancer in Pregnancy

24

Maurício Magalhães Costa and Paula Saldanha

Abstract

Pregnancy-associated breast cancer (PABC) is defined as breast cancer that is diagnosed during gestation, lactation, or the first postpartum year. PABC is rare but extremely serious. The disease puts the lives of both mother and fetus at risk. In addition, PABC typically causes clinical, ethical, and psychological problems as well as doubts related to diagnosis and treatment. Clinical and ethical obstacles are frequently encountered during treatment. The gestational age is critical regarding therapeutic options, causing constant modifications and procedural delays. Surgical treatment can be undertaken during any phase of the pregnancy. Chemotherapy can potentially be administered during the second or third trimester. Radiotherapy is reserved for the postpartum period. Interruption of the gestation does not affect the treatment; however, it undoubtedly facilitates the therapeutic conduct. The indication of this course of action must be undertaken with great consideration and discussed openly with the patient and her family.

Keywords

Breast cancer • Pregnancy • Surgical treatment • Fertility preservation

M. Magalhães Costa, MSc, MD, PhD (✉)
Gynecology Service of the Clementino Fraga Filho Teaching Hospital (UFRJ), Universidade Federal of Rio de Janeiro (UFRJ), Rio de Janeiro, Brazil

Radiumhemmet – Karolinska Institute, Stockholm, Sweden

American Society of Breast Disease (ASBD), Warsaw, IN, USA

SIS Journal – the Electronic Journal of the Senologic International Society (SIS), Warsaw, Poland

Latin American Federation of Mastology, Rio de Janeiro, Brazil

Americas Medical City, Rio de Janeiro, Brazil

Gynecology – Mastology, Universidade Federal do Rio de Janeiro, Rio de Janeiro, Brazil
e-mail: mamcosta@yahoo.com; http://www.cmmc.med.br

P. Saldanha, MD
Clementino Fraga Filho University Hospital (UFRJ), Rio de Janeiro, Brazil

Clínica Maurício Magalhães Costa, Rio de Janeiro, Brazil
e-mail: paulabrantsaldanha@gmail.com

© Springer International Publishing Switzerland 2016
A. Aydiner et al. (eds.), *Breast Disease: Management and Therapies*,
DOI 10.1007/978-3-319-26012-9_24

Introduction

Breast cancer is the most frequent malignant pathology in developed countries. In the United States, it is the second most common cause of death from cancer after lung cancer. Approximately 28 % of cases worldwide are observed in the European region. Between 1950 and 1980, mortality from breast cancer increased in all European countries, with the exception of Norway and Sweden. Since 1990, a drop in this growth was noted, eventually leading to a reduction of cases of deaths [1]. A progressive increase has been observed in the incidence of breast cancer, even in Latin America. In 2020, 70 % of new cases are estimated to occur in emerging countries [2].

In the 1960s and 1970s, the World Health Organization recorded a tenfold increase in the incidence of female breast cancer adjusted by age on the various continents. In relation to most frequent type of cancer worldwide, breast cancer is the most common among women. Breast cancer comprises 22 % of new cancer cases each year. This observation is mainly attributed to the increased longevity of the population during this period [2].

The majority of the increases in the incidence rates have occurred in women over 50 years of age, but the rates also increased among younger patients. These changes in incidence are not only attributed to sociocultural factors because the incidence has also increased in women who migrate from low-risk areas to high-risk areas. These studies suggest that environmental factors have a substantial effect on the risk of breast cancer.

Pregnancy-associated breast cancer (PABC) is defined as breast cancer that is diagnosed during gestation, lactation, or the first postpartum year [3, 4]. PABC is rare, but it is extremely serious. The disease puts the lives of both mother and fetus at risk. PABC typically causes clinical, ethical, and psychological problems as well as doubts related to diagnosis and treatment. PABC was formerly characterized by a poor prognosis and minimally efficacious treatment options due to the worsening promoted by gestation. Today, it is evaluated with less pessimism and is studied more clearly given less alarming data.

History

The first citation regarding PABC was made by Klotz in 1869. Following this landmark, a series of authors committed themselves to studying the disease, persistently emphasizing the very poor prognoses of these patients. In 1929, Kilgore was the first to attribute little importance to the gestational and lactation periods, opposing the idea that the disease's behavior is invariably hopeless. In 1943, Haagensen and Stout studied 29 cases of breast cancer diagnosed during gestation and the postpartum period, and 20 of these cases underwent radical mastectomies. Because a cure was not available and long-term survival was not possible, PABC was considered inoperable [5]. In 1946, Westberg evaluated 224 cases diagnosed as PABC in Sweden and concluded that although gestation did not influence the prognosis, it did delay the diagnosis. In the same study, he observed that interrupting the gestation did not improve the possibility of a cure [6]. In 1967, Haagensen reviewed his initial position in relation to the inoperability attributed to these cases. Since then, most authors have indicated that disease progression depends more on its stage and the compromising of the axilla at the time of diagnosis than on the association with gestation or lactation [7].

Epidemiology

In developing or underdeveloped countries, the incidence of breast cancer varies from low to moderate (20–40 per 100,000 women), with a tendency to increase over time. The incidence has increased yearly, and the International Agency for Research on Cancer estimates an incidence of 120,000 new cases per year in Latin America [8]. Fortunately, PABC is rare. Reviewing the international literature over a period of approximately 100 years, White (1954) noted a PABC rate of 2.8 % among 45,000 cases evaluated [9]. In 1983, Wallack reviewed 32 series of reports of breast cancer and reported PABC rates varying between 0.2 % and 3.8 %

[10]. He also mentioned the incidence of 10–39 cases per 100,000 births. The incidence estimated varies from 1:3,000 to 1:10,000 gestations, with a greater number of cases diagnosed during gestation compared with the postpartum period [4]. This incidence appears to be increasing because women currently delay pregnancy. The case of the youngest patient (16 years old) was reported by Birks in 1973 [11]. In 1984, Richards mentioned an 18-year-old patient with metastases [12]. In principle, one should initially suspect a primary site located in the breast in any pregnant woman who presents with metastatic adenocarcinoma.

Diagnosis

The diagnosis of PABC is always difficult and delayed. The turgidity and the irregularities in the mammary parenchyma during this period make the clinical examination difficult, delaying the indication for a biopsy and consequently the final diagnosis. Max (1983) observed that the mean delay in the detection of the disease during pregnancy ranges from 5 to 15 months compared with patients who are not pregnant [13]. This delay is serious because a delay of 1 month can increase the risk of lymph node metastasis from 1 % to 2 % [14]. These findings could be minimized by prenatal consultations, wherein it is possible to proceed to a more accurate clinical examination as well as self-examination.

Mammography does not appear to reduce the delay in diagnosis. In young, nonpregnant patients (less than 35 years old), mammography may produce false-negative results in up to 50 % of cases. These data appear to be increased in pregnant patients. Ultrasound may also be considered valuable in the diagnosis. In addition to assisting in enhanced characterization of the mammary tumor, ultrasound may be useful in the investigation of abdominal metastases.

Tests involving radiation used to track lesions at a distance, such as radiography and scintigraphy, are contraindicated in most occasions. Nevertheless, the doses associated with these techniques are below the level of danger and appear to be reasonably safe in pregnant women. If scintigraphy is essential, it may be used; however, appropriate hydration and the use of a Foley urinary catheter are important to prevent radiation retention.

Magnetic resonance imaging has been used during pregnancy and may be indicated in cases in which ultrasound is inconclusive. Although no harmful effect has been reported, the National Radiological Protection Board advises that this technique should not be used in the first trimester because insufficient evidence is available for its safe use during the period of organogenesis [15]. In animals, gadolinium has exhibited teratogenic effects, but no reports have been published regarding humans [16].

Fine-needle biopsy is valuable in diagnosis. Although the specificity of mammary cytology is reduced during gestation and lactation due to the hyperplastic and inflammatory phenomena that are characteristic of the period, the increased sensitivity of this technique alerts us to the indication of surgical biopsy. A definitive diagnosis is exclusively obtained through histopathological examination. Surgical biopsy can be safely performed during pregnancy. The procedure occurs under local or general anesthesia via core biopsy or mammotomy.

Regarding the pathological aspects, most cases involve invasive ductal carcinoma, which is similar to that observed in women who are not pregnant. The tumors predominantly exhibit minimal differentiation and are diagnosed at more advanced stages. Hormonal receptor-negative tumors and an increased incidence of HER-2 (human epidermal growth factor receptor 2) overexpression are also frequently observed [17].

Women with a family history or those who carry the BRCA1 and BRCA2 genetic mutations are at greater risk of developing breast cancer at a younger age, a period in which pregnancy is common. Various studies have revealed differential behavior of these mutations in relation to pregnancy. Antoniou et al. compared 457 carriers who developed cancer with 332 carriers who did not develop cancer. The protective effect of gestation was exclusively observed in those women over

40 years of age, and the occurrence of the first gestation at a more advanced age was associated with increased risk of breast cancer in women with the BRCA2 mutation and not in women with the BRCA1 mutation [18]. Cullinane et al. evaluated 1260 multiparous women who carried BRCA1 and BRCA2 mutations compared with multiparous women lacking these mutations. Women with BRCA1 exhibited a reduced risk of breast cancer, whereas those with the BRCA2 mutation exhibited an increased risk. In addition, this study also observed that BRCA2 carriers exhibit an increased risk in the first 2 years postpartum [19].

Treatment

The diagnosis of breast cancer during pregnancy has a strong emotional impact on all those involved because it affects young patients in a special period of their lives. Multidisciplinary evaluation is necessary from the beginning. Psychological assistance should be emphasized with various issues addressed: the maternal prognosis, first and foremost, followed by the effects of the therapy on the fetus and the risk of continuing with the pregnancy. In its early stages, breast cancer does not interfere with the course of the pregnancy. However, advanced-stage breast cancer can lead to cachexia, which causes delayed intrauterine growth and preterm birth.

The course of breast cancer treatment during pregnancy must consider the gestational age and the stage of the disease. In general, the treatment follows the same advice given to cases outside the gestational cycle because no evidence is available suggesting that breast cancer in pregnant women biologically differs from that found in premenopausal women who are not pregnant. Interruption of the pregnancy does not improve survival. Additionally, the possible teratogenic risks of the therapy in isolation do not justify an interruption.

Pregnancy-associated bca should be treated as aggressively as and according to the standards applicable in nonpregnant women; pregnancy after bca does not jeopardize outcome.

The guidelines addressing risks connected to pregnancy and bca lack a high level of evidence for better counseling young women about pregnancy considerations and preventing unnecessary abortions. Ideally, evidence from large prospective randomized trials would set better guidelines, and yet the complexity of such studies limits their feasibility [20].

Surgical Treatment

In 1943, Haagensen asserted that "carcinoma of the breast developing during pregnancy or lactation is so malignant that surgery can not cure it often enough to justify this method of treatment" [5]. At that time, he defended palliative radiotherapy as the only therapy despite the fetal risk [32]. Subsequently, Haagensen modified his criteria and began to surgically treat PABC [7].

The general anesthesia used in surgery is relatively safe for the mother and fetus. Numerous studies have indicated that there is no increase in mortality and that the risk of premature labor in extra-abdominal surgical procedures is minimal [21].

At the time of writing, if evidence does not suggest metastatic disease, the initial therapeutic concept is surgical. Modified radical mastectomy is the technique most often indicated [21, 22]. Even for small tumors, conservative surgery is not indicated because radiotherapy cannot be administered in combination. Studies by Gallenberg et al. (1989) and Willemse et al. [24] indicated that delaying treatment reduces survival. However, in patients in their third trimester with tumors smaller than 4 cm who want conservative treatment, it is possible to perform a segmentectomy with axillary dissection in combination with radiotherapy after the interruption of the pregnancy [23, 24].

Currently, the use of the sentinel lymph node technique with a radiotracer in initial tumors with clinically negative axilla is possible [25]. The procedure's radioactivity and the changes in the lymphatic drainage patterns of the breast during the pregnancy must be evaluated. The use of dyes for researching the sentinel lymph node has not been tested in animals and humans to date and must therefore be avoided. This technique is not indicated in patients with fewer than 30 weeks gestation, and lactation is contraindicated for some days following the procedure due to the excretion of the radioactive substance in the breast milk [26].

Patients whose disease is initially systemic may undergo tumor resection with the palliative objective of cytoreduction. Locally advanced and inflammatory tumors are treated with a combination of chemotherapy, radiotherapy, and surgery. In these cases, the surgery has a hygienic purpose [4].

Radiotherapy

Radiotherapy must be discouraged unless delayed until after the birth because the standard radiation technique for the breast field subjects the fetus to unacceptably high risks. A complete treatment would expose the fetus to doses between 20 and 100 cGy, depending on the field and the fundal height. The risk of malformations increases when the dose of radiation is greater than 10 cGy [23]. Maximum fetal sensitivity occurs during the period of organogenesis and up to the 20th week of gestation. However, in the last trimester, a considerable risk of adverse effects is noted due to the proximity of the fetus to the radiotherapy fields. The sequelae of radiotherapy include loss of pregnancy, malformation, growth and development disorders, and mutagenic and carcinogenic effects in the fetus [17, 27].

Chemotherapy

The primary mechanisms of action of antineoplastic chemotherapies are related to cell growth. Thus, tissues with dividing cells are very sensitive. The cells in the embryo are constantly dividing, making the fetus extremely vulnerable. The risk of teratogenesis depends on the stage of the pregnancy during which the chemotherapy is administered and the type of drug. The most frequent malformations occur in patients who are

exposed to alkylating and antimetabolic agents in the first trimester of gestation. For example, 5-fluorouracil (5-FU), methotrexate, and 6-mercaptopurine are the most teratogenic chemotherapeutic agents.

The risks posed by the association of chemotherapy with pregnancy are not yet clear. Many of the studies have been undertaken using laboratory animals, and research in humans has been restricted to the immediate effects. Thus, information is unavailable regarding the future risk of neoplasias and the risks posed to cognitive development and fertility.

Chemotherapy is indicated in the cases of locally advanced/inflammatory/systemic disease and is neoadjuvant to the primary treatment. In all situations, one must evaluate the risk/benefit of administering chemotherapeutic agents. In the locally advanced and inflammatory disease, chemotherapy is mandatory, generally preoperative. There is urgent need to initiate the therapy, and any delay can result in increased morbidity. A 3- to 6-month delay can increase the risk of metastasis by 5–10 % [14]. Care for the mother takes priority, and the fetal risk is secondary because the mother's life is threatened. In this situation, interruption of the pregnancy may be considered.

Adjuvant chemotherapy is indicated in patients who are treated surgically and those who have a greater risk of developing metastases. The decision to institute treatment must be discussed with the patient, and all the risks of malformations must be explained.

The chemotherapy protocols used in most breast cancer cases include cyclophosphamide/methotrexate/5-FU (CMF) and 5-FU/adriamycin/cyclophosphamide (FAC). Regarding the administration of chemotherapy, methotrexate must be excluded. A study has reported that the weekly administration of doxorubicin in the second and third trimesters resulted in satisfactory results without additional fetal risks of suffering or malformations [28].

The use of any chemotherapeutic agent during the first trimester of pregnancy must be discouraged. FAC or AC may be given with relative safety during the second and third trimesters of pregnancy [29]. Ondansetron, lorazepam, and dexamethasone can be used as part of the pre-chemotherapy antiemetic regimen. Although the use of chemotherapy in the second and third trimesters probably induces few abnormalities, further studies that monitor long-term effects must be performed. Chemotherapy should ideally be postponed until after birth.

In 2010, a review of the literature evaluated 40 cases involving the administration of taxanes during gestation. The taxanes are a group of antineoplastic medications with antimitotic action that improve the prognosis of women with breast cancer, particularly those with affected lymph nodes. Docetaxel and paclitaxel are the most commonly used taxanes. Further studies are needed to evaluate the pharmacokinetics and transplacental passage [30]. If used, the NCCN Panel recommends weekly administration of paclitaxel after the first trimester if clinically indicated by disease status [29].

Trastuzumab (Herceptin) is a human monoclonal antibody that is indicated in tumors that exhibit amplification or overexpression of the HER-2 oncogene. Reports have indicated an association between trastuzumab and gestation, namely, that oligohydramnios is reversible upon suspension during use [31, 32]. The use of trastuzumab is contraindicated during gestation because it can lead to pulmonary hypoplasia and neonatal death. In addition, this drug must not be used by those who are breastfeeding, and breastfeeding is contraindicated up to 6 months after the last dose [32, 33].

Lapatinib, a tyrosine kinase inhibitor that affects both HER-2/neu (erbB-2) and the epithelial growth factor receptor (erbB-1), was approved for use in tumors exhibiting HER-2 overexpression and in patients who do not obtain a satisfactory response through the use of trastuzumab. No studies are available regarding its safe use during pregnancy and lactation. A single case report of 11 weeks of exposure to lapatinib in the first and second trimesters during treatment for breast cancer reported an uncomplicated delivery of a healthy female neonate [34].

Methotrexate is contraindicated in all phases of pregnancy because of its abortive and teratogenic effect [29].

Hormone Therapy

Pregnancy can reduce hormonal receptor levels in the cytoplasm of breast cancer cells, culminating in false-negative results. The high levels of circulating estrogen in pregnant women cause the receptor to translocate to the nucleus. In addition, the circulating estrogen occupies all the cytoplasmic receptors.

The difficulty of defining whether the tumor is hormone receptor positive or negative is an additional obstacle to hormone therapy because it is unknown whether the tumor will respond to hormonal manipulation. In young patients regardless of pregnancy, the tumors are generally undifferentiated and hormonal receptor negative.

The relative increased incidence of malformations, miscarriages, and fetal losses suggests that tamoxifen should not be administered during pregnancy. The principal malformations observed include ambiguous genitalia, hypertrophy of the clitoris, and cleft palate [35].

Summary of the Recommendations for the Treatment of Breast Cancer During Pregnancy

Stages I and II

These tumors are operable. Modified radical mastectomy is the treatment of choice. Segmental resection with axillary dissection and radiotherapy is restricted to those tumors that are up to 4 cm and diagnosed close to term. A sentinel lymph node study may be indicated when the axilla is clinically negative (Pandit-Taskar 2004) [25]. Sentinel node biopsy should not be offered to pregnant women under 30 weeks gestation. Isosulfan blue or methylene blue dye for sentinel node biopsy procedures is discouraged during pregnancy.

The indications for systemic chemotherapy are the same in the pregnant patient as in the nonpregnant patient. Adjuvant chemotherapy may be administered in patients with poor prognosis but only after the 20th week (in the second and third trimester). Chemotherapy during pregnancy should not be given after week 35 of pregnancy or within 3 weeks of planned delivery in order to avoid the complications during delivery.

Stages III and IV

These stages include locally advanced tumors or systemic disease. The initial treatment is clinical via chemotherapy. The surgery indicated (i.e., hygienic mastectomy or tumorectomy) depends on the response to the treatment.

Results

A review of the older literature on breast cancer in pregnancy demonstrates a worse prognosis compared with nonpregnant women [36]. Subsequent studies have revealed similar results when comparing groups with the same stage (Table 24.1). The divergence results from the fact that the diagnosis of breast cancer in pregnant women generally occurs later and at more advanced stages.

Petrek (1991) undertook a retrospective study comparing age and stage in pregnant women with breast cancer and a control group [21]. Nugent (1985) was also associated with this study and compared groups of patients greater and less than 40 years of age [37]. The results demonstrated that age, not pregnancy, is the main predictive factor of a poor prognosis.

Effects on the Fetus and Gestation

The embryonic period lasts up to the ninth week of gestation when the embryo is 4 cm in size and most of the organs are forming. From the tenth week onward, the fetal period begins, which is characterized by the growth and maturation of the newly formed structures. Harm during the embryonic period results in spontaneous miscarriage or significant malformations, whereas deficiencies of growth and development predominate in the fetal period. The susceptibility to teratogenic drugs and radiation reduces as the preg-

Table 24.1 Survival rate of pregnant and nonpregnant women below 40 years of age with breast cancer [37]

Survival (%)			
Stage	Pregnant	Nonpregnant	p
I	4/4 (100)	59/84 (70)	0.57
II	7/14 (50)	27/57 (48)	1.0
III	0/1 (0)	1/14 (7)	1.0
General	11/19 (57)	87/155 (56)	1.0

nancy progresses, and this susceptibility becomes minimal after organogenesis (20 weeks) [38, 39].

Metastases of any kind to the fetus and placenta are rare. At the time of writing, 52 cases are reported in the literature (different sites), including 45 for the placenta and seven for the fetus. Although no case of breast cancer metastasis to the fetus has been reported, four studies have reported breast cancer metastasis to the placenta [40].

Stages I and II do not interfere with the progression of the pregnancy. In advanced and metastatic cases, the general state of the pregnancy may be compromised due to cachexia and consequently delayed intrauterine growth.

The type of birth does not interfere in the progression of the disease. The criteria must be rigorously obstetric.

Lactation

There is no evidence that the suppression of lactation improves the prognosis of patients experiencing breast cancer during the pregnancy-postpartum cycle. Lactation appears to be safe and possible. Breastfeeding from the contralateral breast is not affected.

In patients who receive conservative surgery and subsequent radiotherapy, the production of milk may be affected in the treated breast. Breastfeeding is not recommended from the irradiated breast due to the increased risk of developing mastitis.

The majority of the drugs used to treat breast cancer (mainly the alkylating agents) are excreted in human breast milk. Lactation must be avoided during chemotherapy with trastuzumab and lapatinib and during endocrine therapy [41, 42].

Fertility and Subsequent Pregnancy

The development of modern treatments for malignant tumors allows long survival and preservation of gonadal function [43]. The effect of chemotherapy on ovarian function is similar to that of the radiotherapy, and the probability of ovarian insufficiency is proportional to the cumulative dose and the patient's age. Young patients are less prone to present permanent ovarian insufficiency.

Many women who have been treated for breast cancer wish to become pregnant in the future. Gestations were originally thought to favor tumor relapses due to the high hormonal levels; however, studies by Hoover [44] and Vange (1991) demonstrate that another pregnancy does not influence the prognosis [44, 45]. Petrek (1991) demonstrated increased survival in a group of patients who became pregnant compared with a control group [46].

Although a subsequent gestation does not alter the prognosis, patients are recommended to avoid another pregnancy for 3–5 years following the diagnosis. The highest risk of relapse occurs in the first 2 years, and cancer recurrence in a pregnant woman poses a difficulty for the treatment.

Interruption of the Pregnancy

Formerly, interruption of the pregnancy was routinely indicated as part of the treatment for breast cancer because it was believed that placental hormones stimulated tumor cell growth. Furthermore, in the pregnancy, immunological alterations cause reduced cellular immunity.

Studies by Max et al. (1983), Ribeiro et al. [47], and Hoover [44] demonstrated that interruption of the pregnancy does not influence the prognosis; currently, this practice is exclusively indicated in cases wherein there is risk to the mother's life [13, 44, 47].

Conclusions

Various factors have been implicated in the poor prognosis of PABC, including high hormonal levels, lymphatic and blood vessel vasodilation, and pregnancy-associated immunodeficiency. However, this prognosis does not depend to such an extent on the pregnancy; it is mainly associated with the clinical stage of the disease and these patients' young age.

If there is clinical suspicion of a mammary tumor during pregnancy and lactation, we must never delay the diagnosis. Fine-needle biopsy and ultrasound can be useful; however, negative results do not exclude the need for surgical biopsy. Once the disease is diagnosed, its stage must be established quickly, always bearing in mind the difficulties caused by the gestation.

The treatment frequently encounters clinical and ethical obstacles. The gestational age is fundamental in our therapeutic options, resulting in persistent modifications and procedural delays. Surgical treatment can be undertaken in any phase of the pregnancy. Chemotherapy may possibly be administered in the second or third trimesters. Endocrine therapy and radiation therapy are contraindicated during pregnancy and these treatments are reserved for the postpartum period.

Interruption of the gestation does not affect the treatment; however, it undoubtedly facilitates therapeutic conduct. The indication of this course of action must be undertaken with great consideration and discussed openly with the patient and her family.

References

1. Amant F, Deckers S, Van Calsteren K, Loibl S, Halaska M, Brepoels L, et al. Breast cancer in pregnancy: recommendations of an international consensus meeting. Eur J Cancer. 2010;46(18):3158–68.
2. Matias M. Epidemiologia. In: Magalhães Costa M, Novais Dias E, Salvador Silva H, Figueira A, editors. Câncer de Mama para Ginecologistas. São Paulo: Editora Revinter; 1994.
3. Keinan-Boker L, Lerner-Geva L, Kaufman B, Meirow D. Pregnancy-associated breast cancer. Isr Med Assoc J. 2008;10(10):722–7.
4. Loibl S, Minckwitz GV, Gwyn K, Ellis P, Blohmer JU, Schlegelberger BM, et al. Breast carcinoma during pregnancy. International recommendations from an expert meeting. Cancer. 2006;106(2):237–46.

5. Haagensen CD, Stout AP. Carcinoma of the breast: II. Criteria of operability. Ann Surg. 1943;118(5): 859–70.
6. Westberg SV. Prognosis of breast cancer for pregnant and nursing women. Acta Obstet Gynecol Scand. 1946;25:1–239.
7. Haagensen CD. Cancer of the breast in pregnancy and during lactation. Am J Obstet Gynecol. 1967;98(1):141–9.
8. Brasil. Ministério da Saúde. Instituto Nacional do Câncer. Câncer de Mama. Available at: http://www2. inca.gov.br/wps/wcm/connect/tiposdecancer/site/ home/mama.
9. White TT. Carcinoma of the breast and pregnancy; analysis of 920 cases collected from the literature and 22 new cases. Ann Surg. 1954;139(1):9–18.
10. Wallack MK, Wolf Jr JA, Bedwinek J, Denes AE, Glasgow G, Kumar B, et al. Gestational carcinoma of the female breast. Curr Probl Cancer. 1983;7(9): 1–58.
11. Birks DM, Crawford GM, Ellison LG, Johnstone FR. Carcinoma of the breast in women 30 years of age or less. Surg Gynecol Obstet. 1973;137(1):21–5.
12. Richards SR, Chang F, Moynihan V, O'Shaughnessy R. Metastatic breast cancer complicating pregnancy. J Reprod Med. 1984;29(3):211–3.
13. Max MH, Klamer TW. Pregnancy and breast cancer. South Med J. 1983;76:1008–90.
14. Nettleton J, Long J, Kuban D, Wu R, Shaeffer J, El Mahdi A. Breast cancer during pregnancy: quantifying the risk of treatment delay. Obstet Gynecol. 1996;87(3):414–8.
15. Shellock FG, Crues JV. MR procedures: biologic effects, safety, and patient care. Radiology. 2004;232(3):635–52.
16. Leyendecker JR, Gorengaut V, Brown JJ. MR imaging of maternal diseases of the abdomen and pelvis during pregnancy and the immediate postpartum period. Radiographics. 2004;24(5):1301–16.
17. Dequanter D, Hertens D, Veys I, Nogaret JM. Breast cancer and pregnancy. Review of the literature. Gynecol Obstet Fertil. 2001;29(1):9–14.
18. Antoniou AC, Shenton A, Maher ER, Watson E, Woodward E, Lalloo F, et al. Parity and breast cancer risk among BRCA1 and BRCA2 mutation carriers. Breast Cancer Res. 2006;8(6):R72.
19. Cullinane CA, Lubinski J, Neuhausen SL, Ghadirian P, Lynch HT, Isaacs C, et al. Effect of pregnancy as a risk factor for breast cancer in BRCA1/BRCA2 mutation carriers. Int J Cancer. 2005;117(6):988–91.
20. Raphael J, Trudeau ME, Chan K. Outcome of patients with pregnancy during or after breast cancer: a review of the recent literature. Curr Oncol. 2015;22 Suppl 1:S8–18.
21. Petrek JA. Breast cancer and pregnancy. J Natl Cancer Inst Monogr. 1994;16:113–21.
22. Gemignani ML, Petrek JA, Borgen PI. Breast cancer and pregnancy. Surg Clin N Am. 1999;79(5): 1157–69.
23. Gallenberg MM, Loprinzi CL. Breast cancer and pregnancy. Semin Oncol. 1989;16:369–76.
24. Willemse PH, van der Sijde R, Sleijfer DT. Combination chemotherapy and radiation for stage IV breast cancer during pregnancy. Gynec Obst. 1990;36(2):281–4.
25. Pandit-Taskar N, Dauer LT, Montgomery L, St Germain J, Zanzonico PB, Divgi CR. Organ and fetal absorbed dose estimates from 99mTc-sulfur colloid lymphoscintigraphy and sentinel node localization in breast cancer patients. J Nucl Med. 2006;47(7):1202–8.
26. Filippakis GM, Zografos G. Contraindications of sentinel lymph node biopsy: are there any really? World J Surg Oncol. 2007;5:10.
27. Kal HB, Struikmans H. Radiotherapy during pregnancy: fact and fiction. Lancet Oncol. 2005;6(5): 328–33.
28. Barni S, Ardizzoia A, Zanetta G, Strocchi E, Lissoni P, Tancini G. Weekly doxorubicin chemotherapy for breast cancer in pregnancy. A case report. Tumori. 1992;78(5):349–50.
29. Breast Cancer. v2.2015. http://www.nccn.org/professionals/physician_gls/f_guidelines.asp#site.
30. Mir O, Berveiller P, Goffinet F, Treluyer JM, Serreau R, Goldwasser F, Rouzier R. Taxanes for breast cancer during pregnancy: a systematic review. Ann Oncol. 2010;21(2):425–6.
31. Shrim A, Garcia-Bournissen F, Maxwell C, Farine D, Koren G. Trastuzumab treatment for breast cancer during pregnancy. Can Fam Physician. 2008;54(1): 31–2.
32. Zagouri F, Sergentanis TN, Chrysikos D, Papadimitriou CA, Dimopoulos MA, Bartsch R. Trastuzumab administration during pregnancy: a systematic review and meta-analysis. Breast Cancer Res Treat. 2013;137(2):349–57.
33. http://www2.inca.gov.br/wps/wcm/connect/agencianoticias/site/home/noticias/2013/inca_ministerio_saude_apresentam_estimativas_cancer_2014.
34. Kelly H, Graham M, Humes E, Dorflinger LJ, Boggess KA, O'Neil BH, et al. Delivery of a healthy baby after first-trimester maternal exposure to lapatinib. Clin Breast Cancer. 2006;7(4):339–41.
35. Braems G, Denys H, De Wever O, Cocquyt V, Van den Broecke R. Use of tamoxifen before and during pregnancy. Oncologist. 2011;16(11):1547–51.
36. Barnavon Y, Wallack M. Management of the pregnant patient with carcinoma of the breast. Surg Gynecol Obstet. 1990;171(4):347–52.
37. Nugent P, O Connell T. Breast cancer and pregnancy. Arch Surg. 1985;120(11):1221–4.
38. Epstein RJ. Adjuvant breast cancer chemotherapy during late-trimester pregnancy: not quite a standard of care. BMC Cancer. 2007;7:92.
39. Garber JE. Long-term follow-up of children exposed in utero to antineoplastic agents. Semin Oncol. 1989;16(5):437–44.

40. Potter JF, Schoeneman M. Metastasis of maternal cancer to the placenta and fetus. Cancer. 1970;25(2): 380–8.

41. Moran MS, Colasanto JM, Haffty BG, Wilson LD, Lund MW, Higgins SA. Effects of breast-conserving therapy on lactation after pregnancy. Cancer J. 2005;11(5):399–403.

42. Azim Jr HA, Bellettini G, Gelber S, Peccatori FA. Breast-feeding after breast cancer: if you wish, madam. Breast Cancer Res Treat. 2009;114(1):7–12.

43. Gerber B, Dieterich M, Müller H, Reimer T. Controversies in preservation of ovary function and fertility in patients with breast cancer. Breast Cancer Res Treat. 2008;108(1):1–7.

44. Hoover Jr HC. Breast cancer during pregnancy and lactation. Surg N Am. 1990;70:1151–63.

45. Vange NVD, Dongen JAV. Breast cancer and pregnancy. Eur J Surg Oncol. 1991;17:18.

46. Petrek JA, Dukoff R, Rogatko A. Prognosis of pregnancy associated breast cancer. Cancer. 1991;67(4): 869–72.

47. Ribeiro G, Jones DA, Jones M. Carcinoma of the breast associated with pregnancy. Br J Surg. 1986;73(8):607–9.

Paget's Disease of the Breast

Abdullah İğci, Nihat Aksakal, and Enver Özkurt

Abstract

Paget's disease of the breast is a rare breast tumor that was first identified by Sir James Paget in 1874. It is characterized by eczema-form changes accompanied with erosion and ulceration of the nipple and areolar epidermis. It is mostly correlated with ductal carcinoma in situ (DCIS); additionally, it can be accompanied by invasive ductal carcinoma (IDC). The diagnosis is determined upon microscopically observing Paget cells in a skin biopsy. The width of the lesion is evaluated via mammography and MRI in patients for whom breast-preserving surgery is planned. Depending on the extent of the lesion, sentinel lymph node biopsy and axillary curettage for those having axillary metastases are the treatment alternatives to breast-preserving surgery or mastectomy.

Keywords

Paget carcinoma • Ulceration of the nipple • Eczematous lesions • Central resection

A. İğci, MD, FACS (✉)
Breast Unit, Department of General Surgery,
Istanbul University, Istanbul Medical Faculty,
Istanbul, Turkey
e-mail: aigci@istanbul.edu.tr

N. Aksakal, MD • E. Özkurt, MD
Department of General Surgery, Istanbul University,
Istanbul Medical Faculty, Istanbul, Turkey
e-mail: aksakalnihat@yahoo.com;
doctorenver@gmail.com

Paget's Disease of the Breast

Paget's disease of the breast is a rare breast tumor that was first identified by Sir James Paget in 1874 [1]. It is characterized by eczema-form changes accompanied with erosion and ulceration of the nipple and areolar epidermis. It is mostly correlated with ductal carcinoma in situ (DCIS); additionally, it can be accompanied by invasive ductal carcinoma (IDC). The diagnosis is determined upon microscopically observing Paget cells in a skin biopsy. The width of the lesion is evaluated via mammography and MRI in patients for whom breast-preserving surgery is planned. Based on the extent of the lesion, sentinel lymph node biopsy or axillary curettage for those having axillary metastases are the treatment alternatives with breast-preserving surgery or mastectomy.

Epidemiology

Paget's disease is a less frequent malignant breast tumor than other breast cancers, constituting 0.5–3 % of all breast cancers [2–4]. The incidence of Paget's disease is reported as 1 % clinically, but histologically, the incidence of Paget's disease has been reported to be approximately 5 % in some mastectomy series. It is observed in all decades of life in adult women; however, it is most frequently observed in postmenopausal women in the sixth and seventh decades of life [5, 6]. It develops on the ground of a ductal carcinoma, most frequently on DCIS ground. Rarely, it is observed in men, and its clinical course is similar to that of other breast cancers.

Pathogenesis

The transformation theory and the epidermotropic theory have been suggested for the pathogenesis of Paget's disease. The transformation theory suggests that Paget's disease develops as a result of malign changes of the epidermal keratinocytes on the nipple skin independently from ductal epithelial malignancy. In some cases, it is accompanied by parenchymal breast disease; however, it is suggested that these two tumors are independent from one another because Paget's disease has peripheral localization [7–9]. According to the epidermotropic theory, Paget's disease originates from underlying breast disease. Paget cells develop via the migration of neoplastic ductal epithelial cells toward the epidermis of the nipple through ductal canals. The fact that DCIS and IDC accompany Paget's disease to a great extent supports the accuracy of this theory. Other evidence that confirms the accuracy of this theory includes molecular markers, such as HER2, that

show similarity to Paget's disease and underlying ductal epithelial breast tumors; additionally, Paget cells and ductal epithelial cells show similarity in immunohistochemical (IHC) staining; further, epidermal keratinocytes are not similar to Paget cells [10–12].

Clinic

Paget's disease begins with itching, redness, crusting, and ulceration of the nipple and areola (Fig. 25.1). Erosions and ulcerations imitating eczematous lesions appear around the nipple [13, 14]. At times, hemorrhagic nipple discharge can occur as well. When symptoms such as pain, itching, and burning occur, Paget's disease can easily be confused with benign skin diseases of the nipple. Medical treatment applied is thus the most significant cause of delay in diagnosis. The disease is mostly unilateral, but bilateral cases have also been reported. The involvement of the entire nipple and areola and cutaneous

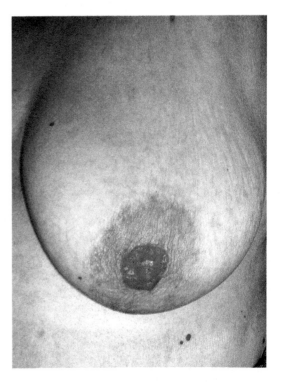

Fig. 25.1 Redness, crusting, and ulcer of the nipple and areola

involvement are rare. Generally, Paget's disease is not accompanied by a mass; however, if it is accompanied with a mass, the possibility that the tumor has evolved into invasive cancer is significantly higher. Although rare, the accompanying retraction of the nipple suggests advanced disease. The time between the development of symptoms and the histopathological diagnosis is approximately 6 months. Because pathologic findings in mammography are rare and because this disease is generally not accompanied by a mass, chronic pathologic findings of the nipple are significant.

Differential Diagnosis

Benign skin diseases such as contact dermatitis and psoriasis, which resemble eczematous lesions, should generally be considered first. When these lesions are considered in differential diagnosis, short-term steroid treatment can be accepted. However, in unilateral and chronic-coursing lesions, Paget's disease should definitely be considered in differential diagnosis. Additionally, some malignant skin lesions such as basal cell carcinoma, superficial spreading malignant melanoma, and Bowen's disease should also be considered in differential diagnosis [7, 15].

Detailed anamnesis is very significant, and whether symptoms such as pain, burning, itching, nipple discharge, and hemorrhage are accompanied by the initiation process of the lesions should be identified. Risk factors should be taken into consideration in terms of individual and familial breast cancer. The breasts should be examined bilaterally, and suspected nipple lesions should be evaluated via biopsy.

Diagnosis

Mammography

In approximately half of Paget patients, mammographic abnormalities such as microcalcifications, masses, and parenchymal distortions are detected. The sensitivity is extremely high in palpable lesions, but it is low in non-palpable lesions. Accompanying parenchymal tumors and extensive microcalcifications may alter surgical treatment alternatives in patients, particularly in those for whom breast-preserving surgery is planned. The presence of multicentric tumors and synchronous tumors in the other breast should be investigated. Thus, patients should be evaluated via bilateral mammography in Paget's disease [16, 17].

Ultrasound (US)

US is a very beneficial complementary imaging method, particularly in patients who are negative mammographically. It is more sensitive in showing a mass or parenchymal distortion, and it is also a good alternative for evaluation of the axilla [18, 19].

Magnetic Resonance Imaging (MRI)

Although MRI has a low sensitivity in terms of DCIS, it is a very sensitive method for the evaluation of IDC. It can show the difference between normal tissue and a nipple-areola complex with a tumor. In non-palpable and preoperative evaluations, it is a very beneficial method in occult lesions in which mammography and US are negative. However, negative MRI findings do not exclude the presence of occult lesions [20, 21].

Biopsy

The definitive diagnosis of Paget's disease is revealed via histopathological examination. A diagnosis can be made with a nipple swab; however, obtaining a tissue sample from the lesion via full-layer wedge biopsy or punch biopsy is generally required. In a microscopic evaluation, Paget cells not invading the basal membrane are observed. These cells consist of hyperchromatic cells with a wide, clear cytoplasm and a prominent nucleolus (Figs. 25.2 and 25.3). They are

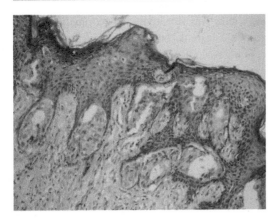

Fig. 25.2 A case of Paget's disease of the nipple: neoplastic glandular cells inside the nipple epidermis (hematoxylin-eosin ×20 original magnification)

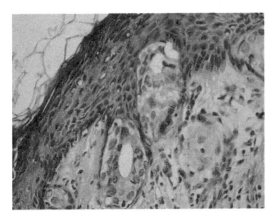

Fig. 25.3 Detailed appearance of neoplastic glandular cells of Paget's disease of the nipple. Note the neoplastic cells are forming apparent glandular structures inside the epidermis (hematoxylin-eosin ×40 original magnification)

present in the nipple epidermis as single cells or in groups. Histologically, these cells can be confused with malignant melanoma because of the presence of epidermal cells, which contain melanin. The presence of cytoplasmic mucin vacuoles may be helpful in the diagnosis. Immunohistochemical tests may be helpful in differential diagnosis. In immunohistochemical tests, positive staining for CEA and negative staining for S100 are differentiating characteristics of malignant melanoma. Positivity for estrogen and progesterone (which is negative in half of the cases) is very beneficial. Hormone receptor

negativity is mostly accompanied with high grades of invasive ductal carcinoma. Cytokeratin positivity with low molecular dominance is a helpful characteristic for differentiating Bowen's disease, which displays cytokeratin positivity with high molecule dominance.

In the absence of typical histopathological findings, CK7 is a very beneficial marker [22, 23].

Staging

Staging is conducted in accordance with the TNM classification of the accompanying breast tumors. The presence of Paget's disease does not change the stage of the tumor. Paget's disease is classified as Tis (Paget) in isolated disease.

Treatment

Determining the treatment of Paget's disease is based on whether or not an accompanying parenchymal pathology exists in the same side. The main factors that determine the treatment approach are the size, invasive characteristics of the accompanying tumor, and whether it is an axillary lymph node or not. Simple mastectomy was a preferred method in the past, but recently, breast-preserving surgery has gained in favor. Paget's disease is more likely to be diagnosed at an advanced stage than conditions not accompanied by a mass [24]. In this condition, mastectomy is required in many patients. In the presence of a palpable mass or mammographic abnormality, breast-preserving surgery which involves nipple-areola complex with negative surgical margin and acceptable cosmesis result can be performed. In this situation, administering radiotherapy to the entire breast is required. Also, a breast-preserving surgery performed with negative surgical margins and reduction of the other breast to provide symmetry and cosmesis can be performed in large breasts.

Simple mastectomy should be preferred in cases with extensive microcalcification, multicentric cancer, or positive histological margins despite re-excision. Despite achieving negative surgical margins, simple mastectomy may be preferred in conditions with poor cosmesis.

In most Paget cases not accompanied by a palpable mass or microcalcification, an underlying carcinoma is the subject. Most of these cases are DCIS; a few are invasive cancers. In this situation, simple mastectomy or breast-preserving surgery involving the nipple-areola complex (central resection) and radiotherapy may be preferred. Local recurrence, disease-free survival, and life expectancy are similar in these two methods [25]. The risk of axillary lymph node metastasis is higher in Paget patients with a palpable mass. The evaluation of axillary lymph node metastasis and the treatment algorithm are similar to those for other cancers of the breast.

Adjuvant Systemic Therapy

Systemic chemotherapy in Paget carcinoma is necessary in cases of invasive cancer and axillary involvement. Endocrine treatment is preferred, as with DCIS.

Prognosis

Tumor stage is the most significant marker that affects the prognosis of Paget's disease. Accompanying invasive ductal cancer and the presence of axillary lymph node metastasis are factors affecting the prognosis. Because the presence of a palpable mass is accompanied by advanced-stage disease, the prognosis is worse than in patients without a mass. Survival in the cases without invasive cancer is similar to DCIS cases. Additionally, the survival of patients who underwent mastectomy is similar to that of patients who were treated with breast-conserving surgery and adjuvant radiotherapy.

References

1. Paget J. On disease of the mammary areola preceding cancer of the mammary gland. St Bartholomew Hosp Rep. 1874;10:87–9.

2. Desai DC, Brennan Jr EJ, Carp NZ. Paget's disease of the male breast. Am Surg. 1996;62(12):1068–72.

3. Caliskan M, Gatti G, Sosnovskikh I, Rotmensz N, Botteri E, Musmeci S, et al. Paget's disease of the breast: the experience of the European Institute of Oncology and review of the literature. Breast Cancer Res Treat. 2008;112:513.

4. Serour F, Birkenfeld S, Amsterdam E, Treshchan O, Krispin M. Paget's disease of the male breast. Cancer. 1988;62(3):601–5.

5. Ortiz-Pagan S, Cunto-Amesty G, Narayan S, Crawford S, Derrick C, Larkin A, et al. Effect of Paget's disease on survival in breast cancer: an exploratory study. Arch Surg. 2011;146(11): 1267–70.

6. Kaelin CM. Paget's disease. In: Harris JR, Lippman ME, Morrow M, Osborne CK, editors. Diseases of the breast. 3rd ed. Philadelphia: Lippincott Williams & Wilkins; 2004. p. 1007–14.

7. Jamali FR, Ricci Jr A, Deckers PJ. Paget's disease of the nipple-areola complex. Surg Clin N Am. 1996;76:365.

8. Kollmorgen DR, Varanasi JS, Edge SB, Carson 3rd WE. Paget's disease of the breast: a 33-year experience. J Am Coll Surg. 1998;187:171.

9. Sagebiel RW. Ultrastructural observations on epidermal cells in Paget's disease of the breast. Am J Pathol. 1969;57:49.

10. Fu W, Lobocki CA, Silberberg BK, Chelladurai M, Young SC. Molecular markers in Paget disease of the breast. J Surg Oncol. 2001;77:171.

11. Kirkham N, Berry N, Jones DB, Taylor-Papadimitriou J. Paget's disease of the nipple. Immunohistochemical localization of milk fat globule membrane antigens. Cancer. 1985;55:1510.

12. Vanstapel MJ, Gatter KC, De Wolf-Peeters C, Millard PR, Desmet VJ, Mason DY. Immunohistochemical study of mammary and extra-mammary Paget's disease. Histopathology. 1984;8:1013.

13. Franceschini G, Masetti R, D'Ugo D, Palumbo F, D'Alba P, Mulè A, et al. Synchronous bilateral Paget's disease of the nipple associated with bilateral breast carcinoma. Breast J. 2005;11:355.

14. Chaudary MA, Millis RR, Lane EB, Miller NA. Paget's disease of the nipple: a ten year review including clinical, pathological, and immunohistochemical findings. Breast Cancer Res Treat. 1986;8:139.

15. Kobayashi TK, Ueda M, Nishino T, Kibe S, Higashida T, Watanabe S. Scrape cytology of pemphigus vulgaris of the nipple, a mimicker of Paget's disease. Diagn Cytopathol. 1997;16:156.

16. Günhan-Bilgen I, Oktay A. Paget's disease of the breast: clinical, mammographic, sonographic and pathologic findings in 52 cases. Eur J Radiol. 2006;60(2):256–63.

17. Ceccherini AF, Evans AJ, Pinder SE, Wilson AR, Ellis IO, Yeoman LJ. Is ipsilateral mammography worthwhile in Paget's disease of the breast? Clin Radiol. 1996;51:35.

18. Tohno E, Cosgrove DO, Sloane JP. Ultrasound diagnosis of breast disease. London: Churchill Livingstone; 1994. p. 76–178.
19. Sakorafas GH, Blanchard K, Sarr MG, Farley DR. Paget's disease of the breast. Cancer Treat Rev. 2001;27:9–18.
20. Tilanus-Linthorst MM, Obdeijn AI, Bontenbal M, Oudkerk M. MRI in patients with axillary metastases of occult breast carcinoma. Breast Cancer Res Treat. 1997;44:179–82.
21. Friedman EP, Hall-Craggs MA, Mumtaz H, Schneidau A. Breast MR. The appearance of normal and abnormal nipple. Clin Radiol. 1997;52:854–61.
22. Gillett CE, Bobrow LG, Millis RR. S100 protein in human mammary tissue immunoreactivity in breast carcinoma, including Paget's disease of the nipple, and value as a marker of myoepithelial cells. J Pathol. 1990;160:19.
23. Yao D, Hoda S, Ying L, Rosen P. Intraepithelial cytokeratin 7 immunoreactive cells in non-neoplastic nipple represents interepithelial extension of lactiferous duct cells (abstract). Mod Pathol. 2001;14:42A.
24. Zakaria S, Pantvaidya G, Ghosh K, Degnim AC. Paget's disease of the breast: accuracy of preoperative assessment. Breast Cancer Res Treat. 2007;102:137.
25. Solin LJ, Kurtz J, Fourquet A, Amalric R, Recht A, Bornstein BA, et al. Fifteen-year results of breast-conserving surgery and definitive breast irradiation for the treatment of ductal carcinoma in situ of the breast. J Clin Oncol. 1996;14:754.

Phyllodes Tumors of the Breast

26

Fatih Aydoğan, Yunus Taşçı, and Yasuaki Sagara

Abstract

Phyllodes tumors, also termed phylloides tumors or cystosarcoma phyllodes, are rare fibroepithelial neoplasms of the breast that remain challenging for both surgeons and pathologists. The World Health Organization (WHO) established the name phyllodes tumor and the histological types: benign, borderline, and malignant. Phyllodes tumors can be observed in all ages, but the majority of patients are in their fifth decade of life. These tumors may present similarity with fibroadenoma. Breast imaging studies may fail to distinguish the phyllodes tumor from a fibroadenoma. A core needle biopsy is preferable to fine-needle aspiration for tissue diagnosis. The common treatment for phyllodes tumors is wide local excision. Mastectomy is indicated for patients with a large lesion. The benefits of adjuvant chemotherapy and radiotherapy are controversial.

Keywords

Phyllodes tumor • Fibroepithelial neoplasms • Breast • Management of phyllodes tumor • Cystosarcoma phyllodes

F. Aydoğan, MD, FEBS (✉)
Division of Breast Disease, Department of General Surgery, Cerrahpasa School of Medicine, Istanbul University, Istanbul, Turkey

Dana Farber/Brigham and Women's Cancer Center, Harvard Medical School, Boston, MA, USA

Division of Breast Disease, Department of Surgery, Istanbul University Cerrahpasa Medical School, Istanbul, Turkey
e-mail: fatihdr@hotmail.com; fatih_aydogan@dfci.harvard.edu

Y. Taşçı, MD
Department of General Surgery, Medical Faculty, Bezmialem Vakif University, Istanbul, Turkey
e-mail: yunustasci@hotmail.com

Y. Sagara, MD
Dana Farber/Brigham and Women's Cancer Center, Harvard Medical School, Boston, MA, USA
e-mail: yasuaki@sagara.or.jp

Introduction

Phyllodes tumors are rare fibroepithelial neoplasms of the breast that comprise <1 % of all breast malignancies and 2–3 % of fibroepithelial neoplasms [1, 2]. Müller first described phyllodes tumors in 1838 as a mass with leaflike projections and cysts [3]. The clinical course for phyllodes tumors can be unpredictable, but these neoplasms are typically benign, unlike their namesake. In the past, these neoplasms have had various names; however, the World Health Organization (WHO) has designated "phyllodes tumors" as the standard nomenclature, with its histological types classified as benign, borderline, and malignant [4]. The malignant form of phyllodes tumors can have an aggressive clinical course with local recurrence and metastatic spread, whereas the benign form is clinically nearly indistinguishable from a benign breast lump. It is important to differentiate a phyllodes tumor from fibroadenomas, which are treated differently. Diagnostic evaluations remain challenging because these tumors have few characteristic findings observed on most imaging modalities. The surgical management of phyllodes tumors typically consists of wide excisions with adequate surgical margins or simple mastectomies.

Epidemiology and Risk Factors

Because of the rarity of these tumors, well-defined risk factors have not been identified. There is some evidence suggesting that there is increased risk for East Asians and for Latina women born in Central or South America but living in the United States [5–7]. For women in the United States, the incidence rate for malignant phyllodes tumors is 2.1 cases per million [5]. In addition, these tumors are clearly more frequent in women, with only a few cases reported in men, which have invariably been associated with gynecomastia [8, 9].

Clinical Presentation and Diagnosis

According to the current literature, the median age of patients diagnosed with phyllodes tumors is 45 years, with age ranging between 9 and 93 years [2, 5, 10, 11]. Although phyllodes tumors can be observed in all ages, the majority of patients are over 40 years old [1, 2, 5]. The most common symptom leading to diagnosis is a rapidly growing mass in the breast (Fig. 26.1). Dilated veins and blue discoloration can also be observed with large tumors (Fig. 26.2); however, nipple retraction and skin ulcerations are uncommon. Bilateral cases are very rare, with an occurrence rate of 1.6 % [8]. The mean tumor size ranges between 5.2 and 7.3 cm [8, 12, 13]. Tumors up to 50 cm in size have been reported in the literature [14, 15]; however, tumor size and growth rates are not often associated with histopathology. Clinical, radiological, and histopathological evaluations of suspected breast lumps are mandatory. Ultrasound imaging typically shows a smooth, lobulated border, a radiolucent halo, and coarse microcalcification, but malignant calcifications are rare. Intramural cysts and an absence of posterior acoustic enhancement can be present. On mammographic imaging, phyllodes tumors typically appear as nonspecific, large, round, or oval masses with well-circumscribed lesions (Fig. 26.3). There is no indicator of malignancy or any characteristic findings observed on ultrasounds or mammography. Phyllodes tumors have higher signal intensities than normal breast parenchyma on T1-weighted images and lower or equal signal intensity on T2-weighted images (Fig. 26.4). The role of magnetic resonance imaging (MRI) in this setting remains under debate, but some authors have found evidence suggesting that MRIs may correlate with the histopathology [2, 16]. A fine-needle aspiration (FNA) biopsy is often inadequate for a clear, differential diagnosis. Ultrasound-guided tru-cut biopsies can be a useful method but can be insufficient in some cases. Differentiating between fibroadenomas and benign phyllodes tumors is more difficult than differentiating between benign and malignant phyllodes tumors. The accuracy of clinical, radiological, and histopathological diagnosis is poor; all three have a low specificity. Both epithelioid and stromal components must be visible to confirm a pathological diagnosis, but only the stromal component determines the biological behavior [17] of phyllodes tumors. Generally, there are no masses in the axillary region. Axillary palpable

Fig. 26.1 Presentation of a giant primary phyllodes tumor

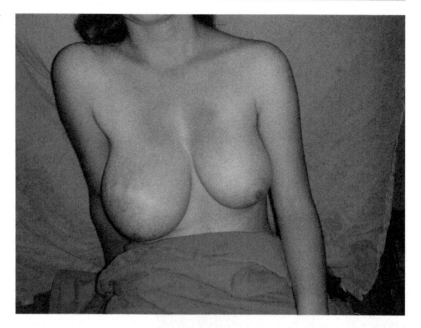

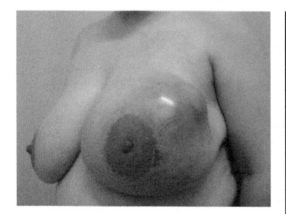

Fig. 26.2 Presentation of a giant recurrent malign phyllodes tumor

nodes observed in 20 % of patients are often reactive in nature [13, 18]. Phyllodes tumors metastasize hematogenously rather than through the lymphatic system; therefore, routine axillary dissection is not recommended [2, 8, 13].

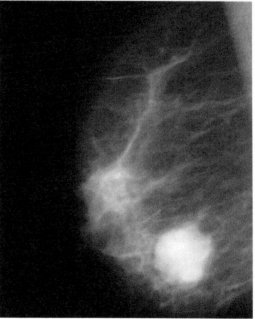

Fig. 26.3 Mediolateral oblique mammography view demonstrating a circumscribed round mass

Pathology

Fibroepithelial neoplasms originate mostly from the stroma in the terminal ducto-lobular unit. Phyllodes tumors are evaluated in fibroepithelial neoplasms, and their microscopic appearance is

widely variable, often mimicking fibroadenoma or sarcoma (Fig. 26.5). Established histological types – benign, borderline, and malignant – are determined by the tumor margin, stromal cellularity, stromal overgrowth, tumor necrosis, cellular atypia, and the number of mitosis per 10 hpf (high-power fields) defined by Azzopardi and Salvadori [10, 19] (Table 26.1). A phyllodes tumor is not a pure sarcomatoid lesion. If there are no epithelial components observed during histological examination, tissue sarcomas [20] should be considered. The clinical appearances of malignant and benign phyllodes tumors are more alike than different; however, tumors of the malignant type often show a more aggressive

course. Today, it is widely accepted that fibroadenomas should be treated conservatively; therefore, it is critical to differentiate between benign phyllodes tumors and fibroadenomas, which display similar clinical, radiological, and cytological findings. Benign phyllodes tumors constitute between 35 % and 64 % of known cases, whereas the malignant form constitutes approximately 25 % of cases [13, 15]. Fibroadenomas and phyllodes tumors can appear synchronously or metasynchronously. Noguchi et al. showed that phyllodes tumors can arise from monoclonal proliferation caused by somatic mutations in a portion of a fibroadenoma [21]. Because of the rarity of this phenomenon, there are no well-described risk factors; however, some genetic factors such as Ki-67, p53, c-myc, c-kit, CD117, and actin expression levels may be helpful to distinguish the malignant from the benign form [22–24].

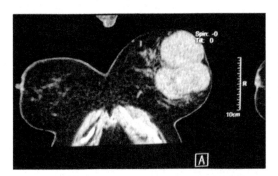

Fig. 26.4 Magnetic resonance imaging of a phyllodes tumor

Treatment

Mastectomy had been the preferred surgical option for several decades; however, breast conservative surgery has recently become widely adopted. Wide excision – with adequate margins – is now the preferred treatment for phyllodes tumors. Large tumors, or tumors occupying the entire breast, can be treated with mastectomy because of the possibility of a poor cosmetic outcome with a wide excision. A 1 cm margin should be obtained, particularly with high-grade malignant phyllodes tumors, because local recurrence and cancer-specific survival are related to both tumor size and margin status [25]. The management for phyllodes tumors is shown in the algorithm (Fig. 26.6). Enucleation or shelling out is not recommended because of the unacceptably

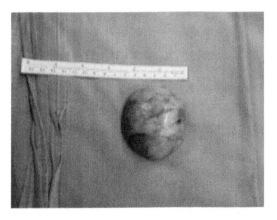

Fig. 26.5 Gross specimen of a phyllodes tumor

Table 26.1 Histologic features used in the classification of phyllodes tumor subtypes

Histological features	Benign	Borderline	Malignant
Tumor margins	Pushing	↔	Infiltrative
Stromal cellular atypia	Mild	Marked	Marked
Mitotic activity	<4 per 10 high-power fields	4–9 per 10 high-power fields	≥10 per 10 high-power fields
Stromal overgrowth	Absent	Absent	Present

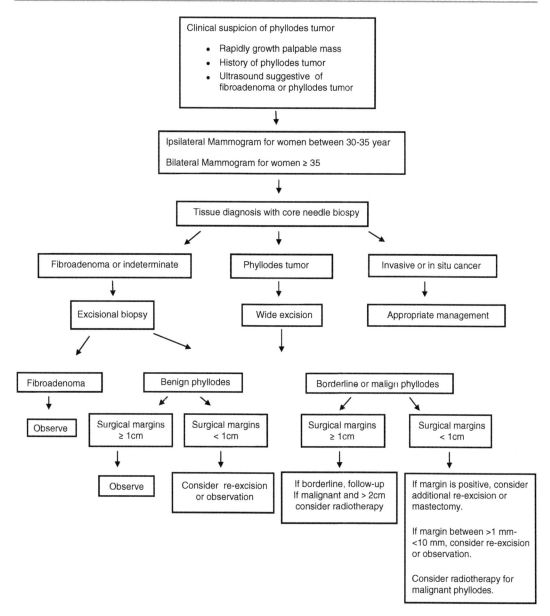

Fig. 26.6 Management algorithm for a phyllodes tumor

high local recurrence rates. Breast reconstruction can be performed in the initial operation if desired. Axillary lymphadenopathy is clinically positive in 10 % of patients, but metastases occur in <1 % of patients [2, 26]. Adjuvant radiotherapy after breast-conserving surgery should be considered for malignant phyllodes tumors larger than 2 cm in diameter [27–29]. There are no prospective randomized data supporting the use of

radiation treatment with phyllodes tumors. However, in settings in which additional recurrences would create significant morbidity (e.g., chest wall recurrence following mastectomy), radiation therapy may be considered following the same principles that are applied to the treatment of soft tissue sarcoma.

There is no evidence that lower distant metastasis rates lead to an increase in overall survival.

Overall survival has a better correlation to malignant phyllodes tumors with inadequate surgical margins [26, 27]. Using adjuvant chemotherapy is more controversial and is generally not recommended. There is no evidence that adjuvant cytotoxic chemotherapy provides benefits in reducing recurrences or death. Although the epithelial component of most phyllodes tumors contains ER (58 %) and/or PR (75 %), endocrine therapy has no proven role in the treatment of phyllodes tumors [30]. Rarely, in some patients who experience a systemic recurrence (usually in the lung), treatment should be recommended similarly to other soft tissue sarcomas.

Twenty percent of phyllodes tumors lead to metastases in distant organs. In most of these cases, the affected organs are the lungs and pleura. Chemotherapy, radiotherapy, and hormonal therapies are all used to treat metastatic disease, but their role and efficacy are unclear.

Local Recurrence and Metastatic Disease

Local recurrence rates ranging between 0 % and 60 % have been previously reported [26, 31]. Local recurrence usually occurs within the first 2 years [31]. For patients with positive surgical margins, the local recurrence rates are as high as 32 % [8]. Distant metastases are very unusual in the benign form, but it has been reported that borderline tumors can metastasize to distant organs [13].

Follow-Up

The most important mode of detecting recurrent disease is clinical evaluation. After treatment for a phyllodes tumor, a clinical assessment should be performed every 6 months. In the vast majority of recurrences, breast phyllodes tumors develop in the excision bed. The 5-year survival rates are approximately 96 %, 74 %, and 66 % for benign, borderline, and malignant types, respectively [2, 31].

References

1. Vorherr H, Vorherr UF, Kutvirt DM, Key CR. Cystosarcoma phyllodes: epidemiology, pathophysiology, pathobiology, diagnosis, therapy and survival. Arch Gynaecol. 1985;236:173–81.
2. Parker SJ, Harries SA. Phyllodes tumours. Postgrad Med J. 2001;77:428–35.
3. Müller J. Uber den feineren Bau und die Formen der krankaften. Geschwilste. 1838;1:54–7.
4. World Health Organisation. Histological typing of breast tumors. Tumori. 1982;68:181–98.
5. Bernstein L, Deapen D, Ross RK. The descriptive epidemiology of malignant cystosarcoma phyllodes tumors of the breast. Cancer. 1993;71:3020–4.
6. Teo JY, Cheong CS, Wong CY. Low local recurrence rates in young Asian patients with phyllodes tumours: less is more. ANZ J Surg. 2012;82:325–8.
7. Chua CL. Cystosarcoma phyllodes: Asian variations. ANZ J Surg. 1988;58:301–5.
8. Spitaleri G, Toesca A, Botteri E, Bottiglieri L, Rotmensz N, Boselli S, et al. Breast phyllodes tumor: a review of literature and a single center retrospective series analysis. Crit Rev Oncol Hematol. 2013;88:427–36.
9. Pantoja E, Llobet RE, Lopez E. Gigantic cystosarcoma phyllodes in a man with gynecomastia. Arch Surg. 1976;111:611.
10. Salvadori B, Cusumano F, Del Bo R, Delledonne V, Grassi M, Rovini D, et al. Surgical treatment of phyllodes tumors of the breast. Cancer. 1989;63:2532–6. 9.
11. Moffat CJ, Pinder SE, Dixon AR, Elston CW, Blamey RW, Ellis IO. Phyllodes tumours of the breast: a clinicopathological review of thirty-two cases. Histopathology. 1995;27:205–18.
12. Tan PH, Jayabaskar T, Chuah KL, Lee HY, Tan Y, Hilmy M, et al. Phyllodes tumors of the breast: the role of pathologic parameters. Am J Clin Pathol. 2005;123:529–40. 13.
13. Reinfuss M, Mitus J, Duda K, Stelmach A, Rys J, Smolak K. The treatment and prognosis of patients with phyllodes tumor of the breast: an analysis of 170 cases. Cancer. 1996;77:910–6.
14. Kumar T, Patel MD, Bhargavan R, Kumar P, Patel MH, Kothari K, et al. Largest phyllodes tumor- case report and brief review article. Indian J Surg Oncol. 2011;2:141–4.
15. Pietruszka M, Barnes L. Cystosarcoma phyllodes. A clinico- pathological analysis of 42 cases. Cancer. 1978;41:1974–83.
16. Yabuuchi H, Soeda H, Matsuo Y, Okafuji T, Eguchi T, Sakai S, et al. Phyllodes tumor of the breast: correlation between MR findings and histologic grade. Radiology. 2006;241:702–9.
17. Aranda FI, Laforga JB, Lopez JL. Phyllodes tumor of the breast. An immunohistochemical study of 28

cases with special attention to the role of myofibro-blast. Pathol Res Pract. 1994;190:474–81.

18. Norris HJ, Taylor HR. Relationship of histological features to behaviour of cystosarcoma phyllodes. Cancer. 1967;20:2090–9.

19. Azzopardi JG. Sarcoma in the breast. In: Benningron J, editor. Problems in breast pathology, vol. II. Philadelphia: WB Saunders; 1979. p. 355–9.

20. Moore MP, Kinne DW. Breast sarcoma. Surg Clin N Am. 1996;76:383–92.

21. Noguchi S, Yokouchi H, Aihara T, Motomura K, Inaji H, Imaoka S, et al. Progression of fibroadenoma to phyllodes tumor demonstrated by clonal analysis. Cancer. 1995;76:1779–85.

22. Chen CM, Chen CJ, Chang CL, Shyu JS, Hsieh HF, Harn HJ. CD34, CD117, and actin expression in phyllodes tumor of the breast. J Surg Res. 2000;94:84–91.

23. Kleer CG, Giordano TJ, Braun T, Oberman HA. Pathologic, immunohistochemical, and molecular features of benign and malignant phyllodes tumors of the breast. Mod Pathol. 2001;14:185–90.

24. Sawyer EJ, Poulsom R, Hunt FT, Jeffery R, Elia G, Ellis IO, et al. Malignant phyllodes tumours show stromal overexpression of c-myc and c-kit. J Pathol. 2003;200:59–64.

25. Kapiris I, Nasiri N, A'Hern R, Healy V, Gui GP. Outcome and predictive factors of local recurrence and distant metastases following primary surgi-cal treatment of high-grade malignant phyllodes tumours of the breast. Eur J Surg Oncol. 2001;27:723–30.

26. Mishra SP, Tiwary SK, Mishra M, Khanna AK. Phyllodes tumor of breast: a review article. ISRN Surg. 2013;2013:361469.

27. Pezner RD, Schultheiss TE, Paz IB. Malignant phyllodes tumor of the breast: local control rates with surgery alone. Int J Radiat Oncol Biol Phys. 2008;1(71):710–3.

28. Gnerlich JL, Williams RT, Yao K, Jaskowiak N, Kulkarni SA. Utilization of radiotherapy for malignant phyllodes tumors: analysis of the National Cancer Data Base, 1998–2009. Ann Surg Oncol. 2014;21:1222–30.

29. Barth Jr RJ, Wells WA, Mitchell SE, Cole BF. A prospective, multi-institutional study of adjuvant radiotherapy after resection of malignant phyllodes tumors. Ann Surg Oncol. 2009;16:2288–94.

30. Tse GM, Lee CS, Kung FY, Scolyer RA, Law BK, Lau TS, Putti TC. Hormonal receptors expression in epithelial cells of mammary phyllodes tumors correlates with pathologic grade of the tumor: a multicenter study of 143 cases. Am J Clin Pathol. 2002;118(4):522–6.

31. Jang JH, Choi MY, Lee SK, Kim S, Kim J, Lee J, et al. Clinicopathologic risk factors for the local recurrence of phyllodes tumors of the breast. Ann Surg Oncol. 2012;19:2612–7.

Nonepithelial Malignancies of the Breast

27

Gürsel Remzi Soybir

Abstract

Breast sarcomas are rare clinical entities. The symptoms are similar to other breast malignancies, and diagnosis depends on conventional triple assessment. However, their biology and prognosis are closer to those of soft tissue sarcomas than to invasive breast cancers. Surgical excision with clear margins is the primary treatment for localized tumors. Lymph node sampling and dissection is not recommended. Adjuvant or neoadjuvant therapy should be considered for high-risk patients. Postoperative radiotherapy shows a small survival advantage, and response rates for systemic therapies are poor. Angiosarcomas are the most common sarcomas of the breast. They can be associated with lymphedema or irradiation. Surgery is the primary treatment, and wide negative margins are essential for a long-term cure. The potential for local recurrence and distant metastasis are high. Leiomyosarcoma, liposarcoma, rhabdomyosarcoma, and fibrosarcoma are the other rare sarcoma subtypes in the breast. Primary breast lymphoma is a rare entity that arises from the periductal and perilobular lymphatic tissue and intramammary lymph nodes. The breast is the first major site of manifestations without any evidence of concurrent systemic disease. A painless, mobile, rapidly enlarging mass is a common clinical presentation. Primary breast lymphomas are sensitive to chemotherapy and radiotherapy. Surgery is limited to biopsy. The clinical stage and histological subtype are the main prognostic factors. Metastatic involvement of the breast most often originates from the contralateral site. The most common malignancy of the body that metastasizes to the breast is malignant melanoma. Hematological malignancies such as leukemia and lymphoma also frequently occur. Comprehensive screening is necessary to identify the origin of the primary tumor.

G.R. Soybir, MD, FALS
Department of General Surgery, Istanbul Memorial Hospital, Istanbul, Turkey
e-mail: gurselr@yahoo.com

© Springer International Publishing Switzerland 2016
A. Aydiner et al. (eds.), *Breast Disease: Management and Therapies*,
DOI 10.1007/978-3-319-26012-9_27

Keywords

Breast • Breast cancer • Sarcoma • Molecular pathogenesis • Postirradiation sarcomas • Post-radiotherapy • Breast lymphoma • Epidemiology • Etiology • Subgroups • Symptoms • Diagnosis • Clinical characteristics • Radiologic imagination • Histological diagnosis • Staging • Treatment • Axillary approach • Surgery • Surgical outcome • Adjuvant therapy • Neoadjuvant therapy • Adjuvant radiotherapy • Adjuvant chemotherapy • Survival • Prognosis • Angiosarcoma • Fibrosarcoma • Leiomyosarcoma • Liposarcoma • Rhabdomyosarcoma • Li-Fraumeni syndrome • Cowden disease • Metastases

Sarcomas

Epidemiology

Breast sarcomas comprise a heterogeneous group of malignant tumors arising from nonepithelial elements of the breast. They are quite rare neoplasms, constituting less than 1 % of breast cancers and less than 5 % of all sarcomas. The increased use of radiotherapy has led to increased breast sarcoma incidence. Breast sarcomas resemble other soft tissue sarcomas of the body. It is very important to differentiate breast sarcomas from other breast cancers because they have substantial biological differences. The phenomenal and predominantly retrospective literature makes it difficult to understand the nature of the disease and to direct disease management. Breast sarcomas are a disease of advanced age, with the median age of breast sarcoma patients between 50 and 60. The disease is more common in women for all subgroups except leiomyosarcomas, for which the incidences are equal in both genders [1–3].

Etiology

The large majority of breast sarcomas have no familiar etiologic factors. While previous radiotherapy and chronic lymphedema are the main etiologic factors, exposure to vinyl chloride and exposure to artificial implants are also risk factors. An incidence of 0.3 % in 15 years has been reported for breast sarcoma. Angiosarcomas appear to be the most common type of radiation-induced sarcoma. Ultimately, breast sarcomas may be part of the spectrum of tumor syndromes such as Li-Fraumeni syndrome that result from genetic mutations [1, 4–6].

Subgroups

Breast sarcomas are generally divided into three distinct groups. The first group is malignant phyllodes tumors, in which the tumor cells originate from epithelial cells. The second and third groups are primary breast sarcomas and postirradiation breast sarcomas, respectively [3]. Breast sarcomas are histologically similar to soft tissue sarcomas and include all subtypes. Although all of the subtypes have been reported to occur in breast, the most common subtypes are malignant fibrous histiocytoma, fibrosarcoma, angiosarcoma, and spindle cell sarcoma. The other rare subtypes are leiomyosarcoma, liposarcoma, rhabdomyosarcoma, hemangiopericytoma, malignant schwannoma, osteogenic sarcoma, chondrosarcoma, and stromal sarcoma [7–12].

Symptoms

Primary sarcomas often present as large, palpable, painless, and rapidly growing masses, whereas secondary angiosarcomas typically present as skin rashes. Advanced breast cancer symptoms such as skin ulcers, discharge, and nipple and skin retractions are unusual manifestations. Axillary lymphatic involvement by the tumor is uncommon [2, 3, 12–14].

Diagnosis

Diagnosis is based on a triple assessment comprising clinical examination, radiologic imaging, and histological evaluation. Core biopsies, which yield more material, are preferred over fine needle aspiration (FNA) biopsies for histological examination [1, 3, 15].

Radiologic Imagination

Three methods—mammography, ultrasonography, and magnetic resonance imaging—are used for radiologic diagnosis and staging. No distinguishing characteristics are found in all three imaging methods in breast sarcomas, except calcification in osteogenic sarcoma. A non-spiculated dense mass with indistinct borders may be the only sign found in mammography. The findings in ultrasonography are usually heterogeneous. Lobulated masses are commonly found. Magnetic resonance imaging may aid in differentiating malignant tumors from benign tumors based on the washout characteristics of the tumor, which will display rapid enhancement [2, 3, 16, 17].

Histological Diagnosis

A biopsy provides a definitive diagnosis. Although there are reports indicating 83 % positive diagnosis by FNA biopsy, breast sarcomas are easily confused with fibroadenomas on cytologic analysis. Furthermore, one report indicated that FNA biopsy was benign for all 28 nonepithelial breast malignancies on which it was performed [18]. A core biopsy should be the definitive diagnostic method of choice in all cases. An open incisional or excisional biopsy may be an alternative method if a core biopsy is not possible. All of the needle pathways should be included in the subsequent wide local excision

area in cases diagnosed with breast sarcoma. Sarcomas are graded according to their cellularity, degree of differentiation, nuclear atypia, and mitotic activity [2, 3, 12].

Staging

To screen for possible remote metastases in patients diagnosed with breast sarcomas, the thorax, abdomen, and pelvis should be scanned by tomography. The staging of breast sarcomas is different from that of breast carcinomas. Tumor grade is one of the decisive factors in staging. Well-differentiated grade I sarcomas are classified as stage I, grade II sarcomas are classified as stage II, and grade III tumors and tumors of any grade with regional lymph node involvement are classified as stage III in the AJCC classification system [1, 2].

Treatment

The management approach to breast sarcomas should be multidisciplinary in nature. The treatment paradigm is the same as for general sarcomas. The mainstay of treatment is surgery.

Surgery

Wide local excision with clear margins is the preferred method for small, localized sarcomas. Mastectomy with reconstruction is the best choice for larger sarcomas for which tumor resection with safe margins or good cosmetic results is not technically feasible [15]. Wide local excision produced the same survival as mastectomy in retrospective trials [19]. However, retrospective trials reported local recurrence rates between 8 and 53 % [20] with wide local excision or mastectomy, and a more radical surgery provided no additional survival advantage [21]. These trials highlight the importance of negative surgical margins and the tumor biology rather than the type of surgery [22]. Although there is a lack of guidelines for surgical margins in the literature, most surgeons agree that 1-cm margins are generally sufficient for breast sarcomas except for angiosarcomas [1, 3, 23].

Axillary Approach

Sarcomas exhibit predominantly hematogenous spreading. Metastatic spreading through the lymphatic route is unusual. Although up to 25 % patients may have palpable nodes, these nodes tend to be reactive. The rate of nodal metastasis is less than 5 % [1, 7, 12, 19, 24]. All patients were reported as node negative in a retrospective trial comprising 34 sarcomas [25]. The rarity of lymph node involvement by a tumor and the considerable additional morbidity discourage the routine performance of lymphatic dissection. Furthermore, axillary dissection is associated with no survival benefits [18–20].

However, nodal metastases may be observed most commonly in patients with significant disseminated end-stage disease and in angiosarcomas. Sentinel lymph node application should be considered in cases with suspicious or palpable lymph nodes [1]. Axillary dissection should only be performed in cases with histologically proven nodal involvement [1–3, 12].

Surgical Outcome

Surgical outcome is affected both by the size and excision margins of the tumor [26, 27]. Tumors larger than 5 cm have a worse prognosis [3]. Higher-grade sarcomas tend to exhibit a worse prognosis, but no consensus has been reached regarding the significance of tumor grade on the surgical outcome, likely due to the low number of patients studied. Patients with tumor enucleation without clear surgical margins experience higher local recurrence rates of up to 85 % [28]. Five-year disease-free survival rates range from 44 to 74 % in patients with adequate surgery.

Neoadjuvant Therapy

In cases of locally advanced disease, neoadjuvant chemotherapy and radiotherapy can be useful to decrease the tumor size, which leads to excision with negative margins and the avoidance of mastectomy [1, 29].

Adjuvant Therapy

Chemotherapy and radiotherapy both have roles in the management of breast sarcomas. Usually, they are provided sequentially in adjuvant therapy protocols; however, concomitant application can also be used [1–3].

A significant survival advantage has been shown with combined regimens, but the role of chemotherapy alone is less clear. However, the combined regimen improved survival without resulting in a complete response in the MD Anderson trial. Several combined regimens have been reported in the literature to produce complete or partial responses [18, 20, 24, 30]; however, none of the reports indicated statistically significant improvements.

Adjuvant Chemotherapy

There are no breast sarcoma-specific data for adjuvant chemotherapy; thus, soft tissue sarcoma indications and protocols are used for breast sarcomas [25]. Patients with small, low-grade tumors and negative excisional margins do not require adjuvant chemotherapy. The absolute indications for adjuvant chemotherapy are as follows: higher-grade tumors (grades II and III), a larger tumor size (>5 cm), and resections with positive margins that cannot be re-excised.

The choice of chemotherapeutic agent is dependent on experiences treating soft tissue sarcomas [31]. Classical sarcoma regimens, including anthracyclines, are initially preferred [1, 2].

Adjuvant Radiotherapy

Adjuvant radiotherapy indications are similar to chemotherapy indications. Additionally, patients with clear margins of less than 2 cm have been reported by some authors to be candidates for adjuvant radiotherapy [2].

The majority of studies in the literature show a trend toward improved survival by radiotherapy [3]. A course of 48 Gy radiotherapy was reported to improve the survival from 50 to 91 % [8]. In a retrospective trial, local failure was decreased from 34 to 13 % by radiotherapy, but the change was not statistically significant [25].

Survival and Prognosis

As for the other soft tissue sarcomas, tumor size, grade, subtype, and surgical margins are predictors of the prognosis of breast sarcoma [7, 11, 32]. The depth of the tumor, which is a predictor of prognosis for sarcomas in other locations, is irrelevant in breast sarcomas because they are usually superficial. Angiosarcomas or postirradiation sarcomas have the worst prognosis [9, 32, 33]. Extending the depth of surgery does not affect survival [8, 10]. The lung is the most commonly reported metastatic site, and the liver, brain, and bones are the next most common sites [2].

Five- and 10-year disease-free survival rates have been reported as 47 % and 42 %, respectively [8]. The 5-year overall survival rates reported in the literature range between 61 and 91 % and are thus better than the disease-free survival rates [20, 24, 30, 34, 35]. The average 10-year overall survival rate is 62 % [32].

Prognosis According to Molecular Pathogenesis

It is not difficult to observe different prognoses in cases within the same histological subtypes. Distinct specific molecular lesions lead to different prognoses for sarcomas. There are a few studies in the literature discussing the specific molecular features of breast sarcomas [1]. However, the molecular pathogenesis of a sarcoma is dependent on the histological subtype and is independent of the primary tumor location.

Based on the currently defined specific molecular lesions of sarcomas, alveolar sarcoma, which is associated with a worse prognosis, is characterized by translocations that fuse the PAX3 or PAX7 gene with the transcription factor POX01. Nevertheless, the same alveolar rhabdomyosarcoma has a much better prognosis, such as that of embryonal rhabdomyosarcoma, when lacking this fusion. Synovial sarcomas, which have been reported to arise in the breast in rare cases, have also been defined by specific translocation-fused genes [36, 37].

Thus, the molecular characterization of sarcomas together with the search for translocations will be helpful to better define the biology of the disease and to develop specific therapies in the future [1].

Novel Treatments

Novel scientific approaches are encouraging for the treatment of sarcomas [3]. Palifosfamide and eribulin are promising new chemotherapeutic agents that are associated with higher-percentage responses in metastatic disease and liposarcomas, respectively. Targeted treatment with new tyrosine kinase inhibitors has been successfully used in sarcomas, but no specific data have been reported in breast sarcomas [38, 39].

Vascular endothelial growth factor (VEGF) is a well-known predictor of angiogenesis and is highly expressed in soft tissue sarcomas and angiosarcomas [40]. VEGF may also be a strong predictor of disease prognosis [41]. Mutant VEGF receptors, which were detected in angiosarcomas, were inhibited by the VEGF receptor inhibitors sorafenib and sunitinib [40].

Angiosarcomas

Epidemiology

Angiosarcomas are the most common nonepithelial sarcomas of the breast, and they account for 15–34 % of all breast sarcomas and 5 % of soft tissue sarcomas [20, 42]. Angiosarcomas occur most often in women in their 60s and 70s [43, 44].

Etiology, Incidence, and Classification

Angiosarcomas are classified according to their occurrence de novo, postirradiation, or in association with lymphedema [12].

The first lymphangiosarcoma was described in the upper extremity of a woman with lymphedema by Stewart and Treves in 1948 [45].

More than 50 % of angiosarcomas arise from the irradiated breast, and 20 % arise from the contralateral breast [12, 20, 34, 46, 47]. The risk of postirradiation malignancy following breast-conserving surgery (BCS) and radiotherapy was reported as 16 % at 10 years [48]. In a large series, the 15-year cumulative incidence of sarcoma was 3.2 per 1,000 irradiated patients. The time between irradiation and the development of sarcoma ranges between 65 months and 17 years with an average of 10 years after radiation [44, 49, 50].

Symptoms

Angiosarcomas can emerge after irradiation on the thoracic wall of patients with mastectomy or in the breasts of patients undergoing breast-conserving surgery [42].

Angiosarcomas are usually dermal or subcutaneous tumors. A rash, cutaneous violaceous non-pigmented nodule, plaque, vesicula, or macula is frequently the initial lesion, but an angiosarcoma may also present as a rapidly growing, painless mass [51]. Atypical vascular skin lesions are rare smaller lesions but may be the precursors to angiosarcomas. All of the detected atypical lesions should be excised with wide margins [52].

Cytology and Classification

Primary angiosarcomas predominantly affect premenopausal women (mean age of 35); 13 % occur in pregnancy, and 21 % involve the contralateral breast [43]. These tumors typically present as a large (average 4–5 cm), painless mass and have a hemorrhagic, spongy cut surface.

Secondary angiosarcomas arise after modified radical mastectomy and lymphedema, after mastectomy and radiotherapy, or after breast-conserving surgery and radiotherapy [53]. Specific diagnostic cytologic findings include hyperchromatic nuclei, a connecting dense vascular network, and vascular elements in the parenchyma.

The histological grading is similar for primary and secondary angiosarcomas. The histological grade is one predictor of prognosis. High-grade tumors are most common in younger patients and have a low survival rate (5 years, 14 %) [42, 43]. Low-grade tumors are usually misdiagnosed as hemangiomas and have better survival rates (5 years, 91 %).

Management

Surgery is the primary treatment, and wide local excision is the recommended procedure. Due to the presence of infiltrative margins, angiosarcomas require larger margins compared with other sarcomas. Some authors recommend up to 3-cm negative margins together with oncoplastic surgery [23]. Wide negative margins are essential for long-term cures in previously irradiated breast because further adjuvant radiotherapy cannot be administered [3]. All detected hemangiomatous lesions around the tumor or in the breast should be included in the excised specimen. Mastectomy is the treatment of choice for tumors that cannot be excised with safe margins [2].

Angiosarcomas can metastasize to regional lymph nodes in 7 % of cases [24]; thus, sentinel lymph node biopsy should be considered, particularly in patients with high-risk factors such as high grade, large tumor, or advanced disease [54].

The adjuvant therapeutic indications for angiosarcomas are similar to those for sarcomas. In addition to conventional chemotherapeutics, angiosarcomas are also sensitive to taxanes and liposomal doxorubicin [55]. Ongoing debate exists regarding whether postirradiation breast sarcomas can be treated similarly by localized radiotherapy. Although most clinicians are reluctant to use more radiotherapy, it has been reported in a retrospective trial that hyper-fractionated accelerated radiotherapy is well tolerated and provides local control in 60 % of patients [1, 5].

Outcome

Angiosarcomas, especially high-grade ones, are highly aggressive tumors. They have high local recurrence rates (50–60 %) and high distant metastatic potential [50, 51]. Bone, lung, ovary, and liver are common sites of metastasis. The 5-year survival rates are 80 % and 20 % for well-differentiated and poorly differentiated tumors, respectively [2, 56].

Fibrosarcoma (Pleomorphic Sarcoma: Malignant Fibrous Histiocytoma)

Fibrosarcoma is one of the rare nonepithelial breast tumors. The definitive diagnosis is made by Tru-Cut biopsy and immunohistochemical staining. Malignant phyllodes tumors and sarcoma with mesenchymal differentiation should be excluded in the differential diagnosis. High-grade types are vulnerable to metastasis, whereas low-grade types are not [57, 58].

Liposarcoma

Liposarcoma is a rare, slow-growing, firm, occasionally painful, nonepithelial breast tumor that does not have any specific clinical features. Tru-Cut biopsy is necessary for the diagnosis of liposarcoma. Malignant phyllodes tumors should be considered in the differential diagnosis. Well-differentiated, myxoid/round cell, poorly differentiated, and pleomorphic types comprise the histological subgroups. Well-differentiated types are less aggressive. Dedifferentiated types have significant metastatic potential. In the case of recurrence, well-differentiated histology can progress to a dedifferentiated type. All of the histological types of liposarcomas tend to recur and metastasize [1, 43, 59, 60].

Leiomyosarcoma

Leiomyosarcoma is a rare type of breast sarcoma. Straight muscle cells in the nipple areola complex can be the origin. Immunohistochemistry is necessary for the differential diagnosis. Recurrence and metastasis frequently occur [43, 61, 62].

Rhabdomyosarcoma

Rhabdomyosarcoma is a rare tumor that occurs more often in adolescent women. Rhabdomyosarcoma is most commonly found as a metastasis from another origin [42]. Rhabdomyosarcomatous differentiation can also be detected in malignant phyllodes tumors and in metaplastic carcinoma of the breast. Alveolar rhabdomyosarcoma is the most frequent histological subtype [63], whereas solid and classic types are the others. Immunohistochemistry is essential for definitive diagnosis. Five-year survival rates have been reported as 90 % in stage I and 30 % in stage IV [43, 64].

Specific Syndromes

Li-Fraumeni Syndrome

Lynch et al. described in detail a complex syndrome with multiple tumors in different anatomical sites of the body, including sarcomas, breast cancer, brain tumors, lung cancer, laryngeal cancer, leukemia, lymphoma, and adrenal cortical carcinoma, which was first described by Li and Fraumeni [65–67]. A P53 gene mutation is characteristic for this syndrome. Breast tumors occur at an early age and tend to recur in this syndrome [68].

Cowden Disease

This syndrome occurs as a result of a PTEN gene mutation, which leads to multiple tumors of the body, including breast cancer, thyroid cancer, female genitourinary tract cancer, and mucocutaneous hamartomas and trichilemmomas [69, 70]. Lesions frequently occur on the face and dorsal and ventral aspects of the hands, feet, and forearms. Breast cancer is observed in 30 % of patients with Cowden disease and is sometimes bilateral. Bilateral prophylactic mastectomy or close surveillance, including monthly breast self-examination, biannual physician examination, biannual mammography, and/or MRI, is usually offered to patients with a PTEN mutation [71, 72]. Virgin hypertrophy, hamartomas, ductal hyperplasia, intraductal papillomatosis, adenosis, fibroadenomas, and fibrocystic mastopathy are not rare. Thyroid lesions such as goiter, adenomas, follicular lesions, and thyroid dysfunction are common. Uterine leiomyomas, brain tumors, gastrointestinal tract hamartomas, and colon cancer have also been reported [65, 66].

Primary Breast Lymphoma

Epidemiology

Lymphoma is the malignant disease of the lymph nodes. Primary extranodal lymphoma is a rare entity that usually originates from B-cells and is of non-Hodgkin's type. The skin, brain, gastrointestinal system, thyroid, testis, and breast are the sites of disease occurrence that have been reported. Diffuse large B-cell lymphoma is the most common type [73]. There are many retrospective studies [74–77] but only one prospective study [78] of primary breast lymphoma in the literature. Breast involvement in Hodgkin's lymphoma has also been reported [79].

Lymphoma in the breast is defined as primary when the breast is the first major site of manifestations without any evidence of a concurrent systemic disease. The disease is considered secondary in the case of breast involvement in addition to a systemic disease. Sometimes it is difficult to determine which is the primary disease when there are both breast involvement and systemic disease, because there is no morphological difference between primary and secondary lymphoma [73].

Primary breast lymphoma arises from the periductal and perilobular lymphatic tissue and intramammary lymph nodes [2]. It accounts for 2.2 % of extranodal lymphomas [80] and 0.1 % of all breast tumors [81–88]. Although it can be observed at all ages, in both genders, and on both sides, it is more frequent in women (95 %) between 50 and 60 and more frequently occurs in the right breast and the upper outer quadrant [83–87]. It tends to be bilateral and exhibits features of Burkitt's lymphoma in young and pregnant women [87, 88].

There are also case reports of primary breast lymphoma induced by implant capsules in the literature [89]. Six cases of anaplastic cell lymphoma in association with silicone breast implants have been reported [90].

Symptoms

A painless, mobile, large, and rapidly enlarging mass is characteristic [73]. Sometimes, the entire breast grows, or pathological lymph nodes in the axilla become palpable as the initial symptom [2]. The tumor is multicentric in 20–30 % of the cases. Locally advanced tumor signs such as skin changes are rare. The tumor is usually misdiagnosed as breast cancer or a benign lesion [91].

Radiology

A mass with clear margins without calcification is the most common sign in radiographic images. However, multiple amorphous masses with diffuse, increased parenchymal density or a spiculated mass may also represent the abnormal findings. Patients may also have normal mammograms.

Ultrasonographic findings are also not specific and cover a wide spectrum, including hypoechogenicity with well-defined borders and without acoustic shadowing.

Enlarged intramammary lymph nodes identified by mammography with increased density, a lack of well-defined borders, and fatty hilum are considered pathological. Lymph nodes are hypoechoic by ultrasonography.

PET has an 89 % sensitivity and 100 % specificity in the differential diagnosis for non-Hodgkin's lymphoma [88].

Diagnosis

The diagnostic criteria for primary breast lymphoma have been defined by an international extranodal lymphoma study group as an extra-nodal lesion as the main symptom with or without lymph node involvement or a tumor limited to a unilateral breast or bilateral breasts with or without lymph node involvement [82, 92, 93]. There are also some specific criteria, such as a primary tumor in the breast, lack of previous lymphoma history, lack of widespread disease, and close histopathological associations with breast tissue. Ipsilateral lymph nodes that develop simultaneously with the primary tumor are not considered exclusion criteria [88]. All other lymphomas that do not meet these criteria are considered secondary breast lymphomas. Clinical and imaging findings are not enough by themselves for the definitive diagnosis. Tru-Cut biopsy and immunohistochemistry staining are necessary [88].

Staging

The Arbor classification [94] is used for the staging, in which stage I indicates disease limited to the breast, stage II indicates disease limited to the breast and ipsilateral axilla, stage III indicates disease limited to the breast but involves both axillae, and stage IV indicates disease limited to the breast with metastasis to the extra-nodular tissue [88].

To accurately stage the disease, chest, abdominal, and pelvic tomography, bone morrow biopsy, and blood tests are mandatory in addition to the assessment of both breasts and axillae [95].

Histopathology

A definitive diagnosis is based on cytologic and histopathological features. Primary breast lymphoma histologically resembles other lymphomas of the body, as well as other breast carcinomas. It is often difficult to distinguish it from poorly differentiated carcinomas. A specific feature of primary breast lymphoma is the infiltration of mammary lobules by uniform malignant lymphoid cells. Adequate tissue sampling is the mainstay for diagnosis; however, immunohistochemistry may also be essential. BOB1 and OCT2 overexpression can be used as immunohistochemical markers [96].

Macroscopically, the mass has a smooth, round shape and a clear surface and does not have a membrane, and the cut surface is pink or gray in color. Most primary breast lymphomas comprise B-cells, and nearly 70 % of cases are diffuse large B-cell lymphoma [97].

Management

Lymphomas are sensitive to chemotherapy and radiotherapy; thus, surgery is limited to Tru-Cut or excisional biopsy [82]. Axillary lymph node excision may be required for the diagnosis, staging, or palliation of palpable large nodes. Mastectomy is not recommended.

The treatment varies widely and depends on the subtype and stage of disease. Systemic chemotherapy, including anthracycline regimens, is usually the standard treatment of choice. Combined RCHOP therapy (rituximab, cyclophosphamide, doxorubicin, vincristine, and prednisone) is the most commonly used regimen in diffuse large B-cell lymphoma. Systemic medical treatment should be combined with radiotherapy. Three cycles of CHOP followed by radiotherapy have been found to be superior to eight cycles of CHOP [88]. Although the optimal treatment for diffuse large B-cell lymphoma has not been defined, several reports have suggested improved survival and local control with radiotherapy following an extensive course of chemotherapy. Radiotherapy can be used as the sole treatment for stage I indolent lymphoma that is limited to the breast [73].

Prognosis

Spontaneous regression of primary breast lymphoma has been reported in the literature [98].

The clinical stage and histological subtypes are the main prognostic factors [73]. The 5- and 10-year survival rates have been reported to be 43–74 % and 51 %, respectively [12].

Synchronous or metachronous contralateral breast involvement should be monitored for up to 10 years. The common relapse sites of primary breast lymphoma have been reported to be the contralateral breast (15 %) and the central nervous system (3 %) [88].

Metastases to the Breast

Epidemiology

Any malignancy may metastasize [99] to the breast; however, metastatic lesions to the breast are rare. Since the first report in 1907, which described ovarian tumors metastasizing to the breast [100], nearly 500 cases have been reported in the literature [101].

The frequency of metastatic involvement of the breast is between 0.4 and 1.3 % [103, 104]. Most breast metastases originate from the contralateral site [8]. Non-mammary metastatic breast neoplasms account for 0.5–6 % of all breast carcinomas [104].

The most common malignancy that metastasizes to the breast is malignant melanoma [105–108]. Both the isolated metastases to the breast [106, 108, 109] and metastases to both the breast and other sites [110] from extramammary cutaneous malignant melanoma have been reported. The detection of bilateral breast metastases from melanoma is highly suggestive of metastatic multiorgan disease and could be useful to address the therapeutic approach [107]. Hematological malignancies such as leukemia and lymphomas [102, 104, 111] are also common. Other malignancies that may metastasize to the breast include oropharynx tumors, ovarian carcinomas, thyroid carcinomas, small bowel carcinoids [102, 111–113], gastrointestinal system malignancies such as esophageal/stomach and colorectal cancers, sarcomas, and, rarely, pulmonary carcinomas [7, 99, 102, 114, 115]. Nineteen colorectal carcinomas that have metastasized to the breast have been

reported in the literature [102, 116]. Twenty-five gastric cancer cases with metastases to the breast have been reported in the literature [4–6, 9, 11], whereas the incidence of metastatic gastric tumors to the breast has been reported as 1–2 % in clinical series [116, 117].

Metastases to the breast usually occur several months after the discovery of the primary tumor; however, in 25–40 % of cases, the metastases are the first sign of the primary tumor [10, 104, 117].

Metastases to the breast are frequently observed in reproductive-aged groups (30–45 years) [117]. The tumors are usually in the upper outer quadrant of the left breast and are superficially located, solitary, discrete lesions. Unlike primary breast cancers, skin or nipple retraction is rare [102, 103, 118]. Metastases are bilateral in 25 % of cases, and concomitant axillary lymph node involvement can be detected in 15 % of cases [7–9].

Clinical and Radiologic Signs

Clinical and radiologic signs are quite polymorphic and vary widely. Furthermore, metastatic lesions can mimic primary breast cancers or even benign lesions [104]. Thus, distinguishing metastatic tumors in the breast from the primary lesion by clinical and radiologic evaluation is extremely difficult [9, 102, 103, 113]. The occurrence of multiple tumor nodules in the breast is rare. Diffuse involvement of the breast is unusual, with the exception of metastases from malignancies of hematological origin [119]. The most common mammographic evidence is often single but sometimes multiple well-circumscribed lesions with smooth margins. Spiculated irregular density can also be observed [4]. Microcalcification is unusual, except for metastases of ovarian papillary carcinomas [102, 112, 113, 117, 120].

Diagnosis

Accurate diagnosis is important because the treatment and outcome for primary breast tumors and metastases to the breast are quite different. There are some specific histopathological features of metastases to the breast. The absence of in situ carcinoma and the presence of sharply circumscribed lesions from the surrounding tissue and elastosis strongly support the diagnosis of metastatic carcinoma [102, 103, 115, 121]. Immunohistochemistry helps to diagnose the majority of cases. Estrogen and progesterone receptors and c-erbB2 are usually negative in metastatic tumors to the breast [1, 101].

Management and Prognosis

Comprehensive screening is necessary to identify the origin of the primary tumor [105], and treatment is modified according to the primary tumor. In most cases, systemic treatment or palliative care is more appropriate than extensive surgery [115]. Most metastases to the breast are correlated with extensive disease and a poor prognosis [115, 117, 122]. Patients usually die within a year of diagnosis [122, 123]. However, considerably improved survival rates have been reported in some patients who were administered effective systemic treatment [122].

References

1. Voutsadakis IA, Zaman K, Leyvraz S. Breast sarcomas: current and future perspectives. Breast. 2001;20:199–204.
2. Nizri E, Merimsky O, Lahat G. Optimal management of sarcomas of the breast: an update. Expert Rev Anticancer Ther. 2014;14:705–10.
3. Pencavel TD, Hayes A. Breast sarcoma – a review of diagnosis and management. Int J Surg. 2009;7:20–3.
4. Balzer BL, Weiss SW. Do bio materials cause implant-associated mesenchymal tumors of the breast? Analysis of 8 new cases and review of the literature. Hum Pathol. 2009;40:1564–70.
5. Yap J, Chuba PJ, Thomas R, Aref A, Lucas D, Severson RK, et al. Sarcoma as a second malignancy after treatment for breast cancer. Int J Rad Oncol Biol Phys. 2002;52:1231–7.
6. Kirova YM, Vilcoq JR, Asselain B, Sastre-Garau X, Fourquet A. Radiation-induced sarcomas after radiotherapy for breast carcinoma. Cancer. 2005;104:856–63.
7. Adem C, Reynolds C, Ingle JN, Nascimento AG. Primary breast sarcoma: clinicopathologic series from the Mayo Clinic and review of the literature. BrJ Cancer. 2004;91:237–41.
8. McGowan TS, Cummings BJ, O'Sullivan B, Catton CN, Miller N, Panzarella T. An analysis of 78 breast sarcoma patients without distant metastases at presentation. Int J Rad Oncol Biol Phys. 2000;46:383–90.
9. Bousquet G, Confavreux C, Magné N, Tunonde LC, Poortmans P, Senkus E, et al. Outcome and prognostic factors in breast sarcoma: a multicenter study from the rare cancer network. Radiother Oncol. 2007;85:355–61.
10. Pandey M, Mathew A, Abraham EK, Rajan B. Primary sarcoma of the breast. J Surg Oncol. 2004;87:121–5.
11. Fields RC, Aft RL, Gillanders WE, Eberlein TJ, Margenthaler JA. Treatment and outcomes of patients with primary breast sarcoma. Am J Surg. 2008;196:559–61.
12. Hunt KK, Newman LA, Copeland III EM, Bland KI. In: Brunicardi FC, Andersen DK, Billiar TR, Dunn DL, Hunter JG, Matthews JB, Pollock RE, editors. Schwartz's principles of surgery. 9th ed. New York: The McGraw-Hill Companies; 2010. p. 423–74.
13. Luini A, Gatti G, Diaz J, Botteri E, Oliveira E, Sahiumde C, Almeida R, et al. Angiosarcoma of the breast: the experience of the European Institute of Oncology and a review of the literature. Breast Cancer Res Treat. 2007;105:81–5.
14. Nakamura R, Nagashima T, Sakakibara M, Nakano S, Tanabe N, Fujimoto H, et al. Angiosarcoma arising in the breast following breast-conserving surgery with radiation for breast carcinoma. Breast Cancer. 2007;14:245–9.
15. Lum YW, Jacobs L. Primary breast sarcoma. Surg Clin N Am. 2008;88:559–70.
16. Yang WT, Muttarak M, HoL W. Non mammary malignancies of the breast: ultrasound, CT, and MRI. Semin Ultrasound CT MR. 2000;21:375–94.
17. Yang WT, Hennessy BT, Dryden MJ, Valero V, Hunt KK, Krishnamurthyb S. Mammary angiosarcomas: imaging findings in 24 patients. Radiology. 2007;242:725–34.
18. Shahbahang M, Franchesci D, Sundaram M, Castillo MH, Moffat FL, Frank DS, et al. Surgical management of primary breast sarcoma. Am Surg. 2007;68:673–7.
19. Gutman H, Pollock RE, Ross MI, Benjamin RS, Johnston DA, Janjan NA, et al. Sarcoma of the breast: implications for extent of therapy. MD Anderson Exp Surg. 1994;116:505–9.
20. Callery CD, Rosen PP, Kinne DW. Sarcoma of the breast: a study of 32 patients with reappraisal of classification and therapy. Ann Surg. 1985;201:527–32.
21. Ciatto S, Bonardi R, Cataliotti L, Cardona G. Sarcomas of the breast: a multicenter series of 70 cases. Neoplasma. 1992;39:375–9.
22. Al-Benna S, Poggemann K, Steinau H-U, Steinstraesser L. Diagnosis and management of primary breast sarcoma. Breast Cancer Res Treat. 2010;122:619–26.

23. Telli ML, Horst KC, Guardino AE, Dirbas FM, Carlson RW. Phyllodes tumours of the breast: natural history, diagnosis, and treatment. J Natl Compr Canc Netw. 2007;5:324–30.

24. Sher T, Hennessy BT, Valero V, Broglio K, Woodward WA, Trent J, et al. Primary angiosarcomas of the breast. Cancer. 2007;110:173–8.

25. Barrow BJ, Janjan NA, Gutman H, Benjamin RS, Allen P, Romsdahl MM, et al. Role of radiotherapy in sarcoma of the breast. A retrospective review of the M.D. Anderson experience. Radiother Oncol. 1999;52:173–8.

26. Kapiris I, Nasiri N, A'Hern R, Healy V, Gui GP. Outcome and predictive factors of local recurrence and distant metastases following primary surgical treatment of high-grade malignant phyllodes tumours of the breast. Eur J Surg Oncol. 2001;27:723–30.

27. Fou A, Schnabel FR, Hamele Bena D, Wei XJ, Cheng B, El Tamer M, et al. Long term outcomes of malignant phyllodes tumors patients: an institutional experience. Am J Surg. 2006;192:492–5.

28. Ben Hassouna J, Damak T, Gamoudi A, Chargui R, Khomsi F, Mahjoub S, et al. Phyllodes tumours of the breast: a case series of 106 patients. Am J Surg. 2006;192:141–7.

29. Reynoso D, Subbiah V, Trent JC, Guadagnolo BA, Lazar AJ, Benjamin R, et al. Neoadjuvant treatment of soft-tissue sarcoma: a multimodality approach. J Surg Oncol. 2010;101:327–33.

30. Parker SJ, Harries SA. Phyllodes tumours. Postgrad Med J. 2001;77:428–35.

31. Grimer R, Athanasiu N, Gerrand C, Judson I, Lewis I, Morton B, Peake D. UK Guidelines for the management of soft tissue sarcomas. Sarcoma. 2010;2010:317462.

32. Zelek L, Llombart Cussacn A, Terrier P, Pivot X, Guinebretiere JM, Le Pechoux C, et al. Prognostic factors in primary breast sarcomas: a series of patients with long-term follow-up. J Clin Oncol. 2010;21:2583–8.

33. Gladdy RA, Qin L-X, Moraco N, Edgar MA, Antonescu CR, Alektiar KM, et al. Do radiation-associated soft tissue sarcomas have the same prognosis as sporadic soft tissue sarcomas? J Clin Oncol. 2010;28:2064–9.

34. Vorburger SA, Xing Y, Hunt KK, Lakin GE, Benjamin RS, Feig BW, et al. Angiosarcoma of the breast. Cancer. 2005;104:2682–8.

35. Barth Jr RJ. Histologic features predict local recurrence after breast conserving therapy of phyllodes tumours. Breast Cancer Res Treat. 1999;57:291–5.

36. Yoshitani K, Kido A, Honoki K, Fujii H, Takakura Y. Pelvic metastasis of breast synovial sarcoma. J Orthop Sci. 2009;14:219–23.

37. Tormo V, Andreu FJ. Primary breast synovial sarcoma: a rare primary breast neoplasia. Clin Transl Oncol. 2009;11:854–5.

38. Verweij J, van Oosterom A, Blay J-Y, Judson I, Rodenhuis S, van der Graaf W, et al. Imatinib mesylate (STI-571 Glivec, Gleevec) is an active agent for gastrointestinal stromal tumours, but does not yield responses in other soft tissue sarcomas that are unselected for a molecular target: results from an EORTC Soft Tissue and Bone Sarcoma Group phase II study. Eur J Cancer. 2003;39:2006–11.

39. Blay J-Y, von Mehren M, Blackstein ME. Perspective on updated treatment guidelines for patients with gastrointestinal stromal tumors. Cancer. 2010;116:5126–37.

40. Antonescu CR, Yoshida A, Guo T, Chang N-E, Zhang L, Agaram NP, et al. KDR activating mutations in human angiosarcomas are sensitive to specific kinase inhibitors. Cancer Res. 2009;69:7175–9.

41. Yudoh K, Kanamori M, Ohmori K, Yasuda T, Aoki M, Kimura T. Concentration of vascular endothelial growth factor in the tumour tissue as a prognostic factor of soft tissue sarcomas. Br J Cancer. 2001;84:1610–5.

42. Blanchard DK, Reynolds CA, Grant CS, Donohue JH. Primary nonphylloides breast sarcomas. Am J Surg. 2003;186:359–61.

43. Wakwlu Jr PE. Mesenchymal neoplasms of the breast. In: Bland KI, Copeland EM, editors. The breast. Comprehensive management of benign and malignant disease. IVth ed. Philadelphia: Saunders/Elsevier; 2009. p. 261–9.

44. Strobbe LJ, Peterse HL, van Tinteren H, Wijnmaalen A, Rutgers EJ. Angiosarcoma of the breast after conservation therapy for invasive cancer, the incidence and outcome. An unforseen sequela. Breast Cancer Res Treat. 1998;47:101–9.

45. Stewart FW, Treves N. Lymphangiosarcoma in post-mastectomy lymphedema. A report of six cases in elephantiasis chirurgica. Cancer. 1948;1:64–81.

46. Kirova YM, Gambotti L, de Rycke Y, Vilcoq JR, Asselain B, Fourque TA. Risk of second malignancies after adjuvant radiotherapy for breast cancer: a large scale, single-institution review. Int J Radiat Oncol Biol Phys. 2007;68:359–63.

47. Fodor J, Orosz Z, Szabo E, Sulyok Z, Polgar C, Zaka Z, et al. Angiosarcoma after conservation treatment for breast carcinoma: our experience and a review of the literature. J Am Acad Dermatol. 2006;54:499–504.

48. Fowble B, Hanlon A, Freedman G, Nicolaou N, Anderson P. Second cancers after conservative surgery and radiation for stage I–II breast cancer: identifying a subset of women at increased risk. Int J Radiat Oncol Biol Phys. 2001;51:679–90.

49. Freedman GM. Radiation complications and their treatment. In: Bland KI, Copeland EM, editors. The breast. Comprehensive management of benign and malignant disease. IVth ed. Philadelphia: Saunders/Elsevier; 2009. p. 1113–22.

50. Billings SD, McKenney JK, Folpe AL, Hardacre MC, Weiss SW. Cutaneous angiosarcoma following

breast-conserving surgery and radiation. An analysis of 27 cases. Am J Surg Pathol. 2004;28:781–8.

51. Montoe AT, Feigenberg SJ, Mendenhall NP. Angiosarcoma after breast-conserving therapy. Cancer. 2003;97:1832–40.

52. Brenn T, Fletcher CDM. Radiation- associated cutaneous atypical vascular lesions and angiosarcoma. Clinicopathologic analysis of 42 cases. Am J Surg Pathol. 2005;29:983–6.

53. Arora TK, Terracina KP, Soong J, Idowu MO, Takabe K. Primary and secondary angiosarcoma of the breast. Gland Surg. 2014;3:28–34.

54. Zeng W, Styblo TM, Li S, Sepulveda JN, Schuster DM. Breast angiosarcoma. FDG PET findings. Clin Nucl Med. 2009;34:443–5.

55. Gambini D, Visintin R, Locatelli E, Bareggi C, Galassi B, Runza L, et al. Secondary breast angiosarcoma and paclitaxel-dependent prolonged disease control: report of two cases and review of the literature. Tumori. 2015. doi:10.5301/tj.5000252 [Epub ahead of print].

56. Rosen PP, Kimmel M, Ernsberge D. Mammary angiosarcoma. The prognostic significance of tumor differentiation. Cancer. 1998;62:2145–51.

57. Kijima Y, Umekita Y, Yoshinaka H, Taguchi S, Owaki T, Funasako Y, et al. Stromal sarcoma with features of giant cell malignant fibrous histiocytoma. Breast Cancer. 2007;14:239–44.

58. Jones MW, Norris HJ, Wargotz ES, Weiss SW. Fibrosarcoma-malignant fibrous histiocytoma of the breast. A clinicopathologic study of 32 cases. Am J Surg Pathol. 1992;16:667–74.

59. Powell CM, Rosen PP. Adipose differentiation in cystosarcoma phyllodes. Am J Surg Pathol. 1994;18:720–7.

60. Charfi L, Driss M, Mrad K, Abbes I, Dhouib R, Sassi S, et al. Primary well differentiated liposarcoma: an unusual tumor in the breast. Breast J. 2009;15:206–7.

61. Falconieri G, Della Libera D, Zanconati F, Bittesini L. Leiomyosarcoma of the female breast. Report of two new cases and review of the literature. Am J Clin Pathol. 1997;108:19–25.

62. Parham DM, Robertson AJ, Hussein KA, Davidson AI. Leiomyosarcoma of the breast: cytological and histological features with a review of the literature. Cytopathology. 1992;3:245–52.

63. Hays DM, Donaldson SS, Shimada H, Crist WM, Newton Jr WA, Andrassy RJ, et al. Primary and metastatic rhabdomyosarcoma in the breast: neoplasms of adolescent females, a report from the Intergroup Rhabdomyosarcoma Study. Med Pediatr Oncol. 1997;29:181–9.

64. Crist WM, Anderson JR, Meza JL, Fryer C, Raney RB, Ruymann FB, et al. Intergroup rhabdomyosarcoma study IV: results for patients with nonmetastatic disease. J Clin Oncol. 2001;19:3091–102.

65. Lynch HT, Marcud JN, Lynch J, Snyder CL, Rubinstein WS. Breast cancer genetics: syndromes, genes, pathology, counseling, testing and treatment. In: Bland KI, Copeland EM, editors. The breast. Comprehensive management of benign and malignant disease. IVth ed. Philadelphia: Saunders/Elsevier; 2009. p. 371–415.

66. Lynch HT, Mulcahy GM, Harris RE, Guirgis HA, Lynch JF. Genetic and pathologic findings in a kindred with hereditary sarcoma, breast cancer, brain tumors, leukemia, lung, laryngeal, and adrenal cortical carcinoma. Cancer. 1978;41:2055–64.

67. Li FP, Fraumeni JF. Soft-tissue sarcomas, breast cancer, and other neoplasms: a familial syndrome? Ann Intern Med. 1969;71:747–52.

68. Lynch HT, McComb RD, Osborn NK, Wolpert PA, Lynch JF, Wszolek ZK, et al. Predominance of brain tumors in an extended Li-Fraumeni (SBLA) kindred including a case of Sturge-Weber syndrome. Cancer. 2000;88:433–9.

69. Liaw D, Marsh DJ, Li J, Dahia PL, Wang SI, Zheng Z, et al. Germline mutations of the PTEN gene in Cowden disease, an inherited breast and thyroid cancer syndrome. Nat Genet. 1997;16:64–7.

70. Nelen MR, van Stavernen WC, Peeters EA, Hassel MB, Gorlin RJ, Hamm H, et al. Germline mutations in the PTEN/MMAC1 gene in patients with Cowden disease. Hum Mol Genet. 1997;6:1383–7.

71. Williard W, Borgen P, Bol R, Tiwari R, Osborne M. Cowden's disease: a case report with analysis at the molecular level. Cancer. 1992;69:2969–74.

72. Schrager CA, Schneider D, Gruener AC, Tsou HC, Peacocke M. Clinical and pathological features of breast disease in Cowden's syndrome: an underrecognized syndrome with an increased risk of breast cancer. Hum Pathol. 1998;29:47–53.

73. Karlin NJ. Breast lymphoma. In: Bland KI, Copeland EM, editors. The breast. Comprehensive management of benign and malignant disease. IVth ed. Philadelphia: Saunders/Elsevier; 2009. p. 315–20.

74. Vignot S, Ledoussal V, Nodio P, Bourguignat A, Janvier M, Mounier N, et al. Non-Hodgkin's lymphoma of the breast. A report of 19 cases and review of the literature. Clin Lymphoma. 2005;6:37–42.

75. Liu MT, Hsieh CY, Wang AY, Pi CP, Chang TH, Huang CC, et al. Primary breast lymphoma: a pooled analysis of prognostic factors and survival in 93 cases. Ann Saudi Med. 2005;25:288–93.

76. Choo SP, Lim ST, Wong EH, Tao M. Breast lymphoma: favorable prognosis after treatment with standard combination chemotherapy. Onkologie. 2006;29:4–18.

77. Ryan GF, Roos DR, Seymour JF. Primary non-Hodgkin's lymphoma of the breast: retrospective analysis of prognosis and patterns of failure in two Australian centers. Clin Lymphoma Myeloma. 2006;6:337–41.

78. Aviles A, Selgado S, Nambo MJ, Neri N, Murillo E, Cleto S. Primary breast lymphoma: results of a controlled clinical trial. Oncology. 2005;69:256–60.

79. Dixon JM, Lumsden AB, Krajewski A, Elton RA, Anderson TJ. Primary lymphoma of the breast. Br J Surg. 1987;74:214–6.

80. Fruchart C, Denoux Y, Chaste J, Peny AM, Boute V, Ollivier JM, et al. High grade primary breast lymphoma: is it a different clinical entity? Breast Cancer Res Treat. 2005;93:91–8.

81. Ganjoo K, Advani R, Mariappan M, McMillan A, Horning S. Non-Hodgkin's lymphoma of the breast. Cancer. 2007;110:25–30.

82. Cheah CY, Campbell BA, Seymour JF. Primary breast lymphoma. Cancer Treat Rev. 2014;40:900–8.

83. Mpallas G, Simatos G, Tadidou A, Patra E, Galateros G, Lakiotis G, et al. Primary breast lymphoma in a male patient. Breast. 2004;13:436–8.

84. Hong JW, Zhong YW. Treatment situation of primary breast lymphoma. Zhongguo Xiandai Putong Waike Jinzhan. 2007;10:513–5.

85. Lyons JA, Myles J, Pohlman B, Macklis RM, Crowe J, Crownover RL. Treatment of prognosis of primary breast lymphoma: a review of 13 cases. Am J Clin Oncol. 2000;23:334–6.

86. Yang WT, Lane DL, Le-Petross HT, Abruzzo LV, Macapinlac HA. Breast lymphoma: imaging findings of 32 tumors in 27 patients. Radiology. 2007;245:692–702.

87. Vasilaki T, Zizi-Sermpetzoglou A, Katsamagkou E, Grammatoglou X, Petrakopoulou N, Glava C. Bilateral primary breast lymphoma. A case report. Eur J Gynae Oncol. 2006;27:623–4.

88. Yang H, Lang RG, Fu L. Primary breast lymphoma (PBL): a literature review. Clin Oncol Cancer Res. 2011;8:128–32.

89. Bishara MR, Ross C, Sur M. Primary anaplastic large cell lymphoma of the breast arising in reconstruction mammoplasty capsule of saline filled breast implant after radical mastectomy for breast cancer: an unusual case presentation. Diagn Pathol. 2009;4:11–6.

90. Newman MK, Zemmel NJ, Bandak AZ, Kaplan BJ. Primary breast lymphoma in a patient with silicone breast implants: a case report and review of the literature. J Plast Reconstr Aestet Surg. 2008;61:822–5.

91. Dan L, Can M, Qingming J. Primary breast diffuse large B cell lymphoma: a clinicopathologic study of twelve cases. Chongqing Yike Daxue Xuebao. 2009;34:650–3.

92. Zucca E, Conconi A, Mughal TI, Sarris AH, Seymour JF, Vitolo U, et al. Patterns of outcome and prognostic factors in primary large-cell lymphoma of the testis in a survey by the International Extranodal Lymphoma Study Group. J Clin Oncol. 2003;21:20–7.

93. Ryan G, Martinelli G, Kuper-Hommel M, Tsang R, Pruneri G, Yuen K, et al. Primary diffuse large B-cell lymphoma of the breast: prognostic factors and outcomes of a study by the International Extranodal Lymphoma Study Group. Ann Oncol. 2008;19:233–41.

94. Giron GL, Hamlin PA, Brogi E, Mendez JE, Sciafani L. Primary lymphoma of the breast: a case of marginal zone B-cell lymphoma. Am Surg. 2004;70:720–5.

95. Woo O, Yong H, Dhin B, Park CM, Kang EY. Synchronous bilateral primary breast lymphoma: MRI and pathologic findings. Breast J. 2007;13:429–30.

96. Kuroaüda H, Tamaru J, Takeuchi I, Ohnisi K, Toyozumi Y, Momose S, et al. Primary diffuse large B-cell lymphoma of the breast. Breast Cancer. 2007;14:317–22.

97. Lamovee J, Jancar J. Primary malignant lymphoma of the breast. Cancer. 1987;60:3033–41.

98. Lihara K, Yamaguchi K, Nishimura Y, Iwasaki T, Suzuki K, Hirabayashi Y. Spontaneous regression of malignant lymphoma of the breast. Pathol Int. 2004;54:537–42.

99. Karim RZ, Scolyer RA, Tse GM, Tan PH, Putti TC, Lee CS. Pathogenic mechanisms in the initiation and progression of mammary phyllodes tumours. Pathology. 2009;41:105–17.

100. Sitzenfrey A. Mammakarzinom zwei jahre nach abdominaler radikal operation wegen doppelseitigen carcinoma ovarii. Prag Med Wochenschr. 1907;32:221–35.

101. Madan AK, Ternovits C, Huber SA, Pei LA, Jaffe BM. Gastrointestinal metastasis to the breast. Surgery. 2002;132:889–93.

102. Maounis N, Chorti M, Legaki S, Ellina E, Emmanouilidou A, Demonakou M, Tsiafaki X. Metastasis to the breast from an adenocarcinoma of the lung with extensive micropapillary component: a case report and review of the literature. Diagn Pathol. 2010;17(5):82.

103. Klingen TA, Klaasen H, Aas H, Chen Y, Akslen LA. Secondary breast cancer: a 5-year population-based study with review of the literature. APMIS. 2009;117:762–7.

104. Magri K, Demoulin G, Millon G, Duvert B. Metastasis to the breast from non mammary metastasis. Clinical, radiological characteristics and diagnostic process. A report of two cases and a review of literature. J Gynecol Obstet Biol Reprod. 2007;36:602–6.

105. Kurul S, Taş F, Büyükbabani N, Mudun A, Baykal C, Camlica H. Different manifestations of malignant melanoma in the breast: a report of 12 cases and a review of the literature. Jpn J Clin Oncol. 2005;35:202–6.

106. Majeski J. Bilateral masses as initial presentation of widely metastatic melanoma. J Surg Oncol. 1999;72:175–7.

107. Moschetta M, Telegrafo M, Lucarelli NM, Martino G, Rella L, Stabile Ianora AA, et al. Metastatic breast disease from cutaneous malignant melanoma. Int J Surg Case Rep. 2014;5:34–6.

108. Ho LW, Wong KP, Chan JH, Chow LW, Leung EY, Leong L. MR appearance of metastatic melanotic melanoma in breast. Clin Radiol. 2000;55:572–3.

109. Mayayo AE, Gomez-Aracil V, Mayayo AR, Azua-Romeo A. Spindle cell malignant melanoma metastatic to the breast from pigmented lesion on the back. A case report. Acta Cytol. 2004;48:387–90.

110. Arora R, Robinson W. Breast metastases from malignant melanoma. J Surg Oncol. 1992;50:27–9.

111. Williams SA, Ehlers RA, Hunt KK, Yi M, Kuerer HM, Singletary SE, et al. Metastases to the breast from nonbreast solid neoplasms: presentation and determinants of survival. Cancer. 2007;110:731–7.

112. Vizcaíno I, Torregrosa A, Higueras V, Morote V, Cremades A, Torres V, et al. Metastasis to the breast from extramammary malignancies: a report of four cases and a review of literature. Eur Radiol. 2001;11:1659–65.

113. Noguera JJ, Martínez-Miravete P, Idoate F, Diaz L, Pina L, Zornoza G, et al. Metastases to the breast: a review of 33 cases. Australas Radiol. 2007;51:133–8.

114. Gómez-Caro A, Piñero A, Roca MJ, Torres J, Ferri B, Galindo PJ, et al. Surgical treatment of solitary metastasis in the male breast from non-small cell lung cancer. Breast J. 2006;12:366–7.

115. Lee AHS. The histological diagnosis of metastases to the breast from extramammary malignancies. J Clin Pathol. 2007;60:1333–41.

116. Hamby LS, McGrath PC, Cibull ML, Schwartz RW. Gastric carcinoma metastatic to the breast. J Surg Oncol. 1991;48:117–21.

117. Boutis AL, Andreadis C, Patakiouta F, Mouratidou D. Gastric signet-ring adenocarcinoma presenting with breast metastasis. World J Gastroenterol. 2006;12:2958–61.

118. Yeh CN, Lin CH, Chen MF. Clinical and ultrasonographic characteristics of breast metastases from extramammary malignancies. Am Surg. 2004;70:287–90.

119. Kwak JY, Kim EK, Oh KK. Radiologic findings of metastatic signet ring cell carcinoma to the breast from stomach. Yonsei Med. 2000;41:669–72.

120. Lee SK, Kim WW, Kim SH, Hur SM, Kim S, Choi JH, et al. Characteristics of metastasis in the breast from extramammary malignancies. J Surg Oncol. 2010;101:137–40.

121. Verger E, Conill C, Velasco M, Sole M. Metastasis in the male breast from a lung adenocarcinoma. Acta Oncol. 1992;31:479.

122. Chaignaud B, Hall TJ, Powers C, Subramony C, Scott-Conner CE. Diagnosis and natural history of extramammary tumors metastatic to the breast. J Am Coll Surg. 1994;179:49–53.

123. Alvarado Cabrero I, Carrera Alvarez M, Perez Montiel D, Tavassoli FA. Metastases to the breast. Eur J Surg Oncol. 2003;29:854–5.

Part V

Evaluation After Primary Therapy and Management of Recurrent Breast Cancer

Surveillance of Patients Following Primary Therapy

Varol Çelik, Tümay Aydoğan,
Mehmet Halit Yilmaz, Nejdet Fatih Yaşar,
and Mahmut Müslümanoğlu

Abstract

Regular and appropriate follow-up of patients after treatment for breast cancer is an important aspect of comprehensive care. Breast cancer survival has increased due to improvements of treatment, leading to a much higher long-term survival of women diagnosed with breast cancer. The primary purpose of follow-up is often regarded as the early detection of recurrence as well as the detection of second primary tumors along with long-term sequelae of breast cancer treatment.

Keywords

Breast cancer • Surveillance of patients • Follow-up • Follow-up program • Survival • Recurrence

V. Çelik, MD
Division of Breast Disease, Department of General Surgery, Cerrahpasa School of Medicine, Istanbul University, Istanbul, Turkey
e-mail: varolcelik@yahoo.com

T. Aydoğan, MD (✉)
Department of Medical Education, Biruni School of Medicine, Biruni University, Istanbul, Turkey

Comprehensive Breast Center, Hallmark Health Medical Associates, Stoneham, MA, USA
e-mail: aydoganmd@gmail.com

M.H. Yilmaz, MD

Department of Radiology, Cerrahpasa School of Medicine, Istanbul University, Istanbul, Turkey
e-mail: mhyilmaz@hotmail.com

N.F. Yaşar, MD
Department of General Surgery, Osmangazi Medical School, Eskişehir Osmangazi University, Eskişehir, Turkey
e-mail: nfyasar@gmail.com

M. Müslümanoğlu, MD
Department of General Surgery, Surgery Department, Istanbul University Medical Faculty, Istanbul Medical School, Istanbul, Turkey; http://mahmutm.istanbul.edu.tr

© Springer International Publishing Switzerland 2016
A. Aydiner et al. (eds.), *Breast Disease: Management and Therapies*,
DOI 10.1007/978-3-319-26012-9_28

Introduction

Regular and appropriate follow-up of patients after treatment for breast cancer is an important aspect of comprehensive care. Breast cancer survival has increased due to improvements of treatment, leading to a much higher long-term survival of women diagnosed with breast cancer. Recent data suggest that women have a 5-year survival of 78–91 % according to Surveillance, Epidemiology, and End Results (SEER) database [1].

The primary purpose of follow-up is often regarded as the early detection of recurrence as well as the detection of second primary tumors along with long-term sequelae of breast cancer treatment. The other goals are to assess and treat the complications of the therapy, evaluate the symptoms that may or may not be related to the disease, encourage compliance with ongoing therapy, provide psychosocial support, and give advice about health decisions like pregnancy that may be influenced by a history of breast cancer.

Follow-up care is provided by specialist oncologists in many countries. There is evidence that follow-up care provided by primary care physician or survivorship programs is equivalent to hospital-based outpatient care in detection of cancer recurrences [2]. This brings a high level of patient satisfaction and greater cost-effectiveness [3, 4].

Although local recurrence is generally seen in the first 3–5 years, it may manifest in 5–10 years and even later in patients with estrogen receptor-positive tumors and who receive adjuvant tamoxifen and/or chemotherapy [5–9]. Recurrences tend to occur more often after breast-conservative surgery compared to mastectomy [10, 11]. The recurrence incidence starts to decline after 5 years [12]. Women with a history of breast cancer are at risk of developing ipsilateral breast recurrence (IBR) or a new cancer in the treated breast and/or collateral breast cancer (CBC). Breast cancer distant metastasis is mostly seen in the bones, lungs, liver, and brain. Site of metastasis can show differences according to the subtypes of the breast cancer [13].

Recommendations for Breast Cancer Follow-Up

History

A careful history should be taken. New symptoms or changes in the symptoms should be noted. Persistent pain, fatigue, sexual dysfunction, hot flushes, weight loss, cough, shortness of breath, abdominal pain, lymph edema, and swelling of the arm are some of the most common symptoms. Forty percent of isolated locoregional relapses are detected in asymptomatic patients during routine controls, whereas the remaining 60 % are detected in self-examination (SE) [14, 15]. Early detection of recurrence in asymptomatic breast cancer patients may decrease the mortality rate by 0.5–0.8 % [16].

Survivors on tamoxifen therapy have two to three times the risk of developing endometrial cancer as age-matched women who are not taking tamoxifen [17]. Women receiving tamoxifen should be advised to report any abnormal vaginal bleeding. Annual gynecologic examination is recommended in all women, but specific screening for endometrial cancer in survivors is not recommended. Transvaginal ultrasound in asymptomatic women taking tamoxifen may be associated with false-positive results due to tamoxifen-induced endometrial proliferation, so it is not advised [18]. Women using tamoxifen should be referred to ophthalmologic examination for symptoms suggestive of retinopathy. The incidence of thromboembolic events such as deep vein thrombosis and pulmonary embolism is also increased by tamoxifen [19]. Patients on chemotherapy and aromatase inhibitors should undergo bone densitometry to detect osteopenia and osteoporosis. Vitamin D, calcium, and bisphosphonates can be recommended. Breast cancer tumor markers such as CEA or CA 15-3 should not be used in screening for breast cancer or as a routine follow-up test. Routine blood tests like complete blood count are not recommended for controls.

Physical Examination

Physical examination should be performed every 3–6 months for the first 3 years, then every 6–12 months for the next 2 years, and then annually. In the physical examination of breasts and lymph nodes, axillary, cervical, and supraclavicular regions next to the chest wall must be checked bilaterally. Examination findings must be noted in the patient's file because some tissue changes, such as tissue necrosis due to injected methylene blue for sentinel lymph node biopsy, may be felt as a new mass causing confusion. Both extremities must be controlled for lymph edema. Physicians should counsel patients about the symptoms of recurrence, including new lumps, bone pain, chest pain, dyspnea, and abdominal pain.

Referral for Genetic Counseling

Women at high risk for familial breast cancer syndromes should be referred for genetic counseling. Five to ten percent of familial breast cancers originate from inherited gene mutations [20]. Among these genes, BRCA1 and BRCA2 are responsible for many hereditary breast and ovarian cancers. Patients with mutations in BRCA1 and BRCA2 have a lifetime risk of breast cancer of 35–87 % and ovarian cancer of 16–60 %, depending on the type of mutation [21–23]. Genetic testing by The American Society of Breast Surgeons is recommended to patients who meet the following criteria: Ashkenazi Jewish heritage; history of ovarian cancer at any age in the patient or any first- or second-degree relatives, any first-degree relative with a history of breast cancer diagnosed before the age of 50; two or more first- or second-degree relatives diagnosed with breast cancer at any age, patient or relative with diagnosis of bilateral breast cancer; and history of breast cancer in a male relative [24].

Breast Self-Examination

All women must be encouraged to perform breast SE monthly. The most convenient time is within 5–7 days after the menstrual period in reproductive ages. Breast self-examination (SE) in women diagnosed with breast cancer is important for early detection of recurrences. Tumors that are detected by SE are often smaller than those detected by screening [25, 26]. However, in a wide study including more than 260,000 Chinese women, SE was shown not to be effective on surveillance. No difference was detected between trained and untrained groups in terms of tumor diameter, TNM staging, and cumulative mortality rates. However, no randomized data have been assessed for the cumulative effects of SE as well as mammography in women who were treated for breast cancer.

Mammography

The incidence of contralateral breast cancer is higher in patients diagnosed with breast cancer, so annual mammographic screening should be performed for the healthy breast. Mammography is the first radiological choice of follow-up after a breast-conserving surgery. A routine screening mammography should be performed bilaterally. Mammographic follow-up protocols may differ between patients with quadrantectomy and lumpectomy. Mammography is performed after 6 months of operation and then every year for both breasts. In breasts that have a cosmetic implant, the mammographic screening technique is different [27]. Mammography screening reduces the mortality of breast cancer by about 15 % [28, 29]. Women treated with breast-conserving surgery should have their first mammogram 6 months later. Subsequent mammograms should be performed every 6–12 months for surveillance of abnormalities.

Breast Ultrasonography

Breast ultrasonography can be used as an adjunct to mammography for dense breasts and in young patients to obtain additional information. Internal structures and the borders of the lump can better be evaluated in ultrasonography than mammography because in ultrasonography there is no superposition of tissues. Ultrasonography is a modality that is user dependent and challenging in detecting microcalcifications, so it cannot be used alone for screening of breast cancer [30–32]. Ultrasonography is the first radiological modality for evaluation of the chest wall in patients with mastectomy. It is also used for differentiation of cystic-solid masses, evaluation of axilla, and biopsies of non-palpable masses. Ultrasonography is used for evaluation of implant integrity. Short performance time and low cost are some of its advantages. The handicap of ultrasonography is its user dependency.

Breast Magnetic Resonance Imaging

Breast magnetic resonance imaging (MRI) gives us useful information for the evaluation of the chest wall in patients who have undergone mastectomy and lesion status assessment [33]. Breast MRI is used in implant patients to distinguish recurrence and scarring after breast-conserving surgery, and it may be used in genetically high-risk patients. The best-known indication of breast MRI is its usage for evaluation of breast parenchyma and the integrity of implants in patients with breast-conserving surgery and silicone implants. Breasts with prostheses can be shown in any axes by MRI, while there is no need to use contrast material to identify the integrity of implants in breasts with prostheses. It is mandatory to use contrast with dynamic MRI in routine follow-up and malignancy detections. In MRI, low-intensity linear lines (collapsed membranes swimming in silicone) are defined as the "linguine sign" and reveal an intracapsular rupture.

Silicone, which can seep out of the capsule, is another sign of capsular rupture.

Other Imaging Studies

Chest X-rays, bone scans, ultrasonography of the liver, CT scanning, fluorodeoxyglucose positron emission-computed tomography (FDG-PET/CT) scanning, and breast MRI are not recommended for routine breast cancer surveillance [34–41]. Recommendations for breast cancer follow-up are shown in Table 28.1.

Most of the patients with axillary lymph node involvement have bone metastases within 10 years after the mastectomy. This incidence increases with time: For the first 3 years, this rate is 8.9 %, 11.2 % for 5 years, and 14.4 % for 10 years. In advanced stages of the disease, 70 % of the patients may develop bone metastases [42]. In large studies, bone scintigraphy was shown to be very sensitive and specific. In a 10-year study conducted by Crippa et al., bone scintigraphy had 98.2 % sensitivity, 95.2 % specificity, and 95.5 % accuracy [43].

FDG-PET scanning is more sensitive in recurrences of breast cancer [44–46]. One study included 60 breast cancer patients with suspicion of relapse. Forty of them had relapse, and the efficiency of PET scan in detecting locoregional and distant metastases was assessed. PET scan and CA 15–3 were compared for detection of the relapses, and PET scan was more sensitive. In a meta-analysis discussing 16 patient-based studies and 8 lesion-based studies, the mean sensitivity and specificity of PET scan were 92.7 % and 81.6 %, respectively [47].

Follow-up can be coordinated by primary care physicians, and further oncology assessment may be considered if needed, especially for patients receiving adjuvant endocrine therapy [34]. Long-term management of breast cancer survivors requires a multidisciplinary approach including psychological health and other health issues [48–50].

Table 28.1 Recommendations for breast cancer follow-up and management in the adjuvant setting

Surveillance	History/physical examination	Regular visits every 3–4 months in the first 2 years, every 6 months from years 3 to 5, and annually thereafter are recommended
	Breast self-examination	Monthly
Imaging	Mammography	Screening mammogram annually
	Breast ultrasound	Annual ipsilateral (after BCT) and/or contralateral mammography with ultrasound is recommended. Ultrasound can also be considered in the follow-up of lobular invasive carcinomas
	Breast MRI	In women with familial breast cancer, with or without proven BRCA mutations, annual screening with MRI of the breast, in combination with mammography, is recommended
	Other imaging studies	Chest X-ray, bone scan, liver ultrasound, CT scanning, and FDG-PET scanning are not recommended for routine breast cancer surveillance
Blood tests	CBC, automated biochemistry, and tumor markers	Not recommended for routine surveillance of patients with breast cancer after primary therapy
Monitoring for late effects	Bone health	Yearly
	Pelvic examination	Yearly
	Lymphedema assessment	Personalized
	Sexual health/fertility	Personalized
Risk reduction	Genetic counseling	Women at high risk for familial breast cancer syndromes

BCT breast-conserving therapy, *CBC* complete blood count, *MRI* magnetic resonance imaging, *FDG-PET* [^{18}F] fluorodeoxyglucose positron emission tomography

Pregnancy

Loss of fertility as a result of treatment is a stressful aspect of breast cancer diagnosis [51–53]. Chemotherapy, tamoxifen, and ovarian ablation can affect fertility. Tamoxifen itself is not a direct cause of infertility, but women are instructed not to get pregnant while taking it. The risk of chemotherapy depends on the therapy regimen, the patient's age, and the ovarian history. Even if menstruation continues during chemotherapy, the patient is likely to experience a premature menopause. Regarding future pregnancy following breast cancer treatment, patients are advised to wait for at least 2 years. According to most of the retrospective studies, there is no significant risk of recurrence due to pregnancy [54–58].

Psychosocial Problems

Younger women are at a greater risk of depression and anxiety because they have a fear about their body image, hair loss, and sexuality. If they have children, they may worry about not seeing them grow up [59–61]. They may have fatigue, which can affect their job. In follow-up, doctors should be careful about signs of depression and refer the patients to psychiatry or a support group if needed.

References

1. DeSantis C, Ma J, Bryan L, Jemal A. Breast cancer statistics, 2013. CA Cancer J Clin. 2014;64:52–62.
2. Rojas MP, Telaro E, Russo A, Fossati R, Confalonieri C, Liberati A. Follow-up strategies for women treated for early breast cancer. Cochrane Database Syst Rev. 2005;(1):CD001768.
3. Grunfeld E, Fitzpatrick R, Mant D, Yudkin P, Adewuyi-Dalton R, Stewart J, et al. Comparison of breast cancer patient satisfaction with follow-up in primary care versus specialist care: results from a randomized controlled trial. Br J Gen Pract. 1999;49:705–10.
4. Grunfeld E, Mant D, Yudkin P, Adewuyi-Dalton R, Cole D, Stewart J, et al. Routine follow up of breast cancer in primary care: randomized trial. BMJ. 1996;313:665–9.
5. Hollowell K, Olmsted CL, Richardson AS, Pittman HK, Bellin L, et al. American Society of Clinical Oncology-recommended surveillance and physician specialty among long term breast cancer survivors. Cancer. 2010;116:2090–8.
6. Chalasani P, Downey L, Stopeck AT. Caring for the breast cancer survivor: a guide for primary care physicians. Am J Med. 2010;123:489–95.
7. Saphner T, Tormey DC, Gray R. Annual hazard rates of recurrence for breast cancer after primary therapy. J Clin Oncol. 1996;14:2738–46.
8. Voogd AC, van Oost FJ, Rutgers EJ, Elkhuizen PH, van Geel AN, Scheijmans LJ, et al. Long-term prognosis of patients with local recurrence after conservative surgery and radiotherapy for early breast cancer. Eur J Cancer. 2005;41:2637–44.
9. Haffty BG, Carter D, Flynn SD, Fischer DB, Brash DE, Simons J, et al. Local recurrence versus new primary: clinical analysis of 82 breast relapses and potential applications for genetic fingerprinting. Int J Radiat Oncol Biol Phys. 1993;27:575–83.
10. van Tienhoven G, Voogd AC, Peterse JL, Nielsen M, Andersen KW, Mignolet F, et al. Prognosis after treatment for loco-regional recurrence after mastectomy or breast conserving therapy in two randomised trials (EORTC 10801 and DBCG-82TM). EORTC Breast Cancer Cooperative Group and the Danish Breast Cancer Cooperative Group. Eur J Cancer. 1999;35:32–8.
11. Francis M, Cakir B, Ung O, Gebski V, Boyages J. Prognosis after breast recurrence following conservative surgery and radiotherapy in patients with node-negative breast cancer. Br J Surg. 1999;86:1556–62.
12. Buist DS, Abraham LA, Barlow WE, Krishnaraj A, Holdridge RC, Sickles EA, Breast Cancer Surveillance Consortium, et al. Diagnosis of second breast cancer events after initial diagnosis of early stage breast cancer. Breast Cancer Res Treat. 2010;124:863–73.
13. Smid M, Wang Y, Zhang Y, Sieuwerts AM, Yu J, Klijn JG, et al. Subtypes of breast cancer show preferential site of relapse. Cancer Res. 2008;68:3108–14.
14. Khatcheressian JL, Wolff AC, Smith TJ, Grunfeld E, Muss HB, Vogel VG, et al. American Society of Clinical Oncology. American Society of Clinical Oncology 2006 update of the breast cancer follow-up and management guidelines in the adjuvant setting. J Clin Oncol. 2006;24:5091–7.
15. de Bock GH, Bonnema J, van der Hage J, Kievit J, van de Velde CJ. Effectiveness of routine visits and routine tests in detecting isolated locoregional recurrences after treatment for early-stage invasive breast cancer: a meta-analysis and systematic review. J Clin Oncol. 2004;22:4010–8.
16. Lu WL, Jansen L, Post WJ, Bonnema J, Van de Velde JC, De Bock GH. Impact on survival of early detection of isolated breast recurrences after the primary treatment for breast cancer: a meta-analysis. Breast Cancer Res Treat. 2009;114:403–128. Hayes DF. Clinical practice. Follow-up of patients with early breast cancer. N Engl J Med. 2007;356:2505–13.
17. American College of Obstetricians and Gynecologists Committee on Gynecologic Practice. ACOG committee opinion. No. 336: tamoxifen and uterine cancer. Obstet Gynecol. 2006;107:1475–8.
18. Hayes DF. Clinical practice. Follow-up of patients with early breast cancer. N Engl J Med. 2007;14(356):2505–13.
19. Deitcher SR, Gomes MP. The risk of venous thromboembolic disease associated with adjuvant hormone therapy for breast carcinoma: a systematic review. Cancer. 2004;101:439–49.
20. Emery J, Lucassen A, Murphy M. Common hereditary cancers and implications for primary care. Lancet. 2001;7(358):56–63.
21. King MC, Marks JH, Mandell JB, New York Breast Cancer Study Group. Breast and ovarian cancer risks due to inherited mutations in BRCA1 and BRCA2. Science. 2003;302:643–6.
22. Antoniou A, Pharoah PD, Narod S, Risch HA, Eyfjord JE, Hopper JL, et al. Average risks of breast and ovarian cancer associated with BRCA1 or BRCA2 mutations detected in case Series unselected for family history: a combined analysis of 22 studies. Am J Hum Genet. 2003;72:1117–30.
23. Fossland VS, Stroop JB, Schwartz RC, Kurtzman SH. Genetic issues in patients with breast cancer. Surg Oncol Clin N Am. 2009;18:53–71.
24. The American Society of Breast Surgeon Position Statement on BRCA genetic testing for patients with and without breast cancer (2012) https://www.breast-surgeons.org/statements/PDF_Statements/BRCA_Testing.pdf. Accessed 26 June 2014.

25. Koibuchi Y, Lino Y, Takei H, Maemura M, Horiguchi J, Yo- Koe T, et al. The effect of mass screening by physical examination combined with regular breast self-examination on clinical stage and course of Japanese women with breast cancer. Oncol Rep. 1998;5:151–5.

26. GIVIO (Interdisciplinary Group for Cancer Care Evaluation). Practice of breast self examination: disease extent at diagnosis and patterns of surgical care. A report from an Italian study. J Epidemiol Community Health. 1991;45:112–6.

27. Yilmaz MH. Imaging and follow-up after breast reconstruction. J Breast Dis. 2012;1:81–4.

28. Gotzsche PC, Jorgensen KJ. Screening for breast cancer with mammography. Cochrane Database Syst Rev. 2013;(6):CD001877.

29. Magnus MC, Ping M, Shen MM, Bourgeois J, Magnus JH. Effectiveness of mammography screening in reducing breast cancer mortality in women aged 39–49 years: a meta-analysis. J Women's Health (Larchmt). 2011;20:845–52.

30. Kim SJ, Moon WK, Cho N, Chang JM. The detection of recurrent breast cancer in patients with a history of breast cancer surgery: comparison of clinical breast examination, mammography and ultrasonography. Acta Radiol. 2011;1(52):15–20.

31. Gweon HM, Son EJ, Youk JH, Kim JA, Chung J. Value of the US BI-RADS final assessment following mastectomy: BI-RADS 4 and 5 lesions. Acta Radiol. 2012;53:255–60.

32. Destounis S, Morgan R, Arieno A, Seifert P, Somerville P, Murphy P. A review of breast imaging following mastectomy with or without reconstruction in an outpatient community center. Breast Cancer. 2011;18:259–67.

33. Yilmaz MH, Esen G, Ayarcan Y, Aydoğan F, Ozgüroğlu M, Demir G, et al. The role of US and MR imaging in detecting local chest wall tumor recurrence after mastectomy. Diagn Interv Radiol. 2007;13:13–8.

34. Khatcheressian JL, Hurley P, Bantug E, Esserman LJ, Grunfeld E, Halberg F, et al. American Society of Clinical Oncology. Breast cancer follow-up and management after primary treatment: American Society of Clinical Oncology clinical practice guideline update. J Clin Oncol. 2013;31:961–5.

35. Lin NU, Thomssen C, Cardoso F, Cameron D, Cufer T, Fallowfield L, et al. European School of Oncology-Metastatic Breast Cancer Task Force. International guidelines for management of metastatic breast cancer (MBC) from the European School of Oncology (ESO)-MBC Task Force: surveillance, staging, and evaluation of patients with early-stage and metastatic breast cancer. Breast. 2013;22:203–10.

36. Salloum RG, Hornbrook MC, Fishman PA, Ritzwoller DP, O'Keeffe Rossetti MC, et al. Adherence to surveillance care guidelines after breast and colorectal cancer treatment with curative intent. Cancer. 2012;118:5644–51.

37. Harris L, Fritsche H, Mennel R, Norton L, Ravdin P, Taube S, et al. American Society of Clinical Oncology. American Society of Clinical Oncology 2007 update of recommendations for the use of tumor markers in breast cancer. J Clin Oncol. 2007;25:5287–312.

38. Tolaney SM, Winer EP. Follow-up care of patients with breast cancer. Breast Suppl. 2007;2: S45–50.

39. Keating NL, Landrum MB, Guadagnoli E, Winer EP, Ayanian JZ. Surveillance testing among survivors of early-stage breast cancer. J Clin Oncol. 2007;25:1074–81.

40. Smith TJ. American Society of Clinical Oncology. The American Society of Clinical Oncology Recommended Breast Cancer Surveillance Guidelines can be done in a routine office visit. J Clin Oncol. 2005;23:6807.

41. Elston Lafata J, Simpkins J, Schultz L, Chase GA, Johnson CC, Yood MU, et al. Routine surveillance care after cancer treatment with curative intent. Med Care. 2005;43:592–9.

42. Coleman SJ, Rubens RD. The clinical course of bone metastasis from breast cancer. Br J Cancer. 1987;55:61–6.

43. Crippa F, Seregni E, Agresti R, Bombardieri E, Buraggi GL. Bone scintigraphy in breast cancer: a ten years follow up study. J Nucl Biol Med. 1993;37:57–61.

44. Manohar K, Mittal BR, Senthil R, Kashyap R, Bhattacharya A, Singh G. Clinical utility of F-18 FDG PET/CT in recurrent breast carcinoma. Nucl Med Commun. 2012;33:591–6.

45. Murakami R, Kumita S, Yoshida T, Ishihara K, Kiriyama T, Hakozaki K, et al. FDG-PET/CT in the diagnosis of recurrent breast cancer. Acta Radiol. 2012;53:12–6.

46. Hodgson NC, Gulenchyn KY. Is there a role for positron emission tomography in breast cancer staging? J Clin Oncol. 2008;26:712–20.

47. Isasi CR, Moadel RM, Blaufox MD. A meta-analysis of FDG-PET for the evaluation of breast cancer recurrence and metastases. Breast Cancer Res Treat. 2005;90:105–12.

48. Granziera E, Guglieri I, Del Bianco P, Capovilla E, Dona' B, Ciccarese AA, et al. A multidisciplinary approach to improve preoperative understanding and reduce anxiety: a randomised study. Eur J Anaesthesiol. 2013;30:734–42.

49. Rajan S, Foreman J, Wallis MG, Caldas C, Britton P. Multidisciplinary decisions in breast cancer: does the patient receive what the team has recommended? Br J Cancer. 2013;108:2442–7.

50. Taylor C, Shewbridge A, Harris J, Green JS. Benefits of multidisciplinary teamwork in the management of breast cancer. Breast Cancer (Dove Med Press). 2013;5:79–85.

51. Bimes J, Oleske DM, Cobleigh MA. Ovarian function in premenopausal women treated with adjuvant chemotherapy for breast cancer. J Clin Oncol. 1996;14:1718–29.

52. Perz J, Ussher J, Gilbert E. Loss, uncertainty, or acceptance: subjective experience of changes to fertility after breast cancer. Eur J Cancer Care (Engl). 2014;23:514–22.

53. Munster PN. Fertility preservation and breast cancer: a complex problem. Oncology (Williston Park). 2013;27:533–9.

54. Sinha G. Pregnancy after breast cancer appears safe. J Natl Cancer Inst. 2012;104:725–6.

55. Pagani O, Partridge A, Korde L, Badve S, Bartlett J, Albain K, et al. Breast International Group; North American Breast Cancer Group Endocrine Working Group. Pregnancy after breast cancer: if you wish, ma'am. Breast Cancer Res Treat. 2011;129:309–17.

56. Azim Jr HA, Santoro L, Pavlidis N, Gelber S, Kroman N, Azim H, et al. Safety of pregnancy following breast cancer diagnosis: a meta-analysis of 14 studies. Eur J Cancer. 2011;47:74–83.

57. Kranick JA, Schaefer C, Rowell S, Desai M, Petrek JA, Hiatt RA, et al. Is pregnancy after breast cancer safe? Breast J. 2010;16:404–11.

58. de Bree E, Makrigiannakis A, Askoxylakis J, Melissas J, Tsiftsis DD. Pregnancy after breast cancer. A comprehensive review. J Surg Oncol. 2010;101:534–42.

59. Peled R, Carmil D, Siboni-Samocha O, Shoham-Vardi I. Breast cancer, psychological distress and life events among young women. BMC Cancer. 2008;8:245.

60. Howard-Anderson J, Ganz PA, Bower JE, Stanton AL. Quality of life, fertility concerns, and behavioral health outcomes in younger breast cancer survivors: a systematic review. J Natl Cancer Inst. 2012;104:386–405.

61. Zainal NZ, Nik-Jaafar NR, Baharudin A, Sabki ZA, Ng CG. Prevalence of depression in breast cancer survivors: a systematic review of observational studies. Asian Pac J Cancer Prev. 2013;14:2649–56.

Surgery for the Primary Tumor in Patients with De Novo Stage IV Breast Cancer

29

Atilla Soran and Serdar Ozbas

Abstract

Breast carcinoma with distant metastases (stage IV) is still considered to be a disease with no cure. Current guidelines advocate primary systemic therapy as the choice of treatment in such patients. Therefore, surgery for the primary tumor is indicated only if it is symptomatic. However, recent encouraging reports challenged this classical approach. Reports of carefully selected patients (retrospective data which are evaluated with or without controls) presenting with stage IV breast carcinoma suggest that surgery on the primary tumor may result in improved survival. The survival advantage of primary surgery remains unproven, and ongoing prospective trials must be completed before a conclusion.

Keywords

Metastatic breast • Cancer • De novo • Primary surgery • Systemic therapy • Survival

Breast cancer (BC) is the most common cancer in women worldwide and the second most common cancer overall. The incidence of synchronized distant metastatic disease in newly diagnosed BC patients is as high as 10 % [1–3]. BC is also the most frequently diagnosed cancer among women in 140 of 184 countries worldwide and represents one in four cancer cases in women [4]. The incidence of BC is increasing worldwide; in 2012, 1.7 million women were diagnosed with BC, and there were 6.3 million women alive who had been diagnosed with BC in the previous 5 years. Based on these statistics, one may estimate as many as 170,000 cases of de novo stage IV BC worldwide in 2012.

A. Soran, MD, MPH, FACS (✉)
Department of Surgery, Division of Surgical Oncology, Magee-Womens Hospital, University of Pittsburgh Medical Center, Pittsburgh, PA, USA
e-mail: asoran@upmc.edu, asoran65@gmail.com

S. Ozbas, MD
Breast and Endocrine Surgery Unit, Ankara Guven Hospital, Simsek Sokak, No:29, Kavaklidere, Ankara 06540, Turkey
e-mail: sozbas@yahoo.com

© Springer International Publishing Switzerland 2016
A. Aydiner et al. (eds.), *Breast Disease: Management and Therapies*,
DOI 10.1007/978-3-319-26012-9_29

In general, BC with distant metastasis is considered incurable, and the traditional goal of primary tumor surgery is to palliate symptoms to improve quality of life. Currently, the role of surgery to remove the primary tumor and its impact on distant metastatic disease and patient survival are controversial. Therefore, surgical treatment of the intact primary tumor is indicated only if it is symptomatic, i.e., it is bleeding or fungating or is associated with ulceration, pain, or hygienic disturbances. These are among the palliative indications for locoregional surgery. Systemic therapy (ST) is the primary treatment for stage IV BC [5]. However, with advances in adjuvant therapies and a better understanding of tumor biology, the survival of stage IV BC patients appears to be improving [6,7]. Furthermore, with advances in sensitive imaging modalities, low-volume metastatic BC is being diagnosed more often; patients with a single metastatic deposit may represent a very different cohort of patients than those with multiple solid organ metastases. By contrast, there is no evidence that local control in the metastatic setting worsens prognosis. The surgical treatment indications of the intact primary tumor are:

(a) Prolonged overall survival
(b) Prolonged progression-free survival
(c) For locoregional control
(d) Palliative

Earlier disease detection with improved adjuvant treatments may enable improved survival [8]. Removing the primary tumor improves survival in other settings, such as metastatic melanoma, renal cell carcinoma, colorectal cancer, and gastric cancer [9–12]. Removal of the primary tumor may have an immunomodulatory effect, decrease the overall tumor burden, remove a "seed source" of new metastases, or decrease the likelihood of the development of potentially resistant cell lines [13,14]. It is also possible that enhanced survival in BC patients treated with surgery may be explained by selection bias [15]. Patients who are offered surgery may be younger, may be healthier, or may have a lower burden of disease, metastases in more favorable locations,

or a more favorable tumor profile than those for whom surgery was not considered (Table 29.1).

Although retrospective studies do not support the hypothesis that the surgical resection of the primary tumor increases the risk of relapse, in animal models, removing the primary tumor can stimulate metastatic growth [16,17]. Two underlying mechanisms have been proposed: angiogenic and proliferative. The angiogenic surge is due either to the removal of inhibitors or the appearance of stimulators or growth factors in response to surgery [18,19]. This activation temporarily causes inactive distant micrometastases to vascularize and consequently enter a rapid growth phase. The data suggest that such stimulated angiogenesis may occur in approximately 20 % of premenopausal patients with node-positive disease. The proliferative mechanism for early relapse, which is also the result of surgery, is the stimulated division of single dormant cells

Table 29.1 Does local surgery increase survival in stage IV BC? Hypotheses based on retrospective and animal studies

Removal of the primary tumor eradicates one of the sources of further metastatic spread
A reduction in the number of cancer cells may lead to increased ST efficacy by decreasing the risk of the emergence of chemoresistant cells and by removing necrotic, avascular tumor tissue that is poorly accessible to drugs
Immunocompetence may be restored because surgery suppresses the growth of metastases by removing primary cancer-associated inflammatory products (hormonal, angiogenic) from circulation
Tumor-induced immunosuppression may be another mechanism of interaction between the primary tumor and metastases
The number of metastatic sites increases as the size and duration of the tumor increase
Endocrine or cytokine-mediated effects may modify the behavior of tumor cells at the metastatic sites
Debulking surgery is clinically effective in other common solid tumors (ovarian, colorectal, gastric, renal cancers, and malignant melanoma (not generalizable))
A single metastatic deposit may be deemed "stage IV" using modern (PET/CT) imaging; thus, "low burden" stage IV disease can be identified
Selection bias may be responsible for the surgery-mediated increase in survival

or even changes in the dynamics maintaining the steady state of dormant or indolent micrometastases, ultimately resulting in angiogenesis and growth [20]. For primary breast tumors smaller than 2 cm, 50 % of all relapses belong to this first wave of relapses, and for larger tumors, 75–83 % of relapses fall in this category. Early relapses among patients receiving no adjuvant treatment due to stimulated angiogenesis occur in the first 10 months after surgery, whereas the adverse events stimulated by rapid changes occur in the first 4 years after surgery, with a peak at 18 months. There is overlap between these two distributions of outcomes. Together, these distributions create an early peak in relapses that occurs sooner than observed otherwise due to a stimulation of growth by surgery.

Retrospective Studies on Survival (Table 29.2)

Several retrospective studies and meta-analyses have indicated that surgery to remove the primary tumor in de novo stage IV BC not only controls locoregional progression but prolongs overall and disease-free survival. A retrospective analysis of the American National Cancer Database (NCDB) indicated that the resection of the primary breast tumor in patients with stage IV BC was associated with a significant survival advantage [21]. Women in whom the primary breast tumor was removed with tumor-free margins had a superior overall prognosis with a hazard ratio of 0.61 compared to women who did not undergo surgery. In a small retrospective study, Carmichael et al. reported a single-institution case series ($n = 20$) of patients who underwent primary tumor resection for stage IV BC at presentation or were diagnosed with metastases within 1 month of surgery [1]. They found that median survival after surgery was 23 months and that half of the patients were alive with no local disease at 20 months. Because there was no control group to compare these results, no evident conclusion about the superiority of local control could be drawn in this study. Gnerlich et al. reviewed SEER data for stage IV BC patients between 1988 and 2003 and found that patients who underwent surgical removal of the primary tumor had better survival than women who did not undergo surgery [2]. This study demonstrated that patients who underwent primary surgery were 37 % less likely to die than those who did not undergo surgery. In 2006, Barbiera et al. reported their institutional findings for a retrospective cohort of 224 patients with stage IV BC and intact primary tumors [22]. They observed that removal of the primary tumor significantly improved progression-free survival in BC patients with distant organ metastases. However, overall survival did not differ between groups.

Table 29.2 Selected retrospective studies of overall survival for surgery or no surgery of the primary tumor

Author	Surgery survival	No surgery survival	HR
Bafford [32]	3.52 years	2.36 years	0.47
Blanchard [3]	27.1 mths	16.8 mths	0.71
Cady [31]	24 mths	24 mths	n/a
Fields [24]	31.9 mths	15.4 mths	0.53
Gnerlich [2]	36 mths	21 mths	0.63
Hazard [26]	26.3 mths	29.2 mths	0.79
Khan [21]	31.9 mths	19.3 mths	0.61
Rapiti [23] [5 year]	27 %	12 %	0.6
Ruiterkamp [27]	31 mths	14 mths	0.62
Shien [36]	27 mths	22 mths	0.049
Leung [37]	25 mths	13 mths	0.004
McGuire [Median 37 mths] [38]	33 %	20 %	0.0012

HR hazard ratio, *mths* months

Rapiti et al. reported another retrospective study of 300 stage IV BC patients from the Geneva Cancer Registry [23]. They reported that women who underwent complete excision of the primary breast tumor with negative surgical margins had a 40 % reduced risk of death compared with women who did not undergo surgery. In another similar study, Blanchard et al. reported a retrospective series of 427 patients with stage IV BC from their institutional registry [3]. Their results revealed that the interval from diagnosis to death was 27 months for patients who underwent surgical resection of the primary tumor but 17 months for the no-surgery group. This difference between groups was significant. Fields et al. reported a retrospective analysis of their institutional cohort of 409 patients with stage IV BC [24]. This study provided additional evidence that BC patients with distant metastases at diagnosis benefit from surgical excision of the primary lesion in terms of improved survival. After controlling for age, comorbidity, tumor grade, histology, and sites of metastasis, patients who underwent surgical resection were 47 % less likely to die than patients who did not undergo surgery for the primary tumor. The median overall survival was significantly longer in patients who had resection (26.8 months vs. 12.6 months). Thus, not only does patient selection contribute to improved survival, but patients do better with a more complete oncological resection. However, the timing of locoregional tumor resection is controversial and varies in all studies. The literature reports from registry data provide limited information about the timing of surgery because patients underwent locoregional resection of the primary tumor at various times after diagnosis. In an evaluation of chest wall disease and its influence on outcome, Arriagada et al. found that the development of distant metastases was related to local failure as a time-dependent covariate [25]. A similar conclusion was reached by Hazard and colleagues, who reported that uncontrolled chest wall disease was associated with decreased overall survival, independent of surgical intervention [26]. Hazard et al. observed that 36 % of women not initially offered surgery required some form of locore-

gional therapy, either surgical or radiotherapeutic, to control chest wall disease. Only 17 % of the nonsurgical group was maintained with asymptomatic, intact tumors in the breast throughout their course. This result supports the theory of reduced seeding or a reduction of potentially resistant cell lines. The number of metastatic sites negatively influences survival, and it can be argued that the primary tumor constitutes an additional metastatic site. This hypothesis is supported by studies indicating improved survival in patients with limited metastatic BC when a single metastatic site is treated aggressively [27]. However, concerns have been raised that surgery to the primary tumor can actually adversely affect survival [28–30]. Cady et al. studied the impact of the sequence of systemic and surgical treatments in stage IV patients. They observed 2-year survival of 90 % in patients receiving chemotherapy first, which was higher than the rate for patients who received chemotherapy simultaneously with or after surgery, suggesting that delaying surgery after an excellent response to initial chemotherapy may be beneficial. The 2-year survival advantage occurred with presurgery chemotherapy for bone metastases, but no difference in survival with or without surgery occurred when these treatments were simultaneous. Among 5-year survivors, the frequency of primary site surgery after an excellent response to ST, breast surgery in stage III patients incorrectly classified as stage IV, and the frequency of oligo-metastases all indicated selection bias [31]. A review of a prospectively maintained database of patients who presented with stage IV BC between 1998 and 2005 was reported by Bafford et al. [32]. Of the 147 women who presented with stage IV BC, 61 (41 %) underwent mastectomy or lumpectomy, and the median unadjusted overall survival was 3.52 years for surgery versus 2.36 years for no surgery ($p = 0.093$). The ER and Her2neu status and central nervous system and liver metastases were predictors of survival, and multivariate analysis revealed that survival was significantly superior in the surgery group (HR: $0.47 p = 0.003$, mean 4.13 years vs. 2.36 years). In women undergoing surgery, 36 were diagnosed with metastatic disease postoperatively, and 25 were diagnosed preoperatively. These groups had median survival durations of 4.0 years and 2.4 years, respectively, comparable to the median survival of the no surgery group (2.36 years, $p = 0.18$). They concluded that breast surgery is associated with improved survival in stage IV BC. However, this benefit is only realized among patients operated on before the diagnosis of metastatic disease and is likely a consequence of stage migration bias [32]. Ruiterkamp et al. obtained similar results, and in their study, removing the primary tumor in patients with primary distant metastatic disease was associated with an approximately 40 % reduction of mortality risk [33]. The association was independent of age, the presence of comorbidities, and other potential confounders. The median survival of patients who underwent surgery for their primary tumor was significantly longer than that for patients who did not have surgery (31 vs. 14 months), and the 5-year survival rates were 24.5 % and 13.1 %, respectively ($p < 0.0001$). In a multivariate Cox regression analysis, adjusting for age, period of diagnosis, T-classification, number of metastatic sites, comorbidity, use of LRT, and use of ST, surgery appeared to be an independent prognostic factor for overall survival [33].

These studies were all subject to selection biases due to their retrospective nature. It was evident that surgeons were inclined to use surgery in patients with more favorable features (i.e., younger age, smaller tumor size, less evident axillary involvement, fewer sites of metastasis). Therefore, these studies should be interpreted with caution. Further limitations of these trials, such as a lack of information regarding radiation/ ST, histopathological features, and the timing of surgery to remove the intact primary tumor, were obvious. To eliminate selection biases, randomized clinical trials should be designed to compare locoregional treatment for the primary tumor with no intervention to the primary tumor; two trials with such a design and other ongoing studies will be discussed later in this chapter.

Regarding axillary disease control in stage IV BC patients, in the NCDB study, although the extent of nodal disease was not significantly associated with survival, women undergoing total mastectomy were expected to have nodal dissection to some extent. Nodal dissection may have contributed to the survival advantage observed in the total mastectomy group [6]. In the Geneva study, a trend toward improved survival was observed for women who had both a tumor-free surgical margin and axillary clearance [23]. Previous studies have lacked regional radiotherapy (RT) data. In the Geneva registry study, administration of whole-breast RT to patients who underwent BCS increased the hazard of death independently [23].

Harris et al. published a meta-analysis of nine retrospective cohort studies and one case control study in 2013 [34] (Table 29.1). Seven studies covered the period 1988–2005; three of the smaller studies included results dating to the 1970s, and all were multicenter studies. This meta-analysis suggested that appropriately selected patients may derive a survival benefit from resection of the primary tumor. Collated data from 28,693 patients demonstrated that patients undergoing surgery on the primary tumor had improved 3-year survival times (40 %) compared with those treated with ST alone (22 %). However, there are some limitations to this meta-analysis and its conclusions; the data presented are limited to retrospective studies, and surgical patients had a more favorable profile before operative intervention. Selection biases, lack of intervention at metastatic sites, and stage migration are limiting factors that could contribute to the better outcome in retrospective studies. However, even if the published meta-analysis failed to demonstrate any survival benefit of neoadjuvant versus adjuvant chemotherapy, it is unclear from these studies whether patients received chemotherapy in a neoadjuvant setting rather than an adjuvant setting [35]. Her2 data are also limited in many of the studies, and therefore, it is difficult to achieve any meaningful conclusions regarding the role of primary excision in the setting of Her2-positive stage IV disease. Ongoing randomized clinical trials will determine the optimal timing, most favorable tumor biology, and indications for surgery to remove the primary tumor.

A retrospective study from Japan evaluating the prognostic impact of local surgery and other clinicopathological features in patients with de novo stage IV BC found that overall survival was prolonged with local surgery, younger age, and bone or soft tissue metastases ($p < 0.05$). Furthermore, they found that local surgery did not improve overall survival in older patients (>51 years old) or patients with visceral or bone/soft tissue-only metastases ($p > 0.05$). The authors concluded that local surgery should be considered for younger and fewer patients [36].

Randomized Clinical Trials (RCTs) (Table 29.3 and Fig. 29.1)

Currently, there are eight randomized, controlled trials in progress that will address and hopefully clarify the role of primary tumor excision in the setting of stage IV BC. Two RCTs were presented at the San Antonio Breast Cancer Conference in 2013. A group in India conducted a prospective randomized trial to assess the impact of locoregional treatment on outcome in women with metastatic BC at initial diagnosis [39]. In this RCT, anthracyclines ± taxane-based chemotherapy was initially administered for all de novo stage IV BC, and patients who exhibited regression of the primary tumor were randomized to receive surgery or no surgery. The mean ages were 47 and 48, respectively, and 74 % of the patients had three or more metastases in both

groups. None of the patients received trastuzumab, although it was generally expected that 20 % of the patients were Her2 (+). However, the presenter stated that they included all patients in this study, even though their medical condition was not considered. The overall survival hazard ratio for surgery was 1.04 (95 % CI; 0.80–1.34; $p = 0.79$); however, the local progression-free survival hazard ratio was 0.16 (95 % CI; 0.10–1.26; $p = 0.00$), which is additional evidence that locoregional intervention in the metastatic setting provides a reduction of progression of the primary tumor of >80 %. According to the data presented from India, locoregional treatment of the primary tumor did not result in any benefit in overall survival. In fact, surgical removal of the primary tumor may even encourage the growth of distant metastases, lending support to the argument that less is more. This unexpected result should be evaluated in other studies and will remain controversial in the absence of appropriate ST and good patient selection.

The early results of a Turkish trial (MF07-01) with a similar objective to assess whether early surgical treatment of primary BC in women presenting with stage IV disease affects overall survival were also presented at the San Antonio Breast Cancer Conference in 2013 [40]. The MF07-01 trial is a phase III, multicentric, randomized controlled clinical trial comparing locoregional treatment (complete resection of the primary tumor and, when necessary, axillary clearance and RT to the whole breast, thoracic wall,

Table 29.3 Randomized clinical trials evaluating the importance of surgery of the primary tumor in de novo stage IV breast cancer

Country	Clinical trials.gov identifier	Initial therapy	Study period	Sample size	Status
India	NCT00193778	CT	2005–2012	350	Completed
Japan	JCOG	ST	2011–2016	410	Recruiting
USA adjusted	NCT01242800	ST	2010–2016	368	Recruiting
Thailand	NCT01906112	ST	2013–2019	476	No record
Turkey (MF07-01)	NCT00557986	Surgery	2008–2012	278	Completed
Turkey (BOMET)	NCT02125630	Surgery	2014–2017	288	Recruiting
Netherlands	NCT01392586	Surgery	2011–2016	516	Terminated
Austria	NCT01015625	Surgery	2010–2019	254	Recruiting

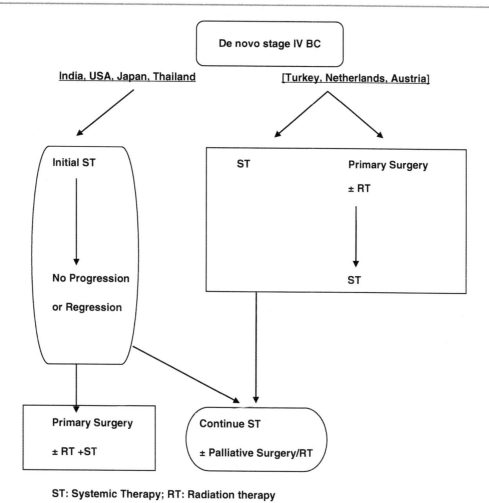

ST: Systemic Therapy; RT: Radiation therapy

Fig. 29.1 Hypothesis testing of the importance of surgery of the primary tumor in de novo. *ST* systemic therapy, *RT* radiation therapy

and/or regional lymph basins) with no locoregional treatment in stage IV BC patients. The protocol differed from the previous trial in that locoregional therapy is performed before initiating ST. All patients receive ST regardless of their study assignment. In the locoregional treatment arm, ST is administered after surgical extirpation of the intact primary tumor, whereas in the no locoregional treatment arm, ST is given immediately after randomization. The hypothesis of this trial is that adequate locoregional treatment of the primary tumor as described above prolongs overall survival compared with no locoregional treatment in stage IV BC patients. Locoregional treatment consists of complete resection of the primary

tumor (either as mastectomy or breast-conserving surgery (BCS)) if axillary nodes are involved and level I–II axillary clearance and RT to the whole breast after BCS. All patients who are clinically node positive undergo standard level I–II axillary clearance. However, in clinically node-negative patients, SLN biopsy is used to assess axillary involvement. Axillary clearance is not required in patients with negative SLN. These patients remain N0. In SLN-positive patients, level I–II axillary clearance is required. All patients who undergo BCS receive RT to the whole breast for 30 days (including 5 days of boost delivery) as indicated for early-stage BC. In the no-locoregional treatment group, primary tumor resection is only allowed when the tumor requires palliation (in conditions such as bleeding, ulceration, and pain). Patients who are assigned to the no-locoregional treatment arm receive ST immediately after randomization, whereas patients who are randomized to the locoregional treatment arm receive ST after their primary tumor is resected. No statistical difference in overall survival was observed at early follow-up. Although longer follow-up is needed to reach a final conclusion, this early analysis demonstrated that LR progression was five times higher in the ST group than in the surgery group (3.6 % vs. 0.7 %, respectively), and potentially important subgroup differences were identified. Trends toward prolonged survival were observed for bone-only metastases, solitary bone metastases, and younger patients (<55) with initial surgery. Patients with aggressive phenotypes appear to derive less benefit from early surgical intervention, and patients with multiple liver and/or pulmonary metastases had a significantly worse prognosis with initial surgery. The overall 30-day mortality rate did not differ between the surgery and ST groups; there were two deaths (1.4 %) in the surgery group and two deaths (1.5 %) in the ST group ($p=0.98$). Mortality was observed in patients with multiple bone metastases ($n=1$), one visceral metastasis without bone metastasis ($n=2$), and multiple visceral metastases ($n=1$) (unpublished data).

Surgery Versus RT

Similar to surgery, the use of radical locoregional therapy (LRT) with surgery or radiation therapy (RT) alone is controversial. To examine the effect of LRT on survival in patients with stage IV BC at diagnosis, Nguyen et al. searched the database to identify women with clinical or pathological M1 BC at diagnosis [41]. They included women in whom the M1 disease was identified at the same time as or within 4 months of the initial diagnosis of primary BC ($n=733$). Women with supraclavicular metastasis but no evidence of distant disease were also excluded from the study. The median follow-up time was 1.9 years, and LRT consisted of surgery alone in 67 % of

patients, RT alone in 22 %, and both surgery and RT in 11 %. ST was administered to 92 % of patients who underwent LRT and 85 % of patients who did not. The 5-year OS rates were 21 % for patients treated with LRT and 14 % for patients treated without LRT ($p<0.001$), and the rates of locoregional progression-free survival were 72 % and 46 %, respectively ($p<0.001$). Multivariable analysis indicated that treatment-related variables associated with improved overall survival were LRT (hazard ratio [HR] 0.78; 95 % confidence interval [CI], 0.64e0.94; $p=0.009$), clear resection margins (HR 0.63; 95 % CI, 0.49 0.81; $p<0.001$), chemotherapy (HR 0.82; 95 % CI, 0.69e0.97; $p=0.02$), and hormone therapy (HR 0.66; 95 % CI, 0.53e0.82; $p<0.001$). The authors concluded that locoregional treatment of primary disease is associated with improved survival in some women with stage IV BC at diagnosis. Among those treated with LRT, the most favorable rates of survival were observed in the subsets with young age and good performance.

In another retrospective study of 581 eligible patients by Le Scodan et al., 320 received LRT, and 261 received no LRT. LRT consisted of exclusive LRR in 249 patients (78 %), surgery of the primary tumor with adjuvant LRR in 41 patients (13 %), and surgery alone in 30 patients (9 %) [42]. At a median follow-up time of 39 months, the 3-year OS rates were 43.4 % and 26.7 % with LRT and without LRT ($p<0.001$), respectively. The association between LRT and improved survival was particularly marked in women with visceral metastases. LRT was an independent prognostic factor in multivariate analysis (hazard ratio [HR]$=0.70$; 95 % CI, 0.58–0.85; $p<0.001$). The adjusted HR for late death (>1 year) was 0.76 (95 % CI, 0.61–0.96; $p=0.02$). The authors concluded that LRT was associated with improved survival in de novo stage IV BC patients and that exclusive LRR may consequently represent an active alternative to surgery.

Although there has been no randomized clinical trial that has evaluated the role of LRT in de novo stage IV BC patients, LRT would be a reasonable alternative approach, particularly in patients with comorbidities for whom surgery may not be indicated.

Uncertainties

As the efficiency of ST increases and local surgery and RT potentially prolong survival, it is unclear how physicians should address issues such as the following:

- Risk and morbidities of surgery and RT
- Quality of life
- Cost
- Reconstruction
- Delay of ST
- Contralateral mastectomy
- Complete response of metastases to ST
- Intervention for metastases

Without a well-designed study covering all of these uncertainties, the physician should address all uncertainties with the patient on a case-by-case basis.

Conclusion

BC outcomes are progressively improving such that BC is beginning to be viewed as a chronic ailment to manage rather than a terminal event and indicating a continually changing role of surgery in the future. The survival advantage of surgery to remove the primary tumor in patients with de novo stage IV BC remains unproven, and ongoing trials must be completed before a conclusion that surgery is either helpful or detrimental to patients with metastatic BC can be reached. Patients with asymptomatic tumors should be informed about ongoing clinical trials. Although more data are needed, the use of primary site local therapy in the two randomized study results demonstrates that primary surgery to remove the tumor provides a local control advantage. If the aim is to control locoregional progression with surgery in this cohort of patients, the patient should have well-controlled distant metastasis and receive ST. In conclusion, there is a need to constantly reevaluate the standards of care to ensure that optimum treatment of BC in all stages is provided.

References

1. Carmichael AR, Anderson EDC, Chetty U, Dixon JM. Does local surgery have a role in the management of stage IV breast cancer? Eur J Surg Oncol. 2003;29:17–9.
2. Gnerlich J, Jeffe DB, Deshpande AD, Beers C, Zander C, Margenthaler JA. Surgical removal of the primary tumor increases overall survival in patients with metastatic breast cancer: analysis of the 1988–2003 SEER data. Ann Surg Oncol. 2007;14:2187–94.
3. Blanchard DK, Bhatia P, Hilsenbeck SG, Elledge RM. Does surgical management of stage IV breast cancer affect outcome? (Abstract 2110). Breast Cancer Res Treat. 2006;100 Suppl 1:S118.
4. WHO international Agency for Reasearch on cancer latest world statistics. 2013. http://www.iarc.fr/en/media-centre/pr/2013/pdfs/pr223_E.pdf.
5. Hortobagyi GN. Treatment of breast cancer. N Eng J Med. 1998;339:974–84.
6. Giordano SH, Buzdar AU, Smith TL, Kau SW, Yang Y, Hortobagyi GN. Is breast cancer survival improving? Cancer. 2004;100(1):44–52.
7. Andre F, Slimane K, Bachelot T, Dunant A, Namer M, Barrelier A, et al. Breast cancer with synchronous metastases: trends in survival during a 14-year period. J Clin Oncol. 2004;22(16):3302–8.
8. Feinstein AR, Sosin DM, Wells CK. The will Rogers phenomenon. Stage migration and new diagnostic techniques as a source of misleading statistics for survival in cancer. N Engl J Med. 1985;312(25):1604–8.
9. Essner R, Lee JH, Wanek LA, Itakura H, Morton DL. Contemporary surgical treatment of advanced-stage melanoma. Arch Surg. 2004;139(9):961–6.
10. Flanigan RC, Salmon SE, Blumenstein BA, Bearman SI, Roy V, McGrath PC, et al. Nephrectomy followed by interferon alfa-2b compared with interferon alfa-2b alone for metastatic renal-cell cancer. N Engl J Med. 2001;345(23):1655–9.
11. Rosen SA, Buell JF, Yoshida A, Kazsuba S, Hurst R, Michelassi F, et al. Initial presentation with stage IV colorectal cancer: how aggressive should we be? Arch Surg. 2000;135(5):530–4.
12. Hallissey MT, Allum WH, Roginski C, Fielding JW. Palliative surgery for gastric cancer. Cancer. 1988;62(2):440–4.
13. Danna EA, Sinha P, Gilbert M, Clements UK, Pulaski BA, Ostrand-Rosenberg S. Surgical removal of primary tumor reverses tumor-induced immunosuppression despite the presence of metastatic disease. Cancer Res. 2004;64:2205–11.
14. Norton L, Massague J. Is cancer a disease of self-seeding? Nat Med. 2006;12(8):875–8.
15. Khan SA. Primary tumor resection in stage IV breast cancer: consistent benefit, or consistent bias? Ann Surg Oncol. 2007;14:3285–7.
16. Retsky M, Demicheli R, Hrushesky W. Premenopausal status accelerates relapse in node positive breast

cancer: hypothesis links angiogenesis, screening controversy. Breast Cancer Res Treat. 2001;65:217–24.

17. Baum M, Chaplain MAJ, Anderson ARA, Douek M, Vaidya JS. Does breast cancer exist in a state of chaos? Eur J Cancer. 1999;35:886–91.

18. O'Reilly MS, Holmgren L, Shing Y, Chen C, Rosenthal RA, Moses M, et al. Angiostatin: a novel angiogenesis inhibitor that mediates the suppression of metastases by a Lewis lung carcinoma. Cell. 1994;79:315–28.

19. Hofer SO, Molema G, Hermens RA, Wanebo HJ, Reichner JS, Hoekstra HJ. The effect of surgical wounding on tumour development. Eur J Surg Oncol. 1999;25:231–43.

20. Naumov GN, MacDonald IC, Weinmeister PM, Kerkvliet N, Nadkarni KV, Wilson SM, et al. Persistence of solitary mammary carcinoma cells in a secondary site: a possible contributor to dormancy. Cancer Res. 2002;62:2162–8.

21. Khan SA, Stewart AK, Morrow M. Does aggressive local therapy improve survival in metastatic breast cancer? Surgery. 2002;132:620–7.

22. Babiera GV, Rao R, Feng L, Meric-Bernstam F, Kuerer HM, Singletary SE, et al. Effect of primary tumor extirpation in breast cancer patients who present with stage IV disease and an intact primary tumor. Ann Surg Oncol. 2006;13:776–82.

23. Rapiti E, Verkooijen HM, Vlastos G, Fioretta G, Neyroud-Caspar I, Sappino AP, et al. Complete excision of primary breast tumor improves survival of patients with metastatic breast cancer at diagnosis. J Clin Oncol. 2006;24:2743–9.

24. Fields RC, Jeffe DB, Trinkaus K, Zhang Q, Arthur C, Aft R, Dietz JR, et al. Surgical resection of the primary tumor is associated with increased long-term survival in patients with stage IV breast cancer after controlling for site of metastasis. Ann Surg Oncol. 2007;14:3345–51.

25. Arriagada R, Rutqvist LE, Mattsson A, Kramar A, Rotstein S. Adequate locoregional treatment for early breast cancer may prevent secondary dissemination. J Clin Oncol. 1995;13(12):2869–78.

26. Hazard HW, Gorla SR, Scholtens D, Kiel K, Gradishar WJ, Khan SA. Surgical resection of the primary tumor, chest wall control, and survival in women with metastatic breast cancer. Cancer. 2008;113(8):2011–9.

27. Nieto Y, Nawaz S, Jones RB, Shpall EJ, Cagnoni PJ, McSweeney PA, et al. Prognostic model for relapse after high-dose chemotherapy with autologous stem-cell transplantation for stage IV oligometastatic breast cancer. J Clin Oncol. 2002;20(3):707–18.

28. Baum M, Demicheli R, Hrushesky W, Retsky M. Does surgery unfavourably perturb the "natural history" of early breast cancer by accelerating the appearance of distant metastases? Eur J Cancer. 2005;41(4):508–15.

29. Coffey JC, Wang JH, Smith MJ, Bouchier-Hayes D, Cotter TG, Redmond HP. Excisional surgery for cancer cure: therapy at a cost. Lancet Oncol. 2003;4(12):760–8.

30. Demicheli R, Valagussa P, Bonadonna G. Does surgery modify growth kinetics of breast cancer micrometastases? Br J Cancer. 2001;85(4):490–2.

31. Cady B, Nathan NR, Michaelson JS, Golshan M, Smith BL. Matched pair analyses of stage IV breast cancer with or without resection of primary breast site. Ann Surg Oncol. 2008;15(12):3384–95.

32. Bafford AC, Burstein HJ, Barkley CR, Smith BL, Lipsitz S, Iglehart JD, et al. Breast surgery in stage IV breast cancer: impact of staging and patient selection on overall survival. Breast Cancer Res Treat. 2009;115(1):7–12.

33. Ruiterkamp J, Ernst MF, van de Poll-Franse LV, Bosscha K, Tjan-Heijnen VC, Voogd AC. Surgical resection of the primary tumour is associated with improved survival in patients with distant metastatic breast cancer at diagnosis. Eur J Surg Oncol. 2009;35(11):1146–51.

34. Harris E, Barry M, Kell MR. Meta-analysis to determine if surgical resection of the primary tumour in the setting of stage IV breast cancer impacts on survival. Ann Surg Oncol. 2013;20:2828–34.

35. Mauri D, Pavlidis N, Ioannidis JP. Neo-adjuvant versus adjuvant systemic treatment in breast cancer: a meta-analysis. J Natl Cancer Inst. 2005;97:188–94.

36. Shien T, Kionoshita T, Shimzu C, Hojo T, Taira N, Doihara H, et al. Primary tumor resection improves the survival of younger patients with metastatic breast cancer. Oncol Rep. 2009;21:827–32.

37. Leung AM, Vu HN, Nguyen KA, Thacker LR, Bear HD. Effects of surgical excision on survival of patients with stage IV breast cancer. J Surg Res. 2010;161:83–8.

38. McGuire KP, Eisen S, Rodriguez A, Meade T, Cox CE, Khakpour N. Factors associated with improved outcome after surgery in metastatic breast cancer patients. Am J Surg. 2009;198:511–5.

39. Badwe RA, Parmar v, Hawaldar R, Nair N, Kaushik R, Siddique S, et al. Surgical removal of primary tumor and axillary lymph nodes in women with metastatic breast cancer at first presentation: A randomized controlled trial. Proceedings of the thirty-sixth annual CTRC-AACR San Antonio Breast Cancer Symposium: 2013 Dec 10-14; San Antonio, TX. Philadelphia (PA): AACR. Cancer Res. 2013;73(24 Suppl):Abstract SABCS13-P4-16-08.

40. Soran A, Ozmen V, Ozbas S, Karanlik H, Muslumanoglu M, Igci A, et al. Early follow up of a randomized trial evaluating resection of the primary breast tumor in women presenting with de novo stage IV breast cancer; Turkish study (protocol MF07-01). Proceedings of the thirty-sixth annual CTRC-AACR San Antonio Breast Cancer Symposium: 2013 Dec 10-14; San Antonio, TX. Philadelphia (PA): AACR. Cancer Res. 2013;73(24 Suppl):Abstract SABCS13-S2-03.

41. Nguyen DHA, Truong PT, Alexander C. Can locoregional treatment of the primary tumor improve outcomes for women with stage IV breast cancer at diagnosis? Int J Radiat Oncol Biol Phys. 2012;84(1):39–45.

42. Le Scoda R, Stevens D, Brain E, Floiras JL, Cohen-Solal C, De La Lande B, et al. Breast cancer with synchronous metastases: survival impact of exclusive locoregional radiotherapy. J Clin Oncol. 2009;27:1375–81.

Neslihan Cabioglu, Enver Özkurt,
and Ayfer Kamali Polat

Abstract

Local recurrence after breast-conservation treatment is most often detected by breast imaging followed by a biopsy for histopathological confirmation. Patients with invasive local recurrence should also undergo a staging workup, mostly by a positron emission tomography-computed tomography (PET-CT), to eliminate the possibility of systemic disease. Although mastectomy is the standard treatment, data are also available regarding a repeat breast-conservation approach with or without reirradiation with accelerated brachytherapy or intraoperative radiotherapy with a potential subsequent increased risk for local recurrence.

Local recurrence after mastectomy as a chest wall recurrence (CWR) is most commonly detected by physical examination and diagnosed by a tissue biopsy for confirmation and for hormone receptor and HER2-neu analysis. A staging workup is necessary to plan the appropriate therapy and is primarily performed by PET-CT. In the absence of distant metastases, CWR should be considered for surgical local excision if the lesion is not fixed to the underlying intercostal bony structures or sternum and if the recurrent lesions are not multiple and diffuse on the chest wall or associated with diffuse skin thickening and erythema requiring neoadjuvant chemotherapy or hormonal therapy. In a patient with an ER/PR-positive HER2-neu (-) local recurrence without distant metastases, adjuvant hormonal therapy followed by surgery for local excision should be primarily

N. Cabioglu, MD, PhD (✉)
Department of General Surgery, Breast Unit,
Istanbul Faculty of Medicine, University of Istanbul,
Istanbul, Turkey
e-mail: neslicab@yahoo.com

E. Özkurt, MD
Department of General Surgery,
Istanbul Medical Faculty, Istanbul University,
Istanbul, Turkey
e-mail: doktorenver@gmail.com

A.K. Polat, MD, FACS
Department of General Surgery,
Ondokuz Mayis University, Samsun, Turkey
e-mail: ayferkp@yahoo.com

© Springer International Publishing Switzerland 2016
A. Aydiner et al. (eds.), *Breast Disease: Management and Therapies*,
DOI 10.1007/978-3-319-26012-9_30

considered. Adjuvant radiotherapy is indicated in patients without prior postmastectomy radiation therapy. CWR in patients with autologous reconstruction should be locally excised without reconstruction or prosthesis removal. Therefore, no standard treatment for patients with CWR is available. Reirradiation for bulky disease may be considered in patients in whom surgery and chemotherapy are not considered. Hyperthermia or photodynamic treatment may also provide alternative therapeutic options for the management of these patients.

A tissue biopsy for diagnosis and hormone receptor and HER2-neu evaluation should be established along with a full metastatic workup. If no distant metastases are noted and the regional recurrence is operable, surgical excision should be considered as the first-line treatment. In hormone receptor (HR)-positive patients, endocrine therapy should be changed or started followed by surgery, whereas chemotherapy should be administered in triple-negative patients followed by surgery. Similarly, anti-HER2-neu therapy with or without chemotherapy and/or endocrine therapy should be considered (e.g., trastuzumab, pertuzumab, lapatinib, TDM-1) in patients with HER2-neu positivity. Therefore, systemic therapies should be personalized to each individual patient.

Keywords

HER2 • True recurrence • New primary • Contrast-enhanced spectral mammography • Uncontrolled local disease • Internal mammary nodes

Introduction

Tumor recurrence can occur in local or regional lymph node areas after the definitive local treatment of breast cancer following either breast-conservation treatment or mastectomy with or without definitive radiation treatment. Local recurrence after breast-conservation treatment may occur in the ipsilateral treated breast, parenchyma, or breast skin. Local recurrence after mastectomy is observed in the ipsilateral chest wall, including the skin. Regional recurrence is defined as the reappearance of cancer involving the local-regional lymph nodes, including mostly ipsilateral axillary or supraclavicular lymph nodes, or less frequently infraclavicular or internal mammary lymph nodes [1]. Local recurrence can be the first manifestation of disease as isolated or solitary recurrence or can occur simultaneously with regional and/or distant metastases.

Local Recurrence After Breast-Conservation Treatment

Contemporary management of early-stage breast cancer decreases the local recurrence rates from 1 % per year to less than 0.5 % per year [2–4]. National Surgical Adjuvant Breast and Bowel Project protocols demonstrated that 37 % of local recurrences were detected in the first 5 years following breast-conservation treatment, whereas the remaining majority of recurrences occur as late recurrence after a 5-year follow-up period [3].

Local recurrences are primarily classified as a true recurrence (TR), which is defined as regrowth of the disease at the tumor bed, and new primary (NP), which is distinct from the index lesion based on histology and location [5–8]. This distinction is commonly made by comparing the characteristics, such as location, pathologic features, and interval to local recurrence, of the initial tumor versus the local recurrence [5–8].

Patients with NP have better clinical outcomes compared with those with TR [5–8]. Distinguishing NP breast carcinomas from TR may be important for the therapeutic management strategies.

Diagnosis

The clinical and radiologic characteristics of recurrent lesions are similar to the initial tumors. Both surgery and radiation treatment may cause some changes, such as a mass-like fibrosis that may be difficult to distinguish clinically or occasionally radiologically from a local recurrence. Any changes noted via physical examination that occur after more than 1–2 years following the completion of radiation treatment must be considered as suspicious. A thorough history along with physical examinations appears to be the most effective method to detect local recurrences [9, 10]. In routine practice, mammography with ultrasound is commonly used for surveillance of the affected breast and to screen the contralateral breast after radiotherapy (Fig. 30.1). A posttreatment mammogram should be obtained 1 year after the initial diagnostic mammogram or 6–12 months after the completion of radiation therapy to establish a new baseline. Posttreatment changes, such as edema, trabecular thickening, and architectural distortion, may remain stable but typically decrease on subsequent annual mammograms. However, any new findings on mammography, such as calcifications, mass, or

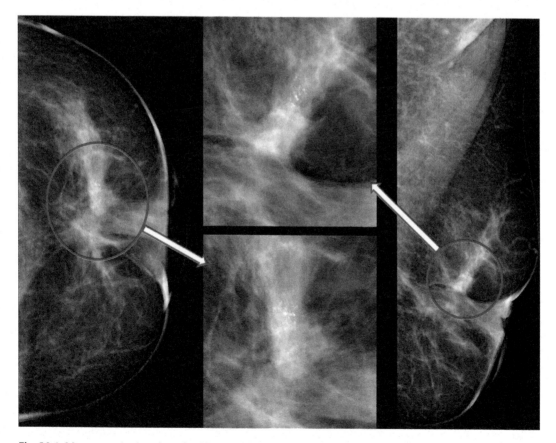

Fig. 30.1 Mammography imaging of a 39-year-old premenopausal patient with a local recurrence 3 years after breast-conservation surgery. *Arrows* show magnified images of a parenchymal distortion together with pleomorphic microcalcifications is noted in the upper-outer quadrant of the left breast. Her biopsy revealed invasive ductal carcinoma that was estrogen receptor and progesterone receptor negative and HER2 positive, which was almost the same as the initial pathology. She received adjuvant chemotherapy, radiotherapy, and trastuzumab for a year after her first operation

increasing architectural distortion, should be evaluated carefully for ipsilateral breast tumor recurrence. In the study by Günhan-Bilgen et al. recurrent tumors were similar in mammographic appearance to primary tumors in 27 (66 %) of 41 cases [11]. Of the 27 primary tumors that initially presented as masses, 19 (70 %) recurred as a mass. Of the six isolated calcifications, five (83 %) recurred as calcifications. Ten (53 %) of the 19 recurrent masses and all 5 recurrent calcifications (100 %) exhibited morphologic features that were similar to those of the primary tumor. In addition, 92 % (11/12) of the recurrences with microcalcifications (isolated or associated with a mass) also contained microcalcifications in the corresponding primary tumor. Seventy-six percent (31/41) of recurrences were located within the lumpectomy quadrant. Furthermore, histologic findings from the primary tumor and the recurrence were identical in 25 (61 %) cases. The majority of recurrent tumors appear to be mammographically similar to primary tumors. Therefore, the researchers concluded that it is important to review preoperative mammograms during follow-up of these patients. In contrast, Weinstein et al. [12] reported that the mammographic appearance of the local recurrence often varied from the appearance of the original breast among 95 patients who developed a recurrence after breast-conservation therapy. The mammographic appearance of the local recurrence often varied from the appearance of the original breast cancer.

Breast sonography is an essential imaging technique that is complementary to mammography in our routine practice to characterize suspicious mammographic findings and identify palpable masses as cystic or solid. Screening sonography has been used to detect mammographically and clinically occult cancers with a higher sensitivity in dense breasts [13]. The role of sonography in addition to mammography in screening has been investigated in the American College of Radiology Imaging Network (ACRIN) trial (protocol 6666) [14]. The study included high-risk patients with dense breast tissue on mammography and sought to determine the detection rate of nonpalpable, mammographically

occult breast cancers identified solely by sonography. From April 2004 to February 2006, 2,809 women, with heterogeneously dense breast tissue, were recruited to undergo mammographic and ultrasonographic examinations. Forty patients (41 breasts) were diagnosed with breast cancer: 8 suspicious on both ultrasound and mammography, 12 on ultrasound alone, 12 on mammography alone, and 8 patients (9 breasts) on neither. The diagnostic yield for mammography was 7.6 per 1,000 women screened (20 of 2,637) and increased to 11.8 per 1,000 (31 of 2,637) for combined mammography plus ultrasound. The diagnostic accuracy for mammography was 0.78 (95 % CI, 0.67–0.87), whereas adding of a single screening ultrasound to mammography increased the accuracy to 0.91 (95 % CI, 0.84–0.96). Of 12 cancers detected by ultrasound alone, 11 (92 %) were invasive cancers with a median size of 10 mm (range, 5–40 mm). The authors concluded that adding a single screening ultrasound to mammography will yield an additional 1.1–7.2 cancers per 1,000 high-risk women.

As another imaging modality, magnetic resonance imaging (MRI) dynamically evaluates the morphology and vascularity of breast lesions after intravenous contrast enhancement. The enhancement pattern on contrast-enhanced MRI is effective in distinguishing posttreatment scars from recurrent cancer in patients with breast-conservation therapy [15]. However, according to the American Cancer Society guidelines, the data are insufficient to recommend routine MRI screening for women after breast-conservation treatment [16].

In the last decade, digital mammography has replaced conventional mammography in many centers due to its enhanced accuracy in dense breasts. Digital breast tomosynthesis (DBT) is also a novel breast imaging tool that is used in three-dimensional planes. Finally, contrast-enhanced spectral mammography (CESM) has been recently introduced as a new breast imaging technique [16, 17]. This technique has been compared with MRI regarding the detection and size estimation of histologically proven breast cancers. Recent studies have demonstrated the enhanced sensitivity of CESM and MRI in breast cancer detection compared with conventional mammography. In addition, contrast-enhanced spectral mammography has promise because it offers comparable results to MRI in the detection of malignant breast lesions [17, 18]. Future studies are needed to determine the role of these new technologies in improving the sensitivity of mammography in distinguishing posttreatment changes from recurrent cancers in patients after breast-conservation treatment.

Management

Various previous studies have demonstrated concurrent distant metastases and/or locally extensive recurrences or regional nodal recurrences in 5–10 % of patients presenting with local recurrences [19–23]. Therefore, staging should be performed, preferably by PET-CT, for patients diagnosed with locally recurrent disease to exclude patients with distant metastases before making decisions regarding the management of these patients. Other studies have demonstrated that local recurrences and distant metastases are independent events that occur at different times [24]. Veronesi et al. evaluated the incidence and associated factors related to local and distant recurrences in patients with BCT ($n=2,233$) at the Milan Cancer Institute from 1970 to 1987. In total, 119 local recurrences, 32 new ipsilateral carcinomas, and 414 distant metastases were detected as first events. The annual probability for local failures was approximately 1 % up to the tenth year. For distant metastases, the annual probability was 5 % in the second year and decreased progressively until the eighth year. In local failure patients, the 5-year overall survival rate was 69 %. Patients with local recurrences exhibited increased risk of distant metastases. In particular, women 35 years old or younger at first diagnosis who had initial peritumoral lymphatic invasion and local recurrence within 2 years are at high risk for distant spread and should be considered candidates for aggressive systemic treatment.

In the study of Shen et al. 120 women who developed isolated IBTR after BCT for stage 0–III breast carcinoma between 1971 and 1996

at the MD Anderson Cancer Center were investigated to identify factors associated with systemic recurrence [25]. At a median follow-up of 80 months after IBTR, 45 patients (37.5 %) exhibited systemic recurrence. Initial lymph node status ($P=0.001$), lymphovascular invasion (LVI) in the primary tumor, time to IBTR ≤48 months, clinical and pathologic IBTR tumor size >1 cm, LVI in the recurrent tumor, and skin involvement at IBTR were identified as significant predictors of systemic recurrence. In a multivariate logistic regression analysis, initial positive lymph node status (relative risk [RR], 5.3; 95 % confidence interval [95 % CI], 1.4–20.1; $P=0.015$) and skin involvement at IBTR (RR, 15.1; 95 % CI, 1.5–153.8; $P=0.022$) remained independent predictors of systemic recurrence. Patients who initially had lymph node-positive disease, skin involvement, or LVI at IBTR represented especially high-risk groups that warranted consideration for aggressive, systemic treatment and novel, targeted therapies after IBTR. In their multicentric study in Japan, Komoike et al. also reported that IBTR significantly correlated with subsequent distant metastases (hazard ratio, 3.93; 95 % CI, 2.676–5.771; $P<0.0001$) [26]. Among the patients who developed IBTR, initial lymph node metastases and a short interval to IBTR were significant risk factors for subsequent distant metastasis. Similar findings were obtained in the study of Doyle et al. which included 93 patients with an invasive local recurrence after BCT. In addition, the interval from diagnosis to local recurrence was predictive of overall survival (OS) at 5 years (≤2 years, 65 % vs. 2.1–5 years, 84 % vs. >5 years, 89 %; $P=0.03$) [27]. However, whether IBTR is an indicator or a cause of subsequent distant metastases remains unclear.

Furthermore, uncontrolled local disease (ULD) following breast conservation is defined as the appearance of clinically manifested invasive cancer in the remaining breast or on the ipsilateral chest wall that could not be eradicated within 3 months of detection [28]. In a cohort of 5,502 patients treated for stage I–II invasive breast cancer with breast-conservation surgery (BCS) from 1976 to 1998 in Stockholm, 307 patients with subsequent IBTR were identified.

At a median follow-up time of 11 years, 50 of 307 patients developed ULD, whereas the 5-year cumulative incidence of ULD following IBTR was 13 %. In multivariate logistic regression analyses, nonsurgical treatment of IBTR, the presence of concurrent distant metastasis with IBTR, initial axillary lymph node metastases, <3 years between breast conservation and IBTR, and no adjuvant endocrine therapy were significant predictors of ULD. Moreover, 88 % of the patients were treated with salvage mastectomy ($n = 207$) or re-excision ($n = 62$). The 5-year cumulative incidence of ULD following salvage mastectomy and salvage re-excision was 10 % and 16 %, respectively, compared with 32 % among patients who were treated nonsurgically. Following IBTR, the 5-year overall survival among patients with local control was 78 % in contrast with 21 % among patients with ULD. Therefore, the authors concluded that patients with IBTR independent of concurrent distant metastases should be recommended for salvage surgery when feasible because it provides superior local control compared with salvage systemic therapy alone.

Mastectomy

The standard treatment for ipsilateral breast tumor recurrence after breast-conservation therapy is mastectomy with/without axillary staging depending on the initial axillary staging procedure [19–23]. Local recurrences have been detected in 3–22 % in patients treated with mastectomy after IBTR [28–30]. Beard et al. investigated the clinical outcome after mastectomy in patients with IBTR ($n = 59$) using a database of 2,101 breast cancer patients with BCT, including Tis (24 %) [29]. IBTR lesions were classified as Tis (20 %), T1 (46 %), T2 (25 %), or T3 (9 %). At a median follow-up of 4.6 years, 13 patients (22 %) developed postmastectomy recurrence (PMR) associated with decreased OS ($P = 0.002$). PMR was more common with larger IBTR tumors ($P = 0.03$), specifically IBTR ≥ T2 ($P = 0.003$). In addition, 85 % of PMR occurred within 2 years of mastectomy. Therefore, patients

with IBTR tumors >2 cm should be considered for adjuvant local and systemic therapies, especially during the first 24 months.

After salvage surgery, the 5- and 10-year disease-specific survival rates after IBTR were 78 % and 67–68 %, respectively, and the 5- and 10-year overall survival rates were 69–89 % and 39–64 %, respectively (Table 30.1) [24, 25, 30–33]. Furthermore, the 5- and 10-year systemic recurrence-free survival rates after IBTR were 61 % and 36–55 %, respectively [25]. Voogd et al. reported the long-term prognosis of 266 patients with isolated IBTR at a median follow-up of 11.2 years [33]. The 10-year OS rate for the 226 patients with invasive local recurrence was 39 % (95 % CI, 32–46). The distant recurrence-free survival rate was 36 % (95 % CI, 29–42), and the local control rate (i.e., survival without subsequent local recurrence or local progression) was 68 % (95 % CI, 62–75). Patients with a local recurrence measuring 1 cm or less exhibited enhanced distant disease-free survival compared with those with larger recurrences, suggesting that early detection of local recurrence can improve the clinical outcome of these patients. Finally, Botteri et al. from the European Institute of Oncology reviewed 282 patients presented with an operable invasive IBTR after BCS between 1997 and 2004 [34]. Of these patients, 161 (57 %) underwent a second conservative surgery, whereas 121 patients (43 %) underwent mastectomy. Recurrences of the mastectomy group were T2–T4 and/or multifocal in 83 cases (68.6 %). With a median follow-up of 5 years after mastectomy, 5-year OS and disease-free survival (DFS) were 73.3 % [95 % CI 65.0–81.6 %] and 50.4 % (95 % CI 40.9–59.8 %), respectively. Based on multivariate analyses, early onset of IBTR, presence of vascular invasion, and Ki67 ≥20 of the recurrent tumor significantly affected both DFS and OS as poor prognostic factors.

Limited data are available for patients with BRCA1/2 mutations who develop local recurrence after BCT. In the study of Turner et al., 8 (15 %) of 52 breast cancer patients with deleterious BRCA mutations had IBTR [37]. The median time to IBTR for patients with BRCA1/2 mutations was

Table 30.1 Outcome of patients detected with IBTR after BCT who were treated by salvage mastectomy or a second breast conservative surgery

Study	Median follow-up	N	5-year DFS	5-year OS	10-year OS	5-year DSS	10-year DSS
Veronesi et al. [24]	nr	119	nr	69 %	nr	nr	nr
Shen et al. [25]	80 months (range, 0.3–331 months)	120	nr	nr	nr	78 %	68 %
Kurtz et al. [30]	nr	178	nr	89 %[a]	nr	nr	nr
Le et al. [31]	138 ± 66 months	105	nr	76 %	56 %	nr	nr
Galpar et al. [32]	85 months	341	nr	81 %	nr	nr	nr
Voogd et al. [33]	134 months (11.2 years)	226	nr	nr	39 %	nr	nr
Botteri et al. [34]	60 months	121	50.4 %	73.3 %	nr	nr	nr
Fodor et al. [35]	165 months (range, 75–240 months)	16[b]	nr	nr	81 %	nr	nr
Albert et al. [36]	166 months (13.8 years)	116	nr	nr	66.7 %	nr	nr

IBTR ipsilateral breast tumor recurrence, *BCT* breast-conservation therapy, *DFS* disease-free survival, *OS* overall survival, *DSS* disease-specific survival, *nr* not reported
[a]Including patients with wide local excision
[b]Patients with ≤2 cm in-breast recurrence

7.8 years compared with 4.7 years for patients without BRCA1/2 mutations (*P* = 0.03). All patients with BRCA1/2 mutations and IBTR underwent successful surgical salvage mastectomy at the time of IBTR and remain alive without evidence of local or systemic progression of disease. However, more studies with larger patient populations are needed to conclude whether local recurrence is not associated with poor prognosis in these patients. Furthermore, in patients with an IBTR in an irradiated breast, mastectomy with a myocutaneous flap reconstruction (i.e., latissimus dorsi flap, transverse rectus abdominis muscle) is the preferred method of reconstruction with improved cosmetic results and lower complication rates compared with implant reconstructions.

Breast-Conservation Therapy

As an alternative to salvage mastectomy, a second conservative treatment has been proposed, namely, either lumpectomy alone or associated with reirradiation of the tumor bed. Between 1983 and 1987, 56 patients developed an isolated local recurrence (ILR) in the chest wall after primary surgery for mastectomy (*n* = 894), and 68 developed an ILR after primary surgery for BCT

(*n* = 415) [35]. The 10-year actuarial rate of cause-specific survival after treatment for ILR is 52 %. On multivariate analysis, operability of recurrence (operable vs. inoperable, relative risk [RR]: 5.9), age at initial diagnosis (>40 vs. ≤40 years, RR: 2.2), and time to ILR (>24 vs. ≤24 months, RR: 2) were identified as independent prognostic factors for OS after ILR. In the conservative surgery (CS) group, the type of salvage surgery (mastectomy vs. repeat complete excision) had no significant impact on survival (*P* = 0.2). The majority (*n* = 44) of CS patients developed ≤2 cm in-breast recurrence, and the 10-year cause-specific survival was 81 % after both salvage excision (*n* = 28) and mastectomy (*n* = 16), suggesting that patients with ≤2 cm in-breast recurrence potentially may undergo a second BCS.

Similarly, Gentilini et al. from the European Institute of Oncology studied 161 patients with invasive IBTR who underwent a second BCS to identify the subset of patients with the best local control [38]. The median follow-up after IBTR was 81 months. The 5-year overall survival after IBTR was 84 % (95 % CI 78–89). The 5-year cumulative incidence of a second local event after IBTR was 29 % (95 % CI 22–37). In the multivariate analysis, IBTR size >2 cm and time to relapse ≤48 months significantly increased the risk of local reappearance (hazard ratio [HR] 3.3, 95 % CI 1.6–7.0; and HR 1.9, 95 % CI 1.1–3.5). The 5-year cumulative incidence of a further local reappearance of the tumor after repeating BCS was 15.2 % in patients with IBTR ≤2 cm. In addition, patients with time to IBTR >48 months were identified as the best candidates for a second BCS, whereas patients with IBTR >2 cm and time to relapse ≤48 months exhibited a 71.2 % 5-year local recurrence rate ($P < 0.001$), indicating that these patients should be considered for a mastectomy after IBTR.

Furthermore, Albert et al. at Yale-New Haven Hospital compared outcomes of salvage mastectomy (SM) and salvage breast-conservation surgery (SBCS) to determine the feasibility of SBCS [36]. Of 2,038 patients treated with BCT, 166 developed IBTR. Patients were considered for SBCS if the recurrence was localized on mammogram and physical examination, was <3 cm pathologic tumor size, was confined to the biopsy site, did not exhibit skin or lymphovascular invasion, and was associated with ≤3 positive nodes. Of the 146 patients who were definitively managed by IBTR, surgery involved SM ($n = 116$) or SBCS ($n = 30$). At a median follow-up time of 13.8 years after IBTR, OS after IBTR was 64.5 % at 10 years, with no significant difference noted between SM (65.7 %) and SBCS (58.0 %). Only two patients in the SBCS cohort subsequently had a second IBTR and were salvaged with mas-

tectomy. Although mastectomy is considered the standard surgical salvage of IBTR, SBCS is feasible, and the prognostic factors are related to favorable tumor biology and early detection (Table 30.2).

Ishitobi et al. further investigated the risk factors associated with local control in patients ($n = 78$) who were treated with repeat lumpectomy after IBTR [40]. At a median follow-up period of 40 months, the 5-year second IBTR-free survival rate was 78.8 %. Multivariate analysis revealed that the ER status of IBTR was a significant independent predictive factor for second IBTR-free survival ($P = 0.0177$). Ishitobi et al. investigated the impact of breast cancer subtype on prognosis after IBTR in 185 patients in another study [41]. A significant difference in distant disease-free survival (DDFS) after IBTR was noted according to breast cancer subtype defined by a Ki67 index cutoff of 20 % ($P = 0.0074$, log-rank test). The 5-year DDFS rates for patients with luminal A, luminal B, triple-negative, and HER2 types were 86.3, 57.1, 56.6, and 65.9 %, respectively.

A PubMed literature review was performed by Hannoun-Levi et al. to assess four different strategies of local treatment options: (a) salvage mastectomy alone, (b) salvage mastectomy with postoperative reirradiation, (c) a second CT with surgery alone, and (d) a second CT with reirradiation [42]. Although the 5-year OS rates after salvage mastectomy and the second CT appeared

Table 30.2 Outcome of patients detected with IBTR after BCT who were treated by a second breast conservative surgery

Study	Median follow-up (months)	N	5-year DFS	10-year DFS	5-year OS	10-year OS
Fodor et al. [35]	165 months (range, 75–240 months)	28[a]	nr	nr	nr	81 %
Gentilini et al. [38]	81 months	161	nr	nr	84 %	nr
Albert et al. [36]	166 months (13.8 years)	30	nr	nr	nr	58 %
Hannoun-Levy et al. [39]	47 months (range, 13–124 months)	217[b]	84.6 %	77.2 %	88.7	76.4

IBTR ipsilateral breast tumor recurrence, *BCT* breast-conservation therapy, *DFS* disease-free survival, *OS* overall survival, *DSS* disease-specific survival, *nr* not reported

[a]Patients with ≤2 cm in-breast recurrence

[b]Patients received partial breast irradiation for IBTR by multicatheter brachytherapy after a repeat breast-conservation surgery

be equivalent ($\approx$75 %), the rate of second local recurrence was approximately 10 % [3–32 %], approximately 25 % [7–36 %], and approximately 10 % [2–26 %], after salvage mastectomy, salvage lumpectomy alone, or salvage lumpectomy in combination with a reirradiation of the tumor bed, respectively. Sedlmayer et al. similarly evaluated the outcome after partial breast reirradiation for IBTR following second BCT by surveying the literature between 2002 and 2012 (PubMed) [43]. Local treatment modalities included partial breast radiotherapy by external beam radiotherapy (EBRT); interstitial brachytherapy (BT) in a low-, high-, and pulse-dose rate technique; combined EBRT/BT; and intraoperative radiotherapy (IORT). The majority of the 310 patients (82 %) were treated by brachytherapy. The selection criteria for a second breast-conservation procedure included T0–T2 recurrent lesions, late onset after primary treatment, and no evidence of metastatic disease before undergoing gross tumor resection with free surgical margins. Treatment doses were similar to those for brachytherapy (LDR 30–55 Gy, HDR 30–34 Gy, PDR 40–50 Gy) and biologically comparable to the only series that exclusively used EBRT (50 Gy). At a follow-up time of 49 months, the oncologic results were similar among the different methods, with local control rates ranging between 76 % and 100 %, and the disease-free and overall survival rates were comparable to the mastectomy series. The GEC-ESTRO working group presented a collaborative analysis on 217 patients at the 35th San Antonio Breast Cancer Meeting treated between 2000 and 2009 in 8 European institutions by brachytherapy (LDR, PDR, and/or HDR) [39]. With a median follow-up of 3.9 year (1.1–10.3) after IBTR retreatment, 5- and 10-year actuarial second local recurrence rates were 5.6 % and 7.2 %, respectively. In comparison to those series with salvage mastectomy series, the outcome of patients with a repeat breast conservative surgery treated by brachytherapy was found to be similar with 5- and 10-year actuarial rates for metastatic recurrence of 9.6 % and 19.1 %, DFS of 84.6 % and 77.2 %, and OS of 88.7 % and 76.4 %, respectively. Acute toxicity was low in

all studies, and major late effects included fibrosis in reirradiated parenchyma as a function of dose and volume, asymmetry (primarily due to double surgery), and breast pain. The cosmetic outcome was satisfactory, with scoring results from excellent to good in 60–80 % of patients. In a highly selected group of patients with IBTR, partial breast irradiation with brachytherapy after second BCS could be safely performed as an alternative to mastectomy to potentially increase breast-conservation rates. Although published data about brachytherapy are more extensive [44–52], there is relatively little information about the oncological safety of other modalities, including PBI via EBRT or novel strategies, such as IORT [53]. All of these studies suggest that repeat BCS may represent a safe and feasible treatment method for isolated ipsilateral breast tumor recurrence in selected patients (Table 30.2).

Limited data about the efficacy of intraoperative radiotherapy in the treatment of IBTR in the previously irradiated breast are available. Trombetta et al. reported their long-term experience with balloon brachytherapy for retreatment of the breast after IBTR [53]. Between 2004 and 2012, 18 patients who had been previously treated with external beam radiotherapy were retreated with the MammoSite (Hologic Corporation, Marlborough, MA), MammoSite ML (Hologic Corporation), or the Contura (Bard Peripheral Vascular, Inc., Tempe, AZ) brachytherapy devices. Sixteen patients were treated for an ipsilateral breast tumor recurrence after breast-conservation surgery and postoperative irradiation (11 of these patients had infiltrating ductal carcinoma [IDC]). The recurrent histology of seven patients was IDC, whereas seven additional patients recurred as DCIS, three recurred as a combination of IDC/DCIS, and one recurred as infiltrating lobular carcinoma. All patients received a twice-daily tumor dose of 3,400 cGy at 340 cGy per fraction. With a mean follow-up of 39.6 months, only two patients developed local recurrence. Both patients were treated locally by salvage mastectomy. The use of balloon brachytherapy devices in the treatment of the previously irradiated breast is feasible and may provide adequate local control in carefully selected patients. However, further studies with larger patient populations are needed for more definitive results. Furthermore, other novel techniques, including radiofrequency (RF) ablation, to treat local recurrence of breast cancer were investigated in various pilot trials; the results indicated insufficient efficacy for recommendations of routine use [54].

Surgical Management of the Axilla

Limited information regarding regional lymphatic recurrence (RLR) after salvage mastectomy or re-excision for IBTR without axillary surgery is available. Therefore, 102 patients who underwent salvage breast surgery without local treatment for the regional lymphatic basin (surgery or radiotherapy) for IBTR after BCT for primary breast cancer were studied [55]. Of these patients, nine (8.8 %) had RLR with a median follow-up period of 3.7 years after breast surgery for IBTR. ER negativity and the presence of lymphovascular invasion of the recurrent breast tumor were significant predictive factors of RLR ($P = 0.04$ and 0.02, respectively). These results suggest that axillary surgery should be performed to determine nodal involvement during salvage surgery for IBTR and provide local-regional control, especially in patients with aggressive ER (-) recurrent cancers or cancers with lymphovascular invasion. Therefore, the feasibility and the clinical impact of performing a second sentinel lymph node biopsy (SLNB) in patients with locally recurrent breast cancer were investigated in two European studies: the "Sentinel Node and Recurrent Breast Cancer (SNARB)" study and a study by Intra et al. from the European Institute of Oncology [56, 57]. A total of 150 patients with locally recurrent breast cancer were subject to lymphatic mapping with SLNB using a dual technique with blue dye and ^{99m}Tc-colloidal albumin. For validation, the surgeons were advised to perform axillary lymph node dissection (ALND) in cases with an intact axillary nodal basin. A total of 41 patients previ-

ously underwent BCT with SLNB. In addition, 82 patients underwent BCT with ALND, and 9 patients were subject to mastectomy with SLNB. Twelve patients underwent mastectomy with ALND. Of these patients, 50 (33 %) had a previous SLNB, 94 (63 %) had a previous ALND, and 6 (4 %) had no axillary surgery. A sentinel lymph node was detected in 95 patients (63.3 %) by preoperative lymphoscintigraphy, and a SLNB was successfully performed in 78 patients (52 %). As expected, extra-axillary lymphatic drainage was observed in 58.9 % of the patients; an increased likelihood of this condition was noted after a previous ALND (79.3 %) compared with a previous SNB (25.0 %) ($P < 0.0001$) by lymphoscintigraphy. In pathologic examination, 18 patients (22.8 %) exhibited a (micro)metastasis, whereas an additional 18 patients had no axillary lymph node metastases. Overall, performing a second SLNB altered the adjuvant treatment plan in 16.5 % of the patients with a successful second SNB. These results suggest that although the detection rates are not satisfactorily high, a SLNB is feasible in approximately half of the patients with a previous axillary surgery as an axillary staging procedure and provides useful information for adjuvant treatment in one of six patients.

A similar study was conducted by Intra et al. in 212 patients with IBTR who were previously treated with BCT, had a negative SLNB, and subsequently underwent salvage breast surgery and a second SLNB from 2001–2011 [57]. Preoperative lymphoscintigraphy demonstrated at least one new axillary sentinel lymph node in 207 patients (97.7 %), whereas no drainage was observed in 5 patients (2.3 %). A SLNB by removal of one or more lymph nodes was accomplished in 196 of 207 patients (95 %). Extra-axillary drainage pathways were identified via lymphoscintigraphy in 17 patients (8 %). At a median follow-up period of 48 months, the 5-year axillary recurrence rate was 3.9 %. All these studies demonstrate that a second SLNB is feasible, accurate, and oncologically safe for selected patients with IBTR who previously underwent a BCT with a negative SLNB finding.

Chest Wall Recurrence After Mastectomy

Chest wall recurrence (CWR) after mastectomy has been noted in up to one-third of cases [58]. In a pooled analysis of randomized trials, Jatoi et al. found that BCS was associated with greater odds of local-regional recurrence (LRR) than mastectomy (pooled odds ratio (OR), 1.56; 95 % CI 1.29–1.89). Moreover, LRR still occurred in 8.5 % of mastectomy patients [59]. LRR after mastectomy tends to occur earlier than in-breast recurrences after breast-conservation treatment [60]. Local recurrences appear in up to 90 % of patients 5 years after mastectomy, with a median interval to LRR of approximately 3 years [61, 62]. However, local recurrences have been reported even decades after the primary surgery. These late recurrences may be NP tumors rather than TRs of the prior cancer. CWR rates of up to 40 % have been reported, depending on the initial treatment and primary tumor characteristics [63]. Even with the addition of adjuvant systemic therapy, CWR remains a significant issue in a considerable proportion of patients.

Prevention

The addition of postmastectomy radiation therapy (PMRT) may reduce the rate of CWR by up to 70 % [64]. Although the British Columbia [65] and Denmark studies [66, 67] were criticized for a variety of reasons, the American Society of Clinical Oncology [68] and the American Society of Therapeutic Radiology and Oncology [69] have both issued guidelines recommending PMRT in patients with four or more positive lymph nodes or with tumors larger than 5 cm. PMRT is not recommended for node-negative patients with tumors smaller than 5 cm, and it remains controversial in the one to three positive-node group. A study of the Early Breast Cancer Trialists' Collaborative Group (EBCTCG) revealed that a 20 % reduction in 5-year local recurrence risk resulted in a 5 % absolute reduction in 15-year breast cancer mortality, thus prompting more widespread use of PMRT in these patients [64].

In a recent meta-analysis by EBCTCG to determine the efficacy of postmastectomy radiotherapy, 8,135 women randomly were assigned to treatment groups from 1964 to 1986 in 22 trials of radiotherapy to the chest wall and regional lymph nodes after mastectomy and axillary surgery versus the same surgery without radiotherapy [70]. Radiotherapy included the chest wall, supraclavicular or axillary fossa (or both), and internal mammary chain. At a follow-up of 10 years for patients with a negative axilla ($n = 700$), radiotherapy showed no significant effect on local-regional recurrence (two-sided significance level [2p] > 0.1), overall recurrence (RR, irradiated vs. not, 1.06, 95 % CI 0.76–1.48, 2p > 0.1), or breast cancer mortality (RR 1.18, 95 % CI 0.89–1.55, 2p > 0.1). However, in patients with one to three positive nodes and ALND ($n = 1,314$), radiotherapy reduced local-regional recurrence (2p < 0.00001), overall recurrence (RR 0.68, 95 % CI 0.57–0.82, 2p = 0.00006), and breast cancer mortality (RR 0.80, 95 % CI 0.67–0.95, 2p = 0.01). As expected, for patients with four or more positive nodes and ALND ($n = 1,772$), radiotherapy also reduced local-regional recurrence (2p < 0.00001), overall recurrence (RR 0.79, 95 % CI 0.69–0.90, 2p = 0.0003), and breast cancer mortality (RR 0.87, 95 % CI 0.77–0.99, 2p = 0.04). The ongoing Medical Research Council (MRC) Selective Use of Postoperative Radiotherapy After Mastectomy (SUPREMO) trial will also provide important information about this important question, and biological markers of tumor aggressiveness and radiosensitivity may be identified that can then help tailor future therapy [71].

Diagnosis

CWR is defined as a breast cancer recurrence in the skin, subcutaneous tissue, nipple-areola complex, muscle, or underlying bone after mastectomy, and this condition requires a high index of suspicion upon physical examination (Fig. 30.2). Regional recurrences occur in the nodal tissue draining the primary tumor, including the supra- and infraclavicular (55 %), axillary (28 %), internal mammary

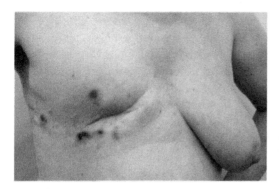

Fig. 30.2 A 58-year-old postmenopausal patient presents with multiple local chest wall recurrences 8 years after modified radical mastectomy. The patient did not receive systemic chemotherapy and chest wall irradiation after her primary surgery. She does not exhibit any nodal involvement or distant metastasis in any of the imaging modalities at the time of chest wall recurrence

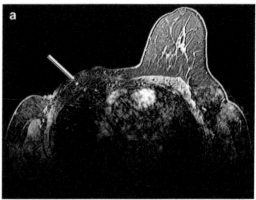
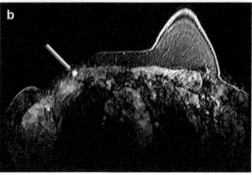

Fig. 30.3 MRI images showing recurrences within the pectoralis major muscle in two different foci (*arrows*) (**a**, **b**) of a 51-year-old postmenopausal patient who underwent MRM 1 year ago with a diagnosis of triple-negative, T4 invasive ductal carcinoma

(2 %), and multiple (15 %) lymph node basins [72]. Numerous CWRs occur within 2–3 years after mastectomy. CWRs have been identified more than 10 years later in a significant number of cases. Therefore, careful surveillance of the chest wall is required after mastectomy. Patients presenting with LRR after mastectomy typically exhibit aggressive progression. Metastatic stage IV disease occurs in almost 33 % of these patients at the time of LRR. Some CWR present as large fungating masses, whereas most are subtle, often presenting with an asymptomatic nodule in the skin or a slight erythematous rash. Over 50 % of all CWR present as a solitary nodule in the skin; the remainder presents as multiple nodules or diffuse disease on the chest wall [73]. Therefore, physical examination is the most important step for early detection of CWR.

Radiologic imaging after the initial treatment using mastectomy rarely demonstrates recurrences that were not suspected clinically. Therefore, routine imaging of the mastectomy site is not recommended. In a group of 827 postmastectomy patients with or without reconstruction, Fajardo et al. [74] found that mammography demonstrated recurrences that were previously clinically suspected based on physical examination findings. Similarly, Propeck and Scanlan [75] studied a group of 185 postmastectomy patients and concluded that routine imaging of this population was not helpful in detecting recurrent disease. However, the contralateral breast should be imaged in the routine fashion. Further workup of the patient, including MRI, thorax CT, bone scintigraphy, PET-CT, and other modalities, may be needed if metastases are suspected (Fig. 30.3).

In 23–70 % of cases, the recurrence appears on the previous mastectomy scar [76–78] (Fig. 30.2a), and CWRs may be mistaken for fat necrosis, radiation-induced injury, or foreign body granuloma [79]. In these cases, histologic confirmation is required and can be obtained with a punch biopsy. The estrogen-receptor status of the primary tumor and that of the subsequent recurrence are the same in approximately 75–85 % of patients.

Prognostic Factors

CWR may be accompanied by the presence of distant metastases in up to 30 % of patients [79]. Numerous factors are associated with improved prognosis in these patients, and a variety of prognostic tools are available to assist clinicians in predicting survival in these patients [76, 80, 81]. The MD Anderson Cancer Center reported that initial node-negative status, time to CWR greater than 24 months, and treatment with radiation therapy for the isolated CWR are independent predictors of improved disease-free and overall survival [82]. Patients with all three favorable features have a median overall survival of 141 months (10-year actuarial survival: 75.4 %). Those with one or two favorable features exhibited a median overall survival of 54 months (10-year actuarial survival: 25.1 %), and those without any favorable features had a median overall survival of 16 months (10-year actuarial survival: 0 %) [81]. These data suggest that patients presenting with CWR are a heterogeneous population, and aggressive management using a multidisciplinary approach is needed for patients anticipating a good prognosis. Haffty et al. [82] reported that positive HER-2/neu status was associated with an increased rate of local-regional disease progression compared with negative HER-2/neu (41 % vs. 8 %, respectively; $P=0.007$) [82].

Fodor et al. found that patients who developed a CWR greater than 24 months from their initial mastectomy and who were initially node negative exhibited enhanced 10-year disease-specific survival [83]. They also found that the prognosis was improved if the recurrence was a single operable lesion in the scar. Subsequent local or regional recurrence after salvage treatment occurs in 25–35 % of treated patients, typically within 5 years of salvage treatment [60].

Surgical Therapy

Surgical resection of CWR is an important issue in the management of patients with CWR because it provides excellent local control in patients with resectable disease. Surgery is particularly useful in patients who have previously undergone radiation therapy or those in whom radiation therapy is inadvisable.

Resection of the CWR is often straightforward for patients with isolated recurrences involving only the skin or the surgical scar. Resection with primary closure is generally favorable and provides excellent local control. Although high response rates are noted with the use of radiation therapy alone for CWR, 60–70 % of patients experience a second failure; thus, surgical resection must be considered for any patient with localized, recurrent disease [83–87]. With more extensive disease, reconstructive procedures, such as coverage with either a skin graft or autologous flap, may be needed [83–87]. The goal of resection should be maintaining a clear margin. Although there is no consensus on what constitutes a "clear margin," wide resection is generally recommended.

Dahlstrom et al. [83] reported 69 patients who underwent wide local excision for local recurrences, and the 5-year actuarial local control rate was 50 % with a 5-year overall survival of 62 %. Pameijer et al. reviewed their experience with full-thickness chest wall resection for CWR of breast cancer ($n=22$) and conducted a meta-analysis to determine patient characteristics and outcomes between 1970 and 2000 [84]. The 5-year DFS was 67 % at City of Hope National Medical Center (COH) and 45 % for the entire group of 400 patients. The 5-year OS was 71 % for the COH group and 45 % for the entire group. Patients with a disease-free interval longer than 24 months exhibited the best prognosis in most studies. In another study by Friedel et al. chest wall resection with a myocutaneous flap was performed in 63 women (mean age, 58 years) with CWR between 1985 and 2006 [85]. The cumulative 5-, 10-, and 15-year OS rates were 46 %, 29 %, and 22 %, respectively, with a median survival of 56 months, whereas mortality was 1.6 %, and morbidity was 25 %.

Local-regional chest wall recurrences with involvement of the ribs and/or sternum after primary breast cancer surgery are associated with a poor outcome. The oncological benefit of extensive CWR, including the ribs and sternum, remains controversial regarding its morbidity. However, various studies have demonstrated good long-term prognosis with full-thickness resections in selected patients. Of 76 patients with isolated sternal or full-thickness chest wall (SCW) recurrences, 44 were treated surgically, and 32 were treated nonsurgically between 1992 and 2011 [86]. No difference in 5-year OS was observed between patients treated with surgery and those who were not (30.6 and 49.6 %, respectively; P=0.52). Patients who were selected for surgery had more advanced and biologically aggressive disease and were more likely to have triple-negative breast cancer at recurrence (52 vs. 17 %; P=0.006). Complications related to radical surgical resection occurred in 25 % of patients. For hormone receptor-positive recurrence, the 5-year progression-free survival was significantly increased among surgical patients (46.3 vs. 14.5 %; P=0.01). Similarly, prognostic factors predicting survival after chest wall resection and reconstruction (CWRR) were investigated in 28 patients at the H. Lee Moffitt Cancer Center between 1999 and 2007 [87]. The postoperative morbidity and mortality rates were 21 % and 0 %, respectively, and the 5-year OS rate was 18 %. The 1-, 2-, and 5-year OS rates for the triple-negative phenotype were 38 %, 23 %, and 0 %, respectively. In contrast, the 1-, 2-, and 5-year OS rates for the non-triple-negative phenotype were 100 %, 70 %, and 39 %, respectively. These findings suggest that patients with isolated SCW recurrence and hormone receptor-positive recurrence are associated with improved survival, whereas the clinical outcome is poor in patients with triple-negative recurrent cancers.

With increased use of skin-sparing mastectomy and nipple-sparing mastectomy (total skin-sparing mastectomy) with immediate reconstruction, various concerns regarding the incidence, detection, and management of CWR have been noted. Evidence does not suggest any difference in local recurrence rates following skin-sparing or nipple-sparing versus conventional mastectomy in terms of the incidence of CWR [88–94]. Furthermore, the incidence of CWR does not vary with the type of reconstruction [88]. Langstein et al. demonstrated that most CWRs following skin-sparing mastectomy with reconstruction occur under the skin (72 %) and are easily palpable on clinical examination [88]. Although the length of time between mastectomy and identifying CWR may be slightly longer in patients with reconstruction, the prognosis between these patients and those who develop a CWR after a conventional mastectomy does not significantly differ [95]. The management of CWR in patients with a reconstructed breast does not necessarily mandate a takedown of the reconstruction [95, 96].

In patients experiencing recurrence at the reconstruction site, such as latissimus flap reconstruction or rectus abdominis musculocutaneous (TRAM), the CWR can often be resected with local flap rearrangement to preserve the breast mound. In patients with implant-based reconstruction, however, removal of the implant is often warranted to facilitate subsequent radiation therapy.

Little information regarding the feasibility and potential clinical benefit of lymph node evaluation in CWR patients is available. Axillary surgery is often required to obtain local control. Sentinel node biopsy is feasible in the setting of recurrent breast cancer [56, 57], and some researchers are also investigating the feasibility of sentinel node biopsy following mastectomy [97].

Radiation Therapy

When treating CWR, radiation therapy is an independent factor leading to improved prognosis [81]. In general, large-field radiotherapy encompassing the entire chest wall is preferable to less extensive radiation. Approximately 93 % of recurrences are controlled within 2 months of the completion of radiotherapy [98]. In a study of 224 patients with CWR, Halverson et al. found that the 5- and 10-year disease-free survival rates of patients treated with large-field radiation were 75 % and 63 %, respectively, compared with 36 % and 18 %, respectively, when smaller fields were used [99]. Subsequent supraclavicular metastases were also significantly reduced with the use of radiation therapy (16 % vs. 6 % without radiation therapy). For recurrences that were completely excised, good local control could be achieved with doses ranging from 4,500 to 7,000 cGy.[99] Recurrences 1–3 cm in diameter were best controlled with a dose of at least 6,000 cGy. However, larger tumors exhibited worse local control (50 %) despite the use of 7,000-cGy doses.

Hastings et al. studied risk factors for LRR after mastectomy in over 1,259 T1 N0 breast cancer patients and identified a small subgroup of patients with grade three disease and a close or positive margin (≤3 mm) who exhibit an increased risk of LRR. These authors concluded that these patients may benefit from the administration of PMRT [100].

In terms of the value of reirradiation, data were previously limited for patients who had previously been treated with radiation therapy to the chest wall. A recent multi-institutional study of reirradiation in the setting of CWR reviewed 81 patients who presented with a local recurrence after a median dose of 60 Gy [101]. Thirty-one of these patients originally had a mastectomy with PMRT and subsequently presented with a CWR. This study found that a second course of radiation at the time of the local recurrence (median: 48 Gy) was not associated with significant grade 3–4 toxicity and was associated with a 57 % overall complete response rate. Factors correlating with an improved 1-year disease-free survival included greater dose of radiation therapy at the time of recurrence, a longer interval from initial radiation therapy, and the use of concurrent chemotherapy.

Other Treatment Modalities

Hyperthermia involves heating the tumor bed to a temperature of 40–45° along with delivery of radiation. Hyperthermia in conjunction with radiation therapy has been evaluated by a number of studies. Although no significant difference was noted in terms of complete response rates between radiation therapy alone and radiation combined with hyperthermia in four studies, two other trials reported a benefit regarding the addition of hyperthermia [79]. A meta-analysis revealed a benefit for hyperthermia with a complete response rate of 59 % versus 41 % in patients treated with radiation therapy alone (OR, 2.3; 95 % Cl, 1.4–3.8; $P=0.007$) [102]. This benefit was particularly noted in those who had undergone previous radiation therapy and was maintained in follow-up. In another prospective randomized controlled trial of hyperthermia and radiation therapy for superficial tumors in 99 of 109 patients, 70 of whom had CWRs, the complete response rate for hyperthermia and radiation was 66 % versus 42 % for radiation therapy alone. Again, previously irradiated patients exhibited the greatest benefit (68.2 % vs. 23.5 %, respectively).

Other modalities used in the treatment of CWR include photodynamic therapy and intra-arterial chemotherapy [79]. However, both of these modalities result in transient responses. A few studies demonstrated that injection of interferon into the recurrent tumor (with or without concomitant radiation therapy) yields reasonable results [79]. When surgical excision of CWR is not possible, topical chemotherapy and electrochemotherapy might also provide a safe, efficient, and noninvasive local-regional treatment approach for CWRs [103, 104]. Electrochemotherapy can be performed either with cisplatin injected intratumorally or via the intratumorally or intravenously administration of bleomycin [103]. Furthermore, novel modalities, including cryotherapy, radiofrequency ablation, laser, and microwave therapy, might be investigated in future studies regarding the management of CWR.

Regional Lymph Node Recurrence

Regional nodal recurrence (RNR) or regional events are defined as breast cancer in ipsilateral lymph nodes based on Maastricht Delphi consensus on event definitions for the classification of recurrence in breast cancer research [105]. The incidence of isolated RNR is generally low (<4 %)

[2, 106]. This condition generally presents as an asymptomatic mass, but specific symptoms are occasionally evident in a minority of patients [107]. MRI may be helpful in this setting [108].

With the increasing use of PET/CT imaging, many RNR are nonpalpable axillary, supraclavicular, infraclavicular, and internal mammary lymph nodes (Fig. 30.4). Although nodal recurrence generally exhibits a poorer prognosis than local recurrence, it remains curable if adequately resected. Nonpalpable masses must be localized either preoperatively with a radioactive seed or a wire guide. These masses can also be localized intraoperatively with ultrasound.

RNR generally have poor prognosis, and the risk of distant metastasis is high (>50 %). Supraclavicular, internal mammary, or multiple sites of nodal disease are correlated with a worse overall prognosis than isolated axillary recurrences [109].

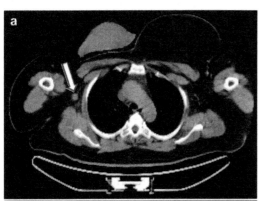

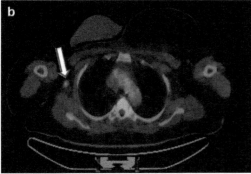

Fig. 30.4 CT and PET fusion imaging (**a, b**) of a 45-year-old woman with an isolated axillary nodal recurrence (*arrows*) 3 years after mastectomy with a negative SLNB. PET-CT modality revealed an increased uptake value of F-18 fluorodeoxyglucose (SUV max: 16.2)

Axillary Nodal Recurrences

In one study, axillary recurrence was observed in 1.2 % (2/162) of positive-sentinel node patients and 0.8 % (5/625) of negative-sentinel node patients [110]. The management of axillary recurrences is typically limited by the extent of disease and the previous therapies that the patient received. Complete level I–II axillary dissection is warranted if a patient had an axillary regional recurrence after SLNB. In patients who undergo ALND with or without axillary radiation, redissection is generally not a technically viable option, but axillary exploration and resection of gross disease may be considered for small, mobile, isolated recurrences. The sentinel node can be identified in approximately 87 % of cases when ten or less lymph nodes were removed during the original surgery in the reoperative setting [111]. Repeat surgical assessment of the axilla may provide prognostic information that is useful in guiding management decisions for recurrences. Given the altered drainage patterns in these patients, particularly in those patients with ten or more lymph nodes removed, clinicians should utilize a preoperative lymphoscintigram when considering repeat surgical axillary assessment [112]. In a recent study, repeat sentinel node biopsy was performed in greater than 150 patients with locally recurrent breast cancer. Aberrant drainage pathways were visualized in 58.9 % of the patients, and this result was significantly more frequently observed after a previous ALND (79.3 %) compared with a previous SNB (25.0 %) (*P* < 0.0001). Overall, the result of their repeat SNB led to a change in the adjuvant treatment plan in 16.5 % of the patients with a successful repeat SNB. These authors conclude that repeat SNB is technically feasible and provides reliable results in patients with locally recurrent breast cancer, leading to change in management in one of six patients [56].

Technological advancements in the delivery of radiation, such as the use of intraoperative electron beam therapy, have facilitated promising preliminary investigations of reirradiation of the axilla [113]. Nevertheless, this technique warrants further investigation prior to its routine use in patients with RNR.

Supraclavicular Nodal Recurrences

The majority of supraclavicular nodal recurrences are associated with a poor prognosis. In addition, the overall survival and outcomes of regional relapses in the supraclavicular fossa are worse compared with those in the axilla [114]. In a large series of supraclavicular recurrences involving 305 patients with an isolated supraclavicular recurrence with or without other local-regional metastases but no distant metastases, additional sites of synchronous local-regional disease were present in 38 % of the patients. In addition, 19 % underwent excisional biopsy of the tumor, 33 % had curative radiation, 26 % had combined local-regional treatment and systemic therapy, and only 10 % underwent surgery plus radiation. Combined local-regional and systemic therapy resulted in the highest rate of initial remission (67 %) compared with either local-regional therapy alone (64 %) or systemic therapy alone (40 %), but the 5-year progression-free and overall survival rates were only 15 % and 24 % percent, respectively. In addition, the only significant predictor of favorable outcomes on multivariate analysis was the receipt of combined local-regional and systemic therapy [115]. In some retrospective series, patients with isolated supraclavicular recurrences have long-term disease-free survival rates ranging from 15 % to 30 % with the utilization of multimodality therapies [116]. Another more recent study by Kong M and Hong SE involving N1 breast cancer patients ($n = 113$) reported 5- and 10-year actuarial supraclavicular lymph node recurrence rates of 9.3 % and 11.2 %, respectively [117]. Factors associated with supraclavicular lymph node recurrence based on multivariate analysis revealed that the patient group with grade 3 and extracapsular extension exhibited a significantly increased rate of supraclavicular lymph node recurrence compared with the remainders (5-year SCLR rate; 71.4 % vs. 4.0 %, respectively, $P < 0.001$). Thus, the researchers mentioned that supraclavicular nodal RT is necessary in N1 breast cancer patients featuring histologic grade 3 and extracapsular extension [117]. Therefore, patients with isolated supraclavicular recurrences without distant metastases should be considered for curative multimodality therapy whenever possible.

Regional reirradiation with therapeutic doses is generally not considered safe if a patient had an isolated nodal recurrence in a previously irradiated field. In this case, limited field reirradiation may be considered as a salvage option in patients who are unresponsive to systemic treatment or those with unresectable disease. Particularly for supraclavicular and axillary recurrences, the utilization of standard external beam techniques results in doses to the normal structures that are well beyond threshold (i.e., brachial plexus).

Internal Mammary Nodal Recurrences

The increased proportion of screening-detected cancers, improved imaging, and techniques (i.e., lymphoscintigraphy for radio-guided SLNB) make it possible to visualize lymphatic drainage to the internal mammary nodes (IMNs). IMN drainage is noted in approximately 18–30 % of breast cancer patients [118, 119]. Although IMNs act as a secondary lymph node drainage basin for breast cancer, nodal recurrence in the IMN chain is rare. This condition is typically not intentionally treated after definitive surgery in most breast cancer patients. In a PET/CT study by Oh et al., 3,561 PET/CT scans were performed in 1,906 postoperative breast cancer patients. Fifty-seven patients (2.99 %) demonstrated isolated extra-axillary nodal recurrences ($n = 85$) on PET/CT (28 IMN recurrences, 24 supraclavicular, 4 infraclavicular, 8 interpectoral, 12 cervical, and 9 mediastinal) [120]. With IMN recurrence rates <2 % after definitive treatment [121], data regarding the effects of surgical resection, systemic therapy, and/or radiation therapy in this setting are limited. One of the largest series of IMN recurrences in breast cancer describes 133 patients with IMN failure after definitive treatment. The 5-year overall survival rate of patients with IMN recurrences was approximately 30 %, whereas the rate for those with isolated IMN recurrence was generally increased (approximately 45 %) [122]. Endocrine therapy for ER/PR+ patients (HR 0.2, 95 % CI, 0.1–0.5; $P=0.001$), radiotherapy delivered to the IMN area after recurrence (HR 0.3, 95 % CI, 0.1–0.9; $P=0.026$), and no concurrent distant metastases (HR 0.7, 95 % CI, 0.4–0.9; $P=0.031$) were significantly correlated with improved disease-free survival rates after IMN recurrence on multivariate analysis. Although surgical resection of an isolated IMN recurrence has been described utilizing various techniques and appears to be associated with a low mortality rate, the surgery itself is typically very extensive in some cases, requiring en bloc resection of the recurrence, surrounding chest wall, ribs, sternum, and previously radiated areas, and often requires reconstruction of the chest wall defect [123]. Recently, a less invasive technique for treating IMN recurrence using a thoracoscopic approaches was described [124]. For patients who have not previously received radiation to the IMN region, the mainstay of treatment for recurrences is radiation therapy, typically with doses of 40–60 Gy.

Systemic Therapy for Local-Regional Recurrence

Local recurrences after mastectomy or BCT or local-regional recurrences are frequently accompanied by distant metastases, so systemic therapy is generally part of the multidisciplinary management of these patients. Although local control is generally the aim of surgery and radiation therapy, various studies have reported a trend toward improved survival using systemic chemotherapy after adequate resection of local recurrence after mastectomy and radiation therapy [77]. The use of hormonal therapy is also associated with an improved prognosis in patients with an estrogen-receptor-positive CWR [97]. Borner et al. reported a significant reduction in second local failures at 5 years in a multicenter trial in which estrogen-receptor-positive patients with isolated CWR were randomized to tamoxifen or placebo after complete local excision and radiation therapy [125]. Overall

survival, however, was not significantly altered [125]. Given the potential usefulness of hormonal therapy and because the estrogen-receptor status is the same as the original tumor in only 75–85 % of cases, the hormone receptor status of the CWR should be ascertained.

As recently published, the CALOR trial is a randomized trial that investigated the efficacy of adjuvant chemotherapy in patients with completely excised isolated local-regional recurrences (ILRR) with negative margins after a mastectomy or lumpectomy for a primary breast cancer [126]. Eligible patients were randomized (1:1) to chemotherapy (type selected by the investigator; multidrug for at least four courses recommended) or no chemotherapy. Patients with ER-positive ILRR received adjuvant endocrine therapy. Radiation therapy was mandated for patients with microscopically involved surgical margins, and anti-HER2 therapy was optional. From Aug 22, 2003, to Jan 31, 2010, 85 patients were randomly assigned to receive chemotherapy, and 77 were assigned to no chemotherapy. At a median follow-up of 4·9 years, the 5-year disease-free survival was 69 % (95 % CI 56–79) with chemotherapy versus 57 % [44–67] without chemotherapy (hazard ratio 0.59 [95 % CI 0.35–0.99]; $P=0.046$). Adjuvant chemotherapy was significantly more effective for women with ER-negative ILRR (p interaction $=0.046$). In conclusion, adjuvant chemotherapy should be recommended for breast cancer patients with completely resected ILRR, especially if the recurrence is ER negative.

The ongoing Breast International Group (BIG) 1-02, the International Breast Cancer Study Group (IBCSG) 27-02, and the National Surgical Adjuvant Breast and Bowel Project (NSABP) B-37 Study (BIG 1-02/IBCSG 27-02/NSABP B-37 are investigating whether cytotoxic chemotherapy is needed in patients with a resected CWR [127]. In this trial, 977 patients with locally recurrent breast cancer will be randomized to receive chemotherapy or no chemotherapy along with radiation therapy, trastuzumab, and hormonal therapy. This study will also hopefully answer the question of whether these patients will benefit from cytotoxic chemotherapy.

In HR-positive patients, endocrine therapy should be changed or started following surgery, whereas chemotherapy with or without anti-HER2-neu therapy (e.g., trastuzumab and pertuzumab, lapatinib, TDM-1) should be considered in HER2-neu-positive or triple-negative patients followed by surgery. Therefore, systemic therapies should be personalized to the individual patient.

Conclusion

Local-regional recurrences following BCT or mastectomy are challenging clinical problems that require a multidisciplinary approach. Although LRRs are considered as a poor prognostic factor and some of these patients will be diagnosed with concurrent systemic disease, patients with LRRs constitute a heterogeneous population. Patients who develop their LRRs more than 2 years from their previous surgery for mastectomy or BCT and were originally node negative exhibit long-term survival, particularly if they can be treated with aggressively with surgery, radiation, and systemic therapy. By understanding the molecular biology of LRRs and developing personalized tailored approaches to systemic therapies along with emerging newer biological agents, systemic therapies for LRRs will also evolve. Finally, the potential utility of genomic expression tests in estimating the benefit of chemotherapeutic agents might also provide useful information for tailoring both local and systemic therapies [128]. Further study is needed to delineate the optimal management of these patients.

References

1. Solin LJ, Harris EER, Weinstein SP, DeMichele A, Tchou J. Local-regional recurrence after breast-conservation treatment or mastectomy. In: Harris JR, Lipmann ME, Morrow M, Osborne CK, editors. Diseases of the breast. 4th ed. Philadelphia: Lippincott Williams & Wilkins; 2010. p. 840–55.
2. Fisher B, Jeong JH, Anderson S, Bryant J, Fisher ER, Wolmark N. Twenty-five year follow-up of a randomized trial comparing radical mastectomy total mastectomy followed by irradiation. N Engl J Med. 2002;347:567–75.
3. Anderson SJ, Wapnir I, Dignam JJ, Fisher B, Mamounas EP, Jeong JH, et al. Prognosis after ipsilateral breast tumor recurrence and locoregional recurrences in patients treated by breast-conserving therapy in five National Surgical Adjuvant Breast and Bowel Project protocols of node-negative breast cancer. J Clin Oncol. 2009;27:2466–73.
4. Cabioglu N, Hunt KK, Buchholz TA, Mirza N, Singletary SE, Kuerer HM, Babiera GV, Ames FC, Sahin AA, Meric-Bernstam F. Improving local control with breast-conserving therapy: a 27-year single-institution experience. Cancer. 2005;104:20–9.
5. Hwang E, Buchholz TA, Meric-Bernstam F, Krisnamurthy S, Mirza NQ, et al. Classifying local disease recurrences after breast conservation therapy based on location and histology. Cancer. 2002;95:2059–67.
6. Komoike Y, Akiyama F, Iino Y, Ikeda T, Tanaka-Akashi S, Ohsumi S. Analysis of ipsilateral breast tumor recurrences after breast-conserving treatment based on the classification of true recurrences and new primary tumors. Breast Cancer. 2005;12:104–11.
7. Panet-Raymond V, Truong PT, McDonald RE, Alexander C, Ross L, Ryhorchuk A, Watson PH. True recurrence versus new primary: an analysis of ipsilateral breast tumor recurrences after breast-conserving therapy. Int J Radiat Oncol Biol Phys. 2011;81:409–17.
8. Yi M, Buchholz TA, Meric-Bernstam F, Bedrosian I, Hwang RF, Ross MI, et al. Classification of ipsilateral breast tumor recurrences after breast conservation therapy can predict patient prognosis and facilitate treatment planning. Ann Surg. 2011;253:572–9.
9. Pivot X, Asmar L, Hortobagyi GN, Theriault R, Pastorini F, Buzdar A. A retrospective study of first indicators of breast cancer recurrence. Oncology. 2000;58:185–90.
10. Aebi S, Wapnir I. Management of locoregional recurrence. In: Winchester DJ, Winchester DP, Hudis CA, Norton L, eds. Breast Cancer, 2nd ed. BC Decker Inc.: Hamilton, Ontario. 2006; p. 511–523.
11. Günhan-Bilgen I, Oktay A. Mammographic features of local recurrence after conservative surgery and radiation therapy: comparison with that of the primary tumor. Acta Radiol. 2007;48:390–7.
12. Weinstein SP, Orel SG, Pinnamaneni P, Tchou J, Czerniecki B, Boraas M, et al. Mammographic appearance of recurrent breast cancer after breast conservation therapy. Acad Radiol. 2008;15:240–4.
13. Leconte I, Feger C, Galant C, Berlière M, Berg BV, D'Hoore W, et al. Mammography and subsequent whole-breast sonography of nonpalpable breast cancers: the importance of radiologic breast density. AJR Am J Roentgenol. 2003;180:1675–9.
14. Berg WA, Blume JD, Cormack JB, Mendelson EB, Lehrer D, Böhm-Vélez M, ACRIN 6666 Investigators, et al. Combined screening with ultrasound and mammography vs mammography alone

in women at elevated risk of breast cancer. JAMA. 2008;299:2151–63.

15. Preda L, Villa G, Rizzo S, Bazzi L, Origgi D, Cassano E, et al. Magnetic resonance mammography in the evaluation of recurrence at the prior lumpectomy site after conservative surgery and radiotherapy. Breast Cancer Res. 2006;8:R53.

16. Saslow D, Boetes C, Burke W, Harms S, Leach MO, Lehman CD, American Cancer Society Breast Cancer Advisory Group, et al. American Cancer Society guidelines for breast screening with MR1 as an adjunct to mammography. CA Cancer J Clin. 2007;57:75–89.

17. Fallenberg EM, Dromain C, Diekmann F, Engelken F, Krohn M, Singh JM, et al. Contrast-enhanced spectral mammography versus MRI: initial results in the detection of breast cancer and assessment of tumour size. Eur Radiol. 2014;24:256–64.

18. Łuczyńska E, Heinze-Paluchowska S, Hendrick E, Dyczek S, Ryś J, Herman K, et al. Comparison between breast MRI and contrast-enhanced spectral mammography. Med Sci Monit. 2015;21:1358–67.

19. Leung S, Otmezguine Y, Calitchi E, Mazeron JJ, Le Bourgeois JP, Pierquin B. Locoregional recurrences following radical external beam irradiation and interstitial implantation for operable breast cancer – a twenty three year experience. Radiother Oncol. 1986;5:1–10.

20. Dalberg K, Mattsson A, Sandelin K, Rutqvist LE, et al. Outcome of treatment for ipsilateral breast tumor recurrence in early-stage breast cancer. Breast Cancer Res Treat. 1998;49:69–78.

21. Fowble B, Solin L, Schultz D, Rubenstein J, Goodman RL. Breast recurrence following conservative surgery and radiation: patterns of failure, prognosis, and pathologic findings from mastectomy specimens with implications for treatment. Int J Radiat Oncol Biol Phys. 1990;19:833–42.

22. Haffty BG, Fischer D, Beinfield M, McKhann C. Prognosis following local recurrence in the conservatively treated breast cancer patient. Int J Radiat Oncol Biol Phys. 1991;21:293–8.

23. Recht A, Schnitt SJ, Connolly JL, Rose MA, Silver B, Come S, et al. Prognosis following local or regional recurrence after conservative surgery and radiotherapy for early stage breast carcinoma. Int J Radiat Oncol Biol Phys. 1989;16:3–9.

24. Veronesi U, Marubini E, Del Vecchio M, Manzari A, Andreola S, Greco M, et al. Local recurrences and distant metastases after conservative breast cancer treatments: partly independent events. J Natl Cancer Inst. 1995;87:19–27.

25. Shen J, Hunt KK, Mirza NQ, Buchholz TA, Babiera GV, Kuerer HM, Bedrosian I, Ross MI, Ames FC, Feig BW, Singletary SE, Cristofanilli M, Meric-Bernstam F. Predictors of systemic recurrence and disease-specific survival after ipsilateral breast tumor recurrence. Cancer. 2005;104:479–90.

26. Komoike Y, Akiyama F, Iino Y, Ikeda T, Akashi-Tanaka S, Ohsumi S, et al. Ipsilateral breast tumor recurrence (IBTR) after breast-conserving treatment for early breast cancer: risk factors and impact on distant metastases. Cancer. 2006;106:35–41.

27. Doyle T, Schultz DJ, Peters C, Harris E, Solin LJ, et al. Long-term results of local recurrence after breast conservation treatment for invasive breast cancer. Int J Radiat Oncol Biol Phys. 2001;51:74–80.

28. Dalberg K, Liedberg A, Johansson U, Rutqvist LE. Uncontrolled local disease after salvage treatment for ipsilateral breast tumour recurrence. Eur J Surg Oncol. 2003;29:143–54.

29. Beard HR, Cantrell EF, Russell GB, Howard-McNatt M, Shen P, Levine EA. Outcome after mastectomy for ipsilateral breast tumor recurrence after breast conserving surgery. Am Surg. 2010;76:829–34.

30. Kurtz JM, Spitalier J-M, Amalric R, Brandone H, Ayme Y, Jacquemier J, et al. The prognostic significance of late local recurrence after breast-conserving therapy. Int J Radiat Oncol Biol Phys. 1990;18:87–93.

31. Le MG, Arriagada R, Spielmann M, Guinebretière JM, Rochard F. Prognostic factors for death after an isolated local recurrence in patients with early-stage breast carcinoma. Cancer. 2002;94:2813–20.

32. Galper S, Blood E, Gelman R, Abner A, Recht A, Kohli A, et al. Prognosis after local recurrence after conservative surgery and radiation for early-stage breast cancer. Int J Radiat Oncol Biol Phys. 2005;61:348–57.

33. Voogd AC, van Oost FJ, Rutgers EJT, Elkhuizen PH, van Geel AN, Scheijmans LJ, et al. Long-term prognosis of patients with local recurrence after conservative surgery and radiotherapy for early breast cancer. Eur J Cancer. 2005;41:2637–44.

34. Botteri E, Rotmensz N, Sangalli C, Toesca A, Peradze N, De Oliveira Filho HR, et al. Unavoidable mastectomy for ipsilateral breast tumour recurrence after conservative surgery: patient outcome. Ann Oncol. 2009;20:1008–12.

35. Fodor J, Major T, Polgar C, Orosz Z, Sulyok Z, Kásler M. Prognosis of patients with local recurrence after mastectomy or conservative surgery for early-stage invasive breast cancer. Breast. 2008; I7:302–8.

36. Alpert TE, Kuerer HM, Arthur DW, Lannin DR, Haffty BG. Ipsilateral breast tumor recurrence after breast conservation therapy: outcomes of salvage mastectomy vs. salvage breast-conserving surgery and prognostic factors for salvage breast preservation. Int J Radiat Oncol Biol Phys. 2005;63:845–51.

37. Turner BC, Harrold E, Matloff E, Smith T, Gumbs AA, Beinfield M, et al. BRCA1/BRCA2 germline mutations in locally recurrent breast cancer patients after lumpectomy and radiation therapy: implications for breast-conserving management in patients with BRCA1/BRCA2 mutations. J Clin Oncol. 1999;17:3017–24.

38. Gentilini O, Botteri E, Veronesi P, Sangalli C, Del Castillo A, Ballardini B, et al. Repeating conservative surgery after ipsilateral breast tumor reappear-

ance: criteria for selecting the best candidates. Ann Surg Oncol. 2012;19:3771–6.

39. Hannoun-Levy JM, Resch A, Gal J, Kauer-Dorner D, Strnad V, Niehoff P, et al. Second conservative treatment for ipsilateral breast tumor recurrence: GEC-ESTRO Breast WG study. Cancer Res. 2012;72(24 Suppl). Abstract No. P4-15-01.

40. Ishitobi M, Komoike Y, Nakahara S, Motomura K, Koyama H, Inaji H. Repeat lumpectomy for ipsilateral breast tumor recurrence after breast-conserving treatment. Oncology. 2011;81:381–6.

41. Ishitobi M, Okumura Y, Arima N, Yoshida A, Nakatsukasa K, Iwase T, et al. Breast cancer subtype and distant recurrence after ipsilateral breast tumor recurrence. Ann Surg Oncol. 2013;20:1886–92.

42. Hannoun-Levi JM, Ihrai T, Courdi A. Local treatment options for ipsilateral breast tumour recurrence. Cancer Treat Rev. 2013;39:737–41.

43. Sedlmayer F, Zehentmayr F, Fastner G. Partial breast re-irradiation for local recurrence of breast carcinoma: benefit and long term side effects. Breast. 2013;22 Suppl 2:S141–6.

44. Adkison JB, Kuske RR, Patel RR. Breast conserving surgery and accelerated partial breast irradiation after prior breast radiation therapy. Am J Clin Oncol. 2010;33:427–31.

45. Trombetta M, Julian TB, Werts ED, Colonias A, Betler J, Kotinsley K, Kim Y, Parda D. Comparison of conservative management techniques in the retreatment of ipsilateral breast tumor recurrence. Brachytherapy. 2011;10:74–80.

46. Hannoun-Levi JM, Castelli J, Plesu A, Courdi A, Raoust I, Lallement M, Flipo B, Ettore F, Chapelier C, Follana P, Ferrero JM, Figl A. Second conservative treatment for ipsilateral breast cancer recurrence using high-dose rate interstitial brachytherapy: preliminary clinical results and evaluation of patient satisfaction. Brachytherapy. 2011;10:171–7.

47. Chadha M, Feldman S, Boolbol S, Wang L, Harrison LB. The feasibility of a second lumpectomy and breast brachytherapy for localized cancer in a breast previously treated with lumpectomy and radiation therapy for breast cancer. Brachytherapy. 2008;7:22–8.

48. Hannoun-Levi JM, Houvenaeghel G, Ellis S, Teissier E, Alzieu C, Lallement M, Cowen D. Partial breast irradiation as second conservative treatment for local breast cancer recurrence. Int J Radiat Oncol Biol Phys. 2004;60:1385–92.

49. Hannoun-Levi JM, Resch A, Gal J, Kauer-Dorner D, Strnad V, Niehoff P, GEC-ESTRO Breast Cancer Working Group, et al. Accelerated partial breast irradiation with interstitial brachytherapy as second conservative treatment for ipsilateral breast tumour recurrence: multicentric study of the GEC-ESTRO Breast Cancer Working Group. Radiother Oncol. 2013;108:226–31.

50. Shah C, Wilkinson JB, Jawad M, Wobb J, Berry S, Mitchell C, et al. Outcome after ipsilateral breast tumor recurrence in patients with early-stage breast cancer treated with accelerated partial breast irradiation. Clin Breast Cancer. 2012;12:392–7.

51. Kauer-Dorner D, Pötter R, Resch A, Handl-Zeller L, Kirchheiner K, Meyer-Schell K, et al. Partial breast irradiation for locally recurrent breast cancer within a second breast conserving treatment: alternative to mastectomy? Results from a prospective trial. Radiother Oncol. 2012;102:96–101.

52. Burger AE, Pain SJ, Peley G. Treatment of recurrent breast cancer following breast conserving surgery. Breast J. 2013;19:310–8.

53. Trombetta M, Hall M, Julian TB. Long-term followup of breast preservation by re-excision and balloon brachytherapy after ipsilateral breast tumor recurrence. Brachytherapy. 2014;13:488–92.

54. Garbay JR, Mathieu MC, Lamuraglia M, Lassau N, Balleyguier C, Rouzier R. Radiofrequency thermal ablation of breast cancer local recurrence: a phase II clinical trial. Ann Surg Oncol. 2008; 15:3222–6.

55. Ishitobi M, Matsushita A, Nakayama T, Motomura K, Koyama H, Tamaki Y. Regional lymphatic recurrence after salvage surgery for ipsilateral breast tumor recurrence of breast cancer without local treatment for regional lymphatic basin. J Surg Oncol. 2014;110:265–9.

56. Maaskant-Braat AJ, Roumen RM, Voogd AC, Pijpers R, Luiten EJ, Rutgers EJ, et al. Sentinel Node and Recurrent Breast Cancer (SNARB): results of a nationwide registration study. Ann Surg Oncol. 2013;20:620–6.

57. Intra M, Viale G, Vila J, Grana CM, Toesca A, Gentilini O, et al. Second axillary sentinel lymph node biopsy for breast tumor recurrence: experience of the European Institute of Oncology. Ann Surg Oncol. 2015;22:2372–7.

58. Chagpar AB. Management of local recurrence after mastectomy. In: Kuerer HM, editor. Kuerer's breast surgical oncology. The McGraw-Hill Company, Inc.; NY, USA. 2010; p. 731–6.

59. Jatoi I, Proschan MA. Randomized trials of breast-conserving therapy versus mastectomy for primary breast cancer: a pooled analysis of updated results. Am J Clin Oncol. 2005;28:289–94.

60. van Tienhoven G, Voogd AC, Peterse JL, Nielsen M, Andersen KW, Mignolet F, et al. Prognosis after treatment for loco-regional recurrence after mastectomy or breast conserving therapy in two randomised trials (EORTC 10801 and DBCG-82TM). EORTC Breast Cancer Cooperative Group and the Danish Breast Cancer Cooperative Group. Eur J Cancer. 1999;35:32–8.

61. Janni W, Dimpfl T, Braun S, Knobbe A, Peschers U, Rjosk D, et al. Radiotherapy of the chest wall following mastectomy for early-stage breast cancer: impact on local recurrence and overall survival. Int J Radiat Oncol Biol Phys. 2000;48:967–75.

62. Tennvall-Nittby L, Tenegrup I, Landberg T. The total incidence of loco-regional recurrence in a randomized trial of breast cancer TNM stage II: the

South Sweden Breast Cancer Trial. Acta Oncol. 1993;32:641–6.

63. Chagpar A, Kuerer HM, Hunt KK, Strom EA, Buchholz TA. Outcome of treatment for breast cancer patients with chest wall recurrence according to initial stage: implications for post-mastectomy radiation therapy. Int J Radiat Oncol Biol Phys. 2003;57:128–35.

64. Clarke M, Collins R, Darby S, Davies C, Elphinstone P, Evans E, et al. Effects of radiotherapy and of differences in the extent of surgery for early breast cancer on local recurrence and 15-year survival: an overview of the randomised trials. Lancet. 2005;366:2087–106.

65. Ragaz J, Jackson SM, Le N, Plenderleith IH, Spinelli JJ, Basco VE, et al. Adjuvant radiotherapy and chemotherapy in node-positive premenopausal women with breast cancer. N Engl J Med. 1997;337:956–62.

66. Overgaard M, Hansen PS, Overgaard J, Rose C, Andersson M, Bach F, et al. Postoperative radiotherapy in high-risk premenopausal women with breast cancer who receive adjuvant chemotherapy. Danish Breast Cancer Cooperative Group 82b Trial. N Engl J Med. 1997;337:949–55.

67. Overgaard M, Jensen MB, Overgaard J, Hansen PS, Rose C, Andersson M, et al. Postoperative radiotherapy in high-risk postmenopausal breast-cancer patients given adjuvant tamoxifen: Danish Breast Cancer Cooperative Group DBCG 82c randomised trial. Lancet. 1999;353:1641–8.

68. Recht A, Edge SB, Solin LJ, Robinson DS, Estabrook A, Fine RE, American Society of Clinical Oncology, et al. Postmastectomy radiotherapy: clinical practice guidelines of the American Society of Clinical Oncology. J Clin Oncol. 2001;19:1539–69.

69. Harris JR, Halpin-Murphy P, McNeese M, et al. Consensus statement on postmastectomy radiation therapy. Int J Radiat Oncol Biol Phys. 1999;44:989–90.

70. EBCTCG (Early Breast Cancer Trialists' Collaborative Group), McGale P, Taylor C, Correa C, Cutter D, Duane F, Ewertz M, et al. Effect of radiotherapy after mastectomy and axillary surgery on 10-year recurrence and 20-year breast cancer mortality: meta-analysis of individual patient data for 8135 women in 22 randomised trials. Lancet. 2014;383:2127–35.

71. Kunkler IH, Canney P, van Tienhoven G, Russell NS, MRC/EORTC (BIG 2-04) SUPREMO Trial Management Group. Elucidating the role of chest wall irradiation in 'intermediate-risk' breast cancer: the MRC/EORTC SUPREMO trial. Clin Oncol (R Coll Radiol). 2008;20:31–4.

72. Wallgren A, Bonetti M, Gelber RD, Booser DJ, Ames F, Strom E, et al. Risk factors for locoregional recurrence among breast cancer patients: results from International Breast Cancer Study Group Trials I through VII. Clin Oncol. 2003;21:1205–13.

73. Freedman GM, Fowble BL. Local recurrence after mastectomy or breast-conserving surgery and radiation. Oncology (Williston Park). 2000;14:1561–81.

74. Fajardo LL, Roberts CC, Hunt KR. Mammographic surveillance of breast cancer patients: should the mastectomy site be imaged? AJR Am J Roentgenol. 1993;161:953–5.

75. Propeck PA, Scanlan KA. Utility of axillary views in postmastectomy patients. Radiology. 1993;187:769–71.

76. Willner J, Kiricuta IC, Kolbl O. Locoregional recurrence of breast cancer following mastectomy: always a fatal event? Results of univariate and multivariate analysis. Int J Radiat Oncol Biol Phys. 1997;37:853–63.

77. Schwaibold F, Fowble BL, Solin LJ, Schultz DJ, Goodman RL. The results of radiation therapy for isolated local regional recurrence after mastectomy. Int J Radiat Oncol Biol Phys. 1991;21:299–310.

78. Donegan WL, Perez-Mesa CM, Watson FR. A biostatistical study of locally recurrent breast carcinoma. Surg Gynecol Obstet. 1966;122:529–40.

79. Recht A, Come S, Troyan SL, Sadowsky N. Management of recurrent breast cancer. In: Harris JR, Lippman ME, Morrow M, Osborne CK, editors. Diseases of the breast. 2nd ed. Philadelphia: Lippincott Williams & Wilkins; 2000. p. 731–48.

80. Kamby C, Sengelov L. Pattern of dissemination and survival following isolated locoregional recurrence of breast cancer. A prospective study with more than 10 years of follow up. Breast Cancer Res Treat. 1997;45:181–92.

81. Chagpar A, Meric-Bernstam F, Hunt KK, Ross MI, Cristofanilli M, Singletary SE, et al. Chest wall recurrence after mastectomy does not always portend a dismal outcome. Ann Surg Oncol. 2003;10:628–34.

82. Haffty BG, Hauser A, Choi DH, et al. Molecular markers for prognosis after isolated postmastectomy chest wall recurrence. Cancer. 2004;100:252–63.

83. Dahlstrom KK, Andersson AP, Andersen M, Krag C. Wide local excision of recurrent breast cancer in the thoracic wall. Cancer. 1993;72:774–7.

84. Pameijer CR, Smith D, McCahill LE, Bimston DN, Wagman LD, Ellenhorn JD. Full-thickness chest wall resection for recurrent breast carcinoma: an institutional review and metaanalysis. Am Surg. 2005;71:711–5.

85. Friedel G, Kuipers T, Dippon J, Al-Kammash F, Walles T, Kyriss T, et al. Full-thickness resection with myocutaneous flap reconstruction for locally recurrent breast cancer. Ann Thorac Surg. 2008;85:1894–900.

86. Shen MC, Massarweh NN, Lari SA, Vaporciyan AA, Selber JC, Mittendorf EA, MacGregor MC, Smith BD, Kuerer HM. Clinical course of breast cancer patients with isolated sternal and full-thickness chest wall recurrences treated with and without radical surgery. Ann Surg Oncol. 2013;20:4153–60.

87. Santillan AA, Kiluk JV, Cox JM, Meade TL, Allred N, Ramos D, et al. Outcomes of locoregional recurrence after surgical chest wall resection and reconstruction for breast cancer. Ann Surg Oncol. 2008;15:1322–9.

88. Langstein HN, Cheng MH, Singletary SE, Robb GL, Hoy E, Smith TL, et al. Breast cancer recurrence after immediate reconstruction: patterns and significance. Plast Reconstr Surg. 2003;111:712–20.

89. Murphy Jr RX, Wahhab S, Rovito PF, Harper G, Kimmel SR, Kleinman LC, et al. Impact of immediate reconstruction on the local recurrence of breast cancer after mastectomy. Ann Plast Surg. 2003;50:333–8.

90. Missana MC, Laurent I, Germain M, Lucas S, Barreau L. Long-term oncological results after 400 skin-sparing mastectomies. J Visc Surg. 2013;150:313–20.

91. Warren Peled A, Foster RD, Stover AC, Itakura K, Ewing CA, Alvarado M, et al. Outcomes after total skin-sparing mastectomy and immediate reconstruction in 657 breasts. Ann Surg Oncol. 2012;19:3402–9.

92. Kneubil MC, Lohsiriwat V, Curigliano G, Brollo J, Botteri E, Rotmensz N, et al. Risk of locoregional recurrence in patients with false-negative frozen section or close margins of retroareolar specimen in nipple-sparing mastectomy. Ann Surg Oncol. 2012;19:4117–23.

93. Stanec Z, Žic R, Budi S, Stanec S, Milanović R, Vlajčić Z, et al. Skin and nipple-areola complex sparing mastectomy in breast cancer patients: 15-year experience. Ann Plast Surg. 2014;73:485–91.

94. Patterson SG, Teller P, Iyengar R, Carlson GW, Gabram-Mendola SG, Losken A, et al. Locoregional recurrence after mastectomy with immediate transverse rectus abdominis myocutaneous (TRAM) flap reconstruction. Ann Surg Oncol. 2012;19:2679–84.

95. Chagpar A, Langstein HN, Kronowitz SJ, Singletary SE, Ross MI, Buchholz TA, et al. Treatment and outcome of patients with chest wall recurrence after mastectomy and breast reconstruction. Am J Surg. 2004;187:164–9.

96. Howard MA, Polo K, Pusic AL, Cordeiro PG, Hidalgo DA, Mehrara B, et al. Breast cancer local recurrence after mastectomy and TRAM flap reconstruction: incidence and treatment options. Plast Reconstr Surg. 2006;117:1381–6.

97. Intra M, Veronesi P, Gentilini OD, Trifirò G, Berrettini A, Cecilio R, et al. Sentinel lymph node biopsy is feasible even after total mastectomy. J Surg Oncol. 2007;95(2):175–9.

98. Schuck A, Konemann S, Matthees B, Rübe CE, Reinartz G, Hesselmann S, et al. Radiotherapy in the treatment of locoregional relapses of breast cancer. Br J Radiol. 2002;75:663–9.

99. Halverson KJ, Perez CA, Kuske RR, Garcia DM, Simpson JR, Fineberg B. Isolated local-regional recurrence of breast cancer following mastectomy: radiotherapeutic management. Int J Radiat Oncol Biol Phys. 1990;19:851–8.

100. Hastings J, Iganej S, Huang C, Huang R, Slezak J. Risk factors for locoregional recurrence after mastectomy in stage T1 N0 breast cancer. Am J Clin Oncol. 2014;37:486–91.

101. Wahl AO, Rademaker A, Kiel KD, Jones EL, Marks LB, Croog V, et al. Multi-institutional review of repeat irradiation of chest wall and breast for recurrent breast cancer. Int J Radiat Oncol Biol Phys. 2008;70:477–84.

102. Vernon CC, Hand JW, Field SB, Machin D, Whaley JB, van der Zee J, et al. Radiotherapy with or without hyperthermia in the treatment of superficial localized breast cancer: results from five randomized controlled trials. International Collaborative Hyperthermia Group. Int J Radiat Oncol Biol Phys. 1996;35:731–44.

103. Jones EL, Oleson JR, Prosnitz LR, Samulski TV, Vujaskovic Z, Yu D, et al. Randomized trial of hyperthermia and radiation for superficial tumors. J Clin Oncol. 2005;23:3079–85.

104. Sersa G, Cufer T, Paulin SM, Cemazar M, Snoj M. Electrochemotherapy of chest wall breast cancer recurrence. Cancer Treat Rev. 2011;38:379–86.

105. Moossdorff M, van Roozendaal LM, Strobbe LJ, Aebi S, Cameron DA, Dixon JM, et al. Maastricht Delphi consensus on event definitions for classification of recurrence in breast cancer research. J Natl Cancer Inst. 2014;106:1–7.

106. Siponen ET, Vaalavirta LA, Joensuu H, Leidenius MH. Axillary and supraclavicular recurrences are rare after axillary lymph node dissection in breast cancer. World J Surg. 2012;36:295–302.

107. Recht A, Pierce SM, Abner A, Vicini F, Osteen RT, Love SM, et al. Regional nodal failure after conservative surgery and radiotherapy for early-stage breast carcinoma. J Clin Oncol. 1991;9:988–96.

108. Moran MS, Chagpar AB, Mayer EL. Management of local regional recurrences after primary breast cancer treatment. In: Harris JR, Lipmann ME, Morrow M, Osborne CK, editors. Diseases of the breast. 5th ed. Philadelphia: Wolters Kluwer Health; 2014. p. 891–904.

109. Port E, Garcia-Etienne C, Park J, Park J, Fey J, Borgen PI, et al. Reoperative sentinel lymph node biopsy: a new frontier in the management of ipsilateral breast tumor recurrence. Ann Surg Oncol. 2007;14:2209–14.

110. García Fernández A, Chabrera C, García Font M, Fraile M, Lain JM, Barco I, et al. Positive versus negative sentinel nodes in early breast cancer patients: axillary or loco-regional relapse and survival. A study spanning 2000–2012. Breast. 2013;22:902–7.

111. Chadha M, Mehta P, Feldman S, Boolbol SK, Harrison LB. Intraoperative high-dose-rate brachytherapy-a novel technique in the surgical management of axillary recurrence. Breast J. 2009;15:140–5.

112. Bartella L, Smith C, Dershaw D, Liberman L. Imaging breast cancer. Radiol Clin N Am. 2007;45:45–67.

113. Willner J, Kiricuta IC, Kolbl O, Bohndorf W. The prognostic relevance of locoregional recurrence following mastectomy in breast carcinoma. Strahlenther Onkol. 1991;167:465–71.

114. Pedersen AN, Moller S, Steffensen KD, Haahr V, Jensen M, Kempel MM, et al. Supraclavicular recurrence after early breast cancer: a curable condition? Breast Cancer Res Treat. 2011;125:815–22.

115. Chen SC, Chang HK, Lin YC, Leung WM, Tsai CS, Cheung YC, et al. Prognosis of breast cancer after supraclavicular lymph node metastasis: not a distant metastasis. Ann Surg Oncol. 2006;13:1457–65.

116. Overgaard M. Overview of randomized trials in high risk breast cancer patients treated with adjuvant systemic therapy with or without postmastectomy irradiation. Semin Radiat Oncol. 1999;9:292–9.

117. Kong M, Hong SE. Predictive factors for supraclavicular lymph node recurrence in N1 breast cancer patients. Asian Pac J Cancer Prev. 2013;14:2509–14.

118. Manca G, Volterrani D, Mazzarri S, Duce V, Svirydenka A, Giuliano A, Mariani G. Sentinel lymph node mapping in breast cancer: a critical reappraisal of the internal mammary chain issue. Q J Nucl Med Mol Imaging. 2014;58:114–26.

119. Kong AL, Tereffe W, Hunt KK, Yi M, Kang T, Weatherspoon K, et al. Impact of internal mammary lymph node drainage identified by preoperative lymphoscintigraphy on outcomes in patients with stage I to III breast cancer. Cancer. 2012;118:6287–96.

120. Oh JK, Chung YA, Kim YS, Jeon HM, Kim SH, Park YH, Chung SK. Value of F-18 FDG PET/CT in detection and prognostication of isolated extra-axillary lymph node recurrences in postoperative breast cancer. Biomed Mater Eng. 2014;24:1173–84.

121. Chen L, Gu Y, Leaw S, Wang Z, Wang P, Hu X, et al. Internal mammary lymph node recurrence: rare but characteristic metastasis site in breast cancer. BMC Cancer. 2010;10:4789.

122. Noble J, Sirohi B, Ashley S, et al. Sternal/parasternal resection for parasternal local recurrence in breast cancer. Breast. 2010;19:350–4.

123. van Geel AN, Wouters MW, van der Pol C, Schmitz PI, Lans T. Chest wall resection for internal mammary lymph node metastases of breast cancer. Breast. 2009;18:94–9.

124. Abrão FC, Tamagno MF, Abreu IR, Alfinito FS, Piato JR, Silva LM, et al. Thoracoscopic approach of the internal thoracic lymphatic chain. Innovations (Phila). 2013;8:215–8.

125. Borner M, Bacchi M, Goldhirsch A, Greiner R, Harder F, Castiglione M, et al. First isolated locoregional recurrence following mastectomy for breast cancer: results of a phase III multicenter study comparing systemic treatment with observation after excision and radiation. Swiss Group for Clinical Cancer Research. J Clin Oncol. 1994;12:2071–7.

126. Aebi S, Gelber S, Anderson SJ, Láng I, Robidoux A, Martín M, CALOR Investigators, et al. Chemotherapy for isolated locoregional recurrence of breast cancer (CALOR): a randomised trial. Lancet Oncol. 2014;15:156–63.

127. Wapnir IL, Aebi S, Gelber S, Anderson SJ, Láng I, Robidoux A, et al. Progress on BIG 1-02/IBCSG 27-02/NSABP B-37, a prospective randomized trial evaluating chemotherapy after local therapy for isolated locoregional recurrences of breast cancer. Ann Surg Oncol. 2008;15:3227–31.

128. Fitzal F, Filipits M, Rudas M, Greil R, Dietze O, Samonigg H, et al. The genomic expression test EndoPredict is a prognostic tool for identifying risk of local recurrence in postmenopausal endocrine receptor-positive, HER2neu-negative breast cancer patients randomised within the prospective ABCSG 8 trial. Br J Cancer. 2015;112:1405–10.

Treatment of Metastatic Breast Cancer: Endocrine Therapy

31

Fatma Sen and Adnan Aydiner

Abstract

Estrogen plays a primary role in breast cancer carcinogenesis and functions similarly to growth factors in some subtypes of breast cancer cells, particularly hormone receptor-positive (HR+) cells. Reducing estrogen production and preventing estrogen from interacting with the estrogen receptor pathway have been the focus of several preclinical and clinical trials and are commonly used strategies for treating HR+ breast cancer. Because the ovaries are the main source of estrogen in premenopausal women, ovarian ablation or functional suppression is the primary means of decreasing circulating estrogen. In postmenopausal women, estrogen production by the ovaries is functionally inactive, and the peripheral conversion of androgens to estrogen is the predominant source of estrogen. Thus, the inhibition of the conversion of androgens by an aromatase inhibitor or of the interaction of estrogen with its receptor is the most frequently used approaches to treat postmenopausal women with HR+ breast cancer. Initial endocrine treatment is a relevant option for patients with locally advanced or metastatic HR+ breast cancer who have no or mild symptomatic disease. Patients in whom breast cancer has progressed during the adjuvant or first-line endocrine treatment or within 1 year after adjuvant endocrine treatment termination should be evaluated

F. Sen, MD • A. Aydiner, MD (✉)
Department of Medical Oncology,
Istanbul University,
Istanbul Medical Faculty,
Institute of Oncology,
Istanbul, Turkey
e-mail: fkaragoz_2000@yahoo.com;
adnanaydiner@superonline.com

© Springer International Publishing Switzerland 2016
A. Aydiner et al. (eds.), *Breast Disease: Management and Therapies*,
DOI 10.1007/978-3-319-26012-9_31

for a non-cross-resistant second-line endocrine agent. The concurrent administration of an endocrine agent with a human epidermal growth factor receptor (HER2)-directed agent is also widely accepted for breast cancer patients with both HR and HER2 receptor positivity.

Keywords

Metastatic disease • Breast cancer • Premenopausal • Postmenopausal • Endocrine treatment • Hormone receptor positive

Introduction

Breast cancer is the most frequently diagnosed malignancy in women and one of the leading causes of cancer-related deaths worldwide. Efforts aimed at curing patients with early-stage breast cancer have increased during the last five decades, but approximately 6 % of breast cancer patients present with distant metastasis and more than one-fifth of patients with initial early-stage disease will develop distant metastases that require immediate and appropriate management [1–3]. The main purposes of systemic treatment, including endocrine therapies, for patients with advanced disease are prolonging survival and improving patient symptoms. Therefore, less toxic treatment approaches should be chosen. Endocrine therapies for hormone receptor-positive (HR+) tumors have a lower toxicity potential than other systemic treatment options, including many cytotoxic agents or some targeted drugs. Furthermore, treating metastatic HR+ breast cancer with endocrine therapy is at least as efficacious as chemotherapy, if not more so [4].

In this chapter, initial endocrine therapy, second- and third-line endocrine therapies for HR+ metastatic breast cancer (MBC) in premenopausal and postmenopausal women, and novel agents for endocrine-resistant HR+ breast cancers will be discussed with a review of the literature.

Estrogens and Estrogen Receptors

The responsiveness of a cell to estrogen depends mainly on estrogen receptor (ER) positivity. Estradiol has a high affinity and specificity for the ER. After estradiol binding to the ER, heat shock proteins dissociate from the ER, enabling receptor-receptor dimerization. Dimerized ERs preferentially translocate to the nucleus and bind to estrogen response elements, discrete DNA sequences located in the regulatory parts of target genes. AF1 and AF2 are activation functions (AFs) and activate transcription [5]. Gene activity is regulated by ligand-bound receptors via AFs by recruiting other proteins to the general transcription complex. These proteins act as coactivators or corepressors of estrogen-regulated transcription [6]. The activity of the amino-terminal AF1 is regulated by growth factors acting through the mitogen-activated protein (MAP) kinase signal transduction pathway and is cell type specific. However, the carboxy-terminal AF2 is located in the ligand-binding region of the ER and is activated by estradiol. Full agonist activity requires both AF1 and AF2 to be active [7, 8].

Receptor Status Determination at Metastatic or Recurrent Sites

The HR and human epidermal growth factor receptor 2 (HER2) status of the primary tumor must be determined to determine breast cancer subtypes, prognosis, and the treatment choice. Approximately 80 % of breast cancers are HR+ and are eventually sensitive to endocrine treatments. However, HR positivity varies with patient age; series have demonstrated that the positivity rate is 10 % in patients younger than 19 years and 90 % in patients older than 70 [9]. HR positivity is inversely correlated with tumor grade: it is very high in grade 1 tumors (90 %) but decreases to nearly 40 % in grade 3 tumors [9].

Substantial discordance in receptor positivity between the primary and metastatic site or the recurrence site of breast cancer has been reported [10]. Differences in receptor status in different sites of the tumor may affect the selection of treatment type and thus alter patient prognosis. In a retrospective study, HER2 and HR status were compared in primary and MBCs using immunohistochemistry and/or in situ hybridization [10]. Conversion from HR+ in the primary site to HR negative in the metastatic site was detected in 21 % of patients, and HR- to HR+ conversion occurred in 3.6 % of patients. HER2 status was discordant between primary and metastatic sites in 12 % of patients [10]. In another recently published retrospective study, the rates of discordance between primary and recurrent/metastatic lesions were 19 %, 34 %, and 7 % for ER, progesterone receptor (PR), and HER2, respectively. ER, PR, and HER2 discordance were observed in 20 %, 38 %, and 6.7 % of patients with distant metastasis and in 14 %, 18 %, and 7 % of patients with locoregional recurrence, respectively [11]. Among patients with distant metastasis, ER discordance, ER loss, HER2 discordance, and HER2 loss resulted in worse overall survival (OS) and PRS compared to the respective concordant cases ($p < 0.05$ for all). Unstable ER or HER2 status in breast cancer appears to be clinically significant and correlates with worse prognosis.

Discordance in the HER2 and HR status between primary and metastatic tumors may change the treatment decisions of patients. In a recently published review by Criscitiello C et al., biopsy of recurrent or metastatic sites led to changes in therapy in approximately 15 % of patients [2]. Therefore, although biopsy of all metastatic or recurrent sites is not required before the initiation of treatment, the evaluation of HER2 and HR in metastatic or recurrent tumors should be considered in patients with breast cancer. Although interventional radiology techniques and the ability of minimally invasive techniques to access metastatic sites have improved, performing biopsy from metastatic lesions can be difficult [1]. When the receptor status of the metastatic or recurrent site cannot be determined, treatment should be planned according to the features of the primary tumor.

International oncology guidelines recommend that metastatic disease at presentation or the first recurrence of breast cancer should be biopsied as part of the initial workup for breast cancer patients with disease recurrence or distant metastasis [12]. For recurrent disease, if the receptor status is previously unknown, originally negative or not overexpressed, the receptor status should be determined. In the case of the previously known HR positivity and/or a clinical course consistent with HR+ breast cancer, endocrine therapy can be started without retesting the receptor status.

Definition of Menopause

Before selecting and/or starting endocrine therapy, particularly AIs, clinicians should obtain a detailed menstruation history of the patient. Menopause should be defined carefully because the type of endocrine therapy depends on menopausal status. The discontinuation of menstrual cycles with previously administered chemotherapies does not definitively indicate menopause. Menstrual cycles may return in subsequent months or years. Thus, clinicians should not accept chemotherapy-induced amenorrhea as menopause before serial determination of plasma follicle-stimulating hormone (FSH) and estradiol levels.

Although clinical trials have not featured a clear consensus on the definition of menopause, menopause is defined by NCCN guidelines as a history of bilateral oophorectomy or age older than 60 years. For younger patients (<60 years), women must be amenorrheic for at least 1 year or more without a history of past or ongoing chemotherapy, ovarian function suppression, toremifene, and tamoxifen in addition to having plasma estradiol and FSH levels in the postmenopausal range [12]. Menopausal status cannot be determined accurately according to amenorrhea or based on FSH or plasma estradiol in patients being treated with a luteinizing hormone-releasing hormone (LHRH) agonist or antagonist.

Candidates for Initial Endocrine Treatment in the Metastatic Setting

Chemotherapy alone, endocrine therapy alone, and the concomitant use of chemotherapy and endocrine therapy are all initial treatment options for patients with metastatic HR+ tumors. The management of these patients depends on the patient's general health, age, presence of comorbidities, extent of disease, course of disease, previous anticancer drug history, and patient choices. HER2 positivity should also be considered during the decision of targeted therapy.

Patients without disease-related or severe symptoms and with a long disease-free interval, a limited number of metastatic sites or metastasis, and only soft tissue or bone metastasis are good candidates for initial endocrine therapies without cytotoxic agents. These characteristics, in addition to HR positivity, indicate a favorable prognosis. By contrast, when a patient has symptomatic and/or disseminated bone or visceral metastases and there is high probability of rapid progression carrying the risk of vital organ failure or other catastrophic complications, chemotherapy should be the first choice of treatment. However, the exact symptom criteria as the cutoff to begin chemotherapy rather than endocrine therapy remain controversial.

A prior systematic review performed by the National Collaborating Centre for Cancer compared the activity of endocrine therapy with chemotherapy in treatment-naive patients with advanced hormone-sensitive breast cancer [13]. Wilcken et al. also subsequently performed a systematic review to compare chemotherapy with endocrine treatments. Ten randomized controlled trials were identified as appropriate for the analysis [14]. OS was similar between the two treatment types. Furthermore, chemotherapy resulted in greater toxicity, particularly emesis and alopecia. Thus, endocrine therapy was recommended as the first-line treatment option in the absence of severe symptomatic disease in which an immediate tumor response is necessary [15].

Recently, the American Society of Clinical Oncology published a guideline to determine the optimal systemic treatment approach for HER2-negative breast cancer patients with advanced-stage disease [15]. A systematic review of randomized studies, previous meta-analyses, and systematic reviews published since 1993 was performed. In total, 20 meta-analyses and/or systematic reviews, 30 first-line treatment trials, and 29 second-line and further lines of treatment trials were identified as appropriate for analysis. Progression-free survival (PFS), survival, toxicity, tumor response, and quality of life were investigated as outcomes to establish recommendations. The expert panel reported that in patients with hormone-sensitive MBC, endocrine therapy is the preferred first-line treatment option instead of chemotherapy in the absence of life-threatening disease that requires sudden improvement with cytotoxics. When chemotherapy is indicated, a single agent should be chosen instead of a combination. The optimal chemotherapeutic agent as the first line and subsequent treatment lines could not be determined, but the number of agents and type of agent depend on the characteristics of the patient and tumor, including previous types of therapy, severity of adverse reactions, performance status, medical comorbidities, and patient choice. A single agent may be administered for long durations; however, toxicity should be balanced with effectiveness. No consensus has been reached on bevacizumab, and the present evidence is insufficient to support the use of other targeted agents in combination with other chemotherapeutic agents in breast cancer patients with HER2-negative disease [15]. However, the expert panel explained the limitations of the review and emphasized that more data about these important issues from randomized trials would be valuable [15].

Endocrine Treatment History for Local or Locally Advanced Breast Cancer

A patient who develops metastasis after or during adjuvant treatment should be evaluated for previous endocrine treatment, including type and duration of treatment and time since cessation of treatment. If progression occurred more than 1 year after the termination of adjuvant therapy, the patient should be accepted and treated as an endocrine treatment-naive patient. However, if the disease progresses or reoccurs under adjuvant endocrine treatment, under first-line endocrine treatment in a metastatic setting, or within 1 year after adjuvant endocrine treatment ended, eligible patients should be evaluated for subsequent endocrine treatment.

HER2-Negative Hormone Receptor-Positive Metastatic Breast Cancer

Premenopausal: Ovarian Ablation/Suppression, Tamoxifen, Selective Estrogen Receptor Modulators, AIs, Tamoxifen Plus Ovarian Suppression, Tamoxifen Versus Ovarian Suppression

Ovarian Ablation/Suppression

The role of hormones in the growth of some tumors was first discovered when tumor regression was observed after ovariectomy in a patient with metastatic breast carcinoma more than a century ago [16]. Estradiol has subsequently been identified as the most powerful hormone stimulator of breast cancer. Thus, medical or surgical deprivation and/or antagonism of estradiol is important in HR+ breast cancer.

In premenopausal patients with advanced breast cancer, bilateral oophorectomy has long been performed as a classical endocrine manipulation. Bilateral adrenalectomy in the 1950s and hypophysectomy in the 1960s were important advances in endocrine therapy for breast cancer patients aimed at the depletion of estrogen biosynthesis.

In addition to oophorectomy, ovarian ablation can be accomplished by irradiation. During the 1970s, based on the positive results of a clinical trial, the practice in Europe was to recommend ovarian irradiation to all premenopausal women and to women within 3 years of menopause at the time of the initial diagnosis of breast cancer [17]. Patients received endocrine treatment when they were not suitable for ovarian irradiation. Patients within 5 years of menopause were administered androgens with or without a chemotherapeutic agent; however, patients who were 5 years or more past menopause were treated with estrogens. The patients in whom breast cancer occurred during perimenopause had the worst response rate to endocrine therapy [17].

The development of HR measurements has allowed clinicians to identify patients who will most likely to respond to endocrine therapy [18]. This development was followed by many preclinical and clinical trials examining antiestrogens, progestins, LHRH agonists, LHRH antagonists, and inhibitors of estrogen synthesis [19].

Ovarian function suppression with an LHRH agonist subsequently became a noninvasive alternative to bilateral oophorectomy. In premenopausal women, pulses of LHRH stimulate the pituitary gland, resulting in pulsatile secretion of gonadotropins and establishing menstrual cycles. Treatment with a long-term depot formulation of an LHRH agonist initially stimulates gonadotropin release and subsequently leads to a reduction in gonadotropin secretion and circulating estrogen to postmenopausal ranges [20]. Despite in vitro studies demonstrating direct antitumor effects of LHRH agonists and evidence of specific binding sites for LHRH in primary breast cancer tissue, the key role of LHRH agonists remains medical castration [21, 22]. In an intergroup trial, 138 premenopausal patients with HR+ MBC were randomized to 3.6 mg of goserelin administered every 4 weeks ($n = 69$) versus surgical oophorectomy ($n = 67$). Failure-free survival and OS were similar between the two treatment arms. The death hazard ratio for goserelin/oophorectomy was 0.80 (95 % confidence interval [CI], 0.53–1.20). Serum estradiol levels were reduced to postmenopausal levels by goserelin treatment. The tumor flare rate (16 vs. 3 %) and rate of hot flashes (75 vs. 46 %) were higher in patients treated with goserelin than in those treated with surgical oophorectomy, but neither of the treatment arms was associated with severe toxicities [23].

Tamoxifen

Development of Tamoxifen

Tamoxifen (Nolvadex, Imperial Chemical Industries, DE 46,474), a nonsteroidal antiestrogenic compound synthesized in 1966 in Great Britain, was initially developed for antifertility. However, it was later demonstrated to stimulate ovulation in infertile women [24–26] and suppress carcinogen-induced rat mammary tumors [27]. Cole et al. were the first to report the clinical efficacy of tamoxifen for metastatic breast cancer in 1971 at Christ Hospital [28]. Following a pharmacological and clinical evaluation of tamoxifen in Great Britain and the United States, the Committee on the Safety of Medicine approved it for the treatment of MBC in postmenopausal women in 1973, and in 1977, the Food and Drug Administration also approved it for same indication. Tamoxifen was also approved in premenopausal women and in men with HR+ advanced breast cancer as a first-line endocrine therapy. Tamoxifen has also become an important form of systemic adjuvant therapy for early breast cancer [24].

Mechanisms of Action of Tamoxifen

In vitro studies suggest that the main antiproliferative effects of tamoxifen are mediated by competition with estrogen to bind cytoplasmic ER. After the formation of a complex with the ER, tamoxifen subsequently inhibits many actions of endogenous estrogen within tumor cells [29]. The inhibition of tumor growth by tamoxifen and its active metabolite correlates with the potency with which they bind to the ER [24]. The tamoxifen/ER complex prevents estrogen/ER-mediated gene transcription, DNA synthesis, and tumor cell growth and increases autocrine polypeptides, such as transforming growth factor-alpha, epidermal growth factor, insulin-like growth factor-II, and other growth factors that may be involved in cell proliferation [30, 31]. By contrast, estrogen stimulates the production of the PR and plasminogen activator and decreases the level of transforming growth factor-beta, an inhibitory factor of epithelial cells, including breast carcinoma [32]. In vitro studies of the effects of tamoxifen on cell cycle kinetics demonstrated that tamoxifen prevents the transition of cells from the early **GI** phase to the mid-G1 phase and leads to the accumulation of cells in the early **GI** phase of the cell cycle and to the reduction of cells in the **S** and G2 plus M phases [33]. These shifts have cytostatic effects. Thus, tamoxifen has been considered a chemosuppressive agent [33]. The continuous administration of tamoxifen to animals inoculated with breast tumor cells prevents tumor growth, whereas the discontinuation of therapy results in the appearance of tumors [34]. Although some studies suggest that tamoxifen has cytocidal activity, the lethal effect of tamoxifen on breast tumor growth in addition to its cytostatic effects is controversial [35].

In tissue culture, the inhibitory effect of tamoxifen on hormone-sensitive breast cancer cell growth is dose dependent. At low concentrations, the cytostatic effect of tamoxifen mediated through ERs can be completely blocked by estradiol [36]. At higher concentrations of tamoxifen, the cytostatic effect is not reversible by estrogens [37]. Tamoxifen may also inhibit cell replication by mechanisms other than the events mediated by ERs. Tamoxifen binds to the antiestrogen-binding site, a microsomal protein, with high affinity [38]. The functional importance of this protein in mediating the clinical effects of tamoxifen is unknown. In addition, tamoxifen inhibits protein kinase C and blocks the activation of calmodulin, a protein that may play a role in tumor promotion [39, 40]. Tamoxifen also induces antibody formation, enhances natural killer cell activity, and inhibits suppressor T-cell lymphocytes [41]. These non-ER-mediated actions of tamoxifen, heterogeneity of ER content within a tumor, or variability of receptor assay methodology may explain the inhibition of tumor growth by tamoxifen in 10–15 % of ER-negative tumors. Tamoxifen also inhibits angiogenesis; this inhibition is not altered in the presence of excess estrogen, suggesting that the antiangiogenic activity of the drug is mediated through a mechanism other than inhibition of estrogen action [24]. Further studies are necessary to characterize the antiangiogenic activity of tamoxifen.

Finally, tamoxifen may also increase serum high-density lipoprotein cholesterol, reduce antithrombin III activity, and inhibit prostaglandins D, F, and E, which may be involved in bone resorption [45]. Whether these effects are crucial to antitumor action remains unknown. Tamoxifen does not appear to have unwanted effects on bone mineral content [42].

The mechanism of action of tamoxifen, particularly its antiproliferative activity, may differ in ER-negative and ER+ cell lines. Unfortunately, data about treatment of ER-negative tumor cell lines with tamoxifen are limited and indicate a reduction in the proportion of cells in GO to G1 phases and an increased percentage of cells in S and G2 plus M phases [43].

Tamoxifen is currently the most widely prescribed agent for the treatment of breast cancer patients in the United States and Great Britain. However, it has several frequently observed side effects, including mild nausea, vaginal bleeding or discharge, menstrual irregularity, fluid retention, and hot flashes, particularly in premenopausal women. Nonspecific central nervous system symptoms such as depression, irritability, headache, dizziness, nervousness, inability to concentrate, sleep disturbance, lethargy, and fatigue have been observed rarely in women receiving tamoxifen [44, 45].

Tamoxifen Versus Ovarian Suppression

The National Cancer Institute of Canada Clinical Trials Group performed a randomized crossover trial named MA.1 that compared 40 mg of tamoxifen daily with ovarian ablation in premenopausal breast cancer patients with advanced disease. They reported objective responses in 25 % of the patients treated with tamoxifen and 16 % of the patients treated with ovarian ablation ($p=0.69$). The overall response, including stable disease, was 60 % in the tamoxifen arm and 42 % in the ovarian ablation arm ($p=0.34$). The median time to progression was 184 days in the tamoxifen arm and 126 days in the ovarian ablation arm ($p=0.40$, odds ratio (OR) for progression, 0.71). OS was also similar in the two groups (median: 2.35 years in the tamoxifen group vs. 2.46 in the ovarian ablation group; $p=0.98$, OR for death,

1.07). The most frequent side effects of tamoxifen were hot flashes and menstrual abnormalities. These side effects did not result in a dose reduction except in one patient. Although it was a small study, tamoxifen was associated with response rates, response durations, and survival times similar to those observed with ovarian ablation [46].

In 1997, Crump et al. [47] performed an individual patient-based meta-analysis to compare tamoxifen with ovarian ablation as a first-line endocrine therapy in premenopausal women with MBC. Ovarian ablation was performed by either bilateral oophorectomy or ovarian irradiation. Four randomized trials were eligible for analysis, and the individual patient data for eligible patients ($n=220$) were updated to June 1992. The patients were required to have ER+ or unknown breast cancer. No difference in the overall response rate was observed between the tamoxifen arm and the oophorectomy arm among the four trials ($p=0.94$). The odds reductions for progression ($p=0.32$) and the odds reductions for mortality ($p=0.72$) did not significantly favor tamoxifen treatment. Although the patients were allowed to cross over to the other treatment arm in all four trials, only 54/111 patients initially treated with ovarian ablation and 34/109 patients receiving tamoxifen as their primary therapy actually crossed over to the other arm at the time of disease progression. The response to the initial treatment type was predictive of the response to subsequent treatment arms ($p<0.05$). The authors concluded that the activity of tamoxifen is similar to that of ovarian ablation obtained by either surgery or radiation in premenopausal ER+ MBC as first-line therapy and was unlikely to be substantially inferior.

Tamoxifen Plus Ovarian Suppression

The purpose of combining an LHRH agonist with tamoxifen in premenopausal women is to inhibit tamoxifen-induced stimulation of pituitary-ovarian function. LHRH agonists are as effective as surgical castration. In 2001, Klijn et al. performed a meta-analysis that combined the findings of four randomized trials and compared OS, PFS, and the objective response for combination therapy or an LHRH agonist alone in premenopausal women with advanced-stage breast cancer [48]. A total of 506 women were randomized in those trials. The overall response rate was significantly higher for combination therapy with a median follow-up of 6.8 years; a significant survival benefit ($p = 0.02$; hazard ratio, 0.78) and PFS benefit ($p = 0.0003$; hazard ratio, 0.70) favoring combination therapy ($p = 0.03$; OR, 0.67) were demonstrated.

Based on the findings of this meta-analysis, the combined administration of an LHRH agonist with tamoxifen has been recommended as the new standard treatment option; however, tamoxifen alone was not compared with combination treatment in the analysis. The Adjuvant Breast Cancer Trials Collaborative Group performed an international study in an adjuvant setting. Pre- and perimenopausal patients who had been treated with prolonged (5 years) tamoxifen with or without chemotherapy were randomized to ovarian ablation or suppression versus no ovarian ablation or suppression [49]. Ovarian ablation or functional suppression were achieved by bilateral oophorectomy, irradiation of the ovaries, or administration of an LHRH agonist. The authors did not observe any additive activity of ovarian ablation or functional suppression on relapse-free survival or OS. However, further study is required to demonstrate the role of ovarian ablation or suppression in premenopausal women younger than 40 years with HR+ breast cancer, particularly those without previous chemotherapy administration. SOFT is the largest trial of ovarian suppression in premenopausal women with early-stage breast cancer. A total of 3,066 premenopausal women were randomized to 5 years of tamoxifen, tamoxifen plus ovarian suppression, or exemestane plus ovarian suppression. Women who were randomly assigned to ovarian suppression in either arm had the choice of monthly injections of triptorelin, surgical removal of the ovaries, or radiation. Women who had undergone chemotherapy entered the trial 8 months post chemotherapy, whereas those who did not undergo chemotherapy entered the trial soon after surgery. The

estimated disease-free survival rate at 5 years was reported to be found as 84.7 % in the tamoxifen alone group and 86.6 % in the tamoxifen plus ovarian suppression group with a median 67 months follow-up (hazard ratio for disease recurrence, second invasive cancer, or death, 0.83; 95 % CI, 0.66–1.04; $p = 0.10$). A multivariable allowance for prognostic factors indicated that tamoxifen plus ovarian suppression has higher treatment effect than with that for tamoxifen alone (hazard ratio, 0.78; 95 % CI, 0.62–0.98). Most recurrences occurred in patients with prior chemotherapy history, among whom the rate of freedom from breast cancer at 5 years was 82.5 % in the tamoxifen-ovarian suppression group and 78.0 % in the tamoxifen group (hazard ratio for recurrence, 0.78; 95 % CI, 0.60–1.02). The rate of freedom from breast cancer at 5 years was found to be 85.7 % in the exemestane plus ovarian suppression group (hazard ratio for recurrence vs. tamoxifen, 0.65; 95 % CI, 0.49–0.87). Authors concluded that for women who were at sufficient risk for recurrence to warrant adjuvant chemotherapy and who remained premenopausal, disease outcomes were improved with the addition of ovarian suppression [50]. Unfortunately, whether combination therapy with LHRH agonists and tamoxifen is superior to single-agent tamoxifen in a metastatic setting remains unknown.

Endocrine therapy for patients with advanced breast cancer should be planned as the sequential administration of single agents. However, combination therapy with an LHRH agonist and tamoxifen was observed to be superior to single-agent therapy in clinical trials [51]. Jonat et al. investigated the activity of goserelin with or without tamoxifen in 318 pre- and perimenopausal women with advanced breast cancer in a randomized multicenter trial [51]. Statistically similar objective responses were obtained in the goserelin treatment arm (31 %) and in combination arm (38 %) ($p = 0.24$). A modest benefit in time to progression (median: 23 weeks in the goserelin alone arm vs. 127 weeks in the combination arm, $p = 0.03$) favoring the combination treatment was reported, but no survival benefit favoring any arm was observed (median survival: 28 weeks in the goserelin alone group vs. 140 weeks in the combination group; $p = 0.25$). The response rate, time to progression, and survival were significantly different in favor of the combination group in patients with skeletal metastases only ($n = 115$). The tolerability and safety of both treatment arms were similar. Therefore, tamoxifen in combination with ovarian function suppression or ablation was deemed superior to tamoxifen monotherapy as a first-line treatment for metastatic or recurrent HR+ disease [51].

Other Selective Estrogen Receptor Modulators

The role of estrogen receptor modifiers (SERMs) in breast cancer treatment is now well established. The antiestrogen MER 25 was first introduced more than five decades ago [52], and 10 years after MER25, tamoxifen, and several antiestrogens with diverse chemical structures were reported [53, 54]. The first SERM to be introduced, tamoxifen, provided a revolutionary new treatment strategy for HR+ breast cancer patients. Currently, tamoxifen is one of the most widely used endocrine therapy drugs in both metastatic and adjuvant settings. Tamoxifen was subsequently shown to decrease breast cancer incidence in healthy women at high risk of developing breast cancer, and raloxifene has been demonstrated to prevent osteoporosis [55, 56]. The therapeutic success of tamoxifen has motivated considerable efforts to synthesize and investigate new-generation antiestrogens for breast cancer therapy.

Although many analogs of tamoxifen, including chlorotamoxifen, idoxifene, and droloxifene, have been described, only a few have been marketed for patients with breast cancer [57–59]. The chemical and pharmacological properties of these agents are similar and include partial agonist activity, a triphenylethylene backbone, and a nonsteroidal structure. Compared to tamoxifen, droloxifene (3-OH-tamoxifen citrate) has higher affinity for ER, a lower estrogenic to antiestrogenic activity ratio, and faster pharmacokinetics.

In a double-blind randomized multicenter dose-finding phase II trial, droloxifene was administered in doses of 20, 40, or 100 mg once daily to 369 postmenopausal women with HR+ or HR unknown locally advanced or advanced breast cancer. Sixty women were ineligible because of violation of entry criteria, 20 were inevaluable, and 15 still await a definitive response evaluation. Thus, 234 patients have been evaluated for response. The overall complete plus partial response rate was 39.3 %: 31 % (23/74) for 20 mg, 44.6 % (33/74) for 40 mg, and 42 % (36/86) for 100 mg (not significantly different within this dose range). The time to progression was similar between the three doses, and toxicity was mild at all doses. The preliminary results of this study demonstrated that droloxifene is active against advanced breast cancer. The outstanding preclinical characteristics of this drug support a large-scale clinical investigation [59].

Several nonsteroidal agents with antiestrogenic effects have been developed, such as substituted tetrahydronaphthalenes (e.g., nafoxidine; trioxifene), indole derivatives (e.g., zindoxifene, ZK 119010), benzothiophenes (e.g., LY117018, keoxifene), and benzopyrans [60]. These nonsteroidal agents have partial-agonist activity with pharmacological characteristics similar to those of tamoxifen. Therefore, although they inhibit the trophic action of estrogens, their activities are incomplete because of their intrinsic agonist activity in vivo. The effects of drug treatment depend on the balance between agonist and antagonist activities.

Toremifene is another SERM that has been widely administered to HR+ breast cancer patients for decades. The structure of toremifene differs from that of tamoxifen by the replacement of one of the hydrogen atoms in the ethyl side chain with a chlorine atom. This difference may modify the metabolism of toremifene by preventing or reducing DNA adduct formation. Several prospective randomized phase III trials comparing toremifene with tamoxifen have established the efficacy of toremifene [61]. Although many studies have demonstrated therapeutic equivalence of tamoxifen and toremifene in terms of response rate (24 vs. 25 %), time to treatment failure (4.9 vs. 5.3 months), and survival (31.0 vs. 33.1 month), some studies reported an advantage for toremifene. Furthermore, toremifene has been associated with less serious vascular events and uterine neoplasms and a better effect on serum lipids than tamoxifen. The safety and tolerability of the initially registered dose (60 mg per day) has been greatly increased to 240 mg per day [61, 62]. NCCN breast cancer guidelines version 2015 recommends toremifene as one of the subsequent endocrine treatment options for both premenopausal and postmenopausal HR+ recurrent or metastatic breast cancer. However, toremifene is cross-resistant with tamoxifen and is therefore ineffective as sequential therapy in patients who are refractory to tamoxifen.

Fulvestrant

The development and mode of action of fulvestrant will be discussed in detail in the section about endocrine therapy in postmenopausal women. Although it has an attractive mode of action, studies of fulvestrant that include premenopausal women have been limited. Currently, a randomized phase II study is investigating the activity of fulvestrant+goserelin in premenopausal women with HR+ recurrent or metastatic breast cancer compared with anastrozole+goserelin and goserelin alone (ClinicalTrials.gov identifier NCT01266213).

Aromatase Inhibitors

During the last five decades, tamoxifen has been widely used for the treatment of patients with breast cancer; it reduces or delays recurrences and incidence of contralateral breast cancer. Because it has both estrogen agonist and antagonist action in different tissue types, the prolonged use of tamoxifen may cause adverse reactions or events. Patients are at an increased risk of stroke and endometrial cancer. In the early 1970s, many alternate agents were studied to prevent the agonist effects of antiestrogens and increase their efficacy and safety [63, 64]. The main purpose of treatment with estrogen biosynthesis inhibitors is to reduce circulating estrogen levels, and studies of these inhibitors highlighted the importance of the enzyme aromatase as an important endocrine agent for the effective and selective treatment of hormone-sensitive breast cancer [65, 66].

Aromatase, a member of the cytochrome P450 enzyme system, catalyzes the final enzymatic step of estrogen biosynthesis and converts androstenedione to estrone and testosterone to estradiol, thereby increasing estrogen levels both in pre- and postmenopausal women (Fig. 31.1). A xenograft tumor model named MCF-7Ca was developed using human ER+ breast cancer cells stably transfected with the human aromatase gene. MCF-7Ca cells were grown as neoplasms in ovariectomized, immunosuppressed mice [67, 68]. These tumors act as autocrine sources of

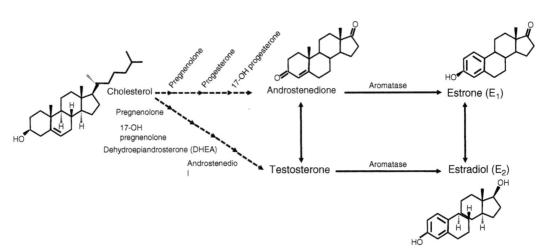

Fig. 31.1 The estrogen synthesis pathway (Miller et al. [163])

estrogen produced by aromatization. Because these mice did not have the ability to produce adrenal androgens, androstenedione was administered throughout the experiment. The xenografts were not only sensitive to the antiproliferative effects of aromatase inhibitors (AIs) but were also sensitive to the antiproliferative effects of antiestrogens [67, 68]. AIs block the conversion of androgens to estrogens but lack partial agonist effects, supporting aromatase as an attractive therapeutic target.

According to chronological order of development, AIs are grouped into three classes: first, second, and third generation. Testolactone and aminoglutethimide are pioneer drugs of this type, i.e., first-generation AIs. Testolactone has been administered to postmenopausal breast cancer women with a modest response rate for 20 years and was later shown to inhibit aromatase irreversibly with very low potency [69]. Aminoglutethimide is a nonsteroidal, reversible, nonspecific, and competitive AI. The clinical use of aminoglutethimide as an anticonvulsant serendipitously revealed its endocrine characteristics [70]. Because of the limited efficacy or tolerability of these agents in postmenopausal breast cancer, many studies were conducted in the 1980s to identify more potent, specific, and safer AIs. Fadrozole, formestane, and rogletimide were developed as second-generation AIs, and letrozole, anastrozole, and exemestane were subsequently produced as third-generation AIs [71, 72].

In premenopausal women, the ovaries are the primary source of estrogen, and the primary type of estrogen is estradiol. By contrast, in postmenopausal women, estrogen in circulation is mainly produced by the aromatization of androgens (androstenedione and testosterone) in the adrenals and ovaries to estrogens (estrone and estradiol) and by aromatase, which is located in peripheral tissues comprising muscle and body fat. Aromatase inhibition alone is not recommended in premenopausal women because inhibition of the hypothalamus pituitary aromatase increases gonadotropin, which in turn stimulates ovarian follicular growth, producing high levels of circulating estrogen, which can thereby induce mammary tumor proliferation [73]. AIs have therefore been studied in phase II trials in combination with ovarian suppression with promising results.

Carlson et al. [74] investigated the antitumor activity of anastrozole in the treatment of premenopausal women with HR+ MBC whose ovaries were functionally suppressed by goserelin, an LHRH agonist, in a prospective, multicenter, single-arm phase II trial. Goserelin was administered subcutaneously in a dose of 3.6 mg every month, and 21 days after the first injection of goserelin, the patients were allowed to receive 1 mg of anastrozole peroral daily. The treatment was terminated if disease progressed or any unacceptable toxicity developed. Of the 35 patients who were initially enrolled in the study, 32 were available for response and toxicity. Estradiol suppression was assessed at 3 and 6 months (mean estradiol levels = 18.7 pg/mL and 14.8 pg/mL, respectively). Three percent of the patients experienced a complete response, 34 % experienced a partial response, and the remaining 34 % had stable disease for 6 months or longer, resulting in a clinical benefit rate of 72 %. The median time to progression was 8.3 months (2–63 months), and at the time of analysis, the median survival was not reached (11–63 months). The commonly observed toxicities were hot flashes (59 %), arthralgias (53 %), and fatigue (50 %). No grade 4–5 toxicity was reported.

In another phase II trial, 73 patients with HR+ MBC (35 premenopausal and 38 postmenopausal) were treated with letrozole (2.5 mg orally daily) as first-line endocrine therapy [75]. Premenopausal women were rendered postmenopausal by administration of goserelin (3.6 mg every 28 days). The baseline characteristics of the premenopausal and postmenopausal women were similar, with the exception of older age (median, 41 vs. 53 years; $p < 0.001$) and a longer disease-free interval (median, 1.8 vs. 3.3 years; $p = 0.03$) in the postmenopausal patients. The clinical benefit rates of the two groups were similar (77 vs. 74 %). The median time to progression was not different between the premenopausal and postmenopausal patients at the median follow-up of 27.4 months (9.5 months vs. 8.9 months). Letrozole (± goserelin) resulted in a greater loss of bone mineral density at 6 months in patients who did not receive bisphosphonate compared to patients who received bisphosphonate (at the lumbar spine: premenopausal patients, −16.7 vs. 53.9 %; $p=0.002$, and postmenopausal patients, −13.3 vs. 17.4 %; $p=0.04$). The clinical efficacies of combination therapy with letrozole and goserelin in premenopausal MBC women were comparable to single-agent letrozole in postmenopausal patients. Although letrozole (± goserelin) was shown to modestly increase bone resorption, concurrent administration of bisphosphonate with endocrine therapy prevented bone resorption at 6 months.

In UpToDate, the authors considered the use of ovarian suppression plus AIs investigational because the benefit of combined treatment compared with ovarian suppression alone is unknown [76].

Postmenopausal Women: Progestins and Tamoxifen, AIs, Switching Between Third-Generation AIs, Fulvestrant

For postmenopausal patients with HR+ MBC who have not received endocrine therapy previously, present with disease progression after 12 months from the end of adjuvant therapy, or present with de novo MBC, the options of endocrine therapy include an AI, SERM, or fulvestrant [76].

Progestins and Tamoxifen

The progestins used for breast cancer therapy are megestrol acetate and medroxyprogesterone. The response rate for megestrol acetate is approximately 30 %, and activity similar to that of tamoxifen was obtained in patients treated with megestrol acetate [77]. Unfortunately, megestrol acetate is associated with important adverse effects such as weight gain at the standard dose of 160 mg daily [78]. Dose escalation did not improve the outcome of megestrol acetate [78]. With the development of new agents such as the AIs and fulvestrant, progestins are now usually administered in later lines of endocrine therapy.

Tamoxifen was initially evaluated in postmenopausal women with MBC [28] at doses of 20–40 mg daily. Tamoxifen was subsequently used in the adjuvant setting, and the current standard recommended dose for early-stage breast cancer is 20 mg daily.

Tamoxifen has also been compared to other endocrine therapies, such as diethylstilbestrol and progestins, including megestrol acetate and medroxyprogesterone, for this indication. Petru and Schmähl [79] evaluated the findings of clinical trials reported between 1971 and 1986 that studied the therapeutic efficacy of endocrine monotherapy with tamoxifen, aminoglutethimide, and medroxyprogesterone acetate in MBC. A total of 7,000 patients were enrolled in those studies. The overall response rates obtained with these endocrine single agents at various dose levels were 31–42 %. When only ER+ patients were evaluated, the response rates of tamoxifen or aminoglutethimide were approximately 41–54 %. The duration of response was 12 months in patients treated with tamoxifen and aminoglutethimide and 6–16 months in patients treated with medroxyprogesterone acetate. The overall mean survival, which was defined as the time from the initiation of the endocrine agent to death from any cause, was 20 months in tamoxifen- and aminoglutethimide-treated patients, whereas information concerning overall survival was obtained only in a minority of patients treated with medroxyprogesterone acetate. When the response was evaluated based on the site of metastatic lesions, all three drugs resulted in a higher degree of remission in the soft tissue than in visceral disease. Although the response rates and OS rates were similar among these endocrine agents, tamoxifen was most tolerable [24, 80].

Because the sequential administration of various endocrine therapies can produce repeated tumor regressions, efforts have been made to increase the antitumor activity of tamoxifen by simultaneous administration with endocrine agents such as DES, MPA, aminoglutethimide, and corticosteroids. However, the objective response rate is not significantly higher, and the durations of response and OS are not improved compared to tamoxifen monotherapy. In a collaborative double-blind randomized trial designed by the North Central Cancer Treatment Group and the Mayo Clinic, the superiority of tamoxifen+prednisolone to tamoxifen alone was investigated in postmenopausal MBC patients [81]. The objective response rates, median time to disease progression, and median survival time were statistically similar between the treatment arms. There was no association between treatment and outcome in the covariate analyses. Tamoxifen+prednisolone was associated with a significantly higher rate of weight gain and edema. Combining prednisolone with tamoxifen did not provide any advantage over tamoxifen alone in postmenopausal patients with MBC.

Limited data suggest a higher response rate and/or a longer time to progression without a survival advantage in postmenopausal women with MBC treated with fluoxymesterone in combination with tamoxifen compared to tamoxifen alone [82, 83].

In conclusion, the routine clinical use of tamoxifen concurrently with other endocrine agents is not justified given the lack of improvement in survival and the significant toxicity associated with multiple endocrine agents.

Simultaneous Administration of Tamoxifen with Cytotoxics

Because all breast tumors are heterogeneous (i.e., composed of hormone-dependent and hormone-independent cells), trials of tamoxifen with chemotherapy have been performed with the aim of killing the ER+ component of the tumor plus the rapidly dividing ER-negative cells. Tamoxifen administered as single-agent therapy has been compared to tamoxifen plus combination chemotherapy administered sequentially or simultaneously in postmenopausal women with disseminated breast cancer. In some of these studies, an increase in the initial response rate was demonstrated when tamoxifen was added to chemotherapy compared to tamoxifen alone [24, 84, 85] However, the median durations of response and overall survival were similar between the two treatment strategies [84, 86, 87]. Cavalli et al. randomized postmenopausal women with advanced breast cancer into two groups to be treated with either tamoxifen alone followed by chemotherapy after disease progression or concurrent administration of tamoxifen with chemotherapy initially [84]. No difference in survival was observed between the two treatment arms. However, in the subgroup of low-risk postmenopausal patients, the survival rate was significantly higher in the tamoxifen arm than the tamoxifen and chemotherapy arm. The Australian and New Zealand Breast Cancer Trials Group demonstrated that tamoxifen followed by chemotherapy on disease progression is as effective as chemotherapy and tamoxifen administered simultaneously in postmenopausal women in terms of overall response rate and survival [85]. Moreover, tamoxifen administered simultaneously or sequentially with chemotherapy produces a higher response rate, although without significant differences in survival, compared to chemotherapy alone [88–90].

It is appropriate to use tamoxifen alone instead of tamoxifen plus chemotherapy as the initial treatment in postmenopausal patients with advanced breast cancer who are candidates for hormonal manipulation. Chemotherapy should be reserved for patients who have failed to respond to endocrine therapy or whose disease is severely symptomatic and requires an immediate response. To improve the effectiveness of phase-specific cytotoxic agents, attempts have been made to exploit cell cycle arrest using tamoxifen to synchronize tumor cells and then estrogen to prime the cells in S phase.

Estrogens and Androgens

Estrogenic compounds can be used for patients with MBC, although there are no clinically significant data on the impact on treatment outcomes compared to placebo. Prior to the introduction of tamoxifen, high-dose estrogen resulted in a secondary response defined as the "withdrawal response" in 25–35 % of patients after estrogen was ceased at disease progression. This withdrawal response provided palliation over 12 months [76]. Patients treated with other endocrine therapies (AIs, tamoxifen, megestrol acetate) may occasionally respond to estrogen therapy as well [76]. If estrogen therapy is used, estradiol should be the preferred estrogen option. Although high doses of estrogen (30 mg of estradiol daily in divided doses) have been typically administered, lower doses, such as 6 mg of estradiol daily in divided doses, may be just as effective with less toxicity.

As with progestins, estrogen is contraindicated if the patient has a thromboembolic disorder or other risk factors for thromboembolic events. Progestins should be given to patients who have vaginal bleeding because of estrogen. In addition, patients should be treated with bisphosphonates before the administration of estradiol to prevent hypercalcemia.

Androgens are inferior to high-dose estrogen and are rarely used for MBC. Testosterone, fluoxymesterone, and danazol are the most frequently prescribed agents for this indication. The major side effects of androgens are virilization, edema, and jaundice.

Aromatase Inhibitors

Postmenopausal women continue to have low circulating estrogen concentrations even though the ovaries fail to synthesize estrogen during menopause. Circulating estrogen in postmenopausal women was previously believed to derive from adrenal glandular synthesis, but it has since been well established that the adrenals only contribute plasma androgens. Estrogens are produced by conversion from androgens in various body compartments such as the liver, muscle, skin, and connective tissue in postmenopausal women [91]. As emphasized previously, estrogen ablation in postmenopausal women via adrenalectomy and hypophysectomy became an attractive approach in the 1950s [92–95]. Because adrenalectomy and hypophysectomy are associated with high morbidity, trials of "medical adrenalectomy" led to the evaluation of glucocorticoids and inhibitors of adrenal enzymes such as ketoconazole [96–99]. Although the tumor response obtained with these drugs is inferior to surgical adrenalectomy and hypophysectomy, these efforts have opened the way for aminoglutethimide followed by aromatase inhibition for breast cancer therapy.

Although there is a single aromatase gene, at least ten different promoters are present in the gene [100]. In different tissue types, different promoters and ligands regulate estrogen synthesis [101, 102]. These promoters have different key roles in benign and malignant breast tissue. The main activator is the 1.4 promoter in normal breast tissue, whereas promoters II, 1.3, and 1.7, in addition to 1.4, play a role in breast cancer tissue [100]. However, the different promoters encode similar proteins. Aromatase can convert testosterone into estradiol and androstenedione into estrone. Although plasma androstenedione and testosterone are derived from the adrenals in postmenopausal women, the ovary is reported to contribute circulating testosterone at minor, albeit significant, levels [103, 104]. These plasma androgens are taken up by various body compartments for subsequent aromatization.

The benefits of tamoxifen are mainly attributed to ER blockade, which eliminates the stimulus to continue proliferation, resulting in tumor regression. However, tamoxifen therapy does not result in the maximal inhibition of the effects of estrogen because it has a weak or partial agonist effect on ER. For nearly three decades, tamoxifen has been the mainstay of endocrine therapy in breast cancer, but now third-generation AIs are emerging as potential alternatives with higher clinical efficacy and a better overall safety profile than tamoxifen [105].

Two classes of third-generation AIs, steroidal (e.g., formestane, exemestane) and nonsteroidal (e.g., fadrozole, anastrozole, and letrozole), are currently available. The pharmacokinetic properties, selectivity, and potency of these agents differ, although all third-generation AIs are more selective than aminoglutethimide [51]. Steroidal AIs are analogs of androstenedione, which is the substrate of natural aromatase and irreversibly inactivates the enzyme by binding covalently to the substrate-binding site of aromatase. Nonsteroidal AIs such as letrozole and anastrozole, however, inhibit aromatase in a reversible manner by binding to the heme moiety of the enzyme. In this way, nonsteroidal AIs prevent androgens from binding to the catalytic site [106]. Therefore, the steroidal nonreversible AIs are also known as aromatase inactivators, whereas nonsteroidal AIs are reversible inhibitors of aromatase. For third-generation AIs, 98 % inhibition of total body aromatization has been reported, whereas for first- and second-generation AIs, only inhibition <90 % has been achieved [107].

Folkerd et al. suggested that the level of estradiol and estrone sulfate suppression depends on body mass index in postmenopausal women with early-stage ER+ breast cancer who were previously treated with AIs [108]. These data provide a basis for the improved outcome of AIs compared to tamoxifen in lean patients but not obese patients, which may enable individualized treatment with AIs by regulation of the AI dose depending on the circulating estradiol and estrone sulfate concentrations. Although the measurement of AIs is not difficult using mass spectrometry, the measurement of estrogens, particularly estradiol, is quite challenging.

AIs are associated with less frequent vaginal bleeding and thromboembolic events compared to tamoxifen, although they are known to affect bone turnover and possibly lipid metabolism. The adverse effects profiles between and within these two AI classes may also differ. Because available AIs have similar efficacy, it is likely that their safety and tolerability profiles will affect agent selection in clinical practice. Therefore, the elucidation of the differences in the safety profiles of third-generation AIs is critical.

Nonsteroidal AIs

Third-generation AIs were initially compared to megestrol acetate as a second-line therapy. Two randomized, multicenter trials were designed identically to compare the tolerability and efficacy of anastrozole and megestrol acetate for the treatment of postmenopausal women with advanced breast carcinoma after progression with tamoxifen [49]. Anastrozole was used at doses of 1 or 10 mg once daily, and megestrol acetate was administered in doses of 40 mg four times daily. Both studies were double blind for anastrozole and open label for megestrol acetate. Buzdar et al. performed a combined analysis of the two studies, which enrolled a total of 764 patients. At a median follow-up of 31 months for survival, 1 mg of anastrozole daily exhibited a statistically significant survival benefit over megestrol acetate (HR, 0.78, $p<0.025$) and longer median survival (27 months) compared to the megestrol acetate group (22 months). A dose of 10 mg of anastrozole also resulted in a survival advantage over the megestrol acetate group (HR, 0.8, $p=0.09$). Both doses of anastrozole (56.1 and 54.6 %) were associated with higher 2-year survival rates than megestrol acetate therapy (46.3 %) [109]. This combined analysis clearly demonstrates that anastrozole treatment at a dose of 1 mg once daily results in a statistically and clinically significant benefit over megestrol acetate after disease progression with tamoxifen. In addition to the good tolerability profile of anastrozole, this clinical benefit supports the administration of anastrozole as a valuable new treatment option for this patient population.

Two doses of letrozole (0.5 and 2.5 mg) were compared to megestrol acetate (40 mg qid) in postmenopausal women with advanced breast cancer who had previously received antiestrogens in a double-blind, randomized, multicenter, multinational study [110]. Patients with breast cancer whose disease had progressed during adjuvant antiestrogen therapy, within 12 months of the end of adjuvant antiestrogen therapy received for at least 6 months, or while receiving antiestrogen therapy for advanced disease were enrolled in the study. Their breast cancers had to have ER and/or PR positivity or unknown status. The primary efficacy variable was confirmed with an objective response rate. The performance status according to Karnofsky and quality-of-life assessments according to the European Organization for Research and Treatment of Cancer were evaluated for 1 year. The median duration of treatment was longer in the 0.5 mg letrozole treatment arm (171 days) than the 2.5 mg letrozole (120 days) and megestrol acetate arms (136 days). However, the overall objective tumor response was similar among the three treatment groups. Patients who received 0.5 mg of letrozole had a longer median time to progression compared to the other treatment arms (6 months vs. 3 months). The patients who received 0.5 mg of letrozole had a lower risk of disease progression than the patients who received megestrol acetate (HR, 0.80; $p = 0.044$). Administration of 0.5 mg of letrozole improved disease progression ($p = 0.044$) and decreased the risk of treatment failure ($p = 0.018$) compared to megestrol acetate. The time to progression between the three treatment groups was not statistically significant. Administration of 0.5 mg of letrozole produced a trend ($p = 0.053$) for survival advantage compared to megestrol acetate. Megestrol acetate resulted in a higher incidence of weight gain, vaginal bleeding, and dyspnea, and letrozole at both doses was more likely to cause headache, hair thinning, and diarrhea. Thus, letrozole is equivalent to megestrol acetate based on its favorable tolerability profile, once-daily dosing, and evidence of a clinically relevant benefit. Similar to anastrozole, letrozole should be considered for use as an alternative endocrine therapy in postmenopausal women with advanced breast cancer after treatment failure with antiestrogens.

AIs were subsequently studied as a first-line therapy compared to tamoxifen based on the positive findings obtained in the second-line setting [111–114] (Table 31.1). Bonneterre et al. [111] performed a randomized, double-blind, multicenter study in which the efficacy and tolerability of 1 mg of anastrozole once daily was compared to 20 mg of tamoxifen once daily in postmenopausal patients with advanced breast cancer as a first-line therapy. The tumors were required to be HR+ or of unknown receptor status. The time to progression, overall response rate, and tolerability were planned as primary end points. In total, 668 patients were randomized to the anastrozole arm (340 patients) and the tamoxifen arm (328 patients) and were followed up for a median of 19 months. Both treatment arms resulted in a similar median time to progression (8.2 months in the anastrozole arm and 8.3 months in the tamoxifen arm, hazard ratio for tamoxifen; anastrozole, 0.99). Anastrozole also produced a similar overall response rate compared to tamoxifen (32.9 vs. 32.6 %). The clinical benefit (CR + PR + disease stabilization ≥24 weeks) rates were 56.2 % in the anastrozole arm and 55.5 % in the tamoxifen arm. These findings support the equivalent efficacy of anastrozole and tamoxifen. Although both treatments were well tolerated, fewer thromboembolic events and vaginal bleeding were reported in patients treated with anastrozole compared to those treated with tamoxifen (4.8 vs. 7.3 % [thromboembolic events] and 1.2 % vs. 2.4 % [vaginal bleeding], respectively).

Table 31.1 Comparison of various aromatase inhibitors with tamoxifen as first-line hormonal therapy in hormone receptor-positive advanced breast cancer

	Treatment arms		Overall response rate		Clinical benefit rate[a]		Time to progression/ progression-free survival	
	Agent	No. of patients	%	p value	%	p value	%	p value
Bonneterre et al. 2000 [112] (TARGET study)	Anastrozole	340	33	0.787	56		8.2	0.941
	Tamoxifen	328	33		55		8.3	
Nabholtz et al. 2000 [111] (The North American trial)	Anastrozole	171	21		59	0.0098	11.1	0.005
	Tamoxifen	182	17		46		5.6	
Mouridsen et al. 2003 [114] Phase III trial	Letrozole	453	32	0.0002	50	0.0004	9.4	<0.0001
	Tamoxifen	453	21		38		6	
Paridaens et al. 2008 [115] (EORTC-BCCG)	Exemestane	182	46	0.005	Unknown		9.9	0.121
	Tamoxifen	189	31		Unknown		5.8	

[a]Clinical benefit rate: complete response + partial response + stable disease for at least 6 months

Because the predefined criteria were satisfied, anastrozole was accepted to have at least equivalent efficacy with tamoxifen. Furthermore, based on the lower incidence of certain side effects such as thromboembolic events and vaginal bleeding, anastrozole has been considered as first-line therapy for postmenopausal women with advanced breast cancer [111].

In the same time period, another randomized, double-blind, multicenter trial was conducted by Nabholtz et al. in North America with a similar design as the study conducted by Bonneterre et al. [112]. Again, anastrozole was demonstrated to be as effective as tamoxifen in terms of OR (21 % vs. 17 %, respectively), with a clinical benefit in 59 % of anastrozole-treated patients and 46 % of tamoxifen-treated patients (two-sided $p=0.0098$, retrospective analysis). The median time to progression was significantly longer in the anastrozole arm than the tamoxifen arm (11 vs. 5.6 months, respectively; two-sided $p=0.005$, tamoxifen/anastrozole hazard ratio, 1.44). The safety profiles were also similar to those observed by Bonneterre et al. In this study, anastrozole also satisfied the predefined criteria for equivalence to tamoxifen [112].

Overall, the efficacy of AIs is at least equivalent to that of tamoxifen; thus, they are currently one of the standard first-line treatment options for postmenopausal women with HR+ MBC.

Steroidal AIs

Exemestane is the only third-generation steroidal AI. Its efficacy has been demonstrated as a first-line treatment option in MBC. Therefore, exemestane could be considered a valid first-line therapeutic option or for use in second-line or further situations. This AI has been studied in the neoadjuvant setting as a presurgical treatment and even as chemoprevention in high-risk healthy postmenopausal women. Exemestane may reverse the side effects of tamoxifen, such as endometrial changes and thromboembolic disease, but may also cause inconvenient side effects. In addition, exemestane and nonsteroidal AIs do not exhibit total cross-resistance with respect to antitumoral efficacy; moreover, the two classes of AIs display a non-total overlapping toxicity profile. Therefore, exemestane is a useful treatment option at all stages of breast cancer.

Clinical studies have found that 25 mg/day of exemestane administered orally is the minimum effective dose to produce maximum estrogen suppression [115, 116]. The mean maximum suppression of aromatase by exemestane is 97.9 % [117]. Third-generation AIs achieve 98 % inhibition of total body aromatization, whereas first- and second-generation AIs achieve only 90 % inhibition [107]. Exemestane, similar to other AIs, is associated with increased bone turnover, loss of bone mineral density, and an increased incidence of fractures, thus requiring close observation and treatment if necessary.

The Exemestane Study Group evaluated the efficacy, pharmacodynamics, and safety of exemestane versus megestrol acetate in 769 postmenopausal women with advanced breast cancer whose disease progressed after tamoxifen in a phase III, double-blind, randomized, multicenter trial [118]. A total of 366 postmenopausal women received 25 mg/day of exemestane, and 403 patients received 40 mg of megestrol acetate four times daily. The overall objective response rates were higher in the exemestane arm than the megestrol acetate arm (15 vs. 12.4 %); similar results were observed in patients with visceral metastases (13.5 vs. 10.5 %). Median survival was longer in the exemestane arm (median not reached) than the megestrol acetate arm (123 weeks; $p=0.039$). In addition, the median duration of the overall response (60 vs. 49 weeks; $p=0.025$), time to tumor progression (20.3 vs. 16.6 weeks; $p=0.037$), and time to treatment failure (16.3 vs. 15.7 weeks; $p=0.042$) were also superior in the exemestane arm. Pain, tumor-related signs and symptoms, and quality of life were similar in the two arms or were improved with exemestane compared to megestrol acetate. Both drugs were well tolerated, but grade 3 or 4 weight changes were more common with megestrol acetate (17.1 vs. 7.6 %; $p=0.001$). Based on these findings, including the prolongation of survival, time to progression, and time to treatment failure by exemestane compared to megestrol, exemestane offers a well-tolerated treatment option for postmenopausal women with advanced breast cancer who experienced disease progression under or after tamoxifen treatment.

Although exemestane is often used as a second-line treatment, its efficacy as a first-line treatment has also been demonstrated in clinical trials [114]. The European Organization for the Research and Treatment of Cancer Breast Cancer Cooperative Group undertook a phase III randomized open-label clinical trial to investigate the efficacy and tolerability of exemestane compared to tamoxifen in 371 postmenopausal patients with hormone-sensitive MBC. The overall response rate was higher in the exemestane treatment arm than the tamoxifen arm, whereas OS was similar between the two treatment arms. OS was not significantly different from that for tamoxifen in the different individual trials of the three third-generation AIs, but a meta-analysis indicated an OS benefit of AIs compared to tamoxifen as a first-line therapy for HR+ breast cancer [119]. Thus, AIs can be considered more efficacious than tamoxifen as first-line therapy, which is very significant for quality of life in palliative settings. AIs are also superior to megestrol acetate. Megestrol acetate was previously administered as a standard second-line hormonal therapy in patients resistant to tamoxifen, but these findings indicate that the overall ORRs were higher for exemestane than for megestrol acetate as second-line treatment following tamoxifen failure [118, 120].

Comparing Steroidal AIs with Nonsteroidal AIs

An indirect comparison revealed that exemestane administered at 25 mg daily appeared to inhibit aromatization as efficiently as anastrozole administered at 1 mg daily [121]. Furthermore, 2.5 mg of letrozole daily appeared to be a more potent AI than either exemestane or anastrozole [122]. These results should be interpreted carefully in light of plasma estrogen level measurements. Because the methods to evaluate such low plasma estrogen levels in patients require high sensitivity, obtaining measurements in vivo is very difficult. Assays with a sensitivity limit of 5–7 pM for estrone and 1–2 pM for E2 are required to detect more than 90 % inhibition in vivo. Pauwels et al.

developed a sensitive liquid chromatography-tandem mass spectrometry method for measuring low estrogen levels [123]. The limit of quantification was 1.2 and 1.3 ng/l for estrone and E2, respectively. Exemestane, however, is metabolized into several steroidal compounds. These steroidal molecules may interact nonspecifically during the measurement of estrogen levels and consequently cause cross-contamination [115]. As a result, chromatographic sample purification is required.

There are a limited number of randomized clinical studies comparing two different classes of AIs as first-line or sequential endocrine therapy for patients with hormone-dependent MBC. In one trial, 130 postmenopausal women were randomized to receive anastrozole or exemestane for at least 8 weeks. Another trial randomized 103 postmenopausal women with advanced breast cancer to anastrozole or exemestane until disease progression. Both studies demonstrated no difference in clinical efficacy between exemestane and anastrozole [124, 125].

A systematic review performed by Riemsma et al. indirectly compared different first-line AIs, including anastrozole, letrozole, and exemestane, in postmenopausal women with HR+ (± ErbB2 positivity) advanced breast cancer [126]. Four of 25 randomized controlled trials met the inclusion criteria. A narrative synthesis analysis was used when a meta-analysis using direct or indirect comparisons was not suitable for some or all of the data. These three AIs were compared to tamoxifen based on available data and to each other using a network meta-analysis. Based on direct evidence, the time to progression was significantly better in the letrozole arm than the tamoxifen arm (hazard ratio, 0.70 with 95 % CI, 0.60–0.82). Furthermore, a better overall response rate (RR, 0.65 with 95 % CI, 0.52–0.82) and quality-adjusted time without symptoms or toxicity (Q-Twist difference = 1.5; $p < 0.001$) were obtained. Exemestane was significantly superior to tamoxifen in terms of the objective response rate (RR, 0.68; 95 % CI, 0.53–0.89). Anastrozole was significantly superior to tamoxifen in terms of the time to tumor progression in one trial (hazard ratio, 1.42; 95 % CI, 1.15-NR) but not the other (hazard ratio, 1.01; 95 % CI, 0.87-NR). There were no significant differences in adverse events between letrozole and tamoxifen. However, tamoxifen caused more serious adverse events than exemestane (OR, 0.61; 95 % CI, 0.38–0.97), whereas exemestane was associated with more arthralgia than tamoxifen (OR = 2.33). Anastrozole resulted in a higher incidence of total adverse events (OR = 1.04) and hot flashes (OR = 1.39) compared to tamoxifen in one trial [126]. The indirect comparison of AIs with one another in postmenopausal women with HR+ advanced breast cancer demonstrated that letrozole and exemestane were superior to anastrozole in terms of the objective response rate, whereas OS and PFS, the more clinically relevant outcomes, did not differ significantly among AIs. A class effect of all AIs may explain the similar survival rates.

Although these are the best available data, these findings should be interpreted with appropriate caution because the basic assumptions of homogeneity, similarity, and consistency were not fulfilled for this network analysis and the findings are based on indirect comparisons. Head-to-head comparisons of these three AIs in patients with MBC in first-line settings are warranted.

Taken together, these data indicate that exemestane as a first-line treatment is effective, is well tolerated, and can be considered, similarly to NSAIs, as a valid first-line option for the treatment of HR+ cancers in postmenopausal women. As far as hormonal suppression is concerned, exemestane appears slightly less efficacious compared to the other AIs, whereas the clinical antitumoral efficacy of NSAIs and SAIs appears to be similar. In second-line treatment, the sequence of AIs appears to be irrelevant due to the total lack of cross-resistance.

Switching Between Third-Generation AIs

As emphasized previously, steroidal AIs bind irreversibly to the active site of aromatase; thus, new enzyme production is required for estrogen synthesis. However, nonsteroidal AIs reversibly bind to the active site of aromatase. Although the clinical relevance of these differences is unclear, a lack of cross-resistance between steroidal and nonsteroidal AIs was suggested. Thus, upon the progression of metastatic disease following treatment with NSAIs, exemestane may be effective as sequential hormone therapy or vice versa [127–130]. The subsequent findings of several trials demonstrated that breast cancer patients who have become resistant to NSAIs may experience benefit from SAIs [131–135]. The clinical benefit of exemestane after progression on a nonsteroidal AI is supported by the findings of a systemic review published in 2011 [136]. On average, 25–30 % of patients in the crossover studies experienced an objective response or stable disease for 6 months or more. In addition, the administration of NSAIs after failing SAIs appears to be effective. Several potential mechanisms have been suggested to underlie this non-total cross-resistance, and studies to confirm these mechanisms are eagerly awaited [127–136].

Fulvestrant

Tamoxifen and its derivatives have partial agonist activity on ERs located in certain tissues in addition to having antagonistic activity on ERs. The well-defined agonist effects that limit their clinical efficacy are endometrial stimulation and the induction of tumor growth after previous response to tamoxifen [47]. Fulvestrant (ICI 182,780 Faslodex produced by AstraZeneca Cheshire, United Kingdom) is a novel, steroidal estrogen antagonist and is devoid of the estrogen agonist effect to block uterotrophic activities characteristic of ER agonists and of partial agonists such as tamoxifen and raloxifene. Fulvestrant has been investigated in several in vitro and in vivo preclinical studies. In animals, fulvestrant has 100 times greater affinity for the ER than tamoxifen, and it significantly reduces the ability of the ER to stimulate or inhibit gene transcription possibly by impairing dimerization, increasing ER turnover, and disrupting nuclear localization. In addition, fulvestrant cannot cross the blood-brain barrier in animal models and is neutral with respect to lipids and bone.

Fulvestrant was also assessed clinically in patients with breast carcinoma preoperatively or after the failure of tamoxifen or a nonsteroidal AI and in patients who underwent hysterectomy for benign conditions [47, 137]. The findings of preclinical and clinical studies demonstrated that fulvestrant functionally blocks and decreases cellular ER levels; thus, ERs become unavailable or unresponsive to estrogen or estrogen agonists in breast cancer. Therefore, fulvestrant is now known as a selective ER downregulator. In addition, fulvestrant is not cross-resistant with tamoxifen or the ER-agonist activity associated with tamoxifen.

Although fulvestrant has been studied in postmenopausal patients with HR+ inoperable locally advanced or advanced breast cancer in several phase II and III trials, the dosage, line of therapy, and comparison groups were not uniform. Initially, a dose-response effect of fulvestrant in the dose range of 50–250 mg for intramuscular use was demonstrated, but later trials evaluating the clinical activity of 125 mg of fulvestrant did not show any objective tumor response after 3 months of treatment [138]. Therefore, the subsequent clinical development of fulvestrant in advanced breast cancer was performed with monthly dosages of 250 mg, although 500 mg was later tested and compared to 250 mg [139].

Fulvestrant Versus Tamoxifen

Howell et al. conducted a multicenter, double-blind, randomized trial to compare the efficacy and tolerability of fulvestrant with tamoxifen as a first-line endocrine therapy in postmenopausal women with advanced breast cancer [140]. The tumors of the patients were required to be ER+ and/or PR+ or of unknown receptor status. Patients were randomized to 250 mg of fulvestrant (once-monthly intramuscular injection; $n=313$) or 20 mg of tamoxifen (once-daily oral tablets; $n=274$). In 2004, with a median follow-up of 14.5 months, the median time to progression was similar between fulvestrant and tamoxifen (6.8 months and 8.3 months, respectively; HR, 1.18; 95 % CI, 0.98–1.44; $p=0.088$). A prospectively planned subgroup analysis of patients with known HR+ tumors (78 %) revealed that the median time to progression was also similar between the two treatment arms (8.2 months

for fulvestrant and 8.3 months for tamoxifen; HR, 1.10; 95 % CI, 0.89–1.36; $p=0.39$). For the overall population, the objective response rate was 31.6 % with fulvestrant and 33.9 % with tamoxifen, and in the known HR+ subgroup, the objective response rate was similar between the two treatment arms (33.2 % and 31.1 %, respectively, OR, 1.10; 95 % CI, 0.74–1.63; $p=0.64$). In addition, the clinical benefit rate was similar among the treatment arms (57 % for fulvestrant, 62.7 % for tamoxifen; OR, 0.79; 95 % CI, −15.01–3.19; $p=0.22$). Both tamoxifen and fulvestrant were well tolerated. The median time to treatment failure was longer in patients who were treated with tamoxifen than in fulvestrant-treated patients (7.8 months vs. 5.9 months; HR, 1.24; 95 % CI, 1.03–1.50; $p=0.026$). Among patients with HR+ breast cancer, the median time to treatment failure was similar between the treatment arms (7.5 months for fulvestrant and 8 months for tamoxifen: HR, 1.15; 95 % CI, 0.93–1.42; $p=0.19$) [140]. The median survival was longer in the tamoxifen arm than in the fulvestrant arm (38.7 months vs. 36.9 months, respectively; HR, 1.29; 95 % CI, 1.01–1.64; $p=0.04$) according to the planned analysis with adjustments for baseline covariates. However, when the analysis was unadjusted for baseline covariates, survival did not differ between the two groups (HR, 1.21; 95 % CI, 0.95–1.54; $p=0.12$). Among the patients with HR+ tumors, the median survival was 39.3 months in the fulvestrant group and 40.7 months in the tamoxifen group (HR, 1.16; 95 % CI, 0.88–1.54; $p=0.30$). The upper limit of the 95 % CI was 1.54, which did not satisfy the predefined criterion (≤ 1.25) to conclude noninferiority of fulvestrant compared to tamoxifen. In total, 12 % of the fulvestrant-treated patients and 11 % of the tamoxifen-treated patients died without "breast cancer," and these deaths represented approximately a quarter of all deaths in both treatment arms [140].

The results from this trial indicate that differences in efficacy favored tamoxifen, and in the first-line setting, the noninferiority of fulvestrant could not be demonstrated. Nevertheless, in patients with potentially hormone-sensitive breast cancer (HR+ tumors), the efficacy of fulvestrant was at least similar efficacy to that of tamoxifen, without significant differences between end points and a favorable overall tolerability profile. The survival analysis revealed similar results for time to progression, i.e., patients with both ER+ and PR+ breast cancer appeared to gain the most benefit from fulvestrant.

Fulvestrant Versus Anastrozole

A phase III clinical trial (trial 0020) was performed to compare the efficacy and tolerability of fulvestrant at a dose of 250 mg in a once-monthly intramuscular injection with anastrozole at a dose of 1 mg once daily in tablets in postmenopausal women with advanced breast cancer whose disease had progressed after prior endocrine therapy [36]. Trial 0020 was an open-label, non-blinded, randomized, multicenter, parallel-group study conducted in South Africa, Europe, and Australia. The time to progression was the primary end point, and overall response rates, duration of response, and tolerability were determined as secondary end points. The median time to disease progression was similar between the fulvestrant and anastrozole arms (5.5 months and 5.1 months, respectively; HR, 0.98; 95 % CI, 0.80–1.21; $p=0.84$) with a median follow-up of 14.4 months. Although the overall response rates indicated a numerical benefit of fulvestrant (20.7 %) over anastrozole (15.7 %), this difference did not reach statistical significance (OR, 1.38; 95 % CI, 0.84–2.29; $p=0.20$). The clinical benefit rates were 44.6 % in the fulvestrant arm and 45.0 % in the anastrozole arm. The median duration of response was also similar in the two groups (14.3 months for fulvestrant and 14 months for anastrozole). Both fulvestrant and tamoxifen were well tolerated; treatment was terminated because of an adverse event in 3.2 % of fulvestrant-treated patients and 1.3 % of anastrozole-treated patients [141].

Another phase III, randomized, double-blind trial entitled "trial 0021" was conducted in North America concurrently with trial 0020 [142]. The main aim of the trial was to compare two doses of monthly fulvestrant (125 mg and 250 mg) as an intramuscular injection with anastrozole (1 mg/d

oral dose) in the treatment of patients with advanced breast cancer whose disease had progressed during prior endocrine therapy. The end points of this study were the same as those of trial 0020. To determine the clinical activity of 125 mg of fulvestrant, a planned preliminary data summary and an interim analysis were conducted. After the first 30 patients in the fulvestrant 125 mg group (combined from both trials) were enrolled into the studies and followed up for 3 months, both trials conducted a preliminary data summary. This interim assessment demonstrated insufficient evidence for 125 mg of fulvestrant in terms of clinical activity without any objective tumor response at 3 months. Thus, the independent data monitoring committee offered to stop recruitment to the fulvestrant 125 mg treatment arm. The patients who were already randomized into the 125 mg arm in trial 0021 were permitted to continue the 125 mg of fulvestrant or to withdraw from the trial and receive the other treatments at the discretion of the clinician. These patients were not monitored further for efficacy. As a consequence, the protocol for the study was amended to compare 250 mg of fulvestrant with 1 mg of anastrozole [142].

With a median follow-up of 16.8 months, fulvestrant was shown to be as effective as anastrozole with respect to time to progression (5.4 months with fulvestrant vs. 3.4 months with anastrozole: HR, 0.92; 95.14 % CI, 0.74–1.14; $p=0.43$). Both treatments resulted in 17.5 % overall response rates and statistically similar clinical benefit rates (42.2 % for fulvestrant and 36.1 % for anastrozole; 95 % CI, −4.00–16.41 %; $p=0.26$). In all patients, fulvestrant caused a longer duration of response compared to anastrozole (ratio of average response durations: 1.35; 95 % CI, 1.10–1.67; $p<0.01$). In responding patients, the median duration of response was 19 months for fulvestrant and 10.8 months for anastrozole. Both treatments were shown to be well tolerated [142].

In 2003, the authors performed the prospectively planned combined analysis of data from these two phase III trials comparing 250 mg of fulvestrant monthly ($n=428$) and 1 mg of anastrozole daily ($n=423$) in postmenopausal women with advanced breast carcinoma whose disease had previously progressed after receiving endocrine therapy [143]. The main aim of both trials was to demonstrate the superiority of fulvestrant over anastrozole. At a median follow-up of 15 months, disease progression occurred in approximately 83 % of patients in each arm. The median time to progression (5.5 months in the fulvestrant arm and 4.1 months in the anastrozole arm; HR, 0.95; 95.14 % CI, 0.82–1.10; $p = 0.48$) and overall response rates (19.2 % for fulvestrant and 16.5 % for anastrozole; 95.14 % CI, 2.27–9.05 %; $p = 0.31$) were similar between the two treatment arms. In responding patients, to obtain more complete information on the duration of response, further follow-up (median of 22.1 months) was performed; the median duration of response was determined (from randomization to disease progression). A statistical analysis of all randomized patients revealed a significantly longer duration of response in fulvestrant-treated patients compared to anastrozole-treated patients. Both drugs were well tolerated with few withdrawals due to drug-related adverse events (0.9 % in the fulvestrant group and 1.2 % in the anastrozole group). However, there was a lower incidence of joint disorders in the fulvestrant arm ($p = 0.0036$). These data further supported the use of fulvestrant as an additional, effective, and well-tolerated treatment option in postmenopausal women whose disease progressed during prior endocrine therapy, with efficacy end points slightly favoring fulvestrant [143].

Fulvestrant Plus Anastrozole Versus Anastrozole

Some patients eventually become resistant to single-agent endocrine therapy and experience disease progression, as observed for many other cancer therapies. It was hypothesized that fulvestrant combined with an AI might lead to better outcomes compared to anastrozole alone in patients with HR+ MBC. Subsequent, preclinical work precluded the potential synergy of fulvestrant with AI therapy to delay the development of endocrine resistance.

Bergh et al. performed an open-label randomized phase III clinical trial entitled "FACT" to compare the efficacy of anastrozole with that of combined fulvestrant and anastrozole therapy in women who had experienced a first relapse of breast cancer after the primary treatment of early disease [144]. Postmenopausal women or premenopausal women receiving an LHRH agonist were included. A total of 514 patients were randomized to receive fulvestrant (initiated with a loading dose followed by monthly injections) plus anastrozole (1 mg daily and $n = 258$) or to anastrozole (1 mg daily, $n = 256$) alone. Although two-thirds of the patients had been treated with adjuvant antiestrogens, only eight women had received an AI. The median time to progression, which was the primary end point of the study, was similar in the experimental and standard arms (10.8 vs. 10.2 months, respectively; hazard ratio, 0.99; 95 % CI, 0.81–1.20; $p = 0.91$). The median OS was also similar among the two treatment groups (37.8 and 38.2 months, respectively; hazard ratio, 1.0; 95 % CI, 0.76–1.32; $p = 1.00$). The incidences of prespecified adverse events were also similar. Hot flashes were more common in the experimental arm than in the standard arm (24.6 vs. 13.8 %, $p = 0.0023$). Death due to adverse events occurred in 4.3 % of the patients treated with the experimental regimen and 2 % of the patients in the standard arm [144].

The Southwest Oncology Group (SWOG) performed a similarly designed randomized phase III trial [145]. Treatment-naive postmenopausal women with MBC were randomized to receive either anastrozole (group 1) (1 mg orally every day with permission to cross over to fulvestrant alone as disease progressed) or anastrozole in combination with fulvestrant (group 2). The stratification was performed based on the absence or presence of prior adjuvant tamoxifen therapy. Fulvestrant was administered at a dose of 500 mg on day 1 and 250 mg on days 14 and 28 and monthly thereafter as an intramuscular injection. The clinical benefit rate was 73 % for the combination therapy and 70 % for single-agent anastrozole ($p = 0.39$). Stable disease was the most frequent response type. In patients who had measurable disease, the overall response rate was similar in the two arms (27 % for combination therapy vs. 22 % for anastrozole alone; $p = 0.26$). Three deaths in group 2 were potentially attributable to the treatment. The median PFS was 13.5 months in the anastrozole-alone arm and 15 months in the combination arm (hazard ratio for progression or death with combination therapy: 0.80; 95 % CI, 0.68–0.94; $p = 0.007$). The combination therapy provided a longer median overall survival (41.3 months vs. 47.7 months for anastrozole vs. the combination; hazard ratio, 0.81; 95 % CI, 0.65–1.00; $p = 0.05$); however, after progression, 41 % of the patients in the anastrozole group crossed over to fulvestrant. In general, combination therapy was more effective than single-agent anastrozole in all subgroups, without significant interactions. There was a similar rate of serious side effects between the two groups [145]. These findings indicated that combined use of anastrozole and fulvestrant was superior to anastrozole alone or the sequential administration of anastrozole with fulvestrant for the treatment of HR+ MBC, although the dose of fulvestrant in this trial was below the current standard.

In subgroup analyses that were not prespecified, among 414 women (59.7 %) who were not treated with prior tamoxifen, the median PFS was longer with combination therapy (12.6 months vs. 17 months in groups 1 and 2, respectively; hazard ratio for progression or death with combination arm: 0.74; 95 % CI, 0.59–0.92; $P = 0.006$) [145]. Among women with a prior tamoxifen history, the estimated median PFS was similar (14.1 months vs. 13.5 months, respectively; hazard ratio, 0.89; 95 % CI, 0.69–1.15; $P = 0.37$). There was no significant interaction between therapy and a history of prior adjuvant tamoxifen. Among women without prior tamoxifen, the OS was significantly different between the groups with a hazard ratio for death with the combination therapy of 0.74 (95 % CI, 0.56–0.98; $p = 0.04$); however, OS was similar among women with prior tamoxifen history (hazard ratio, 0.91; 95 % CI, 0.65–1.28; $p = 0.59$), and the combination therapy resulted in a benefit for both groups [145].

A possible explanation for the conflicting results in terms of efficacy between the FACT and SWOG S0226 studies is that the primary end point of FACT was time to disease progression, whereas the primary end point of SWOG S0226 was PFS. Although these end points appear similar, death without progression would only be captured in the SWOG S0226 study, thereby potentially increasing the progression numbers. Furthermore, the percentage of patients without a history of endocrine therapy was higher in the SWOG S0226 study than in the FACT study (59.7 % vs. 32.2 %, respectively) [145, 146].

Tan et al. performed a meta-analysis of these prospective randomized clinical trials and compared the effectiveness of fulvestrant+anastrozole with anastrozole alone as first-line treatment in postmenopausal women with HR+, HER2-negative MBC [147]. The pooled hazard ratio for PFS was 0.88 (95 % CI, 0.72–1.09; 95 % PI, 0.65–1.21), the pooled OS was 0.88 (95 % CI, 0.72–1.08; 95 % PI, 0.68–1.14) and the pooled odds ratio for the response rate was 1.13 (95 % CI, 0.79–1.63; 95 % PI, 0.78–1.65). A nonsignificant trend of marginal superiority was observed for anastrozole+fulvestrant compared to anastrozole alone for the end points of PFS, OS, and response rates.

Based on these data, the evidence for combining monthly fulvestrant at a dose of 250 mg with anastrozole is insufficient to recommend this combination as a first-line therapy for all women with postmenopausal HR+ breast cancer.

In 2013, Al-Mubarak et al. [138] performed a systematic review of eight randomized trials comparing fulvestrant versus other endocrine therapies. The hazard ratios for time to progression and the odds ratios for serious adverse events, drug discontinuation because of toxicity, and commonly observed toxicities were pooled in this meta-analysis. The meta-regression analysis was conducted to explore the heterogeneity of the study populations and fulvestrant dosing. No significant differences were observed in the time to progression between fulvestrant and the other treatment groups (HR, 0.94; $p = 0.18$). The meta-regression analysis demonstrated that fulvestrant, when used as a first-line treatment, reduced the hazard ratios for time to progression compared to AIs in studies in which fewer patients were administered adjuvant endocrine therapy and at higher doses. The rates of serious adverse events and treatment discontinuation were similar between the fulvestrant and other groups, but fulvestrant monotherapy was associated with less frequent arthralgia (OR, 0.73; $p=0.02$). Combining fulvestrant with AI did not improve the time to progression, but it did increase toxicity. Fulvestrant monotherapy was associated with similar efficacy but reduced arthralgia compared to other endocrine therapy options in unselected patient populations. High-dose fulvestrant monotherapy, when used as a first-line treatment or in patients with limited prior exposure to adjuvant endocrine therapy, may delay progression compared to AIs [138].

Another mode of action of fulvestrant that differs from that of other currently used antiestrogens is that fulvestrant consistently reduces PR levels in the tumor in a dose-dependent manner.

Similar to many other antiestrogens, resistance to fulvestrant occurs in the majority of patients with advanced breast cancer after prolonged therapy, although the underlying mechanisms are poorly understood and may include overexpression of the microRNA miR-221/222.

HER2-Positive Hormone Receptor-Positive Metastatic Breast Cancer

Premenopausal and Postmenopausal

Several studies have demonstrated the mutual effects of ER and HER2. In experimental models, despite initially lacking EGFR or HER2, hormone-sensitive ER+ breast cancer cells usually develop endocrine resistance over time via the enhanced expression of receptors involved in cross-talk with ER [148, 149]. Therefore, the overexpression of HER2 results in resistance to established endocrine therapies [150]. Combined therapeutic strategies might enhance endocrine effectiveness in patients with HR+, HER2+ breast cancer and delay disease progression for those with HR+, HER2-negative tumors at risk of early relapse. This treatment strategy has been evaluated in many clinical studies.

Endocrine Treatment with or Without Trastuzumab

Mackey and colleagues compared the AI anastrozole with combination anastrozole+trastuzumab in an open-label, multicenter, two-arm phase III trial [151]. A total of 208 HER2+, ER+ patients were randomized to receive either anastrozole alone (1 mg daily) or anastrozole (1 mg daily) + trastuzumab (4 mg/kg loading dose followed by 2 mg/kg weekly) until disease progression. Patients who had not received prior chemotherapy in the metastatic setting were also included. Patients who received tamoxifen either in the adjuvant or first-line metastatic setting were included. PFS was the primary end point. The median PFS was twofold longer in the anastrozole+trastuzumab arm: 4.8 months vs. 2.4 months with anastrozole alone ($p=0.0016$). More than 15 % of the patients in the anastrozole+trastuzumab arm had PFS exceeding 2 years. The overall response rate was significantly better in the anastrozole+trastuzumab arm (58 %) than the anastrozole-alone arm (45 %), although the individual rates were similar [151]. In the anastrozole-alone arm, 70 % of the patients were allowed to proceed to trastuzumab later in the course of disease. OS, although not statistically significant, was numerically superior in the combination arm (28.5 vs. 23.9 months, $p=0.325$). Treatment with anastrozole+trastuzumab was associated with manageable toxicity with no unexpected adverse events, although the frequency of common adverse events was increased [151].

Kaufman et al. investigated endocrine therapy in combination with anti-HER2 therapy in a randomized trial entitled "The Trastuzumab and Anastrozole Directed Against ER+ HER2+ Mammary Carcinoma (TAnDEM)" [152]. Postmenopausal women with HR+ and HER2+ MBC were randomized to receive anastrozole alone ($n=104$) or combination therapy with anastrozole and trastuzumab ($n=103$), and patients treated with anastrozole alone were allowed to cross over to the combination therapy after disease progression in the anastrozole arm. Approximately two-thirds of the patients on anastrozole alone received the combination treatment at progression. At the central laboratory, receptor analyses were repeated, and HR positivity was confirmed in 150 patients (77 in the trastuzumab+anastrozole arm; 73 in the anastrozole-alone arm). However, 44 patients (21 in the trastuzumab+anastrozole arm; 23 in the anastrozole-alone arm) were identified as ER/PR negative by the central laboratory [152]. Treatment with trastuzumab+anastrozole resulted in significantly longer PFS compared to treatment with anastrozole alone (4.8 vs. 2.4 months, respectively; hazard ratio 0.63; 95 % CI, 0.47–0.8; log-rank $p=0.0016$). Among patients with centrally confirmed HR positivity, the median PFS was 5.6 months in the combination arm and 3.8 months in the anastrozole-alone arm (log-rank $p=0.006$) [152]. However, the median OS was statistically similar between the two treatment groups in either the overall or centrally confirmed HR+ subgroups, which may be attributable in part to the high crossover rate [152].

The addition of an AI to HER2-targeted therapy may delay the use of chemotherapy in some patients and provides an important advantage. Based on these positive results, trastuzumab used concurrently with an AI has been approved for the treatment of postmenopausal patients with HR+ and HER2+ MBC who have not received prior trastuzumab. Based on the results of clinical trials, nonsteroidal AIs have become one of the standard treatment options in this patient population; however, there is no reason to believe a different result would be obtained with a steroidal AI.

Endocrine Treatment with or Without Lapatinib

In the first-line setting, the combination of lapatinib with letrozole was compared to letrozole+placebo in 1,286 patients with HR+ MBC [107]. In HER2+ patients, lapatinib+letrozole led to a longer median PFS than letrozole+placebo (8.2 vs. 3 months; HR, 0.71; 95 % CI, 0.53–0.96; $p=0.019$) [153]. In patients with centrally confirmed HR+, HER2-negative disease ($n=952$), lapatinib+letrozole did not improve PFS [153].

In 2012, a systematic review analyzed outcomes including OS, PFS, time to progression, and ORR of first-line hormone therapy in combination with an anti-HER2 agent in HR+, HER2+ MBC patients [154]. Relevant interventions were combination

regimens with endocrine agents including AIs (letrozole, anastrozole, and exemestane), tamoxifen, and an anti-HER2 agent (lapatinib or trastuzumab). They searched randomized controlled clinical trials reported in six databases until January 2009 to assess the safety and efficacy of first-line treatments for postmenopausal women with HR+ and HER2+ MBC without prior therapy for advanced or metastatic disease. Eighteen studies (62 papers) were included in the systematic analysis. Lapatinib+letrozole was significantly superior to letrozole alone based on a direct head-to-head study in terms of PFS/time to progression and overall response rate. In terms of PFS/time to progression and ORR, tamoxifen (hazard ratio, 0.45 [95 % CI, 0.32–0.65]) and anastrozole (hazard ratio, 0.53 [95 % CI, 0.36–0.80]) were significantly worse (tamoxifen, OR, 0.25 [95 % CI, 0.12–0.53]; anastrozole, OR, 0.27 [95 % CI, 0.12, 0.58]) compared to lapatinib+letrozole. The combination also appeared significantly superior to exemestane in terms of PFS/time to progression (hazard ratio, 0.52 [95 % CI, 0.34, 0.79]). Lapatinib+letrozole was also superior, although not significantly, in terms of OS to tamoxifen, hazard ratio, 0.74 (0.49, 1.12); anastrozole, hazard ratio, 0.71 (0.45, 1.14); and exemestane, hazard ratio, 0.65 (0.39, 1.11). Although the p value was statistically nonsignificant, when compared to trastuzumab+anastrozole, lapatinib+letrozole was superior in terms of OS (hazard ratio, 0.85 [0.47, 1.54]), PFS/time to progression (hazard ratio, 0.89 [0.54, 1.47]), and ORR (OR, 0.92 [0.24, 3.48]). Based on a direct head-to-head study, lapatinib+letrozole was significantly superior to letrozole in terms of PFS/time to progression and ORR. Consequently, indirect comparisons appeared to favor lapatinib+letrozole versus other first-line treatments in this patient population in terms of three main outcomes: OS, PFS/time to progression, and ORR.

The FDA approved lapatinib+letrozole for the treatment of postmenopausal women with HR+ MBC overexpressing the HER2 receptor for whom hormonal therapy is indicated. However, it is important to note that lapatinib in combination with an AI has not yet been compared to a trastuzumab-containing chemotherapy regimen for the treatment of MBC.

The results of the CALGB 40302 trial were recently published. The authors investigated whether lapatinib improved PFS among women with HR+ MBC treated with fulvestrant [155]. Eligible women had ER+ and/or PR+ tumors, regardless of HER2 positivity and prior AI treatment. Five hundred milligrams of fulvestrant was administered to patients intramuscularly on day 1, followed by 250 mg on days 15 and 28 and every 4 weeks thereafter with either 1,500 mg of lapatinib or placebo daily. The study planned to accrue 324 patients and was powered for a 50 % improvement in PFS with lapatinib from 5 to 7.5 months. At the third planned interim analysis, the futility boundary was crossed, and the data and safety monitoring board recommended study closure, having accrued 295 patients. No difference was detected in PFS (hazard ratio of placebo to lapatinib: 1.04; 95 % CI, 0.82–1.33; $p = 0.37$); the median PFS was 4.7 months for fulvestrant+lapatinib versus 3.8 months for fulvestrant+placebo at the final analysis. There was no difference in OS (hazard ratio, 0.91; 95 % CI, 0.68–1.21; $p = 0.25$). The median PFS was similar among the treatment arms (4.1 vs. 3.8 months for HER2-normal tumors) in HER2+ MBC patients, and lapatinib was associated with longer median PFS (5.9 vs. 3.3 months), but the differential treatment effect by HER2 status was not significant ($p = 0.53$). Diarrhea, fatigue, and rash were the most frequently experienced toxicities associated with lapatinib. Adding lapatinib to fulvestrant did not improve PFS or OS in ER+ advanced breast cancer and increased toxicity [155].

In premenopausal women with HR+ HER2+ breast cancer, data are insufficient to conclude the overall benefit of tamoxifen therapy in combination with an anti HER2 agent. However, based on the data obtained in postmenopausal women, tamoxifen+trastuzumab is widely used in premenopausal breast cancer patients. In conclusion, the combination of an anti-HER2 agent with endocrine therapy is an active and safe method with favorable response rates and survival advantages in patients with HR+ and HER2+ advanced breast cancer.

Targeted Agents for Endocrine-Resistant Hormone Receptor-Positive Breast Cancer

Preclinical studies have suggested that acquired AI resistance may be a result of the upregulation of several growth factor receptors such as HER2 and IGFR1. The increased expression of these receptors may promote the activation of downstream protein kinases such as mitogen-activated protein kinase and AKT, which, in turn, could result in increased ER phosphorylation and activation and sensitization of tumor cells to estrogen. The combination of endocrine agents with a molecular-targeted agent continues to be explored in several currently active or recently finalized clinical trials with the aim of overcoming endocrine resistance.

PI3K-AKT-MTOR Signaling Pathway

The development of resistance to endocrine therapy in breast cancer has been linked to activation of the PI3K-Akt-mTOR signaling pathway. The inhibition of proliferation could be synergistically enhanced by the addition of an mTOR inhibitor to endocrine treatment [156]. The Breast Cancer Trials of Oral Everolimus-2 (BOLERO-2) study investigated the safety and efficacy of the mTOR inhibitor everolimus in combination with exemestane in breast cancer patients who had been previously treated with NSAIs [157]. Patients were randomly assigned to receive 25 mg of exemestane daily or exemestane plus 10 mg of everolimus daily. The study demonstrated that concomitant use prolonged PFS (median of 7 vs. 3 months; hazard ratio for mortality: 0.43, 95 % CI, 0.35–0.54) and provided a higher overall response rate (9.5 vs. 0.4 %). Nonetheless, combination therapy was associated with a higher incidence of serious adverse events including stomatitis (8 %), dyspnea (4 %), noninfectious pneumonitis (3 %), and elevated liver enzymes (3 %) compared to exemestane monotherapy. However, combination therapy led to a higher percentage of treatment discontinuation [158].

The combination of everolimus with tamoxifen was studied by the Groupe d'Investigateurs

Nationaux pour l'Etude des Cancers Ovariens et du sein (GINECO) [159]. Postmenopausal women ($n=111$) who had progression on an AI were randomly assigned to receive tamoxifen with or without everolimus. The combination therapy resulted in an improved time to progression (median of 9 vs. 5 months; hazard ratio, 0.54; 95 % CI, 0.36–0.81) and in risk of death (hazard ratio, 0.45; 95 % CI, 0.24–0.81). However, the overall response rates of the two arms were similar (14 vs. 13 %). Furthermore, grade 3–4 stomatitis (11 vs. 0 %), anorexia (7 vs. 4 %), and the incidence of pneumonitis were higher in the combination therapy arm.

Insulin-Like Growth Factors (IGF-1 AND IGF-2)

The binding of insulin-like growth factors (IGF-1 and IGF-2) to the IGF-1 receptor (IGF-1R) enhances cell proliferation and prolongs cell survival. Ganitumab is a monoclonal IgG1 antibody that blocks IGF-1R. In a phase II double-blind randomized controlled trial, the efficacy and safety of ganitumab in combination with endocrine therapy was investigated in postmenopausal patients with HR+ locally advanced or MBC previously treated with endocrine agents [160]. The median PFS was similar between the ganitumab and placebo arms (3.9 months vs. 5.7 months; $p=0.44$). However, OS was shorter in the ganitumab arm than in the placebo arm (HR, 1.78; 80 % CI, 1.27–2.50; $p=0.025$). With the exception of hyperglycemia (11 vs. 0 %), adverse events were generally similar between the groups. Because the addition of ganitumab to endocrine treatment in women with previously treated HR+ locally advanced or MBC did not improve outcomes, further studies of ganitumab in this patient subgroup have not been designed.

Class I Histone Deacetylases Inhibitors

Entinostat is a small-molecule inhibitor of class I histone deacetylases that plays a key function in the control of gene expression. It exerts antiproliferative effects and promotes apoptosis in breast cancer cell lines and has been evaluated as a second or later line of therapy in women with ER+ breast cancer. In the ENtinostat Combinations Overcoming REsistance (ENCORE 301) randomized phase II trial, 130 women who had previously progressed on AI therapy were randomly assigned to receive 25 mg of exemestane daily with 5 mg of entinostat daily or with placebo [161]. The patients included in the trial had undergone multiple prior lines of therapy including chemotherapy and endocrine agents. The preliminary findings demonstrated that exemestane+entinostat therapy improved PFS (median of 4 vs. 2 months) at the expense of more fatigue (46 vs. 26 %) and uncomplicated neutropenia (25 vs. 0 %).

Cyclin-Dependent Kinases 4 and 6 Inhibitor

PD 0332991, called palbociclib, is a highly selective, orally administered inhibitor of cyclin-dependent kinases 4 and 6 (CDK 4/6). Preclinical studies demonstrated that palbociclib inhibits the proliferation of ER+ breast cancer cell lines, and early clinical trials suggested that it improves PFS when combined with an endocrine agent [162]. PALOMA3 trial is a phase III randomized trial which included patients with HR+ and HER2- advanced breast cancer to compare palbociclib plus fulvestrant with placebo plus fulvestrant. The study was stopped early due to significant efficacy results reported at interim analysis favoring fulvestrant plus palbociclib (median PFS: 9.2 versus 3.8 months; HR:0.42, 95 % CI 0.32–0.56; p < 0.001). Although longer follow-up is required to obtain the impact of combination therapy on OS, available PFS data support the use of plabociclib in combination with fulvestrant.

In conclusion, endocrine therapy should be considered for patients with hormone-sensitive advanced breast cancer without life-threatening visceral involvement. Premenopausal women with HR+ advanced breast cancer should receive ovarian ablation or functional suppression therapy in combination with other endocrine agents recommended to postmenopausal women. Nonsteroidal AIs comprising anastrozole and

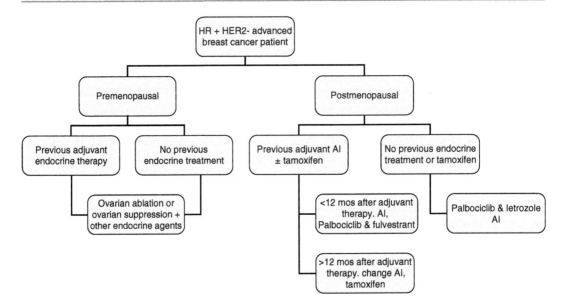

Fig. 31.2 Summary of treatment algorithms for hormone receptor-positive (HR+) and HER2-negative (HER2-) metastatic breast cancer

letrozole, steroidal AIs (exemestane), fulvestrant, tamoxifen or toremifene, progestins such as megestrol acetate and fluoxymesterone, and estrogens such as ethinyl estradiol can be used sequentially. Exemestane in combination with everolimus may be offered to patients whose disease progressed under nonsteroidal AIs. Trastuzumab or lapatinib can be combined with other endocrine agents, particularly AIs or tamoxifen, in patients with both HER2- and HR-positive breast cancer. Several targeted agents are currently being studied in patients with HR+ and endocrine-resistant disease, and in the near feature, there may be many other treatment options for HR+ endocrine therapy-resistant advanced breast cancer. A summary of treatment algorithms is presented in Fig. 31.2.

References

1. Gennari A, Conte P, Rosso R, Orlandini C, Bruzzi P. Survival of metastatic breast carcinoma patients over a 20-year period: a retrospective analysis based on individual patient data from six consecutive studies. Cancer. 2005;104(8):1742–50.
2. Criscitiello C, Andre F, Thompson AM, De Laurentiis M, Esposito A, Gelao L, et al. Biopsy confirmation of metastatic sites in breast cancer patients: clinical impact and future perspectives. Breast Cancer Res. 2014;16(2):205.
3. Early Breast Cancer Trialists' Collaborative Group (EBCTCG). Effects of chemotherapy and hormonal therapy for early breast cancer on recurrence and 15-year survival: an overview of the randomised trials. Lancet. 2005;365:1687–717.
4. Lu J, Steeg PS, Price JE, Krishnamurthy S, Mani SA, Reuben J, et al. Breast cancer metastasis: challenges and opportunities. Cancer Res. 2009;69(12):4951–3.
5. Tsai MJ, O'Malley BW. Molecular mechanisms of action of steroid/thyroid receptor superfamily members. Annu Rev Biochem. 1994;63:451–86.
6. Horwitz KB, Jackson TA, Bain DL, Richer JK, Takimoto GS, Tung L, et al. Nuclear receptor coactivators and corepressors. Mol Endocrinol. 1996;10(10):1167–77.
7. Huet G, Mérot Y, Le Dily F, Kern L, Ferrière F, Saligaut C, et al. Loss of E-cadherin-mediated cell contacts reduces estrogen receptor alpha (ER alpha) transcriptional efficiency by affecting the respective contribution exerted by AF1 and AF2 transactivation functions. Biochem Biophys Res Commun. 2008;365(2):304–9.
8. Kato S, Endoh H, Masuhiro Y, Kitamoto T, Uchiyama S, Sasaki H, et al. Activation of the estrogen receptor through phosphorylation by mitogen-activated protein kinase. Science. 1995;270(5241):1491–4.
9. Parikh PM, Gupta S, Dawood S, Rugo H, Bhattacharyya GS, Agarwal A, et al. ICON 2013: practical consensus recommendations for hormone receptor-positive Her2-negative advanced

or metastatic breastcancer. Indian J Cancer. 2014;51(1):73–9.

10. Yang YF, Liao YY, Yang M, Peng NF, Xie SR, Xie YF, et al. Discordances in ER, PR and HER2 receptors between primary and recurrent/metastatic lesions and their impact on survival in breast cancer patients. Med Oncol. 2014;31(10):214.

11. Chang HJ, Han SW, Oh DY, Im SA, Jeon YK, Park IA, et al. Discordant human epidermal growth factor receptor 2 and HR status in primary and MBC and response to trastuzumab. Jpn J Clin Oncol. 2011;41(5):593–9.

12. National Comprehensive Cancer Network Clinical Practice Guidelines in Oncology: Breast Cancer, Version 3, 2014. http://www.nccn.org/professionals/physiciangls/pdf/breast.pdf.

13. National Collaborating Centre for Cancer (UK). Advanced breast cancer: diagnosis and treatment. Cardiff, United Kingdom, National Collaborating Centre for Cancer (UK), 2009;90–332.

14. Wilcken N, Hornbuckle J, Ghersi D. Chemotherapy alone versus endocrine therapy alone for metastatic breast cancer. Cochrane Database of Systematic Rev;(2):2003. Art. No.: CD002747. DOI: 10.1002/14651858.CD002747.

15. Partridge AH, Rumble RB, Carey LA, Come SE, Davidson NE, Di Leo A, et al. Chemotherapy and targeted therapy for women with human epidermal growth factor receptor 2-negative (or unknown) advanced breast cancer: American Society of Clinical Oncology Clinical Practice Guideline. J Clin Oncol. 2014;32(29):3307–29.

16. Dutta U, Pant K. AIs: past, present and future in breast cancer therapy. Med Oncol. 2008;25:113–24.

17. Paterson R, Russel MH. Clinical trials in malignant disease. Part II-breast cancer: value of irradiation of the ovaries. J Fac Radiol. 1959;10:130–3.

18. Beatson GT. On the treatment of inoperable cases of carcinoma of the mamma: suggestion for a new method of treatment, with illustrative cases. Lancet. 1896;2:104–7.

19. Jensen EV, Greene GL, Closs LE, DeSombre ER, Nadji M. Receptors reconsidered: a 20-year perspective. Rec Prog Horm Res. 1982;38:1–40.

20. Blamey RW, Jonat W, Kaufmann M, Bianco AR, Namer M. Goserelin depot in the treatment of premenopausal advanced breast cancer. Eur J Cancer. 1992;28:810–4.

21. Foekens JA, Henkelman ME, Fukkink JF, Blankenstein MA, Klijn JG. Combined effects of buserelin, estradiol and tamoxifen on the growth of MCF-7 human breast cancer cells in vitro. Biochem Biophys Res Commun. 1986;140:550–6.

22. Klijn JGM, Berns PM, Bontenbal M, Alexieva-Figusch J, Foekens JA. Clinical breast cancer, new developments in selection and endocrine treatment of patients. J Steroid Biochem Mol Biol. 1992;43:211–21.

23. Taylor CW, Green S, Dalton WS, Martino S, Rector D, Ingle JN, et al. Multicenter randomized clinical trial of goserelin versus surgical oophorectomy in premenopausal patients with receptor-positive MBC: an intergroup study. J Clin Oncol. 1998;16(3):994–9.

24. Jaiyesimi IA, Buzdar AU, Decker DA, Hortobagyi GN. Use of tamoxifen for breast cancer: twenty-eight years later. J Clin Oncol. 1995;13(2):513–29.

25. Klopper A, Hall M. New synthetic agent for the induction of ovulation: preliminary trial in women. Br Med J. 1971;2:152–4.

26. Williamson JG, Ellis JD. The induction of ovulation by tamoxifen. J Obstet Gynaecol Br Commonw. 1973;80:844–7.

27. Nicholson RI, Golder MP. The effect of synthetic antioestrogens on the growth and biochemistry of rat mammary tumours. Eur J Cancer. 1975;11:571–9.

28. Cole MP, Jones CTA, Todd IDH. A new antioestrogenic agent in late breast cancer: an early clinical appraisal of ICI 46,474. Br J Cancer. 1971;25:270–5.

29. Heel RC, Brogden RN, Speight TM, Avery GS. Tamoxifen: a review of its pharmacological properties and therapeutic use in the treatment of breast cancer. Drugs. 1978;16(1):1–24.

30. Imai Y, Leung CKH, Friesen HG, Shiu RP. Epidermal growth factor receptors and effect of epidermal growth factor on growth of human breast cancer cells in long term tissue culture. Cancer Res. 1982;42:4394–8.

31. Osborne CK, Coronado EB, Kitten LJ, Arteaga CI, Fuqua SA, Ramasharma K, et al. Insulin like growth factor-II (IGF-II): a potential autocrine/paracrine growth factor for human breast cancer acting via IGF-1 receptor. Mol Endocrinol. 1989;3:1701–9.

32. Sporn MB, Roberts AB. Transforming growth factor-beta. Multiple actions and potential clinical applications. JAMA. 1989;262:938–41.

33. Osborne CK, Boldt DH, Clark GM, Trent JM. Effects of tamoxifen on human breast cancer cell cycle kinetics: accumulation of cells in early G1 phase. Cancer Res. 1983;43(8):3583–5.

34. Jordan VC. Long-term tamoxifen therapy to control or to prevent breast cancer: laboratory concept to clinical trials. Prog Clin Biol Res. 1988;262:105–23.

35. Sutherland RL, Hall RE, Taylor IW. Cell proliferation kinetics of MCF-7 human mammary carcinoma cells in culture and effects of tamoxifen on exponentially growing and plateau-phase cells. Cancer Res. 1983;43(9):3998–4006.

36. Lippman M, Bolan G, Huff K. The effects of estrogens and antiestrogens on hormone-responsive human breast cancer in long-term tissue culture. Cancer Res. 1976;36:4595–601.

37. Darbre PD, Curtis S, King RJ. Effects of estradiol and tamoxifen on human breast cancer cells in serum-free culture. Cancer Res. 1984;44:2790–3.

38. Sutherland RL, Murphy LC, Foo MS, Green MD, Whybourne AM, Krozowski ZS. High affinity antioestrogen binding site distinct from the oestrogen receptor. Nature. 1980;288:273–5.

39. Horgan K, Cooke E, Hallett MB, Mansel RE. Inhibition of protein kinase C mediated signal

transduction by tamoxifen. Importance for antitumour activity. Biochem Pharmacol. 1986;35(24):4463–5.

40. Gulino A, Barrera G, Vacca A, Farina A, Ferretti C, Screpanti I, et al. Calmodulin antagonism and growth-inhibiting activity of triphenylethylene antiestrogens in MCF-7 human breast cancer cells. Cancer Res. 1986;46(1):6274–8.

41. Berry J, Green BJ, Matheson DS. Modulation of natural killer cell activity by tamoxifen in stage I postmenopausal breast cancer. Eur J Cancer Clin Oncol. 1987;23(5):517–20.

42. Love RR, Mazess RB, Barden HS, Epstein S, Newcomb PA, Jordan VC, et al. Effects of tamoxifen on bone mineral density in postmenopausal women with breast cancer. N Engl J Med. 1992;326(13):852–6.

43. Reddel RR, Murphy LC, Hall RE, Sutherland RL. Differential sensitivity of human breast cancer cell lines to the growth-inhibitory effects of tamoxifen. Cancer Res. 1985;45(4):1525–31.

44. Margreiter R, Wiegle J. Tamoxifen (Nolvadex) for premenopausal patients with advanced breast cancer. Breast Cancer Res Treat. 1984;4:45–84.

45. Sawka CA, Pritchard KI, Paterson AHG, Sutherland DJ, Thomson DB, Shelley WE, et al. Role and mechanism of action of tamoxifen in premenopausal women with metastatic breast carcinoma. Cancer Res. 1986;46:3152–6.

46. Sawka CA, Pritchard KI, Shelley W, DeBoer G, Paterson AII, Meakin JW, et al. A randomized crossover trial of tamoxifen versus ovarian ablation for MBC in premenopausal women: a report of the National Cancer Institute of Canada Clinical Trials Group (NCIC CTG) trial MA.1. Breast Cancer Res Treat. 1997;44(3):211–5.

47. Crump M, Sawka CA, DeBoer G, Buchanan RB, Ingle JN, Forbes J, et al. An individual patient-based meta-analysis of tamoxifen versus ovarian ablation as first line endocrine therapy for premenopausal women with MBC. Breast Cancer Res Treat. 1997;44(3):201–10.

48. Klijn JG, Blamey RW, Boccardo F, Tominaga T, Duchateau L, Sylvester R. Combined Hormone Agents Trialists' Group and the European Organization for Research and Treatment of Cancer. Combined tamoxifen and luteinizing hormone-releasing hormone (LHRH) agonist versus LHRH agonist alone in premenopausal advanced breast cancer: a meta-analysis of four randomized trials. J Clin Oncol. 2001;19(2):343–53.

49. Adjuvant Breast Cancer Trials Collaborative Group. Ovarian ablation or suppression in premenopausal early breast cancer: results from the international adjuvant breast cancer ovarian ablation or suppression randomized trial. J Natl Cancer Inst. 2007;99(7):516–25.

50. Francis PA, Regan MM, Fleming GF, Láng I, Ciruelos E, Bellet M, et al. Adjuvant ovarian suppression in premenopausal breast cancer. N Engl J Med. 2015;372:436–46.

51. Jonat W, Kaufmann M, Blamey RW, Howell A, Collins JP, Coates A, et al. A randomised study to compare the effect of the luteinising hormone releasing hormone (LHRH) analogue goserelin with or without tamoxifen in pre- and perimenopausal patients with advanced breast cancer. Eur J Cancer. 1995;31(2):137–42.

52. Lerner LJ, Holthaus FJ, Thompson CR. A non-steroidal estrogen antiagonist 1-(p-2-diethylaminoethoxyphenyl)-1-phenyl-2-p-methoxyphenyl ethanol. Endocrinology. 1958;63(3):295–318.

53. Harper MJ, Walpole AL. A new derivative of triphenylethylene: effect on implantation and mode of action in rats. J Reprod Fertil. 1967;13(1):101–19.

54. Harper MJ, Walpole AL. Mode of action of I.C.I. 46,474 in preventing implantation in rats. J Endocrinol. 1967;37(1):83–92.

55. Fisher B, Costantino JP, Wickerham DL, Redmond CK, Kavanah M, Cronin WM, et al. Tamoxifen for prevention of breast cancer: report of the National Surgical Adjuvant Breast and Bowel Project P-1 Study. J Natl Cancer Inst. 1998;90(18):1371–88.

56. Bryant HU, Dere WH. Selective estrogen receptor modulators: an alternative to hormone replacement therapy. Proc Soc Exp Biol Med. 1998;217(1):45–52.

57. Szamel I, Vincze B, Hindy I, Kerpel-Fronius S, Eckhardt S, Mäenpää J, et al. Hormonal effects of toremifene in breast cancer patients. J Steroid Biochem. 1990;36(3):243–7.

58. Coombes RC, Haynes BP, Dowsett M, Quigley M, English J, Judson IR, et al. Idoxifene: report of a phase I study in patients with MBC. Cancer Res. 1995;55(5):1070–4.

59. Bruning PF. Droloxifene, a new anti-oestrogen in postmenopausal advanced breast cancer: preliminary results of a double-blind dose-finding phase II trial. Eur J Cancer. 1992;28(8–9):1404–7.

60. Wakeling AE. Hormone therapy in breast and prostate cancer. Jordan VC, Furr B JA, editors. Chapter 7: Pure antiestrogens. Humana press totowa, New Jersey; 2002. p. 162.

61. Mika VJ. Mustonen, Seppo Pyrhönen, Pirkko-Liisa Kellokumpu-Lehtinen. Toremifene in the treatment of breast cancer. World J Clin Oncol. 2014;5(3):393–405.

62. Mao C, Yang ZY, He BF, Liu S, Zhou JH, Luo RC, et al. Toremifene versus tamoxifen for advanced breast cancer. Cochrane Database Syst Rev;(7):2012. Art. No.: CD008926. DOI: 10.1002/14651858. CD008926.pub2.

63. Schwarzel WC, Kruggel W, Brodie HJ, Liu S, Zhou JH, Luo RC. Studies on the mechanism of estrogen biosynthesis. VII. The development of inhibitors of the enzyme system in the human placenta. Endocrinol. 1973;92:866–80.

64. Brodie AMH, Schwarzel WC, Shaikh AA, Brodie HJ. The effect of an AI, 4-hydroxy-4-androstene-3, 17-dione, on estrogen dependent processes in reproduction and breast cancer. Endocrinol. 1977;100:1684–94.

65. Lombardi P. Exemestane, a new steroidal AI of clinical relevance. Biochim Biophys Acta. 2002;1587(2–3):326–37.
66. Santen RJ. Potential clinical role of new AIs. Steroids. 1977;50:575–93.
67. Yue W, Zhou DJ, Chen S, Brodie A. A new nude mouse model for postmenopausal breast cancer using MCF-7 cells transfected with the human aromatase gene. Cancer Res. 1994;54:5092–5.
68. Yue W, Wang J, Savinov A, Brodie A. Effect of AIs on the growth of mammary tumors in a nude mouse model. Cancer Res. 1995;55:3073–7.
69. Various Authors. Proceedings of the conference aromatase: new perspectives for breast cancer. Cancer Res. 1982;42S.
70. Barone RM, Shamonki IM, Siiteri PK, Judd HL. Inhibition of peripheral aromatization of androstenedione to estrone in postmenopausal women with breast cancer using D1-testololactone. J Clin Endocrinol Metab. 1979;49:672–6.
71. Griffiths CT, Hall TC, Saba Z, Barlow JJ, Nevinny HB. Preliminary trial of aminoglutethimide in breast cancer. Cancer. 1973;32:31–7.
72. Harvey HA. AIs in clinical practice: current status and a look to the future. Semin Oncol. 1996;23:33–8.
73. De Jong PC, Blijham GH. New AIs for the treatment of advanced breast cancer in postmenopausal women. Neth J Med. 1999;55:50–8.
74. Rao RD, Cobleigh MA. Adjuvant endocrine therapy for breast cancer. Oncology. 2012;26(6):541–7.
75. Carlson RW, Theriault R, Schurman CM, Rivera E, Chung CT, Phan SC, et al. Phase II trial of anastrozole plus goserelin in the treatment of HR+, metastatic carcinoma of the breast in premenopausal women. J Clin Oncol. 2010;28(25):3917–21.
76. Park IH, Ro J, Lee KS, Kim EA, Kwon Y, Nam BH, et al. Phase II parallel group study showing comparable efficacy between premenopausal MBC patients treated with letrozole plus goserelin and postmenopausal patients treated with letrozole alone as first-line hormone therapy. J Clin Oncol. 2010;28(16):2705–11.
77. Ellis M, Naughton MJ, Ma CX. Treatment approach to metastatic hormone receptor-positive breast cancer: endocrine therapy. Uptodate. Section Editor: Hayes DF, Deputy Editor: Dizon DS, 2014; p. 1–17.
78. Espie M. Megestrol acetate in advanced breast carcinoma. Oncology. 1994;51(1):8–12.
79. Abrams J, Aisner J, Cirrincione C, Berry DA, Muss HB, Cooper MR, et al. Dose- response trial of megestrol acetate in advanced breast cancer: cancer and leukemia group B phase III study 8741. J Clin Oncol. 1999;17:64–73.
80. Petru E, Schmähl D. On the role of additive hormone monotherapy with tamoxifen, medroxyprogesterone acetate and aminoglutethimide, in advanced breast cancer. Klin Wochenschr. 1987;65(20):959–66.
81. Cardoso F, Bischoff J, Brain E, Zotano ÁG, Lück HJ, Tjan-Heijnen VC, et al. A review of the treatment of endocrine responsive MBC in postmenopausal women. Cancer Treat Rev. 2013;39(5):457–65.
82. Ingle JN, Mailliard JA, Schaid DJ, Krook JE, Gesme Jr DH, Windschitl HE, et al. A double-blind trial of tamoxifen plus prednisolone versus tamoxifen plus placebo in postmenopausal women with MBC. A collaborative trial of the North Central Cancer Treatment Group and Mayo Clinic. Cancer. 1991;68(1):34–9.
83. Tormey DC, Lippman ME, Edwards BK, Cassidy JG. Evaluation of tamoxifen doses with and without fluoxymesterone in advanced breast cancer. Ann Intern Med. 1983;98:139–44.
84. Ingle JN, Twito DI, Schaid DJ, Cullinan SA, Krook JE, Mailliard JA, et al. Randomized clinical trial of tamoxifen alone or combined with fluoxymesterone in postmenopausal women with MBC. J Clin Oncol. 1988;6:825–31.
85. Cavalli F, Beer M, Martz G, Jungi WF, Alberto P, Obrecht JP, et al. Concurrent or sequential use of cytotoxic chemotherapy and hormone treatment in advanced breast cancer: report of the Swiss Group for Clinical Cancer Research. Br Med J. 1983;286:5–8.
86. Australian and New Zealand Breast Cancer Trials Group. A randomized trial in postmenopausal patients with advanced breast cancer comparing endocrine and cytotoxic therapy given sequentially or in combination. J Clin Oncol. 1986;4:186–93.
87. Glick JH, Creech RH, Torri S, Holroyde C, Brodovsky H, Catalano RB, et al. Tamoxifen plus sequential CMF chemotherapy versus tamoxifen alone in postmenopausal patients with advanced breast cancer: a randomized trial. Cancer. 1980;45:735–41.
88. Bezwoda WR, Derman D, DeMoor NG, Lange M, Levin J. Treatment of MBC in estrogen receptor positive patients: a randomized trial comparing tamoxifen alone versus tamoxifen plus CMF. Cancer. 1982;50:2747–50.
89. Mouridsen HT, Rose C, Engelsman E, Sylvester R, Rotmensz N. Combined cytotoxic and endocrine therapy in postmenopausal patients with advanced breast cancer. A randomized study of CMF vs CMF plus tamoxifen. Eur J Cancer Clin Oncol. 1985;21:291–9.
90. Cocconi G, Delisi V, Boni C, Mori P, Malacarne P, Amadori D, et al. Chemotherapy versus combination of chemotherapy and endocrine therapy in advanced breast cancer. A prospective randomized study. Cancer. 1983;51:581–8.
91. Bocccardo F, Rubagotti A, Rosso R, Santi L. Chemotherapy with or without tamoxifen in postmenopausal patients with late breast cancer: a randomized study. J Steroid Biochem. 1985;23:1123–7.
92. Lønning PE, Dowsett M, Powles TJ. Postmenopausal estrogen synthesis and metabolism: alterations caused by AIs used for the treatment of breast cancer. J Steroid Biochem. 1990;35:355–66.
93. Luft R, Olivecrona H, Sjögren B. Hypophysectomy in man. Nord Med. 1952;14:351–4.
94. Huggins C, Dao TLY. Adrenalectomy and oophorectomy in treatment of advanced carcinoma of the breast. J Am Med Assoc. 1953;151:1388–94.

95. Fracchia AA, Randall HT, Farrow JH. The results of adrenalectomy in advanced breast cancer in 500 consecutive patients. Surg Gynecol Obstet. 1967;125:747–56.

96. Fracchia AA, Farrow JH, Miller TR, Tollefsen RH, Greenberg EJ, Knapper WH. Hypophysectomy as compared with adrenalectomy in the treatment of advanced carcinoma of the breast. Surg Gynecol Obstet. 1971;133:241–6.

97. Kofman S, Nagamani D, Buenger RF, Taylor SG. The use of prednisolone in the treatment of disseminated breast carcinoma. Cancer. 1958;11:226–32.

98. Lemon HM. Prednisone therapy of advanced mammary cancer. Cancer. 1959;12:93–107.

99. Harris AL, Cantwell BMJ, Dowsett M. High dose ketoconazole: endocrine and therapeutic effects in postmenopausal breast cancer. Br J Cancer. 1998;58:493–6.

100. Geisler J, Lonning PE. Aromatase inhibition: translation into a successful therapeutic approach. Clin Cancer Res. 2005;11:2809–21.

101. Bulun SE, Sebastian S, Takayama K, Suzuki T, Sasano H, Shozu M. The human CYP19 (aromatase P450) gene: update on physiologic roles and genomic organization of promoters. J Steroid Biochem Mol Biol. 2003;86:219–24.

102. Agarwal VR, Bulun SE, Leitch M, Rohrich R, Simpson ER. Use of alternative promoters to express the aromatase cytochrome p450 (CYP19) gene in breast adipose tissues of cancer-free and breast cancer patients. J Clin Endocrinol Metab. 1996;81:3843–9.

103. Mendelson CR, Jiang B, Shelton JM, Richardson JA, Hinshelwood MM. Transcriptional regulation of aromatase in placenta and ovary. J Steroid Biochem Mol Biol. 2005;95:25–33.

104. Dowsett M, Cantwell B, Lal A, Jeffcoate SL, Harris AL. Suppression of postmenopausal ovarian steroidogenesis with the luteinizing hormone- releasing hormone agonist goserelin. J Clin Endocrinol Metab. 1988;66:672–7.

105. Couzinet B, Meduri G, Lecce M, Young J, Brailly S, Loosfelt H, et al. The postmenopausal ovary is not a major androgen-producing gland. J Clin Endocrinol Metab. 2001;86:5060–6.

106. Johnson PE, Buzdar A. Are differences in the available AIs and inactivators significant? Clin Cancer Res. 2001;7(12):4360–8.

107. Van Asten K, Neven P, Lintermans A, Wildiers H, Paridaens R. AIs in the breast cancer clinic: focus on exemestane. Endocrinol Relat Cancer. 2014;21(1):31–49.

108. Lønning PE, Eikesdal HP. Aromatase inhibition 2013: clinical state of the art and questions that remain to be solved. Endocrinol Relat Cancer. 2013;20(4):183–201.

109. Folkerd EJ, Dixon JM, Renshaw L, A'Hern RP, Dowsett M. Suppression of plasma estrogen levels by letrozole and anastrozole is related to body mass index in patients with breast cancer. J Clin Oncol. 2012;30:2977–80.

110. Buzdar AU, Jonat W, Howell A, Jones SE, Blomqvist CP, Vogel CL, et al. Anastrozole versus megestrol acetate in the treatment of postmenopausal women with advanced breast carcinoma: results of a survival update based on a combined analysis of data from two mature phase III trials. Arimidex Study Group. Cancer. 1998;83(6):1142–52.

111. Buzdar A, Douma J, Davidson N, Elledge R, Morgan M, Smith R, et al. Phase III, multicenter, double-blind, randomized study of letrozole, an AI, for advanced breast cancer versus megestrol acetate. J Clin Oncol. 2001;19(14):3357–66.

112. Bonneterre J, Thurlimann B, Robertson JF, Krzakowski M, Mauriac L, Koralewski P, et al. Anastrozole versus tamoxifen as first-line therapy for advanced breast cancer in 668 postmenopausal women: results of the Tamoxifen or Arimidex Randomized Group Efficacy and Tolerability study. J Clin Oncol. 2000;18:3748–57.

113. Nabholtz JM, Buzdar A, Pollak M, Harwin W, Burton G, Mangalik A, et al. Anastrozole is superior to tamoxifen as first-line therapy for advanced breast cancer in postmenopausal women: results of a North American multicenter randomized trial. Arimidex Study Group. J Clin Oncol. 2001;18:3758–67.

114. Mouridsen H, Gershanovich M, Sun Y, Perez-Carrion R, Boni C, Monnier A, et al. Phase III study of letrozole versus tamoxifen as first-line therapy of advanced breast cancer in postmenopausal women: analysis of survival and update of efficacy from the International Letrozole Breast Cancer Group. J Clin Oncol. 2003;21:2101–9.

115. Paridaens RJ, Dirix LY, Beex LV, Nooij M, Cameron DA, Cufer T, et al. Phase III study comparing exemestane with tamoxifen as first-line hormonal treatment of MBC in postmenopausal women: the European Organisation for Research and Treatment of Cancer Breast Cancer Cooperative Group. J Clin Oncol. 2008;26:4883–90.

116. Johannessen DC, Engan T, Di Salle E, Zurlo MG, Paolini J, Ornati G, et al. Endocrine and clinical effects of exemestane (PNU 155971), a novel steroidal AI, in postmenopausal breast cancer patients: a phase I study. Clin Cancer Res. 1997;3(7):1101–8.

117. Evans TR, Di Salle E, Ornati G, Lassus M, Benedetti MS, Pianezzola E, et al. Phase I and endocrine study of exemestane (FCE 24304), a new AI, in postmenopausal women. Cancer Res. 1992;52(21):5933–9.

118. Geisler J, King N, Anker G, Ornati G, Di Salle E, Lønning PE, et al. In vivo inhibition of aromatization by exemestane, a novel irreversible AI, in postmenopausal breast cancer patients. Clin Cancer Res. 1998;4(9):2089–93.

119. Kaufmann M, Bajetta E, Dirix LY, Fein LE, Jones SE, Zilembo N, et al. Exemestane is superior to megestrol acetate after tamoxifen failure in postmenopausal women with advanced breast cancer: results of a phase III randomized double-blind trial. The Exemestane Study Group. J Clin Oncol. 2000;18(7):1399–411.

120. Mauri D, Pavlidis N, Polyzos NP, Ioannidis JP. Survival with aromatase inhibitors and inactivators versus standard hormonal therapy in advanced breast cancer: meta-analysis. J Natl Cancer Inst. 2006;98(18):1285–91.

121. Walker G, Xenophontos M, Chen L, Cheung K. Long-term efficacy and safety of exemestane in the treatment of breast cancer. Patient Prefer Adherence. 2013;7:245–58.

122. Lønning PE, Geisler J. Evaluation of plasma and tissue estrogen suppression with third-generation AIs: of relevance to clinical understanding? J Steroid Biochem Mol Biol. 2010;118(4–5):288–93.

123. Geisler J, Haynes B, Anker G, Dowsett M, Lønning PE. Influence of letrozole and anastrozole on total body aromatization and plasma estrogen levels in postmenopausal breast cancer patients evaluated in a randomized, cross-over study. J Clin Oncol. 2002;20(3):751–7.

124. Pauwels S, Antonio L, Jans I, Lintermans A, Neven P, Claessens F, et al. Sensitive routine liquid chromatography-tandem mass spectrometry method for serum estradiol and estrone without derivatization. Anal Bioanal Chem. 2013;405(26):8569–77.

125. Campos SM, Guastalla JP, Subar M, Abreu P, Winer EP, Cameron DA. A comparative study of exemestane versus anastrozole in patients with postmenopausal breast cancer with visceral metastases. Clin Breast Cancer. 2009;9(1):39–44.

126. Llombart-Cussac A, Ruiz A, Antón A, Barnadas A, Antolín S, Alés-Martínez JE, et al. Exemestane versus anastrozole as front-line endocrine therapy in postmenopausal patients with HR+, advanced breast cancer: final results from the Spanish Breast Cancer Group 2001-03 phase 2 randomized trial. Cancer. 2012;118(1):241–7.

127. Riemsma R, Forbes CA, Kessels A, Lykopoulos K, Amonkar MM, Rea DW, et al. Systematic review of AIs in the first-line treatment for hormone sensitive advanced or MBC. Breast Cancer Res Treat. 2010;123(1):9–24.

128. Lønning PE. Clinico-pharmacological aspects of different hormone treatments. Eur J Cancer. 2010;36(4):81–2.

129. Kim SH, Park IH, Lee H, Lee KS, Nam BH, Ro J. Efficacy of exemestane after nonsteroidal aromatase inhibitor use in metastatic breast cancer patients. Asian Pac J Cancer Prev. 2012;13(3):979–83.

130. Bertelli G, Garrone O, Merlano M, Occelli M, Bertolotti L, Castiglione F, et al. Sequential treatment with exemestane and non-steroidal aromatase inhibitors in advanced breast cancer. Oncology. 2005;69(6):471–7.

131. Steele N, Zekri J, Coleman R, Leonard R, Dunn K, Bowman A, et al. Exemestane in metastatic breast cancer: effective therapy after third-generation non-steroidal aromatase inhibitor failure. Breast. 2006;15(3):430–6.

132. Gennatas C, Michalaki V, Carvounis E, Psychogios J, Poulakaki N, Katsiamis G, et al. Third-line hormonal treatment with exemestane in postmenopausal patients with advanced breast cancer progressing on letrozole or anastrozole. A phase II trial conducted by the Hellenic Group of Oncology (HELGO). Tumori. 2006;92(1):13–7.

133. Chin YS, Beresford MJ, Ravichandran D, Makris A. Exemestane after non-steroidal aromatase inhibitors for post-menopausal women with advanced breast cancer. Breast. 2007;16(4):436–9.

134. Chia S, Gradishar W, Mauriac L, Bines J, Amant F, Federico M, et al. Double-blind, randomized placebo controlled trial of fulvestrant compared with exemestane after prior nonsteroidal aromatase inhibitor therapy in postmenopausal women with hormone receptor-positive, advanced breast cancer: results from EFECT. J Clin Oncol. 2008;26(10):1664–70.

135. Mauriac L, Romieu G, Bines J. Activity of fulvestrant versus exemestane in advanced breast cancer patients with or without visceral metastases: data from the EFECT trial. Breast Cancer Res Treat. 2009;117(1):69–75.

136. Iaffaioli RV, Formato R, Tortoriello A, Del Prete S, Caraglia M, Pappagallo G, et al. Phase II study of sequential hormonal therapy with anastrozole/exemestane in advanced and metastatic breast cancer. Br J Cancer. 2005;92(9):1621–5.

137. Beresford M, Tumur I, Chakrabarti J, Barden J, Rao N, Makris A. A qualitative systematic review of the evidence base for non-cross-resistance between steroidal and non-steroidal aromatase inhibitors in metastatic breast cancer. Clin Oncol (R Coll Radiol). 2011;23(3):209–15.

138. Howell A, Osborne CK, Morris C, Wakeling AE. ICI 182,780 (Faslodex): development of a novel, "pure" antiestrogen. Cancer. 2000;89(4):817–25.

139. Al-Mubarak M, Sacher AG, Ocana A, Vera-Badillo F, Seruga B, Amir E. Fulvestrant for advanced breast cancer: a meta-analysis. Cancer Treat Rev. 2013;39(7):753–8.

140. Robertson JF, Nicholson RI, Bundred NJ, Anderson E, Rayter Z, Dowsett M, et al. Comparison of the short-term biological effects of 7alpha-[9-(4,4,5,5,5-pentafluoropentylsulfinyl)-nonyl]estra-1,3,5, (10)-triene-3,17beta-diol (Faslodex) versus tamoxifen in postmenopausal women with primary breast cancer. Cancer Res. 2001;61(18):6739–46.

141. Ciruelos E, Pascual T, Arroyo Vozmediano ML, Blanco M, Manso L, Parrilla L, et al. The therapeutic role of fulvestrant in the management of patients with HR+ breast cancer. Breast. 2014;23(3):201–8.

142. Howell A, Robertson JF, Abram P, Lichinitser MR, Elledge R, Bajetta E, et al. Comparison of fulvestrant versus tamoxifen for the treatment of advanced breast cancer in postmenopausal women previously untreated with endocrine therapy: a multinational, double-blind, randomized trial. J Clin Oncol. 2004;22(9):1605–13.

143. Howell A, Robertson JF, Quaresma Albano J, Aschermannova A, Mauriac L, Kleeberg UR, et al.

Fulvestrant, formerly ICI 182,780, is as effective as anastrozole in postmenopausal women with advanced breast cancer progressing after prior endocrine treatment. J Clin Oncol. 2002;20(16):3396–403.

144. Osborne CK, Pippen J, Jones SE, Parker LM, Ellis M, Come S, et al. Double-blind, randomized trial comparing the efficacy and tolerability of fulvestrant versus anastrozole in postmenopausal women with advanced breast cancer progressing on prior endocrine therapy: results of a North American trial. J Clin Oncol. 2002;20(16):3386–95.

145. Robertson JF, Osborne CK, Howell A, Jones SE, Mauriac L, Ellis M, et al. Fulvestrant versus anastrozole for the treatment of advanced breast carcinoma in postmenopausal women: a prospective combined analysis of two multicenter trials. Cancer. 2003;98(2):229–38.

146. Bergh J, Jönsson PE, Lidbrink EK, Trudeau M, Eiermann W, Brattström D, et al. FACT: an open-label randomized phase III study of fulvestrant and anastrozole in combination compared with anastrozole alone as first-line therapy for patients with receptor-positive postmenopausal breast cancer. J Clin Oncol. 2012;30(16):1919–25.

147. Mehta RS, Barlow WE, Albain KS, Vandenberg TA, Dakhil SR, Tirumali NR, et al. Combination anastrozole and fulvestrant in MBC. N Engl J Med. 2012;367(5):435–44.

148. Tan PS, Haaland B, Montero AJ, Lopes G. A meta-analysis of anastrozole in combination with fulvestrant in the first line treatment of HR+ advanced breast cancer. Breast Cancer Res Treat. 2013;138(3):961–5.

149. Knowlden JM, Hutcheson IR, Jones HE. Elevated levels of epidermal growth factor receptor/cerbB2 heterodimers mediate an autocrine growth regulatory pathway in tamoxifen-resistant MCF-7 cells. Endocrinology. 2013;144:1032–44.

150. Massarweh S, Osborne CK, Jiang S, Wakeling AE, Rimawi M, Mohsin SK, et al. Mechanisms of tumor regression and resistance to estrogen deprivation and fulvestrant in a model of estrogen receptor-positive, HER-2/neu-positive breast cancer. Cancer Res. 2006;66:8266–77.

151. Shin I, Miller T, Arteaga CL. ErbB receptor signaling and therapeutic resistance to AIs. Clin Cancer Res. 2006;12:1008–12.

152. Mackey JR, Kaufman B, Clemens MR, Bapsy PP, Vaid A, Wardley A, et al. Trastuzumab prolongs progression-free survival in hormone-dependent and HER2+ MBC. Breast Cancer Res Treat. 2006;100:5.

153. Kaufman B, Mackey JR, Clemens MR, Bapsy PP, Vaid A, Wardley A, et al. Trastuzumab plus anastrozole versus anastrozole alone for the treatment of postmenopausal women with human epidermal growth factor receptor 2- positive, HR+ MBC: results from the randomized phase III TAnDEM study. J Clin Oncol. 2009;27:5529–37.

154. Johnston S, Pippen JJ, Pivot X, Lichinitser M, Sadeghi S, Dieras V, et al. Lapatinib combined with letrozole versus letrozole and placebo as first-line therapy for postmenopausal HR+ MBC. J Clin Oncol. 2009;27:5538–46.

155. Riemsma R, Forbes CA, Amonkar MM, Lykopoulos K, Diaz JR, Kleijnen J, et al. Systematic review of lapatinib in combination with letrozole compared with other first-line treatments for HR+(HR+) and HER2+ advanced or MBC (MBC). Curr Med Res Opin. 2012;28(8):1263–79.

156. Burstein HJ, Cirrincione CT, Barry WT, Chew HK, Tolaney SM, Lake DE, et al. Endocrine therapy with or without inhibition of epidermal growth factor receptor and human epidermal growth factor receptor 2: a randomized, double-blind, placebo-controlled phase III trial of fulvestrant with or without lapatinib for postmenopausal women with HR+ advanced breast cancer-CALGB 40302 (Alliance). J Clin Oncol. 2014;32(35):3959–66.

157. Boulay A, Rudloff J, Ye J, Zumstein-Mecker S, O'Reilly T, Evans DB, et al. Dual inhibition of mTOR and estrogen receptor signaling in vitro induces cell death in models of breast cancer. Clin Cancer Res. 2005;11(14):5319–28.

158. Baselga J, Campone M, Piccart M, Burris 3rd HA, Rugo HS, Sahmoud T, et al. Everolimus in postmenopausal hormone-receptor-positive advanced breast cancer. N Engl J Med. 2012;366(6):520–9.

159. Dhillon S. Everolimus in combination with exemestane: a review of its use in the treatment of patients with postmenopausal hormone receptor-positive, HER2-negative advanced breast cancer. Drugs. 2013;73(5):475–85.

160. Bachelot T, McCool R, Duffy S, Glanville J, Varley D, Fleetwood K, et al. Comparative efficacy of everolimus plus exemestane versus fulvestrant for hormone-receptor-positive advanced breast cancer following progression/recurrence after endocrine therapy: a network meta-analysis. Breast Cancer Res Treat. 2014;143(1):125–33.

161. Yardley DA, Ismail-Khan RR, Melichar B, Lichinitser M, Munster PN, Klein PM, et al. Randomized phase II, double-blind, placebo-controlled study of exemestane with or without entinostat in postmenopausal women with locally recurrent or metastatic estrogen receptor-positive breast cancer progressing on treatment with a nonsteroidal aromatase inhibitor. J Clin Oncol. 2013;31(17):2128–35.

162. Finn RS, Dering J, Conklin D, Kalous O, Cohen DJ, Desai AJ, et al. PD 0332991, a selective cyclin D kinase 4/6 inhibitor, preferentially inhibits proliferation of luminal estrogen receptor-positive human breast cancer cell lines in vitro. Breast Cancer Res. 2009;11(5):77.

163. Miller WR, Bartlett J, Brodie AM, Brueggemeier RW, di Salle E, Lønning PE, et al. Aromatase inhibitors: are there differences between steroidal and nonsteroidal aromatase inhibitors and do they matter? Oncologist. 2008;13(8):829–37.

Treatment of Metastatic Breast Cancer: Chemotherapy

32

Saveri Bhattacharya and Shannon L. Puhalla

Abstract

There is no prespecified treatment algorithm for patients with metastatic breast cancer and treatment is tailored to each patient's tumor biology as well as tolerance of side effects. Comorbidities, receptor status, and sites of metastasis are all taken into account when devising a treatment plan for each patient. Anthracyclines and taxanes continue to remain at the core of all treatment plans and both are equally efficacious in patients with metastatic breast cancer. The management of metastatic breast cancer aims at prolonging survival while maintaining quality of life.

Keywords

Metastatic breast cancer • Chemotherapy • Personalized therapy • Anthracyclines • Taxanes

S. Bhattacharya, DO
Hematology/Oncology, University of Pittsburgh, Pittsburgh, PA, USA
e-mail: Bhattacharyas3@upmc.edu

S.L. Puhalla, MD (✉)
Division of Hematology/Oncology, Magee Womens Cancer Program, University of Pittsburgh Cancer Institute, Pittsburgh, PA, USA

Division of Hematology/Oncology, Magee-Womens Hospital of UPMC, University of Pittsburgh School of Medicine, Pittsburgh, PA, USA
e-mail: puhallasl@mail.magee.edu

Introduction

The aim when treating metastatic breast cancer is not curing the disease but rather prolonging survival, alleviating symptoms, and maintaining quality of life. The advent of newer systemic chemotherapies has improved the median overall survival to approximately 18–24 months [1]. However, survival ranges from a few months to years. Factors that affect a patient's overall survival include the specific biology of tumor (e.g., hormone receptor positive, triple negative, or HER2 positive), sites of metastasis, and the burden of metastatic disease. Early-stage breast cancer has a 5-year survival rate of 97 %. However, for patients with metastatic disease, the 5-year survival rate ranges from 17 to 28 % [2]. Hormone receptor status and HER2 overexpression are some of the most important predictors of treatment response in patients with metastatic breast cancer. Patients with either HER2 overexpression or triple-negative metastatic breast cancer historically exhibit a reduced median survival. However, the advent of new therapies, such as pertuzumab in combination with trastuzumab and chemotherapy, is greatly improving survival rates for patients with HER2+ disease. For example, the likelihood of response is 70 % in patients with tumors expressing estrogen receptor (ER) and progesterone receptor (PR) versus 40 % in ER-positive/PR-negative or ER-negative/PR-positive versus less than 10 % in ER-negative/PR-negative tumors [3]. Estrogen receptor-positive and progesterone receptor-positive patients can receive endocrine therapy, which tends to be associated with fewer side effects than chemotherapy and helps maintain quality of life. However, if the tumor does not respond to endocrine therapy or once resistance develops, systemic chemotherapy will ultimately be required.

Principles of Metastatic Breast Cancer Treatment

No ideal sequence of chemotherapy for patients with metastatic breast cancer is available given the sheer volume of agents available. The treatment plan is tailored to the patient, and medical oncologists must weigh the risks and benefits of single-agent chemotherapy, combination chemotherapy, endocrine therapy, and biologic agents when evaluating a patient with metastatic breast cancer. Other clinical factors, such as symptoms, medical comorbidities, performance status, previous exposure to chemotherapy, and premenopausal or postmenopausal status, are also carefully considered before choosing a regimen.

Each patient's tumor burden, or the extent of disease observed on imaging studies, is carefully examined and impacts the decision to start with single or combination therapy. Single-agent chemotherapy is typically reserved for patients with more limited tumor burden and minimal symptoms.

Combination therapy is administered to patients who are symptomatic with high tumor burden and rapidly progressive disease. Combination therapy is generally more toxic than single-agent therapy. However, combination therapy has a higher response rate and may be indicated in patients with rapidly growing tumors that are causing severe symptoms [4]. In the majority of circumstances, sequential single-agent therapy is preferred. Various trials have demonstrated improved survival with combination therapy, but other trials have not reported similar results. For example, in a trial by Albain et al., paclitaxel was compared with gemcitabine in combination with paclitaxel in patients who relapsed after adjuvant anthracycline therapy. A total of 255 patients were randomly assigned to each arm of the study. The median survival in the GT arm (gemcitabine and paclitaxel) was 18.6 months versus 15.8 months ($p=0.0187$) in the paclitaxel only arm. Additionally, the time to progression was increased in the GT arm (6.14 months vs. 3.98 months) [5].

Other trials have demonstrated that single-agent and combination therapy appear to have similar overall survival [6]. The Eastern Cooperative Group (ECOG) 1193 trial assigned over 700 patients to doxorubicin and paclitaxel (AP), single-agent doxorubicin, or single-agent paclitaxel. The results revealed an increased overall response rate for combination therapy compared with single-agent therapy (47 % vs. 36 % for single-agent doxorubicin or 34 % for single-agent paclitaxel). However, no difference in overall survival (22 months for combination, 19 months for single-agent doxorubicin, and 22 months for single-agent paclitaxel) was noted. Little data are available regarding the benefit of combination therapy in the second- or third-line setting.

Additionally, the location of metastatic disease can affect survival. Patients with metastatic lesions in the chest wall, bones, or lymph nodes may have prolonged progression-free survival compared with those with hepatic and/or lymphangitic pulmonary disease who tend to have reduced progression-free survival and overall survival [7]. The term "visceral crisis" is used to describe patients with lymphangitic lung metastases, bone marrow replacement, carcinomatous meningitis, or significant liver metastases [8]. Combination therapy is generally used in visceral crisis.

Patient preferences must be considered. For example, in patients who prefer to avoid alopecia, capecitabine can limit hair loss. Additionally, patients who prefer chemotherapy to be administered infrequently because they live a great distance from an infusion center can opt for therapies that are administered every 3 or 4 weeks, such as liposomal doxorubicin or ixabepilone, rather than weekly treatments, such as vinorelbine or gemcitabine.

The benefit of treatment with systemic chemotherapy must be balanced with effects on quality of life and tolerability. Chemotherapy is indicated for patients with hormone-insensitive breast cancer and patients with aggressive hormone-positive cancer. Patients with HER2-positive tumors should be administered anti-HER2 biologic therapy, i.e., trastuzumab, in combination with systemic therapy. Therapy with single agents versus combination agents is a matter of debate, but combination therapy should generally be pursued when the patient is highly symptomatic or in patients with rapidly progressive visceral metastasis. In the majority of patients, sequential single-agent therapy is preferred.

Additionally, in contrast to other malignancies, there is no predetermined duration of therapy. Treatment duration is individualized to the specific goals of each patient and dependent on disease progression and treatment toxicity. Additionally, there is an option to continue maintenance chemotherapy if a patient can tolerate it. Data suggest that maintenance chemotherapy may improve disease-free survival in patients who tolerate chemotherapy. In a phase III trial published by Park et al., 324 patients were randomized to maintenance chemotherapy or observation until progression. Patients in the maintenance arm exhibited increased median progression-free survival (approximately 7.5 months) compared with those in the observation group (3.8 months, $p = 0.026$). Additionally, the median overall survival was increased in the maintenance arm, with a survival of 32.3 months versus 23.5 months ($p = 0.047$) [9].

Taxanes

The taxanes are some of the most active agents in the setting of metastatic breast cancer. Taxanes, including docetaxel, paclitaxel, and nab-paclitaxel, function by stabilizing microtubules, leading to mitotic arrest [10]. The overall response rates are 21–62 % [11], and this class of drugs rivals the anthracyclines in terms of response rates and time to disease progression. Taxanes are frequently used as first-line chemotherapy for patients with metastatic breast cancer who are naive to treatment, have previously been treated with anthracyclines, or have contraindications for anthracyclines (e.g., in a patient with heart failure) [11].

Taxanes may be used as single agents or in combination with other agents. Monotherapy includes paclitaxel weekly or triweekly, docetaxel on a weekly or triweekly schedule, or nab-paclitaxel administered on a triweekly schedule in the dose regimens highlighted above (see Table 32.1). Combination therapies include taxanes with an anthracycline, gemcitabine, capecitabine, vinorelbine, or carboplatin in the dose regimens highlighted above (see Table 32.2). A report of the Intergroup trial by Sledge et al. compared doxorubicin with paclitaxel or the combination of both in metastatic disease [12]. In this study, equal response and survival rates were noted for patients receiving single-agent and combination therapy. Additionally, overall survival with combination therapy was equivalent to treatment with either single-agent alone [12].

The frequency of chemotherapy administration has been analyzed in a number of studies. A meta-analysis of randomized controlled trials comparing weekly and thrice weekly administration of taxanes in advanced breast cancer revealed that weekly 80–100 mg/m^2 paclitaxel exhibited a survival benefit compared with triweekly paclitaxel at 175 mg/m^2 (1471 patients, HR of 0.78, and $p = 0.001$). The toxicity profiles differed; worse sensory neuropathy was noted with weekly paclitaxel, but less myelosuppression was observed [13]. In the CALGB 9840 trial, weekly paclitaxel was compared with triweekly paclitaxel at a dose of 175 mg/m^2. In this study, the weekly dose of paclitaxel was reduced from 100 to 80 mg/m^2 due

Table 32.1 Single-agent taxane therapies in metastatic breast cancer

Regimens	Dosing	Overall response rate	Toxicity	References
Paclitaxel monotherapy weekly or triweekly	Weekly: 80–100 mg/m^2 Triweekly: 175 mg/m^2	21.5 % (95 % CI 15.4–27.5 %)	Allergic reactions Neuropathy Myalgia Fatigue	Perez et al. [48]
Docetaxel monotherapy weekly or triweekly	Weekly: 30–40 mg/m^2 Triweekly: 80–100 mg/m^2	30–42 %	Fluid retention GI toxicity Stomatitis Febrile neutropenia	Burris et al. [49]
Abraxane (nab-paclitaxel)	175 mg/m^2 every 3 weeks	33 % response rate compared with paclitaxel (19 %)	GI toxicity Neuropathy Flushing Neutropenia Fewer allergic reactions	Gradishar et al. [50]

Table 32.2 Taxane combination regimens in metastatic breast cancer

Regimen	Dosing	Progression-free survival	Toxicity	References
Docetaxel/ capecitabine (DC)	Docetaxel 75 mg/m^2 IV day 1 + capecitabine 950 mg/m^2 PO BID days 1–14, cycled 21 days	11 months vs. 10.6 months with docetaxel and epirubicin (DE)	Neutropenia Hand-foot syndrome Anemia Asthenia	Mavroudis et al. [51]
Paclitaxel/ gemcitabine	Paclitaxel 175 mg/m^2 on day 1 and gemcitabine 1250 mg/m^2 IV days 1 and 8 every 21 days	18.6 months vs. 15.8 months with single-agent paclitaxel	Neutropenia Fatigue Neuropathy	Albain et al. [5]
Paclitaxel/ bevacizumab	Paclitaxel 90 mg/m^2 by 1 h IV days 1, 8, and 15; bevacizumab 10 mg/kg IV days 1 and 15; cycled every 28 days	11.9 months vs. 5.9 months (paclitaxel alone)	Hypertension Proteinuria Headache Cerebrovascular ischemia	Miller et al. [52]

to a 30 % incidence of grade 3 sensory neuropathy. The weekly regimen was superior to the triweekly regimen in terms of RR (42 % vs. 29 %, $p=0.004$), time to progression (9 months vs. 5 months, $p<0.001$), and overall survival (24 months vs. 12 months, $p=0.0092$) [14]. These results are similar to the results in the adjuvant setting, demonstrating that weekly paclitaxel after standard doxorubicin and cyclophosphamide improved disease-free and overall survival compared with dosing every 3 weeks [15].

The safety profiles differ among taxanes, but data comparing taxanes against each other are limited. Paclitaxel has an increased risk of neuropathy and myalgia compared with docetaxel. Docetaxel cannot be administered in the setting of hepatic dysfunction, but paclitaxel can be administered in the setting of moderate hepatic dysfunction. Docetaxel toxicities include febrile neutropenia, edema, and GI toxicities. Dexamethasone is often administered as a premedication to help retain fluid and can also add to the side effect profile. In the TAX-311 multicenter open-label phase III study of 499 patients with advanced breast cancer who progressed after an anthracycline, docetaxel compared with paclitaxel produced a significantly better median time to progression (5.7 vs. 3.6 months, respectively; $p<0.0001$) and overall survival (15.4 vs. 12.7 months, respectively; $p=0.03$). However, the hematologic and non-hematologic toxicity profile associated with docetaxel was much worse than paclitaxel [16].

Paclitaxel, nab-paclitaxel, and the agent ixabepilone were compared as first-line agents (with or without bevacizumab) in a trial conducted by the Cancer and Leukemia Group B (CALGB) and the North Central Clinical Trials Group (NCCTG). Preliminary results were presented at the 2012 ASCO meeting and included 799 patients who were randomly assigned to weekly treatment with paclitaxel (90 mg/m^2) or nab-paclitaxel (150 mg/m^2) on a 3-week on, 1-week off schedule. An additional arm assessed weekly ixabepilone (16 mg/m^2). No difference in progression-free survival (10 months in both arms, HR 0.94, 95 % CI 0.73–1.22) and overall survival (27 vs. 26 months, 95 % CI 0.75–1.38) was noted between paclitaxel and nab-paclitaxel, respectively. However, nab-paclitaxel resulted in an increased rate of serious toxicity, including sensory neuropathy (25 % vs. 16 %, respectively) and hematologic toxicity (51 % vs. 21 %, respectively) [17].

Anthracyclines

Anthracyclines were first used in the 1980s for the treatment of metastatic breast cancer and have significantly advanced the treatment of metastatic breast cancer. Patient outcome is heavily based on the extent of metastatic disease, performance status, and prior chemotherapy exposure [11]; response rates are 35–50 % in patients who are anthracycline-naive and in those who develop metastatic disease more than 12 months after receiving anthracycline therapy [12, 18]. In the combination drug setting, anthracycline-based chemotherapy regimens are associated with response rates of up to 60 % in patients who have not previously been treated [19]. The most popular regimens used are highlighted in Table 32.3.

Anthracyclines are derived from the fungus *Streptomyces peucetius* and commonly intercalate into DNA, directly affecting transcription and replication. These agents form a tripartite

Table 32.3 Anthracycline-containing therapies for metastatic breast cancer

Regimens	Dosing	Overall response rate	Toxicities	References
Doxorubicin monotherapy	60–75 mg/m^2 IV day 1 every 21 days or 20 mg/m^2 weekly	30–47 %	GI toxicities Fatigue Neutropenia Alopecia	Norris et al. [53]; Andersson et al. [54]
Pegylated liposomal doxorubicin monotherapy	50 mg/m^2 IV day 1 every 28 days	10–33 %	Plantar erythrodysesthesia Stomatitis Mucositis	O'Brien et al. [22]; Keller et al. [55]
Epirubicin monotherapy	60–90 mg/m^2 IV day 1 every 21 days	42–50 %	Fatigue Alopecia Neutropenia	Joensuu et al. [56]
Cyclophosphamide, doxorubicin, fluorouracil (CAF)	5-fluorouracil 500 mg/m^2 IV days 1 and 8; doxorubicin 50 mg/m^2 IV day 1; cyclophosphamide 500 mg/m^2 IV day 1 every 21 days	76 %	GI toxicity Alopecia Fatigue	Hortobagyi et al. [57]
Doxorubicin/ cyclophosphamide (AC)	Doxorubicin 60 mg/m^2 IV on day 1 and cyclophosphamide 600 mg/m^2 IV on day 1 cycled every 21 days	47 %	Febrile neutropenia Infections	Nabholtz et al. [58]
Epirubicin/ cyclophosphamide (EC)	Epirubicin 75 mg/m^2 IV day 1 and cyclophosphamide 600 mg/m^2 IV day 1 cycled every 21 days	55 %	Alopecia Infection GI toxicity	Langley et al. [59]

complex with topoisomerase II and DNA, producing a double-strand break at the 3′-phosphate backbone and allowing strand passage and uncoiling of supercoiled DNA. Doxorubicin and epirubicin are commonly used to treat solid human tumors [20]. Doxorubicin is available for intravenous infusion and administered at 60–75 mg/m^2 every 3 weeks or 20 mg/m^2 weekly. Epirubicin is administered at 75–100 mg/m^2 every 3 weeks or 20–30 mg/m^2 weekly. Epirubicin exhibits similar efficacy and is somewhat less toxic compared with doxorubicin. Side effects of anthracyclines include nausea, vomiting, myelosuppression, and alopecia. One potential limitation of using anthracyclines involves the risk for cardiac toxicity with cumulative doses. Although the incidence is rare based on the limited doses used in the adjuvant setting (less than 360 mg/m^2), the risk of cardiac toxicity is as high as 18 % in doses greater than 700 mg/m^2 [21]. Dexrazoxane may minimize the risk of cardiac toxicity in doses greater than 300 mg/m^2; however, this drug is not widely used.

Another consideration is a patient's comorbidities. Liposomal doxorubicin may be considered for use in a patient with heart failure. In a trial by O'Brien et al., pegylated liposomal doxorubicin was compared with doxorubicin and exhibited equivalent progression-free survival (6.9 vs. 7.8 months, respectively) and overall survival (21 vs. 22 months, respectively) but a significantly lower risk of cardiotoxicity (HR=3.16, 95 % CI 1.58–6.31). However, the ORR was slightly increased in the doxorubicin group (38 % vs. 33 %). Additionally, fewer toxicities, including alopecia, nausea, vomiting, and neutropenia, were associated with pegylated liposomal doxorubicin. Patients administered pegylated doxorubicin exhibited increased plantar-plantar erythrodysesthesia, stomatitis, and mucositis [22].

Currently, no evidence suggests that anthracyclines are superior to taxanes in the setting of metastatic breast cancer. In 2008, a meta-analysis of the data from 919 patients reported that treatment with an anthracycline was associated with improved ORR (38 % vs. 33 %) and progression-free survival (7 vs. 5 months) compared with taxanes. However, the analysis was limited due to the heterogeneity and differing schedules for administration of chemotherapy among the trials [23]. It is difficult to draw conclusions from this meta-analysis without a prospective randomized trial. Both anthracyclines and taxanes are reasonable choices for the first-line treatment of metastatic breast cancer; however, taxanes may be the more practical choice given the reduced risk for cumulative cardiac toxicity.

Antimetabolites

Capecitabine

Capecitabine is an oral fluoropyrimidine prodrug that is enzymatically activated to 5-fluorouracil by thymidine phosphorylase at the site of the tumor [24]. This drug provides increased directed cytotoxicity and leads to less direct release of fluorouracil into the bowel, potentially reducing the incidence of diarrhea. In 1998, capecitabine was first approved as a single-agent therapy for patients with anthracycline and taxane resistance. Clinically, its activity is similar to its parent drug, 5-fluorouracil, a continuous infusion drug that has been used historically in the treatment of breast cancer [11].

Single-agent capecitabine (1000–1250 mg/m^2 twice daily for 14 days followed by 7 days of rest) is a good first-line choice for patients with metastatic breast cancer, especially those with bony disease and those with estrogen receptor-positive disease who have progressed despite endocrine therapy. Additionally, capecitabine is orally available and reduces the need for frequent doctor visits. Capecitabine also crosses the blood-brain barrier and can be used in patients with brain metastases [25]. Common side effects of capecitabine include hand-foot syndrome, nausea, and diarrhea, and these symptoms are typically improved by dose reduction [26]. Unlike most drugs for metastatic breast cancer, capecitabine causes minimal alopecia and neuropathy.

The first study of capecitabine in metastatic breast cancer was performed by Blum and colleagues and involved patients who had been previously treated with paclitaxel and anthracycline for metastatic disease. Capecitabine was administered for 14 days followed by 1 week of rest. Of the 135 patients, 27 (20 %) of these subjects demonstrated complete ($N=3$) or partial

($N=24$) responses. The median duration of response was 8.1 months, and the median survival time was 12.8 months [27]. The benefit of capecitabine was further demonstrated in a study performed by Fumoleau et al. in a phase II multicenter trial involving 126 patients who had been pretreated with an anthracycline or taxane. The patients were subsequently treated with 1250 mg/m² capecitabine. In this study, the time to progression was 5 months, and the ORR was 28 %, with a median overall survival of 15 months [28]. In another phase II open-label study by O'Shaughnessy et al. in 2001, 95 patients were randomized to either intermittent oral capecitabine at 1250 mg/m² twice daily for 2 weeks or intravenous CMF (cyclophosphamide, methotrexate, 5-fluorouracil) administered every 3 weeks. In the study, the median TTP was similar between the two groups (4 vs. 3 months, respectively); however, capecitabine resulted in a longer median overall survival (20 vs. 17 months, respectively) [29].

Capecitabine has also been studied in combination with other chemotherapy drugs, albeit with an increase in toxicity. O'Shaughnessy et al. conducted a phase III study with patients treated in the first-line setting with capecitabine plus docetaxel combination therapy. In anthracycline-pretreated patients, capecitabine/docetaxel exhibited an additive effect and resulted in superior efficacy in time to disease progression (6.1 vs. 4.2 months, CI of 0.545–0.780, $p=0.0001$), overall survival (14.5 vs. 11.5 months, $p=0.0126$), and objective tumor response rate (42 % vs. 30 %, $p=0.006$) when compared with docetaxel alone [30].

Gemcitabine

In 2004, gemcitabine was first approved for first-line treatment of metastatic breast cancer. This drug is a nucleoside analog that is generally well tolerated. Single-agent response rates range from 14 to 37 % in metastatic breast cancer patients [31, 32]. Gemcitabine can also be used in combination with paclitaxel (1000 mg/m² days 1 and 8 of a 21-day cycle) in the first-line setting; however, it is most frequently used as a single agent. Chemotherapy-naive patients can generally tolerate doses of 1000–1250 mg/m²/week on days 1, 8, and 15 every 28 days. Reducing the dose in subsequent cycles or omitting the day 15 dose can improve a patient's ability to tolerate future cycles. Thrombocytopenia is a common side effect and can be dose limiting, especially in pretreated patients [33]. Gemcitabine is well tolerated in patients, and its side effects, such as alopecia, GI toxicity, and neuropathy, are quite mild compared with taxanes and anthracyclines.

A phase II trial conducted by Charmichael et al. studied the efficacy of gemcitabine administered once per week at a dose of 800 mg/m² for 3 weeks followed by a 1-week rest every 4 weeks. Overall, the response rate was 25 % with a median survival time of 11.5 months. Neutropenia was a major side effect; and 23.3 % and 7 % of patients suffered from grade 3 and 4 neutropenia, respectively [32]. A phase II study conducted by Blackstein et al. revealed that women with metastatic breast cancer treated in the first-line setting with gemcitabine at 1200 mg/m² on days 1, 8, and 15 of a 3-week cycle every 28 days for a maximum of eight cycles exhibited an overall response rate of 37.1 % (95 % confidence interval 21.5–55.1 %), with 2 complete responses and 11 partial responses. The median time to progression was 5.1 months, and the median survival time was 21.1 months. The most common toxicity was nausea/vomiting (10 %). Grade 3 neutropenia occurred in 30.3 % of patients, and thrombocytopenia occurred in 6.3 % of patients [31].

Gemcitabine monotherapy appears to be effective as a salvage therapy in patients who have been previously treated with doxorubicin and taxane therapy. In a study by Rha et al., the efficacy and tolerability of gemcitabine were assessed in a set of 41 patients. The patients underwent a total of 178 cycles of gemcitabine at 850 mg/m² for 30 min for 3 of every 4 weeks. The median response duration was 9 months, and the overall survival was 11 months. In patients treated in the third-line setting, the overall survival was 12 months. However, in the fourth-line setting, survival was approximately 7 months. The toxicities experienced were mild, including grade 3 neutropenia and grade 3 or 4 thrombocytopenia without clinical symptoms [33].

In the first-line setting, gemcitabine is inferior to epirubicin. In a phase III multicenter study conducted by Feher et al., 198 postmenopausal women (older than 60 years of age) received gemcitabine

(1200 mg/m^2) and 199 patients received epirubicin (35 mg/m^2) on days 1, 8, and 15 of a 28-day cycle. A total of 185 and 192 cycles were administered in the gemcitabine and epirubicin groups. The epirubicin group demonstrated superior time to progression (6.1 months vs. 3.4 months, $p=0.0001$) and improved overall survival (19.1 months vs. 11.8 months, $p=0.0004$) when compared with the gemcitabine group, suggesting that anthracyclines remain important drugs in the first-line setting [34].

Microtubule Inhibitors

Ixabepilone

Ixabepilone (Ixempra) is an epothilone analog that binds to microtubules and causes microtubule stabilization and mitotic arrest. Ixabepilone is used as a single agent and in combination with capecitabine, and it was approved in 2007 for treatment of metastatic breast cancer patients who were resistant to anthracycline and taxane treatment or those contraindicated for anthracyclines. Additionally, it is indicated for use in patients who are resistant to capecitabine [11]. The dose should be adjusted in patients with liver function test abnormalities. Side effects of fatigue, anemia, and peripheral neuropathy are the most debilitating and are often dose limiting. In fact, this drug is not approved for use in Europe due to the risk of peripheral neuropathy.

A phase II trial conducted by Perez, EA., and colleagues demonstrated that ixabepilone is safe to use in metastatic breast cancer patients who are resistant to taxanes, anthracyclines, and capecitabine. In this trial, 126 patients were treated, and 113 were assessable for response. Of these 113 patients, 88 % received at least two lines of prior chemotherapy in the metastatic setting with an ORR of 11.5 % (95 % CI 6.3–18.9 %). The median overall survival was 8.6 months, and the ORR was 19 % with a median duration of response of 5.7 months. Peripheral neuropathy was the primary side effect, occurring in approximately 14 % of patients [35].

In the first-line setting for patients with metastatic breast cancer, ixabepilone may not be as effective as taxanes. In the CALGB 40502 trial, weekly ixabepilone resulted in shorter median progression-free survival when compared with taxanes (7.6 months vs. 10 months, respectively), as well as inferior overall survival (21 months vs. 26 months with paclitaxel and 27 months with nab-paclitaxel). However, this study showed that the incidence of hematologic toxicity was much lower in the ixabepilone arm (12 %) versus the taxane arm (21 % with paclitaxel and 51 % with nab-paclitaxel). The rate of peripheral neuropathy was similar between ixabepilone and nab-paclitaxel (25 %) [17].

Vinorelbine

Vinorelbine, also known as Navelbine, is a semisynthetic vinca alkaloid that interferes with microtubule assembly. The main side effects include neutropenia, pain with infusion, flu-like symptoms, and gastrointestinal symptoms, such as nausea and constipation. Response rates for first-line vinorelbine therapy range from 35 to 53 %, and second-line therapy response rates range from 20 to 30 % [36]. Zelek et al. found that weekly vinorelbine at a dose of 25 mg/m^2 had a 25 % response rate in patients whose disease had progressed following taxane or anthracycline therapy [37].

Vinorelbine may be particularly well tolerated in elderly patients. In a study by Vogel et al., patients 60 years of age or older were treated with 30 mg/m^2 vinorelbine as a weekly infusion. The objective response rate was 38 %, and approximately 4 % of patients obtained complete responses. The median duration of response was approximately 9 months. The dose-limiting toxicity was neutropenia, and approximately 80 % of patients suffered from grade 3 or 4 granulocytopenia [38].

Eribulin

Eribulin inhibits the polymerization of tubulin and microtubules and is administered at a dose of 1.4 mg/m^2 on days 1 and 8 of a 21-day cycle. Eribulin can be administered in the setting of mild to moderate hepatic dysfunction and may also result in less neuropathy than other microtubule inhibitors. The EMBRACE trial by Cortes et al. was a phase III open-label trial that led to the approval of eribulin for metastatic breast cancer in pretreated individuals. Patients in this study previously received between two and five lines of chemotherapy. In this trial, 762 women were randomly allotted to eribulin (508) versus the physician's choice

(254). Patients treated with the physician's choice were treated with vinorelbine (25 %), gemcitabine (19 %), capecitabine (18 %), taxanes (15 %), anthracyclines (10 %), or other chemotherapies (10 %). Overall survival was significantly improved with eribulin (13.1 months, 95 % CI 11.8–14.3) compared with the physician's choice (10.6 months). Peripheral neuropathy was the most common side effect leading to eribulin discontinuation and occurred in 5 % of the patients. Other side effects included fatigue (54 %) and neutropenia (52 %) [39]. Capecitabine and eribulin have also been compared against each other in a trial. No difference in eribulin and capecitabine in terms of progression-free survival (4 months) or overall survival (11 vs. 11.5 months, respectively) was noted [40].

Cyclophosphamide

Cyclophosphamide is metabolized by the liver to 4-hydroxy-cyclophosphamide, which decomposes into an alkylating agent, chloroacetalde-hyde, and acrolein. Liver disease can impair drug activation. Cyclophosphamide is most often used as part of combination therapy for metastatic breast cancer, as outlined in Table 32.5.

Cyclophosphamide can also be used alone and is administered in a metronomic manner. In this strategy, cytotoxic chemotherapy is administered at a very low dose in close intervals. In a phase II trial conducted by Licchetta et al., daily cyclophosphamide (50 mg/daily days 1 through 21 in a 28-day cycle) and twice daily megestrol acetate (80 mg twice daily) were administered to patients with metastatic breast cancer. The overall response rate was 31 %, and the disease control rate was 41.3 % with a mean time to tumor progression of 7.4 months and mean overall survival of 13.4 months [41].

Cisplatin/Carboplatin

Cisplatin inhibits DNA synthesis by forming DNA intra-strand cross-links, denaturing the double helix, binding covalently to DNA bases, and disrupting DNA function. Additionally, it binds to RNA and proteins. The primary dose-limiting toxicity of cisplatin is nephrotoxicity. A 30–50 % loss of GFR is a commonly reported adverse reaction with the use of platinum-based chemotherapies. Carboplatin was subsequently developed to avoid the nephrotoxicity of cisplatin while main-

taining the antitumor effect [42]. Other common toxicities include hearing loss and neurotoxicity, including stocking-and-glove sensorimotor neuropathy; however, these toxicities are less commonly reported for the use of carboplatin.

Historically, platinum salts had limited use as single agents in the treatment of metastatic breast cancer. In the third-line setting, cisplatin and carboplatin exhibit a limited response, typically approximately 10 % [11]. The response to platinum agents is reportedly less than 10 % when used as a third-line therapy and beyond. A limited number of clinical trials reported response rates of 50 % in chemotherapy-naive patients. However, the toxicities associated with platinum regimens resulted in their use being limited primarily to the salvage setting [43].

Interest in platinum-based therapy has been renewed in patients harboring germ-line BRCA mutations and patients with triple-negative breast cancer. In a recent publication by Isakoff et al., patients with metastatic triple-negative breast cancer were treated with cisplatin or carboplatin in the first- or second-line setting. In total, 86 patients were enrolled in this trial, and an equal number of patients received cisplatin ($n=43$) or carboplatin ($n=43$). Patients harboring BRCA1 or BRCA2 mutations had a cisplatin or carboplatin response of 54.5 %. In patients who did not harbor a BRCA mutation, a DNA instability signature defined who responded to therapy. Thus, platinum-based therapies may be beneficial in patients with BRCA1 or BRCA2 mutations and in non-BRCA carrier patients who lack DNA repair functions [44]. Triple-negative breast cancers appear to have a defect in DNA repair processes, such as an allelic imbalance in copy-number alterations, rendering them more sensitive to platinum-based regimens. Watkins et al. found that the meiotic gene HORMAD1 is a driver of homologous recombination deficiency in patients with triple-negative breast cancer and is associated with the response to platinum-based chemotherapies [45].

The TNT trial by Tutt et al. that was presented at the 2014 San Antonio Breast Cancer Symposium compared single-agent carboplatin with single-agent docetaxel and found that the response rates were similar with both agents.

Among the triple-negative patients with a BRCA1 or BRCA2 mutation, carboplatin resulted in increased progression-free survival. Among the 43 patients who were BRCA positive, a 68 % response to carboplatin was noted compared with a 33 % response with docetaxel; this result was significant ($p = 0.03$). BRCA mutation patients treated with carboplatin had a median progression-free survival of 6.8 months versus 3.1 months for non-BRCA-mutated patients treated with carboplatin [46].

Table 32.5 Chemotherapy combinations in the setting of metastatic breast cancer [47]

CAF/FAC (cyclophosphamide/doxorubicin/fluorouracil)
FEC (fluorouracil/epirubicin/cyclophosphamide)
AC (doxorubicin/cyclophosphamide)
EC (epirubicin/cyclophosphamide)
Docetaxel/capecitabine
GT (gemcitabine/paclitaxel)
Gemcitabine/carboplatin
Paclitaxel/bevacizumab

Summary

A number of treatment options are available for patients with metastatic breast cancer. There is no set algorithm for therapy, and treatment is tailored to the individual patient's preferences, including toxicities to avoid, frequency of therapy, and the duration of treatment as highlighted in Tables 32.4 and 32.5. Anthracyclines and taxanes remain the most potent drugs and are used quite frequently in the first-line setting. Unlike other solid tumors with only second- or third-line therapy options, numerous options are available for patients after progression before hospice is considered.

Table 32.4 Single-agent chemotherapy in the setting of metastatic breast cancer [47]

Doxorubicin
Pegylated liposomal doxorubicin
Paclitaxel
Capecitabine
Gemcitabine
Vinorelbine
Eribulin
Cyclophosphamide
Carboplatin
Docetaxel
Albumin-bound paclitaxel
Cisplatin
Epirubicin
Ixabepilone

*Please note that italicized items are preferred first-line single agents

References

1. Greenberg PA, Hortobagyi GN, Smith TL, Ziegler LD, Frye DK, Buzdar AU. Long-term follow-up of patients with complete remission following combination chemotherapy for metastatic breast cancer. J Clin Oncol. 1996;14(8):2197–205.
2. American Cancer Society. Breast cancer facts and figures 2007–2008. Atlanta: American Cancer Society; 2009.
3. Osborne CK, Yochmowitz MG, Knight 3rd WA, McGuire WL. The value of estrogen and progesterone receptors in the treatment of breast cancer. Cancer. 1980;46(12 Suppl):2884–8.
4. Carrick S, Parker S, Thornton CE, Ghersi D, Simes J, Wilcken N. Single agent versus combination chemotherapy for metastatic breast cancer. Cochrane Database Syst Rev. 2009;(2):CD003372.
5. Albain KS, Nag SM, Calderillo-Ruiz G, Jordaan JP, Llombart AC, Pluzanska A, et al. Gemcitabine plus Paclitaxel versus Paclitaxel monotherapy in patients with metastatic breast cancer and prior anthracycline treatment. J Clin Oncol. 2008;26(24):3950–7.
6. Dear RF, McGeechan K, Jenkins MC, Barratt A, Tattersall MH, Wilcken N. Combination versus sequential single agent chemotherapy for metastatic breast cancer. Cochrane Database Syst Rev. 2013;(12): CD008792.
7. Hortobagyi GN, Smith TL, Legha SS, Swenerton KD, Gehan EA, Yap HY, et al. Multivariate analysis of prognostic factors in metastatic breast cancer. J Clin Oncol. 1983;1(12):776–86.
8. Barrios CH, Sampaio C, Vinholes J, Caponero R. What is the role of chemotherapy in estrogen receptor-positive, advanced breast cancer? Ann Oncol. 2009;20(7): 1157–62.
9. Park YH, Jung KH, Im SA, Sohn JH, Ro J, Ahn JH, et al. Phase III, multicenter, randomized trial of maintenance chemotherapy versus observation in patients with metastatic breast cancer after achieving disease control with six cycles of gemcitabine plus paclitaxel as first-line chemotherapy: KCSG-BR07-02. J Clin Oncol. 2013;31(14):1732–9.
10. Valero V, Jones SE, Von Hoff DD, Booser DJ, Mennel RG, Ravdin PM, et al. A phase II study of docetaxel in

patients with paclitaxel-resistant metastatic breast cancer. J Clin Oncol. 1998;16(10):3362–8.

11. Kantarajan HM, Wolff RA, Koller C. The MD Anderson manual of clinical oncology. 2nd ed. New York: McGraw-Hill; 2011.

12. Sledge GW, Neuberg D, Bernardo P, Ingle JN, Martino S, Rowinsky EK, Wood WC. Phase III trial of doxorubicin, paclitaxel and the combination of doxorubicin and paclitaxel as front-line chemotherapy for metastatic breast cancer: an Intergroup trial (E1193). J Clin Oncol. 2003;21(4):588–92.

13. Mauri D, Kamposioras K, Tsali L, Bristianou M, Valachis A, Karathanasi I, et al. Overall survival benefit for weekly vs. three-weekly taxanes regimens in advanced breast cancer: a meta-analysis. Cancer Treat Rev. 2010;36(1):69–74.

14. Winer EP, Berry DA, Woolf S, Duggan D, Kornblith A, Harris LN, et al. Failure of higher-dose paclitaxel to improve outcome in patients with metastatic breast cancer; cancer and leukemia group B trial 9342. J Clin Oncol. 2004;22(11):2061–8.

15. Sparano JA, Wang M, Martino S, Jones V, Perez EA, Saphner T, et al. Weekly paclitaxel in the adjuvant treatment of breast cancer. N Engl J Med. 2008;358(16): 1663–71.

16. Jones S, Erban J, Overmoyer B, et al. Randomized phase III study of docetaxel compared with paclitaxel in metastatic breast cancer. J Clin Oncol. 2005;23(24): 5542–51.

17. Rugo HS, Barry WT, Moreno-Aspitia A. CALGB 40502/NCCTG N063H: randomized phase III trial of weekly paclitaxel (P) compared to weekly nanoparticle albumin bound nab-paclitaxel (NP) or ixabepilone (Ix) with or without bevacizumab (B) as first-line therapy for locally recurrent or metastatic breast cancer (MBC). J Clin Oncol. 2012;30(suppl; abstr CRA1002).

18. Yu KD, Huang S, Zhang JX, Liu GY, Shao ZM. Association between delayed initiation of adjuvant CMF or anthracycline-based chemotherapy and survival in breast cancer: a systematic review and meta-analysis. BMC Cancer. 2013;13:240.

19. Falkson G, Tormey DC, Carey P, Witte R, Falkson HC. Long-term survival of patients treated with combination chemotherapy for metastatic breast cancer. Eur J Cancer. 1991;27(8):973–7.

20. Brunton L, Lazo J, Parker K. Goodman and Gilman's, the pharmacological basis or therapeutics. New York: McGraw-Hill; 2012.

21. Weiss RB. The anthracyclines: will we ever find a better doxorubicin? Semi Oncol. 1992;19:670–86.

22. O'Brien ME, Wigler N, Inbar M, Rosso R, Grischke E, Santoro A, et al. Reduced cardiotoxicity and comparable efficacy in a phase III trial of pegylated liposomal doxorubicin HCl (CAELYX/Doxil) versus conventional doxorubicin for first-line treatment of metastatic breast cancer. Ann Oncol. 2004;15(3):440–9.

23. Piccart-Gebhart MJ, Burzykowski T, Buyse M, Sledge G, Carmichael J, Lück HJ, et al. Taxanes alone or in combination with anthracyclines as first-line therapy of patients with metastatic breast cancer. J Clin Oncol. 2008;26(12):1980–6.

24. Singletary SE, Robb GL, Hortobagyi GN. Advanced therapy of breast disease. BC Decker: Hamilton, Ontario; 2004.

25. Bachelot T, Romieu G, Campone M, Diéras V, Cropet C, Dalenc F, et al. Lapatinib plus capecitabine in patients with previously untreated brain metastases from HER2-positive metastatic breast cancer (LANDSCAPE): a single-group phase 2 study. Lancet Oncol. 2013;14(1): 64–71.

26. Talbot DC, Moiseyenko V, Van Belle S, O'Reilly SM, Alba Conejo E, Ackland S, et al. Randomised phase II trial comparing oral capecitabine (Xeloda) with Paclitaxel in patients with metastatic/advanced breast cancer pretreated with anthracyclines. Br J Cancer. 2002;86(9):1367–72.

27. Blum JL, Jones SE, Buzdar AU, LoRusso PM, Kuter I, Vogel C, et al. Multicenter phase II study of capecitabine in paclitaxel-refractory metastatic breast cancer. J Clin Oncol. 1999;17(2):485–93.

28. Fumoleau P, Largillier R, Clippe C, Dièras V, Orfeuvre H, Lesimple T, et al. Multicentre, phase II study evaluating capecitabine monotherapy in patients with anthracycline and taxane pretreated metastatic breast cancer. Eur J Cancer. 2004;40(4):536–42.

29. O'Shaughnessy JA, Blum J, Moiseyenko V, Jones SE, Miles D, Bell D, et al. Randomized, open-label, phase II trial of oral capecitabine (Xeloda) vs. a reference arm of intravenous CMF (cyclophosphamide, methotrexate and 5-fluorouracil) as first-line therapy for advanced/metastatic breast cancer. Ann Oncol. 2001;12(9):1247–54.

30. O'Shaughnessy J, Miles D, Vukelja S, Moiseyenko V, Ayoub JP, Cervantes G, et al. Superior survival with capecitabine plus docetaxel combination therapy in anthracycline-pretreated patients with advanced breast cancer: phase III trial results. J Clin Oncol. 2002;20(12):2812–23.

31. Blackstein M, Vogel CL, Ambinder R, Cowan J, Iglesias J, Melemed A. Gemcitabine as first-line therapy in patients with metastatic breast cancer: a phase II trial. Oncology. 2002;62(1):2–8.

32. Carmichael J, Possinger K, Phillip P, Beykirch M, Kerr H, Walling J, Harris AL. Advanced breast cancer: a phase II trial with gemcitabine. J Clin Oncol. 1995;13(11):2731–6.

33. Rha SY, Moon YH, Jeung HC, Kim YT, Sohn JH, Yang WI, et al. Gemcitabine monotherapy as salvage chemotherapy in heavily pretreated metastatic breast cancer. Breast Cancer Res Treat. 2005;90(3): 215–21.

34. Feher O, Vodvarka P, Jassem J, Morack G, Advani SH, Khoo KS, et al. First-line gemcitabine versus epirubicin in postmenopausal women aged 60 or older with metastatic breast cancer: a multicenter, randomized, phase III study. Ann Oncol. 2005;16(6): 899–908.

35. Perez EA, Lerzo G, Pivot X, Thomas E, Vahdat L, Bosserman L, et al. Efficacy and safety of ixabepilone (BMS-247550) in a phase II study of patients with advanced breast cancer resistant to an anthracycline, a taxane and capecitabine. J Clin Oncol. 2007;25(23): 3407–14.

36. Canobbio L, Boccardo F, Pastorino G, Brema F, Martini C, Resasco M, Santi L. Phase-II study of Navelbine in advanced breast cancer. Semin Oncol. 1989;16(2 Suppl 4):33–6.

37. Zelek L, Barthier S, Riofrio M, Fizazi K, Rixe O, Delord JP, et al. Weekly vinorelbine is an effective palliative regimen after failure with anthracyclines and taxanes in metastatic breast carcinoma. Cancer. 2001;92(9):2267–72.

38. Vogel C, O'Rourke M, Winer E, Hochster H, Chang A, Adamkiewicz B, et al. Vinorelbine as first-line chemotherapy for advanced breast cancer in women 60 years of age or older. Ann Oncol. 1999;10(4):397–402.

39. Cortes J, O'Shaughnessy J, Loesch D, Blum JL, Vahdat LT, Petrakova K, et al. Eribulin monotherapy versus treatment of physician's choice in patients with metastatic breast cancer (EMBRACE): a phase 3 open-label randomized study. Lancet. 2011;377(9769):914–23.

40. Kaufman PA, Awada A, Twelves C, Yelle L, Perez EA, Velikova G, et al. Phase III open-label randomized study of eribulin mesylate versus capecitabine in patients with metastatic breast cancer previously treated with an anthracycline and a taxane. J Clin Oncol. 2015;33(6):594–601.

41. Licchetta A, Correale P, Migali C, Remondo C, Francini E, Pascucci A, et al. Oral metronomic chemo-hormonal-therapy of metastatic breast cancer with cyclophosphamide and megestrol acetate. J Chemother. 2010;22(3):201–4.

42. Lerma E, Nissenson A, Berns J. Acute renal failure from therapeutic agents from current diagnosis and treatment: nephrology and hypertension. Curr Diagn Treat: Nephrol Hypertens. New York: McGraw-Hill; 2009.

43. Martin M. Platinum compounds in the treatment of advanced breast cancer. Clin Breast Cancer. 2001;2(3):190–208; discussion 209.

44. Isakoff SJ, Mayer EL, He L, Traina TA, Carey LA, Krag KJ, et al. TBCRC009: a multicenter phase II clinical trial of platinum monotherapy with biomarker assessment in metastatic, triple-negative breast cancer. J Clin Oncol. 2015;33(17):1902–9.

45. Watkins J, Weekes D, Shah V, Gazinska P, Joshi S, Sidhu B, et al. Genomic complexity profiling reveals that HORMAD1 contributes to homologous recombination deficiency in triple-negative breast cancers. Cancer Discov. 2015;5(5):488–505.

46. Tutt A, Ellis P, Kilburn L, Gilett C, Pinder S, Abraham J, et al. TNT: a randomized phase III trial of carboplatin compared with docetaxel for patients with metastatic or recurrent locally advanced triple negative or BRCA 1/2 breast cancer. Abstract from San Antonio Breast Cancer Symposium. San Antonio: TX; 2014.

47. Gradishar WJ, Anderson BO, et al. NCCN guidelines in oncology: breast cancer. Version 2.2015. J Natl Compr Canc Netw. 2015;13:448–75. http://www.nccn.org/professionals/physician_gls/pdf/breast.pdf

48. Perez EA, Vogel CL, Irwin DH, Kirshner JJ, Patel R. Multicenter phase II trial of weekly paclitaxel in women with metastatic breast cancer. J Clin Oncol 2001;19:4216–23.

49. Burris HA 3rd. Single-agent docetaxel (Taxotere) in randomized phase III trials. Semin Oncol. 1999;26:1–6.

50. Gradishar WJ, Tjulandin S, Davidson N, Shaw H, Desai N, Bhar P, et al. Phase III trial of nanoparticle albumin-bound paclitaxel compared with polyethylated castor oil-based paclitaxel in women with breast cancer. J Clin Oncol. 2005;23:7794–803.

51. Mavroudis D, Papakotoulas P, Ardavanis A, Syrigos K, Kakolyris S, Ziras N, et al. Breast Cancer Investigators of the Hellenic Oncology Research Group. Randomized phase III trial comparing docetaxel plus epirubicin versus docetaxel plus capecitabine as first-line treatment in women with advanced breast cancer. Ann Oncol. 2010;21: 48–54.

52. Miller K, Wang M, Gralow J, Dickler M, Cobleigh M, Perez EA, et al. Paclitaxel plus Bevacizumab versus Paclitaxel Alone for Metastatic Breast Cancer. N Engl J Med. 2007;357:2666–76.

53. Norris B, Pritchard KI, James K, Myles J, Bennett K, Marlin S, et al. Phase III comparative study of vinorelbine combined with doxorubicin versus doxorubicin alone in disseminated metastatic/recurrent breast cancer: National Cancer Institute of Canada Clinical Trials Group Study MA8. J Clin Oncol. 2000;18: 2385–2394.

54. Andersson M, Daugaard S, von der Maase H, Mouridsen HT. Doxorubicin versus mitomycin versus doxorubicin plus mitomycin in advanced breast cancer: a randomized study. Cancer Treat Rep 1986; 70:1181.

55. Keller AM, Mennel RG, Georgoulias VA, Nabholtz JM, Erazo A, Lluch A, et al. Randomized phase III trial of pegylated liposomal doxorubicin versus vinorelbine or mitomycin C plus vinblastine in women with taxane-refractory advanced breast cancer. J Clin Oncol 2004; 22:3893.

56. Joensuu H, Holli K, Heikkinen M, Suonio E, Aro AR, Hietanen P, Huovinen R. Combination chemotherapy versus single-agent therapy as first- and second-line treatment in metastatic breast cancer: a prospective randomized trial. J Clin Oncol 1998; 16:3720.

57. Hortobagyi GN, Blumenschein GR, Tashima CK, Buzdar AU, Burgess MA, Livingston RB, et al. Ftorafur, adriamycin, cyclophosphamide and BCG in the treatment of metastatic breast cancer. Cancer. 1979;44:398–405.

58. Nabholtz JM, Falkson C, Campos D, Szanto J, Martin M, Chan S, et al. Docetaxel and doxorubicin compared with doxorubicin and cyclophosphamide as first-line chemotherapy for metastatic breast cancer: results of a randomized, multicenter, phase III trial. J Clin Oncol 2003;21:968.

59. Langley RE, Carmichael J, Jones AL, Cameron DA, Qian W, Uscinska B, et al. Phase III trial of epirubicin plus paclitaxel compared with epirubicin plus cyclophosphamide as first-line chemotherapy for metastatic breast cancer: United Kingdom National Cancer Research Institute trial AB01. J Clin Oncol. 2005;23:8322–30.

Treatment of HER2-Overexpressing Metastatic Breast Cancer

Adnan Aydiner

Abstract

Metastatic breast cancer (MBC) overexpressing human epidermal growth factor receptor-2 (HER2) once had an overall worse prognosis, but therapies targeting HER2 have altered the natural course of HER2-positive disease. The initial success of trastuzumab in improving survival rates led to the clinical development of lapatinib, pertuzumab, and trastuzumab emtansine (T-DM1). HER2 protein overexpression and/or gene amplification remains the most important predictive factor for response to HER2-targeted therapies. The optimal duration of chemotherapy (CT) is at least 4–6 months (or longer) and/or to the time of maximal response, depending on toxicity and the absence of progression. HER2-targeted therapy can continue until progression or unacceptable toxicity. For patients with estrogen receptor–positive/progesterone receptor–positive breast cancer who are not good candidates for CT or wish to avoid the toxicity of CT, initial therapy with hormone therapy in combination with HER2-targeted therapy is a reasonable option. However, because the addition of HER2 therapy to endocrine therapy does not improve overall survival (OS), patients with low-volume disease, a long disease-free interval, indolent disease, or significant comorbidities are also candidates for endocrine therapy alone. For patients who relapse and were previously treated with adjuvant anti-HER2 therapy, the resumption of systemic treatment that includes HER2 blockade is recommended. As in the first-line setting, multiple choices are available for second- and third-line therapy. Successful targeting of HER2 has improved outcomes in HER2-positive breast cancer,

A. Aydiner, MD
Department of Medical Oncology, Istanbul University
Istanbul Medical Faculty, Institute of Oncology,
Istanbul, Turkey
e-mail: adnanaydiner@superonline.com

© Springer International Publishing Switzerland 2016
A. Aydiner et al. (eds.), *Breast Disease: Management and Therapies*,
DOI 10.1007/978-3-319-26012-9_33

but treatment resistance and brain metastases remain a problem. Ongoing studies are evaluating novel therapeutic approaches to overcome primary and secondary drug resistance in HER2-positive tumors.

Keywords

HER2 • Trastuzumab • Pertuzumab • T-DM1 • Lapatinib • Trastuzumab emtansine • PI3K • PI3KCA • PTEN • Drug resistance • Antibody-drug conjugate • Everolimus • mTOR • Afatinib • Metastatic • EGFR • HER3 • Cardiotoxicity • Leptomeningeal metastases • Brain metastases • RECIST

Introduction

Human epidermal growth factor receptor-2 (HER2) is amplified or overexpressed in 15–25 % of breast cancers. Historically, overexpression of HER2 was associated with an increased risk of disease recurrence and worse overall prognosis. Therapies that target HER2 have become important in the treatment of metastatic breast cancer (MBC) and have altered the natural course of HER2-positive breast cancer. The initial success of trastuzumab in improving survival rates led to the clinical development of lapatinib, pertuzumab, and trastuzumab emtansine (T-D1) [1–3]. Chemotherapy (CT) regimens combined with HER2-targeted therapy can induce high overall response rates (ORR), extend the time to progression (TTP)/progression-free survival (PFS), and prolong overall survival (OS).

HER2 protein overexpression and/or gene amplification remains the most important predictor of response to HER2-targeted therapies. Quality HER2 testing is required for the appropriate identification and management of HER2-positive patients.

HER2- and estrogen-targeted treatment combinations improve PFS but not OS [4, 5]. This combination may be considered for patients who are reluctant to receive CT or have only a low burden of bone metastases. Clinicians should recommend HER2-targeted combinations for first-line treatment, with the exception of a very select group of patients with estrogen receptor (ER)–positive or progesterone receptor (PgR)–positive and HER2-positive disease, for whom clinicians may use endocrine therapy alone.

When the best treatment response has been obtained (usually after 6–12 months of combined therapy), cytotoxic chemotherapy is stopped, and anti-HER2 therapy is continued, although the optimal duration of treatment is unknown. Following discontinuation of chemotherapy, endocrine therapy must be added to HER2-directed therapy of patients whose tumors are also hormone receptor positive. Further treatments for patients with MBC who progress on HER2-directed therapy must be based on individual considerations [1–3].

First-Line Treatment

The trial by Slamon et al. and other randomized controlled trials of trastuzumab observed a benefit for HER2-targeted therapy combinations [6]. Other agents that improve survival include lapatinib and the combination of trastuzumab plus pertuzumab.

There are a number of effective options: single-agent chemotherapy and an anti-HER2 agent. Taxanes [6], vinorelbine [7], and capecitabine [8, 9] are generally preferred regimens with anti-HER2 partners. Double-agent chemotherapy with HER2-targeted agents is generally avoided because PFS is improved at the cost of significantly increased toxicity [10].

Many clinically important randomized trials of first-line treatments for HER2 MBC, including trastuzumab, lapatinib, pertuzumab, trastuzumab emtansine (T-DM1), and mammalian target of rapamycin (mTOR) inhibitor (everolimus), have affected medical practice (Table 33.1).

Table 33.1 First-line randomized phase III studies in HER2-positive metastatic breast cancer patients

Trial	Study arms	ORR		PFS		OS	
		%	p	Months		Months	
Slamon [6]	Trastuzumab + chemotherapy	50	p < 0.001	7.4	RR = 0.51 P < 0.001	25.1	RR = 0.80 p = 0.046
	Chemotherapy	32		4.6		20.3	
NCIC CTG MA-31 Gelmon [19]	Lapatinib + taxane	54	NS	9.0	HR 1.37 p = 0.001	NR	HR 1.28 p = 0.11
	Trastuzumab + taxane	55		11.3		NR	
CLEOPATRA Swain [22]	Pertuzumab + trastuzumab + docetaxel	80.2	p = 0.0001	18.7	HR 0.69 p < 0.0001	56.5	HR 0.66 p = 0.0001
	Placebo + trastuzumab + docetaxel	69.3		12.4		40.8	
MARIANNE Ellis [28]	Trastuzumab + taxane	67.9	NR	13.7	HR 0.91 P = 0.31	NR	HR 0.86 p=NR
	T-DM1 + placebo	59.7		14.1	HR 0.87 P = 0.14	NR	HR:0.82 p=NR
	T-DM1 + pertuzumab	64.2		15.2		NR	
BOLERO-1 Hurvitz [32]	Everolimus + trastuzumab + paclitaxel	NR	NS	15 ER(-) 20.3	HR 0.89 p = 0.11	NR	NR
	Placebo + trastuzumab + paclitaxel	NR		14.5 ER (-) 13.1	ER(-) HR: 0.66 p = 0.049	NR	

ORR objective response rate, *PFS* progression-free survival, *OS* overall survival, *HR* hazard ratio, *RR* relative risk, *ER* estrogen receptor, *NR* not reported, *NS* nonsignificant, *T-DM1* trastuzumab emtansine

Trastuzumab

The HER2 proto-oncogene encodes a 185-kDa transmembrane receptor protein that is structurally related to the epidermal growth factor receptor (EGFR). HER2 in cancer cells can be activated by either heterodimerization with other ligand-bound HER family members (including HER1, HER3, and HER4) or, when overexpressed, by homodimerization. Upon binding, ligand-induced receptor homo- or heterodimerization activates a phosphorylation-signaling cascade, leading to enhanced responsiveness to stromal growth factors and oncogenic transformation. Downstream signaling regulates the transcription of genes responsible for cell proliferation, survival, angiogenesis, invasion, and metastasis [11]. Trastuzumab inhibits the proliferation of human tumor cells that overexpress HER2 in vitro and in animals. Trastuzumab binds to subdomain IV of HER2 to disrupt ligand-independent signaling and mediate antibody-dependent cellular cytotoxicity [11] (Fig. 33.1).

Single-agent trastuzumab treatment may be reasonable when avoiding the cytotoxic side effects of chemotherapy is desirable but may result in poorer outcomes compared with trastuzumab administered in combination with chemotherapy. In the HERTAX trial, patients who were randomly assigned treatment with trastuzumab followed by docetaxel had lower median OS (20 vs. 31 months) and significantly lower ORR (53 % vs. 79 %) than those receiving docetaxel plus trastuzumab [12] However, sequential treatment was associated with lower toxicity. These clinical data suggest that a monoclonal antibody-chemotherapy combination is preferable to initiating treatment with single-agent trastuzumab. This trial did not

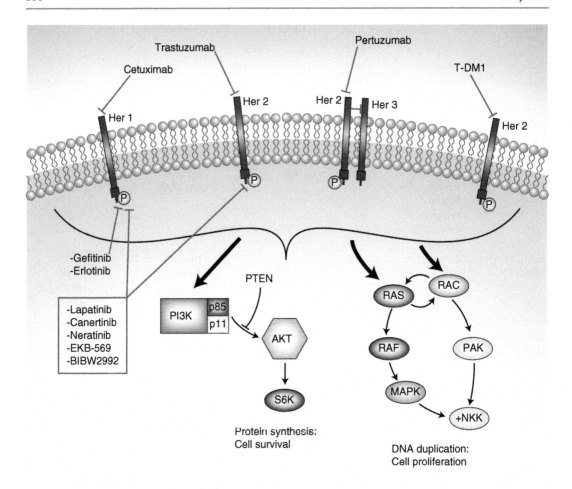

Fig. 33.1 Epidermal growth factor receptor (EGFR) family. The EGFR family is composed of four homologous receptors: ERBB1 (EGFR/HER1), ERBB2 (HER2/neu), ERBB3 (HER3), and ERBB4 (HER4). Three receptors have been implicated in the development of cancer; the role of ERBB4 is less clear. Six different ligands, known as EGF-like ligands, bind to EGFR. After ligand binding, the ERBB receptor is activated by dimerization between two identical receptors (i.e., homodimerization) or between different receptors of the same family (i.e., heterodimerization). Dimerization leads to the phosphorylation of several intracellular catalytic substrates, including members of the Ras/Raf/mitogen-activated protein kinase (MAPK) pathway, the phosphatidylinositol-3-kinase (PI3K)/Akt/PTEN family, and other important signaling pathways that regulate apoptosis, protein synthesis, and cellular proliferation. The morphologies of the extracellular domains of the four EGFRs are nearly identical, but the EGFRs vary considerably in functional activity. For instance, ERBB3 lacks inherent kinase function but can heterodimerize with other ERBB receptors. The ERBB2-ERBB3 dimer, which is considered the most active ERBB signaling dimer, is fundamental for ERBB2-mediated signaling in tumors with ERBB2 amplification (Reprinted from Alvarez et al. [11] with permission from the American Society of Clinical Oncology)

address the efficacy of transitioning from single-agent trastuzumab to trastuzumab plus single-agent chemotherapy at the time of disease progression. If a patient progresses on single-agent trastuzumab therapy, adding single-agent chemotherapy to trastuzumab is an option.

Trastuzumab Plus Chemotherapy

Trastuzumab is more active when used in combination with many chemotherapeutic agents, resulting in significantly improved ORR and OS. In the only first-line phase III trial to compare

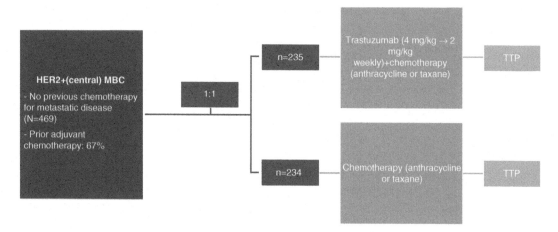

Fig. 33.2 "Trastuzumab plus chemotherapy (anthracycline or taxane)" vs. "chemotherapy (anthracycline or taxane)" (SLAMON) [6]. *HER2* human epidermal growth factor receptor 2, *MBC* metastatic breast cancer, *TTP* time to disease progression

an HER2-targeted therapy plus chemotherapy with chemotherapy alone, Slamon et al. observed improved survival, TTP, and ORR in the trastuzumab arm (Fig. 33.2) [6]. Patients were randomly assigned to receive standard chemotherapy alone or standard chemotherapy plus trastuzumab. Those who had not previously received adjuvant therapy with an anthracycline were treated with an anthracycline and cyclophosphamide with or without trastuzumab. Patients who had previously received adjuvant anthracycline were treated with paclitaxel alone or paclitaxel with trastuzumab. The addition of trastuzumab to chemotherapy was associated with a longer PFS (7.4 vs. 4.6 months; $P<0.001$), a higher ORR (50 % vs. 32 %, $P<0.001$), a longer duration of response (9.1 vs. 6.1 months; $P<0.001$), a lower rate of death at 1 year (22 % vs. 33 %, $P=0.008$), longer survival (25.1 vs. 20.3 months; $P=0.046$), and a 20 % reduction in the risk of death. The most important adverse event was cardiac dysfunction. The addition of trastuzumab was not associated with increases in other chemotherapy-associated toxicities. The cardiac dysfunction was New York Heart Association class III or IV and occurred in 27 % of the group administered an anthracycline, cyclophosphamide, and trastuzumab; 8 % of the group administered an anthracycline and cyclophosphamide alone; 13 % of the group

administered paclitaxel and trastuzumab; and 1 % of the group administered paclitaxel alone. This trial demonstrated that trastuzumab increases the clinical benefit of first-line chemotherapy in metastatic HER2-overexpressing breast cancer. The combination of an anthracycline and trastuzumab is not recommended because of the risk of significant cardiotoxicity [6].

The HERNATA study compared taxane- and non-taxane-based chemotherapy backbones in association with trastuzumab [7]. A total of 284 patients were randomized to trastuzumab plus either docetaxel or vinorelbine. OS was similar in both arms, but vinorelbine was much better tolerated; significantly more patients in the docetaxel arm experienced grade 3–4 toxicities and discontinued therapy. Efficacy was similar. In a smaller study that compared trastuzumab with either vinorelbine or a weekly taxane (paclitaxel or docetaxel), vinorelbine was associated with greater hematological toxicity [13]. Weekly paclitaxel has less toxicity and is better tolerated than three-weekly docetaxel. Data for patients who cannot use a taxane are limited, and the selection of an appropriate chemotherapy agent should be guided by patient and provider preferences.

Trastuzumab is generally not given in combination with multi-agent chemotherapy because of the excess risk of toxicity [14, 15]. No trials have

Table 33.2 Dosage dose modification of trastuzumab based on asymptomatic left ventricular ejection fraction decrease from baseline

Relationship of left ventricular ejection fraction (LVEF) to the lower limit of normal (LLN)	Trastuzumab dose modification based on asymptomatic LVEF decrease from baseline		
	≤10 percentage points	10–15 percentage points	≥15 percentage points
Within a facility's normal limits	Continue	Continue	Hold and repeat MUGA/ECHO after 4 weeks
<6 % below LLN	Continue[a]	Hold and repeat MUGA/ECHO after 4 weeks[a, b]	Hold and repeat MUGA/ECHO after 4 weeks[b, c]
≥6 % below LLN	Continue and repeat MUGA/ECHO after 4 weeks[c]	Hold and repeat MUGA/ECHO after 4 weeks[b, c]	Hold and repeat MUGA/ECHO after 4 weeks[b, c]

[a]Consider cardiac assessment. Cardiotoxicity associated with trastuzumab typically responds to appropriate medical therapy but may be severe and lead to cardiac failure
[b]After two holds, consider permanent trastuzumab discontinuation
[c]Refer to cardiologist

demonstrated that this approach improves OS. Two phase III trials explored the value of combination chemotherapy plus trastuzumab. The Breast Cancer International Research Group 007 study investigated the addition of carboplatin to docetaxel and trastuzumab [14]. The response rates were identical in both arms, with no significant differences in OS.

Robert et al. randomized 196 patients to trastuzumab and paclitaxel with or without carboplatin [15]. The response rate was higher in the triple-therapy arm; no significant difference in OS was observed. The increased toxicity of doublet chemotherapy limits the clinical role of this treatment strategy.

The single most important contraindication to HER2-targeted therapy is decreased left ventricular ejection fraction (LVEF) and/or clinical evidence of congestive heart failure arising from low LVEF [16]. The University of Texas M.D. Anderson Cancer Center evaluated the cardiac safety of long-term trastuzumab therapy in patients with HER2-overexpressing MBC. The median cumulative time of trastuzumab administration was 21.3 months. The median follow-up was 32.6 months (range, 11.8–79.0 months). Among the patients, 28 % experienced a cardiac event (CE): 15.6 % with grade 2 cardiac toxicity and 19 patients (10.9 %) with grade 3 cardiac toxicity. With trastuzumab discontinuation and appropriate therapy, all but three patients

had improved left ventricular ejection fraction (LVEF) or diminished symptoms of congestive heart failure. Baseline LVEF was significantly associated with CEs (HR, 0.94; $P=0.001$). The risk of CE among patients receiving concomitant taxanes was higher early in the follow-up period and subsequently declined. This toxicity was reversible in the majority of patients. Additional treatment with trastuzumab can be considered after recovery of cardiac function among patients who experience CE (Tables 33.2 and 33.3).

In conclusion, HER2-targeted therapy in combination with chemotherapy in the first-line setting is associated with improvements in the response rate, PFS, TTP, and OS when compared with chemotherapy alone. These data support the use of HER2-targeted therapy in combination with chemotherapy for the first-line treatment of MBC.

Lapatinib

Lapatinib is a small-molecule tyrosine kinase inhibitor that dually targets human epidermal growth factor receptors 1 (EGFR) and HER2. In contrast to trastuzumab, lapatinib enters the cell and binds to the intracellular domain of the tyrosine kinase receptor, completely blocking the autophosphorylation site and halting the downstream cascade (Fig. 33.1). After oral administration, lapatinib reaches peak plasma levels within

Table 33.3 Dosage dose modification of trastuzumab and pertuzumab combination based on asymptomatic left ventricular ejection fraction decrease from baseline

Left ventricular ejection fraction	Trastuzumab and pertuzumab		
	Action	LVEF at reassessment	Dose
<40 % and asymptomatic	Pause and repeat MUGA in 3 weeks	>45 % or 40–45 % and <10 % ↓ from baseline	Restart
40–50 %[a] and ≥10 % points below baseline and asymptomatic		<40 % or 40–50 %[a] and ≥10 % points below baseline or symptomatic	Discontinue
Symptomatic	Consider discontinuing	Not applicable	Not applicable

[a]In the CLEOPATRA trial, trastuzumab and pertuzumab treatments were paused if LVEF was 40–45 % and ≥10 % below baseline and asymptomatic. At LVEF reassessment, pertuzumab and trastuzumab may be restarted if LVEF "≥46 %" or "40–45 % and <10 % ↓ from baseline"; otherwise, discontinue

approximately 4 h and steady-state levels within 6–7 days and has a half-life of 24 h [17].

Single-agent lapatinib is not approved. As a second-line combination therapy, lapatinib and capecitabine improve TTP compared with capecitabine monotherapy for the treatment of HER2-positive MBC refractory to anthracycline-, taxane-, and trastuzumab-containing regimens [17]. Lapatinib plus chemotherapy is also active as a first-line treatment compared with chemotherapy alone but may be inferior to trastuzumab-based therapy [18, 19]. Two phase III trials have explored the use of lapatinib in the first-line setting, one of which compared lapatinib against placebo.

Guan et al. randomized patients who had not been treated with chemotherapy for metastatic disease to weekly paclitaxel (80 mg/m² weekly for 3 weeks every 4 weeks) plus either lapatinib (1500 mg daily) or placebo [18]. The addition of lapatinib to paclitaxel significantly improved OS vs. paclitaxel plus placebo (treatment hazard ratio, 0.74; 95 % CI, 0.58–0.94; $P=0.0124$); median OS was 27.8 vs. 20.5 months, respectively. Median PFS was prolonged by 3.2 months, from 6.5 months with placebo plus paclitaxel to 9.7 months with lapatinib plus paclitaxel (hazard ratio, 0.52; 95 % CI, 0.42–0.64; stratified log-rank $P<0.001$). ORR was significantly higher with lapatinib plus paclitaxel compared with placebo plus paclitaxel (69 % vs. 50 %, respectively; $P<0.001$). The incidence of grade 3 and 4

diarrhea and neutropenia was higher in the lapatinib plus paclitaxel arm. Only 4 % of patients in this group reported febrile neutropenia. Cardiac events were low grade, asymptomatic, and mostly reversible. The incidence of hepatic events was similar in both arms. There were no fatal adverse events in the lapatinib plus paclitaxel arm.

The MA.31 trial compared a combination of first-line anti-HER2 therapy (lapatinib or trastuzumab) and taxane therapy (paclitaxel 80 mg/m² weekly or docetaxel 75 mg/m² 3 weekly) for 24 weeks, followed by the same anti-HER2 monotherapy until progression (Fig. 33.3) [19]. A total of 652 patients were accrued, including 537 patients with centrally confirmed HER2-positive tumors. Median follow-up was 21.5 months. Median intention-to-treat (ITT) PFS was 9.0 months with lapatinib and 11.3 months with trastuzumab. ITT analysis indicated that PFS for lapatinib was inferior to trastuzumab, with a stratified hazard ratio of 1.37 (95 % CI, 1.13–1.65; $P=0.001$). In patients with centrally confirmed HER2-positive tumors, median PFS was 9.1 months with lapatinib and 13.6 months with trastuzumab (hazard ratio, 1.48; 95 % CI, 1.20–1.83; $P<0.001$). More grade 3 or 4 diarrhea and rash were observed with lapatinib ($P<0.001$). The PFS results were supported by the secondary end point of overall survival, with an ITT hazard ratio of 1.28 (95 % CI, 0.95–1.72; $P=0.11$); in patients with centrally confirmed HER2-positive tumors, the HR was 1.47 (95 % CI, 1.03–2.09; $P=0.03$).

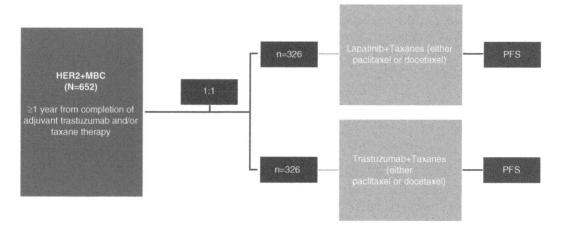

Fig. 33.3 "Taxane plus trastuzumab" vs. "taxane plus lapatinib" (NCIC CTG MA-31) [19]. *HER2* human epidermal growth factor receptor 2, *MBC* metastatic breast cancer, *PFS* progression-free survival

In conclusion, as first-line therapy for HER2-positive MBC, lapatinib combined with taxane was associated with a shorter PFS and more toxicity compared with trastuzumab combined with taxane. Taken together, the evidence suggests that trastuzumab-based regimens should still be considered the standard of care in this setting.

Pertuzumab

The pairing of HER receptors on the cell surface is referred to as dimerization. HER2 dimerizes with the other members of the HER family, including HER1, HER3, and HER4. HER2–HER3 dimerization is believed to produce the strongest mitogenic signal, resulting in the activation of two key pathways that regulate cell survival and growth: mitogen-activated protein kinase (MAPK) and phosphoinositide 3-kinase (PI3K) (Fig. 33.1) [11]. The humanized monoclonal antibody pertuzumab prevents the dimerization of HER2 with other HER receptors, particularly the pairing of the most potent signaling heterodimer HER2/HER3, thus providing a potent strategy for dual HER2 inhibition. Pertuzumab binds to the extracellular domain of HER2 at a different epitope than trastuzumab [20]. Preclinical data indicated that the combination of pertuzumab and trastuzumab was more active than either antibody alone because the antibodies

bind different HER2 epitopes, resulting in a more comprehensive signaling blockade [20]. Phase II studies demonstrated that pertuzumab was generally well tolerated as a single agent or in combination with trastuzumab and/or cytotoxic agents and implied that the combination of pertuzumab and trastuzumab has improved clinical efficacy for early and advanced HER2-positive breast cancer [21].

In the CLEOPATRA trial, the survival of patients with HER2 positive MBC was significantly improved after first-line therapy with pertuzumab, trastuzumab, and docetaxel compared with placebo, trastuzumab, and docetaxel (Fig. 33.4) [22]. In this trial, patients with MBC who had not received previous chemotherapy or anti-HER2 therapy for their metastatic disease were randomly assigned to receive the pertuzumab or placebo combination. The median overall survival was 56.5 months in the group receiving the pertuzumab combination, compared to 40.8 months (95 % CI, 35.8–48.3) in those receiving the placebo combination (hazard ratio favoring the pertuzumab group, 0.68; $P < 0.001$). Median PFS, as assessed by the investigators, improved by 6.3 months in the pertuzumab group (hazard ratio, 0.68; 95 % CI, 0.58–0.80). Pertuzumab extended the median duration of response by 7.7 months, as independently assessed. Dual HER2 blockade did not increase the risk of cardiac toxicity.

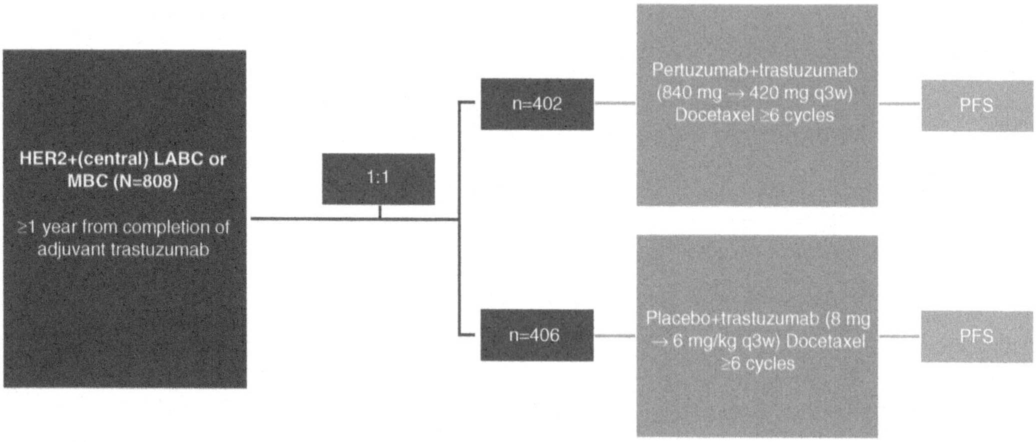

Fig. 33.4 Docetaxel plus trastuzumab vs. docetaxel plus trastuzumab plus pertuzumab (CLEOPATRA) [23]. *HER2* human epidermal growth factor receptor 2, *LABC* locally advanced breast cancer, *MBC* metastatic breast cancer, *q3w* every 3 weeks, *PFS* progression-free survival

Febrile neutropenia was more common with pertuzumab (13.8 % vs.7.6 %), driven mostly by a high incidence in Asian patients (26 % vs. 10 %), for reasons not currently clearly understood. The rate of grade 3 and 4 diarrhea (7.9 % vs. 5.0 %) was increased in the pertuzumab arm. In conclusion, compared with the addition of placebo, the addition of pertuzumab to trastuzumab and docetaxel significantly improved median OS of patients with HER2-positive MBC.

In the CLEOPATRA study, pertuzumab consistently showed a PFS benefit, independent of biomarker subgroups (hazard ratio<1.0), including the estrogen receptor–negative and estrogen receptor–positive subgroups [23]. The prognosis was significantly better for patients with high HER2 protein, high HER2 and HER3 mRNA levels, wild-type phosphatidylinositol-4,5-bisphosphate 3-kinase catalytic subunit alpha (PIK3CA), and low sHER2 ($P<0.05$). PIK3CA was the strongest prognostic indicator, with longer median PFS for patients whose tumors expressed wild-type vs. mutated PIK3CA in both the control (13.8 vs. 8.6 months) and pertuzumab groups (21.8 vs. 12.5 months). The biomarker data demonstrate that HER2 is the only marker suited for patient selection for the trastuzumab plus pertuzumab-based regimen in HER2-positive MBC. HER2, HER3, and PIK3CA were relevant prognostic factors. Interestingly, mutated PIK3CA was associated with worse prognosis when patients were treated with lapatinib plus capecitabine but not with T-DM1, suggesting that T-DM1 might overcome the negative implications of PIK3CA mutations. Novel biomarkers could help refine and optimize therapy for specific subsets of patients in the future.

Antibody-Drug Conjugate (ADC):T-DM1

Most ADC targets are cell surface proteins that are much more abundant on tumor cells than normal cells or tissues. ADCs selectively deliver targeted chemotherapy and could be important components of combination treatment regimens. The three components of ADCs, antibody, linker, and drug must be stable in the circulation for days or weeks. Antibody conjugates are a diverse class of therapeutics comprising a cytotoxic agent linked covalently to an antibody or antibody fragment directed toward a specific cell surface target expressed by tumor cells. Patients whose tumors express high levels of the target antigen are most likely to benefit from treatment. An appropriate antibody for ADC therapeutics allows the antibody-target complex to be internalized by the target cells, followed by drug release (Fig. 33.5) [24].

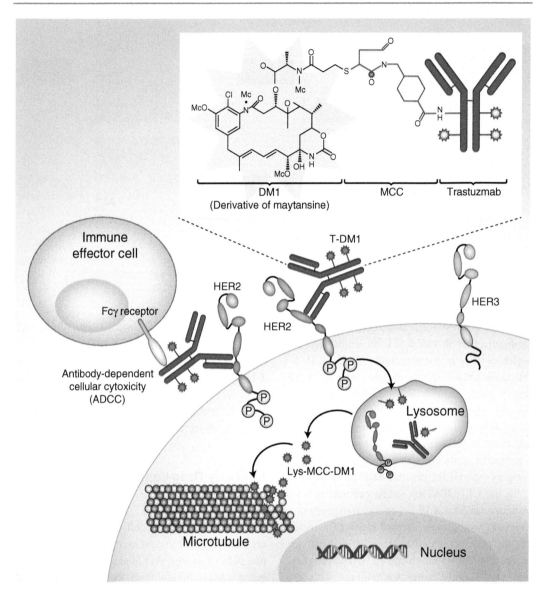

Fig. 33.5 Structure of T-DM1 and mechanisms of action. After T-DM1 binds HER2, the HER2/T-DM1 complex undergoes internalization, followed by lysosomal degradation. This process results in the intracellular release of DM1-containing catabolites that bind to tubulin, preventing microtubule polymerization and suppressing microtubule dynamic instability. T-DM1 retains the mechanisms of action of trastuzumab, including disruption of the HER3/PI3K/AKT signaling pathway and Fcγ receptor–mediated engagement of immune effector cells, which leads to antibody-dependent cellular cytoxicity (Reprinted from LoRusso et al. [26] with permission from the American Association for Cancer Research)

Drugs targeting tubulin or DNA are most often employed to form ADCs. ADCs are an effective method to increase the therapeutic index of these highly potent cytotoxic agents. The drugs used in ADCs must conjugate with a linker that can influence their circulating half-life and safety by minimizing the release of the drug molecule in the circulation. The goal is to optimize the delivery of the conjugate to the target tissue. An underconjugated antibody decreases ADC potency, whereas a highly conjugated antibody markedly decreases circulating half-life and impairs

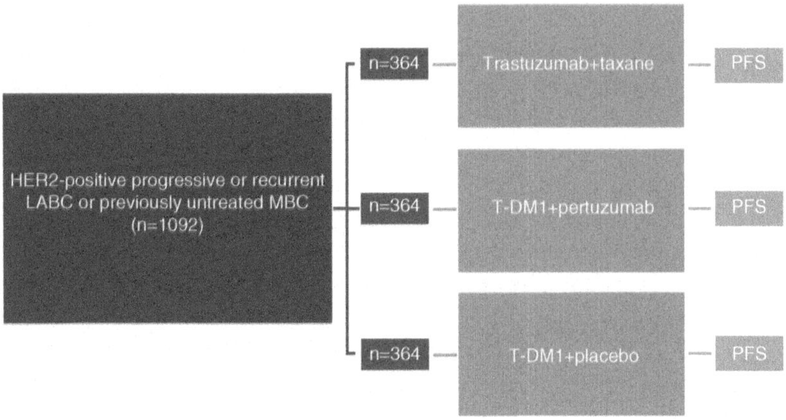

Fig. 33.6 Docetaxel/paclitaxel plus trastuzumab vs. T-DM1 vs. T-DM1 plus pertuzumab (MARIANNE) [28]. *HER2* human epidermal growth factor receptor 2, *LABC* locally advanced breast cancer, *MBC* metastatic breast cancer, *T-DM1* trastuzumab emtansine, *PFS* progression-free survival

binding to the target protein, thus decreasing ADC potency and efficacy [25].

T-DM1 is the first ADC to gain regulatory approval for HER2-positive MBC. T-DM1 binds HER2: the complex is internalized and degraded in lysosomes (Fig. 33.5). This process releases DM1-containing catabolites that bind to tubulin, thereby preventing microtubule polymerization and suppressing microtubule dynamic instability. T-DM1 retains the mechanisms of action of trastuzumab, including disruption of the HER3/PI3K/AKT signaling pathway and Fcγ receptor–mediated engagement of immune effector cells, resulting in antibody-dependent cellular cytotoxicity [26]. The mechanisms of ADC action for T-DM1 include all of the effects of trastuzumab plus the effects of the conjugated maytansine derivative.

Evidence supporting a potential role for T-DM1 comes from a phase II trial involving 137 women with HER2-positive MBC who were randomly assigned to trastuzumab plus docetaxel (HT) or T-DM1 [27]. Median PFS was 9.2 months with HT and 14.2 months with T-DM1 (hazard ratio, 0.59; 95 % CI, 0.36–0.97); median follow-up was approximately 14 months in both arms. ORR was 58.0 % (95 % CI, 45.5–69.2) with HT and 64.2 % (95 % CI, 51.8–74.8) with T-DM1. T-DM1 had a favorable safety profile vs. HT, with fewer grade ≥3 adverse events (adverse events; 46.4 % vs. 90.9 %), adverse events leading to treatment discontinuations (7.2 % vs.

34.8 %), and serious adverse events (20.3 % vs. 25.8 %). Grade 3–4 adverse events included neutropenia (6 % vs. 62 %), febrile neutropenia (0 % vs. 24 %), and epistaxis (1 % vs. 5 %) and were less with T-DM1. T-DM1 was associated with a higher incidence of serious pneumonias (6 % vs. 0 %) and increased liver transaminases (aspartate aminotransferase, 9 % vs. 0 %; alanine aminotransferase, 10 % vs. 0 %). In conclusion, in this randomized phase II study, first-line treatment with T-DM1 for patients with HER2-positive MBC provided a significant improvement in PFS vs. HT with a favorable safety profile.

After obtaining regulatory approval for T-DM1 when progression develops after trastuzumab treatment, the logical next step was to evaluate the efficacy of this novel ADC as a first-line treatment in a phase III randomized study. The MARIANNE (NCT01120184) trial recruited more than 1000 patients with HER2-positive MBC who had not received any chemotherapy in the metastatic setting (Fig. 33.6) [28]. In this phase III study, patients with centrally assessed HER2-positive (IHC3+ or ISH+) progressive/recurrent locally advanced BC or previously untreated MBC with a ≥6-month interval since treatment in the (neo)adjuvant setting with taxanes or vinca alkaloids were randomized 1:1:1 to HT (docetaxel or paclitaxel plus trastuzumab), T-DM1 (T-DM1 plus placebo, hereafter T-DM1), or T-DM1 plus pertuzumab at standard doses. The primary end point was PFS assessed by independent review. Comparisons between HT and T-DM1 or T-DM1 plus pertuzumab were considered separately. In each arm, approximately 31 % of patients had prior (neo)adjuvant treatment with HER2-directed therapy, and approximately 37 % overall had de novo disease. PFS and OS were similar across treatment arms. T-DM1 and T-DM1 plus pertuzumab demonstrated noninferior PFS compared with HT but were not superior to HT. The addition of pertuzumab to T-DM1 did not improve PFS. T-DM1–containing regimens were associated with different toxicity profiles than the control regimen. T-DM1 was better tolerated than HT, with fewer grade 3–4 adverse events and fewer adverse event-related treatment discontinuations. No febrile neutropenia and less neuropathy, diarrhea and alopecia were observed with T-DM1, though these subjects had greater transaminase elevation and thrombocytopenia. Health-related quality of life was maintained for longer with T-DM1. These results suggest that T-DM1 may be an alternative to HT in previously untreated HER2-positive MBC. However, this trial did not include a comparator arm with taxane, trastuzumab, and pertuzumab, which is the standard first-line therapy for HER2-positive MBC.

mTOR Inhibitor: Everolimus

The PI3K/Akt/mammalian target of rapamycin (mTOR) signaling pathway is an established driver of oncogenic activity in human malignancies and regulates cell growth and proliferation [29] (Fig. 33.7). In breast cancer, the PI3K/Akt/mTOR pathway has been associated with resistance to endocrine therapy, HER2-directed therapy and cytotoxic therapy. Therapeutic targeting of this pathway holds significant promise as a treatment strategy. In the BOLERO-2 trial the mTOR inhibitor everolimus is the first of this class of agents approved for the treatment of hormone receptor–positive, HER2-negative advanced breast cancer [30]. In early studies, everolimus showed antitumor activity in breast cancer and synergy with both trastuzumab and paclitaxel [31].

The BOLERO-1 trial is in progress and will evaluate the combination of everolimus with trastuzumab plus paclitaxel as a first-line treatment for women with HER2-positive, locally advanced or MBC (Fig. 33.8) [32]. In this phase 3 randomized trial, women with HER2-positive advanced breast cancer, without prior trastuzumab or chemotherapy for advanced disease, were randomized 2:1 to receive either everolimus (10 mg/day) or placebo and weekly paclitaxel plus trastuzumab. The two primary objectives are to compare the investigator-assessed PFS between everolimus plus trastuzumab plus paclitaxel and placebo plus trastuzumab plus paclitaxel in the full population and the hormone receptor–negative subpopulation. A total of 719 patients were randomized to receive everolimus or placebo. Baseline characteristics/prior therapies were balanced between the two treatment arms. The median age was 53 years; 70.5 % had visceral metastases, and 43.3 % were hormone receptor negative. Prior therapy included trastuzumab (10.8 %) and taxane (24.9 %). The baseline characteristics for the hormone receptor–negative subpopulation were generally balanced between the two treatment arms and similar to the overall population. Median study follow-up at the time of analysis was 41.3 months. The study did not meet its primary objective in the full population: median PFS was 15 months (95 %: 14.6–17.9) in the everolimus arm vs. 14.5 months (95 % CI: 12.3–17.1) in the placebo arm (hazard ratio, 0.89; 95 % CI, 0.73–1.08; $P=0.1166$). The hormone receptor–negative subpopulation ($n=311$) achieved a clinically relevant 7.2 months of benefit in median PFS in the everolimus arm (20.3 months) vs. placebo arm (13.1 months); (hazard ratio = 0.66; 95 % CI: 0.48–0.91; $P=0.0049$), just short of the protocol pre-specified level of statistical significance ($P=0.0044$). An additional sensitivity analysis of PFS without censoring patients at the start of new antineoplastic therapy yielded a hazard ratio consistent with the primary analysis ($P=0.0043$). PFS based on a central assessment corroborated the investigator-assessed PFS in both the full population and in the hormone receptor–negative subpopulation. OS data

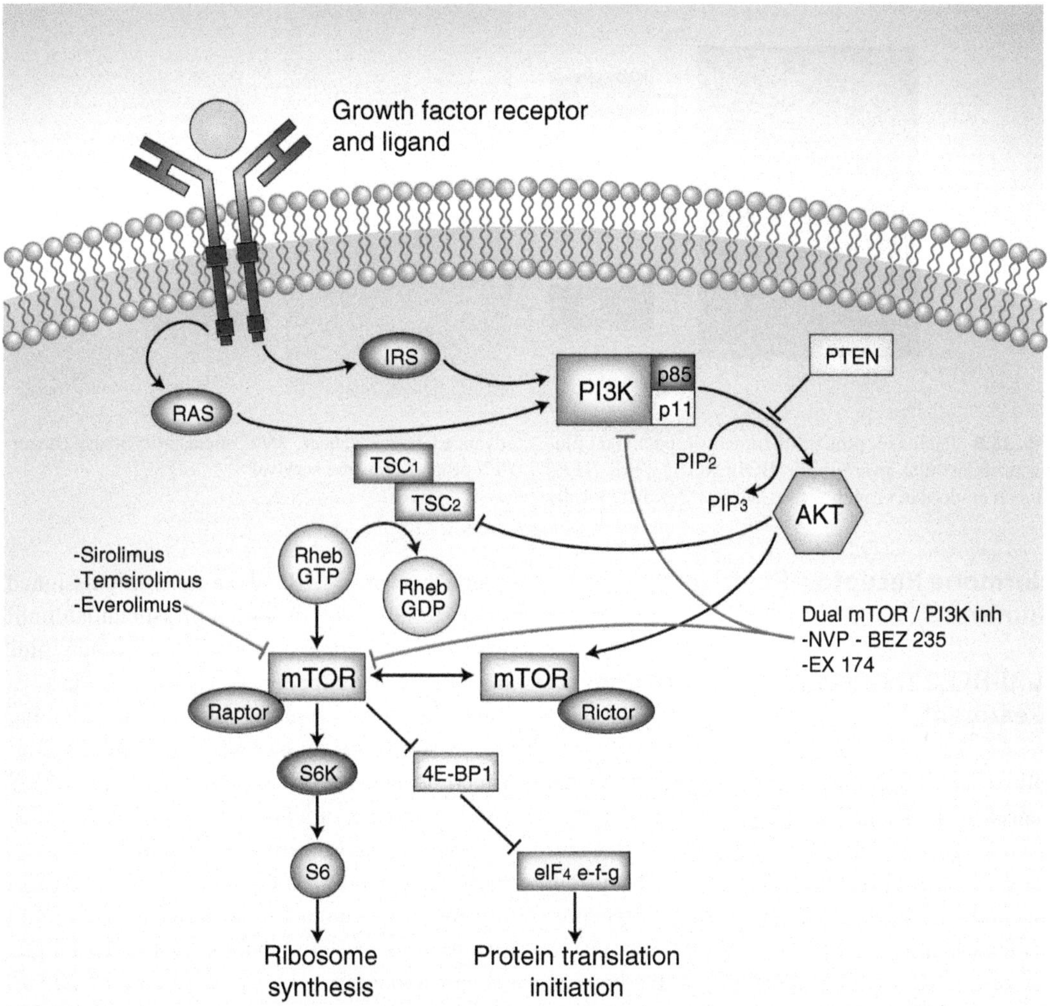

Fig. 33.7 The mammalian target of rapamycin (mTOR) signaling network. mTOR is a highly conserved pathway that regulates cell proliferation and metabolism in response to environmental factors. The growth factor receptor is linked to mTOR signaling via the phosphatidylinositol-3-kinase (PI3K)/Akt family. *PTEN* plays an important role in this pathway; loss of *PTEN* function through mutation, deletion, or epigenetic silencing results in increased activation of Akt and mTOR. The mTOR proteins regulate the activities of the translational regulators 4E-BP1 and p70S6 kinase (S6K). mTOR antagonists have been developed to inhibit mTORC1 (raptor) (Reprinted from Alvarez et al. [11] with permission from the American Society of Clinical Oncology)

were not complete at the time of this publication. The most common adverse events in the everolimus vs. placebo arms were stomatitis (66.5 % vs. 32.4 %), diarrhea (56.6 % vs. 46.6 %), and alopecia (46.8 % vs. 52.5 %). Suspected drug-related serious adverse events were reported for 21.8 % vs. 7.6 %, and on-treatment adverse event-related deaths were reported for 3.6 % vs. 0 % of patients,

respectively. In conclusion, first-line therapy with everolimus plus trastuzumab plus paclitaxel did not show a PFS benefit in patients with HER2-positive advanced breast cancer; the hormone receptor–negative subpopulation derived a clinically robust benefit to median PFS of 7.2 months, suggesting that everolimus may have a role in this patient subpopulation.

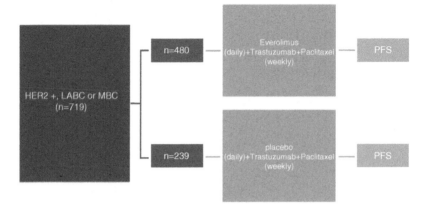

Fig. 33.8 Paclitaxel plus trastuzumab vs. paclitaxel plus trastuzumab plus everolimus (BOLERO-1) [32]. *HER2* human epidermal growth factor receptor 2, *LABC* locally advanced breast cancer, *MBC* metastatic breast cancer, *PFS* progression-free survival

Hormone Receptor–Positive Tumors

Anti-HER2 Treatment Plus Endocrine Treatment

HER2- and hormone receptor–positive breast cancer is a distinct subtype associated with a good prognosis but a lower response to standard chemotherapy plus anti-HER2 agents. Concurrent blockade of the HER2 and estrogen receptor pathways has been a successful strategy to increase ORR and PFS in patients with advanced disease [4, 5].

For select patients with HER2-positive and hormone receptor–positive (ER positive/PgR positive or negative) breast cancer, endocrine treatment with either trastuzumab or lapatinib or endocrine therapy alone may be an acceptable first-line treatment [4, 5]. Endocrine therapy alone is included as an option because trials of endocrine therapy with or without HER2-targeted therapy did not demonstrate an OS advantage. Several trials have examined the addition of HER2-targeted agents to aromatase inhibitors in postmenopausal women [4, 33, 34].

TAnDEM is the first randomized phase III study to combine a hormonal agent and trastuzumab without chemotherapy as treatment for HER2/hormone receptor–positive MBC [4]. Postmenopausal women with HER2/hormone receptor–positive MBC were randomly assigned to anastrozole with or without trastuzumab until progression. Patients in the trastuzumab plus anastrozole arm experienced significant improvements in PFS compared with those receiving anastrozole alone. In patients with centrally confirmed hormone receptor positivity, median PFS was 5.6 and 3.8 months in the trastuzumab plus anastrozole and anastrozole alone arms, respectively (log-rank $P=0.006$). OS did not differ significantly between treatments. The most common toxicities in the combination arm were fatigue (21 %), vomiting (21 %), and diarrhea (20 %). The incidence of grade 3 and 4 adverse events was 23 % and 5 %, respectively, in the trastuzumab plus anastrozole arm, and 15 % and 1 %, respectively, in the anastrozole-only arm.

The eLEcTRA trial compared the efficacy and safety of letrozole combined with trastuzumab to letrozole alone in patients with HER2- and hormone receptor–positive MBC [33]. Patients were randomized to either letrozole alone (arm A, $n=31$) or letrozole plus trastuzumab (arm B, $n=26$) as first-line treatments. An additional 35 patients with HER2-negative and hormone receptor–positive tumors received letrozole alone (arm C). Median time to progression in arm A was 3.3 months compared to 14.1 months in arm B (hazard ratio, 0.67; $P=0.23$) and 15.2 months in arm C (hazard ratio, 0.71; $P=0.03$). The clinical benefit rate was 39 % for arm A compared to

65 % in arm B (odds ratio 2.99, 95 % CI 1.01–8.84) and 77 % in arm C (odds ratio 5.34, 95 % CI 1.83–15.58). The eLEcTRA trial demonstrated that the combination of letrozole and trastuzumab is a safe and effective treatment option for patients with HER2- and hormone receptor–positive MBC.

Both of these trials observed PFS and TTP benefits but no OS benefit in the combination arm. In another more recent trial [34], postmenopausal women with hormone receptor–positive MBC were randomized to daily oral treatment with letrozole plus lapatinib vs. letrozole plus placebo. Of the 1286 patients enrolled in the phase III study, 219 had HER2-positive tumors. In the hormone receptor–positive HER2-positive population, adding lapatinib to letrozole significantly lowered the risk for disease progression compared to letrozole alone (hazard ratio, 0.71; 95 % CI, 0.53–0.96). PFS was 8.2 months vs. 3.0 months. ORR (28 % vs. 15 %) and the clinical benefit rate (48 % vs. 29 %) were also significantly greater in lapatinib-treated women. The most common adverse events in the lapatinib group were diarrhea (68 %) and rash (46 %), primarily grade 1 and 2. In conclusion, the risk for disease progression among women with hormone receptor–positive HER2-positive MBC was a statistically significant 29 % lower risk for treatment with letrozole plus lapatinib compared to letrozole alone. The combination therapy was well tolerated, with primarily grade 1 and 2 toxicities. This trial further confirms that sustained HER2 inhibition benefits patients with HER2-positive MBC. Moreover, the addition of oral lapatinib provides a convenient option for women who receive oral endocrine therapy for an extended time.

There is no clear evidence that the ER/PgR status of patients with HER2-positive advanced breast cancer affects their response to HER2-targeted therapy. No significant difference in OS was observed in first-line treatment trials comparing an HER2-targeted agent plus endocrine therapy to endocrine therapy alone [4, 33, 34]. Although adding HER2-targeted therapy to endocrine therapy does not seem to benefit OS, these studies did show a PFS benefit for the combination therapy groups. Patients with ER-positive breast cancer have also been included in first-line chemotherapy trials, such as CLEOPATRA, which showed an OS benefit from the chemotherapy and HER2-targeted therapy combinations [22].

No studies have directly compared endocrine plus HER2-targeted therapies with chemotherapy plus HER2-targeted therapy. Although the clinician may discuss using endocrine therapy with or without HER2-targeted therapy, most patients will receive chemotherapy plus HER2-targeted therapy. There are no methods for identifying patients who would benefit from combined therapy vs. endocrine therapy alone. When chemotherapy is discontinued, clinicians may recommend that patients start endocrine therapy, which is typically administered in conjunction with HER2-targeted therapy.

In conclusion, initial therapy with endocrine agents is a reasonable option for patients who are not good candidates for chemotherapy or for those who wish to avoid the toxicity of chemotherapy. In most circumstances, endocrine therapy should be administered with HER2-targeted therapy [34]. However, given that the addition of HER2 therapy to endocrine therapy does not improve OS, patients who have low-volume disease, a long disease-free interval, indolent disease or significant comorbidities would be the most appropriate candidates for endocrine therapy alone.

Second-Line Therapy

Multiple phase III clinical trials have demonstrated that continuation of anti-HER2 therapy in the second-line setting improves the clinical outcome of patients whose disease has recurred or progressed on first-line trastuzumab-based therapy (Table 33.4). All studies have demonstrated a benefit of continuing some form of HER2-targeted therapy in the second-line setting as either a combination of HER2-targeted therapy and chemotherapy, a combination of two HER2-targeted therapies, or T-DM1. These therapies were associated with improved outcomes.

Table 33.4 Second-line randomized phase III studies in HER2-positive metastatic breast cancer patients

Trial	Study arms	ORR (CR/PR) %	p	PFS Months	Hazard ratio (95 % CI), p	OS Months	Hazard ratio (95 % CI), p
EMILIA Verma [41]	T-DM1	43.6	<0.001	9.6	HR 0.65 p<0.001	30.9	HR 0.68 p<0.001
	Lapatinib + capecitabine	30.8		6.4		25.1	
BOLERO-3 Andre [39]	Everolimus + trastuzumab + vinorelbine	41	=0.210	7	HR 0.78 (0.65–0.95) p<0.001	NR	
	Trastuzumab + vinorelbine	37		5.8		NR	
TH3RESA[a] Krop [49]	T-DM1	31	=0.0001	6.2	HR 0.53 p<0.0001	NE	HR 0.55 p=0.0034 (NS)
	Physicians' choice[b]	9		3.3		14.9	
EGF 104900 Blackwell [35]	Lapatinib + trastuzumab	NR		11.1	HR 0.74 (0.58–0.94)	14	HR 0.74 (0.57–0.97)
	Lapatinib[c]	NR		8.1		9.5	
LUX Breast I Harbeck [47]	Afatinib + vinorelbine	46.1	=0.851	5.5	p=0.4272	20.5	p=0.0048
	Trastuzumab + vinorelbine	47		5.6		28.6	

MBC metastatic breast cancer, *ORR* objective response rare, *CR* complete response, *PR* partial response, *PFS* progression-free survival, *OS* overall survival, *HR* hazard ratio, *T-DM1* trastuzumab emtansine, *NE* not evaluable, *NS* nonsignificant

[a]In this trial OS (immature)

[b]Physician's choice could have been single-agent chemotherapy, hormonal therapy, or HER2-directed therapy or a combination of HER2-directed therapy with chemotherapy, hormonal therapy, or other HER2-directed therapies: 68.% chemotherapy + trastuzumab, 10.3 % trastuzumab + lapatinib, and 2.7 % chemotherapy + lapatinib

[c]Lapatinib is not approved as a single agent

The evaluated therapeutic options included continuing trastuzumab with a different chemotherapy partner, switching to T-DM1, adding the mTOR pathway inhibitor everolimus, or switching to a regimen of capecitabine plus lapatinib.

Continuing Trastuzumab

The strategy of continuing trastuzumab while switching its chemotherapy partner was evaluated in two phase III trials. Continuation of trastuzumab in conjunction with lapatinib without cytotoxic chemotherapy was investigated in the EGF104900 study (Fig. 33.9) [35]. Heavily pretreated patients were randomized to lapatinib plus trastuzumab or to lapatinib alone. The improvement in response rate was not significant. In the updated final analysis of all patients randomly assigned with strata

($n=291$), lapatinib plus trastuzumab continued to be superior to lapatinib monotherapy in PFS (hazard ratio, 0.74; 95 % CI, 0.58–0.94; $P=0.011$) and offered significant OS benefit (hazard ratio, 0.74; 95 % CI, 0.57–0.97; $P=0.026$). Improvements in absolute OS rates were 10 % at 6 months and 15 % at 12 months in the combination arm compared with the monotherapy arm. Multiple baseline factors, including an Eastern Cooperative Oncology Group (ECOG) performance status of 0, nonvisceral disease, <3 metastatic sites, and shorter time from initial diagnosis to random assignment, were associated with improved OS. The incidence of adverse events was consistent with previously reported rates. These data demonstrated a significant 4.5-month median OS advantage of the lapatinib and trastuzumab combination and support dual HER2 blockade in patients with heavily pretreated HER2-positive MBC.

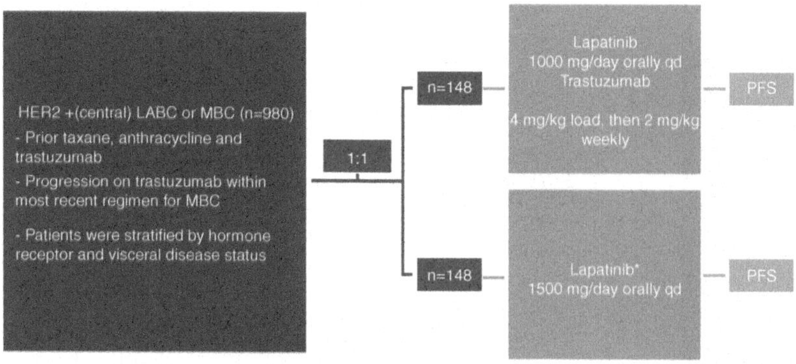

Fig. 33.9 Lapatinib plus trastuzumab vs. lapatinib alone (EGF 104900) [35]. *HER2* human epidermal growth factor receptor 2, *LABC* locally advanced breast cancer, *MBC* metastatic breast cancer, *qd* once daily, *PFS* progression-free survival; *Lapatinib is not approved for use as a single agent

In a German Breast Group/Breast International Group study, 156 patients with HER2-positive breast cancer that progressed during treatment with trastuzumab were randomly assigned to receive capecitabine (2500 mg/m² body-surface area on days 1 through 14 [1250 mg/m² semi-daily]) alone or with continuation of trastuzumab (6 mg/kg body weight) in 3-week cycles [9]. Median times to progression were 5.6 months in the capecitabine group and 8.2 months in the capecitabine-plus-trastuzumab group, with an unadjusted hazard ratio of 0.69 (95 % CI, 0.48–0.97; two-sided log-rank $P=0.0338$). OS was 20.4 months (95 % CI, 17.8–24.7) in the capecitabine group and 25.5 months (95 % CI, 19.0–30.7) in the capecitabine-plus-trastuzumab group ($P=0.257$). ORR was 27.0 % with capecitabine and 48.1 % with capecitabine plus trastuzumab (odds ratio, 2.50; $P=0.0115$). The continuation of trastuzumab beyond progression was not associated with increased toxicity, and the continuation of trastuzumab plus capecitabine resulted in a significant improvement in ORR and TTP compared with capecitabine alone.

Trastuzumab and Pertuzumab Combination

A study of the combination of trastuzumab and capecitabine with or without pertuzumab in patients with HER2-positive MBC (PHEREXA) is ongoing [36]. This randomized, two-arm study will evaluate the efficacy and safety of a combination of trastuzumab and capecitabine with or without pertuzumab in patients with HER2-positive MBC. The study population consists of female patients whose disease has progressed during or following previous trastuzumab therapy for metastatic disease. All patients in Arms A and B receive trastuzumab (8 mg/kg iv as loading dose and then 6 mg/kg iv every 3 weeks thereafter) plus capecitabine oral twice daily for 14 days every 3 weeks (1250 mg/m² twice daily in Arm A and 1000 mg/m² twice daily in Arm B). In addition, patients in Arm B will receive pertuzumab (840 mg iv as a loading dose and then 420 mg iv thereafter) every 3 weeks. The study treatment will continue until disease progression or unacceptable toxicity.

mTOR Inhibitors to Target Resistance

Although HER2-targeted therapy in the clinic has significantly improved patient outcomes, treatment resistance remains a problem. The causes of resistance include pathway redundancy, reactivation, or the utilization of escape pathways [37, 38]. Understanding the mechanisms of resistance can lead to better therapeutic strategies to overcome resistance and optimize outcomes.

In breast cancer, the PI3K/Akt/mTOR pathway has been associated with resistance to

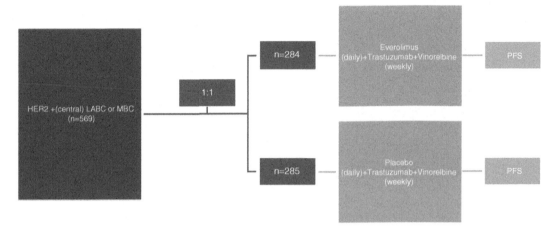

Fig. 33.10 Everolimus in combination with vinorelbine and trastuzumab (BOLERA-3) [39]. *HER2* human epidermal growth factor receptor 2, *LABC* locally advanced breast cancer, *MBC* metastatic breast cancer, *PFS* progression-free survival

endocrine therapy, HER2-directed therapy and cytotoxic therapy [29, 37]. Disease progression in patients with HER2-positive breast cancer receiving trastuzumab might be associated with activation of the PI3K/Akt/mTOR intracellular signaling pathway. Adding the mTOR inhibitor everolimus to trastuzumab might restore sensitivity to trastuzumab (Fig. 33.7) [37, 38].

In the BOLERO-3 trial, women with HER2-positive, trastuzumab-resistant, advanced breast cancer who had previously received taxane therapy were randomized to daily everolimus (5 mg/day) (*n*=284) plus weekly trastuzumab (2 mg/kg) and vinorelbine (25 mg/m²) or to placebo (*n*=285) plus trastuzumab plus vinorelbine in 3-week cycles, stratified by previous lapatinib use (Fig. 33.10) [39]. Median follow-up at the time of analysis was 20.2 months. Median PFS was 7.0 months with everolimus and 5.78 months with placebo (hazard ratio: 0.78; *P*=0.0067). The greatest benefit was to patients with hormone receptor–negative tumors. The most common grade 3–4 adverse events were neutropenia (73 % in the everolimus group vs. 62 % in the placebo group), leukopenia (38 % vs. 29 %), anemia (19 % vs. 6 %), febrile neutropenia (16 % vs. 4 %), stomatitis (13 % vs. 1 %), and fatigue (12 % vs. 4 %). Serious adverse events were reported in 42 % of patients in the everolimus group and 20 % in the placebo group.

T-DM1 is an ideal candidate for combination with agents that, because of overlapping toxicities,

have been difficult to combine with chemotherapy. Ongoing trials are combining T-DM1 with a variety of downstream inhibitors of signaling or other molecular pathways, including inhibitors of heat shock proteins, cyclin-dependent kinases, PI3K/AKT, and mTOR.

Capecitabine Plus Lapatinib

Geyer et al. conducted a phase III study comparing capecitabine plus lapatinib with capecitabine alone in patients who had progressed on prior trastuzumab-based therapy [8, 40]. Patients were randomized to lapatinib (1250 mg/day) plus capecitabine (2000 mg/m²) or capecitabine monotherapy (2500 mg/m²) on days 1–14 of a 21-day cycle. In total, 207 and 201 patients were enrolled to combination therapy and monotherapy, respectively. The median OS was 75.0 weeks for the combination arm and 64.7 weeks for the monotherapy arm (hazard ratio, 0.87; 95 % CI, 0.71–1.08; *P*=0.210). This study showed significant clinical benefits, including a trend toward OS in favor of the combination vs. monotherapy in patients with trastuzumab-pretreated HER2-positive MBC. These results led to the premature termination of accrual to the study, and 36 patients receiving monotherapy were permitted to cross over to combination therapy. A Cox regression analysis considering crossover as a

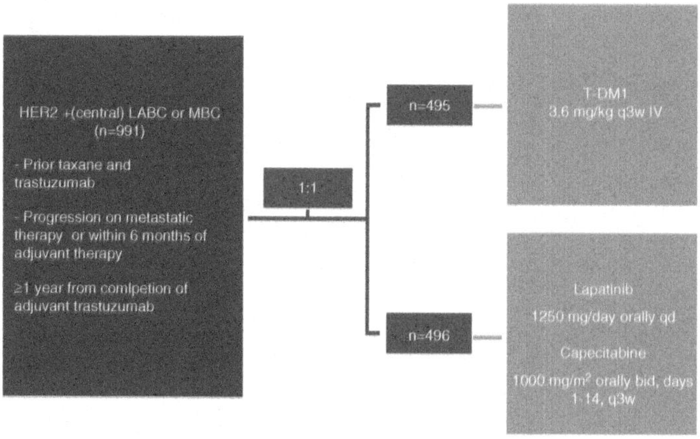

Fig. 33.11 T-DM1 vs. "capecitabine plus lapatinib" (EMILIA) [41]. *HER2* human epidermal growth factor receptor 2, *LABC* locally advanced breast cancer, *MBC* metastatic breast cancer, *T-DM1* trastuzumab emtansine, *q3w* every 3 weeks, *IV* intravenous, *PD* progressive disease, *qd* once daily, *bid* twice daily

time-dependent covariate suggested that there may have been a 20 % lower risk for death in the combination therapy arm (hazard ratio, 0.80; 95 % CI, 0.64–0.99; $P = 0.043$). Although premature termination and crossover resulted in insufficient power to detect an OS benefit, these updated analyses confirm a trend toward an OS advantage in the combination arm. The incidence of diarrhea (60 % vs. 39 %) and rash (27 % vs. 15 %) was higher in the combination arm, but the incidences of severe toxicities were comparable between the two arms. Lapatinib was approved by the FDA for the treatment of HER2-positive breast cancer in combination with capecitabine for patients who progressed after an anthracycline, taxane, and trastuzumab.

T-DM1

T-DM1 is an antibody-drug conjugate incorporating the HER2-targeted antitumor properties of trastuzumab with the cytotoxic activity of the microtubule-inhibitory agent DM1 (Fig. 33.5) [41]. The superiority of T-DM1 to capecitabine plus lapatinib in the second-line setting was established in the EMILIA trial (Fig. 33.11) [41]. Patients with HER2-positive advanced breast cancer who had previously been treated with trastuzumab and a taxane were randomly assigned to

T-DM1 or lapatinib plus capecitabine. Among 991 patients, median PFS as assessed by independent review was 9.6 months for T-DM1 vs. 6.4 months for lapatinib plus capecitabine (hazard ratio for progression or death from any cause, 0.65; $P < 0.001$), and median OS at the second interim analysis crossed the stopping boundary for efficacy (30.9 months vs. 25.1 months; hazard ratio for death from any cause, 0.68; $P < 0.001$). ORR was higher with T-DM1 (43.6 %, vs. 30.8 %; $P < 0.001$). Rates of grade 3 or 4 adverse events were higher with lapatinib plus capecitabine than with T-DM1 (57 % vs. 41 %). The incidences of thrombocytopenia and increased serum aminotransferase levels were higher with T-DM1, whereas the incidences of diarrhea, nausea, vomiting, and palmar-plantar erythrodysesthesia were higher with lapatinib plus capecitabine. The incidence of grade 3 or worse thrombocytopenia was 12.9 % in the T-DM1–treated group and 0.2 % in the lapatinib/capecitabine group. Patients treated with T-DM1 in the EMILIA trial experienced an overall higher rate of bleeding compared with those treated with capecitabine plus lapatinib (30 % vs. 16 %, respectively), although the rate of serious bleeding events was low in both arms (1.4 % vs. 0.8 %). However, the etiology of bleeding was not entirely explained by other risk factors (e.g., the use of anticoagulants or concomitant thrombocytopenia). Platelets do not

Table 33.5 Dosage dose modification of T-DM1 based on asymptomatic left ventricular ejection fraction decrease from baseline

Criteria	Left ventricular ejection fraction (LVEF)	Action	Action at LVEF reassessment
1	>45 %	Continue and follow routine monitoring guidelines	Follow actions based on criteria
2	40–45 % AND <10 % below baseline and asymptomatic	Continue and repeat LVEF in 3 weeks	Discontinue permanently if no recovery. If improved to criteria # 1 (for # 2, 3, or 4) or # 2 (for # 3 or 4), it may be restarted; monitor closely
3	40–45 % AND ≥10 % below baseline, and asymptomatic	Pause and repeat LVEF in 3 weeks	
4	<40 % and asymptomatic		
5	Symptomatic or confirmed CHF	Discontinue	Not applicable

overexpress HER2, and the thrombocytopenia may be mediated in part by DM1-induced impairment of megakaryocytic differentiation. For most patients receiving T-DM1, thrombocytopenia can be monitored without any changes in treatment. T-DM1 can cause liver failure and death. If serum transaminases or total bilirubin are increased, the dose of T-DM1 should be reduced or discontinued. All patients should undergo evaluation of LVEF before and during treatment with T-DM1. If a patient develops a clinically meaningful decrease in left ventricular function, the treatment should be discontinued. Additional treatment with T-DM1 can be considered after recovery of cardiac function among patients who experience cardiac event (Table 33.5).

Patient-reported outcomes from EMILIA have also been published [42]. A secondary endpoint of the EMILIA study was time to symptom worsening, which was delayed in the T-DM1 arm vs. the capecitabine-plus-lapatinib arm (7.1 months vs. 4.6 months, respectively; hazard ratio = 0.796; $P=0.012$). In the T-DM1 arm, 55.3 % of patients developed clinically significant improvement in symptoms from baseline vs. 49.4 % in the capecitabine-plus-lapatinib arm ($P=0.084$). Although similar at baseline, the number of patients reporting diarrhea increased 1.5 to twofold during treatment with capecitabine and lapatinib but remained near baseline levels in the T-DM1 arm. Together with the EMILIA primary data, these results support the view that T-DM1 has greater efficacy and tolerability than capecitabine plus lapatinib, which may translate into improvements in health-related quality of life. Based on the available data, the ASCO guideline recommends the use of anti-HER 2 therapy including T-DM1 in the second-line setting [43].

The ability of ADCs to deliver chemotherapy selectively to the tumor not only offers the potential for greater efficacy and reduced toxicity as monotherapy but also expands the potential for combination regimens. Virtually any agent that one would consider adding to a trastuzumab/chemotherapy backbone could be considered for addition to T-DM1. The order of treatment may be important; in preclinical models, pretreatment with pertuzumab appeared to blunt the efficacy of T-DM1 [44]. Ongoing trials are exploring the potential of combining T-DM1 with a variety of chemotherapy agents, including paclitaxel, docetaxel, and capecitabine, among others. Alternatively, T-DM1 has been substituted for the taxane/trastuzumab portion of adjuvant therapy for high-risk patients in the ongoing KAITLIN trial.

Tyrosine Kinase Inhibitors

Afatinib is an oral ErbB family blocker that covalently binds and irreversibly blocks all kinase-competent ErbB family members. A phase II, open-label, single-arm study explored afatinib activity in HER2-positive breast cancer patients progressing after trastuzumab treatment [45]. Patients had stage IIIB/IV HER2-positive MBC with progression following trastuzumab or trastuzumab intolerance and an ECOG performance status of 0–2. Patients received 50 mg of afatinib once daily until disease progression. The primary endpoint was ORR using RECIST 1–0 (Response Evaluation Criteria in Solid Tumors 1.0) criteria [46]. Forty-one patients who had received a median of three prior chemotherapies (range, 0–15), including 68.3 % who had received trastuzumab for >1 year, were treated. Four patients (10 % of 41 treated; 11 % of evaluable patients) had a partial response. Fifteen patients (37 % of 41) had stable disease as the best response, and 19 (46 % of 41) achieved clinical benefit. Median PFS was 15.1 weeks (95 % CI: 8.1–16.7), and median OS was 61.0 weeks (95 % CI: 56.7–not evaluable). The most frequent grade 3 treatment-related adverse events were diarrhea (24.4 %) and rash (9.8 %).

In the LUX Breast I trial, patients with HER2-positive MBC and failure of one trastuzumab-based regimen (adjuvant/first-line) were randomized 2:1 to afatinib plus vinorelbine (AV) (40 mg/day oral+25 mg/m^2/week iv) or trastuzumab plus vinorelbine (TV) (2 mg/kg/week iv after 4 mg/kg loading dose+25 mg/m^2/week iv). Treatment continued until disease progression or unacceptable adverse events. The primary endpoint was PFS [47]. A total of 508 patients were randomized (AV:339, TV:169). A pre-planned risk/benefit assessment was found unfavorable, and recruitment was stopped. Patients on AV therapy were switched to TV, received A or V monotherapy, or stopped treatment. Median PFS was 5.5 months with AV vs. 5.6 months with TV (hazard ratio, 1.10; $P=0.4272$). ORR was 46.1 % with AV and 47.0 % with TV (odds Ratio 1.04; $P=0.8510$). Median OS was 19.6 months with AV and 28.6 months with TV (hazard ratio, 1.76; 95 % CI 1.20, 2.59; $P=0.0036$). The most common drug-related adverse events were diarrhea (80.1 %), neutropenia (75.1 %) and rash (45.1 %) with AV and neutropenia (78.7 %), leukopenia (37.3 %) and anemia (27.8 %) with TV. Three AV patients died due to treatment-related causes. In conclusion, AV and TV demonstrated similar PFS and ORR, but the OS diverged and was shorter for AV compared to TV in patients with HER2-positive MBC. The safety profile of AV was consistent with the individual monotherapies, but its tolerability compared unfavorably to TV.

Neratinib is a potent irreversible pan-tyrosine kinase inhibitor with antitumor activity. A multinational, open-label, phase I/II trial was conducted to determine the maximum-tolerated dose (MTD) of neratinib plus capecitabine in patients with solid tumors (part one) and to evaluate the safety and efficacy of neratinib plus capecitabine in patients with HER2-positive MBC (part two) [48]. Part one was a 3+3 dose-escalation study in which patients with advanced solid tumors received oral neratinib once per day continuously plus capecitabine twice per day on days 1–14 of a 21-day cycle at predefined dose levels. In part two, patients with trastuzumab-pretreated HER2-positive MBC received neratinib plus capecitabine at the MTD. The primary endpoint of part two was ORR. In part one ($n=33$), the combination of neratinib 240 mg per day plus capecitabine 1500 mg/m^2 per day was defined as the MTD, which was further evaluated in part 2 ($n=72$). The most common drug-related adverse events were diarrhea (88 %) and palmar-plantar erythrodysesthesia (48 %). In part two, ORR was 64 % ($n=39$ of 61) in patients with no prior lapatinib exposure and 57 % ($n=4$ of 7) in patients previously treated with lapatinib. Median PFS was 40.3 and 35.9 weeks, respectively. Neratinib in combination with capecitabine had a manageable toxicity profile and showed promising antitumor activity in patients with HER2-positive MBC pretreated with trastuzumab and lapatinib.

Third-Line Therapy and Beyond

The lapatinib plus trastuzumab study did include a heavily pretreated population and showed a benefit for continuing trastuzumab in combination with lapatinib after progression during previous trastuzumab-containing regimens. These data support the continuation of HER2-targeted therapy in the third-line setting and beyond.

Patients with progressive disease after two or more HER2-directed regimens for recurrent or MBC have few effective therapeutic options. Th3Resa is a phase III trial to specifically address the efficacy of anti-HER2 therapy in this third-line setting (Fig. 33.12) [49]. Patients with progressive HER2-positive advanced breast cancer who had received two or more HER2-directed regimens in the advanced setting, including trastuzumab and lapatinib, and previous taxane therapy in any setting

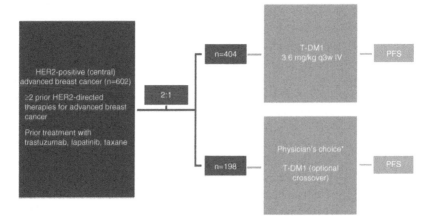

Fig. 33.12 T-DM1 vs. physician treatment of choice (TH3RESA) [49]. *Physician's choice could be single-agent chemotherapy, hormonal therapy, or HER2-directed therapy or a combination of a HER2-directed therapy with chemotherapy, hormonal therapy, or other HER2-directed therapies: 68.% chemotherapy + trastuzumab, 10.3 % trastuzumab + lapatinib, and 2.7 % chemotherapy + lapatinib. *HER2* human epidermal growth factor receptor 2, *T-DM1* trastuzumab emtansine, *IV* intravenous, *q3w* every 3 weeks, *PFS* progression-free survival

were randomly assigned (in a 2:1 ratio) to T-DM1 (3.6 mg/kg intravenously every 21 days) or the physician's choice. A total of 602 patients were randomly assigned (404 to T-DM1 and 198 to physician's choice). At data cutoff, 44 patients assigned to physician's choice had crossed over to T-DM1. After a median follow-up of 7.2 months in the T-DM1 group and 6.5 months in the physician's choice group, PFS was significantly improved with T-DM1 compared with physician's choice (median 6.2 months vs. 3.3 months) (stratified HR 0.53; $P<0.0001$). Interim overall survival analysis showed a trend favoring T-DM1 (stratified HR 0.55; $P=0.0034$). A lower incidence of grade 3 or worse adverse events was reported with T-DM1 than with physician's choice (32 % vs. 43 %). Grade 3 or worse adverse events including neutropenia, diarrhea, and febrile neutropenia were more common in the physician's choice group than in the T-DM1 group. Thrombocytopenia (5 % vs. 2 %) was the principal grade 3 or worse adverse event in the T-DM1 group. Serious adverse events were reported by 18 % of patients in the T-DM1 group and 21 % in the physician's choice group. T-DM1 should be considered as a new standard for patients with HER2-positive advanced breast cancer who have previously received trastuzumab and lapatinib.

The ASCO guidelines for HER2-positive advanced breast cancer recommended anti-HER 2 therapy including T-DM1, pertuzumab, and capecitabine plus lapatinib in the third-line setting, with hormonal therapy in patients with ER-positive and/or PgR-positive disease [43]. Additionally, if a patient's HER2-positive advanced breast cancer has progressed during or after second-line or greater HER2-targeted therapy, clinicians should offer T-DMI if she has not received T-DM1, pertuzumab if she has not received pertuzumab, or third-line or greater HER2-targeted therapy–based treatment if she has received both T-DM1 and pertuzumab. Options include lapatinib plus capecitabine and other combinations of chemotherapy with trastuzumab, lapatinib, and trastuzumab or hormonal therapy (in patients with ER-positive and/or PgR-positive disease). There is insufficient evidence to recommend one regimen over another (Fig. 33.13) [43].

Treatment Influence of Previous HER2 Therapy

First-Line Treatment

For patients who received adjuvant trastuzumab and develop MBC, decisions are based on the time that elapsed from the end of adjuvant treatment to the diagnosis of MBC. For patients with a

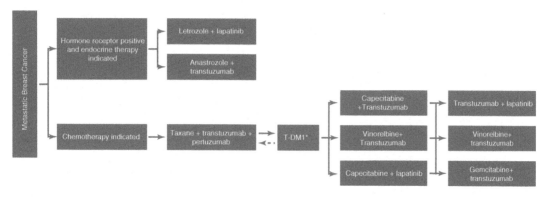

*T-DM1 may be used as front line if the patient develops metastasiz with 6 months of finishing adjuvant therapy

Fig. 33.13 In HER2-positive metastatic breast cancer (MBC), decision pathways provide recommendations based on the best evidence available at the time of this book edition. Because new data from randomized clinical trials are published continuously, decision pathways must be subject to change. ASCO, ESMO, CCO, and NCCN guidelines are continuously updated and revised to reflect new data and clinical information that may add to or alter current clinical practice standards

Table 33.6 Combined usage of cytotoxic drugs with dual anti-Her2 inhibition for HER2-positive advanced breast cancer

Regimen	Drug	Dosage	Route of administration	Frequency of cycles
Trastuzumab plus Pertuzumab with docetaxel	Trastuzumab	8 mg/kg IV day 1 followed by 6 mg/kg	Intravenous	Cycled every 21 days
	Pertuzumab	840 mg IV day 1 followed by 420 mg	Intravenous	Cycled every 21 days
	Docetaxel	75–100 mg/m²	Intravenous	Cycled every 21 days
Trastuzumab plus Pertuzumab with paclitaxel	Trastuzumab	8 mg/kg IV day 1 followed by 6 mg/kg	Intravenous	Cycled every 21 days OR
		4 mg/kg day 1 followed by 2 mg/kg	Intravenous	Weekly
	Pertuzumab	840 mg IV day 1 followed by 420 mg	Intravenous	Cycled every 21 days
	Paclitaxel	175 mg/m²	Intravenous	Cycled every 21 days OR
	Paclitaxel	80–90 mg/m²	Intravenous	Cycled every 7 days

treatment-free interval of 6 months or longer, pertuzumab, trastuzumab, and a taxane can be preferred. For patients with a treatment-free interval of less than 6 months, T-DM1 can be preferred. This recommendation is based on the phase III EMILIA trial, which demonstrated that T-DM1 improves clinical outcomes and is better tolerated than lapatinib plus capecitabine [41]. An alternative trastuzumab-containing regimen or a lapatinib-based combination can be used if T-DM1 is not available (Tables 33.6, 33.7, and 33.8).

1. *For patients with recurrence ≤12 months after adjuvant treatment*:

    If a patient finished trastuzumab-based adjuvant treatment ≤12 months before recurrence, clinicians should follow the second-line HER2-targeted therapy–based treatment recommendations. For patients who progress 6 months or longer after the completion of adjuvant trastuzumab (without pertuzumab), trastuzumab plus pertuzumab in combination with a taxane can also be suggested [43].

Table 33.7 Combined usage of cytotoxic drugs with trastuzumab for Her2-positive advanced breast cancer

Regimen	Drug	Dosage	Route of administration	Frequency of cycles
Trastuzumab plus the following cytotoxic(s)	Trastuzumab	4 mg/kg day 1 followed by 2 mg/kg	Intravenous	Weekly
		8 mg/kg IV day 1 followed by 6 mg/kg	Intravenous	Cycled every 21 days
Paclitaxel/carboplatin	Carboplatin	AUC 6	Intravenous	Day 1 Cycled every 21 days
	Paclitaxel	175 mg/m²	Intravenous	Day 1 Cycled every 21 days
Weekly paclitaxel/ carboplatin	Carboplatin	AUC 2	Intravenous	Days 1, 8, and 15 Cycled every 28 days
	Paclitaxel	80 mg/m²	Intravenous	Days 1, 8, and 15 Cycled every 28 days
Paclitaxel	Paclitaxel	175 mg/m²	Intravenous	Day 1 Cycled every 21 days
	Paclitaxel	80–90 mg/m²	Intravenous	Day 1 Cycled every 7 days
Docetaxel	Docetaxel	80–100 mg/m²	Intravenous	Day 1 Cycled every 21 days
	Docetaxel	35 mg/m²	Intravenous	Day 1 Cycled every week
Vinorelbine	Vinorelbine	25 mg/m²	Intravenous	Day 1 weekly Cycled every 21 days
	Vinorelbine	30–35 mg/m²	Intravenous	Days 1 and 8 Cycled every 21 days
Capecitabine	Capecitabine	1000–1250 mg/m²	Peroral	Twice daily days 1–14 Cycled every 21 days

Table 33.8 Systemic therapy for previously trastuzumab–treated Her2-positive advanced breast cancer patients

Regimen	Drug	Dosage	Route of administration	Frequency of cycles
T-DM1	Ado-trastuzumab emtansine	3.6 mg/kg	Intravenous	Day 1 Cycled every 21 days
Lapatinib + capecitabine	Lapatinib PO daily	1250 mg	Peroral	Days 1–21 Cycled every 21 days
	Capecitabine	1000 mg/m²	Peroral	Twice daily days 1–14 cycled every 21 days
Trastuzumab + capecitabine	Capecitabine	1000–1250 mg/m²	Peroral	Twice daily days 1–14 Cycled every 21 days
	Trastuzumab	4 mg/kg day 1 followed by 2 mg/kg	Intravenous	Weekly
		8 mg/kg IV day 1 followed by 6 mg/kg	Intravenous	Cycled every 21 days
Trastuzumab+ lapatinib (without cytotoxic therapy)	Lapatinib	1000 mg	Peroral	Days 1–21 Cycled every 21 days
	Trastuzumab	4 mg/kg day 1 followed by 2 mg/kg	Intravenous	Weekly
		8 mg/kg IV day 1 followed by 6 mg/kg	Intravenous	Cycled every 21 days

2. *For patients with recurrence >12 months after adjuvant treatment*:

If a patient finished trastuzumab-based adjuvant treatment >12 months before recurrence, clinicians should follow the first-line HER2-targeted therapy–based treatment recommendations [43].

Patients Who Require Second- or Later-Line Treatment

In general, trastuzumab can be continued across treatment regimens for women who experience disease progression on an HER2-directed agent, regardless of the line of treatment. There are no high-quality data available to support the continued use of pertuzumab through multiple lines of therapy.

For patients with HER2-positive MBC who experience disease progression on a regimen that includes an HER2-directed agent, available options include the following (Fig. 33.13):

1. Trastuzumab plus an alternative cytotoxic agent
2. T-DM1, if not previously administered
3. Lapatinib plus capecitabine or trastuzumab, if not previously administered

When lapatinib is administered, it must be combined with another agent (e.g., capecitabine or trastuzumab) because combination therapies have better clinical outcomes than monotherapy. Lapatinib plus capecitabine is an option for patients who experience disease progression on trastuzumab, particularly if they prefer oral medications [43]. The combination of lapatinib and trastuzumab is a chemotherapy-free option for patients with HER2-positive MBC whose disease has progressed on trastuzumab [43].

For patients who progress after initial trastuzumab and a taxane in the metastatic setting or after both trastuzumab- and lapatinib-containing regimens, T-DM1 is an active agent, provided they have not received it previously. This recommendation is based on both the EMILIA trial and the second-phase III TH3RESA trial [41, 49].

The optimal selection of anti-HER2 therapy and personalization of treatment remain active areas of research. Trials to examine the utility of newer agents in various settings are under way and may change our future clinical practice.

Duration of Chemotherapy or HER2-Targeted Therapy

If a patient is receiving an HER2-targeted therapy and chemotherapy combination, the chemotherapy should continue for approximately 4–6 months (or longer) and/or to the time of maximal response, depending on toxicities and the absence of progression. When chemotherapy is stopped, clinicians should continue the HER2-targeted therapy: no further change in the regimen is needed until time of progression or unacceptable toxicities. There are insufficient data to make a single statement on when to stop administering HER2-targeted therapy [43].

In most trials, HER2-targeted therapy was administered until disease progression or until toxic adverse events caused the clinician and patient to decide to discontinue this therapy. For patients who have an optimal treatment response and for whom cytotoxic chemotherapy has been discontinued, the decision to discontinue HER2-directed therapy should be individualized because there are no prospective data to provide guidance. Anti-HER2–directed therapy can be continued for many years in such patients without disease progression. However, the same can be said for patients who discontinue treatment. While continuation of HER2-directed treatment can increase the risk of cumulative toxicity (particularly cardiotoxicity), increase healthcare costs, and may be inconvenient, these considerations must be balanced by the potential benefit of treatment in delaying (or preventing) disease progression [43].

Monitoring Therapy

The receptor status of metastasis or a recurrent tumor can change. Curigliano et al. evaluated the discordance rates of ER, PgR, and HER2 status between the primary tumor and liver metastases, which would potentially impact treatment choices [50]. They identified 255 consecutive patients with matched primary and liver tissue samples and observed changes in ER status in 14.5 % and in PgR status in 48.6 % of cases. Changes in HER2 status were observed in 24 of 172 assessable patients (13.9 %). HER2 status changed from positive to negative in 17 of 54 patients (32 %) and from negative to positive in 7 of 118 patients (6 %). The study also revealed that a change in HER2 status from negative to positive was associated with a certain decrease in ER and PgR expression between the primary tumor and liver biopsy. A discordance in receptor status (ER, PgR, and HER2) between the primary tumor and liver metastases led to a change in therapy in 31 of 255 patients (12.1 %). Biopsy of metastases for reassessment of biological features should be considered in all patients when safe and easy to perform because it is likely to impact treatment choice.

The continuous evaluation of patients during therapy should be individualized according to patient and provider preferences. Careful assessment for response to treatment requires serial clinical examinations, repeat laboratory evaluation (including tumor markers when initially elevated), and radiographic imaging. Although there is no standard schedule for evaluation during treatment, a reasonable approach would be as follows: history and physical exam prior to the start of each treatment cycle, serial assay for serum tumor markers (e.g., cancer antigen [CA] 15-3 or carcinoembryonic antigen [CEA] if they were elevated at baseline), and repeat imaging studies (using the same imaging modality throughout) every two to three cycles of therapy.

Definition of Treatment Failure

This decision is made on the basis of serial changes in tumor markers, evidence of disease progression based on serial imaging, and the clinical status of the patient. We generally use RECIST criteria for the definition of progression (Table 33.9). According to RECIST 1.1, disease

Table 33.9 RECIST 1.1 criteria

Minimum target lesion size	≥10 mm (CT + MRI)
	≥15 mm lymph nodes
	≥20 mm chest X-ray
Measurement	Unidimensional
	Lymph nodes = short axis
Progressive disease	20 % increase in sum of diameter (SOD)
	+ minimum 5-mm increase from nadir
Nonmeasurable assessment	Substantial worsening
	Tumor burden has increased sufficiently
Lymph node measurements	Specific instructions
	≥15 mm, 10–14 mm, <10 mm
PET	May be considered to support CT
	For progressive disease and confirmation of CR

progression on imaging is simply defined as any of the following: the appearance of any new lesions, a 20 % or greater increase in the sum of measurable target lesions compared with the sum previously recorded, or a worsening of existing nontarget lesions such as bone metastases [46].

Overview of RECIST Criteria

RECIST is a set of published rules that define when tumors in cancer patients improve ("respond"), remain the same ("stabilize"), or worsen ("progress") during treatment. Important points of RECIST are summarized as follows:

(a) Measure in the plane of the longest diameter.
(b) Do not measure lesions across normal, nontumor tissue.
(c) Do not necessarily select the largest lesions as targets. Select those that are best defined and reproducibly measurable.
(d) Use consistent imaging quality.
(e) Precise and consistent visualization of lesions is essential. Scanning without intravenous contrast usually is useless in a clinical study and typically makes the patient nonevaluable.

(f) Typically, the same anatomy must be imaged for all time points. Keep it consistent and always scan all anatomy with disease, so the reviewer can make consistent comparisons.

(g) Measure where the target lesion is largest.

(h) A slight increase in existing non-target lesions alone does not justify progressive disease. The progression shall be clear and obvious to determine a substantial worsening.

(i) If a target lesion separates, measure the longest diameter of each lesion separately. The individual longest diameters of all the resulting lesions shall contribute to the sum of diameters (SOD).

(j) If target lesions become confluent, calculate the longest diameter of the resulting lesion.

(k) Include the hypervascular "enhancing rim," if present, in the longest diameter measurement. Measure the longest diameter irrespective of a central necrosis.

(l) Continue measuring target lesions in their longest diameter, even when they develop central cavities or necrosis. If the sum of diameters does not accurately reflect the patient's response assessment, a different assessment may be needed.

Lymph nodes: Identify the longest diameter of a lymph node or nodal mass (e.g., 18 mm), and then measure the longest perpendicular diameter to that as the short axis (e.g., 12 mm). A short axis of 12 mm defines this lymph node as being pathological but not measurable (to be measurable, it must be ≥15 mm). As such it shall be recorded as a nontarget lesion.

Lytic bone lesions, with an identifiable soft tissue component, evaluated by CT or MRI, can be considered as measurable lesions if the soft tissue component otherwise meets the definition of measurability. Blastic bone lesions are nonmeasurable.

MRI has excellent contrast, spatial, and temporal resolution; however, there are many image acquisition variables involved in MRI that greatly impact image quality, lesion conspicuity, and measurement. Chest MRI is not recommended. Measurements are possible on isotropic reconstructions and non-axial MRI planes: sagittal, coronal, or oblique. Always measure in the same plane.

Evaluating a PET-CT for progression: It is sometimes reasonable to incorporate FDG-PET to complement CT scanning in assessment of progression.

Negative PET at baseline with a positive PET at follow-up is progressive disease based on a new lesion.

No PET at baseline and a positive PET at follow-up:

- If the positive PET at follow-up corresponds to a new site of disease on CT, this is progressive disease.
- If the positive PET at follow-up is not confirmed as a new site of disease on CT, additional follow-up CT scans are needed to determine if there is truly progression occurring at that site.
- If the positive PET at follow-up corresponds to a preexisting site of disease on CT that is not progressing on the basis of the anatomic images, this is not progressive disease (See Box 33.1).

Box 33.1: Summary of the Optimal HER2-Targeted Therapy for Advanced Human Epidermal Growth Factor Receptor 2 (HER2)–Positive Breast Cancer

- Clinicians should recommend HER2-targeted therapy–based combinations for first-line treatment. If HER2-positive advanced breast cancer progresses during or after first-line HER2-targeted therapy, clinicians should recommend second-line HER2-targeted therapy–based treatment.
- If HER2-positive advanced breast cancer progresses during or after second-line or greater HER2-targeted treatment, clinicians should recommend third-line or greater HER2-targeted therapy–based treatment.
- If available, the clinicians should recommend the combination of trastuzumab, pertuzumab, and a taxane for first-line and trastuzumab emtansine

(T-DM1) as second-line treatment. If HER2-positive advanced breast cancer progresses during or after second-line or greater HER2-targeted treatment but the patient has not received pertuzumab, clinicians may offer pertuzumab.

- If the patient has already received trastuzumab, pertuzumab, and T-DM1, clinicians should recommend third-line or greater HER2-targeted therapy–based treatment (lapatinib plus chemotherapy, trastuzumab plus lapatinib, trastuzumab plus chemotherapy, trastuzumab or lapatinib plus hormonal therapy in patients with hormone receptor–positive disease).
- If a patient is receiving HER2-targeted therapy and chemotherapy combinations, chemotherapy should continue to the time of maximal response, depending on toxicity and in the absence of progression. When chemotherapy ends, clinicians should continue the HER2-targeted

therapy, and no further change in the regimen is needed until time of progression or unacceptable toxicities.

- If a patient finished trastuzumab-based adjuvant treatment >12 months before recurrence, clinicians should follow the first-line HER2-targeted therapy–based treatment recommendations.
- If a patient's cancer is hormone receptor positive and HER2 positive, clinicians may recommend either HER2-targeted therapy plus chemotherapy or in select cases endocrine therapy plus trastuzumab or lapatinib. Clinicians may add endocrine therapy to the HER2-targeted therapy when chemotherapy ends and/or when the cancer progresses.
- In highly selected patients with special circumstances, such as low disease burden, long disease-free survival, and/or presence of severe comorbidities, clinicians may offer first-line endocrine therapy alone.

Targeting HER2 in Breast Cancer Brain Metastases

Brain metastases occur in one-third of patients with HER2-positive MBC and are responsible for death in half of these patients. Patients with brain metastases should receive appropriate local therapy and systemic therapy. Local therapies include surgery, whole-brain radiotherapy (WBRT), and stereotactic radiosurgery (SRS). Treatments depend on factors such as patient prognosis, presence of symptoms, resectability, number and size of metastases, prior therapy, and whether metastases are diffuse [51]. Other options include systemic therapy, best supportive care, enrollment onto a clinical trial, and/or palliative care. Recommendations in the National Comprehensive Cancer Network (NCCN) guidelines for patients with one to three brain metastases are surgery or SRS, and consider WBRT in advanced systemic disease [1] and, for >3 brain metastases, WBRT, or consider SRS in select cases.

In a retrospective study, 176 breast cancer patients underwent SRS for brain metastases, and median survival time was 16 months for 95 newly diagnosed patients and 11.7 months for 81 patients with recurrent brain metastasis. There was no association between the number of treated brain metastases and survival. Longer survival was associated with age <50 years, Karnofsky performance status >70, primary tumor control, ER positivity, and HER2 overexpression [52].

There are currently no systemic therapies approved to treat patients with breast cancer and brain metastases. Data primarily stem from single-arm prospective trials and from case series and/or retrospective studies. Large monoclonal antibody agents such as trastuzumab, T-DM1, and pertuzumab may not penetrate the blood-brain barrier (BBB) because of their molecular size. A few hours after trastuzumab infusion, the serum levels achieved were, as expected, in the range of 10,000–100,000 ng/mL, whereas cerebrospinal fluid levels were 300-fold lower [53].

However, when metastatic tumors grow and after radiation therapy, the BBB loses those structural features that are critical for its function. The serum- and cerebrospinal fluid-level ratio of trastuzumab is altered in patients with HER2-positive breast cancer and impairment of the BBB. In a study by Stemmler HJ et al., the ratio of median trastuzumab levels in the serum and cerebrospinal fluid was 420:1 before and 76:1 after completion of cranial radiotherapy [54]. With concomitant meningeal carcinomatosis, the trastuzumab serum to cerebrospinal fluid ratio was 49:1 after radiotherapy.

In another small trial, the authors performed a feasibility study to determine the optimal dosage and time of administration of the zirconium-89 ((89)Zr)-trastuzumab monoclonal antibody to enable PET imaging of HER2-positive lesions. The patients underwent at least two PET scans between days 2 and 5 [55]. The results of the study demonstrated that the best time to assess (89)Zr-trastuzumab uptake by tumors was 4–5 days after the injection. PET scanning after administration of (89)Zr-trastuzumab at appropriate doses allows visualization and quantification of uptake by HER2-positive lesions in patients with MBC. This suggests that trastuzumab can cross a disrupted BBB and that continuation of trastuzumab after the development of brain metastases may benefit these patients.

registHER is a prospective, observational study of 1,012 patients with confirmed HER2-positive tumors, including 377 (37.3 %) patients with central nervous system (CNS) metastases [56]. Compared with patients with no CNS metastases, those with CNS metastases were younger and more likely to have hormone receptor–negative disease and a higher disease burden. Median time to CNS progression among patients without CNS disease at initial MBC diagnosis was 13.3 months. Treatment with trastuzumab, chemotherapy, or surgery after CNS diagnosis was associated with a statistically significant improvement in median OS following diagnosis of CNS disease (trastuzumab vs. no trastuzumab, 17.5 vs. 3.8 months; chemotherapy vs. no chemotherapy, 16.4 vs. 3.7 months; and surgery vs. no surgery, 20.3 vs. 11.3 months). The results of

multivariable proportional hazards analyses confirmed the independent significant effects of trastuzumab and chemotherapy (hazard ratio = 0.33, $P < 0.001$; hazard ratio = 0.64, $P = 0.002$, respectively). The effects of surgery and radiotherapy did not reach statistical significance ($P = 0.062$ and $P = 0.898$, respectively). In conclusion, patients with HER2-positive MBC evaluated in registHER survived longer after CNS metastases if treated with trastuzumab, chemotherapy, and surgery.

Lapatinib is the first HER2-directed drug to be validated in preclinical mouse models for activity against brain metastases of breast cancer. Lapatinib belongs to the family of small-molecule tyrosine kinase inhibitors of HER1 and HER2 and can cross the BBB. In a phase II study [57] of 242 patients, eligible patients had HER2-positive breast cancer, progressive brain metastases, prior trastuzumab, and cranial radiotherapy. Objective CNS responses to lapatinib were observed in 6 % of patients. In an exploratory analysis, 21 % of patients experienced a ≥20 % volumetric reduction in their CNS lesions. An association was observed between volumetric reduction and improvement in PFS and neurological signs and symptoms. During disease progression in the same study, 10 of 50 patients (20 %) who received a combination of lapatinib and capecitabine exhibited an objective response in the brain.

In the LANDSCAPE study, a combination of lapatinib plus capecitabine was administered to previously untreated patients with HER2-positive breast cancer and brain metastasis [58]. Twenty-nine patients had an objective CNS response (65.9 %, 95 % CI 50.1–79.5), all of which were partial responses. Twenty-two (49 %) patients had grade 3 or 4 treatment-related adverse events, including diarrhea in nine patients (20 %) and hand-foot syndrome in nine patients (20 %). The median time to RT was 8.3 months. Thirty-six (82 %) patients had received RT to the brain at the time of analysis. Median time to progression was 5.5 months (95 % CI: 4.3–6.0). The 6-month survival rate was 90.9 % (95 % CI: 77.4–956.5), and the median OS was 17 months (95 % CI: 13.7–24.9). At least one severe adverse event was reported by 31 % of patients; treatment was discontinued because of toxicity in four patients. In conclusion, lapatinib plus capecitabine is highly active for untreated brain metastasis, and treatment on this protocol delayed the start of RT.

In the CEREBEL trial, patients without baseline CNS metastases were randomly assigned to receive lapatinib-capecitabine or trastuzumab-capecitabine [59]. The primary endpoint was incidence of CNS metastases as the first site of relapse. The relapse rate was 3 % (8 of 251 patients) for lapatinib-capecitabine and 5 % for trastuzumab-capecitabine ($P=0.360$). PFS and OS were longer with trastuzumab-capecitabine vs. lapatinib-capecitabine (hazard ratio for PFS, 1.30; 95 % CI, 1.04–1.64; hazard ratio for OS, 1.34; 95 % CI, 0.95–1.64). CEREBEL is inconclusive for the primary endpoint, and no difference was detected between lapatinib-capecitabine and trastuzumab-capecitabine for the incidence of CNS metastases. A better outcome was observed with trastuzumab-capecitabine in the overall population.

Results from the phase III CLEOPATRA trial in HER2-positive first-line MBC demonstrated significant improvements in PFS and OS with pertuzumab, trastuzumab, and docetaxel vs. placebo, trastuzumab, and docetaxel [22]. The incidence of CNS metastases as the first site of disease progression was similar (placebo, 12.6 %, pertuzumab, 13.7 %) between the two arms. The median time to development of CNS metastases as the first site of disease progression was 11.9 months in the placebo arm and 15.0 months in the pertuzumab arm (hazard ratio = 0.58, $P=0.0049$). OS in patients who developed CNS metastases as the first site of disease progression showed a trend in favor of pertuzumab, trastuzumab, and docetaxel (hazard ratio = 0.66, 95 % CI 0.39–1.11). Median OS was 26.3 vs. 34.4 months in the placebo and pertuzumab arms, respectively. The differences in the survival curves were not statistically significant in the log-rank test ($P=0.11$) but were significant in the Wilcoxon test ($P=0.04$). While the incidence of CNS metastases was similar between arms, the results suggest that pertuzumab, trastuzumab, and docetaxel delay the onset of CNS disease compared with placebo, trastuzumab, and docetaxel.

In the EMILIA trial [60], patients with HER2-positive advanced breast cancer previously treated with trastuzumab and a taxane were randomized to T-DM1 or capecitabine-lapatinib until disease progression. Among 991 randomized patients, 95 (T-DM1 =45; capecitabine-lapatinib = 50) had CNS metastases at baseline. Among patients with CNS metastases at baseline, a significant improvement in OS was observed in the T-DM1 arm compared with the capecitabine-lapatinib arm [hazard ratio = 0.38; $P=0.008$; 26.8 vs. 12.9 months].

These data strongly support the hypothesis that the best overall treatment also improves survival in cases of brain metastases. Other conventional cytotoxic agents that can cross the BBB may act with anti-HER2 therapy on CNS metastases, and further research is needed.

In a phase I trial combining temozolomide plus lapatinib for the treatment of brain metastases in patients with HER2-positive MBC (LAPTEM trial), 18 patients were enrolled (16 patients with recurrent or progressive brain metastases) [61]. Temozolomide orally once daily at three dose levels, 100, 150, and 200 mg/m^2/day, was given on days 1–5 of a 28-day cycle. Lapatinib was given orally once daily at three dose levels: 1000, 1250, and 1500 mg/day. Both agents were administered until disease progression or intolerable toxicity, with a maximum of six cycles. The most common adverse effects were fatigue, diarrhea, and constipation. Disease stabilization was achieved in 10 of 15 assessable patients. The estimated median survival time for the 16 patients with brain metastases was 10.9 months, and the median PFS was 2.6 months.

Forty patients were enrolled in a phase II trial of neratinib for patients with HER2-positive breast cancer and brain metastases [62]. Neratinib 240 mg orally was given once daily. Follow-up was every 4 weeks, and brain MRI and body CT restaging were performed at week 8. Therapy was continued in CR, PR, and SD. Continued therapy with the addition of trastuzumab is allowed for progressive disease not affecting the CNS. Of the patients, 78 % had prior WBRT. The median number of cycles was 2 (ranges 1–7), and the median PFS was 1.9 months. The most common grade 3 event was diarrhea (23 %), which decreased after loperamide prophylaxis was implemented. There was no complete response, but three patients (8 %) had a partial response. Progressive disease in only the CNS was observed in ten (25 %) patients. Ongoing trials with neratinib include the following: (1) patients undergoing craniotomy receiving neratinib 240 mg peroral daily, with surgical resection to determine neratinib concentrations from a craniotomy specimen, cerebrospinal fluid (CSF), and plasma; (2) patients with no prior lapatinib receiving neratinib 240 mg peroral every day and 750 mg/m^2 capecitabine twice daily (14 days every 21 days); (3) patients with prior lapatinib receiving neratinib 240 mg every day and 750 mg/m^2 capecitabine twice daily (14 days every 21 days).

ONT-380 is a potent selective small-molecule inhibitor of HER2 with minimal EGFR-like side effects. Nine patients with CNS metastases (four with asymptomatic metastases and five with progressive disease) were treated with ONT-380 in combination with other systemic therapies [63]. ONT-380 was given as 300 mg twice daily with approved doses of T-DM1, trastuzumab, or trastuzumab plus capecitabine. There were three partial remissions (two patients with T-DM1, one with trastuzumab plus capecitabine). Four patients had stable disease (two patients with T-DM1, two patients with trastuzumab).

Ongoing studies of patients with HER2-positive breast cancer with brain metastasis include a randomized, phase II study of WBRT with or without lapatinib. This study (NCT01622868) is evaluating lapatinib as a radiosensitizer in combination with WBRT. Other HER2-directed therapies under active investigation in breast cancer with brain metastases include the irreversible HER2 inhibitors neratinib and afatinib. ARRY-380, a HER2-selective inhibitor with some ability to cross the BBB and activity in intracranial tumor models, is undergoing evaluation in combination with trastuzumab [64]. Other ongoing trials for HER2-positive brain metastases include cabazitaxel plus lapatinib (Sarah Cannon); cabozantinib +/− trastuzumab (Tolaney, DFCI); everolimus, trastuzumab, and vinorelbine (Anders, UNC); a phase II trial

of neratinib (Freedman, DFCI); a phase 1b/2 trial using lapatinib, everolimus, and capecitabine (Hurvitz, UCLA); KD019 and trastuzumab (Lin, DFCI); a phase 1b study of ONT-380 combined with T-DM1 (Krop, DFCI); and abemaciclib plus trastuzumab (multicenter).

Intrathecal (IT) Anti-HER2 Treatment

Breast cancer is one of the most common tumors to involve the leptomeninges. Leptomeningeal carcinomatosis (LCM) of HER2-overexpressing breast carcinoma remains potentially sensitive to HER2-type receptor inhibition if the meningeal blood-brain barrier is bypassed. Importantly, the receptor status of a metastasis can change [50]. Several studies and case reports of intrathecal (IT) trastuzumab to treat LCM have been published. Extremely low levels of the antibody are detected in the CSF after intravenous trastuzumab; much higher levels could be reached after intraventricular or IT administration, which might reach therapeutic concentrations.

Seventeen patients were evaluable for the efficacy and safety of IT trastuzumab for the treatment of metastatic cancer in HER2-positive breast cancer patients. The mean age at IT trastuzumab administration was 48 years, and the mean total dose was 400 mg. IT trastuzumab alone or as part of combination therapies seemed to be safe; no serious adverse events were reported in 88 % of cases. In 69 % of cases, there was a significant clinical improvement, whereas 31 % exhibited stabilization or progression of the disease. A CSF response was observed in 67 % of cases. The median OS was 13.5 months, whereas the median CNS-PFS was 7.5 months. In 24 % of cases, IT trastuzumab was administered after CNS progression, with a response observed in 75 % of cases and a CNS-PFS of 9.4 months. The cumulative dose of IT trastuzumab given was 1040 mg (median 1215; range 55–1675). Clinical improvement (hazard ratio 0.14, 95 % CI 0.02–0.91) and cerebrospinal fluid response (hazard ratio 0.09, 95 % CI 0.01–0.89) were associated with longer CNS-PFS [65].

IT trastuzumab might thus be a promising treatment for leptomeningeal involvement in

HER2-positive breast cancer patients, and further studies are warranted to optimize the dose, interval, duration, and combination of drugs for treatment. A role for intrathecal trastuzumab for leptomeningeal metastases in HER2-positive breast cancer is currently being evaluated in a phase II trial in which patients will be treated with 80 mg IT trastuzumab twice a week for 4 weeks and then every 2 weeks. The primary objectives are to determine the radiological, cytological, and clinical responses to IT trastuzumab (Raizer, Northwestern) (See Box 33.2).

Box 33.2: Summary of Recommendations on Disease Management for Patients with Advanced HER2-Positive Breast Cancer and Brain Metastases

- For patients with a favorable prognosis for survival and limited (one to four) metastases, treatment options include ± surgery and radiation therapy (RT) (whole-brain radiation therapy (WBRT) or stereotactic radiosurgery (SRS) or both).
- For other patients with diffuse disease/extensive metastases, options include WBRT and, in select cases, only best supportive care and/or palliative care.
- For patients with leptomeningeal metastases options include involved field RT to bulky disease or symptomatic sites and intratechal treatment for select cases with normal cerebrospinal fluid flow (consider placing ventricular catheter and subcutaneous reservoir).
- For patients whose systemic disease is not progressive at the time of brain metastasis diagnosis, the same systemic therapy should be continued, and for patients whose systemic disease is progressive at the time of brain metastasis diagnosis, clinicians should use the algorithms for treatment of HER2-positive metastatic breast cancer.

Future Directions

Successful targeting of HER2 has improved outcomes in HER2-positive breast cancer, but treatment resistance remains a problem. Many patients have tumors that exhibit de novo or acquired resistance, and most progress within a year. Treatment resistance can be caused by pathway redundancy or reactivation or by escape pathways. The use of combination anti-HER2 treatments for potent inhibition of HER family signaling is biologically sound and offers great clinical promise. ER is a potential resistance pathway for anti-HER2 treatments. Concomitant inhibition of ER with potent HER2 inhibition is being investigated in clinical trials. PI3K pathway activation is also a potential mechanism for resistance and is an attractive therapeutic target to overcome or prevent resistance to anti-HER2 treatment. Other proposed markers of trastuzumab resistance include a truncated form of HER2 (p95), HER2/IGF-IR dimerization, and Src activation [38].

HER2 receptors are present on the surface of breast cancer cells with HER2 gene amplification as monomers, homodimers, and heterodimers with EGFR/HER3. Although HER2 has no known ligands, more than ten different ligands can activate other receptors of this family. HER2 on cancer cells can be activated by either heterodimerization with other ligand-bound HER family members or, when overexpressed, by homodimerization. Upon binding, ligands induce receptor homo- and heterodimerization that activates a phosphorylation-signaling cascade leading to enhanced responsiveness to stromal growth factors and oncogenic transformation. The resulting downstream signaling regulates the transcription of genes responsible for cell proliferation, survival, angiogenesis, invasion, and metastasis [66, 67]. Trastuzumab can inhibit signaling from HER2 homodimers better than heterodimers with HER1 (EGFR) or HER3 [68].

PI3K/AKT pathway aberrations are common in breast cancer. The PI3K/AKT pathway is a powerful downstream signaling pathway activated by HER2 signaling. The resulting downregulation of the PI3K/AKT pathway signaling leads to apoptosis in human tumors. Hyperactivation of the PI3K pathway by activating mutations or loss of PTEN expression has been associated with resistance to trastuzumab-based chemotherapy [69–71]. Metastatic tumors arising in patients who had previously been treated with trastuzumab expressed lower levels of PTEN compared with the primary tumor [69]. Inhibiting the PI3K/AKT pathway (as with anti-HER2 drugs) leads, by feedback mechanisms, to a rebound in HER3 activity, which is one of the main pathways to resistance. Combining targeted therapies (dual HER2 inhibition) with HER3-targeting drugs might inhibit this feedback response. Even with dual HER2 inhibition, a proportion of patients do not respond to therapy, as observed in the CLEOPATRA study [22, 23].

Several PI3 kinase inhibitors are in phase 1/2 stage development. A phase 1/2 study of pilaralisib (SAR245408) in combination with trastuzumab or paclitaxel and trastuzumab in patients with HER2-positive MBC who progressed on a previous trastuzumab-based regimen has been completed. Other PI3 kinase inhibitors are also under investigation. Other ongoing studies are evaluating novel therapeutic approaches to overcome primary and secondary drug resistance in tumors, including inhibition of PI3K/TOR, heat shock protein 90 (HSP90), IGF-IR, and angiogenesis [38].

Trastuzumab can induce antibody-dependent cellular cytotoxicity. HER2 overexpression in breast cancers is associated with higher levels of proliferation, high histological grade, and higher levels of tumor-infiltrating lymphocytes (TILs) compared with HER2-negative tumors. HER2-stimulated immunosuppression and its inhibition by trastuzumab are currently being investigated [71–73].

Tumor-targeting therapy by the anti-HER2 monoclonal antibody is mediated by CD8(+) T-cell responses. Analysis of the tumor microenvironment has demonstrated that tumor tissues are heavily infiltrated by immunosuppressive macrophages and that most tumor-infiltrating T cells, particularly CD8(+) T cells, express high levels of the inhibitory cosignaling receptor programmed death-1 (PD-1). The term "immune evasion" refers to the ability of a tumor to suppress and change the host's antitumor immune responses. The programmed cell death 1 (PD-1) pathway may be engaged by tumor cells to overcome active T-cell immune surveillance. The ligands for PD-1 (PD-L1 and PD-L2) are constitutively expressed or can be induced in various tumors. High expression of these ligands (particularly PD-L1) on tumor cells correlates with poor prognosis and survival. Avoidance of destruction by the host's immune system must contribute importantly to tumor growth and progression. These data suggest that the tumor microenvironment is dominated by immunosuppressive responses that prevent antitumor immunity. Removing inhibitory signals from the tumor microenvironment in combination with other therapies should be a successful tumor therapy [71–73]. Investigating the therapeutic potential of agents that inhibit the suppression of T-cell targeting and combining them with anti-HER2 agents is a promising treatment approach. This approach was confirmed in mouse models of HER2-positive mammary tumors, in which a combination of trastuzumab with anti-PD-1 and anti-PD-L1 antibodies achieved the greatest tumor regression [71, 72]. These observations suggest that the PD-1/PD-L1 pathway plays a critical role in immune evasion by tumors and could be considered an attractive target for therapeutic intervention in several solid organ types.

In an ongoing phase I/II study of HER2-positive disease, the investigators propose to determine whether adding an immunotherapy can reverse trastuzumab resistance and improve clinical outcomes [73]. In this study, the investigators will determine if a monoclonal antibody targeted against PD-1 can reverse trastuzumab resistance in patients previously progressing on trastuzumab. HER2 has also been explored as an antigen for vaccine development in HER2-positive breast cancer in many other trials: the results could change our future clinical practice.

ADCs represent an exciting frontier in cancer medicine [75, 76]. ADCs currently on the market or in clinical trials are predominantly based on two drug classes: auristatins and maytansinoids. Both are tubulin binders and block cell progression through mitosis. A newly developed class of linker-drugs is based on duocarmycins, which are potent DNA-alkylating agents with DNA-alkylating and DNA-binding moieties that bind the minor groove of DNA. SYD985 displayed high antitumor activity in two patient-derived xenograft models of HER2-positive MBCs. These data indicate that this new HER2-targeting ADC has a favorable safety profile and great potential for patients with HER2-positive cancers.

Studies comparing ADCs with different average drug-to-antibody ratios (DARs) have demonstrated that a higher average DAR leads to increased efficacy but also somewhat less favorable physicochemical and toxicological properties. SYD985 combines several favorable properties of unfractionated ADCs with improved homogeneity. SYD985 was selected for further development and recently entered clinical phase I evaluation [74]. Preliminary evidence suggests that SYD985 could have an efficacy superior to that of T-DM1, particularly for tumors that are HER2-negative by fluorescence in situ hybridization and 1+ to 2+ for HER2 by immunohistochemistry [75]. If confirmed in the clinic, this could extend the target population of patients with breast and gastric cancers who may respond to this treatment modality to include those with fluorescence in situ–negative or immunohistochemistry-negative HER2 2-positive and HER2 1-positive disease.

Conclusion

Therapies that target HER2 have altered the natural course of HER2-positive MBC. The initial success of trastuzumab in improving survival rates led to the clinical development of lapatinib, pertuzumab, and T-DM1. HER2 protein overexpression and/or gene amplification remains the most important predictive factor of response to HER2-targeted therapies. Although successful targeting of HER2 has improved outcomes in HER2-positive breast cancer, treatment resistance and brain metastases remain problematic. As in the first-line setting, multiple choices exist for second- and third-line therapies. The choice is often based on patient preferences, prior toxicities, and drug availability. Ongoing studies are evaluating novel therapeutic approaches to overcome primary and secondary drug resistance in tumors (Fig. 33.14).

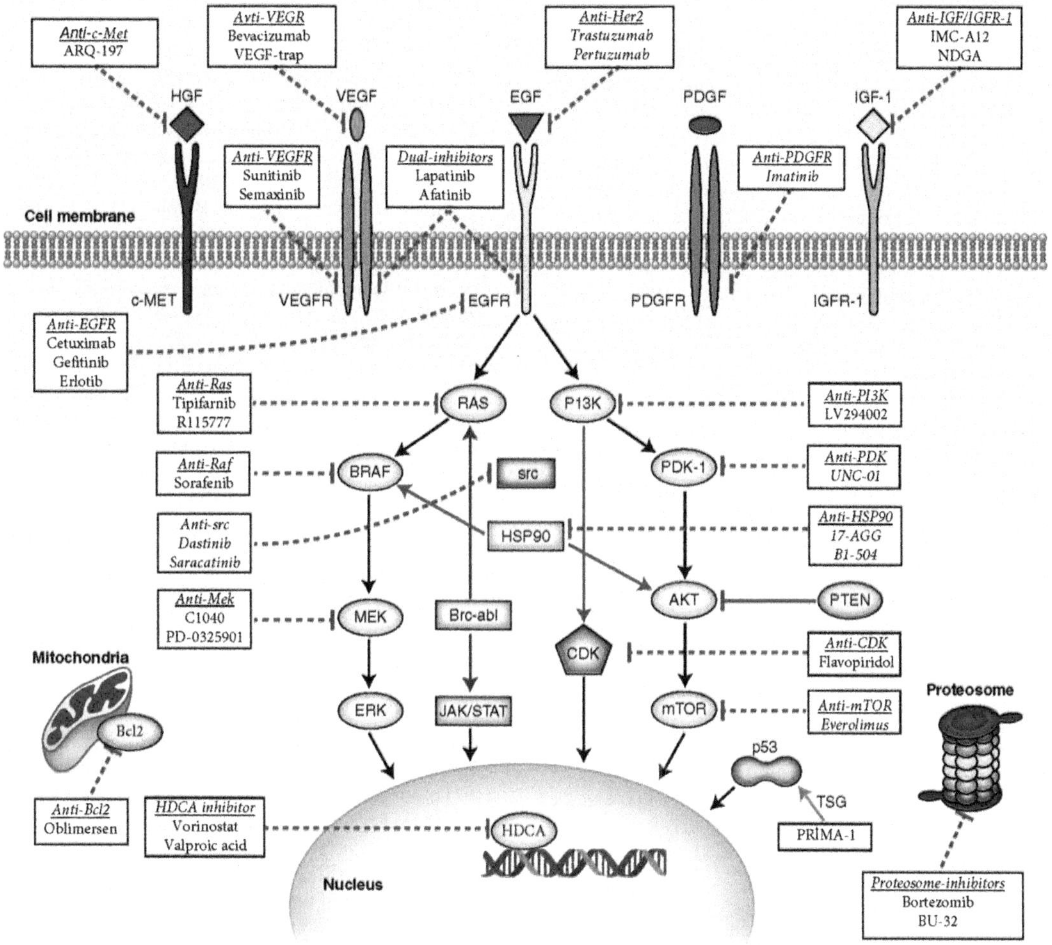

Fig. 33.14 Overview of intracellular signal transduction pathways involved in the proliferation and progression of breast cancer. Targeted therapy agents and their main inhibition targets are illustrated. *EGF* epidermal growth factor, *EGFR* EGF receptor, *HGF* hepatocyte growth factor, *c-MET* mesenchymal-epithelial transition factor, *PDGF* platelet-derived growth factor, *PDGFR* PDGF receptor, *IGF-1* insulin-like growth factor-I, *IGF-1R* IGF-1 receptor, *PI3K* phosphatidylinositol 3-kinase, *Ras* rat sarcoma subfamily of GTPases, *AKT* protein kinases B, *PDK1* pyruvate dehydrogenase kinase isozyme 1, *mTOR* mammalian target of rapamycin, *MEK* mitogen-activated protein kinase kinase, *VEGF* vascular endothelial growth factor, *VEGFR* VEGF receptor, *BRAF* B-type RAF kinase, *src* v-Src (Rous sarcoma virus) tyrosine kinase, *BCR-ABL* Philadelphia chromosome, *JAK/STAT* Janus kinases/signal transducers and activators of transcription, *PTEN* phosphatase and tensin homolog, *HDAC* histone deacetylases (Reprinted from Munagala et al. [76] with permission from the Indian Journal of Pharmacology)

References

1. National Comprehensive Cancer Network. NCCN Clinic Practice Guidelines in Oncology (NCCN Guideline), Breast Cancer. Version 1.0 2016. www.nccn.org.

2. Mustacchi G, Biganzoli L, Pronzato P, Montemurro F, Dambrosio M, Minelli M, et al. HER2-positive metastatic breast cancer: a changing scenario. Crit Rev Oncol Hematol. 2015;95(1):78–87. doi:10.1016/j.critrevonc.2015.02.002. Epub 2015 Feb 20.

3. Esteva FJ, Miller KD, Teicher BA. What can we learn about antibody-drug conjugates from the T-DM1 experience? Am Soc Clin Oncol Educ Book. 2015;35:e117–25.

4. Kaufman B, Mackey JR, Clemens MR, Bapsy PP, Vaid A, Wardley A, et al. Trastuzumab plus anastrozole versus anastrozole alone for the treatment of postmenopausal women with human epidermal growth factor receptor 2-positive, hormone receptor-positive metastatic breast cancer: results from the randomized phase III TAnDEM study. J Clin Oncol. 2009;27(33):5529–37.

5. Johnston S, Pippen Jr J, Pivot X, Lichinitser M, Sadeghi S, Dieras V, et al. Lapatinib combined with letrozole versus letrozole and placebo as first-line therapy for postmenopausal hormone receptor-positive metastatic breast cancer. J Clin Oncol. 2009;27(33):5538–46.

6. Slamon DJ, Leyland-Jones B, Shak S, Fuchs H, Paton V, Bajamonde A, et al. Use of chemotherapy plus a monoclonal antibody against HER2 for metastatic breast cancer that overexpresses HER2. N Engl J Med. 2001;344:783–92.

7. Andersson M, Lidbrink E, Bjerre K, Wist E, Enevoldsen K, Jensen AB, et al. Phase III randomized study comparing docetaxel plus trastuzumab with vinorelbine plus trastuzumab as first-line therapy of metastatic or locally advanced human epidermal growth factor receptor 2-positive breast cancer: the HERNATA study. J Clin Oncol. 2011;29(3):264–71.

8. Geyer CE, Forster J, Lindquist D, Chan S, Romieu CG, Pienkowski T, et al. Lapatinib plus capecitabine for HER2-positive advanced breast cancer. N Engl J Med. 2006;355(26):2733–43.

9. von Minckwitz G, du Bois A, Schmidt M, Maass N, Cufer T, de Jongh FE, et al. Trastuzumab beyond progression in human epidermal growth factor receptor 2-positive advanced breast cancer: a German Breast Group 26/Breast International Group 03–05 study. J Clin Oncol. 2009;27(12):1999–2006.

10. Wardley AM, Pivot X, Morales-Vasquez F, Zetina LM, de Fátima Dias Gaui M, Reyes DO, et al. Randomized phase II trial of first-line trastuzumab plus docetaxel and capecitabine compared with trastuzumab plus docetaxel in HER2-positive metastatic breast cancer. J Clin Oncol. 2010;28(6):976–83.

11. Alvarez RH, Valero V, Hortobagyi GN. Emerging targeted therapies for breast cancer. J Clin Oncol. 2010;28(20):3366–79.

12. Hamberg P, Bos MM, Braun HJ, Stouthard JM, van Deijk GA, Erdkamp FL, et al. Randomized phase II study comparing efficacy and safety of combination-therapy trastuzumab and docetaxel vs. sequential therapy of trastuzumab followed by docetaxel alone at progression as first-line chemotherapy in patients with HER2+ metastatic breast cancer: HERTAX trial. Clin Breast Cancer. 2011;11:103.

13. Burstein HJ, Keshaviah A, Baron AD, Hart RD, Lambert-Falls R, Marcom PK, et al. Trastuzumab plus vinorelbine or taxane chemotherapy for her2-overexpressing metastatic breast cancer: the trastuzumab and vinorelbine or taxane study. Cancer. 2007;110:965–72.

14. Valero V, Forbes J, Pegram MD, Pienkowski T, Eiermann W, von Minckwitz G, et al. Multicenter phase III randomized trial comparing docetaxel and trastuzumab with docetaxel, carboplatin, and trastuzumab as first-line chemotherapy for patients with her2-gene-amplified metastatic breast cancer (BCIRG 007 Study): two highly active therapeutic regimens. J Clin Oncol. 2011;29:149–56.

15. Robert N, Leyland-Jones B, Asmar L, Belt R, Ilegbodu D, Loesch D, et al. Randomized phase III study of trastuzumab, paclitaxel, and carboplatin compared with trastuzumab and paclitaxel in women with her-2-overexpressing metastatic breast cancer. J Clin Oncol. 2006;24:2786–92.

16. Guarneri V, Lenihan DJ, Valero V, Durand JB, Broglio K, Hess KR, et al. Long-term cardiac tolerability of trastuzumab in metastatic breast cancer: the M.D. Anderson Cancer Center experience. J Clin Oncol. 2006;24(25):4107–15.

17. Paul B, Trovato JA, Thompson J. Lapatinib: a dual tyrosine kinase inhibitor for metastatic breast cancer. Am J Health Syst Pharm. 2008;65(18):1703–10.

18. Guan Z, Xu B, DeSilvio ML, Shen Z, Arpornwirat W, Tong Z, et al. Randomized trial of lapatinib versus placebo added to paclitaxel in the treatment of human epidermal growth factor receptor 2–overexpressing metastatic breast cancer. J Clin Oncol. 2013;31:1947–53.

19. Gelmon KA, Boyle FM, Kaufman B, Huntsman DG, Manikhas A, Di Leo A, et al. Lapatinib or trastuzumab plus taxane therapy for human epidermal growth factor receptor 2-positive advanced breast cancer: final results of NCIC CTG MA.31. J Clin Oncol. 2015;33(14):1574–83.

20. Franklin MC, Carey KD, Vajdos FF, Leahy DJ, de Vos AM, Sliwkowski MX. Insights into ErbB signaling from the structure of the ErbB2-pertuzumab complex. Cancer Cell. 2004;5:317–28.

21. Harbeck N, Beckmann MW, Rody A, Schneeweiss A, Müller V, Fehm T, et al. HER2 dimerization inhibitor pertuzumab – mode of action and clinical data in breast cancer. Breast Care (Basel). 2013;8(1):49–55.

22. Swain SM, Baselga J, Kim SB, Ro J, Semiglazov V, Campone M, CLEOPATRA Study Group, et al. Pertuzumab, trastuzumab, and docetaxel in HER2-positive metastatic breast cancer. N Engl J Med. 2015;372(8):724–34.

23. Baselga J, Cortés J, Im SA, Clark E, Ross G, Kiermaier A, et al. Biomarker analyses in CLEOPATRA: a phase III, placebo-controlled study of pertuzumab in human epidermal growth factor receptor 2-positive, first-line metastatic breast cancer. J Clin Oncol. 2014;32(33):3753–61.
24. Panowksi S, Bhakta S, Raab H, Polakis P, Jagath R, Junutula JG. Site-specific antibody drug conjugates for cancer therapy. MAbs. 2014;6(1):34–45.
25. Hamblett KJ, Senter PD, Chace DF, Sun MM, Lenox J, Cerveny CG, et al. Effects of drug loading on the antitumor activity of a monoclonal antibody drug conjugate. Clin Cancer Res. 2004;10:7063–70.
26. LoRusso PM, Weiss D, Guardino E, Girish S, Sliwkowski MX. Trastuzumab emtansine: a unique antibody-drug conjugate in development for human epidermal growth factor receptor 2-positive cancer. Clin Cancer Res. 2011;17(20):6437–47.
27. Hurvitz SA, Dirix L, Kocsis J, Bianchi GV, Lu J, Vinholes J, et al. Phase II randomized study of trastuzumab emtansine versus trastuzumab plus docetaxel in patients with human epidermal growth factor receptor 2-positive metastatic breast cancer. J Clin Oncol. 2013;31:1157.
28. Ellis PA, Barrios CH, Eiermannc W, Toi M, Im YH, Conte PF, et al. Phase III, randomized study of T-DM1 ± pertuzumab (P) vs trastuzumab + taxane (HT) for first-line treatment of HER2-positive MBC: primary results from the MARIANNE study. J Clin Oncol. 33, 2015 (suppl; abstr 507).
29. Paplomata E, O'Regan R. The PI3K/AKT/mTOR pathway in breast cancer: targets, trials and biomarkers. Ther Adv Med Oncol. 2014;6(4):154–66.
30. Yardley DA, Noguchi S, Pritchard KI, Burris 3rd HA, Baselga J, Gnant M, et al. Everolimus plus exemestane in postmenopausal patients with HR(+) breast cancer: BOLERO-2 final progression-free survival analysis. Adv Ther. 2013;30(10):870–84.
31. Hurvitz SA, Dalenc F, Campone M, O'Regan RM, Tjan-Heijnen VC, Gligorov J, et al. A phase 2 study of everolimus combined with trastuzumab and paclitaxel in patients with HER2-overexpressing advanced breast cancer that progressed during prior trastuzumab and taxane therapy. Breast Cancer Res Treat. 2013;141(3):437–46.
32. Hurvitz SA, Andre F, Jiang Z, Shao Z, Neciosup SP, Mano MS, et al. Phase 3, randomized, double-blind, placebo-controlled multicenter trial of daily everolimus plus weekly trastuzumab and paclitaxel as first-line therapy in women with HER2+ advanced breast cancer: BOLERO-1. SABCS December 2014, abs S6-01).
33. Huober J, Fasching PA, Barsoum M, Petruzelka L, Wallwiener D, Thomssen C, et al. Higher efficacy of letrozole in combination with trastuzumab compared to letrozole monotherapy as first-line treatment in patients with HER2-positive, hormone-receptor-positive metastatic breast cancer: results of the eLEcTRA trial. Breast. 2012;21:27–33.
34. Schwartzberg LS, Franco SX, Florance A, O'Rourke L, Maltzman J, Johnston S. Lapatinib plus letrozole as first-line therapy for HER-2 hormone receptor-positive metastatic breast cancer. Oncologist. 2010;15:122–9.
35. Blackwell KL, Burstein HJ, Storniolo AM, Rugo HS, Sledge G, Aktan G, et al. Overall survival benefit with lapatinib in combination with trastuzumab for patients with human epidermal growth factor receptor 2–positive metastatic breast cancer: final results from the EGF104900 study. J Clin Oncol. 2012;30:2585–92.
36. PHEREXA. A study of a combination of trastuzumab and capecitabine with or without pertuzumab in patients with HER2-positive metastatic breast cancer https://clinicaltrials.gov/ct2.
37. Chumsri S, Sabnis G, Tkaczuk K, Brodie A. mTOR inhibitors: changing landscape of endocrine-resistant breast cancer. Future Oncol. 2014;10(3):443–56.
38. Rimawi MF, De Angelis C, Schiff R. Resistance to anti-HER2 therapies in breast cancer. Am Soc Clin Oncol Educ Book. 2015;35:e157–64.
39. André F, O'Regan R, Ozguroglu M, Toi M, Xu B, Jerusalem G, et al. Everolimus for women with trastuzumab-resistant, HER2-positive, advanced breast cancer (BOLERO-3): a randomised, double-blind, placebo-controlled phase 3 trial. Lancet Oncol. 2014;15(6):580–91.
40. Cameron D, Casey M, Oliva C, Newstat B, Imwalle B, Geyer CE. Lapatinib plus capecitabine in women with her-2–positive advanced breast cancer: final survival analysis of a phase III randomized trial. Oncologist. 2010;15:924–34.
41. Verma S, Miles D, Gianni L, Krop IE, Welslau M, Baselga J, et al. T-DM1 for HER2-positive advanced breast cancer. N Engl J Med. 2012;367(19):1783–91.
42. Welslau M, Diéras V, Sohn JH, Hurvitz SA, Lalla D, Fang L, et al. Patient-reported outcomes from EMILIA, a randomized phase 3 study of T-DM1 (T-DM1) versus capecitabine and lapatinib in human epidermal growth factor receptor 2-positive locally advanced or metastatic breast cancer. Cancer. 2014;120(5):642–51.
43. Giordano SH, Temin S, Kirshner JJ, Chandarlapaty S, Crews JR, Davidson NE, on behalf of the American Society of Clinical Oncology, et al. Systemic therapy for patients with advanced human epidermal growth factor receptor 2–positive breast cancer: American Society of Clinical Oncology clinical practice guideline. J Clin Oncol. 2014;32:2078–99.
44. Korkola JE, Liu M, Liby T, Heiser L, Feiler H, Gray JW. Detrimental effects of sequential compared to concurrent treatment of pertuzumab plus T-DM1 in HER2+ breast cancer cell lines. SABCS. 2014, [S6–07].
45. Lin NU, Winer EP, Wheatley D, Carey LA, Houston S, Mendelson D, et al. A phase II study of afatinib (BIBW 2992), an irreversible ErbB family blocker, in patients with HER2-positive metastatic breast cancer progressing after trastuzumab. Breast Cancer Res Treat. 2012;133(3):1057–65.
46. Eisenhauer EA, Therasse P, Bogaerts J, Schwartz LH, Sargent D, Ford R, RECIST CRITERIA, et al. New response evaluation criteria in solid tumours: revised

RECIST guideline (version 1.1). Eur J Cancer. 2009;45:228–47.

47. Harbeck N, Huang CS, Hurvitz S, Harbeck N, Huang CS, Hurvitz S, et al. Randomized phase III trial of afatinib plus vinorelbine versus trastuzumab plus vinorelbine in patients with HER2-overexpressing metastatic breast cancer who had progressed on one prior trastuzumab treatment: LUX-Breast 1. Poster P5-19-01 presented at the San Antonio Breast Cancer Symposium (SABCS) 2014 Congress, San Antonio, Texas. 9–13 December 2014.

48. Saura C, Garcia-Saenz JA, Xu B, Harb W, Moroose R, Pluard T, et al. Safety and efficacy of neratinib in combination with capecitabine in patients with metastatic human epidermal growth factor receptor 2-positive breast cancer. J Clin Oncol. 2014;32(32): 3626–33.

49. Krop IE, Kim SB, González-Martín A, LoRusso PM, Ferrero JM, Smitt M, et al. T-DM1 versus treatment of physician's choice for pretreated HER2-positive advanced breast cancer (TH3RESA): a randomised, open-label, phase 3 trial. Lancet Oncol. 2014;15(7): 689–99.

50. Cwhen G, Bagnardi V, Viale G, Fumagalli L, Rotmensz N, Aurilio G, et al. Should liver metastases of breast cancer be biopsied to improve treatment choice? Ann Oncol. 2011;22:2227–33.

51. Ramakrishna N, Temin S, Chandarlapaty S, Crews JR, Davidson NE, Esteva FJ, et al. Recommendations on disease management for patients with advanced human epidermal growth factor receptor 2–positive breast cancer and brain metastases: American Society of Clinical Oncology Clinical Practice Guideline. J Clin Oncol. 2014;32:2100–8.

52. Kased N, Binder DK, McDermott MW, Nakamura JL, Huang K, Berger MS, et al. Gamma Knife radiosurgery for brain metastases from primary breast cancer. Int J Radiat Oncol Biol Phys. 2009;75(4): 1132–40.

53. Pestalozzi BC, Brignoli S. Trastuzumab in CSF. J Clin Oncol. 2000;18:2349–51.

54. Hans-Joachim S, Manfred S, Amina W, Helga B, Nadia H, Volker H. Ratio of trastuzumab levels in serum and cerebrospinal fluid is altered in HER2-positive breast cancer patients with brain metastases and impairment of blood-brain barrier. Anti-Cancer Drugs. 2007;18:23–8.

55. Dijkers EC, Oude Munnink TH, Kosterink JG, Brouwers AH, Jager PL, de Jong JR, et al. Biodistribution of 89Zr-trastuzumab and PET imaging of HER2-positive lesions in patients with metastatic breast cancer. Clin Pharmacol Ther. 2010; 87:586–92.

56. Brufsky AM, Mayer M, Rugo HS, Kaufman PA, Tan-Chiu E, Tripathy D, et al. Central nervous system metastases in patients with HER2-positive metastatic breast cancer: incidence, treatment, and survival in patients from registHER. Clin Cancer Res. 2011; 17(14):4834–43.

57. Lin NU, Diéras V, Paul D, Lossignol D, Christodoulou C, Stemmler HJ, et al. Multicenter phase II study of lapatinib in patients with brain metastases from HER2-positive breast cancer. Clin Cancer Res. 2009; 15:1452–9.

58. Bachelot T, Romieu G, Campone M, Diéras V, Cropet C, Dalenc F, et al. Lapatinib plus capecitabine in patients with previously untreated brain metastases from HER2-positive metastatic breast cancer (LANDSCAPE): a single-group phase 2 study. Lancet Oncol. 2013;14:64–71.

59. Pivot X, Manikhas A, Żurawski B, Chmielowska E, Karaszewska B, Allerton R, et al. CEREBEL (EGF111438): a phase III, randomized, open-label study of lapatinib plus capecitabine versus trastuzumab plus capecitabine in patients with human epidermal growth factor receptor 2-positive metastatic breast cancer. J Clin Oncol. 2015;33:1564–73.

60. Krop IE, Lin NU, Blackwell K, Guardino E, Huober J, Lu M, et al. T-DM1 (T-DM1) versus lapatinib plus capecitabine in patients with HER2-positive metastatic breast cancer and central nervous system metastases: a retrospective, exploratory analysis in EMILIA. Ann Oncol. 2015;26:113–9.

61. de Azambuja E, Zardavas D, Lemort M, Rossari J, Moulin C, Buttice A, et al. Phase I trial combining temozolomide plus lapatinib for the treatment of brain metastases in patients with HER2-positive metastatic breast cancer: the LAPTEM trial. Ann Oncol. 2013;24:2985–9.

62. Rachel A, Freedman RA, Gelman RS, Wefel JS, KropI IE, Melisko ME, et al. TBCRC 022: phase II trial of neratinib for patients (Pts) with human epidermal growth factor receptor 2 (HER2+) breast cancer and brain metastases (BCBM). J Clin Oncol 32:5s, 2014 (suppl; abstr 528).

63. Ferrario C, Welch S, Chaves JM, Luke N. Walker LN, Ian E, et al. ONT-380 in the treatment of HER2+ breast cancer central nervous system (CNS) metastases (mets). J Clin Oncol. 33; 2015 (suppl; abstr 612).

64. NCT01921335. ARRY-380 + Trastuzumab for breast cancer with brain metastases. https://clinicaltrials.gov/ct2/.

65. Zagouri F, Sergentanis TN, Bartsch R, Berghoff AS, Chrysikos D, de Azambuja E, et al. Intrathecal administration of trastuzumab for the treatment of meningeal carcinomatosis in HER2-positive metastatic breast cancer: a systematic review and pooled analysis. Breast Cancer Res Treat. 2013;139(1):13–22.

66. Citri A, Yarden Y. EGF-ERBB signalling: towards the systems level. Nat Rev Mol Cell Biol. 2006;7:505–16.

67. Arteaga CL. ErbB-targeted therapeutic approaches in human cancer. Exp Cell Res. 2003;284:122–30.

68. Ghosh R, Narasanna A, Wang SE, Liu S, Chakrabarty A, Balko JM, et al. Trastuzumab has preferential activity against breast cancers driven by HER2 homodimers. Cancer Res. 2011;71:1871–82.

69. Berns K, Horlings HM, Hennessy BT, Madiredjo M, Hijmans EM, Beelen K, et al. A functional genetic

approach identifies the PI3K pathway as a major determinant of trastuzumab resistance in breast cancer. Cancer Cell. 2007;12:395–402.

70. Miller TW, Rexer BN, Garrett JT, Arteaga CL. Mutations in the phosphatidylinositol 3-kinase pathway: role in tumor progression and therapeutic implications in breast cancer. Breast Cancer Res. 2011;13:224.

71. Stagg J, Loi S, Divisekera U, Ngiow SF, Duret H, Yagita H, et al. Anti-ErbB-2 mAb therapy requires type I and II interferons and synergizes with anti-PD-1 or anti-CD137 mAb therapy. Proc Natl Acad Sci U S A. 2011;108:7142–7.

72. Loi S. Tumor-infiltrating lymphocytes, breast cancer subtypes and therapeutic efficacy. Oncoimmunology. 2013;2(7), e24720.

73. PANACEA. Anti-PD-1 monoclonal antibody in advanced, Trastuzumab-resistant, HER2-positive breast cancer. https://clinicaltrials.gov/ct2/.

74. Elgersma RC, Coumans RG, Huijbregts T, Menge WM, Joosten JA, Spijker HJ, et al. Design, synthesis, and evaluation of linker-duocarmycin payloads: toward selection of HER2-targeting antibody-drug conjugate SYD985. Mol Pharm. 2015 [Epub ahead of print].

75. Verheijden G, Beusker P, Ubink R, Lee M, Groothuis P, Goedings PJ, et al. Toward clinical development of SYD985, a novel her2-targeting antibody–drug conjugate (adc) [abstract 626]. J Clin Oncol. 2014;32(suppl).

76. Munagala R, Aqil F, Gupta RC. Promising molecular targeted therapies in breast cancer. Indian J Pharmacol. 2011;43(3):236–45.

End-of-Life Considerations in Patients with Breast Cancer

Nazim Serdar Turhal and Faysal Dane

Abstract

Cancer is a leading cause of death worldwide. Terminally ill cancer patients and their families often have some exceptional physical, psychosocial, and spiritual symptoms. Experts who provide care to these patients and their families should widen their assessments to guarantee physical and psychosocial comfort and to detect objectives of care and social and spiritual causes of suffering. Here, some problems frequently faced in dying cancer patients in the last days or weeks of life will be discussed.

Keywords

Breast cancer • Terminal illness • Prognosis • End of life • Hospice • Suffering • Nutrition • Palliation • Bereavement • Grief

Introduction

Most patients in the terminal status of a serious and/or life-threatening illness such as cancer develop remarkable physical and psychosocial symptoms in the last weeks to months before death. Effective treatment may successfully alleviate the majority of symptoms that may arise in terminally ill cancer patients. Here, we will discuss common issues confronted in daily practice during the end of life of advanced cancer patients.

N.S. Turhal (✉)
Department of Medical Oncology, Marmara University, School of Medicine, Istanbul, Turkey

Medical Oncology, Anadolu Medical Center, Cumhuriyet Mh 2255 Sk No 3 Gebze, Kocaeli 41400, Turkey
e-mail: turhal@superonline.com

F. Dane, MD
Department of Medical Oncology, Marmara University, School of Medicine, Istanbul, Turkey
e-mail: faysaldane@yahoo.com

Discussing Prognosis

Prognosis may be defined as the estimation of the likelihood that a particular health event will occur. The prognosis discussion ideally should occur when the patient is not acutely ill and therefore can process the information free of acute distress. Unfortunately, on many occasions, this discussion occurs near the final stages of illness. There is a tendency toward unrealistic aggressive intervention demands that are unlikely to benefit the patient when these discussions are conducted at the final stage [1, 2].

A proper private setting for this conversation is also of utmost importance. Particular attention should be paid to interference, such as cell phones. A typical strategy is to first determine what the other party understands about the situation and begin the conversation at that level, providing small amounts of information and frequently stopping to ensure that the other side grasps the facts [3, 4].

In cancer patients, discussing prognosis may often refer to estimating the expected life span, but this is not the only outcome that the physician is expected to know. The patient or the family may also ask the doctor to estimate the time span for other events such as losing the ability to care for himself/herself. Obviously, the doctor cannot know the course of an illness precisely for a particular patient, but the patient or relatives expect that the doctor has likely faced similar occurrences many times in the past and is thus familiar with the average course and can provide a reasonable estimate. A reasonable estimate allows the patient and family to prepare for the unwanted circumstance in a timely manner. It is important for the physician to reiterate the fact that "every patient is different" and that the exact timing and sequence of events are unknowable. This perspective may also help the patient and the loved ones maintain hope. Several studies have demonstrated that physicians are poor at guessing the life spans of terminally ill patients and even poorer at communicating such estimates frankly to the patient and family [5, 6].

Even though discussions of prognosis are an essential part of a physician's daily tasks, particularly when caring for cancer patients, they represent a miniscule portion of medical education and are not discussed extensively in standard textbooks. This lack of training may also explain why physicians frequently avoid this conversation unless forced by the counterpart or under a sense of obligation as part of good clinical practice [6–8].

Growing interest in palliative care is increasing the importance of grasping the significance of this subject matter by practicing physicians, particularly in the oncology community [6–8].

Every intervention, including laboratory tests for screening and medications, should be guided by the expected prognosis of the patient. The clinical decision-making process may be much easier for the clinician if the patient is also aware of the prognosis. There are no established and commonly agreed upon guidelines for best practices for specific stages of life expectancy [6–8].

Discussing End of Life

When patients approach the end of life and the expected time of death is near, many practical issues regarding patient care surface, particularly if the patient is not fully capable of making decisions on his/her own. There may be some conflict between healthcare providers and family members on subsequent steps. Ideally, the patient's preferences will be discussed in advance to facilitate decision making by the doctor and family. However, such discussions frequently do not occur, and conflicts may arise, particularly if the different parties involved in the patient's care have different expectations. A surrogate is essential under these circumstances to make decisions on the patient's behalf. Detailed advance care planning should be determined long before the crisis arises in the final days or weeks. This approach can prevent arguments both between family members and between loved ones and healthcare providers. The doctor should remember that both the family and the legal surrogate have the right to refuse any further medical interventions, and the doctor must respect that decision [5–8].

Hope

Hope is an important emotion that is highly valued by patients and relatives. Patients or their loved ones frequently reiterate that they did not lose hope or seek traces of hope because of the physician's verbal and nonverbal communication, partly because there is a common belief that success in treatment is not possible if there is no hope on behalf of the patient. Although the correlation between treatment success and hope can work both ways, the physician is frequently expected to speak in a manner that keeps hope "alive" in the patient. We, as physicians, must be honest with our patients about the facts of the disease without doubt. However, emphasizing the positive aspects of the clinical disease course, pathology, or laboratory reports in no way harms the patient and, on the contrary, may increase the patient's cooperation with treatment. An essential distinction is to avoid outright lies to give hope to other parties. The patient or the family's frequent discussion of the hope "issue" may be a strong indicator that this is an issue that must be addressed; thus, the physician should appropriately bring it up during the visit [3–7].

Healing Versus Curing

It is important for the physician to inform the patient about the expected outcome of the intended therapy. The patient may not want to know the full details, and the physician must respect this while demonstrating a readiness to provide answers to the patient's questions anytime they are required. Again, providing information in small chunks and waiting for the information to "sink in" are essential. If the patient does not want to talk about this despite invitation, the physician must respect this decision as well. It is important to know that there is a significant discrepancy between a physician's intentions regarding a particular therapy and how the patient and the family perceive it. Thus, every effort should be made to bring these views closer together. In a developing world healthcare setting, the physician caring for the cancer patient must pitch in to fulfill the role of social worker, psychologist, psychiatrist, and occasionally even chaplain [9, 10].

How to Tell the Children

Every time there is a need to share bad news, there is a dilemma on how to communicate that properly with the patient and/or family, including children. Although there is no one-size-fits-all approach, there are some general rules a practitioner must follow. The explanation must begin at a level the other side currently knows or accepts. In particular, if small children are involved, we must learn about them and their level of understanding, which is of utmost importance. We as doctors must respect whether the patient does not want to know or is ready to hear what we are about to share. Sharing the information in an appropriate setting is also a prerequisite. Giving the facts in honest but small chunks and waiting for the recipients to "come to grips" with what has been said are also important. It may be necessary to stop frequently to answer questions. In addition, the explanation may also take more than one session. Children, particularly at younger ages, may feel guilty about what has happened to their parents or believe that their behavior caused the condition; therefore, this area may require detailed attention to clarify. Concluding the session with a wrap-up of what has been said and the proper communication for the next step for the other party is also important. Perceptions and reactions to bad news can vary widely based on personality and cultural factors, and the above techniques should be adjusted accordingly. However, in general, frankly answering all questions at a level that the other party is ready to understand is essential [11, 12].

Cultural and Religious Considerations

The cultural and religious backgrounds of both the physician and the patient are important aspects of disease perception as well as end-of-life care. The physician must be aware and take proper steps to avoid unnecessary confrontation if background is going to be an important issue at that stage of the patient's care. The physician may not know in full detail how different cultures and/or religions can affect the way that an individual perceives disease and death, but careful observation of the person throughout the duration of care is certainly important and enables an appropriately individualized approach. A proper interpreter if the clinician is not fluent in the patient's language is also an important consideration [12–14].

Care Without Chemotherapy

There are times when the clinical condition requires the patient to be observed and managed for symptoms rather than administering chemotherapy or direct cancer-related treatment. This may cause patient anxiety, although this scenario is not necessarily an issue toward the terminal part of the disease course. Proper communication is also essential when this occurs. The message should not be conveyed as "I have nothing else to offer you." Instead, the physician should state that "I am concentrating on offering you an approach that would put your quality of life above everything else" [13–16].

Hospice Programs

When a patient is admitted to the hospital, the care is based on intervening in most if not all laboratory anomalies. The house staff is trained at detecting these anomalies and correcting them appropriately and immediately. Toward the end of life, this approach may not be in the patient's best interest, and other institutions that concentrate on comforting the patient with dignity rather than correcting chart abnormalities have consequently been established. Although in some developed countries, including the USA, such palliative care teams are available both in the hospital and in hospices, in the developing world, these specialized services do not exist. As major care providers to cancer patients, medical oncologists and staff nurses usually assume this task. Palliative care providers are also an essential part of terminal care, and their presence certainly improves patient satisfaction [17, 18].

Hospices provide terminal care to patients with a life expectancy of less than 6 months. They provide services such as family education, practical support, and counseling. These services are frequently not a top priority in hospitals, which are also not equipped to provide these services. Hospice is also quite costly, and societies with limited resources are inclined to let families handle this difficult task and provide various levels of outside support to ease the work associated with it [17, 19, 20].

Relief of Suffering

Fatigue

Fatigue is the most common and one of the most disregarded and undertreated symptoms in terminally ill cancer patients. The National Comprehensive Cancer Network (NCCN) defines cancer-related fatigue as a "distressing, persistent, subjective sense of physical, emotional, and/or cognitive tiredness or exhaustion related to cancer or cancer treatment that is not proportional to activity and that interferes with usual functioning" [21]. Cancer-related fatigue differs from normal fatigue, which is usually short term and improved by rest. There are many contributing factors that influence fatigue. These factors and the fatigue itself should be assessed and managed appropriately because they significantly affect the quality of life of the patients who are receiving palliative care. Up to 75 % of patients with cancer present with fatigue [21]. At the end of life, its prevalence increases to 85 % in patients with life-threatening illnesses [22].

Some studies have demonstrated an association between fatigue and pain, dyspnea, anorexia, psychological symptoms, and gastrointestinal symptoms such as abdominal discomfort, bloating, abdominal distension, and constipation [23, 24]. The essential factors contributing to cancer-related fatigue are cancer therapy; metabolic/nutritional/hormonal issues such as anemia, poor nutrition, hypothyroidism, menopause, and dehydration; or other comorbidities such as heart problems or pulmonary diseases. Pain and its treatment, emotional distress, and sleep disturbances may also contribute to cancer-related fatigue. Although as a general rule anemia is considered the most important contributor to fatigue in patients experiencing cancer treatment, its importance is diminished toward the end of life for cancer patients. During that stage, other factors, including psychological symptoms such as anxiety and depression, pain, cachexia, adverse effects of medications, physical inactivity, and infection, may play a greater role.

A comprehensive history and physical examination are indicated to identify potentially reversible etiologies. A review of all medications, including alternative therapies, is important to identify side effects and potential drug interactions that may contribute to fatigue. In these cases, altering the dose interval may significantly improve fatigue.

The optimal management of fatigue involves aggressive treatment for potentially treatable etiologies. If a specific reversible etiology cannot be identified, symptomatic treatment is appropriate. There are limited data to support the hypothesis that one pharmacological approach is superior to another for fatigue [25]. Patients who have a high cancer burden with fatigue may be given a 2-week trial of corticosteroids (20–40 mg of prednisone) or megestrol acetate (480–800 mg/day). In cancer patients with severe fatigue who do not respond to steroids or have fatigue that is considered to be related to opioids, methylphenidate or modafinil may be recommended [25]. Moderate exercise, cognitive behavioral therapy, and yoga may be helpful. In most cases of advanced cancer, because of the multidimensional nature of fatigue, a combination of both pharmacological and non-pharmacological interventions may be beneficial.

The increasing cancer burden and declining functional reserve result in fatigue and a decrease in routine daily activities at the end of life. Patients may not be able to even move in their home to access a bedroom or toilet. In such cases, creating space for care on an accessible level or providing a portable toilet may improve patient comfort.

Loss of the ability to move or transfer independently is one of the most significant aspects of functional inadequacy. The period between independent mobility and bed confinement entails a high risk of falls. During this period, assistive equipment may be required. In hospitalized patients, family members should be allowed to stay with the patient for comfort and to promote safety. Bed alarms may help hospital staff to respond to patients' needs promptly to avoid injuries.

A prolonged period of lying on a flat bed on the same part of the body may result in skin ulcers. To decrease these ulcers, turning and repositioning may be beneficial. If these maneuvers are not comfortable for the patient, adequate cushioning may improve comfort.

In Turkey, home healthcare is not widely available. Thus, family members should be educated in transfers, turning, changing, feeding, and other personal care issues to ensure safety.

Insomnia

Insomnia is observed in the majority of terminally ill cancer patients. Insomnia in dying patients may commonly result from undertreated pain, depression, anxiety, delirium, dyspnea, nocturnal hypoxia, nausea and vomiting, or pruritus. Drugs such as steroids and antiemetics may cause insomnia. Apart from adversely affecting the quality of life, insomnia can heighten the intensity and awareness of other symptoms such as pain, anxiety, or fatigue. One study indicated that the most common causes of insomnia in patients receiving palliative care are uncontrolled pain, urinary symptoms, and dyspnea [26]. In this study, 62 % of patients who were prescribed hypnotic drugs reported improvement in sleep disturbance. Another study reported that many terminally ill advanced cancer patients are chronically prescribed hypnotic drugs for unclear indications [27]. In the majority of these patients, discontinuation of the hypnotic drugs may significantly improve cognition without adversely affecting insomnia.

Meta-analyses of randomized, placebo-controlled trials indicate that benzodiazepines are effective in improving sleep duration and sleep quality [28]. A newer class of sleep-promoting medications called non-benzodiazepines such as zaleplon or zolpidem has also been shown to be effective in patients with insomnia [29].

Anecdotal evidence suggests that taking a warm bath or drinking a glass of warm milk prior to bedtime and avoiding caffeinated beverages following dinner may improve the quality of sleep.

Gastrointestinal Symptoms

Nausea and Vomiting

Nausea in palliative care patients with advanced cancer may have many causes. Although there have been many randomized clinical studies in the field of chemotherapy- or radiation treatment-induced nausea and vomiting, evidence is lacking for terminally ill advanced cancer patients who have non-treatment-related nausea [30]. Great effort should be made to identify and manage the treatable etiologies. The correction of metabolic abnormalities, overviewing medications, opioid rotation, rational bowel care, and, in the case of brain involvement, treating the metastasis may provide relief.

If a potentially treatable etiology cannot be identified and if the bowel obstruction is not the cause, symptomatic treatment may be started with a prokinetic agent. In these cases, because of its central antiemetic and peripheral gastric-emptying effects, metoclopramide would be an ideal option for symptomatic treatment [31]. Dexamethasone and other steroids may augment the effects of metoclopramide. In cases in which steroids and metoclopramide are contraindicated, other centrally acting antiemetic agents can be administered. Serotonin antagonists are very useful for chemotherapy-, radiation treatment-, or operation-induced nausea and vomiting. For patients with contraindications for oral administration, metoclopramide, dexamethasone, or haloperidol may be given intravenously. In patients with bowel obstruction, prokinetic agents are contraindicated. In these circumstances, dexamethasone and haloperidol are good options. In addition, because of its reduced effects on gastrointestinal secretions and motility, subcutaneous octreotide may be beneficial in patients with bowel obstruction.

Dry Mouth

More than two-thirds of patients with advanced cancer complain of thirst or dry mouth. Dry mouth in this population is usually a result of opioids and is not because of dehydration and serum sodium; in contrast to healthy individuals, it is unrelieved by fluid therapy [32]. Most palliative care clinicians promote the use of good mouth care and sips of water when desired rather than parenteral hydration in this setting [33].

Decreased Oral Intake

The great majority of patients with advanced stage cancer have reduced oral intake before death. The inability to swallow is a common symptom in these cases. It might occur as a part of weakness or generalized fatigue or as a result of sedation related to medications or metabolic disturbances. The inability to consume sufficient food or fluids generally causes emotional stress for family members and other caregivers. In the final days or weeks of advanced terminal cancer, high caloric intake has not been shown to improve functional status or prolong survival. Thus, parenteral nutrition or tube feeding is not recommended for the nutritional supply of cancer patients in the dying days or hours. Case-based reports and retrospective series support the idea that adequate hydration in terminally ill patients is related to the amelioration of symptoms and a comfortable death. To improve mouth irritation and symptoms of thirst, good mouth care should be performed. In a randomized study, 129 cancer patients were enrolled to receive either 1 l of normal saline over four hours or a placebo (100 ml per day) to determine whether parenteral hydration was superior in improving symptoms of dehydration and delaying the onset or severity of delirium and whether it had any effects on quality of life [34]. The study demonstrated that there was no difference between the treatment and placebo groups in dehydration symptoms, quality of life, or survival.

Loss of Bowel Control

The loss of bowel control in the last days of life may cause incontinence of the urine and/or stool. The incontinence of stool or urine is commonly distressing for the patient and family members. In the case of urinary incontinence, a urinary catheter may minimize the need for frequent cleaning and changing. However, the use of catheters should be considered carefully and may not be used if urine flow is minimal and can be managed with absorbent pads.

Respiratory Symptoms

Upper Airway Secretion

For most patients, problematic airway secretions occur late in the dying process. The loss of the ability to swallow upper airway secretions may result from weakness and decreased neurological function. The gag reflex and clearing of the oropharynx decline, and secretions from the tracheobronchial tree accumulate. Increased airway secretions may interfere with a patient's ability to sleep, worsen dyspnea, precipitate uncomfortable coughing spells, and predispose the patient to infections.

In addition to a professional explaining and reassuring the patient's family, proper positioning and encouraging the family to cleanse the mouth with sponge sticks might be beneficial. Some patients may benefit from suctioning to clear excessive secretions if they have many secretions. However, deep suctioning should be avoided.

A recent review failed to demonstrate that any intervention was superior to placebo in patients with death rattle [35]. Although pharmacological agents have not been demonstrated to be beneficial in these patients, to relieve suffering, clinical judgment must be used to determine whether a pharmacological agent should be used to facilitate drying of secretions. Therefore, for patients managed at home, a scopolamine patch or glycopyrrolate may be recommended. For hospitalized patients, glycopyrrolate may be preferred due to its rapid onset of action and low central nervous system side effects.

Dyspnea in the End of Life

Dyspnea is defined as an uncomfortable awareness of breathing and is observed in approximately 70 % of dying patients [36]. Dyspnea encompasses multiple somatic perceptions that are described as air hunger, increased effort for breathing, chest tightness, rapid breathing, incomplete exhalation, or a feeling of suffocation. Dyspnea is a multidimensional symptom consisting of affective and physical aspects. Dyspnea is a major detriment to quality of life [37]. Dyspnea has prognostic impact for survival, mainly in terminally ill cancer patients [38]. One study found that the presence of dyspnea was associated with a median survival of less than 30 days [39]. The goal in treating dyspnea is to reduce the distress. Among patients receiving palliative care for advanced cancer, the causes of dyspnea are often irreversible. However, if a treatable cause of dyspnea, such as pulmonary emboli, airway obstruction, or pleural effusion, is identified, the specific treatment of the underlying cause may be appropriate depending on the invasiveness of the therapy. Studies of supplemental oxygen for the relief of dyspnea have shown controversial results in hypoxemic patients with cancer. The benefit of oxygen has not been demonstrated in non-hypoxemic patients [40]. A systematic review of controlled trials that included both hypoxemic and non-hypoxemic patients concluded that there was no consistent benefit of oxygen over air inhalation for dyspnea in patients with end-stage cancer [41]. Supplemental oxygen is a standard therapy for the symptomatic management of patients who are hypoxemic on room air. In patients who are not hypoxemic, supplemental oxygen appears no more likely than room air to provide relief of dyspnea. A randomized trial of 239 patients found no difference between oxygen and room air for the treatment of refractory dyspnea in non-hypoxemic adult outpatients [42].

The use of noninvasive positive pressure ventilation (NPPV) at the end of life is a variable practice. In a randomized study, NPPV was shown to improve dyspnea much faster than passive oxygen therapy in 200 hospitalized patients with end-stage cancer and severe respiratory failure [43]. In addition, the dose of morphine required to control dyspnea was significantly less in the NPPV group. Nevertheless, NPPV can be uncomfortable for patients with dyspnea. In addition, decreased mental status is thought to be a contraindication to NPPV because of the risk of aspiration.

Opioid agonists are the best-established pharmacological treatment for the management of dyspnea in patients with advanced disease. Randomized trials and systematic reviews have demonstrated the benefits of opioids in treating dyspnea [44, 45]. In a phase II study, the beneficial dose of sustained-release morphine was 10 mg daily for 70 % of patients, and the benefit at any dose was sustained for 3 months in 53 % of patients [46].

Systematic reviews of a small number of trials have concluded that benzodiazepines do not have a major role in the management of dyspnea in the absence of anxiety [47]. However, benzodiazepines are important drugs when anxiety is significant. Bronchodilators, glucocorticoids, and diuretics may provide relief of dyspnea in some clinical situations.

Psychiatric Disorders in Cancer Patients

Depression and Suicidal Ideation

The prevalence of major depression in cancer patients is as high as 40 % [48]. In cancer patients, depression is the most common mental health problem. Certain cancer drugs, such as steroids and vinca alkaloids, may cause depressive symptoms. Factors that are associated with an increased risk of depression are prior history of depression, young age, and uncontrolled cancer symptoms. If the diagnosis of depression is missed, then the quality of life of dying patients is impaired, and the burden of suffering increases. Individuals who have depression are also at increased risk for suicide. Although depressed mood and sadness are normal responses in patients facing death, feelings of hopelessness, helplessness, loss of interest, excess guilt, and suicidal ideation are among the indicators of depression in advanced cancer patients.

A careful diagnostic interview is the gold standard method for assessing whether patients are clinically depressed. Major depression is a treatable condition, even in terminally ill patients.

The first step in treating depression is to relieve uncontrolled symptoms. For patients with major depression, supportive psychotherapy should be initiated and is sometimes sufficient to treat the condition. However, most experts recommend an approach that combines supportive psychotherapy with patient and family education and the use of antidepressant medication. In terminal care, the psychostimulants methylphenidate, dextroamphetamine, and modafinil have a rapid onset of antidepressant action and are preferred to other agents, such as selective serotonin reuptake inhibitors, which may require weeks to achieve full effectiveness [49].

Delirium

Delirium is one of the most frequent neuropsychiatric disorders observed in patients with advanced cancer [50]. The incidence ranges from 15 % to 75 % depending on the clinical condition. In a study conducted in terminally ill patients, delirium was reported in more than 75 % of patients [51]. Delirium is multifactorial in origin. It might be a result of either the cancer itself or a result of treatments, electrolyte imbalances, or infection, etc. The identification of the reversible causes of delirium is essential because cognitive improvement may occur rapidly with treatment. Symptomatic and supportive therapies such as fluid and electrolyte balance, nutrition, and vitamins are also important. Haloperidol is the drug of choice for delirium in terminally ill patients [52]. Lorazepam plus haloperidol may be more effective than haloperidol alone in sedating the delirious patient.

Stopping Nutrition and Hydration in End-of-Life Care

As mentioned above, the great majority of terminally ill cancer patients have reduced oral intake before death. The reasons for insufficient oral intake include loss of appetite, nausea, vomiting, dysphagia, generalized fatigue, gastrointestinal obstruction, or impaired cognitive function. Family members usually become distressed when the cancer patient is unable to consume sufficient food and fluids, and they fear that the condition will result in more suffering and death [53].

In general, there are no clear indications for artificial nutrition or hydration when supporting palliative care at the end of life. Artificial hydration is the provision of water and electrolytes by any route other than the mouth. Artificial nutrition involves non-oral, enteral, or parenteral delivery of nutrients. Studies suggest that artificial nutrition has no effect on prolonging life or improving functional status in many advanced diseases [54]. Retrospective and case series studies conducted in advanced cancer patients have demonstrated that decreased protein synthesis and increased protein degradation are associated with the release of cytokines [55].

Therefore, providing nutritional supplements by either the enteral or parenteral route does not improve functional status, improve symptoms, or prolong survival in advanced cancer populations. Indeed, there are no randomized trials comparing nutritional support to no nutritional support in patients receiving palliative care for a terminal illness. However, the consistent lack of benefit from retrospective trials argues against the routine use of enteral or parenteral nutrition in patients receiving palliative care.

The practice of administering hydration near the end of life differs widely. Although the majority of cancer patients who die in acute care hospitals receive hydration until death, most patients who die at home receive no fluids. There are conflicting data on the association between symptoms and fluid deficits in terminally ill patients. Decisions regarding the use of hydration should be individualized. Some symptoms, such as delirium, sedation, or myoclonus, are thought to be aggravated by dehydration. In these cases, there may be a role for a trial of a small amount of parenteral fluids. Otherwise, it is inappropriate to routinely use hydration in terminally ill patients.

Palliative Sedation

Palliative sedation aims to relieve severe and refractory symptoms at the end of life. The aim of palliative sedation is to reduce the severity of intolerable suffering for terminally ill patients. It is usually used for the treatment of pain, dyspnea, agitated delirium, and convulsions. In a systematic review of observational studies including more than 1,000 patients, there was no statistically significant difference in survival between patients who underwent sedation and those who did not [56]. The sedative medications used for palliative sedation include midazolam, levomepromazine, chlorpromazine, phenobarbital, and propofol. Once adequate relief has been achieved, dose titration of the sedative drugs may be determined by the clinical situation.

The Final Days

The final days are usually defined as the last few days to weeks of a patient's life. The patient may have many severe symptoms ranging from dyspnea to incontinence, and observing their loved ones suffering from these symptoms may place an unbearable burden on the families.

If the patient is in the hospital, every effort should be made to comfort the patient, and family concerns and demands should be properly addressed. Particular attention should be paid to ensure that the family does not feel "abandoned." This period may be the appropriate time to make arrangements for final visits and for cultural and religious requirements following death [13, 14, 16, 19].

After the Death

The family should be able to spend as much time as needed after the death. Small acts of respect to the family after death, such as offering condolences, may facilitate the acceptance and closure of the process in their own mind [57–59].

Grief and Bereavement

The level of grief may depend on many issues; some are generalizable, such as culture and religion, but some are not, such as personal guilt and coping difficulties. Grief usually begins even before the patient dies; thus, supporting measures should start with the anticipated loss. Suffering should begin to ease by approximately 6 months after the death, but reminders such as anniversaries may remind families of the loss for years after. As resources allow, support for families should continue for at least 1 year after the loss and be available thereafter in case of need. If not supported adequately, grieving individuals are expected to have higher rates of psychiatric illnesses and substance abuse, etc. [57–59].

References

1. Lamont EB, Christakis NA. Complexities in prognostication in advanced cancer: "to help them live their lives the way they want to". JAMA. 2003;290:98.
2. Yourman LC, Lee SJ, Schonberg MA, Widera EW, Smith AK. Prognostic indices for older adults: a systematic review. JAMA. 2012;307:182.
3. Ahalt C, Walter LC, Yourman L, Eng C, Pérez-Stable EJ, Smith AK. "Knowing is better": preferences of diverse older adults for discussing prognosis. J Gen Intern Med. 2012;27:568.
4. Moulton B, King JS. Aligning ethics with medical decision-making: the quest for informed patient choice. J Law Med Ethics. 2010;38:85.
5. Smith AK, Williams BA, Lo B. Discussing overall prognosis with the very elderly. N Engl J Med. 2011;365:2149.
6. Girgis A, Sanson-Fisher RW. Breaking bad news: consensus guidelines for medical practitioners. J Clin Oncol. 1995;13:2449.
7. Butow P, Tattersall MHN, Stockler M. Discussing prognosis and communicating risk. In: Kissane D, Bultz B, Butow P, Finlay I, editors. Handbook of communication in oncology and palliative care. New York: Oxford University Press; 2010.
8. Cheung WY, Neville BA, Cameron DB, Cook EF, Earle CC. Comparisons of patient and physician expectations for cancer survivorship care. J Clin Oncol. 2009;27:2489.
9. Foley E, Baillie A, Huxter M, Price M, Sinclair E. Mindfulness-based cognitive therapy for individuals whose lives have been affected by cancer: a randomized controlled trial. J Consult Clin Psychol. 2010;78(1):72.
10. Ernst E, Pittler MH, Wider B, Boddy K. Complementary/alternative medicine for supportive cancer care: development of the evidence-base. Support Care Cancer. 2007;15(5):565.
11. Muriel AC, Rauch PK. Talking with families and children about the death of a parent. In: Hanks G, Cherny NI, Christakis NA, et al., editors. The Oxford textbook of palliative medicine. 4th ed. Oxford: Oxford University Press; 2009.
12. Danis M. The roles of ethnicity, race, religion, and socioeconomic status in end-of-life care in the ICU. In: Curtis JR, Rubenfeld GD, editors. Managing death in the intensive care unit. Oxford: Oxford University Press; 2001. p. 215.
13. Crawley LM, Marshall PA, Lo B, Koenig BA. Strategies for culturally effective end-of-life. Ann Intern Med. 2002;27(136):673.
14. Koenig B, Gates-Williams J. Understanding cultural differences in caring for dying patients. West J Med. 1995;163:244.
15. Harrington SE, Smith TJ. The role of chemotherapy at the end of life: "When is enough, enough?". JAMA. 2008;299:2667.
16. Searight HR, Gafford J. Cultural diversity at the end of life: issues and guidelines for family physicians. Am Fam Physician. 2005;71:515.
17. Saunders C. The founding philosophy. In: Saunders C, Summers DH, Teller N, editors. Hospice the living idea. Philadelphia: WB Saunders; 1981. p. 4.
18. National Hospice and Palliative Care Organization. Facts and figures: hospice care in America. World Wide Web URL: http://www.nhpco.org/i4a/pages/Index.cfm? page id =3274, 2007.
19. Casarett DJ, Quill TE. "I'm not ready for hospice": strategies for timely and effective hospice discussions. Ann Intern Med. 2007;146:443.
20. Lynn J. Serving patients who may die soon and their families: the role of hospice and other services. JAMA. 2001;85:925.
21. Piper BF, Cella D. Cancer-related fatigue: definitions and clinical subtypes. J Natl Compr Cancer Netw. 2010;8:958.
22. Kutner JS, Kassner CT, Nowels DE. Symptom burden at the end of life: hospice providers' perceptions. J Pain Symptom Manage. 2001;21:473.
23. Stone P, Richards M, A'Hern R, Hardy J. A study to investigate the prevalence, severity and correlates of fatigue among patients with cancer in comparison with a control group of volunteers without cancer. Ann Oncol. 2000;11:561.
24. Hwang SS, Chang VT, Rue M, Kasimis B. Multidimensional independent predictors of cancer-related fatigue. J Pain Symptom Manage. 2003;26:604.
25. Peuckmann V, Elsner F, Krumm N, Trottenberg P, Radbruch L. Pharmacological treatments for fatigue associated with palliative care. Cochrane Database Syst Rev. 2010 Nov 10;(11):CD006788.
26. Hugel H, Ellershaw JE, Cook L, Skinner J, Irvine C. The prevalence, key causes and management of

insomnia in palliative care patients. J Pain Symptom Manage. 2004;27:316.

27. Bruera E, Fainsinger RL, Schoeller T, Ripamonti C. Rapid discontinuation of hypnotics in terminal cancer patients: a prospective study. Ann Oncol. 1996;7:855.

28. Holbrook AM, Crowther R, Lotter A, Cheng C, King D. Meta-analysis of benzodiazepine use in the treatment of insomnia. CMAJ. 2000;162:225.

29. Nowell PD, Mazumdar S, Buysse DJ, Dew MA, Reynolds 3rd CF, Kupfer DJ. Benzodiazepines and zolpidem for chronic insomnia: a meta-analysis of treatment efficacy. JAMA. 1997;278:2170.

30. Davis MP, Hallerberg G, Palliative Medicine Study Group of the Multinational Association of Supportive Care in Cancer. A systematic review of the treatment of nausea and/or vomiting in cancer unrelated to chemotherapy or radiation. J Pain Symptom Manage. 2010;39:756.

31. Bruera E, Seifert L, Watanabe S, Babul N, Darke A, Harsanyi Z, et al. Chronic nausea in advanced cancer patients: a retrospective assessment of a metoclopramide-based antiemetic regimen. J Pain Symptom Manage. 1996;11:147.

32. Huang ZB, Ahronheim JC. Nutrition and hydration in terminally ill patients: an update. Clin Geriatr Med. 2000;16:313.

33. Good P, Cavenagh J, Mather M, Ravenscroft P. Medically assisted hydration for palliative care patients. Cochrane Database Syst Rev. 2008 Apr 16;(2):CD006273.

34. Bruera E, Hui D, Dalal S, Torres-Vigil I, Trumble J, Roosth J, et al. Parenteral hydration in patients with advanced cancer: a multicenter, double-blind, placebo-controlled randomized trial. J Clin Oncol. 2013;31:111.

35. Wee B, Hillier R. Interventions for noisy breathing in patients near to death. Cochrane Database Syst Rev. 2008 Jan 23;(1):CD005177.

36. Ripamonti C, Fulfaro F, Bruera E. Dyspnoea in patients with advanced cancer: incidence, causes and treatments. Cancer Treat Rev. 1998;24:69.

37. Gysels M, Bausewein C, Higginson IJ. Experiences of breathlessness: a systematic review of the qualitative literature. Palliat Support Care. 2007;5:281.

38. Trajkovic-Vidakovic M, de Graeff A, Voest EE, Teunissen SC. Symptoms tell it all: a systematic review of the value of symptom assessment to predict survival in advanced cancer patients. Crit Rev Oncol Hematol. 2012;84:130.

39. Maltoni M, Pirovano M, Scarpi E, Marinari M, Indelli M, Arnoldi E, et al. Prediction of survival of patients terminally ill with cancer. Results of an Italian prospective multicentric study. Cancer. 1995;75:2613.

40. Davidson PM, Johnson MJ. Update on the role of palliative oxygen. Curr Opin Support Palliat Care. 2011;5:87.

41. Cranston JM, Crockett A, Currow D. Oxygen therapy for dyspnoea in adults. Cochrane Database Syst Rev. 2008 Jul 16;(3):CD004769.

42. Abernethy AP, McDonald CF, Frith PA, Clark K, Herndon 2nd JE, Marcello J, et al. Effect of palliative oxygen versus room air in relief of breathlessness in patients with refractory dyspnoea: a double-blind, randomised controlled trial. Lancet. 2010;376:784.

43. Nava S, Ferrer M, Esquinas A, Scala R, Groff P, Cosentini R, et al. Palliative use of non-invasive ventilation in end-of-life patients with solid tumours: a randomised feasibility trial. Lancet Oncol. 2013;14:219.

44. Abernethy AP, Currow DC, Frith P, Fazekas BS, McHugh A, Bui C. Randomised, double blind, placebo controlled crossover trial of sustained release morphine for the management of refractory dyspnoea. BMJ. 2003;327:523.

45. Viola R, Kiteley C, Lloyd NS, Mackay JA, Wilson J, Wong RK. The management of dyspnea in cancer patients: a systematic review. Support Care Cancer. 2008;16:329.

46. Currow DC, McDonald C, Oaten S, Kenny B, Allcroft P, Frith P, et al. Once-daily opioids for chronic dyspnea: a dose increment and pharmacovigilance study. J Pain Symptom Manage. 2011;42:388.

47. Simon ST, Higginson IJ, Booth S, Harding R, Bausewein C. Benzodiazepines for the relief of breathlessness in advanced malignant and nonmalignant diseases in adults. Cochrane Database Syst Rev. 2010 Jan 20;(1):CD007354.

48. Massie MJ. Prevalence of depression in patients with cancer. J Natl Cancer Inst Monogr. 2004;32:57.

49. Fernandez F, Adams F, Holmes VF, Levy JK, Neidhart M. Methylphenidate for depressive disorders in cancer patients. An alternative to standard antidepressants. Psychosomatics. 1987;28:455.

50. Pereira J, Hanson J, Bruera E. The frequency and clinical course of cognitive impairment in patients with terminal cancer. Cancer. 1997;79:835.

51. Massie MJ, Holland J, Glass E. Delirium in terminally ill cancer patients. Am J Psychiatry. 1983;140:1048.

52. Breitbart W, Marotta R, Platt MM, Weisman H, Derevenco M, Grau C, et al. A double-blind trial of haloperidol, chlorpromazine, and lorazepam in the treatment of delirium in hospitalized AIDS patients. Am J Psychiatry. 1996;153:231.

53. Yamagishi A, Morita T, Miyashita M, Sato K, Tsuneto S, Shima Y. The care strategy for families of terminally ill cancer patients who become unable to take nourishment orally: recommendations from a nationwide survey of bereaved family members' experiences. J Pain Symptom Manage. 2010;40:671.

54. Borum ML, Lynn J, Zhong Z, Roth K, Connors Jr AF, Desbiens NA, et al. The effect of nutritional supplementation on survival in seriously ill hospitalized adults: an evaluation of the SUPPORT data. Study to Understand Prognoses and Preferences for Outcomes and Risks of Treatments. J Am Geriatr Soc. 2000;48:S33.

55. Dunlop RJ, Campbell CW. Cytokines and advanced cancer. J Pain Symptom Manage. 2000;20:214.

56. Maltoni M, Scarpi E, Rosati M, Derni S, Fabbri L, Martini F, et al. Palliative sedation in end-of-life care and survival: a systematic review. J Clin Oncol. 2012;30:1378.

57. Osterweis M. Bereavement: reactions, consequences, and care. Washington, DC: National Academy Press; 1984.

58. Maciejewski PK, Zhang B, Block SD, Prigerson HG. An empirical examination of the stage theory of grief. JAMA. 2007;297:716.

59. Bradley EH, Prigerson H, Carlson MD, Cherlin E, Johnson-Hurzeler R, Kasl SV. Depression among surviving caregivers: does length of hospice enrollment matter? Am J Psychiatry. 2004;161:2257.

Part VI

New Breast Cancer Therapeutic Approaches

Angiogenesis Inhibition in Breast Cancer

Kerem Okutur and Gokhan Demir

Abstract

Angiogenesis plays an essential role in tumor development, invasion, and metastasis. In preclinical models, agents that block the vascular endothelial growth factor (VEGF) pathway have been shown to effectively inhibit tumor angiogenesis and growth. Although antiangiogenic therapies, including anti-VEGF antibodies and tyrosine kinase inhibitors, have become important components of the standard of care for the treatment of many solid tumors, the results of clinical trials investigating the efficacy of antiangiogenic agents in breast cancer are contradictory. In this chapter, the importance of angiogenesis inhibition in breast cancer is discussed in light of recent clinical data.

Keywords

Angiogenesis • Tumor angiogenesis • VEGF • Breast cancer • Angiogenesis inhibition • Antiangiogenic agents • Bevacizumab • Tyrosine kinase inhibitors

Introduction

Breast cancer is the most frequently occurring malignant tumor among women. Although there have been many impressive advances in systemic therapies that have translated to significant improvements in survival, postoperative recurrence and distant metastasis remain unsolved problems. Although adjuvant therapies maintain significant decreases in local recurrence and distant metastasis in early-stage breast cancer, nearly one-third of these patients eventually develop metastatic disease. In advanced breast cancer, however, the aim of treatment is palliation, and the mean survival ranges from 24 to 48 months [1].

Angiogenesis is a process with important roles in all stages of cancer, including growth, invasion, progression, and metastasis. Tumors require new

K. Okutur, MD (✉) • G. Demir, MD
Medical Oncology Department, Medical Oncology,
Acibadem University School of Medicine,
Buyukdere Cad. No: 40, Sariyer, Istanbul 34453, Turkey
e-mail: keremokutur@gmail.com; ogdemir@gmail.com

© Springer International Publishing Switzerland 2016
A. Aydiner et al. (eds.), *Breast Disease: Management and Therapies*,
DOI 10.1007/978-3-319-26012-9_35

blood vessel formation to supply oxygen and nutrients. However, tumor-associated angiogenesis shows structural and functional differences from physiological angiogenesis. In tumor-associated new vessel formation, structural anomalies and vascular anarchy are distinctive, and these differences allow increased oxygen and nutrient diffusion and resistance to chemotherapeutic agents and radiation treatment compared with normal tissues [2].

With the shift in cancer treatment from chemotherapeutic agents to targeted treatments in the late 1990s, antiangiogenic strategies were discovered. Since then, preclinical and clinical studies using monoclonal antibodies and small-molecule agents with a role in the angiogenic process have accelerated.

Breast Cancer and Angiogenesis

Tumor angiogenesis is a complex process that involves the interaction of stimulatory and inhibitory factors in multiple steps. The appearance of new vessels during the period of tumor growth (angiogenic switch) occurs when the level of stimulatory factors surpasses the level of inhibitory factors [3]. The vascular endothelial growth factor (VEGF) pathway is the most important pathway; VEGF, as the main element of this pathway, is the most important stimulatory factor in the proliferation of the vascular endothelial cells [4].

There are six molecules in the VEGF family: VEGF-A, VEGF-B, VEGF-C, VEGF-D, VEGF-E, placental growth factor (PGF)-1, and PGF-2 [5]. VEGF receptors (VEGFR) comprise three cell-membrane receptors (VEGFR-1/Flt-1, VEGFR-2/Flt-1 (KDR), and VEGFR-3/Flt-4) and a soluble form of VEGFR-1 (sVEGFR-1). These receptors are mainly expressed by endothelial cells and are activated by VEGF [6]. The VEGF gene is situated on the short arm of the sixth chromosome (6p21.3). There are many factors that stimulate VEGF gene expression, including hypoxia; certain growth factors, such as platelet-derived growth factor (PDGF), fibroblast growth factor (FGF), and epidermal growth factor (EGF); tumor necrosis factor (TNF); transforming growth factor β (TGF-β);

interleukin 1 (IL-1); nitric oxide; tumor suppressor genes, such as p53; oncogenes, such as K-ras, H-Ras, and v-scr; HER-2; and HER-1/EGFR [7]. Among these, the most effective stimulant for angiogenesis is hypoxia.

VEGF receptors contain seven immunoglobulin (Ig)-like domains in the extracellular region, a transmembrane region, and a tyrosine kinase domain. While VEGFR-1 is mainly activated by VEGF-A, VEGF-B, and PIGF, the main stimulant of VEGFR-2 is VEGF-A. The binding of VEGF-C and VEGF-D to VEGFR-3 stimulates lymphangiogenesis [5]. The binding of VEGF to the extracellular domain of the receptor leads to conformational changes in the structure of the receptor and to dimerization. Dimerization of the receptor initiates cytoplasmic catalytic activation, resulting in autophosphorylation of the tyrosine kinase. This autophosphorylation activates the phosphatidylinositol 3-kinase (PI3-K)-Akt pathway and the Ras-Raf-MEK-mitogen-activated protein kinase (MAPK)-dependent pathway [8]. The activation of these pathways triggers many processes that lead to new vessel formation, such as endothelial cell survival, mitogenesis, migration, differentiation, vascular permeability, and endothelial progenitor cell mobilization from the bone marrow into the peripheral circulation.

The first systematic study to draw attention to the importance of angiogenesis in breast cancer came from Folkman and colleagues. From the results of this study, it was determined that angiogenesis is one of the basic requirements for tumor progression (angiogenic switch) [9]. The transfection of breast cancer cells with angiogenic stimulatory peptides increases tumor growth, invasiveness, and metastasis [10]. Furthermore, it has been shown that the inhibition of VEGF in breast cancer cell lines reduces the microvessel density and decreases the infiltration of tumor-related macrophages but, conversely, increases the infiltration of tumor-related neutrophils [11].

Clinical studies show that angiogenesis begins to develop in the early stages of breast cancer and is particularly responsible for progression into an invasive form. In the studies conducted on patients with preinvasive breast lesions (ductal or lobular hyperplasia and carcinoma in situ), angiogenesis and VEGF levels are significantly increased compared with those of normal breast tissue in the preinvasive stage [12]. Similarly, in patients with invasive tumors, angiogenesis and VEGF expression are significantly increased compared with patients with preinvasive lesions [13]. Furthermore, some VEGF polymorphisms significantly increase the risk of developing breast cancer [14]. Increased microvascular density and aggressive biological behavior are linked with breast cancer progression in patients with benign and premalignant lesions [15, 16]; additionally, in cases with higher microvascular density, the risks of distant metastasis and recurrence are higher [17].

A better understanding of the relationship between angiogenesis and tumor development and progression has accelerated the development of treatment strategies targeting these processes. In 1993, VEGF inhibition was shown for the first time to cause an in vivo antitumor effect; this was the start of the studies focused on angiogenesis inhibitors [18]. The angiogenic treatments developed since 1993 can be divided into two groups. The first group comprises antibody treatments targeting VEGF or VEGFR. This group includes the monoclonal anti-VEGF antibody bevacizumab, the VEGF-trap agent aflibercept, and the anti-VEGF agent ramucirumab. The other group features small-molecule tyrosine kinase inhibitors (sunitinib, sorafenib, pazopanib, and others) that exert their effects by binding the tyrosine kinase domain of VEGFR and targeting the intracellular signal transduction system.

Bevacizumab

Bevacizumab is a humanized recombinant IgG1 monoclonal antibody that selectively binds to all isoforms of VEGF. Upon binding, it prevents the VEGF-VEGFR interaction, thereby neutralizing VEGF activity. As a result, the endothelial cells are driven toward apoptosis, and a significant regression in tumor-related abnormal vascularization occurs [19]. The inhibition of VEGF leads not only to a regression of the vascular structure of the tumor but also to a normalization of vasculogenesis by removing the structural and functional anomalies in existing vessels [20]. The normalization of angiogenesis, the removal of tumor-linked vascularization, and the amelioration of bloodstream anomalies all lead to better penetration by chemotherapeutic agents into the tumor tissue, which increases the response rates to and the antitumor efficiency of chemotherapy [21]. Furthermore, the proliferation of endothelial cells and the decrease in migration inhibit new vessel formation by the tumor. VEGFR-1 and VEGFR-2 are expressed on the surface of not only endothelial cells but also tumor cells; therefore, the direct antitumor effect of bevacizumab can be discussed. In the last few years, evidence of the effect of bevacizumab on the immune system has also been found. Bevacizumab increases the activity of B and T lymphocytes and the number of natural killer cells; in particular, as a result of T lymphocyte activation, the antigen presentation capacities of dendritic cells improve, and these changes contribute to the antitumor effects of the drug [22].

The pharmacokinetics of bevacizumab have been evaluated in different studies with doses of 1–20 kg (weekly, once in 2 weeks or 3 weeks). With a dose from 1 to 10 kg, the pharmacokinetic effects of bevacizumab appear to be linear. The half-life of the drug is approximately 20 days. The time to reach a stable plasma concentration is approximately 100 days [23]. The most frequent side effects of bevacizumab are hypertension, proteinuria, and hematuria, and the less frequent but potentially lethal side effects are arterial thrombosis and gastrointestinal perforation [24].

The first FDA approval for bevacizumab was obtained in February 2004 after a study showed that its addition to a first-line treatment regimen in metastatic colorectal cancer including 5-fluorouracil significantly improved overall survival (OS), progression-free survival (PFS), and response rate (RR) [25]. Later, its efficacy as a second-line therapy was also shown [26]. As a result of subsequent studies, it was also approved for the treatment of non-small cell lung cancer with non-squamous cell histology, renal cell carcinoma, ovarian cancer, high-grade glial tumors, and cervical cancer [27–31].

In phase I studies, no serious toxicity of bevacizumab was observed when used as a monotherapy or in combination with other chemotherapeutic agents at a dose ranging from 1 to 10 mg/kg for several tumor types [32–34]. In a phase I–II study that included 75 patients with metastatic breast cancer who received anthracycline and taxane treatment before using bevacizumab at doses of 3 mg/kg, 10 mg/kg, or 20 mg/kg, the overall response rate was 9.3 %, and the median response time was 5.5 months [35]. Four patients left the study because they experienced side effects; hypertension (22 %) was the most frequently observed adverse effect. For subsequent studies, the ideal dosage for bevacizumab was reported to be 10 mg/kg.

Studies in HER2-Negative Advanced Breast Cancer

The results of the XCALIBr study, which was the first multicenter phase II nonrandomized study of the efficacy and safety of bevacizumab in metastatic breast cancer, were presented at the 2007 ASCO annual meeting [36]. In this study, 103 patients with HER2-negative metastatic breast cancer were treated with capecitabine at 100 mg/m^2 twice daily on days 1–14 every 21 days and bevacizumab 15 mg/kg on day 1 every 21 days. The endpoint of the study was set as PFS, and patients who progressed under the study regimen continued their treatment with second-line paclitaxel or vinorelbine combined with bevacizumab. The overall response rate was 38.5 % (stable disease (SD) rate 42.99 %), PFS was 5.7 months, and OS was 10 months. The median time to progression (TTP) was longer in the patients with estrogen receptor-positive than estrogen receptor-negative tumors (8.9 months vs. 4 months, $p < 0.0001$). The treatment was generally well tolerated; the most frequently observed grade III adverse effects that were reported are hand-foot syndrome (13 %) and pain (10 %). Grade IV pulmonary embolism stood out as the most serious side effect in 2 % of the patients. In a phase II study of 56 metastatic breast cancer patients published by Burstein et al., weekly treatment with vinorelbine and bevacizumab

(10 mg/kg every 14 days) was used; the general response rate was 34 %, and the median TTP was 5.5 months [37]. The median TTP was significantly longer in patients with low base-line VEGF levels; therefore, it was reported that the plasma VEGF level could be used as a prognostic parameter for patients receiving anti-VEGF treatment. In another phase II study, 45 metastatic breast cancer patients (NCCTG N0432) were treated with a combination of docetaxel (75 mg/m^2 on day 1 every 21 days), capecitabine (825 mg/m^2 twice daily on days 1–14 every 21 days), and bevacizumab (15 mg/kg on day 1 every 21 days) [38]. The general response rate was 49 %, the median response time was 11.8 months, and the median PFS and OS were 11.1 months and 28.4 months, respectively. Grade II/IV side effects were frequently related to chemotherapy; bevacizumab-related side effects included grade III gastrointestinal bleeding in one patient (2 %), grade III hypertension in two patients (4 %), and grade IV thrombosis in one patient (2 %).

The ATHENA trial, a phase II trial that includes 2,251 patients and involves a median 12.7 month follow-up, is researching the efficacy of bevacizumab addition to the first-line treatment of recurrent or metastatic HER2-negative breast cancer with taxane-based regimens or other non-anthracycline chemotherapeutic agents (capecitabine and vinorelbine) [39]. The median age of the patients in this study is 53, 95 % of the patients who are involved have an ECOG 0–1 performance status, and 65 % of the patients are estrogen receptor positive. Regarding the treatment regimens, 35 % of the patients received paclitaxel, 33 % received docetaxel, and 10 % were given a combination regimen including taxane. The median TTP was 9.5 months, and the ORR was 52 %. TTP in combination with bevacizumab and taxane regimens appeared to be longer (10.9–6.8 months) compared to bevacizumab in regimens lacking taxane. In the triple-negative group, the median TTP was 7.2 months, leading us to believe that the effect of bevacizumab in HER2-related disease is independent of the hormone receptor status. The toxicity observed in the study was consistent with the data from the phase III studies of bevacizumab combined with taxane-based chemotherapy in terms of the side-effect profile. The median OS of the study population after a median of 20 months of follow-up was 25.2 months. The median OS was 18.3 months in the triple-negative group and 20.5 months in the group over 70 years of age. The survival results of triple-negative patients were similar to those of other phase III studies, demonstrating the efficacy of bevacizumab in this subgroup. In the subgroup analysis, the TTP and OS of the patients who continued to use bevacizumab after regression were significantly longer than those of the patients who stopped using bevacizumab before or when chemotherapy was halted (for TTP, median 11.6 months vs. 6.7 months; for OS, median 30 months vs. 18.4 months) [40]. In addition to the longer TTP and OS, prolonged treatment with bevacizumab was also associated with no increase in toxicity. These results raise the question whether bevacizumab can improve the results of metastatic breast cancer in a similar manner as in advanced ovarian cancer. In a few studies that aimed to answer this question, maintenance bevacizumab treatment was tolerated and was linked to a longer period of stabilized disease [41–43]. In the randomized phase III IMELDA trial, 185 patients without disease progression after three to six cycles of first-line docetaxel (75 mg/m^2 every 3 weeks) plus bevacizumab (15 mg/kg) were randomized to receive either capecitabine (1,000 mg/m^2, twice per day on days 1–14 every 21 days) plus bevacizumab (15 mg/kg) or bevacizumab alone [44]. In the maintenance arm, the median PFS and OS were significantly longer in the capecitabine + bevacizumab group (11.9 months vs. 4.3 months, $p < 0.0001$; and 39 months vs. 23.7 months, $p = 0.0003$, respectively). The IMELDA trial confirmed the efficacy of the capecitabine-bevacizumab combination as a maintenance therapy in HER2-negative advanced breast cancer as in metastatic colorectal cancer.

In the first randomized phase III study of breast cancer that included bevacizumab, 462 metastatic breast cancer patients who had been previously treated with anthracycline and taxane were treated with capecitabine alone (2,500 mg/m^2 on days 1–14 every 21 days) or with a combination of capecitabine + bevacizumab (15 mg/kg on day 1 every 21 days) (AVF2119 trial) [45].

HER2-positive patients comprised 20–25 % of the study group, and approximately 75–80 % of the patients has visceral metastases. According to the results of the study, although adding bevacizumab to capecitabine resulted in a twofold increase in the response rate (19.8 % vs. 9.1 %, $p = 0.001$), no change occurred in PFS and OS. Because the increasing response rate did not reflect the primary endpoint of the study, the short response times of the cases that were responsive to bevacizumab and the effect of bevacizumab being masked by previous treatments were emphasized. The authors also suggested that angiogenic pathways become more complex during disease progression; therefore, using antiangiogenic treatments at the earlier stages of metastatic disease (in other words, as the first-line treatment) is likely the best approach.

Directed by this new information, a new phase III study has begun (E200 trial) [46]. In this study, using weekly paclitaxel monotherapy as the first-line treatment of metastatic breast cancer was compared with the same regimen including bevacizumab. HER2-negative cases comprised 90 % of the patients. The primary endpoint of the study was PFS, which was significantly longer in the bevacizumab arm (median 11.8 months vs. 5.8 months, $p < 0.001$). Additionally, the objective response rate was higher in the bevacizumab arm (36.9 % vs. 21.2 %, $p < 0.001$). Conversely, no OS difference was found between the two groups. OS is generally accepted as a reliable cancer endpoint; however, PFS is not accepted by many researchers as an important endpoint in metastatic disease. Nevertheless, the relative benefits of both OS and PFS as primary endpoints are being discussed, especially in cancers, such as breast cancer, that have long post-progression survival times. However, the FDA passed an accelerated approval for bevacizumab in 2008 for the first-line treatment of metastatic HER2-negative breast cancer based on the significant benefit on PFS shown in this study and noting that analyzing the improvement of OS requires a longer period of time for follow-up and larger studies including many more patients.

In the double-blinded, placebo-controlled phase III AVADO (Avastin and docetaxel) study, 736 patients with recurrent, metastatic HER-negative breast cancer who did not receive any treatment were randomized into three groups [47]. The first group received docetaxel and placebo, the second group received docetaxel and bevacizumab (7.5 mg/kg), and the third group received docetaxel and bevacizumab (15 mg/kg). All patients whose disease progressed continued to the second-line treatment, which included bevacizumab. The ORR was 46 % in the placebo group, 55 % in the low-dose bevacizumab (7.5 mg/kg) group, and 64 % in the high-dose bevacizumab (15 mg/kg) group. A significant improvement was observed in PFS in the groups receiving 7.5 mg/kg and 15 mg/kg doses compared with the placebo group (9 months, 10 months, and 8.1 months, respectively). However, this improvement does not reflect the OS because no OS differences were found between treatment groups. The researchers tried to explain this lack of effect on OS as being due to insufficient power of the study for a survival analysis and to one-third of the patients in the placebo group being crossed over to the second-line treatment that included bevacizumab. However, the FDA has withdrawn the previous accelerated approval that it had granted because of the much lower PFS benefit compared with the E2100 study and because no improvement in OS was achieved. In a recently published meta-analysis, the biggest improvement in PFS with bevacizumab was observed in patients who received weekly chemotherapeutic regimens [48]; this may explain why the improvement in PFS observed in the E2100 study is bigger than that in the AVADO trial and in the other trial discussed below, RIBBON-1. According to the newly announced biomarker results of the AVADO study, plasma VEGF-A and VEGFR-2 are potential markers for the efficacy of bevacizumab [49]. The prospective MERiDiaN study has been initiated to conduct detailed biomarker evaluation in HER2-negative disease [50].

The RIBBON-1 trial is a randomized, double-blind, placebo-controlled phase III trial researching the efficacy and safety of bevacizumab in combination with other chemotherapy regimens for the first-line treatment of metastatic breast cancer [51]. A total of 1,237 patients with HER2-negative recurrent or metastatic disease were randomized into two groups. The first group comprised patients who received placebo or bevacizumab added to capecitabine monotherapy, and the other group consisted of patients who received placebo or bevacizumab added to taxane (paclitaxel or docetaxel)-based or anthracycline-based chemotherapy. The dose of bevacizumab was 15 mg/kg, and the endpoint of the study was PFS. A total of 75 % of the patients were hormone receptor positive. In the case of disease progression, patients were provided second-line treatment that included bevacizumab. Similarly to the AVADO study, a significant improvement in PFS was observed in both groups; however, no change in OS was found. Additionally, in this study, nearly half of the patients crossed over to second-line treatment with bevacizumab in the placebo group, which makes OS analysis more difficult.

RIBBON-2 is another randomized, double-blind phase III study that was designed to compare single-agent chemotherapy (taxane, gemcitabine, capecitabine, or vinorelbine) with either bevacizumab (15 mg/kg for three weeks, 10 mg/kg for 2 weeks) or placebo added to the chemotherapeutic regimen [52]. In this study including 684 patients, the ratio of hormone receptor-positive patients was 72 %, the ratio of HER2-negative patients was 85 %, and the ratio of triple-negative patients was approximately 23 %. The addition of bevacizumab to the treatment regimen increased PFS from 5.1 to 7.2 months ($p=0.0072$). The improvement in PFS was most significant in the hormone receptor-negative and triple-negative groups. When investigated with regard to the chemotherapeutic agents, PFS was increased by the addition of bevacizumab in the patients receiving taxane, gemcitabine, and capecitabine, but no improvement was observed in the vinorelbine group. ORR and OS were improved in the bevacizumab arm compared with the placebo arm, but this improvement was not statistically significant. Researchers suggested that in the AVF2119 study, there was no PFS benefit from the addition of bevacizumab to capecitabine because the patient population comprised a majority of heavily pretreated patients with poor prognostic factors. In the open-label phase III TANIA trial, 494 patients with HER2-negative advanced breast cancer who had progressed during/after ≥12 weeks of first-line bevacizumab-containing chemotherapy were randomized to receive second-line single-agent chemotherapy with or without bevacizumab [53]. The primary endpoint of the trial was PFS, and no crossover was allowed. PFS was significantly longer in the bevacizumab arm (6.3 months vs. 4.2 months, $p = 0.0068$).

The TURANDOT (capeciTabine and bevacizUmab Randomized Against avatiN anD taxOl Trial) study is designed to compare the combination regimens of capecitabine + bevacizumab and paclitaxel + bevacizumab as the first-line treatment for metastatic breast cancer in terms of efficacy and safety [54]. The interim results of the TURANDOT study, which is a non-inferiority study, have recently been announced. A total of 564 patients were randomized into two groups receiving paclitaxel (90 mg/m^2 on days 1, 8, and 15 every 4 weeks) plus bevacizumab (10 mg/m^2 on days 1 and 15 every 28 days) or capecitabine 1,000 mg/m^2 twice daily on days 1–14 every 21 days plus bevacizumab 15 mg/m^2 on day 1 every 28 days. The HR for OS was 1.04, and the non-inferiority criteria were not achieved. The objective RR was higher with the paclitaxel-bevacizumab combination compared with the capecitabine-bevacizumab combination (44 % vs. 27 %, $p < 0.0001$). Similarly, PFS in the paclitaxel group was longer compared with the capecitabine group (median 11 months vs. 8.1 months, $p > 0.0052$). The proportion of the patients whose treatment was stopped due to side effects was twofold higher in the capecitabine group than in the paclitaxel group, showing that capecitabine is more tolerable and safer. In the subgroup analysis of the TURANDOT study presented at ASCO 2013, the 1-year OS in the triple-negative patient group was 78 % (with paclitaxel + bevacizumab), which is a very high ratio for triple-negative patients [55]. The high frequency of side effects with paclitaxel + bevacizumab has resulted in the proposal of strategies to reduce toxicity. The first of two studies designed for this purpose and for which results were announced at ASCO 2014 was the phase III SAKK 24/09 study, which was designed in the framework of the following question: "could sufficient antitumor efficacy be ensured with low toxicity by adding metronomic chemotherapy to bevacizumab?" [56]. In this study, a regimen of first-line paclitaxel (90 mg/m^2 on days 1, 8, and 15 every 4 weeks) added to first-line bevacizumab (10 mg/kg, every 2 weeks) (Arm A) was compared with metronomic oral chemotherapy (capecitabine 1,500 mg/day + cyclophosphamide 50 mg/day, continuous) (Arm B) in 147 patients with metastatic HER2-negative breast cancer. No difference was detected between the two arms in terms of ORR and PFS. Additionally, no difference was detected between the two groups in the frequency of grade 3–5 side effects (febrile neutropenia, infection, neuropathy, mucositis, and hand-foot syndrome), which was the primary endpoint of the study. In another phase III study (the AROBASE study), maintenance with exemestane + bevacizumab or treatment and maintenance with paclitaxel + bevacizumab were compared in 113 patients with ER-positive, HER2-negative, locally advanced/metastatic breast cancer previously controlled by first-line paclitaxel + bevacizumab combination therapy [57]. Although the rate of side effects was low with the hormonal therapy + bevacizumab combination, patient recruitment for the study was discontinued due to the failure to achieve a PFS advantage, which was the primary endpoint. The announcement of long-term monitoring results of the study is awaited.

Studies in HER2-Positive Advanced Breast Cancer

In most of the studies that evaluate the efficacy of bevacizumab in metastatic breast cancer, HER2-positive patients are not included; therefore, information on the role of bevacizumab in HER2-positive disease is limited. However, in preclinical studies, an active interaction between angiogenesis and the HER2 signal has been shown [58–60]. In experimental models, HER2 overexpression increases hypoxia-inducible factor (HIF)-α and VEGF mRNA expression [60]. Heregulin and neuregulin, which are HER ligands, increase the synthesis of VEGF in breast cancer cells and thereby increase the migratory and invasive potential [61, 62]. In a cohort study that included 611 breast cancer patients, a significant correlation was established between HER2 and VEGF expression [63]. HER2, by inducing the release of VEGF, upregulates the COX-2 gene, which plays an important role in angiogenesis [64]. Furthermore, in xenograft models of breast cancer, the antitumor effect is significantly increased by the combined blockage of VEGF and HER2 [65].

In a phase II study including 50 patients with HER2-positive metastatic breast cancer that was conducted in light of these preclinical data, trastuzumab and bevacizumab combination therapy was used, and a high OR of 48 % was obtained [66]. Additionally, both agents had safe side-effect profiles. In another phase II study that included 88 patients, bevacizumab 15 mg/kg was added to the combination of capecitabine plus trastuzumab [67]. The response rate in the study was 73 % (77 % complete response (CR) and 66 % partial response (PR)) with a median TTP of 14.4 months and median PFS of 14.4 months. Upon assessing the toxicity profile, ≥ grade 3 side effects were observed in 44 % of the patients, and most of these were related to capecitabine. Treatment was stopped in 13 patients because of side effects, but these patients went on to receive trastuzumab and bevacizumab treatments. In two patients, heart failure was observed. In other phase I–II studies, the concomitant use of bevacizumab with docetaxel + trastuzumab, lapatinib, and lapatinib + trastuzumab was reported to be safe and effective [68–71].

The AVEREL [Avastin (bevacizumab) in combination with hERceptin (trastuzumab)/docetaxEL in patients with HER2-positive metastatic breast cancer] study is the first randomized, open-label phase III study of the efficacy of anti-HER2 + anti-VEGF combination chemotherapy in HER2-positive breast cancer as a first-line treatment [72]. A total of 424 patients were included in the study and were randomized into two arms—the BTH arm (bevacizumab 15 mg/kg, docetaxel 100 mg/m², and trastuzumab 8 mg/kg loading dose followed by 6 mg/kg thereafter) and the TH arm (docetaxel 100 mg/m², trastuzumab 8 mg/kg loading dose followed by 6 mg/kg thereafter). After 26 months of follow-up, the primary endpoint of the study, PFS improvement, was not met (HR 0.82; $p=0.0775$; median PFS 13.7 months for TH vs. 16.5 months

for BTH). The HR for the independent review committee-assessed PFS was 0.72 ($p=0.0162$), with a similar 3-month increase in the median PFS. The ORR was 74 % in the BTH arm and 70 % in the TH arm. No significant difference for the median OS was found between the two groups. The frequencies of grade ≥3 neutropenia and hypertension were higher in the BTH group. According to the biomarker analysis of the study, similarly to the AVADO study, the improvement in PFS was higher in patients with higher plasma VEGF levels.

The ECOG 1105 study is a randomized phase III study designed to test the efficacy of adding bevacizumab (10 mg/kg every 2 weeks) to weekly paclitaxel-trastuzumab combination therapy (days 1, 8, and 15 (±carboplatin) [73]. Patients responding after treatment with six cycles in the bevacizumab arm continued with bevacizumab plus trastuzumab until disease progression or unacceptable toxicity occurred. The study unfortunately ended early because of poor patient accrual. When the 88 patients in the study were analyzed, no differences between the two groups for ORR, PFS, or OS were found. Bevacizumab added to paclitaxel-trastuzumab combination therapy did not increase the toxicity, and the treatment was generally well tolerated.

Taking the results of the AVAREL and ECOG 1105 studies into account, it seems inappropriate at present to use bevacizumab in place of the standard treatment protocols for HER2-positive metastatic disease. Biomarker studies appear to be necessary to define the subgroups that will benefit from bevacizumab in this patient group.

Data regarding the phase III studies of bevacizumab in HER2-negative and HER2-positive advanced breast cancer are summarized in Table 35.1.

Studies in Early-Stage Breast Cancer

After it was shown that angiogenesis develops in the early stages of breast cancer and that within the cases of early-stage breast cancer, the ones with highly angiogenic features have a higher ratio of local recurrence and metastasis, the idea of antiangiogenic agents being effective as adjuvant therapy was promoted, and studies were designed to assess this idea [12, 17]. The ECOG 2014 study was one of the first of these studies and included 226 patients with node-positive, early-stage, HER2-negative breast cancer who had undergone surgery [74]. Patients were randomized into two groups. Group A ($n = 104$) received 4 cycles of dose-dense AC (doxorubicin 60 mg/m^2 and cyclophosphamide 600 mg/m^2, in every 2 weeks) with bevacizumab 10 mg/kg (every 2 weeks) followed by 4 cycles of paclitaxel (175 mg/m^2 every 2 weeks) with bevacizumab (10 mg/kg every 2 weeks) and then 18 cycles of bevacizumab1 0 mg/kg alone (in every 2 weeks). Group B ($n = 122$) received 4 cycles of dose-dense AC without bevacizumab followed by 4 cycles of paclitaxel (175 mg/m^2 every 2 weeks) with bevacizumab (at the same dosage as group A) and then 22 cycles of bevacizumab alone (10 mg/kg every 2 weeks). The primary endpoint of the study was clinically apparent cardiac dysfunction (CHF). When results were evaluated in both groups, three patients had developed CHF. No significant difference between the decrease in left ventricular ejection fraction was found between the two groups. However, in 30 % of the patients, treatment had to be paused due to side effects; these side effects mainly occurred during bevacizumab maintenance. However, grade ≥ 3 side effects related to bevacizumab were rarely observed. Following this phase II pilot ECOG study, a randomized, double-blind, phase III study was initiated. In the ECOG 5103 study, 4,950 node-positive or high-risk, node-negative, operated, early-stage, HER2-negative patients were randomized into three groups [75]. The first group (group A) received four cycles of AC (in every 2–3 weeks) with placebo followed by weekly paclitaxel (days 1, 7, and 15, every 21 days for four cycles) with placebo. Four cycles of AC combined with bevacizumab followed by weekly paclitaxel combined with bevacizumab were applied to the second group (group B). To the third group (group C), the treatment plan for the second group was given followed by bevacizumab maintenance (every 3 weeks for ten cycles). The primary endpoint of the study is disease-free survival (DFS). According to the initial results announced at ASCO 2014, chemotherapy-associated side effects and their frequencies were similar in all three groups. Of the grade 3–5 adverse effects associated with bevacizumab, the frequencies of hypertension, thrombosis, proteinuria, and hemorrhage were 8 %, 3 %, <1 %, and <1 %, respectively. However, a significant portion of patients in the study groups prematurely discontinued bevacizumab (24 % of patients in group B and 55 % of patients in group C); therefore, the period of bevacizumab use in most of the patients was shorter than expected. The cumulative frequencies of clinical cardiac failure detected in month 15 in the study groups were 1 %, 1.9 %, and 3 %, respectively. No differences were detected among the three groups for DFS or OS. The 5-year DFS rates were similar among the groups (77 %, 76 %, and 80 %, respectively).

Another phase III study studying the role of adjuvant bevacizumab in triple-negative breast cancer is BEATRICE [76]. A total of 2,991 patients were randomized to receive ≥ 4 cycles of anthracycline- or taxane-based adjuvant chemotherapy with or without adding a year-long treatment regimen of bevacizumab (5 mg/kg/week). At the end of a median 32 months of follow-up, no DFS improvement, which was the primary endpoint of the study, was obtained (HR 0.87, $p = 0.181$). No difference in fatal adverse effects was found between the bevacizumab and chemotherapy groups; however, the addition of bevacizumab to the adjuvant chemotherapy was correlated with an increased frequency of grade ≥ 3 hypertension (12 % in the bevacizumab arm, 1 % in the chemotherapy arm) and severe cardiac events (1 % in the bevacizumab arm, <0.5 % in the chemotherapy arm). No difference was detected between the two groups for OS (HR 0.86, $p = 0.23$); however, patients with high plasma VEGFR-2 levels may benefit from the addition of bevacizumab to their treatment. An updated analysis of the study showed no difference between the two groups regarding DFS and OS [77].

Adequate data regarding the status of bevacizumab for adjuvant therapy in HER2-positive early-stage breast cancer has not yet been reported.

Table 35.1 Efficacy outcomes from randomized phase III trials of bevacizumab in advanced breast cancer

Trial	Design	Patient population	Patients enrolled	HER2 positive (%)	Chemotherapy regimen	B dose (kg)	Primary endpoint	ORR (%)	Median PFS (months)	Median OS (months)
Miller [45] AVF2119g	Randomized, phase III	Metastatic breast cancer, tax/anthr pretreated	462	26.3	Cape q3w+B vs. Cape alone	15	PFS	19.8 vs. 9.1, p=0.001	4.86 vs. 4.17 (p=0.98)	15.1 vs. 14.5
Miller [46] E2100	Open-label, randomized, phase III	Metastatic breast cancer, first line	722	44.7	Pac weekly+B vs. Pac weekly alone	10	PFS	36.9 vs. 21.2, p<0.001	11.8 vs. 5.9, p<0.001	26.7 vs. 25.2, p=0.16
Miles [47] AVADO	Randomized, double-blind, placebo-controlled phase III	Metastatic or locally recurrent breast cancer, first line	736	0	Docet q3w+B vs. Docet q3w+P	7.5 or 15	PFS	55 vs. 46, p=0.07 64 vs. 46, p<0.001	9.0 vs. 8.2, p=0.12 10.1 vs. 8.2, p=0.006	30.8 vs. 31.9, p=0.72 30.2 vs. 31.9, p=0.85
Robert [51] RIBBON-1	Randomized, double-blind, placebo-controlled phase III	Metastatic or locally recurrent breast cancer, first line	1237	Cape arm: 4.2 Tax/anthr arm: 1.0	Cape q3w+B/ tax q3w or anthr q3w-based regimen+B vs. same regimens+P	15	PFS	Cape+B arm: 35.4 vs. 23.6, p=0.0097 Tax/anthr+ B arm: 51.3 vs. 37.9, p=0.0054	Cape arm: 8.6 vs. 5.7, p<0.001 Tax/anthr arm: 9.2 vs. 8.0, p<0.001	Cape arm: 29.0 vs. 21.2 Tax/anthr arm: 25.2 vs. 23.8
Brufsky [52] RIBBON-2	Randomized, double-blind, placebo-controlled phase III	Metastatic or locally recurrent breast cancer, second line	684	0	Chemo [Cape q3w or tax (docet q3w or pac weekly) or gem weekly or vin q3w-based regimen]+B vs. Same regimens+P	10 or 15	PFS	Chemo+B arm: 39.5 vs. 29.6, p=0.0193	Chemo+B arm: 7.2 vs. 5.1, p=0.0072	Chemo+B arm: 18 vs. 16.4, p=0.0072
Lang [54] TURANDOT [a,b]	Open-label, randomized, phase III, non-inferiority	Metastatic or locally recurrent breast cancer, first line	564	0	Cape q3w+B vs. Pac weekly+B	Cape arm: 15 Pac arm: 10	OS	Cape +B arm: 27 vs. Pac+B arm: 44, p<0.0001	Cape +B arm: 8.1 vs. Pac+B arm: 11, p=0.0052	NR

Arteaga[c] [73] E1105	Randomized, double-blind, placebo-controlled phase III	Metastatic HER2(+) breast cancer, first line	96	100	Pac weekly+T+B vs. Pac+T+P	10	PFS	52 vs. 52, $p>0.05$	12.2 vs. 11.1, $p=0.10$	NR
Gianni [72] AVAREL	Open-label, randomized, controlled phase III	Metastatic or locally recurrent HER2(+) breast cancer, first line	424	100	Docet+T+B q3w vs. docet+T	15	PFS	74 vs. 70, $p=0.3492$	16.5 vs. 13.7, $p=0.0775$	NR
Gligorov [44] IMELDA	Open-label, randomized, phase III, maintenance	Metastatic breast cancer, progression-free after 3–6 cycles of docetaxel+bevacizumab, second line	185	0	Cape q3w+B vs. B alone	15	PFS	86 vs. 77	11.9 vs. 4.3, $p<0.0001$	39.0 vs. 23.7, $p=0.0003$
von Minckwitz [53] TANIA	Open-label, randomized, phase III, beyond-progression	Metastatic or locally recurrent breast cancer, progression during/after ≥12 weeks of bevacizumab+chemotherapy, second line	494	0	Single-agent chemo+B vs. Single-agent chemo alone	10 or 15	PFS	20.9 vs. 16.8, $p=0·3457$	6.3 vs. 4.2, $p=0·0068$	NR

B bevacizumab, *ORR* objective response rate, *PFS* progression-free survival, *OS* overall survival, *tax* taxane, *anthr* anthracycline, *cape* capecitabine, *pac* paclitaxel, *docet* docetaxel, *gem* gemcitabine, *vin* vinorelbine, *T* trastuzumab, *P* placebo, *NR* not reported

[a]Interim analysis

[b]Because the OS data was immature, with events reported in only one-third of the patients, the median OS was not yet determined. The 1-year overall survival was 81 % in the paclitaxel group and 79 % in the capecitabine group; the 2-year overall survival was 60 % in the paclitaxel group and 55 % in the capecitabine group

[c]The study was terminated early due to poor patient accrual

The results of the BETH study, a phase III study in which bevacizumab was added to systemic chemotherapy + trastuzumab combination therapy, which is the standard therapy in this patient group, were recently announced [78]. A total of 3,509 patients were included in the study and were assigned to two treatment groups: six cycles of docetaxel/carboplatin plus trastuzumab (TCH) with or without trastuzumab or three cycles of docetaxel plus trastuzumab with or without bevacizumab followed by three cycles of FEC. In both regimens, patients used trastuzumab (with or without bevacizumab) for a total of 1 year. When all patients were considered or when the TCH and chemotherapy with anthracycline groups were individually analyzed, it was observed that the addition of bevacizumab to the treatment did not cause a significant change in DFS. However, it was also observed that the rates of grade 3–4 adverse effects were higher in the patient group receiving bevacizumab (hypertension 19 % vs. 4 %, $p<0.001$; congestive heart failure 2.1 % vs. 1 %, $p=0.0621$; hemorrhage 2 % vs. <1 %, $p<0.0001$; proteinuria 1 % vs. <1 %, $p<0.0001$; and gastrointestinal perforation 11 cases vs. 1 case, $p=0.0031$).

Neoadjuvant Studies

Many studies have researched the efficacy of adding bevacizumab to systemic chemotherapy in HER2-negative locally advanced breast cancer. In these studies, pathological complete response (pCR) rates range from 9 % to 42 % [79–82]. The results of two large randomized trials based on the data of phase II studies have recently been announced. In the NSABP B40 study, patients were randomized into three groups: docetaxel alone, docetaxel plus capecitabine, and docetaxel plus gemcitabine [83]. After four cycles of chemotherapy, four cycles of AC were applied to all patients. Additionally, the patients in the study were divided into two groups: those who received bevacizumab in their first six cycles of chemotherapy followed by ten cycles of bevacizumab 15 mg/kg postoperatively and those who did not. When the results were evaluated, it was observed that adding bevacizumab to chemotherapy significantly increases the pCR in the breast (28.4 % vs. 34.5 %, $p=0.02$). When both

the breast and axillary nodes were examined in the bevacizumab-treated group, the pCR was higher but did not reach statistical significance (23 % vs. 27.6 % $p=0.08$). When the effect of bevacizumab added to chemotherapy was analyzed according to the hormone receptor status, the pCR rates of the breast and breast + axillary lymph nodes were significantly higher in the hormone receptor-positive group compared with the hormone receptor-negative group. The addition of bevacizumab to chemotherapy increased the frequency of hypertension, left ventricular dysfunction, hand-foot syndrome, and mucositis. Moreover, an apparent increase was also observed in the frequency of postoperative complications (especially in patients with reconstruction administration) [84, 85]. In the survival analysis of the most recently published study, DFS and OS were significantly improved in the bevacizumab group, especially in hormone receptor-positive patients [86].

Another phase III study related to neoadjuvant bevacizumab is the GeparQuinto study designed by von Mincwits et al. [87]. Patients were randomized into two groups, one in which bevacizumab 15 mg/kg was added to four cycles of epirubicin plus cyclophosphamide followed by four cycles of docetaxel and one in which bevacizumab was not added. In the bevacizumab arm, the pCR rate was significantly higher (14.9 % vs. 18.4 %, $p=0.04$). In contrast to the NSABP B40 study, the effect of bevacizumab on pCR was most significant in the triple-negative group (27.9 % vs. 39.3 %, $p=0.003$), whereas bevacizumab was not effective in the hormone receptor-negative group (7.8 % vs. 7.7 %, $p>0.05$). This variation could be the result of differences between the designs, treatment regimens, and patient populations of the NSABP B40 and GeparQuinto studies. Although the frequency of hypertension, mucositis, and febrile neutropenia was higher in the bevacizumab group, no difference in terms of heart failure was found between the two groups. The TORI B-02 study, which is assessing the neoadjuvant efficacy of bevacizumab in combination with TAC, is ongoing [88].

In the CALGB 40603 study, which recruited stage II and stage III triple-negative patients, the effect of carboplatin and/or bevacizumab was examined when added to weekly neoadjuvant paclitaxel and subsequent dose-dense AC [89]. When the results were examined, the addition of carboplatin to neoadjuvant therapy elevated the pCR rate in the breast from 44 % to 60 % ($p = 0.0018$), and the addition of bevacizumab increased the rate from 48 % to 59 % ($p = 0.0089$). The results of a recently published meta-analysis are consistent with the findings that the addition of carboplatin and bevacizumab to neoadjuvant therapy significantly increased the pCR rates in patients with triple-negative breast tumors [90]. However, it remains unknown whether this approach improves survival results.

In the ARTemis study, a phase III study for which the results were announced at ASCO 2014, bevacizumab was added to neoadjuvant chemotherapy with docetaxel and anthracyclinc in HER2-negative patients [91]. In total, 800 patients were randomized in the study, and the pCR rate was higher in the arm treated with bevacizumab (22 % vs. 17 %, $p = 0.03$). When subgroups were analyzed, the groups that benefited most from neoadjuvant therapy with bevacizumab were ER-negative or minimally ER-positive patients. The study results were consistent with the results of the GeparQuinto and CALGB 40603 studies.

Because VEGFR expression was shown to be related to adjuvant anti-hormonal treatment failure, we thought that using antiangiogenic therapy together with hormonal therapy might be effective [92, 93]. In a pilot study of 25 patients, the objective clinic response rate of neoadjuvant letrozole and bevacizumab combination therapy was 68 %, and the pCR rate was 16 % [94]. Neoadjuvant studies including hormone therapy and anti-VEGF treatment combinations in hormone receptor-positive patients are currently being conducted.

Our knowledge regarding neoadjuvant bevacizumab in HER2-positive disease is limited. In a phase II study including 26 patients who received weekly bevacizumab (5 mg/kg) added to weekly neoadjuvant paclitaxel + carboplatin + trastuzumab and who underwent surgery, 14 of the 26 patients had pCR (54 %), but bevacizumab-related complications (most frequently, would healing delay and infections) were observed during neoadjuvant therapy and postoperatively in a significant number of patients [95]; this is most likely linked to the prolonged usage of bevacizumab/trastuzumab. The BEVERLY-2 study is another phase II study that included 52 patients with HER2-positive nonmetastatic inflammatory breast cancer [96]. Patients received FEC + bevacizumab (one to four cycles) and docetaxel + bevacizumab + trastuzumab (five to eight cycles) before surgery and adjuvant radiotherapy trastuzumab and bevacizumab after surgery. The pCR rate with neoadjuvant therapy was 63.5 %; a grade 3 bevacizumab-related side effect (hypertension) was observed in only one patient. In the survival and biomarker analysis of the study, 3-year DFS and OS rates were 68 % and 90 %, respectively, and the pCR and circulating tumor cell presence were predictive of survival [97]. In the AVANTHER study, bevacizumab (15 mg/kg given four times every 3 weeks) was added to weekly neoadjuvant paclitaxel and trastuzumab (12 cycles) [98]. In 18 out of 42 patients, pCR was obtained (42.9 %), and grade 3 side effects (hypertension and mucositis) were observed in only two patients. The AVATAXHER study was designed to evaluate the ability of positron emission tomography (PET) to predict the effect of an early response of the addition of bevacizumab to the treatment regimen in patients who failed to respond to neoadjuvant therapy [99]. Patients were initially administered two cycles of neoadjuvant docetaxel + trastuzumab, and their metabolic responses were assessed by PET immediately before cycles 1 and 2. Patients were assigned to two groups, responders and nonresponders, according to their PET response. In the nonresponder group, bevacizumab was added to the current treatment, and responders continued to receive standard treatment. The pCR response rate was higher in the PET responders group of patients receiving bevacizumab compared with patients not receiving bevacizumab (43.8 % vs. 24 %).

Aflibercept

Aflibercept (VEGF-Trap) is a recombinant protein composed of the VEGFR-1 extracellular domain fused with the VEGFR-3 extracellular domain in combination with the Fc(a) domain of human IgG1. It binds to VEGF-A, VEGF-B, PGF-1, and PGF-2 in circulation [100]. Its fusion protein structure provides many advantages, including binding to VEGF with higher affinity than other anti-VEGF agents (800 times higher than bevacizumab), long plasma half-life (18 days), and the ability to bind to PGF-1 and PGF-2 [101, 102]. In preclinical studies, aflibercept regresses tumor vascularization and simultaneously stimulates the normalization of the existing vascular structure [103, 104]. In phase I studies that include different tumor groups, aflibercept appears to possess clinical antitumor efficiency and to be well tolerated [105–107]. Aflibercept recently received FDA approval for the second-line treatment of metastatic colorectal cancer after its ability to prolong survival was shown [108]. In the only phase II study for aflibercept, metastatic breast cancer patients who received less than two chemotherapy regimens received aflibercept at a dose of 4 mg/kg every 21 days; however, after the partial response rate was found to be 4.8 % and the median PFS was found to be 2.4 months, the trial was closed [109].

Ramucirumab

Ramucirumab (IMC-1121B) is a humanized monoclonal antibody that specifically binds to the extracellular VEGF-binding domain of VEGFR-2 with high affinity. As a result of that binding, it blocks all VEGFs that bind to VEGFR-2, unlike bevacizumab, which only binds to VEGF-A [110, 111]. Its objective antitumoral and antiangiogenic effects were observed in a phase I trial [112]. A phase II trial for ramucirumab in advanced lung cancer as a first-line treatment involved its addition to cisplatin-based chemotherapy; positive effects on PFS were observed [113, 114]. Moreover, in a phase III study (REGARD), it prolonged OS in metastatic gastric cancer when given as a second-line treatment [115]. In a phase III study (TRIO-012) comparing ramucirumab + docetaxel combination therapy with docetaxel alone as a first-line treatment for advanced HER2-negative breast cancer and for which the results have been recently announced, no significant improvement was detected in either PFS or OS upon the addition of docetaxel to ramucirumab [116].

Antiangiogenic Tyrosine Kinase Inhibitors

Small-molecule tyrosine kinase inhibitors have been developed to inhibit the intracellular catalytic function of the VEGF family. Sunitinib, sorafenib, pazopanib, motesanib, vandetanib, vatalanib, and axitinib are among the tyrosine kinase inhibitors for which the efficacy in treating breast cancer is being investigated (Table 35.2).

Sunitinib

Sunitinib is an oral tyrosine inhibitor that blocks not only VEGFR-1, 2, and 3 but also PDGFR-α, PDGFR-β, c-kit, FMS-like tyrosine kinase-3, RET, and colony-stimulating factor-1 receptors [117, 118]. It has received FDA approval for the treatment of advanced renal cell cancer, neuroendocrine cancer, and gastrointestinal stromal tumors. In experimental studies, it has been shown to have significant antitumor activity in breast cancer and bone metastases of breast cancer when given alone; it also enhances the antitumor effects of other chemotherapeutic agents, including taxanes and fluoropyrimidines [119, 120]. In phase I studies in different tumor types, it has been shown that using sunitinib at a dose of 37.5–50 mg/day has a safe toxicity profile [121–123]. The most frequent adverse effects are fatigue, hypertension, and skin changes. In a phase II study that included 64 heavily treated breast cancer patients who had previously received taxane and anthracycline, PR was achieved in 7 patients (11 %), and SD longer than 6 months was obtained in three patients (5 %) [124]. The patients who were responsive were either triple-negative or HER2-positive patients who had previously received trastuzumab. A group study for sunitinib in combination with chemotherapy was then initiated. In a pilot study with 22 advanced breast cancer patients receiving first-line treatment with a paclitaxel-sunitinib combination, an objective response was found in seven patients (two CR and five PR, 38.7 %) [125]. In a phase II study that followed this study, paclitaxel-sunitinib and paclitaxel-bevacizumab combinations were compared [126]. In the interim analysis of this study, which included 485 patients, the study was terminated because of the inferior results of the paclitaxel-sunitinib arm compared with the paclitaxel-bevacizumab arm (median PFS 7.4 months vs. 9.2 months). In both arms, the objective response rate was calculated as 32 %, but the response time was shorter in the sunitinib arm (6.3 months vs. 14.8 months). The SABRE-B study is a phase II dose-escalation study in which sunitinib was added to the paclitaxel-bevacizumab combination therapy [127]. The sunitinib dose began at 25 mg/day and was intended to be increased if the toxicity was tolerable. However, the randomization of the 46 patients included in the study was ended early due to the frequency of serious grade ≥3 side effects in the triple combination therapy arm compared with the paclitaxel-bevacizumab arm (83 % vs. 57 %), and the treatment time required to calculate PFS and OS was not reached because of the side effects. In a phase III study with 296 HER2-negative patients for whom docetaxel-sunitinib combination therapy was compared with docetaxel alone as a first-line treatment, the ORR was found to be higher in the sunitinib arm (55 % vs. 42 %, $p=0.001$), but no difference was found between the two arms in terms of PFS or OS [128]. In an exploratory study that included 26 HER2-positive patients, the objective RR was 76 % with docetaxel-trastuzumab-sunitinib (37.5 mg) combination treatment, which was well tolerated [129]. In another phase III study, HER2-negative advanced breast cancer patients who previously received taxane and anthracycline were randomized to a capecitabine or sunitinib arm for monotherapy, but this study was also closed due to sunitinib having a high side-effect frequency compared with capecitabine and because in terms of PFS, the primary endpoint could not be reached at the first interim analysis [130]. In a recently published phase III study, capecitabine-sunitinib combination therapy and capecitabine monotherapy were compared in breast cancer patients who had received taxane and anthracycline and at least one treatment in a metastatic setting [131]. According to the results, the addition of sunitinib to capecitabine did not result in an advantage in terms of PFS, ORR, or OS, and all side effects except hand-foot syndrome

were more frequent in the sunitinib arm. It appears that adding sunitinib to chemotherapy for breast cancer does not elicit a positive effect. The possible explanations for this situation include the heterogeneity of the patient groups; the changes in the signaling mechanisms of pretreated patients; the fact that antiangiogenic agents sometimes cause hypoxia by inhibiting vascularization more than is necessary, thereby resulting in the formation of more aggressive and invasive cell types; and the uncertainty of both the optimal biological dose of sunitinib and the sequence of drug application. Because side effects occurred in many studies, the optimal dose was never reached, and endpoints were thus affected. The efficacy of sunitinib monotherapy has been evaluated in HER2-negative patients for whom an objective response was achieved with chemotherapy; however, in this study, PFS improvement was not obtained, and toxicity developed in many patients [132]. Sunitinib also led to serious hematological toxicity in a phase II study in which it was used as a neoadjuvant concomitantly with weekly paclitaxel-carboplatin therapy [133]. Additionally, two studies, one in a metastatic setting and the other in a neoadjuvant setting, investigated the combination of sunitinib with exemestane in hormone receptor-positive breast cancer and found that the current regimen was safe [134, 135].

Sorafenib

Sorafenib is an oral multi-kinase inhibitor that inhibits the Ras/Raf/mitogen-activated protein kinase (MAPK) signaling pathway by blocking VEGFR-1, 2, and 3, PDGFR, RET, Flt3, and c-kit [136]. In preclinical studies, its wide-spectrum antitumor activity has been observed [137–139]. Based on the phase II and III studies, it is currently approved for hepatocellular carcinoma and renal cell carcinoma [140–142]. When no response was observed in a phase II study with 23 metastatic breast cancer patients who received anthracycline or taxane before, the study was terminated prematurely [143]. In another phase II trial with 56 patients who received at least one treatment in a metastatic setting, sorafenib monotherapy in one patient (2 %)

Table 35.2 Phase II and III trials of antiangiogenic TKIs in advanced breast cancer

Trial	Design	Patient population	Patient enrolled	HER2 positive (%)	Chemotherapy regimen	TKI dose (day)	Primary endpoint	ORR (%)	Median PFS (months)	Median OS (months)
Burstein [124]	Phase II	Metastatic breast cancer, tax/anthr pretreated	46	19	S (monotherapy)	50	ORR	11	2.3	8.9
Robert [126]	Open-label, randomized, phase III	Metastatic or locally recurrent breast cancer, first line	485[a,b]	0	Pac weekly+S vs. Pac weekly+B	25–37.5	PFS	32.2 vs. 32.1, p=0.525	7.4 vs. 9.2, p=0.999	17.6 vs. NR
Mayer [127] SABRE-B	Open-label, randomized, phase II	Metastatic breast cancer, first line	46	0	Pac weekly+B+S vs. Pac weekly+B	25	PFS	71 vs. 61	NR[c]	NR[c]
Bergh [128]	Open-label, randomized, phase III	Metastatic or locally recurrent breast cancer, first line	296	0	Docet q3w +S vs. Docet q3w alone	37.5	PFS	55 vs. 42, p=0.001	8.6 vs. 8.3, p=0.265	24.8 vs. 25.5, p=0.904
Barrios [130]	Open-label, randomized, phase III	Metastatic or locally recurrent breast cancer, tax/anthr pretreated	482[a,b]	0	S (monotherapy) vs. Cape q3w	37.5	PFS	11 vs. 16, p=0.109	2.8 vs. 4.2, p=0.002	15.3 vs. 24.6, p=0.350
Crown [131]	Open-label, randomized, phase III	Metastatic or locally recurrent breast cancer, tax/anthr pretreated	442	13	Cape q3w+S vs. Cape q3w alone	37.5	PFS	19 vs. 18, p=0.490	5.5 vs. 5.9, p=0.941	16.4 vs. 16.5, p=0.494
Moreno-Aspitia [143] N0336	Phase II	Metastatic breast cancer, tax/anthr pretreated	23	13	Sor (monotherapy)	2×400	RR	0	2.0	NR
Bianchi [144]	Phase II	Metastatic breast cancer, heavily pretreated	56	20	Sor (monotherapy)	2×400	RR	2	1.5	8.6
Baselga [145] SOLTI-0701	Open-label, randomized, placebo-controlled phase IIB	Metastatic or locally advanced breast cancer, first and second line	229	0	Cape q3w+Sor vs. Cape q3w+P	2×400	PFS	38 vs. 31, p=0.25	6.4 vs. 4.1, p=0.001	22.2 vs. 20.9, p=0.42
Gradishar [147]	Randomized, double-blind, placebo-controlled phase IIB	Metastatic or locally recurrent breast cancer, first line	237	0	Pac weekly+Sor vs. Pac weekly+P	2×400	PFS	67 vs. 54, p=0.0468	6.9 vs. 5.6, p=0.0857	16.8 vs. 17.4, p=0.904

Study	Design	Setting	N	N	Treatment arms	N	Endpoint	Results	PFS	OS
Jonhston [157]	Open-label, randomized, phase II	Metastatic/advanced breast cancer, first line	190	100	Lap+Paz vs. Lap alone	400	PDR	36.2 vs. 22.2	36.2 % vs. 38.9 %, $p=0.37$ (PDR at week-12)	NR
Martin [162]	Randomized, double-blind, placebo-controlled phase II	Metastatic or locally recurrent breast cancer, first line		0	Pac weekly+M vs. Pac weekly+B vs. Pac weekly+P	125	RR	49 vs. 41 (placebo arm), $p=0.31$; 49 vs. 52 (B-arm), $p=0.75$	9.5 vs. 9.0 (placebo arm), $p=0.31$; 9.5 vs. 11.5 (B-arm), $p=0.15$	NR
Rugo [166]	Randomized, double-blind, placebo-controlled phase II	Metastatic or locally recurrent breast cancer, first line	168	0	Docet q3w+Ax vs. Docet q3w+P	2×5	TTP	41.1 vs. 23.6, $p=0.011$	8.1 vs. 7.1, $p=0.0091$ (TTP)	NR
Boér [172]	Randomized, double-blind, placebo-controlled phase II	Advanced breast cancer, second line	64	Van-arm: 11 Placebo-arm: 17	Docet q3w+Van vs. Docet q3w+P	100	NPE	40 vs. 17	8.2 vs. 5.6, $p=0.25$	NR

TKI tyrosine kinase inhibitor, *ORR* objective response rate, *PFS* progression-free survival, *OS* overall survival, *tax* taxane, *anthr* anthracycline, *S* sunitinib, *Sor* Sorafenib, *Paz* pazopanib, *M* motesanib, *Ax* axitinib, *Van* vandetanib, *cape* capecitabine, *B* bevacizumab, *Lap* lapatinib, *pac* paclitaxel, *docet* docetaxel, *P* placebo, *PDR* progressive disease rate, *NPE* number of progression events (by the data cutoff), *NR* not reported

[a]Interim analysis

[b]This trial was terminated early because of futility in reaching the primary endpoint, as determined by the independent data monitoring committee during an interim futility analysis

[c]Due to serious toxicity, the study was terminated early. Therefore, follow-up was short, and the median PFS and OS were not reached

achieved a partial response, and stable disease was achieved in 20 patients (37 %) [144]. In both studies, 800 mg/day was well tolerated; fatigue, rash, hand-foot syndrome, and diarrhea were the most common side effects. Because its efficacy is low as monotherapy, combination with chemotherapy has been attempted. In the trial of Baselga et al. (SOLTI-0701 trial), 229 HER2-negative patients were randomized into capecitabine-sorafenib and capecitabine-placebo groups in first- or second-line treatment [145]. Adding sorafenib to capecitabine significantly improved PFS (median 6.4 months vs. 4.1 months, $p=0.001$). However, no difference was shown in terms of ORR (38 % vs. 31 %, $p=0.25$) or OS (median 22.2 vs. 20.9 months, $p=0.42$) between the two groups. In the sorafenib arm, the frequency of side effects such as hand-foot syndrome, rash, mucosal inflammation, neutropenia, and hypertension was significantly higher compared with the placebo arm. Based on these results, a new phase II study (RESILIENCE trial) has started in which the dose of sorafenib added to capecitabine was reduced to 600 mg/day, and a more aggressive treatment for hand-foot syndrome was planned [146]. At an international multicenter phase II study in which paclitaxel-sorafenib and paclitaxel-placebo treatments were compared, the median TTP and ORR were superior in the sorafenib arm (median 8.1 months vs. 5.6 months, $p=0.0343$, and 67 % vs. 54 %, $p=0468$, respectively). However, no difference was shown in terms of PFS or OS between the two groups [147]. In a multi-institutional phase I/II study that included patients showing progression under aromatase inhibitors, PR was achieved by the addition of 800 mg sorafenib to anastrozole treatment in one patient, and SD was achieved in seven patients. However 77 % of the patients required dose reduction, and 31 % had to stop taking sorafenib because of its unacceptable toxicity [148]. A phase II study researching the efficacy of sorafenib-bevacizumab treatment ended early due to serious toxicity [149]. The results of two meta-analyses individually examining the randomized and retrospective studies of sorafenib have shown that sorafenib in combination with chemotherapy improved PFS and TTP compared with chemotherapy alone and had no effect on ORR or OS [150, 151].

Pazopanib

Pazopanib is a small-molecule oral tyrosine kinase inhibitor that exerts its effects by blocking VEGFR-1, 2, and 3, PDGFR, c-kit, and mast-stem cell growth factor receptor [152]. In its phase I study that included many tumor types, it had both antitumor and anti-cytostatic effects [153]. The antitumor effect appeared at a dose of 800 mg/day, and no increase in the plasma concentration was observed at higher doses; therefore, the suggested dose is 800 mg/day. The side effects are generally grade 1 or 2, and the most frequently observed side effects are hypertension, diarrhea, skin hypopigmentation, and nausea. In a phase II study, pazopanib, which has been approved for use in renal cell carcinoma and leiomyosarcoma, was evaluated in 20 recurrent or metastatic breast cancer patients who received two or more treatments (including adjuvant or neoadjuvant); PR was achieved in 1 patient (5 %), and SD was achieved in 11 patients (55 %) (in 4 of the 11 SD patients, the time of response was longer than 6 months) [154]. The median PFS was 5.3 months. In half of the patients, shrinking of the target lesion was observed, and treatment was generally well tolerated. In the neoadjuvant treatment of HER2-negative locally advanced breast cancer, the pCR rate was 17 % with pazopanib added to four cycles of AC and subsequent weekly paclitaxel (9 % in ER-positive patients and 38 % in triple-negative patients) [155].

In a phase I study conducted based on information regarding the additive antitumor effect of anti-HER2 treatment with antiangiogenic treatment, the combination of lapatinib (1,000–1,500 mg) and pazopanib (400–800 mg) had a notable antitumor effect and a safe toxicity profile [156]. However, in subsequent studies of the combination of lapatinib 1,500 mg + pazopanib, serious toxicity and predominant diarrhea were reported [157]. In a phase II study comparing lapatinib 1,000 mg + pazopanib 400 mg in combination with lapatinib 1,500 mg monotherapy, the combination therapy increased the ORR (58 % vs. 47 %) but had no effect on PFS [158]. Furthermore, with the combination therapy, grade ≥ 3 side effects were observed at a high frequency (50 % vs. 17 %).

Motesanib

Motesanib is a small-molecule tyrosine kinase inhibitor that very selectively blocks VEGFR-1, 2, and 3, PDGFR, and c-kit [159]. In preclinical and clinical studies, it has been shown that it has a broad antitumoral effect [159, 160]. In tumor xenograft models of breast cancer, motesanib decreases tumor growth and, when used with tamoxifen or docetaxel, significantly increases the antitumor efficacy [160]. In a phase I study based on these data that included 45 patients, motesanib was added to weekly paclitaxel or docetaxel every 3 weeks [161]. The maximum tolerated dose of motesanib was 125 mg/day. When toxicity was considered, the treatment was generally well tolerated; in seven patients (16 %), motesanib-related grade 3 adverse effects were found (cholecystitis in two patients and hypertension in two patients). The ORR was 56 % with motesanib added to taxane-based chemotherapy. In a phase II study, combinations of paclitaxel-motesanib, paclitaxel-placebo, and paclitaxel-bevacizumab were compared [162]. No difference in terms of ORR was found between the motesanib and placebo groups (49 % vs. 41 %, $p=0.31$). In the bevacizumab arm, ORR was 51 %, which was similar to the motesanib arm. The serious adverse event ratio in patients taking motesanib was higher than that in the other two groups; the most common adverse events were diarrhea, hypertension, fatigue, and peripheral neuropathy.

Axitinib

Axitinib (AG013736) is an oral tyrosine kinase inhibitor that inhibits VEGFR-1, 2, and 3, PDGFR, c-kit, and colony-stimulating factor-1 [163]. Axitinib regresses tumor vasculature in human breast cancer xenograft models and, in parallel, inhibits tumor growth [164]. In a phase I study, axitinib was shown to have a clinical antitumor effect in solid tumors [165]. The suggested dose is 5 mg twice daily. In a phase II study including 168 patients with metastatic breast cancer, axitinib and placebo added to docetaxel were compared [166]. TTP was found to be longer in the axitinib arm compared with the placebo arm (8.1 months vs. 7.1 months), but the difference was not statistically significant. The ORR was significantly higher in the combination arm (41.4 % vs. 23.6 %, $p=0.011$). Adverse effects, including neutropenia, stomatitis, diarrhea, mucositis, and hypertension, were more frequent in the axitinib arm. In the subgroup analysis of the study, TTP in the axitinib arm was significantly better in patients who previously received adjuvant treatment (9.2 months vs. 7.0 months, $p=0.043$).

Vandetanib

Vandetanib (ZD6474) is an oral receptor tyrosine kinase inhibitor that competitively binds to and blocks the ATP-binding site of VEGFR-2 (flk-1/KDR). In contrast to the other antiangiogenic tyrosine kinase inhibitors, vandetanib shows an anti-EGFR effect at sub-micromolar concentrations by simultaneously blocking HER1 [167]. Vandetanib not only inhibits endothelial cell proliferation and angiogenesis but also regresses cancer cell growth by affecting the autocrine EGFR signal [168, 169]. In its phase I study, it was well tolerated at a dose of 300 mg/day, and the most frequent side effects were diarrhea, rash, and hypertension [170]. In a phase II study that included 46 patients with metastatic breast cancer who received anthracycline and taxane, no objective response was observed [171]. The authors proposed that this could be due to changes in the tumor biology that could have made the patients unresponsive to anti-VEGF treatment or to the fact that the adequate plasma concentration for the antitumor effect of vandetanib was not reached. In a small phase II study comparing vandetanib or placebo added to docetaxel, no difference in the risk of disease progression was found between placebo and vandetanib [172]. One of the two studies combining vandetanib and fulvestrant in patients with hormone receptor-positive metastatic breast cancer was discontinued due to low patient participation. In the other study, no significant change was detected in PFS or OS with vandetanib added to fulvestrant compared with placebo in patients with bone-only or bone-predominant metastatic disease [173, 174].

Vatalanib

Vatalanib (PTK787/ZK-222584) is a new class of oral small-molecule tyrosine kinase inhibitor. It blocks all VEGFRs (VEGFR-1 (flt-1), VEGFR-2 (flk-1/KDR), and VEGFR-3 (flt-4)), PDGRF, c-kit, protein tyrosine kinase, and c-fms, but its affinity is highest for VEGFR-1 and 2 [175]. According to preclinical studies, in addition to its antiangiogenic activity, vatalanib also has an aromatase inhibitory effect [176, 177]. In a phase I study, the maximum tolerated dose was 750 mg given twice daily; conversely, the biologically active dose was 1,000 mg twice daily [178]. Phase I/II studies of vatalanib combined with trastuzumab and letrozole were closed prematurely due to low patient enrollment and toxicity [179].

Conclusion

Although targeting tumor angiogenesis represents an active treatment modality for many solid tumors, several studies have indicated that this approach is not an accepted standard treatment for early-stage or advanced breast cancer. There are numerous ongoing trials regarding this issue. In the coming years, the identification of effective combinations and patient subgroups will permit the use of antiangiogenic therapy as a standard treatment option in breast cancer patients.

References

1. Lorusso V. Bevacizumab in the treatment of HER2-negative breast cancer. Biologics. 2008;2:813–21.
2. Bareschino MA, Schettino C, Colantuoni G, Rossi E, Rossi A, Maione P, et al. The role of antiangiogenetic agents in the treatment of breast cancer. Curr Med Chem. 2011;18:5022–32.
3. Azam F, Mehta S, Harris AL. Mechanisms of resistance to antiangiogenesis therapy. Eur J Cancer. 2010;46:1323–32.
4. Gardlik R, Celec P, Bernadic M. Targeting angiogenesis for cancer (gene) therapy. Bratisl Lek Listy. 2011;112:428–34.
5. Tammela T, Enholm B, Alitalo K, Paavonen K. The biology of vascular endothelial growth factors. Cardiovasc Res. 2005;65:550–63.
6. Ferrara N. Role of vascular endothelial growth factor in the regulation of angiogenesis. Kidney Int. 1999;56:794–814.
7. Liekens S, De Clercq E, Neyts J. Angiogenesis: regulators and clinical applications. Biochem Pharmacol. 2001;61:253–70.
8. Koutras AK, Starakis I, Lymperatou D, Kalofonos HP. Angiogenesis as a therapeutic target in breast cancer. Mini Rev Med Chem. 2012;12:1230–8.
9. Folkman J. Tumor angiogenesis: therapeutic implications. N Engl J Med. 1971;285:1182–6.
10. Schneider BP, Miller KD. Angiogenesis of breast cancer. J Clin Oncol. 2005;23:1782–90.
11. Roland CL, Dineen SP, Lynn KD, Sullivan LA, Dellinger MT, Sadegh L, et al. Inhibition of vascular endothelial growth factor reduces angiogenesis and modulates immune cell infiltration of orthotopic breast cancer xenografts. Mol Cancer Ther. 2009; 8:1761–71.
12. Viacava P, Naccarato AG, Bocci G, Fanelli G, Aretini P, Lonobile A, et al. Angiogenesis and VEGF expression in pre-invasive lesions of the human breast. J Pathol. 2004;204:140–6.
13. Bluff JE, Menakuru SR, Cross SS, Higham SE, Balasubramanian SP, Brown NJ, et al. Angiogenesis is associated with the onset of hyperplasia in human ductal breast disease. Br J Cancer. 2009;101:666–72.
14. Schneider BP, Radovich M, Sledge GW, Robarge JD, Li L, Storniolo AM, et al. Association of polymorphisms of angiogenesis genes with breast cancer. Breast Cancer Res Treat. 2008;111:157–63.
15. Guinebretière JM, Lê Monique G, Gavoille A, Bahi J, Contesso G. Angiogenesis and risk of breast cancer in women with fibrocystic disease. J Natl Cancer Inst. 1994;86:635–6.
16. Guidi AJ, Fischer L, Harris JR, Schnitt SJ. Microvessel density and distribution in ductal carcinoma in situ of the breast. J Natl Cancer Inst. 1994;86:614–9.
17. Weidner N, Semple JP, Welch WR, Folkman J. Tumor angiogenesis and metastasis – correlation in invasive breast carcinoma. N Engl J Med. 1991;324:1–8.
18. Kim KJ, Li B, Winer J, Armanini M, Gillett N, Phillips HS, Ferrara N. Inhibition of vascular endothelial growth factor-induced angiogenesis suppresses tumour growth in vivo. Nature. 1993;362:841–4.
19. Inai T, Mancuso M, Hashizume H, Baffert F, Haskell A, Baluk P, et al. Inhibition of vascular endothelial growth factor (VEGF) signaling in cancer causes loss of endothelial fenestrations, regression of tumor vessels, and appearance of basement membrane ghosts. Am J Pathol. 2004;165:35–52.
20. Goel S, Duda DG, Xu L, Munn LL, Boucher Y, Fukumura D, et al. Normalization of the vasculature for treatment of cancer and other diseases. Physiol Rev. 2011;91:1071–121.
21. Wildiers H, Guetens G, De Boeck G, Verbeken E, Landuyt B, Landuyt W, et al. Effect of antivascular endothelial growth factor treatment on the

intratumoral uptake of CPT-11. Br J Cancer. 2003; 88:1979–86.

22. Manzoni M, Rovati B, Ronzoni M, Loupakis F, Mariucci S, Ricci V, et al. Immunological effects of bevacizumab-based treatment in metastatic colorectal cancer. Oncology. 2010;79:187–96.

23. Lu J-F, Bruno R, Eppler S, Novotny W, Lum B, Gaudreault J. Clinical pharmacokinetics of bevacizumab in patients with solid tumors. Cancer Chemother Pharmacol. 2008;62:779–86.

24. Dai F, Shu L, Bian Y, Wang Z, Yang Z, Chu W, Gao S. Safety of bevacizumab in treating metastatic colorectal cancer: a systematic review and meta-analysis of all randomized clinical trials. Clin Drug Investig. 2013;33:779–88.

25. Hurwitz H, Fehrenbacher L, Novotny W, Cartwright T, Hainsworth J, Heim W, et al. Bevacizumab plus irinotecan, fluorouracil, and leucovorin for metastatic colorectal cancer. N Engl J Med. 2004;350:2335–42.

26. Giantonio BJ, Catalano PJ, Meropol NJ, O'Dwyer PJ, Mitchell EP, Alberts SR, Eastern Cooperative Oncology Group Study E3200, et al. Bevacizumab in combination with oxaliplatin, fluorouracil, and leucovorin (FOLFOX4) for previously treated metastatic colorectal cancer: results from the Eastern Cooperative Oncology Group Study E3200. J Clin Oncol. 2007;25:1539–44.

27. Sandler A, Gray R, Perry MC, Brahmer J, Schiller JH, Dowlati A, et al. Paclitaxel-carboplatin alone or with bevacizumab for non-small-cell lung cancer. N Engl J Med. 2006;355:2542–50.

28. Yang JC, Haworth L, Sherry RM, Hwu P, Schwartzentruber DJ, Topalian SL, et al. A randomized trial of bevacizumab, an anti-vascular endothelial growth factor antibody, for metastatic renal cancer. N Engl J Med. 2003;349:427–34.

29. Perren TJ, Swart AM, Pfisterer J, Ledermann JA, Pujade-Lauraine E, Kristensen G, ICON7 Investigators, et al. A phase 3 trial of bevacizumab in ovarian cancer. N Engl J Med. 2011;365:2484–96.

30. Friedman HS, Prados MD, Wen PY, Mikkelsen T, Schiff D, Abrey LE, et al. Bevacizumab alone and in combination with irinotecan in recurrent glioblastoma. J Clin Oncol. 2009;27:4733–40.

31. Tewari KS, Sill M, Long HJ, Ramondetta LM, Landrum LM, Oaknin A, et al. Incorporation of bevacizumab in the treatment of recurrent and metastatic cervical cancer: A phase III randomized trial of the Gynecologic Oncology Group. J Clin Oncol. 2013;31(Suppl):abstr 3.

32. Gordon MS, Margolin K, Talpaz M, Sledge Jr GW, Holmgren E, Benjamin R, et al. Phase I safety and pharmacokinetic study of recombinant human antivascular endothelial growth factor in patients with advanced cancer. J Clin Oncol. 2001;19:843–50.

33. Margolin K, Gordon MS, Holmgren E, Gaudreault J, Novotny W, Fyfe G, et al. Phase Ib trial of intravenous recombinant humanized monoclonal antibody

to vascular endothelial growth factor in combination with chemotherapy in patients with advanced cancer: pharmacologic and long-term safety data. J Clin Oncol. 2001;19:851–6.

34. Jayson GC, Mulatero C, Ranson M, Zweit J, Jackson A, Broughton L, European Organisation for Research and Treatment of Cancer (EORTC), et al. Phase I investigation of recombinant anti-human vascular endothelial growth factor antibody in patients with advanced cancer. Eur J Cancer. 2005;41:555–63.

35. Cobleigh MA, Langmuir VK, Sledge GW, Miller KD, Haney L, Novotny WF, et al. A phase I/II dose-escalation trial of bevacizumab in previously treated metastatic breast cancer. Semin Oncol. 2003;30 Suppl 16:117–24.

36. Sledge G, Miller K, Moisa C, Gradishar W. Safety and efficacy of capecitabine (C) plus bevacizumab (B) as first-line in metastatic breast cancer. J Clin Oncol. 2007;25(Suppl):abstr 1013.

37. Burstein HJ, Chen YH, Parker LM, Savoie J, Younger J, Kuter I, et al. VEGF as a marker for outcome among advanced breast cancer patients receiving anti-VEGF therapy with bevacizumab and vinorelbine chemotherapy. Clin Cancer Res. 2008;14:7871–7.

38. Perez EA, Hillman DW, Dentchev T, Le-Lindqwister NA, Geeraerts LH, Fitch TR, et al. North Central Cancer Treatment Group (NCCTG) N0432: phase II trial of docetaxel with capecitabine and bevacizumab as first-line chemotherapy for patients with metastatic breast cancer. Ann Oncol. 2010;21:269–74.

39. Smith IE, Pierga JY, Biganzoli L, Cortés-Funes H, Thomssen C, Pivot X, ATHENA Study Group, et al. First-line bevacizumab plus taxane-based chemotherapy for locally recurrent or metastatic breast cancer: safety and efficacy in an open-label study in 2,251 patients. Ann Oncol. 2011;22:595–602.

40. Smith I, Pierga JY, Biganzoli L, Cortes-Funes H, Thomssen C, Saracchini S, et al. Final overall survival results and effect of prolonged (≥1 year) first-line bevacizumab-containing therapy for metastatic breast cancer in the ATHENA trial. Breast Cancer Res Treat. 2011;130:133–43.

41. Fabi A, Russillo M, Ferretti G, Metro G, Nisticò C, Papaldo P, et al. Maintenance bevacizumab beyond first-line paclitaxel plus bevacizumab in patients with Her2-negative hormone receptor-positive metastatic breast cancer: efficacy in combination with hormonal therapy. BMC Cancer. 2012;12:482.

42. Bisagni G, Musolino A, Panebianco M, De Matteis A, Nuzzo F, Ardizzoni A, et al. The Breast Avastin Trial: phase II study of bevacizumab maintenance therapy after induction chemotherapy with docetaxel and capecitabine for the first-line treatment of patients with locally recurrent or metastatic breast cancer. Cancer Chemother Pharmacol. 2013;71:1051–7.

43. Militello L, Carli P, Di Lauro V, Spazzapan S, Scalone S, Lombardi D, et al. Bevacizumab as maintenance therapy (mBev) in metastatic breast cancer (MBC). J Clin Oncol. 2013;31(Suppl):abstr e22149.

44. Gligorov J, Doval D, Bines J, Alba E, Cortes P, Pierga JY, et al. Maintenance capecitabine and bevacizumab versus bevacizumab alone after initial first-line bevacizumab and docetaxel for patients with HER2-negative metastatic breast cancer (IMELDA): a randomised, open-label, phase 3 trial. Lancet Oncol. 2014;15:1351–60.

45. Miller KD, Chap LI, Holmes FA, Cobleigh MA, Marcom PK, Fehrenbacher L, et al. Randomized phase III trial of capecitabine compared with bevacizumab plus capecitabine in patients with previously treated metastatic breast cancer. J Clin Oncol. 2005;23:792–9.

46. Miller K, Wang M, Gralow J, Dickler M, Cobleigh M, Perez EA, et al. Paclitaxel plus bevacizumab versus paclitaxel alone for metastatic breast cancer. N Engl J Med. 2007;357:2666–76.

47. Miles DW, Chan A, Dirix LY, Cortés J, Pivot X, Tomczak P, et al. Phase III study of bevacizumab plus docetaxel compared with placebo plus docetaxel for the first-line treatment of human epidermal growth factor receptor 2-negative metastatic breast cancer. J Clin Oncol. 2010;28:3239–47.

48. Chang TY, Dong YH, Lin C, Lin HH, Kuo SH, Lai C, et al. Does chemotherapy schedule matter when combining with bevacizumab? A stratified meta-analysis of randomized controlled trials. J Clin Oncol. 2014;32(suppl; abstr 1076):5s.

49. Miles DW, de Haas SL, Dirix LY, Romieu G, Chan A, Pivot X, et al. Biomarker results from the AVADO phase 3 trial of first-line bevacizumab plus docetaxel for HER2-negative metastatic breast cancer. Br J Cancer. 2013;108:1052–60.

50. Study to evaluate the efficacy and safety of bevacizumab, and associated biomarkers, in combination with paclitaxel compared with paclitaxel plus placebo as first-line treatment of patients with Her2-negative metastatic breast cancer. ClinicalTrials.gov Identifier: NCT01663727.

51. Robert NJ, Diéras V, Glaspy J, Brufsky AM, Bondarenko I, Lipatov ON, et al. RIBBON-1: randomized, double-blind, placebo-controlled, phase III trial of chemotherapy with or without bevacizumab for first-line treatment of human epidermal growth factor receptor 2-negative, locally recurrent or metastatic breast cancer. J Clin Oncol. 2011;29:1252–60.

52. Brufsky AM, Hurvitz S, Perez E, Swamy R, Valero V, O'Neill V, et al. RIBBON-2: a randomized, double-blind, placebo-controlled, phase III trial evaluating the efficacy and safety of bevacizumab in combination with chemotherapy for second-line treatment of human epidermal growth factor receptor 2-negative metastatic breast cancer. J Clin Oncol. 2011;29:4286–93.

53. von Minckwitz G, Puglisi F, Cortes J, Vrdoljak E, Marschner N, Zielinski C, et al. Bevacizumab plus chemotherapy versus chemotherapy alone as second-line treatment for patients with HER2-negative locally recurrent or metastatic breast cancer after first-line treatment with bevacizumab plus chemotherapy (TANIA): an open-label, randomised phase 3 trial. Lancet Oncol. 2014;15:1269–78.

54. Lang I, Brodowicz T, Ryvo L, Kahan Z, Greil R, Beslija S, Central European Cooperative Oncology Group, et al. Bevacizumab plus paclitaxel versus bevacizumab plus capecitabine as first-line treatment for HER2-negative metastatic breast cancer: interim efficacy results of the randomised, open-label, non-inferiority, phase 3 TURANDOT trial. Lancet Oncol. 2013;14:125–33.

55. Inbar MJ, Lang I, Kahan Z, Greil R, Beslija S, Stemmer SM, et al. Central European Cooperative Oncology Group. Efficacy of first-line bevacizumab (BEV)-based therapy for metastatic triple-negative breast cancer (TNBC): subgroup analysis of TURANDOT. J Clin Oncol. 2013;31(Suppl):abstr 1040.

56. Rochlitz C, von Moos R, Bigler M, Zaman K, Anchisi S, Küng M, et al. SAKK 24/09: safety and tolerability of bevacizumab plus paclitaxel versus bevacizumab plus metronomic cyclophosphamide and capecitabine as first-line therapy in patients with HER2-negative advanced stage breast cancer-A multicenter, randomized phase III trial. J Clin Oncol. 2014;32(Suppl):abstr 518.

57. Tredan O, Follana P, Moullet I, Cropet C, Trager-Maury S, Dauba J, et al. Arobase: a phase III trial of exemestane (Exe) and bevacizumab (BEV) as maintenance therapy in patients (pts) with metastatic breast cancer (MBC) treated in first line with paclitaxel (P) and BEV-A Gineco study. J Clin Oncol. 2014;32(Suppl):abstr 501.

58. Yen L, You XL, Al Moustafa AE, Batist G, Hynes NE, Mader S, et al. Heregulin selectively upregulates vascular endothelial growth factor secretion in cancer cells and stimulates angiogenesis. Oncogene. 2000;19:3460–9.

59. Bagheri-Yarmand R, Vadlamudi RK, Wang RA, Mendelsohn J, Kumar R. Vascular endothelial growth factor up-regulation via p21-activated kinase-1 signaling regulates heregulin-beta1-mediated angiogenesis. J Biol Chem. 2000;275:39451–7.

60. Laughner E, Taghavi P, Chiles K, Mahon PC, Semenza GL. HER2 (neu) signaling increases the rate of hypoxia-inducible factor 1alpha (HIF-1alpha) synthesis: novel mechanism for HIF-1-mediated vascular endothelial growth factor expression. Mol Cell Biol. 2001;21:3995–4004.

61. Kumar R, Yarmand-Bagheri R. The role of HER2 in angiogenesis. Semin Oncol. 2001;28 Suppl 16:27–32.

62. Montero JC, Rodríguez-Barrueco R, Ocaña A, Díaz-Rodríguez E, Esparís-Ogando A, Pandiella A. Neuregulins and cancer. Clin Cancer Res. 2008;14:3237–41.

63. Konecny GE, Meng YG, Untch M, Wang HJ, Bauerfeind I, Epstein M, et al. Association between HER-2/neu and vascular endothelial growth factor expression predicts clinical outcome in primary breast cancer patients. Clin Cancer Res. 2004;10:1706–16.

64. Bhattacharjee RN, Timoshenko AV, Cai J, Lala PK. Relationship between cyclooxygenase-2 and human epidermal growth factor receptor 2 in vascular endothelial growth factor C up-regulation and lymphangiogenesis in human breast cancer. Cancer Sci. 2010;101:2026–32.

65. Le XF, Mao W, Lu C, Thornton A, Heymach JV, Sood AK, et al. Specific blockade of VEGF and HER2 pathways results in greater growth inhibition of breast cancer xenografts that overexpress HER2. Cell Cycle. 2008;7:3747–58.

66. Hurvitz S, Pegram M, Lin L, Chan D, Allen H, Dichmann R, et al. Final results of a phase II trial evaluating trastuzumab and bevacizumab as first line treatment of HER2-amplified advanced breast cancer. Cancer Res. 2009;69(24(Suppl)):3.

67. Martín M, Makhson A, Gligorov J, Lichinitser M, Lluch A, Semiglazov V, et al. Phase II study of bevacizumab in combination with trastuzumab and capecitabine as first-line treatment for HER-2-positive locally recurrent or metastatic breast cancer. Oncologist. 2012;17:469–75.

68. Schwartzberg LS, Badarinath S, Keaton MR, Childs BH. Phase II multicenter study of docetaxel and bevacizumab with or without trastuzumab as first-line treatment for patients with metastatic breast cancer. Clin Breast Cancer. 2014;14:161–8.

69. Zhao M, Pan X, Layman R, Lustberg MB, Mrozek E, Macrae ER, et al. A phase II study of bevacizumab in combination with trastuzumab and docetaxel in HER2 positive metastatic breast cancer. Invest New Drugs. 2014;32:1285–94.

70. Rugo HS, Chien AJ, Franco SX, Stopeck AT, Glencer A, Lahiri S, et al. A phase II study of lapatinib and bevacizumab as treatment for HER2-overexpressing metastatic breast cancer. Breast Cancer Res Treat. 2012;134:13–20.

71. Falchook GS, Moulder S, Naing A, Wheler JJ, Hong DS, Piha-Paul SA, et al. A phase I trial of combination trastuzumab, lapatinib, and bevacizumab in patients with advanced cancer. Invest New Drugs. 2015;33:177–86.

72. Gianni L, Romieu GH, Lichinitser M, Serrano SV, Mansutti M, Pivot X, et al. AVEREL: a randomized phase III trial evaluating bevacizumab in combination with docetaxel and trastuzumab as first-line therapy for HER2-positive locally recurrent/metastatic breast cancer. J Clin Oncol. 2013;31:1719–25.

73. Arteaga CL, Mayer IA, O'Neill AM, Swaby RF, Alpaugh RK, Yang XJ, et al. A randomized phase III double-blinded placebo-controlled trial of first-line chemotherapy and trastuzumab with or without bevacizumab for patients with HER2/neu-overexpressing metastatic breast cancer (HER2+ MBC): a trial of the Eastern Cooperative Oncology Group (E1105). J Clin Oncol. 2012;30(Suppl):abstr 605.

74. Miller KD, O'Neill A, Perez EA, Seidman AD, Sledge GW. A phase II pilot trial incorporating bevacizumab into dose-dense doxorubicin and cyclophosphamide

followed by paclitaxel in patients with lymph node positive breast cancer: a trial coordinated by the Eastern Cooperative Oncology Group. Ann Oncol. 2012;23:331–7.

75. Miller K, O'Neill AM, Dang CT, Northfelt DW, Gradishar WJ, Goldstein LJ, et al. Bevacizumab (Bv) in the adjuvant treatment of HER2-negative breast cancer: final results from Eastern Cooperative Oncology Group E5103. J Clin Oncol. 2014;32(Suppl): abstr 500.

76. Cameron D, Brown J, Dent R, Jackisch C, Mackey J, Pivot X, et al. Adjuvant bevacizumab-containing therapy in triple-negative breast cancer (BEATRICE): primary results of a randomised, phase 3 trial. Lancet Oncol. 2013;14:933–42.

77. Bell R, Brown J, Parmar M, Toi M, Suter T, Steger G, et al. Final efficacy and updated safety results of the randomized phase III BEATRICE trial evaluating adjuvant bevacizumab (BEV)-containing therapy for early triple-negative breast cancer (TNBC). 37th Annual San Antonio Breast Cancer Symposium, San Antonio-Texas, 9–13 Dec 2014, abstr: PD2-2.

78. Slamon DJ, Swain SM, Buyse M, Martin M, Geyer CE, Im Y-H, et al. Primary results from BETH, a phase 3 controlled study of adjuvant chemotherapy and trastuzumab ± bevacizumab in patients with HER2-positive, node-positive or high risk node-negative breast cancer. Cancer Res. 2013;73(24 Suppl):abstr S1-03.

79. Greil R, Moik M, Reitsamer R, Ressler S, Stoll M, Namberger K, et al. Neoadjuvant bevacizumab, docetaxel and capecitabine combination therapy for HER2/neu-negative invasive breast cancer: efficacy and safety in a phase II pilot study. Eur J Surg Oncol. 2009;35:1048–54.

80. Rastogi P, Buyse ME, Swain SM, Jacobs SA, Robidoux A, Liepman MK, et al. Concurrent bevacizumab with a sequential regimen of doxorubicin and cyclophosphamide followed by docetaxel and capecitabine as neoadjuvant therapy for HER2-locally advanced breast cancer: a phase II trial of the NSABP Foundation Research Group. Clin Breast Cancer. 2011;11:228–34.

81. Kim HR, Jung KH, Im SA, Im YH, Kang SY, Park KH, et al. Multicentre phase II trial of bevacizumab combined with docetaxel-carboplatin for the neoadjuvant treatment of triple-negative breast cancer (KCSG BR-0905). Ann Oncol. 2013;24:1485–90.

82. Sánchez-Rovira P, Seguí MA, Llombart A, Aranda E, Antón A, Sánchez A, et al. Bevacizumab plus preoperative chemotherapy in operable HER2 negative breast cancer: biomarkers and pathologic response. Clin Transl Oncol. 2013;15:810–7.

83. Bear HD, Tang G, Rastogi P, Geyer Jr CE, Robidoux A, Atkins JN, et al. Bevacizumab added to neoadjuvant chemotherapy for breast cancer. N Engl J Med. 2012;366:310–20.

84. Golshan M, Garber JE, Gelman R, Tung N, Smith BL, Troyan S, et al. Does neoadjuvant bevacizumab

increase surgical complications in breast surgery? Ann Surg Oncol. 2011;18:733–7.

85. Kansal KJ, Dominici LS, Tolaney SM, Isakoff SJ, Smith BL, Jiang W, et al. Neoadjuvant bevacizumab: surgical complications of mastectomy with and without reconstruction. Breast Cancer Res Treat. 2013;141:255–9.

86. Bear HD, Tang G, Rastogi P, Geyer CE, Liu Q, Robidoux A, et al. The effect on overall and disease-free survival (OS & DFS) by adding bevacizumab and/or antimetabolites to standard neoadjuvant chemotherapy: NSABP Protocol B-40. 37th Annual San Antonio Breast Cancer Symposium, San Antonio-Texas, 9–13 Dec 2014, abstr: PD2-1.

87. von Minckwitz G, Eidtmann H, Rezai M, Fasching PA, Tesch H, Eggemann H, German Breast Group, Arbeitsgemeinschaft Gynäkologische Onkologie–Breast Study Groups, et al. Neoadjuvant chemotherapy and bevacizumab for HER2-negative breast cancer. N Engl J Med. 2012;366:299–309.

88. A multicenter, placebo-controlled, double-blind randomized phase II trial of neoadjuvant treatment with single-agent bevacizumab or placebo, followed by six cycles of docetaxel, doxorubicin, and cyclophosphamide (TAC), with or without bevacizumab in patients with stage II or stage III breast cancer. ClinicalTrials.gov Identifier: NCT00203372.

89. Sikov WM, Berry DA, Perou CM, Singh B, Cirrincione CT, Tolaney SM, et al. Impact of the addition of carboplatin and/or bevacizumab to neoadjuvant once-per-week paclitaxel followed by dose-dense doxorubicin and cyclophosphamide on pathologic complete response rates in stage II to III triple-negative breast cancer: CALGB 40603 (alliance). J Clin Oncol. 2015;33:13–21.

90. Chen XS, Yuan Y, Garfield DH, Wu JY, Huang O, Shen KW. Both carboplatin and bevacizumab improve pathological complete remission rate in neoadjuvant treatment of triple negative breast cancer: a meta-analysis. PLoS One. 2014;9, e108405.

91. Earl HM, Hiller L, Blenkinsop C, Grybowicz L, Vallier A, Abraham J, et al, for ARTemis Investigators. ARTemis: a randomised trial of bevacizumab with neoadjuvant chemotherapy (NACT) for patients with HER2-negative early breast cancer-Primary endpoint, pathological complete response (pCR). J Clin Oncol. 2014;32(Suppl):abstr 1014.

92. Rydén L, Stendahl M, Jonsson H, Emdin S, Bengtsson NO, Landberg G. Tumor-specific VEGF-A and VEGFR2 in postmenopausal breast cancer patients with long-term follow-up. Implication of a link between VEGF pathway and tamoxifen response. Breast Cancer Res Treat. 2005;89:135–43.

93. Rydén L, Jirström K, Bendahl PO, Fernö M, Nordenskjöld B, Stål O, et al. Tumor-specific expression of vascular endothelial growth factor receptor 2 but not vascular endothelial growth factor or human epidermal growth factor receptor 2 is associated with impaired response to adjuvant tamoxifen in premenopausal breast cancer. J Clin Oncol. 2005;23:4695–704.

94. Forero-Torres A, Saleh MN, Galleshaw JA, Jones CF, Shah JJ, Percent IJ, et al. Pilot trial of preoperative (neoadjuvant) letrozole in combination with bevacizumab in postmenopausal women with newly diagnosed estrogen receptor- or progesterone receptor-positive breast cancer. Clin Breast Cancer. 2010;10:275–80.

95. Yardley DA, Raefsky E, Castillo R, Lahiry A, Locicero R, Thompson D, et al. Phase II study of neoadjuvant weekly nab-paclitaxel and carboplatin, with bevacizumab and trastuzumab, as treatment for women with locally advanced HER2+ breast cancer. Clin Breast Cancer. 2011;11:297–305.

96. Pierga JY, Petit T, Delozier T, Ferrero JM, Campone M, Gligorov J, et al. Neoadjuvant bevacizumab, trastuzumab, and chemotherapy for primary inflammatory HER2-positive breast cancer (BEVERLY-2): an open-label, single-arm phase 2 study. Lancet Oncol. 2012;13:375–84.

97. Pierga JY, Petit T, Levy C, Ferrero JM, Campone M, Gligorov J, et al. Pathological response and circulating tumor cell count identifies treated HER2+ inflammatory breast cancer patients with excellent prognosis: BEVERLY-2 survival data. Clin Cancer Res. 2015;21(6):1298–304.

98. Fernandez M, Calvo I, Martinez N, Herrero M, Quijano Y, Duran H, et al. Final results of neoadjuvant trial of bevacizumab (B) and trastuzumab (T) in combination with weekly paclitaxel (P) as neoadjuvant treatment in HER2-positive breast cancer: a phase II trial (AVANTHER). Cancer Res. 2012;72 (Suppl):abstr P1-14-10.

99. Coudert B, Pierga JY, Mouret-Reynier MA, Kerrou K, Ferrero JM, Petit T, et al. Use of [(18)F]-FDG PET to predict response to neoadjuvant trastuzumab and docetaxel in patients with HER2-positive breast cancer, and addition of bevacizumab to neoadjuvant trastuzumab and docetaxel in [(18)F]-FDG PET-predicted non-responders (AVATAXHER): an open-label, randomised phase 2 trial. Lancet Oncol. 2014;15:1493–502.

100. Teng LS, Jin KT, He KF, Zhang J, Wang HH, Cao J. Clinical applications of VEGF-trap (aflibercept) in cancer treatment. J Chin Med Assoc. 2010;73: 449–56.

101. Presta LG, Chen H, O'Connor SJ, Chisholm V, Meng YG, Krummen L, et al. Humanization of an anti-vascular endothelial growth factor monoclonal antibody for the therapy of solid tumors and other disorders. Cancer Res. 1997;57:4593–9.

102. Rudge JS, Holash J, Hylton D, Russell M, Jiang S, Leidich R, et al. VEGF Trap complex formation measures production rates of VEGF, providing a biomarker for predicting efficacious angiogenic blockade. Proc Natl Acad Sci U S A. 2007;104: 18363–70.

103. Holash J, Davis S, Papadopoulos N, Croll SD, Ho L, Russell M, et al. VEGF-Trap: a VEGF blocker with potent antitumor effects. Proc Natl Acad Sci U S A. 2002;99:11393–8.

104. Huang J, Frischer JS, Serur A, Kadenhe A, Yokoi A, McCrudden KW, et al. Regression of established tumors and metastases by potent vascular endothelial growth factor blockade. Proc Natl Acad Sci U S A. 2003;100:7785–90.

105. Tew WP, Gordon M, Murren J, Dupont J, Pezzulli S, Aghajanian C, et al. Phase 1 study of aflibercept administered subcutaneously to patients with advanced solid tumors. Clin Cancer Res. 2010;16:358–66.

106. Lockhart AC, Rothenberg ML, Dupont J, Cooper W, Chevalier P, Sternas L, et al. Phase I study of intravenous vascular endothelial growth factor trap, aflibercept, in patients with advanced solid tumors. J Clin Oncol. 2010;28:207–14.

107. Isambert N, Freyer G, Zanetta S, You B, Fumoleau P, Falandry C, et al. Phase I dose-escalation study of intravenous aflibercept in combination with docetaxel in patients with advanced solid tumors. Clin Cancer Res. 2012;18:1743–50.

108. Van Cutsem E, Tabernero J, Lakomy R, Prenen H, Prausová J, Macarulla T, et al. Addition of aflibercept to fluorouracil, leucovorin, and irinotecan improves survival in a phase III randomized trial in patients with metastatic colorectal cancer previously treated with an oxaliplatin-based regimen. J Clin Oncol. 2012;30:3499–506.

109. Sideras K, Dueck AC, Hobday TJ, Rowland Jr KM, Allred JB, Northfelt DW, et al. North central cancer treatment group (NCCTG) N0537: phase II trial of VEGF-trap in patients with metastatic breast cancer previously treated with an anthracycline and/or a taxane. Clin Breast Cancer. 2012;12:387–91.

110. Krupitskaya Y, Wakelee HA. Ramucirumab, a fully human mAb to the transmembrane signaling tyrosine kinase VEGFR-2 for the potential treatment of cancer. Curr Opin Investig Drugs. 2009;10:597–605.

111. Spratlin J. Ramucirumab (IMC-1121B): monoclonal antibody inhibition of vascular endothelial growth factor receptor-2. Curr Oncol Rep. 2011;13:97–102.

112. Spratlin JL, Cohen RB, Eadens M, Gore L, Camidge DR, Diab S, et al. Phase I pharmacologic and biologic study of ramucirumab (IMC-1121B), a fully human immunoglobulin G1 monoclonal antibody targeting the vascular endothelial growth factor receptor-2. J Clin Oncol. 2010;28:780–7.

113. Camidge DR, Ballas MS, Dubey S, Haigentz M, Rosen PJ, Spicer JF, West HJ, et al. A phase II, open-label study of ramucirumab (IMC-1121B), an IgG1 fully human monoclonal antibody (MAb) targeting VEGFR-2, in combination with paclitaxel and carboplatin as first-line therapy in patients (pts) with stage IIIb/IV non-small cell lung cancer (NSCLC). J Clin Oncol. 2010;28(Suppl):abstr 7588.

114. Camidge DR, Doebele RC, Ballas M, Jahan T, Haigentz M, Hoffman D, et al. Final Results of a phase 2, open-label study of Ramucirumab (IMC-1121B; RAM), an IgG1 mab targeting VEGFR-2, with paclitaxel and carboplatin as first-line therapy in patients (pts) with stage IIIB/IV non-small cell lung cancer (NSCLC) (NCT00735696). Ann Oncol. 2012;23 suppl 9:400–46.

115. Fuchs CS, Tomasek J, Cho JY, Dumitru F, Passalacqua R, Goswami C, et al. REGARD: a phase III, randomized, double-blinded trial of ramucirumab and best supportive care (BSC) versus placebo and BSC in the treatment of metastatic gastric or gastroesophageal junction (GEJ) adenocarcinoma following disease progression on first-line platinum- and/or fluoropyrimidine-containing combination therapy. J Clin Oncol. 2012;30(Suppl 34):abstr LBA5.

116. Mackey JR, Ramos-Vazquez M, Lipatov O, McCarthy N, Krasnozhon D, Semiglazov V, et al. Primary results of ROSE/TRIO-12, a randomized placebo-controlled phase III trial evaluating the addition of ramucirumab to first-line docetaxel chemotherapy in metastatic breast cancer. J Clin Oncol. 2015;33:141–8.

117. Patyna S, Laird AD, Mendel DB, O'farrell AM, Liang C, Guan H, et al. SU14813: a novel multiple receptor tyrosine kinase inhibitor with potent antiangiogenic and antitumor activity. Mol Cancer Ther. 2006;5(7):1774–82.

118. Chow LQ, Eckhardt SG. Sunitinib: from rational design to clinical efficacy. J Clin Oncol. 2007;25:884–96.

119. Murray LJ, Abrams TJ, Long KR, Ngai TJ, Olson LM, Hong W, et al. SU11248 inhibits tumor growth and CSF-1R-dependent osteolysis in an experimental breast cancer bone metastasis model. Clin Exp Metastasis. 2003;20:757–66.

120. Abrams TJ, Murray LJ, Pesenti E, Holway VW, Colombo T, Lee LB, et al. Preclinical evaluation of the tyrosine kinase inhibitor SU11248 as a single agent and in combination with "standard of care" therapeutic agents for the treatment of breast cancer. Mol Cancer Ther. 2003;2:1011–21.

121. Faivre S, Delbaldo C, Vera K, Robert C, Lozahic S, Lassau N, et al. Safety, pharmacokinetic, and antitumor activity of SU11248, a novel oral multitarget tyrosine kinase inhibitor, in patients with cancer. J Clin Oncol. 2006;24:25–35.

122. Sweeney CJ, Chiorean EG, Verschraegen CF, Lee FC, Jones S, Royce M, et al. A phase I study of sunitinib plus capecitabine in patients with advanced solid tumors. J Clin Oncol. 2010;28:4513–20.

123. Robert F, Sandler A, Schiller JH, Liu G, Harper K, Verkh L, et al. Sunitinib in combination with docetaxel in patients with advanced solid tumors: a phase I dose-escalation study. Cancer Chemother Pharmacol. 2010;66:669–80.

124. Burstein HJ, Elias AD, Rugo HS, Cobleigh MA, Wolff AC, Eisenberg PD, et al. Phase II study of sunitinib malate, an oral multitargeted tyrosine kinase inhibitor, in patients with metastatic breast cancer previously treated with an anthracycline and a taxane. J Clin Oncol. 2008;26:1810–6.

125. Kozloff M, Chuang E, Starr A, Gowland PA, Cataruozolo PE, Collier M, et al. An exploratory study of sunitinib plus paclitaxel as first-line treatment for patients with advanced breast cancer. Ann Oncol. 2010;21:1436–41.

126. Robert NJ, Saleh MN, Paul D, Generali D, Gressot L, Copur MS, et al. Sunitinib plus paclitaxel versus bevacizumab plus paclitaxel for first-line treatment of patients with advanced breast cancer: a phase III, randomized, open-label trial. Clin Breast Cancer. 2011;11:82–92.

127. Mayer EL, Dhakil S, Patel T, Sundaram S, Fabian C, Kozloff M, et al. SABRE-B: an evaluation of paclitaxel and bevacizumab with or without sunitinib as first-line treatment of metastatic breast cancer. Ann Oncol. 2010;21:2370–6.

128. Bergh J, Bondarenko IM, Lichinitser MR, Liljegren A, Greil R, Voytko NL, et al. First-line treatment of advanced breast cancer with sunitinib in combination with docetaxel versus docetaxel alone: results of a prospective, randomized phase III study. J Clin Oncol. 2012;30:921–9.

129. Cardoso F, Canon JL, Amadori D, Aldrighetti D, Machiels JP, Bouko Y, et al. An exploratory study of sunitinib in combination with docetaxel and trastuzumab as first-line therapy for HER2-positive metastatic breast cancer. Breast. 2012;21:716–23.

130. Barrios CH, Liu MC, Lee SC, Vanlemmens L, Ferrero JM, Tabei T, Pivot X, Iwata H, Aogi K, Lugo-Quintana R, Harbeck N, Brickman MJ, Zhang K, Kern KA, Martin M. Phase III randomized trial of sunitinib versus capecitabine in patients with previously treated HER2-negative advanced breast cancer. Breast Cancer Res Treat. 2010;121:121–31.

131. Crown JP, Diéras V, Staroslawska E, Yardley DA, Bachelot T, Davidson N, et al. Phase III trial of sunitinib in combination with capecitabine versus capecitabine monotherapy for the treatment of patients with pretreated metastatic breast cancer. J Clin Oncol. 2013;31:2870–8.

132. Wildiers H, Fontaine C, Vuylsteke P, Martens M, Canon JL, Wynendaele W, et al. Multicenter phase II randomized trial evaluating antiangiogenic therapy with sunitinib as consolidation after objective response to taxane chemotherapy in women with HER2-negative metastatic breast cancer. Breast Cancer Res Treat. 2010;123:463–9.

133. DA Yardley, NW Peacock, J Peyton, DL Shipley, S Spigel, J Barton, et al. Neoadjuvant sunitinib administered with weekly paclitaxel/carboplatin in patients with locally advanced triple-negative breast cancer: a Sarah Cannon Research Institute Phase I/II Trial. Cancer Res. 2011;71(24 Suppl):Abstract nr P3-14-29.

134. Ahlgren P, Thirlwell M, O'Regan R, Mormont C, Levesque L, Gaspo R, et al. An open-label study of sunitinib (SU) plus exemestane (E) in the first-line treatment of hormone receptor (HR)-positive metastatic breast cancer (MBC). J Clin Oncol. 2009; 27(Suppl):abstr e12019.

135. Pilot/phase II randomised, double blind, placebo controlled multicenter study with biomarker evaluation of neoadjuvant exemestane in combination with sunitinib in post-menopausal women with hormone-sensitive, Her-2 negative primar breast cancer. ClinicalTrials.gov Identifier:NCT00931450.

136. Strumberg D, Richly H, Hilger RA, Schleucher N, Korfee S, Tewes M, et al. Phase I clinical and pharmacokinetic study of the Novel Raf kinase and vascular endothelial growth factor receptor inhibitor BAY 43-9006 in patients with advanced refractory solid tumors. J Clin Oncol. 2005;23:965–72.

137. Wilhelm SM, Carter C, Tang L, Wilkie D, McNabola A, Rong H, et al. BAY 43-9006 exhibits broad spectrum oral antitumor activity and targets the RAF/MEK/ERK pathway and receptor tyrosine kinases involved in tumor progression and angiogenesis. Cancer Res. 2004;64:7099–109.

138. Wilhelm S, Chien DS. BAY 43-9006: preclinical data. Curr Pharm Des. 2002;8:2255–7.

139. Gianpaolo-Ostravage C, Carter C, Hibner B, Bankston D, Natero R, Monahan MC, et al. Antitumor efficacy of the orally active raf kinase inhibitor BAY 43-9006 in human tumor xenograft models. Proc Am Assoc Cancer Res. 2001;42:Abstr 4954.

140. Llovet JM, Ricci S, Mazzaferro V, Hilgard P, Gane E, Blanc JF, SHARP Investigators Study Group, et al. Sorafenib in advanced hepatocellular carcinoma. N Engl J Med. 2008;359:378–90.

141. Escudier B, Eisen T, Stadler WM, Szczylik C, Oudard S, Siebels M, TARGET Study Group, et al. Sorafenib in advanced clear-cell renal-cell carcinoma. N Engl J Med. 2007;356:125–34.

142. Escudier B, Eisen T, Stadler WM, Szczylik C, Oudard S, Staehler M, et al. Sorafenib for treatment of renal cell carcinoma: final efficacy and safety results of the phase III treatment approaches in renal cancer global evaluation trial. J Clin Oncol. 2009;27:3312–8.

143. Moreno-Aspitia A, Morton RF, Hillman DW, Lingle WL, Rowland Jr KM, Wiesenfeld M, et al. Phase II trial of sorafenib in patients with metastatic breast cancer previously exposed to anthracyclines or taxanes: North Central Cancer Treatment Group and Mayo Clinic Trial N0336. J Clin Oncol. 2009; 27:11–5.

144. Bianchi G, Loibl S, Zamagni C, Salvagni S, Raab G, Siena S, et al. Phase II multicenter, uncontrolled trial of sorafenib in patients with metastatic breast cancer. Anticancer Drugs. 2009;20:616–24.

145. Baselga J, Segalla JG, Roché H, Del Giglio A, Pinczowski H, Ciruelos EM, et al. Sorafenib in combination with capecitabine: an oral regimen for patients with HER2-negative locally advanced or metastatic breast cancer. J Clin Oncol. 2012;30: 1484–91.

146. Baselga J, Costa F, Gomez H, Hudis CA, Rapoport B, Roche H, et al. A phase 3 tRial comparing capecitabinE in combination with SorafenIb or pLacebo for treatment of locally advanced or metastatIc HER2-Negative breast CancEr (the RESILIENCE study): study protocol for a randomized controlled trial. Trials. 2013;14:228.

147. Gradishar WJ, Kaklamani V, Sahoo TP, Lokanatha D, Raina V, Bondarde S, et al. A double-blind, randomised, placebo-controlled, phase 2b study evaluating sorafenib

in combination with paclitaxel as a first-line therapy in patients with HER2-negative advanced breast cancer. Eur J Cancer. 2013;49:312–22.

148. Isaacs C, Herbolsheimer P, Liu MC, Wilkinson M, Ottaviano Y, Chung GG, et al. Phase I/II study of sorafenib with anastrozole in patients with hormone receptor positive aromatase inhibitor resistant metastatic breast cancer. Breast Cancer Res Treat. 2011;125:137–43.

149. Mina LA, Yu M, Johnson C, Burkhardt C, Miller KD, Zon R. A phase II study of combined VEGF inhibitor (bevacizumab+sorafenib) in patients with metastatic breast cancer: Hoosier Oncology Group Study BRE06-109. Invest New Drugs. 2013;31: 1307–10.

150. Chen J, Tian CX, Yu M, Lv Q, Cheng NS, Wang Z, et al. Efficacy and safety profile of combining sorafenib with chemotherapy in patients with HER2-negative advanced breast cancer: a meta-analysis. J Breast Cancer. 2014;17:61–8.

151. Tan QX, Qin QH, Lian B, Yang WP, Wei CY. Sorafenib-based therapy in HER2-negative advanced breast cancer: results from a retrospective pooled analysis of randomized controlled trials. Exp Ther Med. 2014;7:1420–6.

152. Sonpavde G, Hutson TE. Pazopanib: a novel multitargeted tyrosine kinase inhibitor. Curr Oncol Rep. 2007;9:115–9.

153. Hurwitz HI, Dowlati A, Saini S, Savage S, Suttle AB, Gibson DM, et al. Phase I trial of pazopanib in patients with advanced cancer. Clin Cancer Res. 2009;15:4220–7.

154. Taylor SK, Chia S, Dent S, Clemons M, Agulnik M, Grenci P, et al. A phase II study of pazopanib in patients with recurrent or metastatic invasive breast carcinoma: a trial of the Princess Margaret Hospital phase II consortium. Oncologist. 2010;15:810–8.

155. Tan AR, Johannes H, Rastogi P, Jacobs SA, Robidoux A, Flynn PJ, et al. Weekly paclitaxel and concurrent pazopanib following doxorubicin and cyclophosphamide as neoadjuvant therapy for HER-negative locally advanced breast cancer: NSABP Foundation FB-6, a phase II study. Breast Cancer Res Treat. 2015;149(1): 163–9.

156. de Jonge MJ, Hamberg P, Verweij J, Savage S, Suttle AB, Hodge J, et al. Phase I and pharmacokinetic study of pazopanib and lapatinib combination therapy in patients with advanced solid tumors. Invest New Drugs. 2013;31:751–9.

157. Johnston SR, Gómez H, Stemmer SM, Richie M, Durante M, Pandite L, et al. A randomized and open-label trial evaluating the addition of pazopanib to lapatinib as first-line therapy in patients with HER2-positive advanced breast cancer. Breast Cancer Res Treat. 2013;137:755–66.

158. Cristofanilli M, Johnston SR, Manikhas A, Gomez HL, Gladkov O, Shao Z, et al. A randomized phase II study of lapatinib + pazopanib versus lapatinib in patients with HER2+ inflammatory breast cancer. Breast Cancer Res Treat. 2013;137:471–82.

159. Rosen LS, Kurzrock R, Mulay M, Van Vugt A, Purdom M, Ng C, et al. Safety, pharmacokinetics, and efficacy of AMG 706, an oral multikinase inhibitor, in patients with advanced solid tumors. J Clin Oncol. 2007;25:2369–76.

160. Coxon A, Bush T, Saffran D, Kaufman S, Belmontes B, Rex K, et al. Broad antitumor activity in breast cancer xenografts by motesanib, a highly selective, oral inhibitor of vascular endothelial growth factor, platelet-derived growth factor, and kit receptors. Clin Cancer Res. 2009;15:110–8.

161. De Boer RH, Kotasek D, White S, Koczwara B, Mainwaring P, Chan A, et al. Phase 1b dose-finding study of motesanib with docetaxel or paclitaxel in patients with metastatic breast cancer. Breast Cancer Res Treat. 2012;135:241–52.

162. Martin M, Roche H, Pinter T, Crown J, Kennedy MJ, Provencher L, TRIO 010 investigators, et al. Motesanib, or open-label bevacizumab, in combination with paclitaxel, as first-line treatment for HER2-negative locally recurrent or metastatic breast cancer: a phase 2, randomised, double-blind, placebo-controlled study. Lancet Oncol. 2011;12:369–76.

163. Choueiri TK. Axitinib, a novel anti-angiogenic drug with promising activity in various solid tumors. Curr Opin Investig Drugs. 2008;9:658–71.

164. Wilmes LJ, Pallavicini MG, Fleming LM, Gibbs J, Wang D, Li KL, et al. AG-013736, a novel inhibitor of VEGF receptor tyrosine kinases, inhibits breast cancer growth and decreases vascular permeability as detected by dynamic contrast-enhanced magnetic resonance imaging. Magn Reson Imaging. 2007; 25:319–27.

165. Rugo HS, Herbst RS, Liu G, Park JW, Kies MS, Steinfeldt HM, et al. Phase I trial of the oral antiangiogenesis agent AG-013736 in patients with advanced solid tumors: pharmacokinetic and clinical results. J Clin Oncol. 2005;23:5474–83.

166. Rugo HS, Stopeck AT, Joy AA, Chan S, Verma S, Lluch A, et al. Randomized, placebo-controlled, double-blind, phase II study of axitinib plus docetaxel versus docetaxel plus placebo in patients with metastatic breast cancer. J Clin Oncol. 2011;29:2459–65.

167. Morabito A, Piccirillo MC, Falasconi F, De Feo G, Del Giudice A, Bryce J, et al. Vandetanib (ZD6474), a dual inhibitor of vascular endothelial growth factor receptor (VEGFR) and epidermal growth factor receptor (EGFR) tyrosine kinases: current status and future directions. Oncologist. 2009;14:378–90.

168. Wedge SR, Ogilvie DJ, Dukes M, Kendrew J, Chester R, Jackson JA, et al. ZD6474 inhibits vascular endothelial growth factor signaling, angiogenesis, and tumor growth following oral administration. Cancer Res. 2002;62:4645–55.

169. Ciardiello F, Caputo R, Damiano V, Caputo R, Troiani T, Vitagliano D, et al. Antitumor effects of ZD6474, a small molecule vascular endothelial growth factor receptor tyrosine kinase inhibitor, with additional activity against epidermal growth factor

receptor tyrosine kinase. Clin Cancer Res. 2003;9: 1546–56.

170. Holden SN, Eckhardt SG, Basser R, de Boer R, Rischin D, Green M, et al. Clinical evaluation of ZD6474, an orally active inhibitor of VEGF and EGF receptor signaling, in patients with solid, malignant tumors. Ann Oncol. 2005;16:1391–7.

171. Miller KD, Trigo JM, Wheeler C, Barge A, Rowbottom J, Sledge G, et al. A multicenter phase II trial of ZD6474, a vascular endothelial growth factor receptor-2 and epidermal growth factor receptor tyrosine kinase inhibitor, in patients with previously treated metastatic breast cancer. Clin Cancer Res. 2005;11:3369–76.

172. Boér K, Láng I, Llombart-Cussac A, Andreasson I, Vivanco GL, Sanders N, et al. Vandetanib with docetaxel as second-line treatment for advanced breast cancer: a double-blind, placebo-controlled, randomized Phase II study. Invest New Drugs. 2012;30:681–7.

173. A randomised, double-blind, parallel- group, multicentre, phase II study to evaluate the safety and pharmacological activity of the combination of vandetanib (100 or 300 MG/ daily or placebo) with fulvestrant (loading dose), in postmenopausal advanced breast cancer patients. ClinicalTrials.gov Identifier: NCT00752986.

174. Clemons MJ, Cochrane B, Pond GR, Califaretti N, Chia SK, Dent RA, et al. Randomised, phase II,

placebo-controlled, trial of fulvestrant plus vandetanib in postmenopausal women with bone only or bone predominant, hormone-receptor-positive metastatic breast cancer (MBC): the OCOG ZAMBONEY study. Breast Cancer Res Treat. 2014;146:153–62.

175. Jost LM, Gschwind HP, Jalava T, Wang Y, Guenther C, Souppart C, et al. Metabolism and disposition of vatalanib (PTK787/ZK-222584) in cancer patients. Drug Metab Dispos. 2006;34:1817–28.

176. Banerjee S, A'Hern R, Detre S, Littlewood-Evans AJ, Evans DB, Dowsett M, et al. Biological evidence for dual antiangiogenic-antiaromatase activity of the VEGFR inhibitor PTK787/ZK222584 in vivo. Clin Cancer Res. 2010;16:4178–87.

177. Banerjee S, Zvelebil M, Furet P, Mueller-Vieira U, Evans DB, Dowsett M, et al. The vascular endothelial growth factor receptor inhibitor PTK787/ZK222584 inhibits aromatase. Cancer Res. 2009;69:4716–23.

178. Thomas AL, Morgan B, Horsfield MA, Higginson A, Kay A, Lee L, et al. Phase I study of the safety, tolerability, pharmacokinetics, and pharmacodynamics of PTK787/ZK 222584 administered twice daily in patients with advanced cancer. J Clin Oncol. 2005;23:4162–71.

179. A phase I/II study of PTK787 in combination with trastuzumab in patients with newly diagnosed HER2 overexpressing locally recurrent or metastatic breast cancer: Hoosier Oncology Group Trial BRE04-80. ClinicalTrials.gov Identifier: NCT00216047.

Tyrosine Kinase Inhibitors

36

Burcu Cakar and Erdem Göker

Abstract

Breast cancer is the most common cancer in women worldwide. Although various subgroups are defined according to the expression of hormones and ErbB family receptors, it is well known that this disease is more heterogeneous than its classification system suggests. As new effective therapeutic choices are developed and used clinically, resistance to these new agents is also being observed. The most promising new anti-HER therapies are T-DM1 and pertuzumab, which has been evaluated in trastuzumab-resistant patients and also in a first-line setting with trastuzumab. The dual blockage of HER seems to be a favorable approach for these patients; however, the downstream signaling steps can be activated to overcome the tyrosine kinase inhibition. Because tumor cells can adapt themselves by using alternative pathways to maintain proliferation, providing a sufficient treatment approach also requires the consideration of possible escape mechanisms in tumor cells. By inhibiting tyrosine kinases combined with another agent that affects downstream factors of the PI3K/AKT/mTOR pathway, drug resistance in breast cancer can be overcome or delayed. In this chapter, we discuss the new tyrosine kinase inhibitors that inhibit more than only HER-2 and discuss some ongoing clinical trials in this area. In so doing, we hope to provide information for overcoming tyrosine kinase drug resistance and to identify the ideal settings for these treatment choices according to recent data.

B. Cakar, MD
Department of Medical Oncology, Tulay Aktaş Oncology Hospital, Ege University Medical Faculty, Kazım Dirik Mahallesi, Bornova, Izmir 35040, Turkey

Medical Oncology Unit, Yunus Emre State Hospital Tepebasi, Eskisehir, Turkey
e-mail: burcu.cakar@gmail.com

E. Göker, MD (✉)
Department of Medical Oncology, Tulay Aktaş Oncology Hospital, Ege University Medical Faculty, Kazım Dirik Mahallesi, Bornova, Izmir 35040, Turkey
e-mail: erdem.goker@gmail.com

© Springer International Publishing Switzerland 2016
A. Aydiner et al. (eds.), *Breast Disease: Management and Therapies*,
DOI 10.1007/978-3-319-26012-9_36

Keywords

T-DM 1 • Pertuzumab • Neratinib • Afatinib • Everolimus • PI3K inhibitors • Pan-HER inhibitors • Gefitinib • Lapatinib

A tyrosine kinase is an enzyme that phosphorylates tyrosine residues in proteins to regulate signaling within a cell. In normal conditions, tyrosine kinase activity is regulated by strict mechanisms; however, this tight control is lost in cancer cells, which results in uncontrolled cell proliferation, differentiation, apoptosis, and invasion [1]. Because tyrosine kinases are the driving step in cell signaling, tyrosine kinase inhibitors (TKIs) can serve as a therapeutic option for breast cancer patients. In this chapter, we will review the monoclonal antibodies targeting tyrosine kinase receptors and the small molecule TKIs that serve as anticancer agents, and we will also discuss the newer therapeutic options developed to overcome drug resistance in breast cancer.

Introduction

Receptor tyrosine kinases have three different major domains—the extracellular domains (domains I–IV), the transmembrane domain, and the juxtamembrane domain. Upon ligand binding, two receptor tyrosine kinases homo- or heterodimerize and tyrosine residues are phosphorylated to activate the downstream signaling cascade. Nearly 90 tyrosine kinases have been identified in humans including receptor tyrosine kinases and cellular tyrosine kinases [2].

Among these, the epidermal growth factor receptor family (EGFR, ErbB) and VEGF are the primary targets studied in breast cancer. Four members of ErbB receptor family have been identified: (1) EGFR (ErbB1), (2) HER-2 (ErbB2), (3) HER-3 (ErbB3), and (4) HER-4 (ErbB4).

Within the ErbB family, HER-2 is the preferred dimerization partner because its kinase catalytic activity is most potent, and it does not require a ligand for dimerization. HER-2 overexpression is observed in 15–30 % of breast cancers

and is associated with poorer prognosis. Trastuzumab, a humanized monoclonal anti-HER-2 antibody, binds to the extracellular domain of HER-2 (subdomain IV) and leads to a conformational change. Previous studies have confirmed that via different mechanisms, including antibody-dependent cell-mediated cytotoxicity, downstream pathway inhibition, and dimerization prevention, trastuzumab exerts antitumor activity. Although the agent achieves its efficacy by various mechanisms, the majority of HER-2-positive tumors develop resistance to treatment. Increased MUC-4 expression, alternative downstream PI3K–AKT pathway activation, PTEN loss, truncated p95 expression, and p27 downregulation are possible reasons for trastuzumab resistance.

The majority of targeted therapy studies have attempted to overcome these resistance mechanisms by targeting various steps of the tyrosine kinase activation cascade or by using a combination of new anti-HER-2 therapies targeting the HER-2 signaling network at multiple points.

Anti-HER-2 Therapies

Lapatinib

Lapatinib is an orally active dual inhibitor of EGFR and HER-2. Preclinical studies demonstrated that lapatinib could inhibit trastuzumab-resistant HER-2(+) breast cancer by binding to truncated p95 [3, 4]. In the metastatic first-line setting, a lapatinib/chemotherapy combination is approved for use following disease progression in patients previously treated with trastuzumab. In this setting, paclitaxel–lapatinib combination therapy significantly improved event-free survival (EFS), the time to progression (TTP), and the clinical benefit rate (CBR) without any overall survival (OS) advantage compared with paclitaxel–placebo in a phase III study [5]. In subsequent settings, lapatinib/capecitabine and lapatinib/trastuzumab are possible therapeutic options [6, 7]. The combination of lapatinib and trastuzumab, by blocking HER-2 through different mechanisms, appears to be a good choice. EGF104900 study data demonstrated that lapatinib plus trastuzumab improved PFS, and the clinical benefit was comparable to lapatinib monotherapy [7, 8]. However, it is not clear whether the sequential or combined use of these agents will establish better results. An ongoing phase III study, NCT00968968, evaluating the efficacy of lapatinib plus trastuzumab versus trastuzumab alone to enable continuous HER-2 suppression after first- or second-line trastuzumab-based chemotherapy combination, will clarify whether dual blockage in maintenance will achieve better results in metastatic setting. Another ongoing phase III study, NCT00667251, which completed patient accrual, is comparing taxane plus trastuzumab or lapatinib combination therapy in untreated HER-2(+) MBC.

In the neoadjuvant setting, although lapatinib/trastuzumab combination therapy significantly improved pCR compared with trastuzumab alone (51.3 % vs. 29.5 %) in the NEO-ALTTO study [9], a head-to-head comparison of trastuzumab and lapatinib with chemotherapy combination therapy in the GeparQuinto study showed that trastuzumab achieved better pCR compared with lapatinib (31.75 % vs. 21.7 %, respectively) [10].. In the randomized phase II CHERLOB trial, preoperative taxane and anthracycline chemotherapy in combination with trastuzumab, lapatinib, or both was evaluated in stage II–IIIA breast cancer patients. The pCR rate was 28 %, 32 %, and 48 % in the trastuzumab, lapatinib, and combination arms, respectively [11]. The present data confirmed that the combination of these agents results in better pCR, whereas single-agent trastuzumab appears to be superior to single-agent lapatinib.

In tumors positive for HER-2 and hormone receptor (HR), inhibiting both the HER-2 and ER pathways might be a more reasonable option. There is crosstalk between these pathways. In lapatinib-exposed cells, continuous inhibition of the PI3K/Akt pathway can lead to upregulation of the transcription factor FOXO3A, which can then increase ER signaling [12]. Two large randomized trials evaluated aromatose inhibition (AI) and anti-HER-2 therapy combinations. In postmenopausal hormone receptor- and HER-2-positive breast cancer patients, lapatinib in combination with letrozole achieved a significantly better median PFS (8.2 months vs. 3 months), ORR (28 % vs. 15 %), and CBR (48 % vs. 29 %) compared with letrozole alone [13]. In the TAnDEM study, trastuzumab and anastrozole combination therapy versus anastrozole alone showed a significantly superior median PFS (4.8 months vs. 2.4 months) and ORR (20.3 % vs. 6.8 %) in metastatic breast cancer [14]. In an ongoing study, NCT01160211, participants are being recruited to compare AI in combination with lapatinib, trastuzumab, or both for the treatment of hormone receptor-positive, HER-2-positive metastatic breast cancer.

Pertuzumab

Pertuzumab is a recombinant humanized monoclonal antibody that binds to the HER-2 extracellular subdomain II and prevents HER-2 dimerization. Unlike trastuzumab, which is effective on HER-2 homodimers, pertuzumab can affect HER-2/EGFR and HER-2/HER-3 interactions (Fig. 36.1). In preclinical studies using pertuzumab as a single agent and in combination with trastuzumab, its activity was confirmed [15]. A subsequent phase II study evaluated the role of pertuzumab–trastuzumab combination therapy in HER-2(+) metastatic breast cancer patients who progressed on prior trastuzumab therapy. The objective response rate (ORR) and CBR were 24 % and 50 %, respectively. The median progression free-survival was 5.5 months [16]. The subsequent phase III CLEOPATRA study compared the efficacy of docetaxel, trastuzumab, and pertuzumab combination therapy with docetaxel, trastuzumab, and placebo in HER-2(+) metastatic breast cancer patients. The majority of the group (90 %) had not previously received an anti-HER-2 agent, and triple combination therapy showed significant improvements in the median PFS and ORR (19 months vs. 12 months; 80 % vs. 69 %, respectively) [17]. Based on this study, pertuzumab received FDA approval in June 2012 for use in the

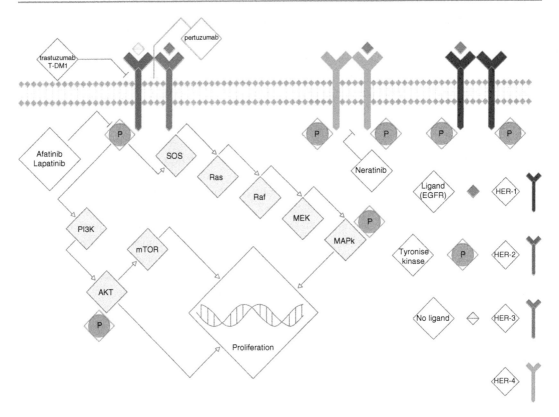

Fig. 36.1 Therapies targeting HER signaling

first-line setting as a combination therapy. The final OS results were presented at the 2014 ESMO Congress in Madrid, Spain. At last follow-up, the median OS was 56.5 versus 40.8 months in the pertuzumab–trastuzumab and trastuzumab only plus chemotherapy arms, respectively.

The role of pertuzumab in second-line setting is not clear. As there is no present study comparing T-DM1 with pertuzumab combinations, the best option for the initial setting in MBC has not been clearly defined.

In neoadjuvant studies, the NEOSPHERE trial randomized operable, locally advanced, or inflammatory HER-2-positive breast cancers to four different treatment groups: (A) docetaxel and trastuzumab; (B) docetaxel, trastuzumab, and pertuzumab; (C) pertuzumab and trastuzumab; and (D) docetaxel and pertuzumab [18]. The pCRs of the four groups were 29 %, 45.8 %, 16.8 %, and 24 %, respectively. In this study, the triple combination showed superior pCR, but a subgroup of arm C also appeared to benefit from dual blockage without chemotherapy. The randomized phase II TRYPHAENA trial compared pertuzumab and trastuzumab (HP) with or without an anthracycline-based chemotherapy regimen in neoadjuvant setting. Fluorouracil, epirubicine, and cyclophosphamide (FEC)–HP followed by docetaxel (D)–HP, FEC followed by D–HP, and docetaxel–carboplatin (DC) with HP were the three treatment arms. The pCR rates were 62 %, 57 %, and 66 % in these three groups, respectively; no significant differences were found [19].

T-DM1

T-DM1 is an antibody drug conjugate comprising trastuzumab and an antimitotic agent derivative maytansine that directly targets HER-2expressing cells [20] (Fig. 36.1). FDA approved the drug in

February 2013 in consequence of EMILIA study results. This phase III study enrolled 978 HER-2(+) MBC patients treated previously with trastuzumab and taxane therapy. The patients were randomized to T-DM1 (3.6 mg/kg IV, D1) OR capecitabine (1,000 mg/m^2 orally twice daily, days 1–14) and lapatinib (1,250 mg orally once daily) combination therapy given every 3 weeks. Significant improvements in the median PFS (10 months vs. 6 months, respectively), OS (31 months vs. 25 months, respectively), and ORR were achieved (44 % vs. 31 %, respectively). In a recent publication evaluating the patient-reported outcomes of the EMILIA study, greater efficacy and tolerability of T-DM 1 were revealed [21].

The THERESA phase 3 trial compared T-DM1 with the physician's treatment of choice in patients with progressive disease following treatment with two or more HER-2-directed regimens for MBC, and this trial revealed that PFS was significantly improved with T-DM1 (median PFS 6.2 months vs. 3.3 months) [22].

Although the approval of the drug is restricted to patients who progressed after trastuzumab therapy, recent studies may confirm the role of T-DM1 in the first-line setting. A recently published phase II study in HER-2(+) MBC/locally advanced patients showed that in the first-line setting, T-DM1 produced a superior median PFS (14.2 months. vs. 9.2 months, respectively) and ORR (64.2 % vs. 58 %, respectively) compared with docetaxel and trastuzumab combination therapy [23]. The phase III MARIANNE study (NCT01120184) completed patient recruitment to compare T-DM1 plus pertuzumab, T-DM1 plus placebo, and trastuzumab plus taxane in HER-2(+) MBC patients without initial therapy in a locally advanced or metastatic setting, but the final results have not been presented. Additionally, an ongoing study, NCT00829166, is comparing the safety and efficacy of T-DM1 with capecitabine plus lapatinib. These studies will identify the therapeutic settings of the new anti-HER-2 drugs and also provide knowledge regarding whether combination therapy will improve the survival endpoints.

These agents mentioned above target HER-1, HER-2, and HER-3 in their dimerization and activation steps; however, various cascades are involved downstream of the ErbB family before the proliferation signals reach the nucleus.

Neratinib

Neratinib is an oral covalent drug that irreversibly inhibits the ATP-binding active site of the ErbB family [24] (Fig. 36.1). In a phase II study, advanced HER-2-positive breast cancer patients received oral neratinib 240 mg once daily. The median PFS was 22.3 or 38.6 weeks for patients with prior trastuzumab therapy or with no prior trastuzumab therapy, respectively. The ORR was 24 % among patients with prior trastuzumab treatment and 56 % in the trastuzumab-naive cohort [25]. In another study comparing neratinib monotherapy versus lapatinib plus capecitabine, the median PFS was 4.5 versus 6.8 months in the neratinib (240 mg/day) arm versus the combination arm. The ORRs were 29 % and 41 %, respectively. The noninferiority of neratinib could not be demonstrated in this study. Another study evaluated neratinib (240 mg/day) and capecitabine combination therapy (1,500 mg/m^2/day) in HER-2(+) breast cancer. The ORRs for patients who had received prior lapatinib treatment and for lapatinib-naive patients were 57 % and 64 %, respectively. The median PFS was superior in the lapatinib-naive group (40.3 vs. 35.9 weeks) [26].

Lessons gained from phase II studies show that neratinib mainly improved responses and survival rates in anti-HER-2-naive patients. Based on the positive results in the metastatic setting, the efficacy of the drug in neoadjuvant and adjuvant settings is being investigated in ongoing trials.

The I-SPY 2 trial evaluated neratinib in combination with weekly paclitaxel with or without trastuzumab followed by doxorubicin and cyclophosphamide (AC) as neoadjuvant therapy for women with HER-2-positive locally advanced breast cancer. The final results were presented at AACR 2014 as an oral presentation. Neratinib plus chemotherapy achieved a pathological complete response rate of 56 % versus 33 % for patients treated with chemotherapy alone [27].

Additionally, an adjuvant study, the ExteNET trial, evaluated neratinib versus placebo after the completion of 1 year of standard trastuzumab therapy in 2,821 patients with HER-2-positive breast cancer. Adjuvant treatment with neratinib extended DFS by 33 % compared with the placebo. The full results have not been presented at a scientific meeting.

The main side effect of neratinib is diarrhea, which is usually of the secretory type without mucositis. Antidiarrheal therapy, including loperamide, can overcome this adverse event.

Afatinib

Afatinib is an oral small molecule inhibitor of the ErbB receptor family that covalently binds and irreversibly blocks ErbB family members (Fig. 36.1). In advanced HER-2(+) breast cancer patients after trastuzumab failure, afatinib 50 mg/day was given to patients once daily until

progression occurred. SD was the best response in 37 % of patients, and 46 % achieved a clinical benefit. The median PFS and OS were 15.1 and 61 weeks, respectively [28]. According to a previous study, the activity appeared to be limited in HER-2(−) patients [29]. A phase 3 randomized study of afatinib in trastuzumab-resistant metastatic breast cancer was halted early due to unfavorable risk–benefit analysis [30].

Dual blocking of tyrosine kinases, pan-HER blocking agents, and drug-conjugated anti-HER-2 agents are being studied in early-phase clinical studies to explain the exact role of these agents in the near future (Table 36.1).

EGFR Inhibitors

EGFR (HER-1) is a member of the ErbB family that enhances tumorigenicity in breast cancer and is also associated with poorer survival and resistance to hormonal therapy [31, 32]. EGFR is not

Table 36.1 Ongoing clinical trials of HER-targeted agents

ClinicalTrials.gov identifier number	Drug description	Patient characteristics	Treatment	Primary endpoint
NCT01304797	MM-302 Nanotherapeutic encapsulation of doxorubicin with attached antibodies	Advanced breast cancer Phase I study	MM-302 30 mg/m² q4w MM-302 40 mg/m² q4w MM-302 50 mg/m² q4w	Maximum tolerated dose
NCT01097460	MM-111 Novel antibody fusion protein targeting HE2/HER-3 heterodimer	Advanced HER-2, heregulin-positive breast cancer Phase I	Dose escalation cohorts	Maximum tolerated dose, safety and tolerability
NCT01569412	Ertumaxomab Hybrid monoclonal antibody targets T cell-CD3 ag and HER-2	Her2-positive advanced solid tumors Phase I–II	Dose escalation	Maximum tolerated dose
NCT00535522	TAK-285 Dual HER2/EGFR inhibitor	Advanced cancer Phase I	Dose escalation cohorts	Maximum tolerated dose
NCT01421472	MM-121	ER-positive or ER-negative	Arm 1:MM-121 plus paclitaxel	pCR
	Fully human anti-HER-3 monoclonal antibody	HER-2-negative locally advanced breast cancer Phase II Neoadjuvant study	Arm 2: paclitaxel	

pCR pathologic complete remission

only related to ER(+) tumors but is also overexpressed in basal-like breast cancers [33]. The small molecule tyrosine kinase inhibitor gefitinib is being investigated in combination with endocrine therapy in hormone receptor-positive tumors, whereas cetuximab is being evaluated in triple-negative patients.

Gefitinib

Gefitinib is a small molecule tyrosine kinase inhibitor that inhibits downstream signaling pathways activated by phosphorylation. The efficacy of the drug could not be demonstrated in monotherapy in taxane- and anthracycline-pretreated metastatic breast cancer patients [34] but was shown to be a reasonable option in the neoadjuvant setting with anastrozole combination therapy in ER(+) and EGFR(+) tumors [35]. A phase II study in the advanced breast cancer setting demonstrated that paclitaxel and carboplatin combined with gefitinib (250 mg/day orally) achieved CR (10.3 %), PR (44.1 %), and SD (30.9 %) in a patient group [36]. In another study, first-line therapy in MBC with gefitinib and docetaxel revealed an ORR of 54 % with better PR and CR in an ER(+) versus ER(−) group (70 % vs. 21 %) [37]. Although various chemotherapeutic combinations had acceptable toxicity profiles, adding gefitinib to chemotherapy as well as to trastuzumab did not achieve a significant improvement in response rates or survival [38–40]. These results carried the drug to be used in a combination with hormonal therapy options.

According to the present data, the addition of gefitinib to anastrozole treatment had no additional clinical effect in a neoadjuvant setting [41]; however, the same combination is associated with improved PFS (17.4 vs. 8.4 months) and CBR (49 % vs. 34 %) compared with anastrozole alone in a metastatic setting [42]. A recent study comparing anastrozole plus gefitinib versus fulvestrant plus gefitinib in postmenopausal HR(+) MBC showed that both combinations have similar clinical benefit rates (44.1 % vs. 41 %, respectively), median PFS (5.3

vs. 5.2 months, respectively), and OS (30.3 vs. 23.9 months, respectively). However, the clinical benefit rates of both combinations are not clearly superior to gefitinib or endocrine therapy alone. Because EGFR expression is related to endocrine resistance, it is rational to hypothesize that gefitinib plus endocrine therapy might overcome hormonal therapy resistance. Additionally, in a phase II study, two patient groups with initial hormonal therapy received gefitinib. Stratum 1 included women with newly diagnosed metastases or who had recurred 1 year after stopping adjuvant therapy with tamoxifen. Stratum 2 involved patients with recurrent disease during or after AI adjuvant therapy or those who progressed after first-line hormonotherapy with AI in a metastatic setting. Patients were randomized to receive tamoxifen plus gefitinib (250 mg/day orally) versus tamoxifen plus placebo. The median PFS (10.9 vs. 8.8 months) was better in the combination arm in Stratum 1. No objective responses were detected in Stratum 2 with combination therapy [43].

These conflicting results reflect that the present data are not sufficient to identify the exact ideal setting of this agent. We believe that in the future, gefitinib can be a part of therapeutic options in HR (+) MBC patients in the initial setting to delay the development of hormone resistance.

Cetuximab

Cetuximab is an epidermal growth factor (EGF) antagonist that specifically binds to EGFR on both normal and tumor cells. The binding of cetuximab to EGFR blocks the phosphorylation and activation of receptor-associated kinases. Signal transduction through EGFR activates k-ras; however, mutant k-ras protein is constitutively active and does not depend on EGFR regulation. The majority of cetuximab studies included triple-negative breast cancers (TNBCs) because they have high EGFR expression. A phase II study evaluating weekly irinotecan/carboplatin with or without cetuximab in patients with metastatic breast cancer showed antitumor activity but also showed significant associated toxicity [44]. The TBCRC001 study evaluated cetuximab and carboplatin combination therapy in metastatic TNBCs; the combination clinical benefit ratio is higher (27 % vs. 10 %), whereas the median PFS was only 2 months in all study groups due to rapid disease progression. BALI-1, the largest EGFR trial in metastatic TNBC, compared cetuximab with cetuximab and cisplatin combination therapies. With combination therapy, the reduction in the risk of progression was 32.5 %, and PFS was longer in the cetuximab arm (3.7 months vs. 1.5 months, HR: 0.67, $p = 0.03$); no significant improvement was found in OS [45].

In addition to these two agents, erlotinib was shown to have minimal activity in unselected previously treated women [46] and limited activity when combined with bevacizumab in MBC after first- or second-line chemotherapy [47]. However, preliminary evidence of anticancer activity was observed with trastuzumab combination therapy [48].

Among the EGFR inhibitors, cetuximab and gefitinib appear to be the most promising drugs according to recent data.

Targeting the PI3K Pathway in Breast Cancer to Overcome TKI Resistance

Phosphoinositide 3-kinases (PI3Ks) are a family of lipid kinases. They function as dimeric enzymes and comprise catalytic (p110 α, β, γ, and δ) and regulatory subunits (p85) in their structures. After a growth factor or a ligand binds to its tyrosine kinase receptor, the inhibitory effect of p85 on p110 is removed, and PI3K is activated. The activated kinases phosphorylate phosphatidylinositol bisphosphate (PIP2) to phosphatidylinositol triphosphate (PIP3), which recruits proteins such as Akt and PDK1 to cellular membranes [49]. Phosphatase and tensin homologue deleted on chromosome ten (PTEN) acts as a catalytic antagonist of PI3K by hydrolyzing PIP3 to PIP2. Class 1 PI3Ks comprise the major subgroup, which is found to be involved in cancer. PI3K mutational activation or overexpression or PTEN inactivation by genetic or epigenetic alterations result in enhanced PI3K signaling. The majority of mutations are in PIK3CA in three hotspots within the p110α catalytic subunit and are gain-of-function mutations. Two of these mutations are helical, and one is on the kinase domain of p110α.

A recent paper published in Nature highlighted the genomic and proteomic features of breast cancer subtypes and showed that PIK3CA mutation was more common in luminal tumors, whereas PTEN mutation/loss was most common in basal-like breast cancers [50]. PIK3CA mutations were found in 49 %, 32 %, 7 %, and 42 % of luminal A, luminal B, basal-like, and HER-2(+) patients, respectively, whereas PTEN mutations/losses were found in 13 %, 24 %, 35 %, and 19 %, respectively.

Previous studies confirmed that PI3KCA mutations could confer favorable clinical outcomes. Because luminal A–B tumors have more frequent mutations with slower disease progression, especially in luminal A tumors, these mutations may be associated with less aggressive disease. However, these mutations are also associated with trastuzumab and lapatinib resistance in HER-2-positive breast cancer and to hormonal therapy resistance in HR-positive tumors by directly inducing ER transcription [51, 52]. Retrospective analyses in HER-2(+) MBC showed that tumors with PIK3CA mutations or PTEN loss are associated with low trastuzumab and lapatinib efficacy and also suggest that anti-HER-2 drug-resistant tumors may still benefit from PI3K inhibitors [53, 54]. In contrast, PTEN-deficient HER-2-positive cells still have upstream input from HER-2; therefore, dual blockage might be effective in this patient group [55].

PI3K pathway inhibitors can be divided into subgroups according to their targets: (1) pan-PI3K inhibitors; (2) mTOR inhibitors; (3) Akt inhibitors; and (4) PI3K/mTOR dual inhibitors. Regarding pan-PI3K inhibitors, phase 1 dose escalation study results in solid tumors have recently been published but will not be mentioned here because phase 2 study results are still pending [56, 57].

mTOR Inhibitors

mTOR is one of the major mediators of cell growth; it acts primarily via two downstream messengers, P70-S6 kinase 1 and 4E-BP1, which exert their activity at the translational level. Because PI3K/Akt/mTOR pathway activation was shown to contribute to trastuzumab and hormonal therapy resistance in previous studies, the addition of mTOR inhibitors to chemotherapy and hormonal therapy options was performed in an attempt to delay resistance in this patient group [58, 59].

Regarding the first studies initiated with temsirolimus, a phase II study exploring the combination of letrozole and temsirolimus compared with letrozole alone showed a longer median PFS in the combination group, but a subsequent phase III study was stopped early due to toxicity issues [60, 61].

Everolimus, with its improved toxicity profile, became the major agent being evaluated in this setting. Everolimus did not achieve a good objective ORR as a monotherapy [62]. However, in HER-2(+) MBC patients, everolimus in combination with paclitaxel plus trastuzumab or vinorelbine with trastuzumab demonstrated efficacy in trastuzumab-pretreated patients [63, 64]. In a phase I/II study, HER-2(+) MBC patients who progressed on trastuzumab-based therapy received everolimus in combination with trastuzumab. Among 47 patients, the combination of everolimus and trastuzumab resulted in PR in seven patients (15 %) and persistent SD (lasting 6 months or longer) in nine patients (19 %), translating to a clinical benefit rate of 34 %. The median PFS was 4.1 months. This study suggests that everolimus may have promising activity in trastuzumab-pretreated patients not receiving cytotoxic chemotherapy [65].

In HR-positive tumors, because endocrine therapy resistance is associated with PI3K/Akt/mTOR pathway activation, the combination of everolimus and hormonal therapy is a rational option to overcome or delay endocrine resistance. The benefit of everolimus plus exemestane was shown in the BOLERO-2 trial in 724 patients who progressed on anastrozole. Patients were randomly assigned to receive either exemestane plus everolimus or exemestane plus placebo [66]. The final study results, with a median 18-month follow-up, show

that the median PFS remained significantly longer with everolimus plus exemestane irrespective of age or metastasis region [investigator review: 7.8 versus 3.2 months, respectively; hazard ratio = 0.45 (95 % confidence interval 0.38–0.54); log-rank $P < 0.0001$; central review: 11.0 versus 4.1 months, respectively; hazard ratio = 0.38 (95 % confidence interval 0.31–0.48); log-rank $P < 0.0001$) [67].

The noninterventional BRAWO study including HR (+) and HER-2(−) MBC patients treated with everolimus and exemestane showed that the median PFS was 8.0 months in the everolimus and exemestane group, with more favorable results in the first-line treatment (PFS:10 months) group; these data were presented at the ESMO 2014 Congress in Spain [68].

In the phase II GINECO study, 111 HR(+), HER-2(−) MBC patients previously treated with aromatase inhibitors were randomly selected to receive tamoxifen alone or tamoxifen in combination with everolimus (10 mg/day). The CBR (61.1 % vs. 42.1 %) and TTP (8.6 months vs. 4.5 months) were significantly improved in the combination group, and the risk of death was reduced by 55 % with tamoxifen plus everolimus versus tamoxifen alone (HR, 0.45; 95 % CI, 0.24–0.81) [69]. When patients were stratified according to primary or secondary hormone resistance, TTP was more improved in secondary hormone-resistant patients who received combination therapy compared with those who received tamoxifen alone (17.5 months vs. 5 months, respectively), whereas TTP was only slightly improved by combination therapy in primary hormone-resistant patients (5.4 months vs. 3.9 months, respectively).

In a phase II study, ER(+) MBC patients who failed AI therapy within 6 months were randomized to receive everolimus 10 mg/day in combination with intramuscular fulvestrant (500 mg D1, 250 mg D14, 250 mg D28, or 250 mg once a month). Although the final results of the study have not been presented, a CBR of 55 % and TTP of 8.6 months were achieved by combination therapy [70].

The present data show that everolimus combined with hormonotherapy might be an ideal therapeutic option in secondary hormone-resistant patients.

The BOLERO-3 trial evaluated the combination of everolimus, vinorelbine, and trastuzumab in women with HER-2-positive, trastuzumab-resistant advanced breast carcinoma who had previously received taxane therapy. Eligible patients were randomly assigned to daily everolimus (5 mg/day) plus weekly trastuzumab (2 mg/kg) and vinorelbine (25 mg/m²) or to placebo plus trastuzumab plus vinorelbine in 3-week cycles [71]. The study revealed that the addition of everolimus to trastuzumab plus vinorelbine prolongs PFS in the patient group [the median PFS was 7.00 months (95 % CI 6.74–8.18) with everolimus and 5.78 months (5.49–6.90) with placebo (hazard ratio 0.78 [95 % CI 0.65–0.95]; $p = 0.0067$)].

An ongoing study, the BOLERO-1 trial (NCT00876395), is evaluating everolimus in combination with trastuzumab and paclitaxel in the first-line setting; the final results have not yet been released.

Everolimus has also evaluated in the neoadjuvant setting in combination with letrozole. Newly diagnosed ER (+) localized breast cancer patients were randomized to receive letrozole 2.5 mg/day plus placebo or letrozole plus everolimus 10 mg/day before surgery. The ORR was found to be 59 % and 68 % in the letrozole and combination arms, respectively [72].

Upon blocking mTOR with everolimus, compensatory Akt activation occurs. Baselga et al. explained in a recent review that this situation was due to reduced S6 following mTOR inhibition and claimed that reduced S6 could not suppress signaling of IGF-1R via supression of IRS-1 anymore. Activated IGF-1R increase PI3K signaling [49].

PI3K Inhibitors

Clinical trials with PI3K inhibitors are ongoing and still in early phases (Table 36.2). Among these inhibitors, XL-765 is a dual mTOR (TORC 1 and 2) and PI3K inhibitor, and XL-147 is a selective inhibitor of PI3K with a potent inhibitory effect on the class I PI3K family. Both agents were designed to be orally administered. Preliminary data from the NCT01082068 trial confirmed that both PI3K inhibitors can be safely

Table 36.2 Ongoing clinical trials of PI3K inhibitors

ClinicalTrials.gov identification number	Patient characteristics	Treatment	Primary endpoint
NCT01629615	Triple-negative MBC	Phase II BKM 120 (PI3K inhibitor) 100 mg daily in cycles of 28 days, until progression	CBR
NCT01816594	HER-2(+) newly diagnosed patients neoadjuvant	Phase II Trastuzumab versus trastuzumab +BKM120 with weekly paclitaxel	pCR
NCT01589861	Trastuzumab-resistant HER-2(+)/PI3K-activated advanced breast cancer	Phase I–II BKM120 plus lapatinib	Maximum tolerated dose-phase I ORR-phase II
NCT00960960	Locally recurrent/metastatic breast cancer	Phase I GDC0941 (PI3K inhibitor) in combination with paclitaxel with or without trastuzumab or bevacizumab	Tolerability and tumor response
NCT01082068	HR(+) HER-2(−) nonsteroidal AI resistant disease	Phase I–II (PI3K inhibitor) XL 147 (SAR245408)+letrozole versus XL 765 (SAR245409)+letrozole	Maximum tolerated dose-phase I PFS-phase II

pCR pathologic complete remission, *ORR* overall response rate, *CBR* clinical benefit rate

combined with letrozole. The phase II studies will clarify whether dual PI3K and mTOR inhibition is better than PI3K inhibition alone.

Concluding Remarks

Targeted therapies in breast cancer have had remarkable effects on patient survival since the first representative drug, trastuzumab, was used in HER-2(+) breast cancer. However, patients develop resistance to these drugs during the treatment period. This is mainly associated with cancer cells finding alternative pathways to maintain proliferative signaling. To delay the development of resistance to these therapies, combined modalities targeting different steps of the signaling cascade have been investigated. The main obstacle to this approach is tumor heterogeneity; because of this, we cannot use simple standard analytical techniques to predict the driving pathway in the tumor that should be blocked. Genomic analyses in recent decades have also confirmed this heterogeneity and revealed that by analyzing tumor characteristics, individualized therapy can be performed for each patient. This direction is also reflected in the ongoing trial protocols, which mainly include patients with demonstrated mutations amenable to treatment with the target drug. The future studies should not only confirm the efficacy of targeted combinations but also stratify the selected patient group for each developed drug.

References

1. Saxena R, Dwivedi A. ErbB family receptor inhibitors as therapeutic agents in breast cancer: current status and future clinical perspective. Med Res Rev. 2012;32(1):166–215. Review.
2. Broekman F, Giovannetti E, Peters GJ. Tyrosine kinase inhibitors: multi-targeted or single-targeted? World J Clin Oncol. 2011;2(2):80–93.
3. Konecny GE, Pegram MD, Venkatesan N, Finn R, Yang G, Rahmeh M, et al. Activity of the dual kinase inhibitor lapatinib (GW572016) against HER-2-overexpressing and trastuzumab-treated breast cancer cells. Cancer Res. 2006;66(3):1630–9.
4. Scaltriti M, Rojo F, Ocana A, Anido J, Guzman M, Cortes J, et al. Expression of p95HER2, a truncated form of the HER2 receptor, and response to anti-HER2 therapies in breast cancer. J Natl Cancer Inst. 2007;99(8):628–38. Research Support, Non-U.S. Gov't.
5. Di Leo A, Gomez HL, Aziz Z, Zvirbule Z, Bines J, Arbushites MC, et al. Phase III, double-blind, randomized study comparing lapatinib plus paclitaxel with placebo plus paclitaxel as first-line treatment for metastatic breast cancer. J Clin Oncol Off J Am Soc Clin Oncol. 2008;26(34):5544–52. Clinical Trial, Phase III Multicenter Study Randomized Controlled Trial Research Support, N.I.H., Extramural Research Support, Non-U.S. Gov't.
6. Cameron D, Casey M, Press M, Lindquist D, Pienkowski T, Romieu CG, et al. A phase III randomized comparison of lapatinib plus capecitabine versus capecitabine alone in women with advanced breast cancer that has progressed on trastuzumab: updated efficacy and biomarker analyses. Breast Cancer Res Treat. 2008;112(3):533–43. Clinical Trial, Phase III Randomized Controlled Trial Research Support, Non-U.S. Gov't.
7. Blackwell KL, Burstein HJ, Storniolo AM, Rugo H, Sledge G, Koehler M, et al. Randomized study of Lapatinib alone or in combination with trastuzumab in women with ErbB2-positive, trastuzumab-refractory metastatic breast cancer. J Clin Oncol Off J Am Soc Clin Oncol. 2010;28(7):1124–30. Clinical Trial, Phase III Multicenter Study Randomized Controlled Trial Research Support, Non-U.S. Gov't.
8. Blackwell KL, Burstein HJ, Storniolo AM, Rugo HS, Sledge G, Aktan G, et al. Overall survival benefit with lapatinib in combination with trastuzumab for patients with human epidermal growth factor receptor 2-positive metastatic breast cancer: final results from the EGF104900 study. J Clin Oncol Off J Am Soc Clin Oncol. 2012;30(21):2585–92. Clinical Trial, Phase III Multicenter Study Randomized Controlled Trial Research Support, Non-U.S. Gov't.
9. Baselga J, Bradbury I, Eidtmann H, Di Cosimo S, de Azambuja E, Aura C, et al. Lapatinib with trastuzumab for HER2-positive early breast cancer (NeoALTTO): a randomised, open-label, multicentre, phase 3 trial. Lancet. 2012;379(9816):633–40. Clinical Trial, Phase III Multicenter Study Randomized Controlled Trial Research Support, Non-U.S. Gov't.
10. Untch M, Loibl S, Bischoff J, Eidtmann H, Kaufmann M, Blohmer JU, et al. Lapatinib versus trastuzumab in combination with neoadjuvant anthracycline-taxane-based chemotherapy (GeparQuinto, GBG 44): a randomised phase 3 trial. Lancet Oncol. 2012;13(2):135–44. Clinical Trial, Phase III Comparative Study Randomized Controlled Trial Research Support, Non-U.S. Gov't.
11. Guarneri V, Frassoldati A, Piacentini F, Jovic G, Giovannelli S, Oliva C, et al. Preoperative chemotherapy plus lapatinib or trastuzumab or both in HER2-positive operable breast cancer (CHERLOB Trial).

Clin Breast Cancer. April 2008. Vol 8 No. 2 192–194. Clinical Trial, Phase II Randomized Controlled Trial Research Support, Non-U.S. Gov't.

12. Xia W, Bacus S, Husain I, Liu L, Zhao S, Liu Z, et al. Resistance to ErbB2 tyrosine kinase inhibitors in breast cancer is mediated by calcium-dependent activation of RelA. Mol Cancer Ther. 2010;9(2):292–9. Research Support, Non-U.S. Gov't.

13. Johnston S, Pippen Jr J, Pivot X, Lichinitser M, Sadeghi S, Dieras V, et al. Lapatinib combined with letrozole versus letrozole and placebo as first-line therapy for postmenopausal hormone receptor-positive metastatic breast cancer. J Clin Oncol Off J Am Soc Clin Oncol. 2009;27(33):5538–46. Clinical Trial, Phase III Comparative Study Multicenter Study Randomized Controlled Trial Research Support, Non-U.S. Gov't.

14. Kaufman B, Mackey JR, Clemens MR, Bapsy PP, Vaid A, Wardley A, et al. Trastuzumab plus anastrozole versus anastrozole alone for the treatment of postmenopausal women with human epidermal growth factor receptor 2-positive, hormone receptor-positive metastatic breast cancer: results from the randomized phase III TAnDEM study. J Clin Oncol Off J Am Soc Clin Oncol. 2009;27(33):5529–37. Clinical Trial, Phase III Comparative Study Multicenter Study Randomized Controlled Trial Research Support, Non-U.S. Gov't.

15. Brockhoff G, Heckel B, Schmidt-Bruecken E, Plander M, Hofstaedter F, Vollmann A, et al. Differential impact of cetuximab, pertuzumab and trastuzumab on BT474 and SK-BR-3 breast cancer cell proliferation. Cell Prolif. 2007;40(4):488–507. Research Support, Non-U.S. Gov't.

16. Baselga J, Gelmon KA, Verma S, Wardley A, Conte P, Miles D, et al. Phase II trial of pertuzumab and trastuzumab in patients with human epidermal growth factor receptor 2-positive metastatic breast cancer that progressed during prior trastuzumab therapy. J Clin Oncol Off J Am Soc Clin Oncol. 2010;28(7):1138–44. Clinical Trial, Phase II Multicenter Study Research Support, Non-U.S. Gov't.

17. Baselga J, Cortes J, Kim SB, Im SA, Hegg R, Im YH, et al. Pertuzumab plus trastuzumab plus docetaxel for metastatic breast cancer. N Engl J Med. 2012;366(2):109–19. Comparative Study Multicenter Study Randomized Controlled Trial Research Support, Non-U.S. Gov't.

18. Gianni L, Pienkowski T, Im YH, Roman L, Tseng LM, Liu MC, et al. Efficacy and safety of neoadjuvant pertuzumab and trastuzumab in women with locally advanced, inflammatory, or early HER2-positive breast cancer (NeoSphere): a randomised multicentre, open-label, phase 2 trial. Lancet Oncol. 2012;13(1):25–32. Clinical Trial, Phase II Multicenter Study Randomized Controlled Trial Research Support, Non-U.S. Gov't.

19. Schneeweiss A, Chia S, Hickish T, Harvey V, Hegg R, Tausch C, et al. Pertuzumab and trastuzumab in combination with an anthracycline-containing or an anthracycline-free standard chemotherapy in the neo-adjuvant treatment of HER2-positive breast cancer (TRYPHAENA). Eur J Cancer. 2012;48:S96–S.

20. Isakoff SJ, Baselga J. Trastuzumab-DM1: building a chemotherapy-free road in the treatment of human epidermal growth factor receptor 2-positive breast cancer. J Clin Oncol Off J Am Soc Clin Oncol. 2011;29(4):351–4. Comment Editorial.

21. Welslau M, Dieras V, Sohn JH, Hurvitz SA, Lalla D, Fang L, et al. Patient-reported outcomes from EMILIA, a randomized phase 3 study of trastuzumab emtansine (T-DM1) versus capecitabine and lapatinib in human epidermal growth factor receptor 2-positive locally advanced or metastatic breast cancer. Cancer. 2014;120(5):642–51. Clinical Trial, Phase III Randomized Controlled Trial Research Support, Non-U.S. Gov't.

22. Krop IE, Kim SB, Gonzalez-Martin A, LoRusso PM, Ferrero JM, Smitt M, et al. Trastuzumab emtansine versus treatment of physician's choice for pretreated HER2-positive advanced breast cancer (TH3RESA): a randomised, open-label, phase 3 trial. Lancet Oncol. 2014;15(7):689–99. Clinical Trial, Phase III Comparative Study Multicenter Study Randomized Controlled Trial Research Support, Non-U.S. Gov't.

23. Hurvitz SA, Dirix L, Kocsis J, Bianchi GV, Lu J, Vinholes J, et al. Phase II randomized study of trastuzumab emtansine versus trastuzumab plus docetaxel in patients with human epidermal growth factor receptor 2-positive metastatic breast cancer. J Clin Oncol Off J Am Soc Clin Oncol. 2013;31(9):1157–63.

24. Lopez-Tarruella S, Jerez Y, Marquez-Rodas I, Martin M. Neratinib (HKI-272) in the treatment of breast cancer. Future Oncol. 2012;8(6):671–81. Review.

25. Burstein HJ, Sun Y, Dirix LY, Jiang Z, Paridaens R, Tan AR, et al. Neratinib, an irreversible ErbB receptor tyrosine kinase inhibitor, in patients with advanced ErbB2-positive breast cancer. J Clin Oncol Off J Am Soc Clin Oncol. 2010;28(8):1301–7. Clinical Trial, Phase II Comparative Study Multicenter Study Research Support, Non-U.S. Gov't.

26. Saura C, Martin M, Moroose R, Harb W, Liem K, Arena F, et al. Safety of neratinib (HKI-272) in combination with capecitabine in patients with solid tumors: a phase 1/2 study. Cancer Res. 2009;69(24):801S–2.

27. Park J, Liu M, Yee D, et al. Neratinib plus standard neoadjuvant chemotherapy for high-risk breast cancer: efficacy results from the I-SPY trial. 2014 AACR Annual Meeting 2014.

28. Lin NU, Winer EP, Wheatley D, Carey LA, Houston S, Mendelson D, et al. A phase II study of afatinib (BIBW 2992), an irreversible ErbB family blocker, in patients with HER2-positive metastatic breast cancer progressing after trastuzumab. Breast Cancer Res Treat. 2012;133(3):1057–65. Clinical Trial, Phase II Multicenter Study Research Support, Non-U.S. Gov't.

29. Schuler M, Awada A, Harter P, Canon JL, Possinger K, Schmidt M, et al. A phase II trial to assess efficacy

and safety of afatinib in extensively pretreated patients with HER2-negative metastatic breast cancer. Breast Cancer Res Treat. 2012;134(3):1149–59. Clinical Trial, Phase II Multicenter Study Research Support, Non-U.S. Gov't.

30. Hurvitz SA, Shatsky R, Harbeck N. Afatinib in the treatment of breast cancer. Expert Opin Investig Drugs. 2014;23(7):1039–47.

31. Tang CK, Gong XQ, Moscatello DK, Wong AJ, Lippman ME. Epidermal growth factor receptor vIII enhances tumorigenicity in human breast cancer. Cancer Res. 2000;60(11):3081–7. Research Support, Non-U.S. Gov't Research Support, U.S. Gov't, P.H.S.

32. Nicholson RI, McClelland RA, Gee JM, Manning DL, Cannon P, Robertson JF, et al. Epidermal growth factor receptor expression in breast cancer: association with response to endocrine therapy. Breast Cancer Res Treat. 1994;29(1):117–25. Clinical Trial Comparative Study Research Support, Non-U.S. Gov't.

33. Nielsen TO, Hsu FD, Jensen K, Cheang M, Karaca G, Hu Z, et al. Immunohistochemical and clinical characterization of the basal-like subtype of invasive breast carcinoma. Clin Cancer Res Off J Am Assoc Cancer Res. 2004;10(16):5367–74. Research Support, U.S. Gov't, P.H.S.

34. von Minckwitz G, Jonat W, Fasching P, du Bois A, Kleeberg U, Luck HJ, et al. A multicentre phase II study on gefitinib in taxane- and anthracycline-pretreated metastatic breast cancer. Breast Cancer Res Treat. 2005;89(2):165–72. Clinical Trial Clinical Trial, Phase II Multicenter Study Research Support, Non-U.S. Gov't.

35. Polychronis A, Sinnett HD, Hadjiminas D, Singhal H, Mansi JL, Shivapatham D, et al. Preoperative gefitinib versus gefitinib and anastrozole in postmenopausal patients with oestrogen-receptor positive and epidermal-growth-factor-receptor-positive primary breast cancer: a double-blind placebo-controlled phase II randomised trial. Lancet Oncol. 2005;6(6):383–91. Clinical Trial Clinical Trial, Phase II Multicenter Study Randomized Controlled Trial Research Support, Non-U.S. Gov't.

36. Fountzilas G, Pectasides D, Kalogera-Fountzila A, Skarlos D, Kalofonos HP, Papadimitriou C, et al. Paclitaxel and carboplatin as first-line chemotherapy combined with gefitinib (IRESSA) in patients with advanced breast cancer: a phase I/II study conducted by the Hellenic Cooperative Oncology Group. Breast Cancer Res Treat. 2005;92(1):1–9. Clinical Trial Clinical Trial, Phase I Clinical Trial, Phase II Multicenter Study Research Support, Non-U.S. Gov't.

37. Ciardiello F, Troiani T, Caputo F, De Laurentiis M, Tortora G, Palmieri G, et al. Phase II study of gefitinib in combination with docetaxel as first-line therapy in metastatic breast cancer. Br J Cancer. 2006;94(11):1604–9. Clinical Trial, Phase II Multicenter Study.

38. Dennison SK, Jacobs SA, Wilson JW, Seeger J, Cescon TP, Raymond JM, et al. A phase II clinical trial of ZD1839 (Iressa) in combination with docetaxel as first-line treatment in patients with advanced breast cancer. Investig New Drugs. 2007;25(6):545–51. Clinical Trial, Phase II Multicenter Study Research Support, N.I.H., Intramural Research Support, Non-U.S. Gov't.

39. Arteaga CL, O'Neill A, Moulder SL, Pins M, Sparano JA, Sledge GW, et al. A phase I-II study of combined blockade of the ErbB receptor network with trastuzumab and gefitinib in patients with HER2 (ErbB2)-overexpressing metastatic breast cancer. Clin Cancer Res Off J Am Assoc Cancer Res. 2008;14(19):6277–83. Clinical Trial, Phase I Clinical Trial, Phase II Research Support, N.I.H., Extramural.

40. Gioulbasanis I, Saridaki Z, Kalykaki A, Vamvakas L, Kalbakis K, Ignatiadis M, et al. Gefitinib in combination with gemcitabine and vinorelbine in patients with metastatic breast cancer pre-treated with taxane and anthracycline chemotherapy: a phase I/II trial. Anticancer Res. 2008;28(5B):3019–25. Clinical Trial, Phase I Clinical Trial, Phase II Research Support, Non-U.S. Gov't.

41. Smith IE, Walsh G, Skene A, Llombart A, Mayordomo JI, Detre S, et al. A phase II placebo-controlled trial of neoadjuvant anastrozole alone or with gefitinib in early breast cancer. J Clin Oncol Off J Am Soc Clin Oncol. 2007;25(25):3816–22. Clinical Trial, Phase II Randomized Controlled Trial Research Support, Non-U.S. Gov't.

42. Cristofanilli M, Valero V, Mangalik A, Royce M, Rabinowitz I, Arena FP, et al. Phase II, randomized trial to compare anastrozole combined with gefitinib or placebo in postmenopausal women with hormone receptor-positive metastatic breast cancer. Clin Cancer Res Off J Am Assoc Cancer Res. 2010;16(6):1904–14. Clinical Trial, Phase II Comparative Study Multicenter Study Randomized Controlled Trial Research Support, N.I.H., Extramural.

43. Osborne CK, Neven P, Dirix LY, Mackey JR, Robert J, Underhill C, et al. Gefitinib or placebo in combination with tamoxifen in patients with hormone receptor-positive metastatic breast cancer: a randomized phase II study. Clin Cancer Res Off J Am Assoc Cancer Res. 2011;17(5):1147–59. Clinical Trial, Phase II Randomized Controlled Trial Research Support, Non-U.S. Gov't.

44. O'Shaughnessy J, Weckstein DJ, Vukelja SJ, McIntyre K, Krekow L, Holmes FA, et al. Preliminary results of a randomized phase II study of weekly irinotecan/carboplatin with or without cetuximab in patients with metastatic breast cancer. Breast Cancer Res Treat. 2007;106:S32–3.

45. Baselga J, Gomez P, Awada A, Greil R, Braga S, Climent MA, et al. The addition of cetuximab to cisplatin increases overall response rate (orr) and progression-free survival (pfs) in metastatic triple-negative breast cancer (tnbc): results of a randomized phase II study (Bali-1). Ann Oncol. 2010; 21:96.

46. Dickler MN, Cobleigh MA, Miller KD, Klein PM, Winer EP. Efficacy and safety of erlotinib in patients with locally advanced or metastatic breast cancer. Breast Cancer Res Treat. 2009;115(1):115–21. Clinical Trial, Phase II Multicenter Study.

47. Dickler MN, Rugo HS, Eberle CA, Brogi E, Caravelli JF, Panageas KS, et al. A phase II trial of erlotinib in combination with bevacizumab in patients with metastatic breast cancer. Clin Cancer Res Off J Am Assoc Cancer Res. 2008;14(23):7878–83. Clinical Trial, Phase II Multicenter Study Research Support, N.I.H., Extramural Research Support, Non-U.S. Gov't.

48. Britten CD, Finn RS, Bosserman LD, Wong SG, Press MF, Malik M, et al. A phase I/II trial of trastuzumab plus erlotinib in metastatic HER2-positive breast cancer: a dual ErbB targeted approach. Clin Breast Cancer. 2009;9(1):16–22. Clinical Trial, Phase I Clinical Trial, Phase II Research Support, N.I.H., Extramural.

49. Baselga J. Targeting the phosphoinositide-3 (PI3) kinase pathway in breast cancer. Oncologist. 2011;16 Suppl 1:12–9. Research Support, Non-U.S. Gov't Review.

50. Ellis MJ, Ding L, Shen D, Luo J, Suman VJ, Wallis JW, et al. Whole-genome analysis informs breast cancer response to aromatase inhibition. Nature. 2012;486(7403):353–60. Research Support, N.I.H., Extramural Research Support, Non-U.S. Gov't.

51. Kalinsky K, Jacks LM, Heguy A, Patil S, Drobnjak M, Bhanot UK, et al. PIK3CA mutation associates with improved outcome in breast cancer. Clin Cancer Res Off J Am Assoc Cancer Res. 2009;15(16):5049–59. Research Support, Non-U.S. Gov't.

52. Eichhorn PJ, Gili M, Scaltriti M, Serra V, Guzman M, Nijkamp W, et al. Phosphatidylinositol 3-kinase hyperactivation results in lapatinib resistance that is reversed by the mTOR/phosphatidylinositol 3-kinase inhibitor NVP-BEZ235. Cancer Res. 2008;68(22):9221–30. Research Support, N.I.H., Extramural Research Support, Non-U.S. Gov't.

53. Wang L, Zhang Q, Zhang J, Sun S, Guo H, Jia Z, et al. PI3K pathway activation results in low efficacy of both trastuzumab and lapatinib. BMC Cancer. 2011;11:248. Clinical Trial Research Support, Non-U.S. Gov't.

54. Esteva FJ, Guo H, Zhang S, Santa-Maria C, Stone S, Lanchbury JS, et al. PTEN, PIK3CA, p-AKT, and p-p70S6K status: association with trastuzumab response and survival in patients with HER2-positive metastatic breast cancer. Am J Pathol. 2010;177(4):1647–56. Research Support, N.I.H., Extramural Research Support, Non-U.S. Gov't Research Support, U.S. Gov't, Non-P.H.S.

55. Miller TW, Rexer BN, Garrett JT, Arteaga CL. Mutations in the phosphatidylinositol 3-kinase pathway: role in tumor progression and therapeutic implications in breast cancer. Breast Cancer Res BCR. 2011;13(6):224. Research Support, N.I.H., Extramural Research Support, Non-U.S. Gov't Review.

56. Ando Y, Inada-Inoue M, Mitsuma A, Yoshino T, Ohtsu A, Suenaga N, et al. Phase I dose-escalation study of buparlisib (BKM120), an oral pan-class I PI3K inhibitor, in Japanese patients with advanced solid tumors. Cancer Sci. 2014;105(3):347–53. Clinical Trial, Phase I Research Support, Non-U.S. Gov't.

57. Shapiro GI, Rodon J, Bedell C, Kwak EL, Baselga J, Brana I, et al. Phase I safety, pharmacokinetic, and pharmacodynamic study of SAR245408 (XL147), an oral pan-class I PI3K inhibitor, in patients with advanced solid tumors. Clin Cancer Res Off J Am Assoc Cancer Res. 2014;20(1):233–45. Clinical Trial, Phase I Research Support, Non-U.S. Gov't.

58. Harari D, Yarden Y. Molecular mechanisms underlying ErbB2/HER2 action in breast cancer. Oncogene. 2000;19(53):6102–14. Research Support, Non-U.S. Gov't Research Support, U.S. Gov't, Non-P.H.S.Research Support, U.S. Gov't, P.H.S. Review.

59. Berns K, Horlings HM, Hennessy BT, Madiredjo M, Hijmans EM, Beelen K, et al. A functional genetic approach identifies the PI3K pathway as a major determinant of trastuzumab resistance in breast cancer. Cancer Cell. 2007;12(4):395–402. Clinical Trial Multicenter Study Research Support, N.I.H., Extramural Research Support, Non-U.S. Gov't.

60. Baselga J, Fumoleau P, Gil M, Colomer R, Roche H, Cortes-Funes H, et al. Phase II, 3-arm study of CCI-779 in combination with letrozole in postmenopausal women with locally advanced or metastatic breast cancer: preliminary results. J Clin Oncol. 2004;22(14):13S–S.

61. Chow LWC, Sun Y, Jassem J, Baselga J, Hayes DF, Wolff AC, et al. Phase 3 study of temsirolimus with letrozole or letrozole alone in postmenopausal women with locally advanced or metastatic breast cancer. Breast Cancer Res Treat. 2006;100:S286–S.

62. Ellard SL, Clemons M, Gelmon KA, Norris B, Kennecke H, Chia S, et al. Randomized phase II study comparing two schedules of everolimus in patients with recurrent/metastatic breast cancer: NCIC Clinical Trials Group IND.163. J Clin Oncol Off J Am Soc Clin Oncol. 2009;27(27):4536–41. Clinical Trial, Phase II Comparative Study Multicenter Study Randomized Controlled Trial Research Support, Non-U.S. Gov't.

63. Andre F, Campone M, O'Regan R, Manlius C, Massacesi C, Sahmoud T, et al. Phase I study of everolimus plus weekly paclitaxel and trastuzumab in patients with metastatic breast cancer pretreated with trastuzumab. J Clin Oncol Off J Am Soc Clin Oncol. 2010;28(34):5110–5. Clinical Trial, Phase I Multicenter Study Research Support, Non-U.S. Gov't.

64. Jerusalem G, Fasolo A, Dieras V, Cardoso F, Bergh J, Vittori L, et al. Phase I trial of oral mTOR inhibitor everolimus in combination with trastuzumab and vinorelbine in pre-treated patients with HER2-overexpressing metastatic breast cancer. Breast Cancer Res Treat. 2011;125(2):447–55. Clinical Trial, Phase I Multicenter Study Research Support, Non-U.S. Gov't.

65. Morrow PK, Wulf GM, Ensor J, Booser DJ, Moore JA, Flores PR, et al. Phase I/II study of trastuzumab in combination with everolimus (RAD001) in patients with HER2-overexpressing metastatic breast cancer who progressed on trastuzumab-based therapy. J Clin Oncol Off J Am Soc Clin Oncol. 2011;29(23):3126–32. Clinical Trial, Phase IClinical Trial, Phase II Multicenter Study Research Support, N.I.H., Extramural Research Support, Non-U.S. Gov't.

66. Beaver JA, Park BH. The BOLERO-2 trial: the addition of everolimus to exemestane in the treatment of postmenopausal hormone receptor-positive advanced breast cancer. Future Oncol. 2012;8(6):651–7. Clinical Trial, Phase III Randomized Controlled Trial.

67. Yardley DA, Noguchi S, Pritchard KI, Burris 3rd HA, Baselga J, Gnant M, et al. Everolimus plus exemestane in postmenopausal patients with HR(+) breast cancer: BOLERO-2 final progression-free survival analysis. Adv Ther. 2013;30(10):870–84. Clinical Trial, Phase III Multicenter Study Randomized Controlled Trial Research Support, Non-U.S. Gov't.

68. Lueftner D, Schuetz F, Grischke EM, Fasching PA. Breast cancer treatment with everolimus and exemestane for ER+ women: results of the first interim analysis of the noninterventional trial BRAWO. Ann Oncol. 2014;25(Supplement 5):v1–41.

69. Bachelot T, Bourgier C, Cropet C, Ray-Coquard I, Ferrero JM, Freyer G, et al. Randomized phase II trial of everolimus in combination with tamoxifen in patients with hormone receptor-positive, human epidermal growth factor receptor 2-negative metastatic breast cancer with prior exposure to aromatase inhibitors: a GINECO study. J Clin Oncol Off J Am Soc Clin Oncol. 2012;30(22):2718–24. Clinical Trial, Phase II Multicenter Study Randomized Controlled Trial Research Support, Non-U.S. Gov't.

70. Barnett CM. Everolimus: targeted therapy on the horizon for the treatment of breast cancer. Pharmacotherapy. 2012;32(4):383–96. Research Support, Non-U.S. Gov't Review.

71. Andre F, Gianni L. BOLERO-3 results: pharmacological activity or pharmacokinetic effect? – authors' reply. Lancet Oncol. 2014;15(8):e304–5. Comment Letter.

72. Baselga J, Semiglazov V, van Dam P, Manikhas A, Bellet M, Mayordomo J, et al. Phase II randomized study of neoadjuvant everolimus plus letrozole compared with placebo plus letrozole in patients with estrogen receptor-positive breast cancer. J Clin Oncol Off J Am Soc Clin Oncol. 2009;27(16):2630–7. Clinical Trial, Phase II Multicenter Study Randomized Controlled Trial Research Support, Non-U.S. Gov't.

Part VII

Site-Specific Therapy of Metastatic Breast Cancer

Şule Karaman and Seden Küçücük

Abstract

Breast cancer is the second most common cause of central nervous system (CNS) metastases and the most common cause of leptomeningeal metastases. The brain, cranial nerves, spinal cord, leptomeninges, and eyes are the parts of the CNS that are at risk for breast cancer metastases. With the advancements in systematic treatment and radiotherapy (RT) techniques, longer overall survival and disease-free survival have been achieved in metastatic brain cancer. Therefore, CNS metastasis has become a clinical problem warranting more attention. Although CNS metastases are not as common as bone and visceral organ metastases, their progressiveness, poor prognosis, and lack of effective, systemic treatment options pose a difficult challenge for the clinician and the patient.

In this section, parenchymal brain metastases and epidural and leptomeningeal metastases of breast cancer and their treatment will be described, and a neurological injury that occurs in breast cancer patients called brachial plexopathy and its treatment will be discussed.

Keywords

Metastatic breast cancer • Brain metastases • Leptomeningeal metastases • Epidural metastases • Stereotactic radiation therapy (SRT) • Whole brain radiotherapy (WBRT) • Radiosurgery • Brain irradiation • Adjuvant WBRT • Hippocampus-sparing radiotherapy

Parenchymal Brain Metastases of Breast Cancer

Ş. Karaman, MD (✉) • S. Küçücük, MD
Radiation Oncology Department, Istanbul University
Institute of Oncology, Çapa, Istanbul, Turkey
e-mail: karamansule@yahoo.com;
seden.kucucuk@gmail.com

Metastases are the most common malignancy (50 %) of the brain parenchyma. They are ten times more common than primary brain tumors [1, 2]. Metastases to the brain (BMs) develop in approximately 20–40 % of all cancers [3, 4], including lung cancer, breast cancer, melanoma, colon cancer, and renal cell tumors [4–8]. In breast cancer patients, the clinical incidence of BM is 10–15 %, whereas in autopsy series, the rate has been reported as 18–30 % [9]. In patients with breast cancer, BMs are diagnosed with localized disease at the time of diagnosis in 2.5 % of patients, in systemic disease in 5–10 % of patients, as a solitary disease in 5–10 % of patients, and metachronous with known systemic disease in ≥80 % of patients. Potential risk factors of metastasis in general have been investigated in many studies, including BM patients. These risk factors include young age, short disease-free survival, the presence of visceral metastases, high-grade, and hormone-negative disease [10]. In the RTOG "Recursive Partitioning Analysis" (RPA) model, which included 1,200 patients, three prognostic categories for BM were identified (Table 37.1). According to this model, the patients with the best prognosis were under 65 years of age, had a Karnofsky performance score (KPS) higher than 70, and had no extracranial disease, and the primary tumor was under control.

There were no differences between solitary and multiple BM models; however, being solitary or multiple BM has extra prognostic value for RPA 1 and RPA 2 [11]. Sperduto et al. updated RTOG's RPA data and proposed a new prognostic scoring system called the "graded prognostic assessment" (GPA) [12]. The GPA scoring system consists of four categories ranging between 2.6 and 11 months (Table 37.2). The GPA system has shown that patients with one to three metastases have a more favorable outcome than patients with >4 metastatic lesions.

If the BM can be controlled or the disease can be eradicated, the GPA scoring system results suggest that patients with a better prognosis can be treated more aggressively. In high-performance patients with a solitary BM, stereotactic radiation therapy (SRT) + whole brain radiotherapy (WBRT) is recommended instead of WBRT (evidence level I).

The CNS metastasis risk is two to four times higher in patients with epidermal growth factor 2-positive (HER-2 (+) breast cancers than those with HER-2 (−) breast cancers. This increase may be due to the aggressive nature of HER-2 (+) breast cancers, but it may also be related to the use of trastuzumab in these patients, which prolongs survival enough for BMs to develop [13] Another hypothesis is that HER-2 positivity activates the

Table 37.1 Median survival in patients treated with WBRT according to the RPA

RPA	Clinical features	Median survival for all primary tumors (months)	Median survival for brain metastatic breast cancer (months)
1	KPS ≥70	7.1 (13.5 with a single BM)	15
	Age <65		
	Primary cancer controlled		
	No extracranial disease		
2	KPS ≥70	4.2 (6 with a single BM)	11
	Age ≥65		
	Primary cancer not controlled or extracranial disease exists		
3	KPS <70	2.3	3

RPA Recursive partitioning analysis score, *KPS* Karnofsky performance status, *BM* Brain metastasis

Table 37.2 GPA score

Score				
(A)				
	0	0.5	1	
Age	>60	50–59	<50	
KPS	<70	70–80	90–100	
Number of CNS metastases	>3	2–3	1	
Extracranial disease	Present	–	none	
(B)				
GPA	0–1	1.5–2	2.5–3	3.5–4
General survival for all primary cancers (months)	3.1	5.4	9.61	6.7
General survival for breast cancer (months)	3.4	7.7	15.1	25.3

KPS Karnofsky performance status, *CNS* Central nervous system, *GPA* Graded prognostic assessment

VEGF pathway and causes a biological predisposition for CNS metastases [14]. Recently, triple-negative breast cancers and HER-2 (+) breast cancers have been shown to have a similar risk of CNS metastases. Lin et al. have reported that 46 % of metastatic triple-negative patients will be diagnosed with a CNS metastasis [15]. In a 2012 study by Sperduto et al. which only included breast cancer patients, tumor subgroup (luminal, A, B, HER-2), KPS (under or over 70), and age (under or over 60) were significant prognostic factors for BM [16, 17].

The diagnosis of BMs begins with a clinical suspicion. The most common symptom is headache (24–48 %) [18]. Mental and cognitive changes, motor deficits, seizures, nausea, and vomiting are some of the other possible symptoms. Contrasted computed tomography (CT) and contrasted brain magnetic resonance imaging (MRI) are used for radiological diagnosis. The most specific diagnostic method for BMs is MRI [19]. In Fig. 37.1a–c, MRI of multiple BMs is shown in three planes. Approximately 20 % of patients with solitary metastases on CT scans have multiple metastases as determined by MRI. Primary brain tumors (benign/malign) should be differentiated from infections, cerebral infarcts, arteriovenous malformations, hemorrhages, demyelinating diseases, and radiation necrosis. To assess the disease status, full systemic scans (such as PET-CT, CT) should be performed simultaneously with BM imaging. There is no survival advantage of early diagnosis when still asymptomatic; however, early diagnosis significantly decreases post-WBRT cerebral deaths.

The aim of breast cancer BM treatment is controlling symptoms, decreasing morbidity caused by potential neurological damage, and increasing local control (LC) and survival without disrupting the quality of life as much as possible.

Treatment methods are symptomatic treatment and treatment of life-threatening problems, such as obstruction or hydrocephalus, with surgery, RT, chemoradiotherapy (CRT), chemotherapy (CT), hormonal treatment (HT), and targeted treatments.

After a diagnosis of BM, the first step is planning symptomatic medical treatment. The aim of symptomatic treatment is to relieve and prevent neurological symptoms caused by edema and to control seizures. Symptomatic patients should immediately be administered steroid treatment (dexamethasone or methylprednisolone). Generally, dexamethasone is chosen because its mineralocorticoid effects are low, it has mild effects on cognitive functions, and it readily penetrates the cerebrospinal fluid (CSF). The only randomized trial to address steroid dosage is Vecht et al.'s trial, which included 96 patients [20]. In this study, the first arm was randomized to 8 mg/day or 16 mg/day doses, which gradually decreased over 4 weeks. The second arm was randomized to 4 mg or 16 mg for 4 weeks, after which the dose was gradually decreased. To prevent gastritis, an H2 receptor agonist was administered simultaneously with dexamethasone. In both arms, there were similar improvements of the KPS on days 7 and 28. The dosing recommendation from this study resulted in a set 4 mg/day dosage with dose tapering over 4 weeks. Starting with a high 16 mg dexamethasone dose and tapering over 4 weeks caused a better improvement in KPS. This effect can be explained by the maximal anti-inflammatory effect of initiating treatment with high doses and the minimization of delayed steroid-related toxicities with dose tapering. In symptomatic patients, treatment can be initiated with an intravenous bolus of 10 mg followed by 4–6 mg of dexamethasone every 6–8 h. In asymptomatic patients with minimal peritumoral edema or mass effect, the steroid dose can be kept at a lower level until neurological symptoms appear. In BM patients, the doses should be arranged individually based on the patient, the clinical features, edema, and mass effect caused by the tumor. Patients presenting with seizures should be given anticonvulsants. Phenytoin, carbamazepine, and sodium valproate are commonly used anticonvulsants. For metastases that are located on the motor cortex and metastases that are concomitant with leptomeningeal metastases, prophylactic anticonvulsant therapy may decrease the risk and frequency of seizures [21]. Valproic acid is the primary anticonvulsant used in chemotherapy patients.

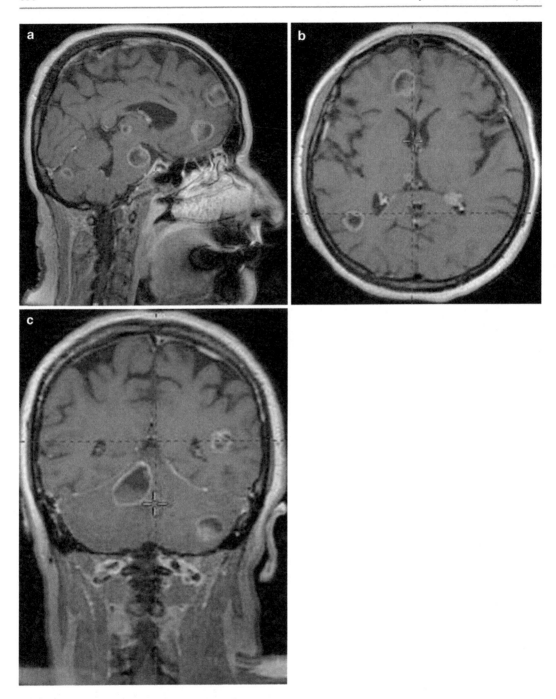

Fig. 37.1 (a–c) MRI of multiple BMs in three planes

In patients with BMs, the median survival with supportive treatment only is 1–3 months. The clinical response rate of WBRT is 50 %, and survival increases twofold (3–6 months). Patients who receive systemic hormonal treatment or chemotherapy after local treatment of the BM have a longer survival than patients who do not receive systemic treatment (7–8 months vs. 3–6 months, respectively) [22]. In oligometastatic disease, the combination of WBRT and local treatments, such as surgery or SRT, results in a higher overall survival rate than WBRT alone.

In our approach to BM treatment, the number and size of the brain lesions, the performance of the patient, and the control of the systemic disease are important factors. If solitary lesions are larger than one centimeter (>1 cm) and there are no signs of extracranial metastatic disease, they are called "solitary metastases"; additionally, if the presence of extracranial metastases is unknown, they are called "single metastases."

A single metastasis is found in 20–30 % of BM patients, two to three oligometastatic metastases are found in 20–30 %, and two third of the patients are polymetastatic and have three or more metastases.

If a solitary metastasis is present, a biopsy should be performed if possible. The diagnosis changes after the biopsy in 11 % of the solitary metastasis. It may be difficult to differentiate these lesions from abscesses, gliomas, and meningiomas, and the incidence of meningiomas is higher in breast cancer patients than in the normal population [23]. CT scans may not be able to detect occult metastases, and incorrect surgical decisions may be made. To avoid this potential problem, preoperative MRI is necessary. The standard treatment for single BMs is surgery. Single small brain lesions suspected to be metastases are treated surgically or are monitored with MRI and treated surgically if growth is detected. The algorithm for the primary treatment of BM is shown in Table 37.3.

WBRT

Although systemic treatment has advantages for the treatment of metastatic breast cancer (MBC), local treatments continue to be more effective in newly diagnosed patients presenting with BMs. Breast cancer metastases to the brain are hematogenous, so there can be micrometastases anywhere in the brain. Therefore, WBRT is the mainstay of the standard treatment of MBC with BM. This treatment has the advantages of preventing or delaying neurological deficits, regaining lost functions, and decreasing steroid

Table 37.3 Primary treatment algorithm of metastatic brain lesions

Number of lesions	Size of lesions	Treatment		
1	<1 cm lesion (asymptomatic, unidentified diagnosis)	Observation or surgery		
		Surgery + WBRT or SRT + WBRT if it grows		
	<1 cm lesion (pathologically verified lesion)	Treated similarly to >1 cm lesions		
	>1 cm lesion	Single	KPS ≥70; if primary is under control	
			Surgery ± WBRT or SRT ± WBRT	
			KPS <70; if primary is not under control	
			WBRT	
		Solitary	KPS <70; if primary is not under control	
			WBRT	
2–3	Any	KPS ≥70; if primary is under control		
		S ± WBRT or SRT ± WBRT		
		KPS <70; if primary is not under control		
		WBRT		
>3	Any	WBRT		

KPS Karnofsky performance score, *RT* Radiotherapy, *SRT* Stereotactic radiotherapy, *cm* Centimeter, *S* Surgery, *WBRT* Whole brain RT

dependency, and it is the best supportive treatment method for BM. Reciprocal and multiple field three-dimensional conformal planning samples are shown in Figs. 37.2 and 37.3.

Randomized trials investigating BM treatments include BM patients in whom BM is caused by various primary cancers. The primary cancer of BM patients in these trials is lung cancer in 50–77 % of the patients and breast cancer in 8–19 % of the patients. In other words, the international guidelines for breast cancer patients are based on only approximately 10 % of the patients in these randomized trials [18]. In addition, low-performance patients (KPS <70) have been excluded from these studies. Because no

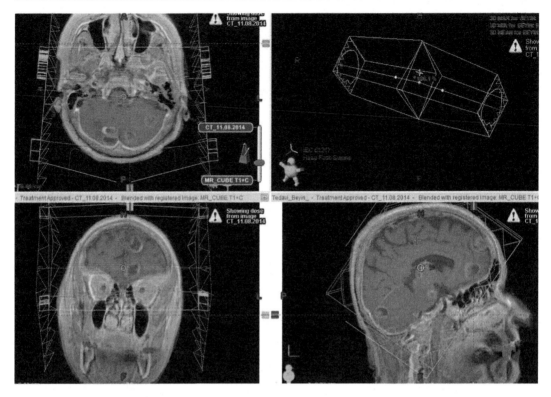

Fig. 37.2 Treatment plan for WBRT with reciprocal fields

randomized trials include only breast cancer BM patients, we must evaluate the characteristics of BMs of lung and breast cancers individually before using the information provided by these randomized trials for the treatment of breast cancer BM. When the epidemiologic data are reviewed, the prognosis of low-performance breast cancer BM (KPS <70) is two times worse than the prognosis of small cell lung cancers. In addition, the probability of the metastasis developing in the brain alone is 20–25 % in breast cancers and 60–75 % in NSCLC [24]. Thus, SRT alone is not always a good option for the treatment of breast cancer BM, and WBRT still plays a very important role.

The studies on breast cancer BM patients who were treated only with WBRT are summarized in Table 37.4 [25–28].

To determine the optimal WBRT dose for BMs, various RT plans, which aimed to increase LC and survival while decreasing delayed side effects, have been compared (Table 37.5)

[29–33]. No difference in general survival and acute toxicity was shown in these studies. Disease-free survival, tumor response rate, and quality of life results were not analyzed. These trials failed to provide a consensus on a single fractionation and dosage. However, fundamental radiation oncology knowledge suggests that plans with lower doses per fraction will result in less delayed neurocognitive side effects. Currently, a commonly used RT plan is 30 Gy, delivered via ten fractions of daily 300 cGy doses. If fractionation is determined according to the patient's prognosis, the long-term side effects of WBRT can be minimized in patients with longer survival expectancy. In RPA III patients who are resistant to chemotherapy, short plans (e.g., 20 Gy/5 fr) may be preferred.

Although chemotherapeutic agents traditionally have a limited role in BM due to their low potential to pass the blood-brain barrier, they have been used in combination with WBRT in some studies. Many randomized trials have investigated

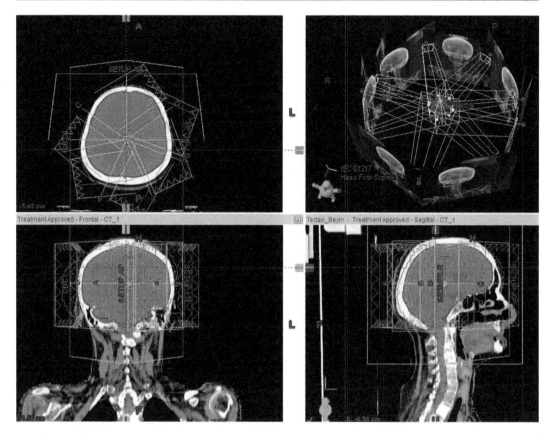

Fig. 37.3 Whole brain radiotherapy planning in multiple fields

Table 37.4 Breast cancer BM studies in which patients were treated with WBRT alone

Study	N	RT plan (Gy/fr)	Response rate (%)	Recurrence rate (%)
Nieder et al. (1997) [25]	46	30/10	65	0
Ogura et al. (2003) [26]	36	30/10	82	32
		50/25		
		10 pts boost RT		
Mahmoud-Ahmed et al. (2002) [27]	116	30/10	NR	50
Le scodan et al. (2007) [28]	117	30/10	NR	42.5

RT Radiotherapy, *Gy* Gray, *fr* Fraction, *pts* Patients, *NR* Not relevant

the use of WBRT in combination with radiation sensitizers, such as misonidazole, motexafin gadolinium (MGd), efaproxiral, thalidomide, and temozolomide (TMZ), for treating the BMs of various primary cancers, most of which were lung cancers [34–37]. However, in most of these studies, the frequency of toxicities had increased, and no difference was found in LC and median survival. In some studies, an increased response rate was observed with radiation sensitizers (especially TMZ) and WBRT [38, 39]. Two randomized trials that compared WBRT alone and with concomitant TMZ use in BMs are summarized in Table 37.6. These trials have shown that TMZ improves LC and delays cerebral progression. However, toxicity was increased, and no change in general survival was reported. The results of these two small trials must be reviewed in larger series. In patients with bulky BMs who are not suitable candidates for SRT, with registration limited to prospective studies, WBRT and concomitant TMZ use may be considered.

In breast cancer patients with BM, treatments targeting the HER-2 receptor are being used in combination with WBRT, and research is ongoing. A retrospective trial including 31 patients has shown that trastuzumab and WBRT combinations are tolerated well, and the responses have been encouraging [40]. Lapatinib combined with WBRT has been tested in HER-2 (+) brain cancer patients in a phase I trial. However, the study did not meet the predefined criteria for feasibility [41]. Further studies are ongoing to determine the use of chemotherapy and targeted treatments in combination with WBRT.

Table 37.5 Some randomized trials on various BM radiotherapy plans

Study	N	RT plan (Gy/fr)	Median survival (w)	P
RTOG 6901	910	30/10	21	NS
Borgelt et al. [29]		30/15	18	
		40/15	18	
		40/20	16	
Haide-Meder et al. [30]	226	25/10	16.8	NS
		36/6	21.2	
Royal College of Radiology [31]	533	30/10	12	NS
		12/2	11	
RTOG 91-04 [32]	429	30/10	18	NS
		54.4/34	18	
Graham et al. [33]	113	40/20	24.4	NS
		20/4	26.4	

RT Radiotherapy, *Gy* Gray, *fr* Fraction, *N* Patient number, *w* Weeks, *NR* Not relevant

In oligometastatic disease, surgery or SRT followed by WBRT has shown no improvement in neurological symptoms and overall survival. This outcome has raised doubts concerning the ability to decrease potential long-term side effects by withholding WBRT and the benefit of initiating treatment of BMs with systemic therapies. Currently, initiating treatment with systemic treatment instead of WBRT is an approach considered in HER-2 (+) breast cancer BM patients because lapatinib has significant efficacy in treating CNS metastases. If life expectancy is longer than 2 years, the long-term side effects of WBRT must be considered. The LANDSCAPE trial results suggested that WBRT can be withheld and that systemic treatment can be initiated in patients with multiple BMs. However, specific patient groups, such as asymptomatic patients at baseline, were also included in the trial. Another randomized trial is warranted to demonstrate the possibility of withholding WBRT in HER-2 (+) BM patients. Advancements that help us to understand the pathobiological processes in BM formation may help us to determine prophylactic strategies to prevent BM formation in high-risk HER-2 (+) or triple-negative breast cancer patients. We previously mentioned that the overexpression of the HER-2 protein is associated with a high brain relapse rate in HER-2 (+) locally advanced breast cancer. Duchnowska et al. reported that 13 gene signatures can be predictive in HER-2 (+) patients and that this feature can be used in further predictive research [42]. Tumor cells cause

Table 37.6 Trials comparing WBRT alone and WBRT + CT in the treatment of breast cancer BMs

Study	N	Primary distribution (%)	Randomization (Gy/fr)	Median survival (m)	Response rate %
Antonadou et al. (2002) [38]	23	Lung: 83	40/20	7	67
		Breast: 11			
	25	Ovaries: 6	40/20 + TMZ	8.6	96
				NS	(*p*: 0.017)
Verger et al. (2005) [39]	41	Lung: 51	30/10	3.1	
		Breast: 16			54
	41	Ovaries: 33	30/10 + TMZ	4.5	72
				NS	(*p*: 0.03)

RT Radiotherapy, *Gy* Gray, *fr* Fraction, *TMZ* Temozolomide, *NS* Nonspecific

brain involvement by integrin-mediated growth along the basal vascular membrane or by inducing neoangiogenesis and nodular growth. An appropriate approach to prevent BM development is suppressing these growth factors with specific drugs (e.g., integrin inhibitors or antiangiogenic drugs). In preclinical animal trials, the intracardiac administration of these drugs prevents the development of BM. The Angle-Celtic VII and Tsarine 0602 trial is an ongoing trial investigating the role of prophylactic brain irradiation in Her-2 (+) breast cancer patients with no BM. However, these trials were not well received by clinicians and patients because of the long-term neurotoxicity caused by RT and were halted due to low patient participation. A more accepted alternative for WBRT planning is hippocampus-sparing PCI. In this approach, better memory preservation is possible. Future trials will be designed to report the results of this technique. An example of hippocampus-sparing conformal WBRT planning is shown in Fig. 37.4.

Surgery

The surgical treatment of BMs provides fast relief of symptoms, LC, and histopathological confirmation of the diagnosis. Developments in cortical mapping and stereotactic techniques and the use of ultrasonography (USG) have made metastatic lesions easily accessible. Surgery is not an appropriate approach in patients with multiple metastases, uncontrolled primary disease, comorbidities, or inaccessible lesions. Three randomized trials have questioned whether WBRT should be used alone or if it should be combined with surgery. One of these randomized trials was from Patchell et al. and included 48 patients, only 10 % of whom were breast cancer patients.

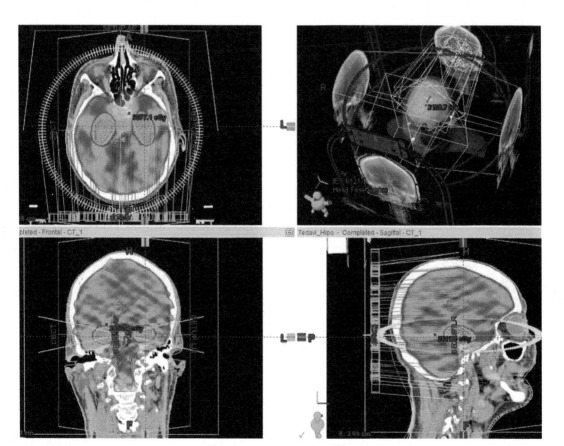

Fig. 37.4 Hippocampus-sparing WBRT planning

Patients were randomized to WBRT alone and surgery with WBRT arms. Functional improvement (38 weeks versus 8 weeks, respectively) and the survival advantages (40 weeks versus 15 weeks, respectively, $p < 0.005$) were significantly better, and recurrence significantly decreased in the combined treatment (surgery + WBRT) arm (20 % versus 52 %, respectively, $p < 0.02$) [43].

The second randomized trial was from Vecht et al. and included 64 BM patients (with primary breast cancer in 19 %) [44]. Similar results with combined treatment were reported in this trial. This study has shown that clinically stable patients without extracranial disease benefit from combined treatment. The median survival was only 5 months in patients with progressive extracranial disease. In a randomized trial by Mintz et al. studying similar arms in 84 patients, no difference in survival was reported [45]. However, 73 % of the patients had extracranial disease and were low performance, and the definition of single metastases was inadequate due to the absence of cranial MRI.

The specifics of the three randomized trials are summarized in Table 37.7. These randomized trials showed that longer survival rates were achieved in patients treated with surgery and WBRT when compared with WBRT alone [43–45]. However, these results were explained by high-performance patients being treated with surgery. All three of these trials suggested that surgical treatment should be limited to high-performance status patients with BMs that can potentially cause life-threatening complications.

In the Cochrane Review of these randomized trials, including 195 patients, an increase in functionally independent survival and a significant decrease in neurological deaths were observed in patients treated with surgery plus WBRT when compared with patients treated with WBRT alone. However, there was no significant difference in overall survival [46].

A postoperative hippocampus-sparing three-dimensional conformal WBRT planning example is shown in Fig. 37.5.

In many retrospective studies, surgery alone has been reported to have more favorable results than WBRT alone [47]. However, surgery patients have high-performance statuses, single metastases, and minimal extracranial diseases. These features are indicative of good prognoses in many multivariate analyses. Surgery alone and WBRT alone have been compared in two randomized trials. In only 10 % of these patients, the primary cancer was breast cancer.

In a study by Patchell et al., the recurrence rates for surgery patients were calculated as 46 % at the initial BM location and 70 % in the whole brain. A total of 44 % of the patients treated with surgery alone died due to neurological symptoms caused by BM recurrence. The similarity of survival rates has led to some studies concluding that surgery alone may be sufficient. However, the primary end point of this trial was recurrence rates, not survival. A statistical analysis of survival results would require 2,000 patients, whereas this trial only included 94 patients. This sample size is not enough for survival analyses [48].

Table 37.7 Randomized trials comparing WBRT and Surgery + WBRT

Study	N #	Randomized arms	RT plan (Gy/fr)	Median survival (m)	FIS
Patel et al. [43]	48	WBRT S + WBRT	36/12	3.4 9.2 $p < 0.01$	–
Vecht et al. [44]	64	WBRT S + WBRT	40/20	6 10 p: 0.04	3.5 7.5 p: 0.06
Mintz et al. [45]	84	WBRT S + WBRT	30/10	6.3 5.6 p: 0.24 (NS)	32 % 32 % (NS)

RT Radiotherapy, *Gy* Gray, *fr* Fraction, *S* Surgery, *WBRT* Whole brain radiotherapy, *NS* Nonspecific, *FIS* Functionally independent survival

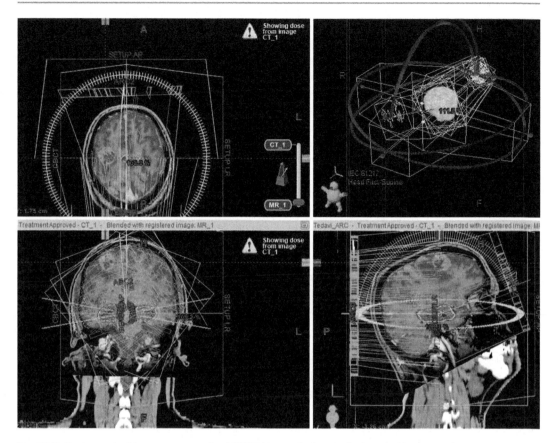

Fig. 37.5 Postoperative hippocampus-sparing WBRT (the surgical cavity is shown with an *arrow*)

The phase III EORTC 22952-26001 trial published in 2001 by Kocher et al. included 359 patients with one to three BMs who were treated with surgery or SRS (20 Gy/1 fr) and were randomized to observation or WBRT (30 Gy/10 fr) arms. LC was 41 % in the surgery group and 73 % in the S and WBRT group. The addition of WBRT decreased intracranial recurrences and neurological deaths but did not increase functionally independent survival or overall survival. Based on the results of this trial, WBRT may be withheld in high-performance patients with stable disease and a limited number of BMs, and these patients may be monitored with frequent imaging studies [49].

In these two trials, no difference in survival was shown in WBRT patients, but brain recurrence rates and neurological deaths decreased. In both trials, less than 50 % of patients had controlled extracranial disease, and subgroups were not analyzed. We can expect a survival advantage in patients with controlled extracranial disease. In addition, the rate of neurological death was significantly higher when RT was delayed. Delayed RT (salvage therapy) seems to be less effective than upfront WBRT.

The surgical approach to single BMs in breast cancer is a treatment option to be considered in patients with a single metastasis, no extracranial disease, and controlled disease. However, this approach is still unclear because the literature about BMs in breast cancer is limited.

With multiple BMs, the role of surgery remains controversial. There are single center results in the literature [47]. In the retrospective data provided by Bindal et al., the postoperative median survival in patients with multiple metastases is 14 months. However, the survival reported by Hazuka et al. in the same patient group was only 5 months. The difference between the data may be due to differences in the distribution of the primary cancers. The surgical approach to multiple BMs of breast cancer is limited due to the morbidity of multiple craniotomies. The use of surgery must be limited to large and symptomatic lesions.

WBRT is one of the treatment options for patients with one to three BMs. WBRT increases LC and intracerebral control but may decrease the quality of life and impair neurocognitive function. Additionally, combined treatment offers no survival benefit. This inadequacy has focused attention on postoperative SRT. With SRT being used in BM, postoperative SRT has been questioned in many retrospective trials. Surgical resection followed by SRT was analyzed by Kelly PJ et al. in 2012 using retrospective data from seven centers. However, there were no BM patients with primary breast cancer among the patients who were evaluated. The median dose was 18 Gy [15–19], and LC was 74–100 %. The median survival was 15 months, and WBRT use could be decreased by 70 %. SRT was administered 4–6 weeks later, with the goal of delivering RT to a smaller cavity after surgery; however, tumor progression may occur during this period. In these series, SRT to the resection cavity was generally offered as an alternative RT option in patients with RPA <3, KPS >70 %, and ≤3 metastases [50].

In the study published in 2012 by Choi et al., SRT was delivered to 120 cavities in 112 patients with a median dose of 20 Gy (12–30 Gy). In 16 % of these patients, the primary of the BM was breast cancer. Univariate analysis showed that LC was better in patients with margins for the target volume. LC is an independent factor for distant metastases (DM) in breast cancer. SRT is suggested as an alternative to WBRT in patients who can be monitored closely [51]. However, no randomized trial with postsurgical WBRT and SRT arms has come to a clear conclusion about these approaches.

SRT

WBRT is the mainstay of treatment for BM. However, serious neurocognitive impairments caused by WBRT have been reported in the last decade [4]. In two randomized trials, the

survival and local control rates of surgery combined with WBRT were better than those for WBRT alone. This improvement has raised hopes that similar results can be achieved when WBRT and SRT are used in combination to treat BM [52]. Examples of photon-based SRT techniques include gamma knife (GK), linear accelerators (LINACs), and CyberKnife. Lars Leksell developed the idea of sending radiation beams to a specific target in the cranium and implemented it using a stereotactic frame. Leksell initially used orthovoltage X-rays, and in 1967, he started using the gamma rays produced by 201 cobalt-60 with Larsson. He named the method "radiosurgery" because it combines surgery and RT and allows the total X-ray dose of classical RT to be delivered to a specific target in one session. The beam he used inspired him to name the system he uses the GammaKnife.

Generally, the tumor diameter must be smaller than 3.5 cm to use the GammaKnife. With increased clinical use of the GammaKnife, LINACs have been modified to the stereotactic RT system to treat tumors of various sizes and locations with stereotactic radiosurgery. In LINAC-based systems, LINAC devices and micro-multileaf collimators or circular collimators are used to shape the beam according to the target volume. The CyberKnife radiosurgery system mainly consists of a linear accelerator generating 6 MV X-rays that is placed on an industrial robot with six joints and a robotic patient bed that can move in six directions. In SRT, the dose that reaches the surrounding brain tissue is clinically insignificant, and a higher dose is delivered to the target volume. SRT has many advantages: the hemorrhaging and infection risks are low, the seeding potential of the tumor is low, and the duration of the hospital stay is shorter, thus reducing hospital costs.

Surgery and SRT have not been compared in any randomized trials. Retrospective studies report controversial results due to patient selection. In a nonrandomized trial by Bindal et al., 31 patients were treated with SRT, and 62 patients were treated with surgery; 16 % of all these patients had primary breast cancer. In the surgery arm, overall survival increased, and neurological deaths decreased [53]. In contrast, no survival advantage was shown in similar groups in a study conducted by the Mayo Clinic [54]. Auchter et al. reported a 1-year local control of 85 % and a median survival of 56 weeks in 122 single BM patients treated with SRT (11 % primary breast cancer) [55]. The results for surgery were similar.

In both studies, the authors concluded that the results for SRT and surgery were equivalent. Due to the lack of randomized data, the decision to treat with SRT or surgery should be made according to the lesion size, current symptoms, and functional status. The neurotoxicity and local failure rates are assumed to increase as the lesion size increases so the use of SRT is suggested for lesions smaller than 3 cm. Surgery should be performed for large and symptomatic lesions that require emergency decompression. For small and asymptomatic lesions, both treatment methods can be used. A planning sample for a patient with a single metastasis is shown in Fig. 37.6.

Three randomized studies and one review have compared WBRT alone and WBRT combined with an SRT boost.

In a randomized study by Kondziolka et al., 27 patients with two to four BMs that were 2.5 cm or smaller were evaluated. WBRT alone and WBRT + SRT were compared. In the WBRT and SRT combined treatment arm, LC and whole brain control results were more favorable, but no difference in survival was reported [56].

In the RTOG 9508 study conducted by Andrews et al., which included 333 patients with one to three BMs, WBRT alone and WBRT + SRT were compared. The WBRT dose was 37.5 Gy/15 fr, and the SRT dose was 15–24 Gy/1 fr. Although 3–4 cm tumors were included in this study, a survival advantage was reported for single metastasis and RPA 1 cases in the WBRT + SRT arm when compared with the WBRT alone arm (6.5 and 4.9 months; p: 0.04; 9.6 and 11.6 months, respectively). This advantage was not demonstrated for multiple metastases. Performance status improved at 6 months (43 % and 27 %, respectively; p: 0.03), and LC

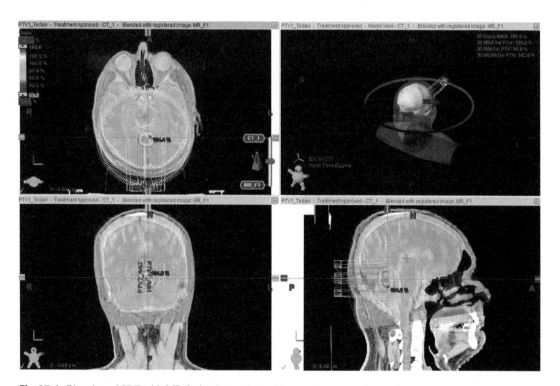

Fig. 37.6 Planning of SRT with MR fusion in a patient with a single metastasis

increased (82 % and 71 %, respectively; *p*: 0.01) in the WBRT + SRT arm when compared with the WBRT alone arm [3].

The results of a randomized trial with three arms by Chagule et al. from Brown University have only been published in summary [57]. Although the survival rates were similar in all three arms, and better LC rates and less brain recurrence were reported, the statistical results were not published. In addition, symptomatic lesions were surgically resected from 51 patients before randomization, and the effect of these patients on the results was not specified as a subgroup in any of the analyses. The patient number was also insufficient for statistically significant results. The SRT doses used were not changed in accordance with the tumor size. The summary of this three armed trial is shown in Table 37.8 [3, 56–58]. It is the only study that has included two arms comparing WBRT and SRT.

The Cochrane Review included three randomized trials that compared WBRT with WBRT + SRT in 385 patients with BM. No difference in overall survival was shown between the two arms. In single BM patients treated with WBRT + SRT, survival significantly increased in comparison with WBRT alone (6.5 months and 4.9 months, respectively; *p*:0.04). When compared with the WBRT arm, local failure rates were lower (HR 0.27; 95 % CI 0.14–0.52), the improvement of performance status was significantly higher (43 % versus 27 %, *p*: 0.05), and steroid dependency decreased (RR 0.64; 95 % CI 0.42–0.97; *p*: 0.03) in the WBRT + SRT arm [58]. In light of these studies, the SRT boost is indicated in single metastases, but it is hard to recommend routine use in patients with multiple metastases.

The results of the three randomized studies and the review on WBRT and WBRT + SRT are shown in Table 37.8.

Three randomized studies have investigated the combination of SRT with WBRT and SRT alone [49, 59, 60]. In the EORTC 22952-26001 study, 359 patients treated with surgery or SRT (20 Gy/1 fr) were randomized to observation or WBRT (30 Gy/10 fr) arms. Patients with stable systemic disease, controlled primary tumors, and high KPS were included in the trial. Compared with observation, the results of adding WBRT showed a decrease in intracranial relapse (surgery 59 % vs. 27 % and SRT 31 % vs. 19 %,

Table 37.8 A summary of the randomized trials and the review that compare WBRT only and WBRT + SRT boost

Study	N #	Randomization	LC (%)	Overall survival (m)	Time to failure (m)	Time to any brain failure (m)	New brain lesion (%)	Performance improvement at 6 months (%)
Kondziolka et al. [56]	27	WBRT + SRT WBRT	96 0 *P*: 0.016	11 7.5 NS	36 6 *P*: 0.005	34 5 *P*: 0.02	–	
Chagule et al. [57]	109	WBRT + SRT WBRT SRT	91 62 87 NS	5 9 7 NS	–		19 23 43 NS	
RTOG 9508 [3]	333	WBRT + SRT WBRT	82 71 *P*: 0.01					43 23 *P*: 0.03
Cochrane [58]	385	WBRT + SRT WBRT	–	Single BM 6.5 4.9 *P*: 0.04	–	–	–	34 27 *P*: 0.05

LC Local control, *WBRT* Whole brain radiotherapy, *SRT* Stereotactic radiotherapy, *BMs* Brain metastases, *NS* Not specified respectively) and death rates due to neurological symptoms. However, no differences were reported in overall survival or functionally independent survival. Just as with surgery, the contribution to disease control in other areas of the brain and overall survival is minimal. In conclusion, in locally treated (SRT) BM patients with one to three metastases, the addition of adjuvant WBRT decreases intracranial relapses and death due to neurological symptoms but makes no difference in functionally independent survival (FIS) and overall survival [49]. In a study by Chang et al., 58 patients with one to three metastases were randomized to SRT followed by WBRT or observation arms [59].

In the JROSG 99-1 study conducted by Aoyama et al., which included the participation of 11 centers in Japan, 132 patients with one to four metastases were randomized to SRT followed by observation or WBRT arms. The 1-year survival rate was significantly higher in the SRT arm compared with the SRT + WBRT arm (76 % and 46.8 %, respectively; $p < 0.001$). In the SRT-alone arm, the brain salvaging treatment requirement was significantly higher in comparison with

that in the SRT + WBRT arm (29 patients and 10 patients, respectively; $p < 0.001$). No differences were observed between the two arms in terms of survival (7.5 and 8 months) and neurological deaths [60].

Tsao et al. updated the Cochrane Review. This update included three randomized trials that compared SRT and SRT + WBRT. Combined therapy increased LC in the whole brain when compared with patients treated with SRT alone but had no effect on overall survival [61].

Until further research is performed, the use of combined SRT and WBRT should be limited to patients with good performance statuses, long life expectancy, and controlled extracranial disease. A sample hippocampus-sparing WBRT and SRT plan for metastases is shown in Fig. 37.7.

The benefit of the addition of SRT to WBRT in multiple BMs is being investigated in four ongoing prospective studies.

No prospective randomized studies have compared surgery + WBRT and SRT + WBRT. In retrospective data, no overall survival difference was noted, apart from one study with patient selection bias.

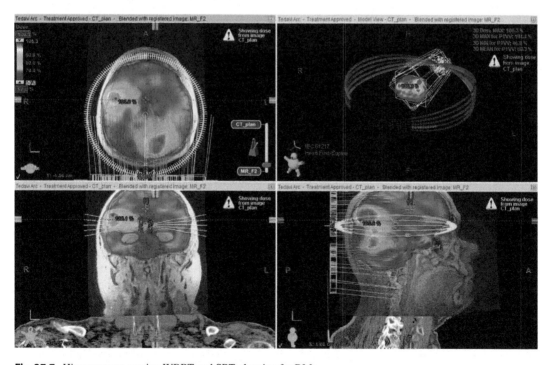

Fig. 37.7 Hippocampus-sparing WBRT and SRT planning for BMs

Adjuvant WBRT After Surgery or SRT

Adjuvant WBRT after surgery or SRT is generally recommended to prevent local recurrence and to target micrometastases that cannot be detected with imaging methods. The basis of this recommendation is the 1998 trial by Patell et al., which demonstrated a larger decrease in local recurrences in patients who received WBRT after surgery than in patients treated only with surgery [48]. The role of surgery followed by WBRT in breast cancer BM has been investigated in many retrospective trials, but no trial has reported a survival benefit. These studies contained heterogeneous groups of BM patients with various primary cancers. In the prospective study by Patell et al., only nine patients had a single BM due to primary breast cancer. In this trial, 95 patients with a single BM were allocated to surgery followed with observation and postoperative WBRT (50.4 Gy/5.5 weeks) arms. In the postoperative WBRT arm, there was a significant decrease in the recurrence (18 % and 70 %, $p < 0.001$) and neurological death rates compared with the surgery followed by observation group (14 % and 44 %, $p = 0.003$, respectively). However, the normal WBRT dose was not used in this study. WBRT has a survival advantage but also increases cognitive side effects. Recent studies have questioned its routine use after SRT and surgery [59, 60, 62, 63].

A Cochrane meta-analysis evaluated 663 patients from five randomized trials comparing SRT with WBRT, surgery, and SRT alone in the treatment of BM. In this meta-analysis, the 1-year intracranial progression risk decreased by 53 % in patients treated with adjuvant WBRT in comparison with patients who were not treated with WBRT ($p < 0.0001$). No differences were shown in overall survival or disease-free survival (p: 0.08 and p: 0.28, respectively) [46]. The effect of WBRT on neurocognitive functions, the quality of life, and neurological events is unclear due to study bias. In light of the five randomized trials on adjuvant RT, following local treatments (SRT, surgery) with adjuvant WBRT should be a standard.

Intracavitary and Interstitial Brain Irradiation

Brachytherapy with the GliaSite Radiation Therapy System has only been approved for the intracavitary treatment of primary brain tumors. One multi-institutional phase II study has defined its use in resectable single BMs. In this study, 62 patients who were at risk for recurrence were treated with a single-use applicator system at doses of 60 Gy RT to a depth of 10 mm. There is a dual silicone balloon at the edge of the applicator. The internal balloon serves as a lotrex (125 I) reservoir, and the external balloon is a backup reservoir. No patients received WBRT, and 43 % of the patients had extracranial disease. In the results of the trial, LR was 82–87 % in MRI follow-ups, and the median survival was 10 months. Thus, the GliaSite results were similar to WBRT for LC, overall survival, and functional independence [64].

Cosgrove et al. treated 14 brain cancer patients with lesions smaller than 3.5 cm with doses of 15 Gy. At the 12 month follow-up, LC was successful in 10 of 13 patients. However, interstitial procedures are not very popular for BM [65].

Second Course Brain Irradiation in Recurrent BMs (Re-irradiation)

If too many recurrent lesions are present for treatment with SRT, the WBRT decision must be made very carefully. As a general principle, SRT must be prioritized and used whenever possible because it preserves normal brain tissue. An SRT planning sample for a patient with a new BM who was previously treated with WBRT 1 year prior is shown in Fig. 37.8.

Wong et al. reported the largest series, which included 86 patients treated with a second course of WBRT. During the first course of WBRT, 30 Gy doses were delivered, and during the second course, an average dose of 20 Gy was delivered. The median survival was 4 months after the second course of irradiation. Among the patients, 27 % experienced full relief of symptoms, 43 % experienced partial relief, and 29 % experienced

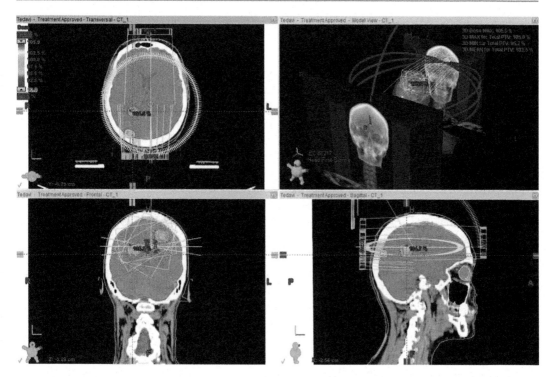

Fig. 37.8 An SRT planning sample for a patient with a new BM, treated with WBRT 1 year prior

worsening symptoms. Multivariate analyses of patients with no extracranial disease showed better survival [66]. In a similar study, 17 patients who were initially treated with 35 Gy were treated with 21 Gy WBRT for brain recurrence. In 80 % of the patients, symptomatic improvements were observed. The median survival was 5.2 months. In patients with stable extracranial disease, the median survival was 19.8 months, and in those with progressive extracranial disease, it was 2.5 months.

For patients who will be irradiated for a second course, SRT or WBRT is chosen according to the systemic disease status, recurrent metastatic brain lesion size, the prior treatment method, and patient performance. The treatment algorithm for recurrent BM patients is shown in Table 37.9.

The RTOG 90-05 trial by Pirzkall et al. is a dose escalation study that included 156 patients with recurrent primary brain tumors or recurrent BMs. This study recommended 24 Gy for ≤2 cm, 18 Gy for 2–3 cm, and 15 Gy for 3–4 cm tumors. Grade 3–5 neurotoxicity was related to tumor

Table 37.9 Salvage treatment during BM treatment

Systemic disease status	Recurrent metastatic brain lesion number	Treatment
None or stable	1–3	SRT if lesions are suitable
		Surgery for mass effect
		WBRT if not performed previously
None or stable	>3	If not delivered before WBRT
		If previously responsive to WBRT, if longer than 4 months has passed since the second WBRT
		Limited field RT
		CT
Progressing	Any	If WBRT was not performed previously, WBRT with accelerated plans (4 Gy ×5 or 3 Gy ×10)
		Supportive treatment
		CT

WBRT Whole brain radiotherapy, *SRT* Stereotactic radiotherapy, *RT* Radiotherapy, *CT* Chemotherapy

size, dose, and KPS [67]. Second WBRT courses should be delivered with a minimum daily dose of 1.8–2 Gy, with a total dose of 20 Gy.

Systemic Treatment

The role of chemotherapy has not been precisely defined in BM. Chemotherapy is rarely part of the BM treatment plan due to the blood-brain barrier (BBB). The agents that penetrate the BBB are temozolomide, topotecan, capecitabine, nitrous urea, thioTEPA, trastuzumab, tamoxifen, liposomal doxorubicin, methotrexate, and gefitinib [68]. Although breast cancer is sensitive to chemotherapy, the contribution of chemotherapy in BM is controversial. Chemotherapy can be used in cases of multiple BMs, extracranial disease, and inadequate local control. Rosner et al. reported 100 breast cancer patients with BM who were treated with cyclophosphamide, fluorouracil, prednisolone, methotrexate, and vincristine. This was the largest series reported [69]. In 50 % of the patients, an objective response was achieved (10 % complete, 40 % partial). The median remission duration was 7 months in partially responsive patients and 10 months in fully responsive patients. The intracranial and extracranial response rates were equivalent. The studies that used systemic chemotherapy protocols that have been proven to be effective in treating CNS metastases of breast cancer are listed in Table 37.10 [69–75]. The most commonly used protocol is CFP (cyclophosphamide, 5-FU, prednisolone). No protocol was superior to the others.

The hormonal therapy agents that can penetrate the BBB in BM are tamoxifen and megestrol acetate. The BBB is disrupted in contrast-enhancing metastases. Targeted treatments with trastuzumab and lapatinib can penetrate the BBB. Lapatinib is a small molecule that can pass the BBB. In a lapatinib study by Lin et al. that included 241 patients, a partial response was reported in 7 patients, and a 20–50 % reduction in tumor volume was achieved in 19 patients [76].

Leptomeningeal Metastases (LMs)

LMs are common complications of BM, and their occurrence rate is gradually increasing. The clinical LM occurrence rate in breast cancer patients is 2–5 %; in autopsy data, this rate is 3–6 %. The approach to LM differs from the approach to parenchymal BMs. In clinical and autopsy series, lobular carcinomas are more likely to spread to the leptomeninges for unknown reasons. In cancers other than breast cancer, LMs generally occur in widespread metastatic stages, whereas in breast cancer, LMs can occur even when the disease is under control and without any systemic metastases. LMs may develop within weeks or up to 15 years after the diagnosis of breast cancer [77].

The most common presentation of LM is spinal symptoms, weakness in the legs, and paresthesia. Sudden multifocal abnormalities in multiple levels of the neuroaxis (cerebellum, cranial nerves, and spine) suggest an LM diagnosis. Neck stiffness is present in 2–13 % of cases. Obstruction of the CSF may cause

Table 37.10 Systemic chemotherapy protocols shown to be active in breast cancer CNS metastases

Study	Protocol	N	Median survival (m)
Rosner et al. [69]	Cyclophosphamide, fluorouracil, prednisone, methotrexate, and vincristine	100	10
Lange [70]	RT + Ifo/BCNU	61	8
Boogerd [71]	Cyclophosphamide, doxorubicin, and fluorouracil	20	6.3
Rivera [72]	Temozolomide + capecitabine	24	3
Kouvaris [73]	Temozolomide + WBRT	33	12
Kurt [74]	Capecitabine	20	7.3
Cocconi [75]	Cisplatin and etoposide	22	14.5

headaches, mental status changes (such as lethargy, confusion, and memory loss), nausea, vomiting, and/or ataxia. Seizures are rare. Mental status changes indicate cerebral dysfunction, and hearing loss is a sign of cranial nerve involvement. To diagnose LM, malignant cells must be found in the CSF. Increased protein levels and mononuclear pleocytosis are often observed in the CSF. Sometimes, the glucose level in the CSF may be <70 % of the normal serum glucose level. Carcinoembryonic antigen (CEA) may be increased in CSF; in this case, the serum CEA levels must also be checked because CEA can penetrate the BBB. Increased CEA in the CSF may be due to increased serum CEA. The extent of the disease must be established with MRI of the whole spinal cord, including the cauda equina and the brain (Fig. 37.9a–e). In these

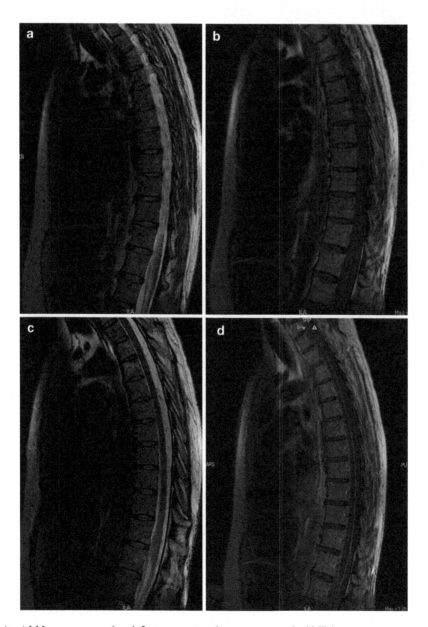

Fig. 37.9 (a–e) LM metastases at t1 and t2; precontrast and postcontrast sagittal MR images

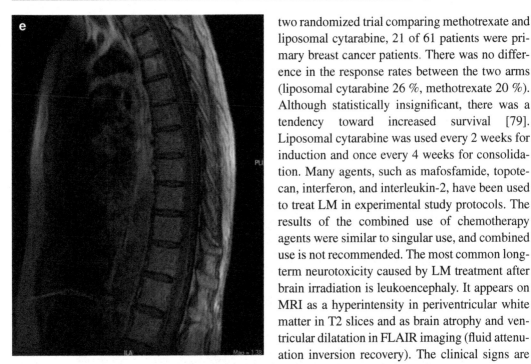

Fig. 37.9 (continued)

patients, cranial MRI must also be performed to scan for BMs.

Whole craniospinal irradiation is not recommended because it can cause myelosuppression. RT is delivered to the area where the bulky or symptomatic lesion is located in the craniospinal axis. After RT, intrathecal (IT) chemotherapy is administered in three phases, induction, consolidation, and protection, by lumbar punctures or an Ommaya reservoir. Administration via an Ommaya reservoir has a lower infection risk. If the CSF flow is blocked, RT may be delivered first and followed with intrathecal chemotherapy. The agents that are frequently used for intrathecal chemotherapy are methotrexate, thioTEPA, and liposomal cytarabine. In a series of 48 breast cancer patients with LM metastases, intrathecal methotrexate was delivered twice a week until CSF was clean and was continued as a protection plan once every 2–4 weeks. In this study, the response rate was 61 %, and the median survival was 7.2 months [78]. Although standard cytarabine has a limited effect on breast cancer metastases, the response rate of liposomal cytarabine is 28 %. In a phase two randomized trial comparing methotrexate and liposomal cytarabine, 21 of 61 patients were primary breast cancer patients. There was no difference in the response rates between the two arms (liposomal cytarabine 26 %, methotrexate 20 %). Although statistically insignificant, there was a tendency toward increased survival [79]. Liposomal cytarabine was used every 2 weeks for induction and once every 4 weeks for consolidation. Many agents, such as mafosfamide, topotecan, interferon, and interleukin-2, have been used to treat LM in experimental study protocols. The results of the combined use of chemotherapy agents were similar to singular use, and combined use is not recommended. The most common long-term neurotoxicity caused by LM treatment after brain irradiation is leukoencephaly. It appears on MRI as a hyperintensity in periventricular white matter in T2 slices and as brain atrophy and ventricular dilatation in FLAIR imaging (fluid attenuation inversion recovery). The clinical signs are cognitive deterioration, behavioral changes, gait abnormalities, and seizures. The use of RT and methotrexate together increases the occurrence of leukoencephalopathy, but in LM patients, it may not be clinically apparent due to poor prognosis. The relationship between the order of RT and chemotherapy administration and the frequency of leukoencephalopathy is not entirely understood. Some studies state that the risk increases when RT is prioritized. Intrathecal chemotherapy may cause aseptic meningitis in 20 % of patients; it presents 12–72 h later with headaches, nausea, vomiting, lethargy, and fever. Other serious complications are neutropenia, sepsis, mental impairment, and increasing myelopathy. The death rate due to treatment is 5 %.

Epidural Metastasis (EM)

EMs are mostly caused by the tumor entering the epidural space from the vertebral column (85 % of cases) and less frequently caused by entry from the paravertebral space. The frequency of epidural spinal compression fractures in breast cancer patients is reported to be 4 %. The vertebral column is the most frequent site of bone metastases.

The frequency is 60 % in brain cancer patients, and approximately 84 % of these patients are advanced-stage breast cancer patients [80]. The epidural spinal cord compression frequency in breast cancer patients is 4 %. Spinal cord damage caused by direct spinal cord compression is more common than damage caused by radicular artery compression. The time between breast cancer diagnosis and EM is 43 months. The median survival is 4–13 months. The most important prognostic factor is discharging the patient in an ambulatory status. Whole spinal canal MRI must be performed (Fig. 37.10). If EMs are left untreated, they may cause paraplegia or quadriplegia, depending on the level of the lesion. If the suspicion of an EM arises, an emergency evaluation is necessary. After diagnosis, steroids and RT must be initiated immediately. In EM patients with no cord compression, patients are given low steroid doses (10 mg dexamethasone); in patients with cord pressure, steroid therapy should be initiated with a bolus dose (100 mg dexamethasone). The continuation steroid dose is 4 mg of dexamethasone every 6 h. It is tapered when radiotherapy is completed or symptoms are stabilized. In progressive or recurrent spinal cord compressions due to the risk of myelopathy caused by a second irradiation course, surgery is recommended. The recommended surgical treatment is "vertebral resection and stabilization with methyl methacrylate cement" [81]. EMs are generally located anterolaterally, and a posterior approach (laminectomy) is not very efficient and may lead to even more weakness. The results of IGRT and SRT trials in EM are expected to be similar to the results of SRT in intracranial lesions [82].

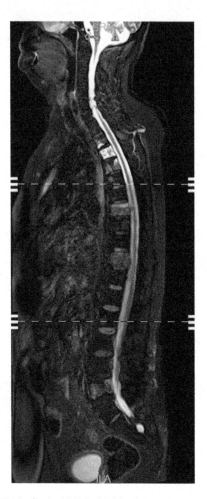

Fig, 37.10 Sagittal MRI of epidural metastases

Brachial Plexopathy

The neoplastic invasion of the brachial plexus is quite rare, but it is still a common cause of plexopathies. MBCs and lung cancers are the second most common causes of nontraumatic brachial plexopathies. Brachial plexus lesions are caused by the direct extension of the tumor to the plexus (Pancoast tumor) or are secondary to a neoplasia that metastasizes from the axillary lymph nodes to the plexus. The axilla apex is one of the lymphatic drainage locations of the breast; thus, brachial plexus involvement is not rare in MBCs. It may develop as a result of neoplastic invasion, but it may also develop as a long-term side effect of breast cancer RT if the treatment falls in the supraclavicular or axillary treatment zones. RT causes the fibrosis of tissues surrounding the brachial plexus, which may result in the compression of nerve fibers and a loss of function (Fig. 37.11a–c). When RT is being planned, the brachial plexus must be defined, and the doses it receives must be evaluated and recorded carefully, as for every organ that is at risk of RT damage [83].

In retrospective reviews, the RT dose, treatment technique, and chemotherapy administration affect the development of brachial plexopathy. In a study by Pierce et al., the risk of brachial plexopathy was 3 % when the axillary dose was <50 Gy and 8 % when the dose was >50 Gy. Approximately 20 % of the brachial plexopathy cases were permanent [84].

Brachial plexopathy is a progressive and potentially permanent clinical picture that disrupts the quality of life, consisting of severe shoulder pain and pain radiating to the medial areas of the hand and forearm. Symptoms may be diffuse, but they frequently include symptoms of the C8–T1 dermatome and myotomes and imitate ulnar neuropathy and C8–T1 radiculopathy. The incidence is less than 0.5 % [85].

Nerve damage in the plexus is determined in a neurological examination and EMG, and the plexopathy is graded. Imaging methods such as CT, MRI, and PETCT can be used in the diagnosis and differential diagnosis (Fig. 37.10). Visually guided fine-needle aspiration biopsy may be performed. Steroids, nonsteroidal anti-inflammatory drugs, tricyclic antidepressants and physical therapy can be used in the treatment.

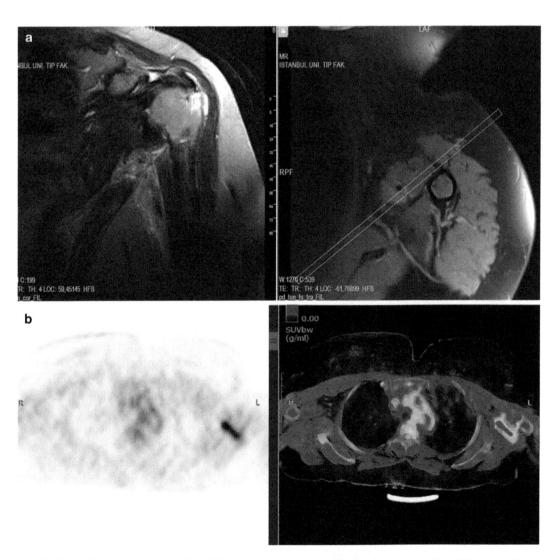

Fig. 37.11 (a) Coronary and axial view of brachial plexopathy in MRI. (b) Axial view of brachial plexopathy in PETCT. (c) Coronary view of brachial plexopathy in PET-CT

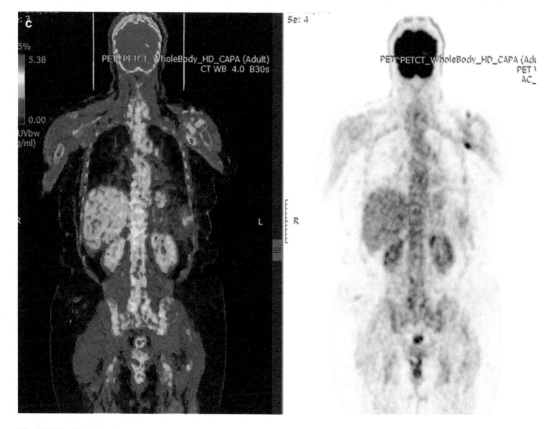

Fig. 37.11 (continued)

References

1. Barnholtz-Sloan JS, Sloan AE, Davis FG, Vigneau FD, Lai P, Sawaya RE. Incidence proportions of brain metastases in patients diagnosed (1973 to 2001) in the Metropolitan Detroit Cancer Surveillance System. J Clin Oncol. 2004;22:2865–72.
2. Counsell C, Grant R. Incidence studies of primary and secondary intracranial tumors: A systematic review of their methodology and results. J Neuro-Oncol. 1998;37:241–50.
3. Andrews DW, Scott CB, Sperduto PW, Flanders AE, Gaspar LE, Schell MC, et al. Whole-brain radiation therapy with or without stereotactic radiosurgery boost for patients with one to three brain metastases: phase III results of the RTOG 9508 randomised trial. Lancet. 2004;363:1665–72.
4. Hasegawa T, Kondziolka D, Flickinger JC, Germanwala A, Lunsford LD. Brain metastases treated with radiosurgery alone: an alternative to whole brain radiotherapy? Neurosurgery. 2003;52:1318–25.
5. Chidel MA, Suh JH, Reddy CA, Chao ST, Lundbeck MF, Barnett GH. Application of recursive partitioning analysis and evaluation of the use of whole brain radiation among patients treated with stereotactic radiosurgery for newly diagnosed brain metastases. Int J Radiat Oncol Biol Phys. 2000;47:993–9.
6. Flickinger JC, Kondziolka D, Lunsford LD, Coffey RJ, Goodman ML, Shaw EG, et al. A multi-institutional experience with stereotactic radiosurgery for solitary brain metastases. Int J Radiat Oncol Biol Phys. 1994;28:797–802.
7. Zimm S, Wampler GL, Stablein D, Hazra D, Young HF. Intracerebral metastases in solid-tumor patients: natural history and results of treatment. Cancer. 1981;48:384–94.
8. Pirzkall A, Debus J, Lohr F, Fuss M, Rhein B, Engenhart-Cabillic R, et al. Radiosurgery alone or in combination with whole-brain radiotherapy for brain metastases. J Clin Oncol. 1998;16:3563–9.
9. Tsukada Y, Fouad A, Pickren JW, Lane WW. Central nervous system metastasis from breast carcinoma. Autopsy study. Cancer. 1983;52(12):2349–54.
10. Sparrow GE, Rubens RD. Brain metastases from breast cancer: clinical course, prognosis and influence of treatment. Clin Oncol. 1982;7(4):291–301.
11. Regine WF, Rogozinska A, Kryscio RJ, Tibbs PA, Young AB, Patchell RA. Recursive partitioning analysis classification I and II: applicability evaluated in a randomized trial for resected single brain metastases. Am J Clin Oncol. 2002;12:417–25.

12. Stemmler HJ, Schmitt M, Willems A, Bernhard H, Harbeck N, Heinemann V. Ratio of trastuzumab levels in serum and cerebrospinal fluid is altered in HER2-positive breast cancer patients with brain metastases and impairment of blood–brain barrier. Anti-Cancer Drugs. 2007;18:23–8.

13. Lin NU, Winer EP. Brain metastases: the HER2 paradigm. Clin Cancer Res. 2007;13:1648–55.

14. Lin NU, Claus E, Sohl J, Razzak AR, Arnaout A, Winer EP. Sites of distant relapse and clinical outcomes in patients with metastatic triple-negative breast cancer: high incidence of central nervous system metastases. Cancer. 2008;113(10):2638–45.

15. Sperduto PW, Kased N, Roberge D, Xu Z, Shanley R, Luo X, ve ark Sneed PK. Effect of tumor subtype on survival and the graded prognostic assessment for patients with breast cancer and brain metastases. Int J Radiat Oncol Biol Phys. 2012;82(5):2111–7.

16. Anders CK, Carey LA. Biology, metastatic patterns, and treatment of patients with triple-negative breast cancer. Clin Breast Cancer. 2009;9(2):73–81.

17. Saip P, Cicin I, Eralp Y, Karagol H, Kucucuk S, Cosar AR, et al. Identification of patients who may benefit from the prophylactic cranial radiotherapy among breast cancer patients with brain metastasis. J Neurooncol. 2009;93(2):243–51.

18. Nussbaum ES, Djalilian HR, Cho KH, Hall WA. Brain metastases. Histology, multiplicity, surgery, and survival. Cancer. 1996;78(8):1781–8.

19. Schaefer PW, Budzik Jr RF, Gonzalez RG. Imaging of cerebral metastases. Neurosurg Clin N Am. 1996;7(3):393–423.

20. Vecht CJ, Hovestadt A, Verbiest HB, van Vliet JJ, van Putten WL. Dose-effect relationship of dexamethasone on Karnofsky performance in metastatic brain tumors. Neurology. 1994;44(4):675–80.

21. Soffietti R, Rudā R, Mutani R. Management of brain metastases. J Neurol. 2002;249(10):1357–69.

22. Niwinska A, Murawska M, Pogoda K. Breast cancer brain metastases: differences in survival depending on biological subtype, RPA RTOG prognostic class and systemic treatment after whole-brain radiotherapy. Ann Oncol. 2010;21:942–8.

23. Bonito D, Giarelli L, Falconieri G, Bonifacio-Gori D, Tomasic G, Vielh P. Association of breast cancer and meningioma. Report of 12 new cases and review of the literature. Pathol Res Pract. 1993;189(4):399–404.

24. Aoyama H. Radiation therapy for brain metastases in breast cancer patients. Breast Cancer. 2011;18:244–51.

25. Nieder C, Berberich W, Schnabel K. Tumor-related prognostic factors for remission of brain metastases after radiotherapy. Int J Radiat Oncol Biol Phys. 1997;39:25–30.

26. Ogura M, Mitsumori M, Okumura S, Yamauchi C, Kawamura S, Oya N, Nagata Y, Hiraoka M. Radiation therapy for brain metastases from breast cancer. Breast Cancer. 2003;10:349–55.

27. Mahmoud-Ahmed AS, Suh JH, Lee SY, Crownover RL, Barnett GH. Results of whole brain radiotherapy in patients with brain metastases from breast cancer: a retrospective study. Int J Radiat Oncol Biol Phys. 2002;54:810–7.

28. Le Scodan R, Massard C, Mouret-Fourme E, Guinebretierre JM, Cohen-Solal C, De Lalande B, et al. Brain metastases from breast carcinoma: validation of the radiation therapy oncology group recursive partitioning analysis classification and proposition of a new prognostic score. Int J Radiat Oncol Biol Phys. 2007;69:839–45.

29. Borgelt B, Gelber R, Larson M, Hendrickson F, Griffin T, Roth R. Ultra-rapid high dose irradiation schedules for the palliation of brain metastases: final results of the first two studies by the Radiation Therapy Oncology Group. Int J Radiat Oncol Biol Phys. 1981;7(12):1633–8.

30. Haie-Meder C, Pellae-Cosset B, Laplanche A, Lagrange JL, Tuchais C, Nogues C, et al. Results of a randomized clinical trial comparing two radiation schedules in the palliative treatment of brain metastases. Radiother Oncol. 1993;26(2):111–6.

31. Priestman TJ, Dunn J, Brada M, Rampling R, Baker PG. Final results of the Royal College of Radiologists' trial comparing two different radiotherapy schedules in the treatment of cerebral metastases. Clin Oncol (R Coll Radiol). 1996;8(5):308–15.

32. Murray KJ, Scott C, Greenberg HM, Emami B, Seider M, Vora NL, et al. A randomized phase III study of accelerated hyperfractionation versus standard in patients with unresected brain metastases: a report of the Radiation Therapy Oncology Group (RTOG) 9104. Int J Radiat Oncol Biol Phys. 1997;39(3):571–4.

33. Graham PH, Bucci J, Browne L. Randomized comparison of whole brain radiotherapy, 20 Gy in four daily fractions versus 40 Gy in 20 twice-daily fractions, for brain metastases. Int J Radiat Oncol Biol Phys. 2010;77(3):648–54.

34. Komarnicky LT, Phillips TL, Martz K, Asbell S, Isaacson S, Urtasun R. A randomized phase III protocol for the evaluation of misonidazole combined with radiation in the treatment of patients with brain metastases (RTOG-7916). Int J Radiat Oncol Biol Phys. 1991;20:53–8.

35. Mehta MP, Rodrigus P, Terhaard CH, Rao A, Suh J, Roa W, et al. Survival and neurologic outcomes in a randomized trial of motexafin gadolinium and whole-brain radiation therapy in brain metastases. J Clin Oncol. 2003;21:2529–36.

36. Knisely JP, Berkey B, Chakravarti A. A phase III study of conventional radiation therapy plus thalidomide vs. conventional radiation therapy for multiple brain metastases (RTOG 0118). Int J Radiat Oncol Biol Phys. 2008;71:79–86.

37. Scott C, Suh J, Stea B, Nabid A, Hackman J. Improved survival, quality of life, and quality-adjusted survival in breast cancer patients treated with efaproxiral (Efaproxyn) plus whole-brain radiation therapy for brain metastases. Am J Clin Oncol. 2007;30:580–7.

38. Antonadou D, Paraskevaidis M, Sarris G, Coliarakis N, Economou I, Karageorgis P, Throuvalas N. Phase

II randomized trial of temozolomide and concurrent radiotherapy in patients with brain metastases. J Clin Oncol. 2002;20:3644–50.

39. Verger E, Gil M, Yaya R, Viñolas N, Villà S, Pujol T, Quintó L, Graus F. Temozolomide and concomitant whole brain radiotherapy in patients with brain metastases: a phase II randomized trial. Int J Radiat Oncol Biol Phys. 2005;61:185–91.

40. Chargari C, Idrissi HR, Pierga JY, Bollet MA, Diéras V, Campana F, et al. Preliminary results of whole brain radiotherapy with concurrent trastuzumab for treatment of brain metastases in breast cancer patients. Int J Radiat Oncol Biol Phys. 2011;88:631–6.

41. Lin NU, Freedman RA, Ramakrishna N, Younger J, Storniolo AM, Bellon JR, et al. A phase I study of lapatinib with whole brain radiotherapy in patients with human epidermal growth factor receptor 2 (HER2)-positive breast cancer brain metastases. Breast Cancer Res Treat. 2013;142:405–14.

42. Duchnowska R, Jassem J, Goswami CP, Gokem-Polar Y, Thorat MA, Flores N, et al. 13-gene signature to predict rapid development of brain metastases in patients with HER-2-positive advanced breast cancer. J Clin Oncol. 2012;30(15):505.

43. Patchell RA, Tibbs PA, Walsh JW, Dempsey RJ, Maruyama Y, Kryscio RJ, et al. A randomized trial of surgery in the treatment of single metastases to the brain. N Engl J Med. 1990;322:494–500.

44. Vecht CJ, Haaxma-Reiche H, Noordijk EM, Padberg GW, Voormolen JH, Hoekstra FH, et al. Treatment of single brain metastasis: radiotherapy alone or combined with neurosurgery? Ann Neurol. 1993;33:583–90.

45. Mintz AH, Kestle J, Rathbone MP, Gaspar L, Hugenholtz H, Fisher B, et al. A randomized trial to assess the efficacy of surgery in addition to radiotherapy in patients with a single cerebral metastasis. Cancer. 1996;78:1470–6.

46. Soon YY, Tham IW, Lim KH, Koh WY, Lu JJ. Surgery or radiosurgery plus whole brain radiotherapy versus surgery or radiosurgery alone for brain metastases. Cochrane Database Syst Rev. 2014;3:CD009454.

47. Bindal RK, Sawaya R, Leavens ME, Lee JJ. Surgical treatment of multiple brain metastases. J Neurosurg. 1993;79(2):210–6.

48. Patchell RA, Tibbs PA, Regine W, Dempsey R, Mohiuddin M, Kryscio R, et al. Postoperative radiotherapy in the treatment of single metastases to the brain. J Am Med Assoc. 1998;280(17):1485–9.

49. Kocher M, Soffietti R, Abacioglu U, Villa S, Fauchon F, Baumert B, et al. Adjuvant whole-brain radiotherapy versus -observation after radiosurgery or surgical resection of one to three cerebral metastases: results of the EORTC 22952–26001 Study. J Clin Oncol. 2011;29(2):134–41.

50. Kelly PJ, Lin YB, Yu AY, Alexander BM, Hacker F, Marcus KJ, Weiss SE. Stereotactic irradiation of the postoperative resection cavity for brain metastasis: a frameless linear accelerator-based case series and review of the technique. Int J Radiat Oncol Biol Phys. 2012;82(1):95–101.

51. Choi CY, Chang SD, Gibbs IC, Adler JR, Harsh GR, Lieberson RE, et al. Stereotactic radiosurgery of the postoperative resection cavity for brain metastases: prospective evaluation of target margin on tumor control. Int J Radiat Oncol Biol Phys. 2012;84(2):336–42.

52. Sneed PK, Lamborn KR, Forstner JM, McDermott MW, Chang S, Park E, Gutin PH, Phillips TL, Wara WM, Larson DA. Radiosurgery for brain metastases: is whole brain radiotherapy necessary? Int J Radiat Oncol Biol Phys. 1999;43(3):549–58.

53. Bindal AK, Bindal RK, Hess KR, Shiu A, Hassenbusch SJ, Shi WM, Sawaya R. Surgery versus radiosurgery in the treatment of brain metastasis. J Neurosurg. 1996;84(5):748–54.

54. O'Neill BP, Iturria NJ, Link MJ, Pollock BE, Ballman KV, O'Fallon JR. A comparison of surgical resection and stereotactic radiosurgery in the treatment of solitary brain metastases. Int J Radiat Oncol Biol Phys. 2003;55(5):1169–76.

55. Auchter RM, Lamond JP, Alexander E, Buatti JM, Chappell R, Friedman WA, et al. A multiinstitutional outcome and prognostic factor analysis of radiosurgery for resectable single brain metastasis. Int J Radiat Oncol Biol Phys. 1996;35(1):27–35.

56. Kondziolka D, Patel A, Lunsford LD, Kassam A, Flickinger JC. Stereotactic radiosurgery plus whole brain radiotherapy versus radiotherapy alone for patients with multiple brain metastases. Int J Radiat Oncol Biol Phys. 1999;45(2):427–34.

57. Chougule PB, Burton-Williams M, Saris S, Zheng Z, Ponte B, Noren G, et al. Randomized treatment of brain metastasis with gamma knife radiosurgery, whole brain radiotherapy or both. Int J Radiat Oncol Biol Phys. 2000;48(3S):114.

58. Patil CG, Pricola K, Sarmiento JM, Garg SK, Bryant A, Black KL. Whole brain radiation therapy (WBRT) alone versus WBRT and radiosurgery for the treatment of brain metastases. Cochrane Database Syst Rev. 2012;9:CD006121.

59. Chang E, Wefel J, Hess K, Allen P, Lang F, Kornguth D, et al. Neurocognition in patients with brain metastases treated with radiosurgery or radiosurgery plus whole-brain irradiation: a randomised controlled trial. Lancet Oncol. 2009;10(11):1037–44.

60. Aoyama H, Shirato H, Tago M, Nakagawa K, Toyoda T, Hatano K, et al. Stereotactic radiosurgery plus whole-brain radiation therapy vs stereotactiv radiosurgery alone for treatment of brain metastases. J Am Med Assoc. 2006;295(21):2483–90.

61. Tsao MN, Lloyd N, Wong RKS, Chow E, Rakovitch E, Laperriere N, et al. Whole brain radiotherapy for the treatment of newly diagnosed multiple brain metastases. Cochrane Database Syst Rev. 2012;(4):58–60.

62. Roos D, Writh A, Burmeister B, Spry N, Drummond K, Beresford J, et al. Whole brain irradiation following surgery or radiosurgery for solitary brain metastases: mature results of a prematurely closed randomized Trans- Tasman Radiation Oncology Group trial (TROG 98.05). Radiother Oncol. 2006;80(3): 318–22.

63. Soffietti R, Kocher M, Abacioglu U, Villa S, Fauchon F, Baumert B, et al. A European Organization for Research and Treatment of Cancer phase III trial of adjuvant whole brain radiotherapy versus observation in patients with one to three brain metastases from solid tumors after surgical resection or radiosurgery: quality of life results. J Clin Oncol. 2013;31:65–72.

64. Rogers LR, Rock JP, Sills AK, Vogelbaum MA, Suh JH, Ellis TL, et al. Results of a phase II trial of the GliaSite radiation therapy system for the treatment of newly diagnosed, resected single brain metastases. J Neurosurg. 2006;105(3):375–84.

65. Cosgrove GR, Hochberg FH, Zervas NT, Pardo FS, Valenzuela RF, Chapman P. Interstitial irradiation of brain tumors, using a miniature radiosurgery device: initial experience. Neurosurgery. 1997;40(3):518–23.

66. Wong WW, Schild SE, Sawyer TE, Shaw EG. Analysis of outcome in patients reirradiated for brain metastases. Int J Radiat Oncol Biol Phys. 1996;34(3):585–90.

67. Shaw E, Scott C, Souhami L, Dinapoli R, Kline R, Loeffler J, et al. Single dose radiosurgical treatment of recurrent previously irradiated primary brain tumors and brain metastases: final report of RTOG protocol 90-05. Int J Radiat Oncol Biol Phys. 2000;47(2): 291–8.

68. Lin NU, Bellon JR, Winer EP. CNS metastases in breast cancer. J Clin Oncol. 2004;22(17):3608–17.

69. Rosner D, Nemoto T, Lane WW. Chemotherapy induces regression of brain metastases in breast carcinoma. Cancer. 1986;58(4):832–9.

70. Lange OF, Scheef W, Haase KD. Palliative radio-chemotherapy with ifosfamide and BCNU for breast cancer patients with cerebral metastases. Cancer Chemother Pharmacol. 1990;26(1):78–80.

71. Boogerd W, Dalesio O, Bais EM, et al. Response of brain metastases from breast cancer to systemic chemotherapy. Cancer. 1992;69(4):972–80.

72. Rivera E, Meyers C, Groves M, et al. Phase I study of capecitabine in combination with temozolomide in the treatment of patients with brain metastases from breast carcinoma. Cancer. 2006;107(6):1348–54.

73. Kouvaris JR, Miliadou A, Kouloulias VE, Kolokouris D, Balafouta MJ, Papacharalampous XN, Vlahos LJ. Phase II study of temozolomide and concomitant whole-brain radiotherapy in patients with brain metastases from solid tumors. Onkologie. 2007; 30(7):361–6.

74. Kurt M, Aksoy S, Hayran M, Guler N. A retrospective review of breast cancer patients with central nervous system metastasis treated with capecitabine. J Clin Oncol. 2007;256:1098.

75. Cocconi G, Lottici R, Bisagni G, Bacchi M, Tonato M, Passalacqua R, et al. Combination therapy with platinum and etoposide of brain metastases from breast carcinoma. Cancer Invest. 1990;8:327–34.

76. Lin NU, Diéras V, Paul D, Lossignol D, Christodoulou C, Stemmler HJ, et al. Multicenter phase II study of lapatinib in patients with brain metastases from HER2-positive breast cancer. Clin Cancer Res. 2009;15(4):1452–9.

77. Yap HY, Yap BS, Rasmussen S, Levens ME, Hortobagyi GN, Blumenschein GR. Treatment for meningeal carcinomatosis in breast cancer. Cancer. 1982;50(2):219–22.

78. Chamberlain MC, Kormanik PR. Carcinomatous meningitis secondary to breast cancer: predictors of response to combined modality therapy. J Neurooncol. 1997;35(1):55–64.

79. Glantz MJ, Jaeckle KA, Chamberlain MC, Phuphanich S, Recht L, Swinnen LJ, et al. A randomized controlled trial comparing intrathecal sustained-release cytarabine (DepoCyt) to intrathecal methotrexate in patients with neoplastic meningitis from solid tumors. Clin Cancer Res. 1999;5(11):3394–402.

80. Fornasier VL, Horne JG. Metastases to the vertebral column. Cancer. 1975;36(2):590–4.

81. Siemionow K, Lieberman IH. Surgical approaches to metastatic spine disease. Curr Opin Support Palliat Care. 2008;2(3):192–6.

82. Park HK, Chang JC. Review of stereotactic radiosurgery for intramedullary spinal lesions. Korean J Spine. 2013;10(1):1–6.

83. Wood JJ, Gawler J, Whittle RJ, Staunton MD. Brachial plexopathy in breast carcinoma-an unsolved problem. Eur J Surg Oncol. 1991;17:265–9.

84. Pierce SM, Recht A, Lingos TI, Abner A, Viccini F, Silver B, et al. Long-term radiation complications following conservative surgery (CS) and radiation therapy (RT) in patients with early stage breast cancer. Int J Radiat Oncol Biol Phys. 1992;23(5):915–23.

85. Cherny NI, Foley KM. Brachial plexopathy in patients with breast cancer. In: Harris JR, Hellman S, Henderson IC, Kinne DW, editors. Breast diseases. 1st ed. Philadelphia: JB Lippincott; 1996. p. 722–39.

Ocular Metastases

Nergiz Dagoglu and Anand Mahadevan

Abstract

Although ocular metastasis from breast cancer is a rare entity, metastasis to the eye is the most common ocular neoplasm, and among these neoplasms, breast cancer is the primary site for most of these cases. Treatment requires an individualized approach in which both tumor and patient characteristics are considered. Metastatic disease to the eye from the breast was first described by Johann Friedrich Horner in 1864. Since then, reports of ocular involvement have steadily increased. Prompt treatment with radiotherapy (RT) typically results in a higher probability of better vision and organ retention, making RT the standard treatment. Moreover, some patients benefit from chemotherapy (CT) or hormone therapy (HT). Given the increasing survival rates of cancer patients, the incidence of ocular metastasis is expected to increase. This point brings up the need for more focused attention on the importance of the patient quality of life.

Keywords

Ocular metastasis • Cryotherapy • Plaque brachytherapy • Radiotherapy

Introduction

Metastatic carcinoma of the eye is the most common malignant ocular neoplasm [1]. Among all cases, breast cancer is responsible for most of these metastases, making it a significant sequel [2]. Breast cancer as a cause is followed by lung carcinoma and carcinoma of an unknown primary. Gastrointestinal, genitourinary, and other carcinomas are infrequently responsible for ocular metastasis (Table 38.1) [3, 4]. Metastatic disease to the eye from the breast was first described

N. Dagoglu, MD (✉)
Department of Radiation Oncology, Istanbul University, Istanbul Faculty of Medicine, Çapa-Fatih, Istanbul 34093, Turkey
e-mail: ranedag@yahoo.com

A. Mahadevan, MBBS, MD, FRCS, FRCR
Department of Radiation Oncology,
Beth Israel Deaconess Medical Center,
Harvard Medical School,
330 Brookline Avenue, Boston,
MA 02215-5400, USA
e-mail: amahadev@bidmc.harvard.edu

© Springer International Publishing Switzerland 2016
A. Aydiner et al. (eds.), *Breast Disease: Management and Therapies*,
DOI 10.1007/978-3-319-26012-9_38

by Johann Friedrich Horner in 1864 [5]. Since then, reports of ocular involvement have steadily increased in living patients as well as in histopathological studies on postmortem subjects. However, the true incidence of ocular metastases is underestimated because subclinical disease is frequently overlooked, especially in patients with metastatic disease in other life-threatening organs that affect the patient's performance status [1].

Because of differences in the diagnostic rate, the prevalence of ocular metastases in patients with breast carcinoma shows a large range between 10 % and 38 % [6, 7]. In a study of 250 patients with breast carcinoma, 38 % of 152 patients with ocular symptoms and 9 % of 98 asymptomatic patients had ocular metastases [7]. All asymptomatic patients had stage IV disease. Bilateral involvement is common and ranges between 20 % and 40 % [8]. Multifocal involvement of a single eye is also common, occurring in 20–28 % of affected eyes [9, 10].

Table 38.1 Primary sites for patients with ocular metastases [4]

Breast	47 %
Lung	21 %
Gastrointestinal	4 %
Kidney	2 %
Skin	2 %
Prostate	2 %
Unknown	17 %
Other	5 %

The globe itself is the anatomic structure that is most frequently diagnosed with an ocular metastasis. In the globe, the uveal tract of the eye, which is composed of the iris, the ciliary body, and the choroidal layer with its rich vascular network, is involved in the large majority of ocular metastatic disease (Fig. 38.1) [3, 4].

The reasons for the propensity of breast carcinoma to cause ocular metastases rather than other tumors are unclear. Possible hypotheses include the ability of such cells to survive in relatively inhospitable microenvironments, the tendency to cause metastases many years after the diagnosis of the primary tumor, and the prolonged survival of many patients with metastatic disease [7, 10, 11].

Ocular metastasis from breast cancer usually occurs or is diagnosed after metastasis to other organs, primarily the lungs. At the time of ocular metastasis diagnosis, 85 % of patients also have pulmonary involvement. The reported interval from breast cancer diagnosis to ocular metastasis is 2–5 years [10, 12], and the interval from the detection of non-ocular metastases to the detection of ocular metastasis is 10 months in most cases. In rare cases, ocular metastasis can be perceived as the first sign of metastatic spread in breast cancer [13] or may be the initial indication of breast carcinoma [14].

The expected median survival time of patients with ocular metastases is short and ranges between 4 and 12 months [15, 16]. Breast cancer patients with ocular metastases survive significantly

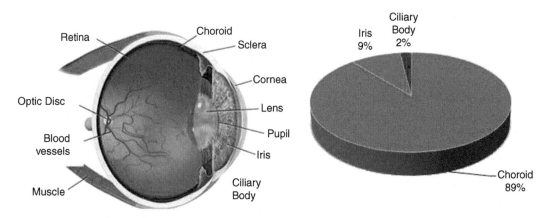

Fig. 38.1 Anatomic structures of the eye and anatomic locations of ocular metastases [4]

longer than patients with other primary tumors because 10 % of these patients survive more than 5 years. This survival correlates with the results of modern multimodality therapy strategies for breast cancer [16, 17].

Given the increasing survival rates of cancer patients, the incidence of ocular metastasis is expected to increase. This point brings up the need for more focused attention on the importance of the patient quality of life.

Symptoms and Signs

The most common presenting symptom recorded in patients with ocular metastasis is blurred vision [18]. In contrast, either proptosis or visual loss frequently is the first complaint for most other ocular neoplasms [19]. However, this difference rarely assists the differential diagnosis.

More specific symptoms and signs may be present depending on the affected area. For example, choroidal involvement may induce blurry vision or vision field loss because these tumors cause retinal detachment, which leads to lens and iris displacement and secondary angle-closure glaucoma [20]. Optic disc metastases often produce rapid, profound visual loss. Iris metastases frequently cause secondary open-angle glaucoma when the trabecular meshwork becomes clogged with tumor cells [21]. Although some authors have stressed pain as a typical symptom for metastatic lesions, any primary malignancy that has perineural invasion and some benign processes will present with pain [22, 23].

The differential diagnosis with ocular melanoma or other ocular lesions can be made by clinical evaluation, including a previous cancer history. The standard workup includes direct ophthalmoscopy, Goldmann perimetry, and ultrasonography (USG) [3, 24]. Computed tomography (CAT), magnetic resonance imaging (MRI), and single photon emission computed tomography (SPECT) imaging are also utilized [25–27].

USG is useful for determining the extent of retinal detachment and outlining any underlying choroidal masses. MRI has several advantages, such as distinguishing small metastases or choroidal masses that can often be missed with other modalities. Additionally, it may provide some indication regarding tissue specificity and therefore be helpful in distinguishing between benign and malignant lesions. Nevertheless, incorporating MRI or a CAT scan of the brain as a part of the initial evaluation is also essential because the risk of synchronous brain metastases for these patients is 25–30 % [25, 26].

SPECT imaging with technetium-99m-MIBI is another method that can be used if more conventional techniques fail to distinguish between malignant and benign lesions. It is a highly sensitive technique (92 %) for detecting malignant ocular tumors [27].

The majority of intraocular tumors can be diagnosed based on clinical examination and radiographic features, which lessens the need for diagnostic ophthalmic fine needle aspiration biopsy (FNAB). In general, the diagnostic precision of ophthalmic FNAB is high but still limited because cellularity can confound the results. Furthermore, surgical biopsy may cause a significant risk of visual loss or other ocular morbidity and presents a significant risk of seeding along the biopsy track [28].

Treatment

If ocular metastasis is detected early enough, it can be treated effectively to prevent vision loss and thus maintain quality of life [3]. The short-term prognosis for vision is usually good, but the systemic prognosis is poor. Treatment requires an individualized approach in which both the tumor and patient characteristics are considered. Tumor characteristics include the size, extent, and location of the tumor; the number of tumors; the laterality of involvement; and the effects on normal intraocular tissues. Patient characteristics involve the visual status of the affected eye or eyes, the visual status of the contralateral eye in unilateral cases, the extent of primary disease, and the age and general health of the patient [29].

Treatment requires a multidisciplinary approach with close communication between the patient's ophthalmologist, medical oncologist, radiation oncologist, and neuroradiologist. Indications for treatment of uveal metastases include visual symptoms attributable to the lesion (e.g., blurred vision, scotoma, flashes, floaters, and dysmorphopsia), lesions close to the optic nerve or macula with signs of active disease, enlargement despite systemic chemotherapy, and painful lesions [30].

Since its first application in 1979, radiotherapy (RT) has become a well-established and widely available treatment for uveal metastases [31]. RT can be applied as a conventional external beam RT (EBRT), plaque brachytherapy, stereotactic body RT (SBRT), or proton beam. Other local therapies include intravitreal injection, laser therapy, and cryotherapy.

Though timely treatment with RT typically anticipates a higher probability for better vision and organ preservation, some patients with hormone-sensitive lesions may benefit from chemotherapy (CT) or hormone therapy (HT) [32]. Manquez et al. [33] found choroidal metastasis regression with aromatase inhibitor treatment in 10 of 17 patients with hormone receptor-positive breast cancer over a mean follow-up of 20 months.

In patients who are already on CT or HT when the metastatic carcinoma of the eye is detected, a regimen change may be recommended. An appropriate drug regimen often produces satisfactory regression of all tumors and preservation or recovery of useful vision in the affected eye or eyes [34].

Because the choroid is the most common site of ocular metastasis and has a vascular structure, anti-vascular endothelial growth factor (anti-VEGF) has been tested as part of the treatment in several case reports. Preliminary results support the use of anti-VEGF [35, 36], emphasizing the ease of administration and the minimal time commitment required. However, there are still many uncertainties, such as the optimal dose, the interval and number of injections, the indications for use, and maintenance therapy.

Surgical resection can be reserved for a minority of carefully chosen patients [34]. Resection may be indicated particularly when the metastases cause pain or proptosis and if RT, CT, or management approaches fail to relieve symptoms [37].

The optimal therapy for asymptomatic ocular metastases is controversial. Data in the literature regarding the treatment of asymptomatic metastasis are rare, and the best time for treatment initiation is arguable. A careful "watchful waiting" strategy and systemic CT in patients with breast cancer seem reasonable [22, 23, 38].

Radiotherapy Doses

RT is effective in relieving symptoms and controlling tumor growth. Though the reported series address the application of different techniques and doses, more current protocols suggest a total dose of 30–40 Gy, delivered in fractionated doses of 2–5 Gy [23, 39].

Doses of less than 30 Gy are less effective. Maor et al. reported that none of the nine patients in their study who received 30 Gy in ten fractions had tumor regrowth after therapy, but two of ten patients treated with 25 Gy in ten fractions had tumor regrowth [40]. In another series reported by Reddy et al. [41], 30 % of tumors did not respond to treatment with doses of 21–30 Gy. Importantly, for most patients, the benefit in vision produced by RT lasted for the remainder of their lives.

Rudoler et al. [8] reported the results of the largest series of 188 patients with 233 ocular metastases over a 23-year time period. A wide range of doses, from 4 to 63 Gy, were used, but most (72 %) patients were treated with 30–40 Gy total doses in 2–3 Gy fraction sizes. Their results showed an improvement or stabilization of visual acuity in 57 % of all patients.

One of the most recent reports evaluating a more uniform treatment was presented by Wiegel et al. [22, 23]. They evaluated 65 eyes that were treated with a total dose of 40 Gy in 20 fractions that was applied with asymmetric fields, resulting in increased visual acuity for 36 % of the patients. This was thought to correspond with the finding that doses higher than 30 Gy were strongly correlated with better or more stable visual acuity because almost 90 % of the patients showed an increase or stabilization during their lifetime.

However, doses higher than 40 Gy are not used because of the possible increase in side effects.

A total of 15–20 % of patients with unilateral metastasis develop symptomatic contralateral metastasis later. Additionally [22, 23, 42, 43], a unilateral field for unilateral choroidal metastasis without sparing the contralateral choroid is an effective technique in destroying possible contralateral micrometastasis and may lower the risk of late side effects compared with bilateral fields.

Radiotherapy Techniques

Most metastatic carcinomas are responsive to RT delivered by the external beam (EB) or plaque methods. These tumors generally show rapid regression after RT, and vision in the eye is frequently stabilized, if not improved [32].

EBRT is particularly applicable to patients with large tumors that involve the optic nerve or macula and either cause substantial visual disturbance or affect multiple areas in both eyes. Unilateral RT with a lateral electron portal of sufficient energy is adequate to treat most ocular metastases. The anterior border should be placed just behind the anterior chamber of the eye, and a posterior tilt should be utilized to avoid the lens. For bilateral metastases, posteriorly tilted opposing photon fields may be an option [44, 45].

Furthermore, single small-to-medium-sized tumors can occasionally be treated effectively by radioactive plaque therapy. This treatment consists of suturing a radioactive device (plaque) to the sclera directly overlying the intraocular tumor. The plaque is left in place for several days, generally until a radiation dose of 40–50 Gy has been delivered to the apex of the tumor, and then, the plaque is removed [46, 47].

Considering the risk of ocular toxicity, other techniques, such as SBRT [48] or proton beam RT [49], that promise less toxicity or shorter treatment times are applied to choroidal metastases.

Side Effects

The rate of severe late side effects after EBRT is low. Approximately 30–50 % of the patients died after 5–7 months; therefore, late side effects did not appear [50]. Referring to data from Wills Eye Hospital [32], patients who live significantly longer seem to have more late side effects, as expected. The small number of side effects, however, did not allow multivariate analysis of possible risk factors.

Radiation-induced ocular side effects have been well described. Thus far, cataracts, keratopathy, retinopathy, neovascularization of the iris, and optic neuropathy have been described [51]. Mild skin erythema and conjunctivitis occur frequently. Cataracts are particularly common in patients with irradiation of anterior segment metastases.

The retinal vasculature may also be damaged by RT [52]. Clinical manifestations are typically delayed in onset for a median of approximately 8 months after treatment and are progressive. The incidence of radiation-induced retinopathy and papillopathy is 8 %. The severity of retinopathy does not correlate with the RT dose and occurs with exposures as low as 50 cGy.

In particular, a significant influence of additional chemotherapy on retinopathy could not be demonstrated.

Course and Outcome

If untreated, most ocular metastases are progressive [22, 23]. They tend to grow faster when compared with primary malignant intraocular neoplasms. If the patient survives long enough, many of the untreated metastatic carcinomas ultimately yield to blindness and pain. Factors used to predict the potential for the preservation or recovery of vision in the affected eye or eyes include the number and size of tumors, their locations relative to the optic disc and fovea, the severity of their effects on the retina and other ocular tissues, and their response to treatment. Moreover, the treatment response is also dependent on the site of the primary tumor and its pathological features.

Ocular metastases do not affect overall survival because the eye is not a vital structure. The prognosis for a patient's survival is dependent on the presence and extent of metastatic tumors in vital organs.

Conclusion

As the survival time of breast cancer patients increases, the incidence of ocular metastasis is expected to rise. With the new therapeutic regimes used in the modern treatment of breast cancer, the range of ocular and visual problems that may be observed will undoubtedly increase. Both ophthalmologists and oncologists should be aware of the range of disorders that may be directly or indirectly caused by breast cancer, not only for the palliation of symptoms but also because the first signs of breast cancer may present as eye symptoms in some cases. Early diagnosis may positively affect the long-term prognosis for patients.

Physicians who treat patients with breast cancer should maintain a high degree of suspicion of ocular metastases. Because patients with breast cancer often have prolonged survival after the diagnosis of ocular metastases, early diagnosis and treatment of this lesion is a primary concern to maximize their quality of life [10].

References

1. Kreusel KM, Bechrakis NE, Krause L, Wiegel T, Foerster MH. Incidence and clinical characteristics of symptomatic choroidal metastasis from breast cancer. Acta Ophthalmol Scand. 2007;85:298–302.
2. Weiss L. Analysis of the incidence of intraocular metastasis. Br J Ophthalmol. 1993;77:1149–51.
3. McCormick B, Abramson D. Breast cancer metastases to the eye. In: Piccart M, Wood WC, Hung CM, Solin LJ, Cardosa F, editors. Breast cancer management and molecular medicine. New York: Springer; 2006. p. 565–7.
4. Shields CL, Shields JA, Gross NE, Schwartz GP, Lally SE. Survey of 520 eyes with uveal metastases. Ophthalmology. 1997;104:1265–76.
5. Horner F. Carcinoma der dura mater exophthalmus. Klin Monatsbl Augenheilkd. 1864;2:186–90.
6. Albert DM, Rubenstein RA, Scheie HG. Tumor metastasis to the eye, part I. Incidence in 213 adult patients with generalized malignancy. Am J Ophthalmol. 1967;63:723–6.
7. Ferry AP, Font RL. Carcinoma metastatic to the eye and orbit. I. A clinicopathologic study of 227 cases. Arch Ophthalmol. 1974;92:276–86.
8. Rudoler SB, Shields CL, Corn BW, De Potter P, Hyslop T, Curran Jr WJ, Shields JA. Functional vision

9. is improved in the majority of patients treated with external-beam radiotherapy for choroid metastases: a multivariate analysis of 188 patients. J Clin Oncol. 1997;15:1244–51.
9. Mewis L, Young SE. Breast carcinoma metastatic to the choroid analysis of 67 patients. Ophthalmology. 1982;89:147–51.
10. Merrill CF, Kaufman DI, Dimitrov NV. Breast cancer metastatic to the eye is a common entity. Cancer. 1991;68:623–7.
11. Font RL, Ferry AP. Carcinoma metastatic to the eye and orbit: III. A clinicopathologic study of 28 cases metastatic to the orbit. Cancer. 1976;38:1326–35.
12. Ferry AP. Metastatic carcinoma of the eye and ocular adnexa. Int Ophthalmol Clin. 1967;7:615–58.
13. Eckardt AM, Rana M, Essig H, Gellrich NC. Orbital metastases as first sign of metastatic spread in breast cancer: case report and review of the literature. Head Neck Oncol. 2011;22:37. doi:10.1186/1758-3284-3-37.
14. Demirci H, Shields CL, Chao AN, Shields JA. Uveal metastasis from breast cancer in 264 patients. Am J Ophthalmol. 2003;36:264–71.
15. Ratanatharathorn V, Powers W, Grimm J, Steverson N, Han I, Ahmad K, Lattin PB. Eye metastases from carcinoma of the breast: diagnosis, radiation treatment and results. Cancer Treat Rev. 1991;18:261–76.
16. Jang RW, Doherty M, Hopkins JJ, Warner E. A case of prolonged disease-free survival in a patient with choroidal metastasis from breast cancer. nature clinical practice. Nat Clin Pract Oncol. 2009;6:118–21.
17. Freedman MI, Folk JC. Metastatic tumors to the eye and orbit: patient survival and clinical characteristics. Arch Ophthalmol. 1987;105:1215–9.
18. Shields JA, Shields CL. Metastatic tumors to uvea and retina. In: Shields JA, Shields CL, editors. Diagnosis and management of intraocular tumors. Philadelphia: WB Saunders; 1992. p. 207–38.
19. Shields JA. Metastatic tumors to uvea. Int Ophthalmol Clin. 1993;33:155–61.
20. Chong JT, Mick A. Choroidal metastasis: case reports and review of the literature. Optometry. 2005;76:293–301.
21. Shields JA, Shields CL, Singh AD. Metastatic neoplasms in the optic disc: the 1999 Bjerrum Lecture. Part 2. Arch Ophthalmol. 2000;118:217–24.
22. Wiegel T, Bornfeld N, Kreusel KM, Guttenberger R, Hinkelbein W. Radiotherapy for choroidal metastases: interim analysis of a prospective study of the ARO(ARO 95-08). Front Radiat Ther Oncol. 1997;30:154–9.
23. Wiegel T, Bottke D, Kreusel KM, Schmidt S, Bornfeld N, Foerster MH, Hinkelbein W, German Cancer Society. External beam radiotherapy of choroidal metastases – final results of a prospective study of the German Cancer Society (ARO 95-08). Radiother Oncol. 2002;64:13–8.
24. Smith JA, Gragoudas ES, Dreyer EB. Uveal metastases. Int Ophthalmol Clin. 1997;37:183–99.

25. Bottke D, Wiegel T, Kreusel KM, Höcht S, Hinkelbein W. Is a diagnostic CT of the brain indicated in patients with choroidal metastases before radiotherapy? Strahlenther Onkol. 2005;181:251–4.

26. Peyster RG, Augsburger JJ, Shields JA, Hershey BL, Eagle Jr R, Haskin ME. Intraocular tumors: evaluation with MR imaging. Radiology. 1988;168:773–9.

27. Alonso O, Núñez M, Cánepa J, Guisoli P, Mut F, Lago G, Touya E. Evaluation of ocular tumors with technetium-99m-MIBI: planar pinhole technique or SPECT? J Nucl Med Technol. 2000;28:85–7.

28. Singh AD, Biscotti CV. Fine needle aspiration biopsy of ophthalmic tumors. Saudi J Ophthalmol. 2012;26:117–23.

29. Stephens RF, Shields JA. Diagnosis and management of cancer metastatic to the uvea: a study of 70 cases. Ophthalmology. 1979;86:1336–49.

30. Kanthan GL, Jayamohan J, Yip D, Conway RM. Management of metastatic carcinoma of the uveal tract: an evidence-based analysis. Clin Exp Ophthalmol. 2007;35:553–65.

31. Guangyan J, Lei X, Jianbo H, Lingquan K, Ziwei W, Guosheng R, et al. Clinical study on eye metastasis in patients with breast cancer. Chin Med J. 2014;127:961–7.

32. Finger PT. Radiation therapy for orbital tumors:concepts, current use, and ophthalmic radiation side effects. Surv Ophthalmol. 2009;54:545–68.

33. Manquez ME, Brown MM, Shields CL, Shields JA. Management of choroidal metastases from breast carcinomas using aromatase inhibitors. Curr Opin Ophthalmol. 2006;17:251–6.

34. Ausburger JJ, Guthoff RF. Metastatic cancer to the eye. In: Yanoff M, Duker JS, editors. Ophthalmology. 2nd ed. St. Louis: Mosby; 2004. p. 1064–9.

35. Mansour AM, Alameddine R. Intravitreal bevacizumab for consecutive multiple choroidal breast metastatic lesions. BMJ Case Rep. 2012. doi:10.1136/bcr.03.2012.6124.

36. Augustine H, Munro M, Adatia F, Webster M, Fielden M. Treatment of ocular metastasis with anti-VEGF: a literature review and case report. Can J Ophthalmol. 2014;49:458–63.

37. Goldberg RA, Rootman J, Cline RA. Tumors metastatic to the orbit: a changing picture. Surv Ophthalmol. 1990;35:1–24.

38. Wiegel T, Kreusel KM, Bornfeld N, Bottke D, Stange M, Foerster MH, et al. Frequency of asymptomatic choroidal metastasis in patients with disseminated breast cancer: results of a prospective screening programme. Br J Ophthalmol. 1998;82:1159–61.

39. Schwartz DL, Kim SK, Ang KK. Metastasis to the orbit. In: Cox J, Ang KK, editors. Radiation oncology: rationale, technique, results. 9th ed. Philadelphia: Mosby; 2010. p. 315–6.

40. Maor M, Chan RC, Young SE. Radiotherapy of choroidal metastases: breast cancer as primary site. Cancer. 1977;40:2081–6.

41. Reddy S, Saxena VS, Hendrickson F, Deutsch W. Malignant metastatic disease of the eye: management of an uncommon complication. Cancer. 1981;47:810–2.

42. Wiegel T, Kreusel KM, Schmidt S, Bornfeld N, Foerster MH, Hinkelbein W. Radiotherapy of unilateral choroidal metastasis: unilateral irradiation or bilateral irradiation for sterilization of suspected contralateral disease? Radiother Oncol. 1999;53:139–41.

43. Tkocz HJ, Hoffmann S, Schnabel K, Ruprecht KW, Schmidt W, Mink D. Bilateral radiotherapy in cases of one-sided choroidal metastases. Front Radiat Ther Oncol. 1997;30:160–4.

44. Chu FCH, Huh SH, Nisce LZ, Simpson LD. Radiation therapy of choroid metastasis from breast cancer. Int J Radiat Oncol Biol Phys. 1977;2:273–9.

45. Hoogenhout J, Brink HMA, Verbeek AM, van Gasteren JJ, Beex LV. Radiotherapy of choroidal metastases. Strahlenther Onkol. 1989;165:375–9.

46. Shields CL, Shields JA, De Potter P, Quaranta M, Freire J, Brady LW, et al. Plaque radiotherapy for the management of uveal metastasis. Arch Ophthalmol. 1997;115:203–9.

47. Shields CL. Plaque radiotherapy for the management of uveal metastasis. Curr Opin Ophthalmol. 1998;9:31–7.

48. Bellmann C, Fuss M, Holz FG, Debus J, Rohrschneider K, Völcker HE, et al. Stereotactic radiation therapy for malignant choroidal tumors: preliminary, short-term results. Ophthalmology. 2000;107:358–65.

49. Tsina EK, Lane AM, Zacks DN, Munzenrider JE, Collier M, Gragoudas ES. Treatment of metastatic tumours of the choroid with proton beam irradiation. Ophthalmology. 2005;112:337–43.

50. Parsons JT, Bova FJ, Fitzgerald CR, Mendenhall WM, Million RR. Severe dry-eye syndrome following external beam irradiation. Int J Radiat Oncol Biol Phys. 1994;30:775–80.

51. Brady LW, Shields J, Augusburger J, Markoe A, Karlsson UL. Complications from radiation therapy to the eye. Front Radiat Ther Oncol. 1989;23:238–50.

52. Parsons JT, Bova FJ, Fitzgerald CR, Mendenhall WM, Million RR. Radiation retinopathy after external-beam irradiation: analysis of time-dose factors. Int J Radiat Oncol Biol Phys. 1994;30:765–73.

Management of Malignant Pleural Effusions in Breast Cancer

39

Jelena Grusina-Ujumaza and Alper Toker

Abstract

Carcinomatous pleurisy is often a manifestation of malignant disease and an indicator of the terminal stage of disease. Breast carcinoma is one of the most common neoplasms and causes approximately one-third of all malignant pleural effusions (MPE). The ideal treatment is to remove the fluid and to prevent its re-accumulation. Various methods such as thoracentesis, chest tube drainage, permanent catheter placement, talc or other adhesive molecule use, and video-assisted thoracoscopic surgery (VATS) have been used to create pleural symphysis. Repeated thoracentesis controls less than 15 % of the effusions. A tunneled indwelling pleural catheter (TIPC) may improve symptoms for patients with MPE and does not appear to be associated with major complications; additionally, this method does not require hospitalization. TIPC also prevents the pain and complications that are associated with chemical agents. Pleurodesis with VATS has a very high efficacy in terms of effusion control if preoperative indications (complete pulmonary expansion) are respected. The advantage of pleurodesis with VATS is the possibility of conducting the procedure in direct view and achieving uniform talc distribution, even in the most inaccessible areas. Bedside talc pleurodesis has a high success rate when thoracoscopy is unavailable.

J. Grusina-Ujumaza, MD
Department of Thoracic Surgery, Pauls Stradins
Clinical University Hospital,
Pilsona 13, Riga LV1002, Latvia
e-mail: elena.uyumaz@gmail.com

A. Toker, MD (✉)
Department of Thoracic Surgery, Group Florence
Nightingale Hospitals, Istanbul, Turkey

Department of Thoracic Surgery, Istanbul Medical
School, Istanbul University, Millet Caddesi, Çapa,
Fatih, Istanbul 34390, Turkey
e-mail: aetoker@superonline.com

© Springer International Publishing Switzerland 2016
A. Aydiner et al. (eds.), *Breast Disease: Management and Therapies*,
DOI 10.1007/978-3-319-26012-9_39

Keywords

Breast carcinoma • Thoracentesis • Chest tube drainage • Permanent catheters • Talc poudrage • Pleurodesis • Thoracoscopy • Re-accumulation • Lung re-expansion • Trapped lung • Talc pleurodesis • Sclerosing agent • Doxycycline pleurodesis • Bleomycin • Erythromycin • *c-ErbB-2* (a type of receptor tyrosine kinase) • Malignant pleural effusions (MPE) • Video-assisted thoracoscopic surgery (VATS) • Tunneled indwelling pleural catheter (TIPC)

Introduction

Carcinomatous pleurisy often manifests in malignant disease as an indicator of the terminal stage of disease. However, the optimal strategy for palliation of the malignant pleural effusion (MPE) is not well understood. This partially depends on the nature of the cancer and the performance status of the patients. Breast carcinoma is one of the most common neoplasms and causes approximately one-third of all MPEs. It has been reported that the majority of patients with recurrent MPE die within 6 months [1, 2], whereas patients with pleural effusion due to breast carcinoma have a longer median survival time, ranging from 6 to 36 months [3, 4]. A clinical cohort study that included 145 breast carcinoma patients with MPE also showed that the mean survival after the diagnosis of MPE was 6 months; survival was especially shortened in patients with triple-negative breast carcinoma and in those who tested positive for malignant cells in the pleural fluid [5].

Although there are exceptions such as the studies mentioned, the long life expectancy has generally led to the development of surgical strategies and palliative strategies for controlling dyspnea during the first intervention in MPE associated with breast cancer [6, 7]. Pleural progression-free survival in breast carcinoma patients is better if patients received systemic therapy following initial pleurodesis rather than systemic therapy alone [8].

The ideal treatment is to remove fluid and to prevent re-accumulation. Among the methods tried in the past, none has been demonstrated as the most effective. Various methods such as thoracentesis, chest tube drainage, permanent catheter placement, talc or other molecule use, and video-assisted thoracoscopic surgery (VATS) have been used to create pleural symphysis. Whole chest radiotherapy, decortication, and pleurectomy have also been considered in previous years [9].

The outcome of pleurodesis might depend on the tumor type: Bielsa and colleagues [10] demonstrated that the pleurodesis outcome is better for breast carcinoma patients than for lung cancer or mesothelioma patients.

Symptoms

Dyspnea is one of the most widespread symptoms, and it decreases the quality of life. Medical treatment does not have any effect on dyspnea linked to pleural effusion. Less than 30 % of the patients with metastatic pleural effusion from breast carcinoma will benefit from hormonal or chemotherapeutic treatment. The remaining patients with long-lasting pleural effusion or who experienced incomplete re-expansion due to insufficient thoracentesis can develop a peel and a trapped lung. These patients are often the most difficult to treat.

Treatment with Nonsurgical Methods

Patients treated with nonsurgical methods, especially repeated thoracentesis, may live for a considerable length of time, but their quality of life is suboptimal due to recurring effusions. Furthermore, this modality leads to a low percentage of success, with possible complications that may worsen the symptomatology. Repeated thoracentesis controls less than 15 % of the effusions. In addition to the risk of empyema, loss of function of the lung due to incomplete expansion and the persistence of symptoms may occur.

Treatment with Thin Pleural Catheters

Because the long-term benefit of thoracentesis is low, chronic TIPC use has gained popularity in the past two decades. Van Meter and colleagues [11] analyzed 19 studies with a total of 1,370 patients and concluded that TIPC may improve the symptoms of patients with MPE and does not appear to be related to major complications. This method does not require hospitalization and also prevents the pain and complications that are unique to chemical agents [12]. Spontaneous pleurodesis can occur in up to 50 % of the patients [13, 14] and is more likely in patients with primary breast or gynecologic tumors [15]. However, in the absence of enough data, the longer time for pleurodesis, risk of infection, and potential for nutritional loss that can occur with ongoing drainage decrease the evidence supporting TIPC use. Furthermore, some patients may develop unpleasant feelings due to a distorted body image and the extra responsibility faced by them or their family members. In 2003, Ohm and colleagues [16] performed a study in MPE patients. They divided their patients into two groups. They performed VATS and talc pleurodesis on patients with an expanded lung and used TIPC for those with a trapped lung. TIPC patients experienced a shorter hospital stay. The authors concluded that TIPC is safe and effective and has a role in the treatment of patients with a trapped lung [16].

TIPC patients also had better survival with effusion control at 30 days compared with those who underwent bedside talc pleurodesis (82 % vs. 52 %, respectively; $p = 0.024$) [17]. Sioris and colleagues [18] recommended the use of the indwelling pleural catheter as a safe alternative for patients with MPE who are unsuitable for talc pleurodesis.

The most popular TIPC drainage systems that are currently used are the PleurX and Jackson Pratt systems. The PleurX (CareFusion Corporation, San Diego, CA, USA) tunneled pleural catheter system was developed to control symptomatic, recurrent MPE and trapped lung syndrome. The PleurX comprises a fenestrated silicone catheter (15.5 Fr diameter) with a valve mechanism and a polyester cuff. It shows good results for spontaneous pleurodesis and relieves patients of dyspnea [15]. Another type of TIPC is the Jackson Pratt 10 Fr drain, which is easily and effectively used in breast cancer MPE and shows good results in patients with a trapped lung [19].

Chemical Pleurodesis

Chemical pleurodesis by the instillation of asbestos-free talc has been shown to be an effective and safe procedure for the palliation of symptoms related to metastatic pleural effusion [20, 21], and it is strongly recommended in patients with an expected median survival greater than 6 months [22, 23]. Studies comparing chemicals for use in pleurodesis have been performed for more than two decades. Talc has been demonstrated to be the most effective and widely used sclerosing agent. However, talc has side effects, including severe and fatal complications. It has been demonstrated that recent chemotherapy, oxygen supplementation, and peripheral edema were independent prognostic factors for the development of complications [24]. Such patients are recommended to be reserved for TIPC. One of the most interesting studies compared doxycycline pleurodesis versus TIPC; in this study, the initial success rate with doxycycline was 68 %, whereas it was 97 % with TIPC [12]. Recurrence rates of 21 % and 13 % have been reported in doxycycline and TIPC patients, respectively.

Chest Tube Drainage and Pleurodesis

Talc poudrage and pleurodesis via chest tube drainage have lower success rates, with risks associated with infection of the pleural cavity. Thus, they should only be used in cases with poor prognosis and for a short period of time. Large particle talc, which is available in the market from Bryan Corporation, is reported to cause less deposition in the lung and liver than normal or mixed particle talc [25].

Other sclerosing agents—tetracycline and bleomycin—are available, with different success rates and side effects such as fever and pleuritic chest pain [26]. Sedrakyan and colleagues [27] analyzed 46 randomized clinical trials and concluded that talc tended to be associated with fewer recurrences compared to bleomycin and, with less certainty, to tetracycline. Tetracycline (or doxycycline) was not superior to bleomycin.

Furthermore, Balassoulis and colleagues [28] recommended intrapleural erythromycin as an effective and safe sclerosing agent for pleurodesis. They observed a complete response rate (no re-accumulation of pleural fluid after 90 days) for erythromycin pleurodesis of 79.4 %, but all patients suffered chest pain.

VATS Technique

The aim of this technique is to differentiate the ideal candidates for a complete lung expansion and to employ talc pleurodesis. Those patients whose lungs do not have the ability to completely expand could either undergo VATS decortication, if possible, or receive a TIPC.

In our practice, we often use VATS for the management of MPE, and we have developed an optimal surgical technique to obtain successful results.

We perform all VATS procedures under general anesthesia by single lumenal tube intubation or under sedation. Patients are placed in the lateral decubitus position. Two thoracoscopic ports are opened: one port for the camera and one port for biopsies and instrumentation. We use a 30-degree optical camera to assess the pleura and the lung surface by asking the anesthesiologist to keep the patient in an apneic state. Before the apneic state is achieved, it is expected that the anesthesiologist will ventilate the patient with 100 % FiO2 for a period of time to allow for apnea if the patient is intubated. At least four different biopsy specimens are obtained, including

2×2-cm specimens from abnormal areas, and a frozen section examination is performed by collecting the remainder of the specimens for further pathological evaluation. If intraoperative complete lung re-expansion is achieved with contact between the parietal and visceral pleura, talc poudrage is accomplished under direct vision by the nebulization into the pleural cavity of 4–6 g of asbestos-free sterilized talc when the lung is deflated. At the end of the procedure, one chest tube is kept in site through the thoracoscopic access ports to drain both the apex and the base of the pleural cavity. If lung re-expansion is not completely achieved or if a partial expansion in the apex but not in the basal part of the hemithoracic cavity is achieved, we consider the following two options: first, the performance of a VATS decortication and second, leaving a TIPC. By observing the lung re-expansion by postoperative chest x-ray, we can remove the silicon catheter. We do not recommend prescribing anti-inflammatory medication, which could possibly prevent adhesions.

Another primary advantage of the surgical approach is the possibility of obtaining significant surgical specimens, thereby enabling complete tumor characterization at the final pathologic evaluation with reassessment of the estrogen, progesterone, and c-ErbB2 status [29]. Pleural biopsy performed under optic vision had 100 % diagnostic accuracy.

Pleurodesis with VATS has a very high efficacy in terms of effusion control if preoperative indications (complete pulmonary expansion) are respected. The advantage of the pleurodesis in VATS is the possibility of conducting the procedure in direct view, which permits the distribution of talc in a uniform manner, even in the most inaccessible areas. Additionally, talc pleurodesis has a high success rate when thoracoscopy is unavailable [27].

This VATS approach has a success rate of approximately 90 % with the first attempt. Evacuative thoracentesis or drainage of the pleural cavity and the consequent assessment of pulmonary re-expansion was a predictive factor of the success of the procedure [30]. Re-expansion capacity may be observed during surgery by inflating the lung with 30 cm H_2O. Recurrent pleural effusion with bulky mediastinal lymph node involvement and lymphangitic pulmonary carcinomatosis demonstrated by computerized tomography may indicate unsuccessful surgical performance. The cytologic analysis of pleural effusion almost always depends on the quantity/quality ratio of the material; generally, the obtained effusion is not sufficient to perform immunohistochemical analysis [23].

Moreover, the biological patterns of the tumor in breast carcinoma may be useful to obtain new, updated information to predict the response to specific drugs. High hormone receptor expression levels (negative in primary breast carcinoma) represented a determining factor in prescribing endocrine agents [29], and the presence of c-ErbB2 overexpression was a determining factor in prescribing monoclonal antibodies such as trastuzumab [31]. Completely new information might also be obtained when the diagnosis is performed in a rural area where efficient diagnostic modalities are absent (histological exam lost or not available).

In some series with VATS and chemical pleurodesis, an overall median survival time of 17 months was obtained [30]. These data are more sensitive than the median survival times reported by Fentiman et al. [4] (105 patients) and Raju and Kardinal [3] (122 patients) of 13 and 6 months, respectively. Chi-square test analysis of tumor characteristics did not show any significant prognostic effect of pleural effusion recurrence. In addition, the survival time was negatively affected by the number of metastatic sites. In patients with a single metastatic site (pleura) at the time of recurrent pleural effusion, the median survival was 20 months, compared with 12 months in those with multiple sites of metastatic disease ($p = 0.0003$).

Conclusions

Pleurodesis via VATS is a safe and effective procedure to treat pleural effusion that is associated with a low recurrence rate, and this method should be considered the standard treatment to achieve complete lung re-expansion. Pleural biopsy was a determining factor to

assess high hormone receptor expression levels together with the presence of c-ErbB2 overexpression. In breast carcinoma patients, this information may be useful in predicting the response to specific drugs such as endocrine agents and trastuzumab. The management of MPE is palliative for patients with terminal-stage disease, and our goal is to choose the most effective and adequate way to help these patients.

References

1. Putnam Jr JB. Malignant pleural effusions. Surg Clin North Am. 2002;82:867–83.
2. Perrone F, Carlomagno C, De Placido S. First-line systemic therapy for metastatic breast cancer and management of pleural effusion. Ann Oncol. 1995;6:1033–43.
3. Raju R, Kardinal C. Pleural effusion in breast carcinoma: analysis of 122 cases. Cancer. 1981;48:2524–7.
4. Fentiman IS, Millis R, Sexton S, Hayward JL. Pleural effusion in breast cancer. A review of 105 cases. Cancer. 1981;47:2087–92.
5. Santos GT, Prolla JC, Camillo ND, Zavalhia LS, Ranzi AD, Bica CG. Clinical and pathological factors influencing the survival of breast cancer patients with malignant pleural effusion. J Bras Pneumol. 2012;38(4):487–93.
6. Sahn SA. Management of malignant pleural effusions. Monaldi Arch Chest Dis. 2011;56:394–9.
7. Anderson CB, Philpott GW, Ferguson TB. The treatment of malignant pleural effusion. Cancer. 1974;33:916–22.
8. Hirata T, Yonemori K, Hirakawa A, Shimizu C, Tamura K, Ando M. Efficacy of pleurodesis for malignant pleural effusions in breast cancer patients. Eur Respir J. 2011;38(6):1425–30.
9. Reshad K, Inui K, Takahashi Y, Hitomi S. Treatment of malignant pleural effusion. Chest. 1985;88:392–7.
10. Bielsa S, Hernandez P, Rodriguez-Panadero F, Taberner T, Salud A, Porcel JM. Tumor type influences the effectiveness of pleurodesis in malignant effusions. Lung. 2011;189(2):151–5.
11. Van Meter ME, McKee KY, Kohlwes RJ. Efficacy and safety of tunneled pleural catheters in adults with malignant pleural effusions: a systematic review. J Gen Intern Med. 2011;26(1):70–6.
12. Putnam Jr JB, Light RW, Rodriguez RM, Ponn R, Olak J, Pollak JS. A randomized comparison of indwelling pleural catheter and doxycycline pleurodesis in the management of malignant pleural effusion. Cancer. 1999;86:1992–9.
13. Tremblay A, Michaud G. Single-center experience with 250 tunnelled pleural catheter insertions for malignant pleural effusion. Chest. 2006;129(2):362–8.

14. Spector M, Pollak JS. Management of malignant pleural effusions. Semin Respir Crit Care Med. 2008;29(4):405–13.
15. Warren WH, Kim AW, Liptav MJ. Identification of clinical factors predicting Pleurx catheter removal in patients treated for malignant pleural effusion. Eur J Cardiothorac Surg. 2008;33(1):89–94.
16. Ohm C, Park D, Vogen M, Bendick P, Welsh R, Pursel S, Chmielevski G. Use of an indwelling pleural catheter compared with thoracoscopic talc pleurodesis in the management of malignant pleural effusions. Am Surg. 2003;69(3):198–202.
17. Demmy TL, Gu L, Burkhalter JE, Toloza EM, D'Amico TA, Sutherland S. Optimal management of malignant pleural effusions (results of CALGB 30102). J Natl Compr Cancer Netw. 2012;10(8):975–82.
18. Sioris T, Sihvo E, Salo J, Räsänen J, Knuuttila A. Long-term indwelling pleural catheter (PleurX) for malignant pleural effusion unsuitable for talc pleurodesis. Eur J Surg Oncol. 2009;35(5):546–51.
19. Demirhan O, Ordu C, Toker A. Prolonged pleural catheters in the management of pleural effusion due to breast cancer. J Thorac Dis. 2014;6(2):74–8.
20. De Campos JR, Vargas FS, De Campos Werebe E, Cardoso P, Teixeira LR, Jatene FB. Thoracoscopy talc poudrage: a 15-year experience. Chest. 2001;119:801–6.
21. Cardillo G, Facciolo F, Carbone L, Regal M, Corzani F, Ricci A. Long-term follow up of video-assisted talc pleurodesis in malignant recurrent pleural effusions. Eur J Cardiothorac Surg. 2002;21:302–5.
22. Pearson FG, MacGregor DC. Talc poudrage for malignant pleural effusion. J Thorac Cardiovasc Surg. 1996;51:732–8.
23. Viallat JR, Rey F, Astoul P, Boutin C. Thoracoscopic talc poudrage pleurodesis for malignant effusions. A review of 360 cases. Chest. 1996;110:1387–93.
24. Kuzniar TJ, Blum MG, Kasibowska-Kuzniar K, Mutlu GM. Predictors of acute lung injury and severe hypoxemia in patients undergoing operative talc pleurodesis. Ann Thorac Surg. 2006;82: 1976–81.
25. Ferrer J, Montes JF, Villarino MA, Light RW, Garcia Valero J. Influence of particle size on extrapleural talc dissemination after talc slurry pleurodesis. Chest. 2002;122:1018–27.
26. Antunes G, Neville E, Duffy. BTS guidelines for the management of malignant pleural effusions. Thorax. 2003;58(Suppl II):ii29–38.
27. Sedrakyan A, Browne J, Swift S, Tan C. The evidence on the effectiveness of management for malignant pleural effusion: a systematic review. Eur J Cardiothorac Surg. 2006;29(5):829–38.
28. Balassoulis G, Sichletidis L, Spyratos D, Chloros D, Zarogoulidis K, Kontakiotis T. Efficacy and safety of erythromycin as sclerosing agent in patients with recurrent malignant pleural effusion. Am J Clin Oncol. 2008;31(4):384–9.
29. Colleoni M, Minchella I, Mazzarol G, Nolè F, Peruzzotti G, Rocca A. Response to primary chemotherapy in breast cancer patients with tumors not expressing estrogen and progesterone receptors. Ann Oncol. 2000;11:1057–9.
30. Gasparri R, Leo F, Veronessi G, De Pas T, Colleoni M, Maisonneuve P, Pelosi G. Video-assisted management of malignant pleural effusion in breast carcinoma. Cancer. 2006;106:271–6.
31. Kubo M, Morisaki T, Kuroki H, Tasaki A, Yamanaka N, Matsumoto K, Nakamura K. Combination of adoptive immunotherapy with Herceptin for patients with HER2-expressing breast cancer. Anticancer Res. 2003;23:4443–9.

Management of Discrete Pulmonary Nodules

40

Sukru Dilege, Yusuf Bayrak, and Serhan Tanju

Abstract

In the case of a pulmonary nodule on preoperative examination or during postoperative follow-up of breast cancer patients, it can be difficult to distinguish between primary lung cancer, a metastatic pulmonary tumor, and a benign pulmonary lesion. The size, morphology, and number of nodules are helpful parameters for differential diagnoses in many cases, whereas more interventional methods are required to clarify the etiology of progression at follow-up. Benign lesions such as atypical pneumonia, tuberculosis, atypical mycobacteria, inflammatory granuloma, rheumatoid nodules, and atypical bronchoalveolar hyperplasia are also common in immunocompromised patients who underwent multiple cycles of chemotherapy.

Keywords

Metastasectomy • Pulmonary nodule • Solitary pulmonary lesion

S. Dilege, MD (✉)
Department of Thoracic Surgery, Koc University School of Medicine, Rumeli Feneriyolu-Sariyer, Istanbul, Turkey
e-mail: sdilege@ku.edu.tr

Y. Bayrak, MD
Department of Thoracic Surgery, Vehbi Koc Foundation, American Hospital, Istanbul, Turkey
e-mail: yusufb@amerikanhastanesi.org

S. Tanju, MD
Department of Thoracic Surgery, Koc University School of Medicine, Istanbul, Turkey
e-mail: stanju@ku.edu.tr

Introduction

Pulmonary metastases following surgery for breast cancer usually present as multiple lesions and/or pleural effusion or lymphatic carcinomatosis. When chemotherapy fails to show adequate efficacy in a patient with multiple pulmonary lesions that were thought to be metastases, the possibility of changes in the molecular biological properties of the metastatic tumor and the possibility of a (second) primary lung cancer should be considered. The immunohistochemical profiles of cytokeratins such as CK7 and CK20 along with TTF-1 and the breast cancer marker

GCDFP-15 are useful in determining the origin of cancer. Solitary pulmonary lesions in breast cancer patients are candidates for transthoracic fine needle aspiration or wedge resection for accurate tissue diagnosis, and treatment should be planned after a final diagnosis is made. Nevertheless, we suggest that patients with primary breast cancer and indeterminate pulmonary nodules or questionable metastases be offered treatment with curative intent.

There is a broad spectrum of thoracic manifestations in patients with breast cancer [1]. The thorax is a common site for metastasis, which can include local or regional recurrence, bone metastases, spinal cord compression, solitary or multiple pulmonary nodules with or without cavitation, an airspace pattern (lepidic), endobronchial metastasis, lymph node metastasis, and pleural or pericardial involvement complicated by their effusions. Treatment-related complications are numerous, and modalities such as chemo- and radiotherapy may adversely affect the cardiopulmonary system, presenting as pneumonitis, cardiotoxicity, and pericardial effusion. Taken together, physicians dealing with this disease should be familiar with pulmonary/thoracic radiology. In contrast to this issue, the American Society of Clinical Oncology (ASCO) does not recommend chest radiographs or CT scans for routine follow-up in an otherwise asymptomatic patient with no specific findings on clinical examination [2].

The topic of this chapter is the isolation of pulmonary nodules from all other thoracic manifestations.

Diagnosis

Breast cancer progresses from local tumor invasion to axillary lymph nodes and then to organs such as the brain, bone, liver, and lungs. Once a breast cancer case presents with a pulmonary mass, it must be evaluated for metastatic disease [3]. We must not forget that most lung metastases are asymptomatic and are found incidentally. Symptoms occur in 15–20 % of patients and usually reflect proximity to the central airways; these symptoms include cough, hemoptysis, or dyspnea [4]. A chest CT is the recommended diagnostic tool to evaluate a pulmonary nodule and is best performed within 4 weeks of resection. However, positron emission tomography is helpful to determine if there is evidence of other metastatic disease not detected on physical examination or other imaging [5, 6].

Histological diagnosis is important in disease management because of the possibility of primary lung cancer or a benign, inflammatory, or infectious pulmonary process. Although results vary between series of breast cancer patients with pulmonary nodules, most nodules are metastatic lesions (34.2–75 %), 11.5–48 % are primary lung cancer, and 13.5–17.7 % are benign lesions [7, 8]. There are also many case reports that present examples of the possible combination of two distinct diseases in the same organ, especially in patients in whom the pulmonary nodule increases in size during anticancer therapies [9, 10]. The probable reactivation of tuberculosis should be kept in mind even in people without tuberculosis symptoms and not only from endemic regions [11].

Although lymphangitic metastasis was the most frequently observed pulmonary manifestation in a series of patients who died of disseminated breast cancer [12, 13], it is not easy to distinguish a median value of the incidence of pulmonary nodules found in breast cancer patients. This is in contrast to the increasing number of patients with other cancers who undergo routine staging using CT or PET-CT; only a subset of (802/1578) patients were assessed with CT scans in a large series of breast cancer patients [14]. Evangelista showed that the inclusion of PET-CT in the diagnostic algorithm of evaluated patients helped to avoid unnecessary overtreatment in 12 of 29 patients [15].

Additional valuable data are sometimes provided during radiotherapy. Simulation CT scans for three-dimensional radiotherapy planning offer clinical information, including the postoperative status of the breast, lungs, and liver [16]. Because simulation CT scans are of poorer image quality than diagnostic scans due to lower resolution, no enhancement, and thicker image slices, and because they are not routinely interpreted by diagnostic radiologists, the incidence of incidental findings in that study is reportedly low; however, they recommend that the suspicious findings be further evaluated [16].

Among breast cancer patients with pulmonary nodules, biopsy was performed in 30 of 54 patients; breast cancer was presumed in 21, but biopsy showed primary lung cancer in 12 [17]. These two groups did not differ in age, stage, breast tumor size, nodal involvement, or estrogen receptor positivity. In conclusion, it was valuable to evaluate patients with one or more pulmonary lesions without evidence of other metastatic disease. Aggressive workup can allow for the treatment of lung cancer and can impact survival.

Transthoracic fine needle aspiration biopsy is the most frequently used method for histological diagnosis when multiple nodules are present that are not eligible for resection. They occur via hematogenous tumor spreading and are generally spherical or ovoid, vary in size, are sharply marginated, and are mostly peripherally located [18]. Among CT findings, presence of a solid opacity, well-defined tumor, and absence of an air bronchogram were significantly associated with metastatic breast tumor [19].

Okasaka reported the evaluation of pulmonary nodules that appeared in 48 patients after mastectomy [20]. Differential diagnosis was obtained by morphopathological methods alone in 32 patients and by immunohistochemical and molecular marker examination in the remaining 16. The molecular marker mammaglobin 1 was used for differential diagnosis. The final diagnosis was metastatic breast cancer in 40 patients (83.3 %) and primary lung cancer in 8 patients (16.7 %).

A total of 1,703 patients with primary breast cancer were reviewed to investigate the clinical value of preoperative chest CT in detecting lung and liver metastases [21]. Abnormal CT findings, including suspected metastases and indeterminate nodules in the lung or liver, were found in 266 patients (15.6 %). True metastases were found in 26 patients (1.5 % of all patients and 9.8 % of patients with abnormal CT findings), including 17 in the lungs, 3 in the liver, and 6 in both. The largest group having true metastases comprised 24 patients with stage III disease. The sensitivity, specificity, and positive predictive value of chest CT were 100 %, 89.1 %, and 11.3 %, respectively, for lung metastasis and 100 %, 97.6 %, and 18.4 %, respectively, for liver metastasis. All true metastatic lung lesions were small nodules, ranging from 0.2 to 1.5 cm, that could not be detected on chest X-rays. It was not possible to demonstrate the usefulness of routine preoperative chest CT in detecting asymptomatic liver and lung metastasis in patients with early breast cancer. However, chest CT upstaged 6.0 % of stage III patients to stage IV.

Immunohistochemistry staining is performed in nearly all cases to distinguish between primary and metastatic lesions and to compare the hormonal receptor status with the tumor resected from the breast. Thyroid transcription factor-1 (TTF-1) is a sensitive marker for thyroid and pulmonary adenocarcinomas as well as a highly specific method in the differential diagnosis of primary and metastatic lung adenocarcinomas [22].

There are many studies in the literature in which the authors simply resect the pulmonary nodule without conducting a biopsy. Kitada reported 1,226 patients who had breast cancer surgery [23]. A total of 49 patients had pulmonary nodules before or after surgery, and 14 of them had video-assisted thoracoscopic surgery to remove this solitary pulmonary nodule for diagnosis. Evaluation of the immunohistochemical cytokeratin profile and the TTF-1 and GCDFP-15 levels of the lesion was useful when distinguishing between pulmonary cancer and a metastatic pulmonary tumor.

Treatment

In the case of pulmonary metastases in breast cancer patients, resection is advocated if there are no other distant metastases, if the primary tumor is under control, if complete resection can be performed, and if the disease-free interval is longer than 36 months [24]. Estrogen, progesterone, and Her-2 receptor positivity are also good prognostic and predictive factors that enable the continuation

Table 40.1 Pulmonary metastasectomy in breast cancer patients

Author	Number of patients	Median survival (months)	5-year overall survival (%)
Mountain, 1978	21	27	14
Mc Cormick, 1978	28	20	15
Lanza, 1992	37	47	49.5
Staren, 1992	33	58 (single lesion)	36
McDonald, 1994	60	42	37.8
Girard, 1994	32	–	–
Friedel, 1994	91	–	27
Livartowski, 1998	40	70	54
Murabito, 2000	62 (28 CR)	79 CR,15.5 IR	80 CR
Friedel, 2002	467	35	35
Ludwig, 2003	21	96.9	53
Planchard, 2004	125	50	45
Tanaka, 2005	39	32	30.8
Rena, 2007	27	–	38
Welter, 2008	47	32	36

CR complete resection, *IR* incomplete resection

of endocrine therapy and/or anti-Her2 therapy after metastasectomy.

Table 40.1 shows the different series of breast cancer patients, indicating the series that are retrospective and those in which complete resection was mostly associated with long-term survival. Staren evaluated 5,143 patients with breast cancer [25] and found that 284 patients had metastases, including lung metastasis; 63 (1.2 %) had only lung metastasis. Furthermore, 33 patients had resection of the metastatic pulmonary nodule, and 23 patients were given adjuvant chemotherapy. The 5-year survival of the metastasectomy group was 36 %, whereas that of the non-resection group was 11 %. The Mayo Clinic reported their experience in 13,502 breast cancer patients, of whom 60 (0.4 %) were metastatic only to the lungs [26]. Patients with complete resection achieved 42 % 5-year survival in contrast to those with incomplete resection, who achieved 36 %. The study, however, did not mention the other potential prognostic factors related to prolonged survival. The largest series reporting lung metastasectomy in breast cancer patients included 467 patients; complete resection was performed in 84 %, and the median survival was 37 months compared with 25 months in incompletely resected patients [27]. Complete resection and a disease-free interval of more than 36 months were the two most significant factors associated with prolonged survival.

After complete resection of all visible metastases is achieved (NED: no evidence of disease), there are no prospective data regarding the addition of chemotherapy to improve survival. The goal of systemic therapy should be to fight against micrometastasis. Studies from the MD Anderson Cancer Center that summarize and update the data from the last 30 years note that the addition of newer chemotherapy agents may improve long-term survival after recurrence. Hanrahan showed that patients who receive anthracycline-based chemotherapy at primary diagnosis could benefit from the local treatment of isolated recurrences followed by docetaxel-based chemotherapy [28]. The median follow-up for this docetaxel-based trial ($n = 26$ patients) was 45 months. The early outcomes of this study are promising. The median disease-free survival (DFS) was 44 months, and the 3-year DFS and overall survival (OS) rates were 58 % and 87 %, respectively.

Conclusion

The major goal of pulmonary resection (metastasectomy) is to differentiate the primary tumor from metastatic disease and to reevaluate the hormonal status and biological changes of breast cancer. Although there are no prospective data, radical resection may lead to long-term survival for selected patients with good prognostic factors.

Algorithm from the Perspective of a Thoracic Surgeon

Approach to a discrete pulmonary nodule in a breast cancer patient.

Breast cancer patient with pulmonary nodule in chest X-Ray (CT or PET-CT?)

Extrapulmonary metastatic site?

If yes, go on with medical oncology and follow the nodule after chemotherapeutic response.

If no, define the lesion.

(i) One nodule with FDG(+), SUVmax >5 without mediastinal FDG uptake: perform sublobar resection (lobectomy, if primary)

(ii) One nodule with low FDG (SUVmax <5) without mediastinal FDG uptake: consider Noguchi classification [28], follow or perform resection

(iii) At least two nodules: diagnose with bronchoscopy/transthoracic biopsy/wedge resection

(iv) Single nodule with mediastinal enlarged lymph nodes (FDG+): perform endobronchial ultrasonography (EBUS) or mediastinoscopy

(v) Cavitary nodule in a smoker: perform sublobar resection (lobectomy, if primary)

(vi) Calcified, popcorn-shaped single lesion: radiologic follow-up

(vii) Nodule increasing in size during chemotherapy: perform sublobar resection (lobectomy, if primary)

(viii) Nodule with pleural effusion: perform VATS-wedge resection/biopsy with/without talc pleurodesis

References

1. Jung JI, Kim HH, Park SH, Song SW, Song SW, Chung MH, Kim HS, et al. Thoracic manifestations of breast cancer and its therapy. Radiographics. 2004;24:1269–85.
2. Khatcheressian JL, Hurley P, Bantug E, Esserman LJ, Grunfeld E, Halberg F, et al. Breast cancer follow-up and management after primary treatment: American Society of Clinical Oncology clinical practice guideline update. J Clin Oncol. 2013;31:961–5.
3. Rashid OM, Takabe K. The evolution of the role of surgery in the management of breast cancer lung metastasis. J Thorac Dis. 2012;4:420–4.
4. Rusch VW. Pulmonary metastasectomy. Current indications. Chest. 1995;107:322S–31.
5. Detterbeck FC, Grodzki T, Gleeson F, Robert JH. Imaging requirements in the practice of pulmonary metastasectomy. J Thorac Oncol. 2010;5:S134–9.
6. Nichols FC. Pulmonary metastasectomy. Thorac Surg Clin. 2012;22:91–9.
7. Rena O, Papalia E, Ruffini E, Filosso PL, Oliaro A, Maggi G, et al. The role of surgery in the management of solitary pulmonary nodule in breast cancer patients. Eur J Surg Oncol. 2007;33:546–50.
8. Tanaka F, Li M, Hanaoka N, Bando T, Fukuse T, Hasegawa S, et al. Surgery for pulmonary nodules in breast cancer patients. Ann Thorac Surg. 2005;79:1711–4; discussion 1714–1715.
9. Endri M, Cartei G, Zustovich F, Serino FS, Fassina A. Differential diagnosis of lung nodules: breast cancer metastases and lung tuberculosis. Infez Med. 2010;1:39–42.
10. Ou KW, Hsu KF, Cheng YL, Hsu GC, Hsu HM, Yu JC. Asymptomatic pulmonary nodules in a patient with early-stage breast cancer: Cryptococcus infection. Int J Infect Dis. 2010;14:e77–80.
11. Kaplan MH, Armstrong D, Rosen P. Tuberculosis complicating neoplastic disease: a review of 201 cases. Cancer. 1974;33:850–8.
12. Kreisman H, Wolkove N, Finkelstein HS, Cohen C, Margolese R, Frank H. Breast cancer and thoracic metastases: review of 119 patients. Thorax. 1983;38:175–9.

13. Connolly Jr JE, Erasmus JJ, Patz Jr EF. Thoracic manifestations of breast carcinoma: metastatic disease and complications of treatment. Clin Radiol. 1999;54:487–94.

14. Lee B, Lim A, Lalvani A, Deschamps MJ, Leonard R, Nallamala S, et al. The clinical significance of radiologically detected silent pulmonary nodules in early breast cancer. Ann Oncol. 2008;19:2001–6.

15. Evangelista L, Panunzio A, Cervino AR, Vinante L, Al-Nahhas A, Rubello D, Muzzio PC, Polverosi R. Indeterminate pulmonary nodules on CT images of breast cancer patient: the additional value of 18F-FDG PET-CT. J Med Imaging Radiat Oncol. 2012;56:417–24.

16. Park JS, Choi DH, Huh SJ, Park W, Nam SJ, Lee JE, Kil WH, Lee KS. Incidental findings on simulation CT images for adjuvant radiotherapy in breast cancer patients. Technol Cancer Res Treat. 2015;14:525–9.

17. Chang EY, Johnson W, Karamlou K, Khaki A, Komanapalli C, Walts D, Mahin D, Johnson N. The evaluation and treatment implications of isolated pulmonary nodules in patients with a recent history of breast cancer. Am J Surg. 2006;191:641–5.

18. Seo JB, Im J, Goo JM, Chung MJ. Atypical pulmonary metastases: spectrum of radiologic findings. RadioGraphics. 2001;21:403–17.

19. Kinoshita T, Yoshida J, Ishii G, Hishida T, Wada M, Aokage K, et al. The availability of pre- and intraoperative evaluation of a solitary pulmonary nodule in breast cancer patients. Ann Thorac Cardiovasc Surg. 2015;21:31–6.

20. Okasaka T, Usami N, Mitsudomi T, Yatabe Y, Matsuo K, Yokoi K. Stepwise examination for differential diagnosis of primary lung cancer and breast cancer relapse presenting as a solitary pulmonary nodule in patients after mastectomy. J Surg Oncol. 2008;98:510–4.

21. Kim H, Han W, Moon HG, Min J, Ahn SK, Kim TY, et al. The value of preoperative staging chest computed tomography to detect asymptomatic lung and liver metastasis in patients with primary breast carcinoma. Breast Cancer Res Treat. 2011;126:637–41.

22. Moldvay J, Jackel M, Bogos K, Soltesz I, Agocs L, Kovacs G, et al. The role of TTF-1 in differentiating primary and metastatic lung adenocarcinomas. Pathol Oncol Res. 2004;10:85–8.

23. Kitada M, Sato K, Matsuda Y, Hayashi S, Miyokawa N, Sasajima T. Role of treatment for solitary pulmonary nodule in breast cancer patients. World J Surg Oncol. 2011;9:124.

24. Kycler W, Laski P. Surgical approach to pulmonary metastases from breast cancer. Brest J. 2012;18:52–7.

25. Staren ED, Salerno C, Rangione A. Pulmonary resection for metastatic breast cancer. Arch Surg. 1992;127:1282–4.

26. Mc Donald ML, Deschamps C, Ilstrup DM. Pulmonary resection for metastatic breast cancer. Ann Thorac Surg. 1994;58:1599–602.

27. Friedel G, Pastorino U, Ginsberg RJ. Results of lung metastasectomy from breast cancer: prognostic criteria on the basis of 467 cases of the International Registry of Lung Metastases. Eur J Cardiothorac. 2002;22:335–44.

28. Hanrahan EO, Broglio KR, Buzdar AU, Theriault RL, Valero V, Cristofanilli M, et al. Combined-modality treatment for isolated recurrences of breast carcinoma: update on 30 years of experience at the University of Texas M.D. Anderson Cancer Center and assessment of prognostic factors. Cancer. 2005;104:1158–71.

Management of Isolated Liver Metastasis

Abdullah İğci and Enver Özkurt

Abstract

A solitary first metastasis to the liver in breast cancer is an uncommon presentation. Nearly half of all patients with metastatic breast cancer develop liver metastases [1–3], but a minority of patients present with metastatic breast cancer limited to the liver (5–12 %) [3–6]. Among patients who have died of breast cancer, hepatic metastases are found in 55–75 % of autopsies [7]. Overall, the 5-year survival of patients with stage IV breast cancer is currently 23 % [8] and drops to 8.5 % for those patients with liver metastases [4].

Hepatic metastases generally occur at later stages of disseminated disease and carry a very poor prognosis, with a median survival of 6 months [9]. However, the median survival of patients with isolated liver metastases is approximately 1 year if untreated [10]. Even with systemic chemotherapy, the median survival time is approximately 19 months for patients with metastatic breast cancer to the liver only or with limited disease elsewhere [11].

Published studies have evaluated the safety and benefit of hepatic resection, radiofrequency ablation (RFA), transarterial chemoembolization (TACE) or intra-arterial chemotherapy, stereotactic body radiation therapy (SBRT), and interstitial laser therapy (ILT) to treat liver metastases from breast cancer. Because no randomized controlled trials have been performed, the comparative efficacies of these approaches remain controversial. Moreover, identifying appropriate patients for treatment remains a challenge [3, 12, 13], and the carefully selected patients in these published series may represent good prognosis subgroups independent of the therapeutic approach.

A. İğci, MD, FACS (✉)
Breast Unit, Department of General Surgery,
Istanbul University, Istanbul Medical Faculty,
Istanbul, Turkey
e-mail: aigci@istanbul.edu.tr

E. Özkurt, MD
Department of General Surgery, Istanbul Medical
Faculty, Istanbul University, Istanbul, Turkey

© Springer International Publishing Switzerland 2016
A. Aydiner et al. (eds.), *Breast Disease: Management and Therapies*,
DOI 10.1007/978-3-319-26012-9_41

Keywords

Breast cancer • Liver metastasis • Radiofrequency ablation • Metastasectomy

Management of Isolated Liver Metastases

A solitary first metastasis of the liver in breast cancer is an uncommon presentation. Nearly half of all patients with metastatic breast cancer develop liver metastases [1–3], but a minority of patients present with metastatic breast cancer limited to the liver (5–12 %) [3–6]. Among patients who have died of breast cancer, hepatic metastases are found in 55–75 % of autopsies [7]. Overall, the 5-year survival of patients with stage IV breast cancer is currently 23 % [8] and drops to 8.5 % for those patients with liver metastases [4].

Hepatic metastases generally occur at later stages of disseminated disease and carry a very poor prognosis, with a median survival of 6 months [9]. However, the median survival of patients with isolated liver metastases is approximately 1 year, if untreated [10]. Even with systemic chemotherapy, the median survival time is approximately 19 months for patients with metastatic breast cancer to the liver only or with limited disease elsewhere [11].

Published studies have evaluated the safety and benefit of hepatic resection, radiofrequency ablation (RFA), transarterial chemoembolization (TACE) or intra-arterial chemotherapy, stereotactic body radiation therapy (SBRT), and interstitial laser therapy (ILT) to treat liver metastases from breast cancer. Because no randomized controlled trials have been performed, the comparative efficacies of these approaches remain controversial. Moreover, identifying appropriate patients for treatment remains a challenge [3, 12, 13], and the carefully selected patients in published series may represent good prognosis subgroups independent of the therapeutic approach.

Patient Selection Criteria

Palliative liver-directed therapy may be beneficial if the hepatic disease adversely affects the patient's quality of life. Most oncologists consider this a palliative situation in which surgical treatment is reserved for symptomatic cases only. The risks and benefits of liver-directed therapies should be compared with systemic treatment options [5]. However, various retrospective studies have noted a survival benefit for aggressive local treatment of the primary tumor in select patients even in the presence of distant metastases [14–16].

In particular, candidates should have limited metastatic disease in the liver, controlled primary disease, a younger age, longer disease-free intervals, and a higher performance status [3, 5, 17–20]. The presence of extrahepatic metastatic or residual primary breast cancer is commonly [21, 22], but not always [23, 24], considered a contraindication to liver-directed therapy.

To aid in risk assessment and decision making, the pre-procedure work-up should define the extent of disease and its responsiveness to systemic therapy. For this critical decision making, a pathologic examination and some imaging modalities should be performed. A computed tomography (CT) scan of the abdomen and pelvis should be used to evaluate the number and location of liver metastases to facilitate procedure planning and to rule out other intra-abdominal diseases. Further, CT imaging of the chest should be performed to rule out pulmonary and mediastinal disease. Additionally, a bone scan should be undertaken to rule out bone metastases, and a positron emission tomography (PET) scan may be useful to identify extrahepatic disease.

Surgical Treatment Options

Liver resection for metastases that derive from non-portal vein-associated organs is still controversial even though it is widely accepted in colorectal cancer and neuroendocrine tumors. In those cases, liver metastases may be regarded as a sign of systemic tumor spread that is only amenable to systemic chemotherapy [25]. Increasing evidence suggests that patients with breast cancer liver metastases (BCLMs) may receive survival benefits from liver metastasectomy associated with systemic treatment [26]. Moreover, the 5-year survival rate is comparable to that after colorectal cancer liver metastasis resection [27].

Most published studies are designed as retrospective single-arm and single-center analyses. The limited number of eligible cases in these centers leads to an average caseload of two to three patients per year [8]. Independent prognostic factors that are predictive of survival are still not clearly defined. Because only patients with a limited number of liver lesions seem to benefit from surgical therapy, liver resection is rarely performed [8]. If the patients' physical performance is good enough for surgery, perioperative morbidity and mortality rates are low [21, 28–30].

Candidates for Surgical Treatment

Patient selection and operative criteria for hepatic resection remain controversial. The important criteria seem to be that patients have fewer than four hepatic metastases, no extrahepatic disease, and demonstrated disease regression or stability with systemic therapy before resection [31]. At a minimum, a patient should have a normal performance status and normal hepatic function tests [32]. Pocard and Selzner indicated that the size and number of hepatic metastases was an important factor [17]. Patients in whom hepatic metastases were found more than 1 year after resection of the primary cancer had significantly better outcomes than those with early (<1 year after resection) metastatic disease. Younger patients with a limited number of tumor locations seem to be good candidates for this option, and hepatic metastasectomy may lead to prolonged survival [33].

Increasing evidence in the literature also suggests that patients with oligometastases (metastases limited to one organ with a small number of lesions) may be good candidates for surgical therapy. Furthermore, the pattern of oligometastases may result from a distinct biological behavior with a specific gene expression and tumor metabolism [34].

Chua et al. indicated that the response to chemotherapy might predict a better outcome for patients who undergo liver resection for hepatic metastases [8]. To select patients who will benefit from surgical treatment, a better understanding of the individual biological behavior of BCLM is warranted. This study should include molecular markers, metabolic activity, and the response to chemotherapy [35, 36].

Presurgical Evaluation

Before hepatic resection, patients should be examined to rule out extrahepatic, intra-abdominal disease. Metachronous metastases must be regarded as tumor recurrence. There is a broad variety of secondary tumor growth in distant organ systems, most frequently in the bone, liver, lungs, and brain. Among these different metastatic locations, the liver is the second most frequent site of metachronous metastases (40–50 %) [33]. Intraoperative ultrasound (US) may be beneficial for identifying additional liver lesions and determining the exact location of the lesions concurrently with their proximity to venous structures.

Hepatic resection candidates must have enough liver remnant after resection of the lesion(s). Because the function and architecture of the liver are integrated, adequate liver function can be maintained if there is a critical volume of intact liver and a contiguous bile duct system (20 % of a normal liver, 40 % of the liver if steatosis is present). If a small liver remnant is anticipated, the patient may benefit from preoperative portal vein embolization of the lobe to be resected. This embolization causes hypertrophy of the opposite lobe that will be the remnant, thereby decreasing the risk of postoperative hepatic insufficiency [37].

In the absence of prospective data, the role and effectiveness of hepatic metastasectomy in BCLM has not been defined. In terms of safety, mortality was 0 % in the large majority of studies [18, 21, 26, 29–31, 38–42], and morbidity ranged between 0 % [43] and 35.9 % [44]. Regarding survival, the median survival after hepatectomy ranged between 27 and 63 months (Table 41.1) [43]. Other authors have also noted that repeat hepatectomy for BCLM is associated with improved survival [31]. Large disease-free intervals between primary breast cancer surgery and liver metastases diagnosis [18, 20], positive hormone receptor status [38], response to chemotherapy, and R0 resection [29] are all favorable prognostic factors in patients with BCLM [45,

Table 41.1 The 5-year survival rates after curative liver resection

Reference	Number of patients	5-year survival rate (%)	Median survival (months)
Raab et al. [43]	34	18 %	27
Carlini et al. [50]	17	46 %	53
Arena and Ferrero [51]	17	41 %	–
Vlastos et al. [21]	31	61 %	63
Sakamoto et al. [28]	34	21 %	36
Yedibela et al. [52]	17	50 %	62
Adam et al. [31]	85	43 %	43
Elias and Di Pietroantonio [53]	54	34 %	34
Thelen et al. [29]	39	61 %	73
Hoffmann et al. [46]	41	48 %	58
Dittmar et al. [41]	21	38 %	52

Reprinted from Ref. [41] with permission of Springer Science and Business Media ©Springer-Verlag Berlin Heidelberg 2013

46]. The variables associated with poor outcomes after liver resection for BCLM include the presence of the extrahepatic disease at the time of resection [28], multiple liver metastases, and estrogen receptor (ER)-negative status [30, 47].

Vlastos et al. studied the long-term survival of 31 patients with breast cancer with metastases limited to the liver who underwent hepatic resection at the MD Anderson Cancer Center [21]. The hepatic metastases had developed after a median of 22 months from the initial diagnosis. Solitary hepatic metastases were found in 20 patients, and multiple hepatic metastases were found in 11 patients. Major hepatic resections (three or more segments resected) were performed in 14 patients, and minor resections (fewer than three segments resected) with or without radiofrequency ablation were performed in 17 patients. The median size of the largest hepatic metastasis was 2.9 cm. A total of 87 % of the patients received either pre- or postoperative systemic therapy, with a median survival of 63 months. The overall 2- and 5-year survival rates were 86 % and 61 %, respectively, while the 2- and 5-year disease-free survival rates were 39 % and 31 %, respectively. Vlastos et al. were unable to identify any treatment- or patient-specific variables associated with the survival rates. They concluded that in select patients with hepatic metastases from breast cancer, an aggressive surgical approach was associated with favorable long-term survival and that hepatic resection should be considered as a component of the multimodality treatment of breast cancer in these patients.

In a prospective study of 50 patients with hepatic metastases of breast cancer, 34 patients underwent laparotomy with the intention of undergoing a curative liver resection [41]. Liver resection was performed in 34 patients. Resection margins were clear in 21 cases (R0). Nine patients with clear resection margins lived for more than 60 months after liver resection. The observed 5-year survival rate was 21 % for all 50 patients, 28 % for resected patients, and 38 % after R0 resection. On univariate analysis of their results, the survival rates of the resected patients were significantly influenced by

R classification, age, extrahepatic tumor at the time of liver resection, size of metastases, and HER2 expression of liver metastases. Multivariate analysis revealed an absence of HER2 expression, the presence of extrahepatic tumor, and a patient's age ≥50 years as independent factors of poor prognosis. They concluded that breast cancer patients who were younger than 50 years with technically resectable hepatic metastases, minimal extrahepatic tumor, and positive HER2 expression appear to be suitable candidates for liver resection with curative intent, and an aggressive multidisciplinary management of those patients, including surgical treatment, may improve long-term survival.

In another single-center study from Bucharest, Romania [48], 52 female patients underwent surgery for BCLM between 2002 and 2013. Only patients with liver resections ($n=43$) were included in their analysis. The median survival of the 43 patients with liver resection was 32.2 months. The factors that were significantly associated with overall post-hepatectomy survival were estrogen/progesterone receptor (ER/PR) status ($p=0.002$), node involvement of the primary tumor ($p=0.049$), and the size ($p=0.005$) and number ($p=0.006$) of the metastatic lesions. The 1-, 3-, and 5-year survival rates after curative liver resection were 93.02 %, 74.42 %, and 58.14 %, respectively. They emphasized that BCLM resection is a safe procedure and offers a survival benefit, especially in patients with reduced liver metastatic burden (solitary metastases, diameter of the metastases <5 cm) and positive ER/PR status.

Polistina et al. retrospectively reviewed 26 women with isolated BCLM and without any sign of disease progression after a cycle of chemotherapy [49]. Women were treated with hepatic resection for unilobar disease or surgical "open" RFA for bilobar disease. The overall survival from the breast cancer diagnosis was 47.69±22.25 months (range 33–84, median 45.5 months); these rates were 52.25±14.57 months (range 33–84, median 48.5 months) for the hepatic resection patients and 43.79±27.14 months (range 9–101, median 39 months) for the RFA patients. Overall survival from the BCLM treatment was 21.12±12.78 months (range 9–64, median 15.5 months);

specifically, it was 29.42±14.53 months (range 12–64, median 29.5 months) for the resected patients and 14±4.45 months (range 9–24, median 13.5 months) for patients treated with RFA, with a strongly significant survival difference for surgically treated patients ($p=0.001$). The overall disease-free survival from BCLM was 15.96±13.16 months (range 3–64, median 12 months), disease-free survival for resected patients was 23.22±16.2 months (range 8–64, median 18.5 months), and for patients treated by RFA was 9.64±4.22 months (range 3–18, median 9 months). The overall 1-, 2-, and 5-year (actuarial) survival rates were, respectively, 80.7, 57, and 31 %. When calculated for the two groups, these rates were, respectively, 100, 66.6, and 34 % (actuarial) for the resected group patients and 64.2, 21.4, and 11.5 % (actuarial) for the RFA patients. These data indicate that aggressive treatment of isolated BCLMs may improve survival for these patients.

Finally, in a systemic review about hepatic resection for metastatic breast cancer, Terence et al. searched the MEDLINE and PubMed databases (January 2000–January 2011) to identify studies that reported the outcomes of hepatectomy for BCLM [8]. Nineteen studies were examined, comprising 553 patients. Hepatectomy for BCLM was performed at a rate of 1.8 (range, 0.7–7.7) cases per year in the reported series. The median time to liver metastases occurred at a median of 40 (range, 23–77) months. The median mortality and complication rates were 0 % (range, 0–6 %) and 21 % (range, 0–44 %), respectively. The median overall survival was 40 (range, 15–74) months, and the median 5-year survival rate was 40 % (range, 21–80 %). Potential prognostic factors associated with a poorer overall survival include a positive liver surgical margin and hormone refractory disease. Consequently, the authors indicated that, for selected patients with isolated liver metastases and in those with well-controlled minimal extrahepatic disease, hepatectomy has a superior 5-year survival. Thus, to evaluate its efficacy and control for selection bias, a randomized trial of standard chemotherapy with or without hepatectomy for BCLM is warranted.

When we reviewed all of the studies of the surgical treatment of isolated BCLM, we confirmed that hepatic resection has not been compared in a randomized trial with systemic chemotherapy or with nonsurgical, liver-directed options (Table 41.1) [21, 28, 29, 31, 41, 43, 46, 50–53]. This lack of comparison could be due to a low number of cases per year. Nevertheless, multicenter prospective randomized studies are needed to specify the exact efficacy of surgery among this specific group of patients.

Nonsurgical Treatment Options

BCLM usually indicates the presence of hematogenous disseminated cancer with a very poor prognosis [54]. Apart from hepatic resections, minimally invasive therapy methods, such as RFA, TACE, SBRT, and ILT, have been used for effective and relatively simple treatment of BCLM for patients who are not good candidates for resection or do not desire surgical procedures [55–60].

Radiofrequency Ablation Therapy

Radiofrequency ablation uses a high-frequency electrical current (375–480 kHz) that is applied through one or more needle electrodes that are electrically insulated along all but the distal 1–3 cm of the shaft. The radiofrequency current produces ionic agitation that leads to heat production. Heating results in cellular destruction and protein denaturation at temperatures above 50 °C when applied for 4–6 min and within a few seconds at temperatures above 75 °C [61]. Temperatures higher than 100 °C may result in tissue water boiling and gas formation within the target. Although these bubbles allow visualization using B-mode diagnostic US imaging, it may retard the transmission of the radiofrequency current. Most work has been performed using simple monopolar radiofrequency probes that consist of an electric generator, needle electrode(s), and a grounding pad attached to the skin of the patient.

Surgical resection with or without chemotherapy is considered the best treatment option in selected cases with solitary BCLM and has a low surgical risk. Solitary liver metastases in breast cancer patients are rare, occurring in only approximately 5 % of all cases. Most patients are unsuitable for surgery because of their poor general condition or the stage of disease. RFA is an alternative to resection and the preferred adjunctive treatment (instead of surgery) to systemic chemotherapy for hepatic metastases and in patients with hepatic disease after chemotherapy [62]. Many patients are not eligible for surgery, and a review of the major surgical studies shows that RFA of hepatic metastases has a lower mortality and periprocedural complication rate compared with surgery. Additionally, RFA offers clear advantages with regard to the length of hospital stay and costs compared with surgery. However, due to the poor local effectiveness of RFA in treating metastases larger than 3 cm in diameter, surgery remains better for larger lesions [63].

RFA is a relatively simple technique that constitutes an effective local treatment for hepatic metastases, with minimal invasiveness and few adverse events [62]. Hepatic RFA has been primarily used to treat hepatocellular carcinoma and metastases from colorectal cancer, but a small number of reports also concern metastases from the breast, stomach, kidney, and lung carcinoma and from cholangiocarcinoma and melanoma [64].

Veltri et al. analyzed 45 patients (mean age 55 years) with 87 metastases (mean size 23 mm), examining adverse events, complete ablation at the initial follow-up assessment and during the subsequent follow-up (mean 30 months), time to progression, and survival [63]. They investigated the correlation between local effectiveness and metastasis size. They also analyzed possible predictors of 3-year survival, including the local effectiveness of RFA (complete ablation maintained at 1 year versus treatment failure). Nine adverse events occurred in their series (two major complications, 2.3 %). Complete ablation at initial follow-up was obtained in 90 % of patients; in 19.7 %, the complete ablation relapsed, with a time to progression of 8 months. The difference between the mean diameter of maintained complete ablation (22 mm) and that of the treatment failures (30 mm) was highly significant ($p = 0.0005$), as was the 30 mm threshold ($p = 0.0062$). The overall survival rates at years 1, 2, and 3 were 90, 58, and 44 %. In the univariate analysis, the local effectiveness of RFA did not reach significance, so the authors concluded that RFA of hepatic metastases from breast cancer has high local effectiveness in tumors up to 30 mm but that it is not relevant in determining survival.

In another study from Italy [65] that aimed to evaluate the effectiveness of RFA of liver metastases from breast cancer and its impact on survival, 13 female patients (age range 36–82 years; median 54.5 years) underwent RFA for the treatment of 21 liver metastases from breast cancer. The procedures were performed under ultrasound guidance using an RF 2000 or RF 3000 generator system and Le Veen monopolar needle electrodes. Follow-up was performed by CT after 1, 3, 6, and 12 months. The technical success was 100 %. No major or minor complications occurred at the end of the procedure. In their series, 7/21 lesions in 7/13 patients increased in size at 7, 18, 19, and 38 months. This increase resulted in a mean disease-free interval of 16.6 months. The mean overall survival after RFA was 10.9 months. The authors noted that RFA appears to be a useful adjunct to systemic chemotherapy and/or hormone therapy in the locoregional treatment of hepatic metastases from breast cancer. RFA may also be a less invasive alternative to surgery in the locoregional treatment of liver metastases from breast cancer.

After a median follow-up of 16 months, 64 % of patients were alive in a group of 14 patients with 16 tumors who were treated with RFA [66]. In a larger case series of 24 breast cancer patients with 64 liver metastases treated with RFA and followed for a median of 19 months, 58 % developed new metastases, the majority of which occurred in the liver (71 %) [56]. However, most patients with disease limited to the liver were disease free at the last follow-up.

Sites that are treated with RFA frequently cavitate after the procedure, forming a distinctive scar band. The risk of complications increases with proximity to the porta hepatis. Hepatitis, infection, and injury to larger bile ducts and nearby bowels rarely occur. Patients with preexisting liver damage, such as cirrhosis, and those with larger tumors are more likely to experience complications [67]. Although it is uncommon, needle track seeding has been reported [68]. Aside from the risks mentioned above, RFA can be performed as an outpatient procedure.

In most reported cases for metastatic breast cancer, RFA was used in combination with systemic chemotherapy, and very few side effects (mild right upper quadrant discomfort and asymptomatic pleural effusion) were noted; however, none required specific treatment [24, 66]. RFA has also been combined with surgical resection [21].

Even in light of the lack of correlation between local effectiveness and survival, hepatic RFA should not be used as the only treatment for metastatic breast cancer. To produce a positive effect on medium-term survival, a systemic therapeutic approach is required. Nonetheless, RFA may be proposed as an alternative to surgery in the context of a multimodal strategy because it is safe and effective in achieving local control of limited disease, especially when the burden of systemic therapy needs to be decreased, in part to improve the quality of life of the patient. Based on these data and the experience with other malignancies, RFA for metastatic breast cancer limited to the liver may be beneficial for select patients.

Transarterial Chemoembolization and Intra-arterial Chemotherapy

TACE is a local, catheter-based, minimally invasive therapeutic option for unresectable liver tumors and is defined as the selective administration of chemotherapy, usually in combination with embolization of the vascular supply of the tumor [69]. In contrast with the normal liver parenchyma, which is primarily fed by the portal vein, tumors in the liver are supplied by the hepatic artery. TACE takes advantage of this blood supply pattern by instilling cytotoxic agents mixed with iodized oil into the hepatic artery feeding the tumor and then embolizing this vessel (often with gelatin sponge particles) to cut off the tumor blood supply [70].

The technical success of TACE is demonstrated by the presence of hyper-attenuating iodized oil within the tumor on unenhanced CT [71]. Because of the size of the liver, the tumor may not change after liver-directed therapy [72]; thus, the European Association for the Study of the Liver (EASL) has been proposed as an alternative to the Response Evaluation Criteria in Solid Tumors (RECIST). A surrogate end point for response is the apparent diffusion coefficient (ADC), which measures the mobility of water in tissues: viable tumor cells restrict the mobility of water, while necrotic tumor cells allow increased diffusion [71]. In one study of TACE for patients with metastatic breast cancer ($n = 14$, prospective chart review), no tumors met the RECIST criteria for complete response, but the ADC increased by a mean of 27 % after treatment [71].

Indications for TACE

Indications for the TACE treatment of liver metastases in patients with breast cancer were primarily palliative or symptomatic. During the course of treatment in some patients, the indication changed to neoadjuvant. Palliative chemoembolization was defined as therapy for asymptomatic patients intended mainly to prolong survival and to preserve and improve the quality of life without curing the disease. Symptomatic treatment was defined as a therapy intended to alleviate or decrease tumor-related symptoms (e.g., pain or bulk-related symptoms). Neoadjuvant TACE was defined as a clinical scenario in which TACE resulted in a relevant downsizing of the size and number of metastases, resulting in a situation where the criteria for local thermal ablation via laser-induced thermotherapy (LITT) were met. These criteria were defined as ≤5 metastases and ≤5 cm in diameter. Patients who met such inclusion criteria for LITT treatment before chemoembolization also received chemoembolization before LITT to decrease the tumor activity and to decrease tumor vascularity (based on findings of contrast-enhanced magnetic resonance imaging [MRI] performed at first

presentation) to maximize the ablative effect of the LITT on the tumor [73].

Contraindications for TACE

Contraindications for treatment with TACE were poor performance status (Karnofsky status, ≤70 %), nutritional impairment, the presence of marked ascites, high serum total bilirubin level [>3 mg/dL (51.3 μmol/L)], poor hepatic synthesis [serum albumin level <2.0 mg/dL (20 g/L)], and renal failure [serum creatinine level >2 mg/dL (176.8 μmol/L)]. Partial or complete thrombosis of the main portal vein was a further exclusion criterion for the procedure, as were cardiovascular or respiratory failure. The tumor load of the liver was restricted to not more than 70 % of the total liver volume [73].

A chart review of eight patients treated with TACE demonstrated a median overall survival of 6 months, with no patient surviving longer than 14 months [72]. A study of 14 patients with 27 lesions using MRI showed a median survival of 25 months and a 35 % overall survival at 3 years [71].

Li et al. [74] compared the results of TACE ($n = 28$) and systemic chemotherapy ($n = 20$) and concluded that there was a significant difference between the two groups in terms of response rates and survival rates. The 1-, 2-, and 3-year survival rates for the TACE group were 63.04, 30.35, and 13.01 %, whereas those for the systemic chemotherapy group were 33.88, 11.29, and 0 %.

In another study, 208 patients (mean age 56.4 years, range 29–81) with unresectable hepatic metastases from breast cancer were repeatedly treated with TACE at 4-week intervals [73]. In total, 1,068 chemoembolizations were performed with Lipiodol and starch microspheres. Tumor response was evaluated by MRI according to the RECIST criteria. For all protocols, local tumor control was defined as a partial response in 13 % (27/208), stable disease in 50.5 % (105/208), and progressive disease 3 in 6.5 % (76/208) of patients. The 1-, 2-, and 3-year survival rates after TACE were 69 %, 40 %, and 33 %, respectively. The median and mean survival times from the start of TACE were 18.5 and

30.7 months, respectively. Treatment with mitomycin-C only showed median and mean survival times of 13.3 and 24 months, respectively; with gemcitabine only, they were 11 and 22.3 months, and with a combination of mitomycin-C and gemcitabine, they increased to 24.8 and 35.5 months, respectively. These authors emphasized that TACE is an optional therapy for the treatment of liver metastases in breast cancer patients with better results from the combined chemotherapy protocol.

An open-label, prospective non-randomized single-center phase II study evaluated the efficacy and tolerability of transarterial chemoembolization with gemcitabine in patients with inoperable BCLM [75]. Forty-three patients were enrolled. Tumor response was evaluated by MRI and CT imaging. All patients tolerated the treatment well, with no dose-limiting toxicities. Imaging follow-up according to the RECIST criteria revealed a partial response in 3 patients, stable disease in 16 patients, and progression in 22 patients. The progression-free survival was 3.3 months. A significant correlation existed only with vascularization: strongly vascularized tumors show a significantly worse response. Patients with complete or partial response and the main fraction of the stable disease group showed only moderate vascularization in the MRI and angiography. The resulting estimate of the total survival rate amounts to a median of 10.2 months. The authors concluded that transarterial chemoembolization with gemcitabine is well tolerated and provides an alternative treatment method for patients with liver metastases of breast cancer.

Overall treatment efficacy may be improved by combining TACE with other localized treatments, such as RFA [76] and SBRT. Once again, it is difficult to establish a survival benefit for TACE in the absence of randomized, controlled trials.

Stereotactic Body Radiation Therapy

SBRT is similar to central nervous system stereotactic radiosurgery, except that it addresses tumors outside of the central nervous system. A

stereotactic radiation treatment for the body means that a specially designed coordinate system is used for the exact localization of the tumors in the body to treat it with limited but highly precise treatment fields. SBRT involves the delivery of a single high-dose radiation treatment or a few fractionated radiation treatments (usually up to five treatments). A highly potent biological dose of radiation is delivered to the tumor, improving the cure rates for the tumor, in a manner that was not previously achievable by standard conventional radiation therapy.

SBRT for liver lesions must be performed cautiously, given the challenges of the low toxicity tolerance of the neighboring liver tissue and organ motion. Because SBRT relies on imaging to precisely define the target lesion or lesions to accommodate physiologic motion, candidates for this approach should have tumors with well-delineated borders and must also be willing and able to have fiducials placed. The primary size limitation for SBRT is the size of the remaining liver after treatment. This critical liver volume is approximately one-third of the liver (approximately 500–700 cm^3) [77, 78], and damaging more than this amount may cause liver failure [79]. Early CT follow-up to assess the response after SBRT can be hindered by a zone of hypodensity corresponding to the normal tissue volume that received approximately 30 Gy [77, 80].

Data for the SBRT of breast cancer metastatic to the liver are limited. However, several prospective trials of SBRT have included a mix of primary tumor types, including metastatic breast cancer. After retrospective results showed promise for SBRT [79, 81], 37 patients with 60 lesions (4 primary liver tumors and 56 metastatic tumors, 14 of which were from breast cancer) were prospectively treated with a single fraction of SBRT (dose escalated from 14 to 25 Gy) [82]. No major complications were reported, and the actuarial freedom from local failure rate at 18 months was 67 %, with failures mainly occurring in patients who were treated with lower doses. However, an updated report with long-term follow-up showed high rates of recurrence [83].

A higher dose (approximately 30 Gy in three fractions) was used in a series of 23 patients who received SBRT for liver metastases, 6 (26 %) of which were metastatic breast cancer, and this dose achieved actuarial local control rates at 1 and 2 years of 76 % and 61 %, respectively [84]. Although there was one case of self-limited grade 2 hepatitis at 6 weeks, no patient experienced a grade 3 or higher toxicity.

A prospective SBRT study of 69 patients (16 [23 %] with metastatic breast cancer) with a total of 174 metastases in the liver achieved a local control rate of 57 % at 20 months and a median survival of 14.5 months [85]. Subsequent subset analysis suggested that breast cancer lesions had better survival and control compared with metastases from other primary sites: 2- and 4-year survival rates were 72 % and 64 %, respectively, in patients with breast cancer compared with 38 % and 18 %, respectively, for other primary sites [85]. With the high radiation doses, SBRT may offer a benefit to selected patients.

Early results from a phase II trial for SBRT of one to three metastases in the liver have been reported by Scorsetti et al. [86]. A total of 61 patients (76 lesions) were treated in three fractions of up to 75 Gy using volumetric modulated arc therapy by RapidArc (Varian, Palo Alto, CA). After a median of 12 months, the in-field local control rate was 94 %, the median overall survival was 19 months, and the actuarial survival at 12 months was 83.5 %. No acute toxicity higher than G3 (one patient) and no radiation-induced liver disease were observed. The authors noted that SBRT for unresectable liver metastases can be considered an effective, safe, and noninvasive therapeutic option, with excellent rates of local control and low treatment-related toxicity.

A randomized study comparing the major nonsurgical ablative techniques, namely, SBRT and RFA, is still lacking. However, outcomes in terms of local tumor recurrence rates from recent published trials compare very favorably with RFA [87]. A prospective comparison of RFA versus SBRT is being addressed by a currently ongoing trial (Radiofrequency Ablation Versus Stereotactic Radiotherapy Trial) [88].

Interstitial Laser Therapy

Localized tumor destruction can also be achieved through hyperthermic coagulative necrosis caused by laser light delivered through quartz-diffusing laser fibers that are placed directly in the tumor [57]. ILT has been used to treat tumors up to 5 cm and can be performed through a variety of modalities: percutaneously with local anesthesia in the outpatient setting, laparoscopically, or intraoperatively [57]. Accurate positioning of the laser can be ensured using real-time imaging; MRI is preferred over CT and ultrasonography due to the heat sensitivity of the MRI sequence and its ability to demonstrate the degree of necrosis by rapidly depicting temperature changes. Monitoring with MRI also minimizes radiation exposure, thereby increasing safety [57].

Previous studies have already focused on ablative methods such as ILT and their survival data, particularly for hepatic metastases from colorectal cancer [89, 90]. However, no studies have addressed patients with other non-colorectal primary tumors; only a few briefly focused on breast cancer [57, 91].

The largest published study with ILT for metastatic breast cancer was published by Mack et al. and included 232 patients with 578 liver metastases from breast cancer. The mean survival rate for all treated patients, with calculation started on the date of diagnosis of the metastases that would be treated with ILT, was 4.9 years (95 % confidence interval: 4.3, 5.4). The median survival was 4.3 years, with 1-, 2-, 3-, and 5-year survivals of 96 %, 80 %, 63 %, and 41 %, respectively. The mean survival after the first ILT treatment was 4.2 years (95 % confidence interval: 3.6, 4.8) [57]. Although ILT may be promising, data are limited for BCLM.

Vogl et al. designed a study that evaluated prognostic factors for long-term survival and progression-free survival after the treatment of non-colorectal cancer liver metastases through MR-guided ILT [92]. They included 401 patients (mean age, 57.3 years) with liver metastases from different primary tumors who were treated with ILT. The median survival was 37.6 months starting from the date of ILT. The 1-, 2-, 3-, 4-, and 5-year survival rates were 86.5 %, 67.2 %, 51.9 %, 39.9 %, and 33.4 %, respectively. The median progression-free survival was 12.2 months. The 1-, 2-, 3-, 4-, and 5-year progression-free survival rates were 50.6 %, 33.8 %, 26 %, 20.4 %, and 17 %, respectively. The initial number of metastases, the volumes of metastases, and the quotient of the volumes of metastases and necroses influenced the long-term and progression-free survival. The authors stated that ILT shows good results in long-term survival and progression-free survival. The initial number of metastases and their volume are the most important prognostic factors. The status of the lymph nodes, the existence of other extrahepatic metastases, the location of the primary tumor, and different neoadjuvant therapies have no prognostic value.

Minimally invasive ablation treatments such as ILT have limits. For example, numerous hepatic lesions with excessively large dimensions make it impossible to induce sufficient necrotic areas. For these cases, TACE is the most common treatment with good results. In one study, repeated TACE in 161 patients with liver metastases resulted in a reduction of approximately 27 % in the tumor size [93]. Based on those insights, neoadjuvant TACE is a budding possibility for effective downsizing and reduction of the number of metastases, thus making the patients eligible for ILT [94].

References

1. Viadana E, Cotter R, Pickren JW, Bross ID. An autopsy study of metastatic sites of breast cancer. Cancer Res. 1973;33:179–81.
2. Winston CB, Hadar O, Teitcher JB, Caravelli JF, Sklarin NT, Panicek DM, et al. Metastatic lobular carcinoma of the breast: patterns of spread in the chest, abdomen, and pelvis on CT. AJR Am J Roentgenol. 2000;175:795–800.
3. Atalay G, Biganzoli L, Renard F, Paridaens R, Cufer T, Coleman R, et al. Clinical outcome of breast cancer patients with liver metastases alone in the anthracycline-taxane era: a retrospective analysis of two prospective randomized metastatic breast cancer trials. Eur J Cancer. 2003;39:2439–49.
4. Pentheroudakis G, Fountzilas G, Bafaloukos D, Koutsoukou V, Pectasides D, Skarlos D, et al. Metastatic breast cancer with liver metastases: a registry analysis of clinicopathologic, management and outcome characteristics of 500 women. Breast Cancer Res Treat. 2006;97:237–44.
5. Wyld L, Gutteridge E, Pinder SE, James JJ, Chan SY, Cheung KL, et al. Prognostic factors for patients with hepatic metastases from breast cancer. Br J Cancer. 2003;89:284–90.
6. Zinser JW, Hortobagyi GN, Buzdar AU, Smith TL, Fraschini G. Clinical course of breast cancer patients with liver metastases. J Clin Oncol. 1987;5:773–82.
7. Schneebaum S, Walker MJ, Young D, Farrar WB, Minton JP. The regional treatment of liver metastases from breast cancer. J Surg Oncol. 1994;55:26–32.
8. Chua TC, Saxena A, Liauw W, Chu F, Morris DL. Hepatic resection for metastatic breast cancer: a systematic review. Eur J Cancer. 2011;47(15):2282–90.
9. Cutler SJ, Asire AJ, Taylor SG. Classification of patients with disseminated cancer of the breast. Cancer. 1969;24:861–9.
10. Largillier R, Ferrero JM, Doyen J, Barriere J, Namer M, Mari V, et al. Prognostic factors in 1,038 women with metastatic breast cancer. Ann Oncol. 2008;19(12):2012–9.
11. Atalay G, Biganzoli L, Renard F, Paridaens R, Cufer T, Coleman R, et al. Clinical outcome of breast: cancer patients with liver metastases in the anthracycline-taxane era. Breast Cancer Res Treat. 2002;76 suppl 1:S47.
12. Eichbaum MH, Kaltwasser M, Bruckner T, de Rossi TM, Schneeweiss A, Sohn C. Prognostic factors for patients with liver metastases from breast cancer. Breast Cancer Res Treat. 2006;96:53–62.
13. Hortobagyi GN. Progress in systemic chemotherapy of primary breast cancer: an overview. J Natl Cancer Inst. 2001;30:72–9.
14. Blanchard DK, Shetty PB, Hilsenbeck SG, Elledge RM. Association of surgery with improved survival in stage IV breast cancer patients. Ann Surg. 2008;247(5):732–8.
15. Fields RC, Jeffe DB, Trinkaus K, Zhang Q, Arthur C, Aft R, et al. Surgical resection of the primary tumor is associated with increased long-term survival in patients with stage IV breast cancer after controlling for site of metastasis. Ann Surg Oncol. 2007;14(12):3345–51.
16. Ruiterkamp J, Ernst MF, van de Poll-Franse LV, Bosscha K, Tjan-Heijnen VC, Voogd AC. Surgical resection of the primary tumor is associated with

improved survival in patients with distant metastatic breast cancer at diagnosis. Eur J Surg Oncol. 2009;35(11):1146-51.

17. Selzner M, Morse MA, Vredenburgh JJ, Meyers WC, Clavien PA. Liver metastases from breast cancer: long-term survival after curative resection. Surgery. 2000;127(4):383–9.

18. Pocard M, Pouillart P, Asselain B, Salmon R. Hepatic resection in metastatic breast cancer: results and prognostic factors. Eur J Surg Oncol. 2000;26:155–9.

19. d'Annibale M, Piovanello P, Cerasoli V, Campioni N. Liver metastases from breast cancer: the role of surgical-treatment. Hepatogastroenterology. 2005;52:1858–62.

20. Maksan SM, Lehnert T, Bastert G, Herfarth C. Curative liver resection for metastatic breast cancer. Eur J Surg Oncol. 2000;26:209–12.

21. Vlastos G, Smith DL, Singletary SE, Mirza NQ, Tuttle TM, Popat RJ, et al. Long-term survival after an aggressive surgical approach in patients with breast cancer hepatic metastases. Ann Surg Oncol. 2004;11:869–74.

22. Elias D, Baton O, Sideris L, Matsuhisa T, Pocard M, Lasser P. Local recurrences after intraoperative radiofrequency ablation of liver metastases: a comparative study with anatomic and wedge resections. Ann Surg Oncol. 2004;11:500–5.

23. Hoyer M, Roed H, Traberg Hansen A, Ohlhuis L, Petersen J, Nellemann H, et al. Phase II study on stereotactic body radiotherapy of colorectal metastases. Acta Oncol. 2006;45:823–30.

24. Sofocleous CT, Nascimento RG, Gonen M, Theodoulou M, Covey AM, Brody LA, et al. Radiofrequency ablation in the management of liver metastases from breast cancer. AJR Am J Roentgenol. 2007;189:883–9.

25. O'Rourke TR, Tekkis P, Yeung S, Fawcett J, Lynch S, Strong R, et al. Long-term results of liver resection for non-colorectal, non-neuroendocrine metastases. Ann Surg Oncol. 2008;15(1):207–18.

26. Lubrano J, Roman H, Tarrab S, Resch B, Marpeau L, Scotte M. Liver resection for breast cancer metastasis: does it improve survival? Surg Today. 2008;38:293–9.

27. Rees M, Tekkis PP, Welsh FK, O'Rourke T, John TG. Evaluation of long-term survival after hepatic resection for metastatic colorectal cancer: a multifactorial model of 929 patients. Ann Surg. 2008;247:125–35.

28. Sakamoto Y, Yamamoto J, Yoshimoto M, Kasumi F, Kosuge T, Kokudo N, et al. Hepatic resection for metastatic breast cancer: prognostic analysis of 34 patients. World J Surg. 2005;29(4):524–7.

29. Thelen A, Benckert C, Jonas S, Lopez-Hänninen E, Sehouli J, Neumann U, et al. Liver resection for metastases from breast cancer. J Surg Oncol. 2008;97(1):25–9.

30. Elias D, Maisonnette F, Druet-Cabanac M, Ouellet JF, Guinebretiere JM, Spielmann M, et al. An attempt to

clarify indications for hepatectomy for liver metastases from breast cancer. Am J Surg. 2003;185(2):158–64.

31. Adam R, Aloia T, Krissat J, Bralet MP, Paule B, Giacchetti S, et al. Is liver resection justified for patients with hepatic metastases from breast cancer? Ann Surg. 2006;244(6):897–907.

32. Singletary SE, Walsh G, Vauthey JN, Curley S, Sawaya R, Weber KL, et al. A role for curative surgery in the treatment of selected patients with metastatic breast cancer. Oncologist. 2003;8:241–51.

33. Ruiterkamp J, Ernst MF. The role of surgery in metastatic breast cancer. Eur J Cancer. 2011;47 Suppl 3:S6–22.

34. Iwata H. Future treatment strategies for metastatic breast cancer: curable or incurable? Breast Cancer. 2012;19(3):200–5.

35. Fang L, Barekati Z, Zhang B, Liu Z, Zhong X. Targeted therapy in breast cancer: what's new? Swiss Med Wkly. 2011;141:w13231.

36. Marme F, Schneeweiss A. Personalized therapy in breast cancer. Onkologie. 2012;35 Suppl 1:28–33.

37. Hemming AW, Reed AI, Howard RJ, Fujita S, Hochwald SN, Caridi JG, et al. Preoperative portal vein embolization for extended hepatectomy. Ann Surg. 2003;237:686–91.

38. van Walsum GA, de Ridder JA, Verhoef C, Bosscha K, van Gulik TM, Hesselink EJ, et al. Resection of liver metastases in patients with breast cancer: survival and prognostic factors. Eur J Surg Oncol. 2012;38:910–7.

39. Belda T, Montalva EM, Lopez-Andujar R, Rosell E, Moya A, Gómez I, Mir J. Role of resection surgery in breast cancer liver metastases. Experience over the last 10 years in a reference hospital. Cir Esp. 2010;88:167–73.

40. Caralt M, Bilbao I, Cortes J, Escartín A, Lázaro JL, Dopazo C, et al. Hepatic resection for liver metastases as part of the "oncosurgical" treatment of metastatic breast cancer. Ann Surg Oncol. 2008;15:2804–10.

41. Dittmar Y, Altendorf-Hofmann A, Schule S, Schüle S, Ardelt M, Dirsch O, et al. Liver resection in selected patients with metastatic breast cancer: a single-centre analysis and review of literature. J Cancer Res Clin Oncol. 2013;139:1317–25.

42. Ercolani G, Grazi GL, Ravaioli M, Ramacciato G, Cescon M, Varotti G, et al. The role of liver resections for non-colorectal, non-neuroendocrine metastases: experience with 142 observed cases. Ann Surg Oncol. 2005;12:459–66.

43. Raab R, Nussbaum KT, Behrend M, Weimann A. Liver metastases of breast cancer: results of liver resection. Anticancer Res. 1998;18:2231–3.

44. Kostov DV, Kobakov GL, Yankov DV. Prognostic factors related to surgical outcome of liver metastases of breast cancer. J Breast Cancer. 2013;16:184–92.

45. Adam R, Chiche L, Aloia T, Elias D, Salmon R, Rivoire M, et al. Hepatic resection for non-colorectal non-endocrine liver metastases: analysis of 1,452

patients and development of a prognostic model. Ann Surg. 2006;244:524–35.

46. Hoffmann K, Franz C, Hinz U, Schirmacher P, Herfarth C, Eichbaum M, et al. Liver resection for multimodal treatment of breast cancer metastases: identification of prognostic factors. Ann Surg Oncol. 2010;17:1546–54.

47. Abbott DE, Brouquet A, Mittendorf EA, Andreou A, Meric-Bernstam F, Valero V, et al. Resection of liver metastases from breast cancer: estrogen receptor status and response to chemotherapy before metastasectomy define outcome. Surgery. 2012;151:710–6.

48. Bacalbasa N, Dima SO, Purtan-Purnichescu R, Herlea V, Popescu I. Role of surgical treatment in breast cancer liver metastases – a single center experience. Anticancer Res. 2014;34(10):5563–8.

49. Polistina F, Costantin G, Febbraro A, Robusto E, Ambrosino G. Aggressive treatment for hepatic metastases from breast cancer – results from a single center. World J Surg. 2013;37(6):1322–32.

50. Carlini M, Lonardo MT, Carboni F, Petric M, Vitucci C, Santoro R, Lepiane P, Ettorre GM, Santoro E. Liver metastases from breast cancer. Results of surgical resection. Hepatogastroenterology. 2002;49(48): 1597–601.

51. Arena E, Ferrero S. Surgical treatment of liver metastases from breast cancer. Minerva Chir. 2004; 59(1):7–15.

52. Yedibela S, Gohl J, Graz V, Pfaffenberger MK, Merkel S, Hohenberger W, et al. Changes in indication and results after resection of hepatic metastases from non-colorectal primary tumors: a single-institutional review. Ann Surg Oncol. 2005; 12(10):778–85.

53. Elias D, Di Pietroantonio D. Surgery for liver metastases from breast cancer. HPB (Oxford). 2006;8(2):97–9.

54. Hoe AL, Royle GT, Taylor I. Breast liver metastases-incidence, diagnosis and outcome. J R Soc Med. 1991;84(12):714–6.

55. Vogl TJ, Mack MG, Straub R, Engelmann K, Zangos S, Eichler K. Interventional laser-induced thermotherapy of hepatic metastases from breast cancer. Method and clinical outcome. Gynakologe. 1999;32:666–74.

56. Livraghi T, Goldberg SN, Solbiati L, Meloni F, Ierace T, Gazzelle GS. Percutaneous radio-frequency ablation of liver metastases from breast cancer: initial experience in 24 patients. Radiology. 2001;220(1):145–9.

57. Mack MG, Straub R, Eichler K, Söllner O, Lehnert T, Vogl TJ. Breast cancer metastases in liver: laser-induced interstitial thermotherapy-local tumor control rate and survival data. Radiology. 2004;233(2): 400–9.

58. Brown DB, Geschwind J-FH, Soulen MC, Millward SF, Sacks D. Society of Interventional Radiology position statement on chemoembolization of hepatic malignancies. J Vasc Interv Radiol. 2006;17:217–23.

59. Germer CT, Buhr HJ, Isbert C. Nonoperative ablation for liver metastases. Possibilities and limitations as a curative treatment. Chirurg. 2005;76(6):552–4. 556–563.

60. Liapi E, Geschwind JF. Transcatheter and ablative therapeutic approaches for solid malignancies. J Clin Oncol. 2007;25(8):978–86.

61. Goldberg SN, Gazelle GS, Halpern EF, Rittman WJ, Mueller PR, Rosenthal DI. Radiofrequency tissue ablation: importance of local temperature along the electrode tip exposure in determining lesion shape and size. Acad Radiol. 1996;3:212e218.

62. Lawes D, Chopada A, Gillams A, Lees W, Taylor I. Radiofrequency ablation (RFA) as a cytoreductive strategy for hepatic metastasis from breast cancer. Ann R Coll Surg Engl. 2006;88:639–42.

63. Veltri A, Gazzera C, Barrera M, Busso M, Solitro F, Filippini C, et al. Radiofrequency thermal ablation (RFA) of hepatic metastases (METS) from breast cancer (BC) – an adjunctive tool in the multimodal treatment of advanced disease. Radiol Med. 2014;119(5): 327–33.

64. Yun BL, Lee JM, Baek JH, Kim SH, Lee JY, Han JK, et al. Radiofrequency ablation for treating liver metastases from a non-colorectal origin. Korean J Radiol. 2011;12:579–87.

65. Carrafiello G, Fontana F, Cotta E, Petullà M, Brunese L, Mangini M, et al. Ultrasound-guided thermal radiofrequency ablation (RFA) as an adjunct to systemic chemotherapy for breast cancer liver metastases. Radiol Med. 2011;116(7):1059–66.

66. Gunabushanam G, Sharma S, Thulkar S, Srivastava DN, Rath GK, Julka PK, et al. Radiofrequency ablation of liver metastases from breast cancer: results in 14 patients. J Vasc Interv Radiol. 2007;18:67–72.

67. Kondo S, Katoh H, Omi M, Hirano S, Ambo Y, Tanaka E, et al. Hepatectomy for metastases from breast cancer offers the survival benefit similar to that in hepatic metastases from colorectal cancer. Hepatogastroenterology. 2000;47:1501–3.

68. Poon RT, Ng KK, Lam CM, Ai V, Yuen J, Fan ST. Radiofrequency ablation for subcapsular hepatocellular carcinoma. Ann Surg Oncol. 2004;11:281–9.

69. Brown DB, Cardella JF, Sacks D, Goldberg SN, Gervais DA, Rajan DK, et al. Quality improvement guidelines for transhepatic arterial chemoembolization, embolization, and chemotherapeutic infusion for hepatic malignancy. J Vasc Inter Radiol. 2006; 17:225–32.

70. Poon RT, Fan ST, Tsang FH, Wong J. Locoregional therapies for hepatocellular carcinoma: a critical review from the surgeon's perspective. Ann Surg. 2002;235:466–86.

71. Buijs M, Kamel IR, Vossen JA, Georgiades CS, Hong K, Geschwind JF. Assessment of metastatic breast cancer response to chemoembolization with contrast agent enhanced and diffusion-weighted MR imaging. J Vasc Interv Radiol. 2007;18:957–63.

72. Giroux MF, Baum RA, Soulen MC. Chemoembolization of liver metastasis from breast carcinoma. J Vasc Interv Radiol. 2004;15:289–91.

73. Vogl TJ, Naguib NN, Nour-Eldin NE, Eichler K, Zangos S, Gruber-Rouh T. Transarterial chemoembolization (TACE) with mitomycin C and gemcitabine for liver metastases in breast cancer. Eur Radiol. 2010;20(1):173–80.

74. Li X, Meng Z, Guo W, Li J. Treatment for liver metastases from breast cancer: results and prognostic factors. World J Gastroenterol. 2005;11(24):3782–7.

75. Eichler K, Jakobi S, Gruber-Rouh T, Hammerstingl R, Vogl TJ, Zangos S. Transarterial chemoembolization (TACE) with gemcitabine – phase II study in patients with liver metastases of breast cancer. Eur J Radiol. 2013;82(12):e816–22.

76. Vogl TJ, Mack MG, Balzer JO, Engelmann K, Straub R, Eichler K, et al. Liver metastases: neoadjuvant downsizing with transarterial chemoembolization before laser-induced thermotherapy. Radiology. 2003;229:457–64.

77. Kavanagh BD, McGarry RC, Timmerman RD. Extracranial radiosurgery (stereotactic body radiation therapy) for oligometastases. Semin Radiat Oncol. 2006;16:77–84.

78. Kavanagh BD, Bradley J, Timmerman RD. Stereotactic irradiation of tumors outside the central nervous system. In: Halperin E, Perez C, Brady L, et al., editors. Perez and Brady's principles and practice of radiation oncology. Baltimore: Lippincott Williams & Wilkins; 2007. p. 389–96.

79. Blomgren H, Lax I, Goranson H, et al. Radiosurgery for tumors in the body: clinical experience using a new method. J Radiosurg. 1998;1:63–74.

80. Herfarth KK, Hof H, Bahner ML, Lohr F, Höss A, Van Kaick G, et al. Assessment of focal liver reaction by multiphasic CT after stereotactic single-dose radiotherapy of liver tumors. Int J Radiat Oncol Biol Phys. 2003;57:444–51.

81. Blomgren H, Lax I, Naslund I, Svanström R. Stereotactic high dose fraction radiation therapy of extracranial tumors using an accelerator. Clinical experience of the first thirty-one patients. Acta Oncol. 1995;34:861–70.

82. Herfarth KK, Debus J, Lohr F, Bahner ML, Rhein B, Fritz P, et al. Stereotactic single-dose radiation therapy of liver tumors: results of a phase I/II trial. J Clin Oncol. 2001;19:164–70.

83. Herfarth KK, Debus J, Wannenmacher M. Stereotactic radiation therapy of fiver metastases: update of the initial phase I/II trial. Front Radiat Ther Oncol. 2004;38:100–5.

84. Wulf J, Hadinger U, Oppit U, Thiele W, Ness-Dourdoumas R, Flentje M. Stereotactic radiotherapy of targets in the lung and liver. Strahlenther Onkol. 2001;177:645–55.

85. Katz AW, Carey-Sampson M, Muhs AG, Milano MT, Schell MC, Okunieff P. Hypofractionated stereotactic body radiation therapy (SBRT) for limited hepatic metastases. Int J Radiat Oncol Biol Phys. 2007;67:793–8.

86. Scorsetti M, Arcangeli S, Tozzi A, Comito T, Alongi F, Navarria P, et al. Is stereotactic body radiation therapy an attractive option for unresectable liver metastases – A preliminary report from a phase 2 trial. Int J Radiat Oncol Biol Phys. 2013;86(2):336–42.

87. Alongi F, Arcangeli S, Filippi AR, Ricardi U, Scorsetti M. Review and uses of stereotactic body radiation therapy for oligometastases. Oncologist. 2012;17:1100–7.

88. Radiofrequency ablation versus stereotactic radiotherapy in colorectal liver metastases (RAS01). Clinical Trials.gov NCT01233544. Last Updated: 20 Mar 2012.

89. Pathak S, Jones R, Tang JM, Parmar C, Fenwick S, Malik H, Poston G, et al. Ablative therapies for colorectal liver metastases: a systematic review. Colorectal Dis. 2011;9:252Y265.

90. Eickmeyer F, Schwarzmaier H, Müller FP, Nakic Z, Yang Q, Fiedler V. Langzeitüberleben nach laserinduzierter interstitieller Thermotherapie kolorektaler LebermetastasenVein Vergleich erster klinischer Erfahrungen mit aktuellen Behandlungsergebnissen. Röfo. 2008;1:35Y41.

91. Meloni MF, Andreano A, Laeseke PF, Livraghi T, Sironi S, Lee Jr FT. Breast cancer liver metastases: US-guided percutaneous radiofrequency ablation-intermediate and long-term survival rates. Radiology. 2009;253(3):861–9.

92. Vogl TJ, Freier V, Nour-Eldin NE, et al. Magnetic resonance guided laser-induced interstitial thermotherapy of breast cancer liver metastases and other noncolorectal cancer liver metastases. An analysis of prognostic factors for long-term survival and progression-free survival. Invest Radiol. 2013;48(6):406–12.

93. Vogl TJ, Naguib NN, Nour-Eldin NA, et al. Repeated chemoembolization followed by laser-induced thermotherapy for liver metastasis of breast cancer. AJR Am J Roentgenol. 2011;196(1):W66–72.

94. Ritz J, Lehmann K, Isbert C, et al. Effectivity of laser-induced thermotherapy: in vivo comparison of arterial microembolization and complete hepatic inflow occlusion. Lasers Surg Med. 2005;36(3):238–44.

Bone-Directed Therapy and Breast Cancer: Bisphosphonates, Monoclonal Antibodies, and Radionuclides

42

Bulent Erdogan and Irfan Cicin

Abstract

Breast cancer bone metastasis causes severe morbidity and is commonly encountered in daily clinical practice. It causes pain, pathologic fractures, spinal cord and other nerve compression syndromes and life-threatening hypercalcemia. Breast cancer metastasizes to the bone through a complicated process that involves numerous molecules. Metastatic cells disrupt normal bone turnover and create a vicious cycle. All treatment effort is directed to breaking this vicious cycle. Bisphosphonates have been used safely for more than two decades. As a group, bisphosphonates delay the time to the first skeletal-related event and reduce pain. However, they do not prevent the development of bone metastasis in patients with no bone metastasis and do not prolong survival. The receptor activator for nuclear factor κB ligand inhibitor denosumab also delays the time to the first skeletal-related event and reduces the skeletal morbidity rate. Radionuclides are another treatment option for bone pain.

B. Erdogan, MD (✉)
Department of Medical Oncology,
Faculty of Medicine, Balkan Oncology Hospital,
Trakya University of Medicine, Edirne 22030, Turkey
e-mail: bulenterdogan@trakya.edu.tr

I. Cicin, MD
Department of Medical Oncology,
Faculty of Medicine, Balkan Oncology Hospital,
Trakya University of Medicine, Edirne 22030, Turkey

Trakya Üniversitesi Hastanesi Medikal Onkoloji
Bilim Dalı, Edirne 22030, Turkey
e-mail: irfancicin@trakya.edu.tr

© Springer International Publishing Switzerland 2016
A. Aydiner et al. (eds.), *Breast Disease: Management and Therapies*,
DOI 10.1007/978-3-319-26012-9_42

Keywords

Macrophage colony-stimulating factor (M-CSF) • Parathyroid hormone-related peptide (PTHrP) • Prostaglandin F2 (PGE2) • Interleukin 6 (IL-6) • Interleukin 11 (IL-11) • Intracellular adhesion molecule (ICAM-1) • Vascular cell adhesion molecule (VCAM-1) • P-selectin • E-selectin • $\alpha\nu\beta3$ integrin • Cadherin-11 • Insulin-like growth factor 1 (IGF1) • Mevalonate pathway • Bisphosphonate • Prenylation • Farnesyl pyrophosphate synthase enzyme • Clodronate • Pamidronate • Zoledronic acid • Ibandronate • Denosumab • Nephrotoxicity • Osteonecrosis of the jaw (ONJ) • Hypocalcemia • Conjunctivitis • Uveitis • Scleritis • Episcleritis • Iritis. Strontium-89 hydrochloride (Sr-89) • Samarium-153 lexidronam (Sm-153) • Rhenium-186 hydroxyethylidene diphosphonate (Re-186) • Radionuclide • Phosphorus-32 (P-32) • Src • Dasatinib • Saracatinib • Odanacatib • Cathepsin K

Introduction

The bone is the most common site of breast cancer metastasis, and up to two-thirds of patients who die of breast cancer have bone metastases [1]. Breast cancer patients with only bone metastases have a good prognosis relative to visceral organ metastases [1]. However, bone metastasis seriously impairs the quality of life because patients with bone metastases subsequently develop complications related to the bone metastases and generally need medical and surgical intervention. These skeletal-related complications, also called skeletal-related events (SREs), include pain, pathologic fractures, spinal cord and other nerve compression syndromes, and life-threatening hypercalcemia, and they are sources of devastating morbidity.

All metastases develop in a stepwise fashion. First, the proliferation and invasion of cancer cells occur at the breast. Then, cancer cells migrate and attach to the bone. Following attachment, cancer cells colonize the bone and cause destruction. All of these steps are very complicated and not yet completely understood. However, we know that epithelial cell adhesion molecules, matrix metalloproteinases (MMPs), integrins, chemokines, and several growth factors play crucial roles in this complicated process. More than 100 years ago, Paget [2] proposed that cancer cells metastasize to organs in which the microenvironment is appropriate for their survival. This theory is called the seed-and-soil hypothesis and still remains valid. Bone is a metabolically active tissue. Therefore, it has a huge source of growth factors, cell adhesion molecules, and cytokines that make it fertile soil for the survival of metastasized breast cancer cells.

Normal Bone Physiology

The bones give shape and support to the body and protect vital organs from external damage. Bone is essentially composed of collagen that is mineralized with hydroxyapatite crystals. To protect its strength and renew minor damage that occurs throughout life, bone constantly undergoes remodeling. Under normal conditions, osteoclast-mediated bone resorption and osteoblast-mediated bone formation continue in equilibrium.

The precursors of osteoblasts are multipotent mesenchymal stem cells. Under the influence of growth factors, including fibroblast growth factor (FGF), platelet-derived growth factor (PDGF), transforming growth factor beta (TGF-β), and bone morphogenetic proteins (BMPs), mesenchymal stem cells proliferate and differentiate to form osteoblasts. In addition to new bone formation, they also control osteoclast formation by expressing receptor activator for nuclear factor κB ligand

(RANKL) and producing osteoprotegerin (OPG). Osteoclastogenesis occurs under the influence of RANKL, which is produced by osteoblasts and stromal cells, and macrophage colony-stimulating factor (M-CSF). These two molecules are necessary for the development and survival of osteoclasts. The binding of RANKL to the RANK receptor, which is found on the surface of mononuclear precursors of the monocyte/macrophage lineage, in the presence of M-CSF promotes the fusion of mononuclear precursors to form osteoclasts [3]. OPG, a decoy receptor for RANKL, inhibits osteoclast differentiation by competitively binding to RANKL [4]. The balance between RANKL and OPG determines osteoclastic activity and the extent of bone resorption. Parathyroid hormone, parathyroid hormone-related peptide (PTHrP), prostaglandin E2 (PGE2) through the receptor EP4, interleukin 6 (IL-6), and IL-11 also stimulate osteoclast production [5–7]. Activated osteoclasts adhere to the bone and degrade bone matrix by secreting acid and lysosomal enzymes. The life-span of an osteoclast ends with apoptosis.

Metastasis of Breast Cells to the Bone

Red marrow-containing bones and bones with a rich vascular supply, including the vertebrae, and the metaphysis of long bones and ribs are generally the preferred sites for metastasis. In this metaphyseal bone, the vascular bed is composed of specialized sinusoids that aid the passage of hematopoietic and blood cells in and out of bone marrow. These sinusoids lie in a close proximity with trabecular bone. Endothelial cells lining the sinusoids express cell adhesion molecules, including intracellular adhesion molecule (ICAM-1), vascular cell adhesion molecule (VCAM-1), P-selectin, and E-selectin, without any inflammatory stimulus [8]. This sinusoidal structure and the pooling of blood in the sinusoids provide an advantage to cancer cells for extravasation and homing [9].

Not all breast cancer cells have the ability to metastasize to the bone. Breast cancer cells that express specific adhesion molecules for bone matrix proteins preferentially metastasize to the bone. Integrins are transmembrane glycoproteins that mediate cell-cell and cell-extracellular matrix interactions. Integrin $\alpha\nu\beta3$, which is expressed by breast cancer cells, mediates the attachment to trabecular bone by binding matrix proteins, including vitronectin, osteopontin, and bone sialoprotein [10]. Pecheur et al. [11] suggested that breast cancer cells expressing integrin $\alpha\nu\beta3$ have an increased ability to invade and adhere to mineralized bone; therefore, these cells accelerate bone metastasis. Another transmembrane protein, cadherin-11, is expressed in stromal osteoblastic cells in the bone marrow and mediates homophilic cell-cell adhesion. Breast cancer cells also express cadherin-11. Cadherin-11-expressing breast cancer cells interact with stromal osteoblastic cells, thus enhancing invasion and adhesion. Cadherin-11 expression may be a sign of more aggressive, bone-metastasizing tumors [12].

Under normal physiological conditions, bone matrix production and degradation are well balanced. When breast cancer cells settle in the bone, this balance is impaired in favor of bone degradation. Tumor-secreted PTHrP is the main regulator of excess bone degradation. It triggers a vicious cycle that causes osteoclastogenesis, osteolysis, and improved malignant cell survival and proliferation [13]. Breast cancer cells indirectly activate stromal cells and osteoblasts to produce RANKL through the stimulation of parathyroid hormone receptor 1 (PTHR1) by tumor-derived PTHrP; concurrently, the OPG level decreases. Together, the RANKL-RANK interaction and decreased OPG levels induce osteoclast production. Then, mature osteoclasts begin to degrade the bone. As bone degradation occurs, bone-stored growth factors, including insulin-like growth factor 1 (IGF1) and TGF-β, are released into the bone microenvironment [14]. IGF-1 plays an important role in stimulating breast cancer cell migration and growth. The TGF-β-TGF-β receptor interaction facilitates PTHrP production by tumor cells [15]. IL-6, IL-11, PGE2, M-CSF, tumor necrosis factor

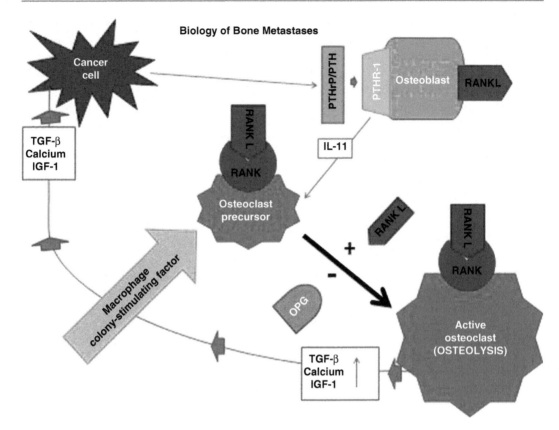

Fig. 42.1 PTHrP produced by cancer cells induces the RANKL-RANK pathway. Specifically, the TGF-β, calcium, and IGF-1 that increased as a result of bone degradation stimulate cancer cells. The vicious cycle is mainly created by PTHrP (*PTH* parathyroid hormone, *PTHrP* parathyroid hormone-related peptide, *TGF-β* transforming growth factor beta, *RANK* receptor activator for nuclear factor κB, *RANKL* receptor activator for nuclear factor κB ligand, *OPG* osteoprotegerin, *IGF1* insulin-like growth factor 1, *IL-11* interleukin 11)

alpha (TNF-α), and PDGF produced by cancer cells or released in the course of osteolysis all contribute to the enhancement and continuation of this vicious cycle (Fig. 42.1). Infect this process is much more complicated, and several other molecules are involved. All medical treatment modalities are directed to breaking this vicious cycle (Fig. 42.1).

Bone-Directed Therapy

Bisphosphonates

Structure and Mode of Action

As the name implies, bisphosphonates contain two phosphorous atoms that are attached to a central carbon atom (P-C-P) (Fig. 42.2) and thus are analogs of inorganic pyrophosphate, in which the phosphorus atoms attach to a central oxygen atom. Based on this similarity, bisphosphonates can affect various enzymes and metabolic activities in the bone. The P-C-P structure makes up the backbone of a bisphosphonate molecule. This backbone is highly resistant to hydrolysis; therefore, bisphosphonates are resistant to biological degradation. In addition to the phosphorus molecules, two side chains, the R1 and R2 groups, also bind to the central carbon atom. These side chains distinguish the different bisphosphonates, which have different biochemical properties based on the side chains bound to the central carbon atom [16] (Fig. 42.2).

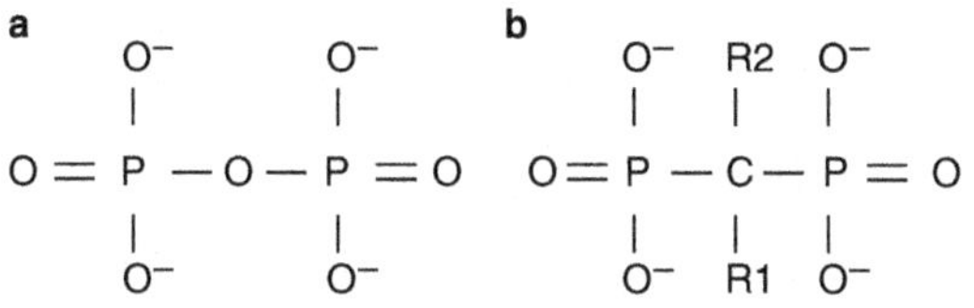

Fig. 42.2 (a) Structure of pyrophosphate, (b) structure of the bisphosphonate backbone

Table 42.1 Bisphosphonates

Non-nitrogen containing	Nitrogen containing
Etidronate	Pamidronate
Clodronate	Zoledronate
Tiludronate	Ibandronate
	Alendronate
	Risedronate
	Olpadronate

The main role of bisphosphonates is to inhibit bone degradation. They are also used in several benign diseases, including osteoporosis, Paget's disease of bone, primary hyperparathyroidism, and osteogenesis imperfecta. Based on the nitrogen content of the side chain, bisphosphonates are divided into two classes, including non-nitrogen containing and nitrogen containing (Table 42.1) [17].

When bisphosphonates are administered, they selectively bind to bone mineral. The acidic environment provided by osteoclastic activity causes dissolution of the bisphosphonate molecules. Dissociated bisphosphonate molecules are taken up by osteoclasts via endocytosis [18]. Non-nitrogen-containing bisphosphonates are metabolized to nonhydrolyzable ATP analogs that cause osteoclast dysfunction and apoptosis [19]. Nitrogen-containing bisphosphonates inhibit the mevalonate pathway, which produces important molecules for the posttranslational modification (prenylation) of GTP-binding signaling proteins, including Ras, Rho, Rab, and Rac [20]. The main target of nitrogen-containing bisphosphonates in this pathway is farnesyl pyrophosphate synthase enzyme. The prenylation of the signaling proteins is essential for osteoclast function and survival. Defective signaling proteins and an excess accumulation of metabolites, which occur due to the blockage of farnesyl pyrophosphate synthase enzyme, lead to osteoclast dysfunction and induce apoptosis [17].

Efficacy of Bisphosphonates in Metastatic Disease

Historically, several studies have suggested that bisphosphonates have beneficial effects in skeletal metastasis of breast cancer [21, 22]. The first placebo-controlled, double-blind randomized study to evaluate the efficacy of oral clodronate in breast cancer patients with bone metastasis was published by Paterson et al. in 1993 [23]. They compared 1,600 mg daily oral clodronate (85 patients) with placebo (88 patients) in 173 patients with breast cancer bone metastasis. After a median 14 months of follow-up, there was a significant reduction (27 %) in cumulative SREs, including hypercalcemia, radiotherapy needed for bone pain, and vertebral and nonvertebral fractures with the use of clodronate ($P<0.001$), and there was no survival difference. Two other similar trials have also demonstrated the beneficial effect of clodronate [24, 25]. In these three trials, clodronate therapy significantly delayed the time to the first SRE. Pamidronate is another nitrogen-containing bisphosphonate that is beneficial in breast cancer patients with osteolytic bone metastasis. In two large multicenter, randomized, placebo-controlled studies, the addition of intravenous pamidronate (90 mg 3–4 weeks intravenous) to patients receiving cytotoxic therapy or patients receiving hormonal therapy reduced skeletal morbidity and delayed the time to the first SRE [26, 27]. A combined follow-up of these two studies at 24 months demonstrated that pamidronate compared to placebo significantly reduced the skeletal morbidity rate (2.4 events vs. 3.7 events, $P<0.001$) and skeletal complications (51 % vs. 64 %, $P<0.001$). The median time to the first SRE was significantly longer (12.7 months vs. 7.0 months, $P<0.001$), and pain scores were significantly better in the pamidronate arm. The addition of pamidronate to systemic therapy is well tolerated and effective in preventing SRE and symptomatic palliation [28]. Administration of 60 mg pamidronate (four times, given weekly) was also effective in reducing SREs and improving the quality of life of patients with breast cancer bone metastasis [29]. Even lower doses of pamidronate (45 mg every 3 weeks) are beneficial in prolonging the time to progression of bone lesion. In this placebo-controlled trial, marked pain relief has also been achieved [30]. Unfortunately, the researchers did not evaluate its effect on SREs. Although effective at lower doses, the recommended dose is 2 h intravenous infusions of 90 mg pamidronate every 3–4 weeks.

Rosen et al. [31] compared the effects of 4 or 8 mg zoledronic acid with 90 mg pamidronate in patients with breast cancer bone metastasis or multiple myeloma. They analyzed 1,130 patients with breast cancer bone metastasis [32]. The 8 mg zoledronic acid dose was reduced to 4 mg, and the infusion time was increased to 15 min because of nephrotoxicity. At the end of 13 months, the proportion of patients with an SRE was similar in both treatment arms. In patients with lytic bone metastasis, 4 mg zoledronic acid achieved a 17 % relative reduction in the proportion of patients with an SRE compared with pamidronate; however, this difference was not significant (48 % vs. 58 %, respectively, $P=0.058$). Although the primary end point was not reached, 4 mg zoledronic acid delayed the time to first SRE (310 days vs. 174 days, respectively, $P=0.013$) and yielded a 20 % reduction in the risk of SRE (HR, 0.801; $P=0.037$) compared with pamidronate in this trial. This trial was extended to 24 months, and 412 patients with breast cancer were involved in the extended study [33]. In a subset analysis of patients with breast cancer, the proportion of patients with at least one SRE was still similar in both groups at the end of the extended phase. In multiple event analysis, 4 mg zoledronic acid achieved an additional 20 % reduction in the risk of developing SREs compared with pamidronate (RR, 0.799; 95 % CI, 0.657–0.972; $P=0.025$). Zoledronic acid (4 mg, administered via a 15-min intravenous infusion) was as well tolerated as pamidronate (90 mg 2 h intravenous infusion), and the SRE risk was significantly reduced.

Ibandronate is a relatively new bisphosphonate that is effective in the treatment of bone metastasis. It can be given orally or via an intravenous route.

The efficacy of intravenous ibandronate was shown in a placebo-controlled phase III trial. Six milligrams of ibandronate every 3–4 weeks for 2 years was superior to the placebo in terms of the skeletal morbidity period rate, new SREs, and delaying the time to the first new SRE, and it also reduced pain scores [34]. In another study that used the same dose and schedule of ibandronate, the proportion of patients who developed an SRE was significantly reduced compared with placebo (36 % vs. 48 %, respectively; $P=0.027$) [35]. Oral administration is also effective. In a pooled analysis of two randomized, placebo-controlled studies, 50 mg oral ibandronate administered daily reduced the risk of an SRE compared with placebo (HR 0.62; 95 % CI, 0.48–0.79; $P=0.0001$). The need for radiotherapy (0.73 vs. 0.98, respectively, $P<0.001$) and surgery (0.47 vs. 0.53, respectively, $P=0.037$) was significantly less in the ibandronate group, and it was well tolerated except for slight adverse upper gastrointestinal effects [36].

In a mixed treatment analysis of 17 studies, the annual SRE rate was lowest in breast cancer patients treated with zoledronic acid (1.6). The annual SRE rates for oral and intravenous ibandronate were 1.67 and 1.7, respectively. The highest SRE rates were observed with pamidronate (2.07) and clodronate (2.29). According to this analysis, zoledronic acid is the most effective bisphosphonate that reduce the risk of SREs [37].

All of these large randomized clinical trials suggest that the addition of bisphosphonates to systemic therapy, either chemotherapy or hormone therapy, reduces the risk of developing SREs and delays the time to the first SRE in breast cancer patients with bone metastasis. The oral administration of ibandronate can be advantageous for patients who do not want parenteral drugs (Table 42.2).

Denosumab

Denosumab prevents the RANKL-RANK interaction through binding to RANKL. It is a fully human IgG2 monoclonal antibody that was designed to specifically bind RANKL. The inhibition of the

Table 42.2 Select important clinical trials

Study	Protocol	Important results
Paterson et al. [23]	1,600 mg daily oral clodronate vs. placebo	27 % reduction in cumulative SRE ($P<0.001$)
Kristensen et al. [24]	800 mg daily oral clodronate vs. control	Delayed the time to the first SRE ($P=0.015$)
		Reduced the occurrence of fractures ($P=0.023$)
Tubina-Hulin et al. [25]	1,600 daily oral clodronate vs. placebo	Delayed the time to the first SRE ($P=0.05$)
		Reduced the pain intensity and analgesic need ($P=0.01$)
Hortobagyi et al. [26]	90 mg iv. pamidronate every 3–4 weeks vs. placebo	Delayed time to the first SRE ($P<0.001$)
		Reduced the rate of SREs ($P<0.001$)
Theriault et al. [27]	90 mg iv. pamidronate every 4 weeks vs. placebo	Delayed time to the first SRE ($P=0.049$)
		Reduced the skeletal morbidity rate ($P=0.008$)
Lipton et al. [28] (Pooled analysis of two pamidronate trials at 24 months)	90 mg iv. pamidronate every 3–4 weeks vs. placebo	Delayed time to the first SRE ($P<0.001$)
		Reduced the skeletal morbidity rate ($P<0.001$)
Rosen et al. [33]	4–8 mg iv. zoledronic acid vs. 90 mg iv. pamidronate every 3–4 weeks	20 % risk reduction for developing SRE compared with pamidronate ($P=0.025$)
Body et al. [34]	2 mg iv. ibandronate for 3–4 weeks vs. 6 mg iv. ibandronate for 3–4 weeks vs. placebo	6 mg iv. reduced the skeletal morbidity period rate ($P=0.004$ vs. placebo)
		6 mg iv. delayed time to first the SRE ($P=0.018$ vs. placebo)
		6 mg iv. 38 % reduction in the number of new bone events vs. both 2 mg and placebo
Body et al. [36]	50 mg daily oral ibandronate vs. placebo	Reduced mean skeletal morbidity period rate ($P=0.004$)
		Reduced risk of SRE ($P=0.0001$)
Stopeck et al. [39]	4 mg iv. zoledronic acid vs. sc. placebo vs. 120 mg sc. denosumab vs. iv. placebo	Denosumab delayed time to first in-study SRE ($P<0.001$ for noninferiority; $P=0.01$ for superiority)
		Denosumab reduced risk of multiple SREs ($P=0.001$)
		Denosumab reduced skeletal morbidity rate ($P=0.004$)

iv intravenous, *sc* subcutaneous

RANKL-RANK interaction prevents osteoclast formation and survival [18]. In a phase II study, five different doses of denosumab were compared with intravenous bisphosphonates in patients with breast cancer bone metastasis. At the end of 13 weeks, denosumab was similar in reducing SREs and suppressing bone turnover when compared with bisphosphonates. The incidence of adverse events was also similar. The most effective course for suppressing bone turnover was four weekly 120 mg administrations of denosumab [38]. The largest clinical trial (2,046 patients with breast cancer bone metastasis) that compared denosumab with zoledronic acid was published in 2010 by Stopeck et al. [39]. Denosumab was superior to zoledronic acid in delaying the time to first in-study SRE (HR, 0.82; 95 % CI, 0.71–0.95; $P<0.001$ for noninferiority; $P=0.01$ for superiority) and in reducing the risk of multiple SREs (rate ratio, 0.77; 95 % CI, 0.66–0.89; $P=0.001$). Denosumab also significantly reduced the skeletal morbidity rate ($P=0.004$). Overall survival was not different (HR, 0.95; 95 % CI, 0.81–1.11; $P=0.49$) between the groups.

Clinical Use of Bone-Modifying Agents

To initiate the administration of a bone-modifying agent, the bone metastasis should be documented with plain radiographs or with other imaging methods (e.g., bone scan, CT scan, or MRI). The American Clinical Society of Oncology (ASCO) considers it reasonable to begin administering bone-modifying agents when bone metastasis is documented with an abnormal bone scan and an abnormal CT or MRI, with a normal plain radiograph. Initiating bone-modifying therapy based only on abnormal findings on bone scan without any evidence of bone metastasis on plain radiograph, CT scan, or MRI outside of a clinical trial is not recommended by ASCO. Even if an extraskeletal metastasis is present, ASCO does not recommend starting a bone-modifying agent in the absence of documented bone metastasis [40]. In patients with metastatic breast cancer without bone metastasis, bisphosphonates did not reduce the incidence of bone metastasis in a Cochrane meta-analysis (RR 0.99; 95 % CI, 0.67–1.47; $P=0.97$) [41]. If bone metastasis is detected with PET/CT, bone scintigraphy may not be needed [42].

The optimal duration and schedule of treatment have not been defined. Generally, clinical trials have evaluated the bone-modifying agents up to 2 years or until there is unacceptable toxicity. Therefore, the ASCO guideline recommends continuing bone-modifying agent until evidence of a substantial decline in the patient's performance status. Bone-modifying agents also reduce the time to the first and subsequent SREs [39]. Therefore, the development of an SRE is not an indication to stop the administration of a bone-modifying agent. Another controversial issue is switching to another bisphosphonate after an SRE develops. In two phase II studies, patients with skeletal progression or the development of an SRE while on clodronate or pamidronate were switched to the more potent bisphosphonate zoledronic acid or ibandronate, which may provide pain palliation and also reduce the expression bone turnover markers [43, 44]. In another phase II study that evaluated switching, switching to denosumab reduced uNTx levels significantly more than continuing zoledronic acid in patients in whom urinary N-telopeptide (uNTx) levels were still elevated despite zoledronic acid treatment, and patients in the switch arm also experienced fewer SREs [45]. These trials do not provide enough evidence to recommend changing bone-modifying agent in cases of treatment failure. However, switching to a more potent agent can be reasonable. Clinicians should decide whether switching to an alternative agent is warranted based on the individual patient.

Apart from delaying the time to SRE, bone-modifying agents also provide bone pain palliation in patients with breast cancer bone metastasis. All approved bisphosphonates and denosumab can decrease the bone pain caused by breast cancer bone metastasis to some degree. Denosumab and zoledronic acid have similar effects in palliating pain; however, denosumab significantly delays pain worsening in patients who have no or mild pain [46]. Different pain assessment tools and treatment protocols were used in these clinical trials; therefore, it is not possible to determine which one is better [40]. The current standard care for cancer pain must be applied to all patients with bone pain. Bone-modifying agents are recommended as an adjunctive therapy for bone pain control and not as a first-line treatment by the ASCO guideline [40]. Bisphosphonates and denosumab do not provide any survival advantage in patients with breast cancer bone metastasis [41].

Safety

Osteonecrosis of the Jaw

The incidence of osteonecrosis of the jaw (ONJ) ranges from 0.6 to 6.2 % in breast cancer patients who are treated with bisphosphonate. In patients treated with denosumab, the ONJ incidence is similar to that observed with zoledronic acid treatment (2–1.4 %, respectively, $P = 0.39$) [39]. A longer duration of therapy, higher cumulative doses, treatment with more potent bisphosphonates (e.g., zoledronic acid and pamidronate), a history of recent alveolar trauma, and inflammatory dental disease are known risk factors for ONJ [47, 48]. Glucocorticoid treatment or anti-angiogenic therapy may also contribute to ONJ development [49]. The inhibition of bone remodeling and wound healing through the inhibition of osteoclastic activity are some of the proposed mechanisms of ONJ development. Infection and exposed necrotic bone in the jaw or maxilla are the usual clinical presentations. Pain, suppuration, mucosal swelling, and ulceration may precede clinical presentation. Mild cases are generally controlled with systemic or local antimicrobial therapy and oral rinses. Surgical intervention may be needed for refractory or severe cases [49]. Bisphosphonates accumulate in the bone, and the effect of denosumab on the bone becomes reversible after several months. Therefore, the beneficial effect of stopping a bone-modifying agent is unclear in the case of ONJ. This decision should be made based on the individual patient after a multidisciplinary assessment of the risk-benefit ratio. ASCO recommends a dental examination and any necessary preventive dentistry before the initiation of bone-directed therapy. If invasive manipulations that affect bone are indicated, the initiation of bone-directed therapy should be delayed for 2–3 weeks. After the initiation of a bone-modifying agent, good oral hygiene should be maintained, and invasive dental procedures should be avoided as much as possible [40].

Nephrotoxicity

Nephrotoxicity is an important adverse event observed with bisphosphonate treatment. Renal toxicity ranges from acute kidney injury with acute renal failure to slowly progressing or non-progressing renal insufficiency [50]. Pamidronate may cause nephrotic syndrome [51, 52]. In a trial that compared 4 and 8 mg zoledronic acid with 90 mg pamidronate, the infusion time for zoledronic acid was extended from 5 to 15 min, and the 8 mg dose was reduced to 4 mg due to the high incidence of nephrotoxicity [31]. Bisphosphonate-related nephrotoxicity depends on the infusion time and dose. Zoledronic acid and pamidronate should not be administered in less than the advised durations of 15 min and 2 h, respectively. Further extension of the infusion time does not provide extra protection [53]. Dose adjustment should be made according to the calculated creatinine clearance (CrCl) in patients with mild to moderate renal failure (CrCl between 30 and 60 ml/min) who will be treated with zoledronic acid. Both zoledronic acid and pamidronate are not recommended for patients with renal failure (CrCl <30 ml/min). Serum creatinine should be monitored prior to every dose of pamidronate or zoledronic acid, and electrolytes, calcium, magnesium, and hemoglobin should also be monitored regularly. If renal function deteriorates during therapy, the drug should be withheld until renal function returns to within 10 % of the baseline [40]. In ibandronate studies, including both intravenous and oral administration, the renal adverse effects of treatment were similar with placebo, and no one experienced renal failure [34–36]. Denosumab is a monoclonal antibody; therefore, it is mostly cleared through the reticuloendothelial system and not through the kidney. Although renal-associated adverse effects are nearly equal between zoledronic acid and denosumab, severe renal-associated adverse events (1.5 % vs. 0.2 %, respectively) and renal failure (1.5 % vs. 0.2 %, respectively) are more frequent with zoledronic acid [39]. In a meta-analysis, the risk of renal adverse events was significantly higher with zoledronic acid in patients with breast cancer, prostate cancer, and other solid tumors (RR 0.76; 95 % CI, 0.59–0.98) [54]. In a small trial involving patients with renal function ranging from normal to dialysis-dependent renal failure, the pharmacokinetics and pharmacodynamics of denosumab (subcutaneous 60 mg single dose) were not affected by renal function. Therefore, dose adjustment is not required. In this trial, the most common adverse event was hypocalcemia. Denosumab may be cautiously given to a patient with renal impairment, and the patient should be closely monitored for hypocalcemia.

Hypocalcemia and Other Adverse Effects

Bone-modifying drugs disrupt bone calcium homeostasis by inhibiting osteoclastic activity. Parathyroid hormone protects the patient from hypocalcemia after the administration of bone-modifying drugs. If any condition that affects parathyroid hormone secretion or calcium metabolism (e.g., surgical hypoparathyroidism, hypomagnesemic hypoparathyroidism, vitamin D deficiency, and renal failure) is present, the patients become prone to hypocalcemia [55, 56]. Hypocalcemia and hypophosphatemia are more common with denosumab [39, 57]. Calcium and vitamin D supplementation were added to treatment protocols in nearly all clinical trials. If no contraindication is present, calcium and vitamin D supplementation is recommended to all patients receiving bone-modifying agents with breast cancer bone metastasis to prevent hypocalcemia.

An acute phase response may occur up to 3 days after the administration of intravenous nitrogen-containing bisphosphonate due to increased cytokine production in 15–30 % of patients [58]. Generally, bisphosphonate-naïve patients experience influenza-like symptoms, including fever, chills, myalgia, headache, nausea, and arthralgia, after the first dose. This adverse event is self-limited, resolves after several days, and is not encountered after subsequent doses. Therefore, symptomatic management with anti-inflammatory drugs and acetaminophen is enough [59]. Apart from the acute phase response, severe musculoskeletal pain may occur days or years after initiating bisphosphonate. Discontinuing the causative agent may provide immediate improvement but may not lead to complete improvement [59]. All bisphospho-

nates, especially pamidronate, may cause ocular inflammation, including conjunctivitis, uveitis, scleritis, episcleritis, and iritis. All patients with ocular inflammation must be evaluated and treated by an ophthalmologist. Conjunctivitis is treated with topical NSAIDs; episcleritis is treated with topical steroid eye drops. The prognosis for both is good, and bisphosphonate treatment can continue. Uveitis, scleritis, and global orbital inflammation are severe conditions and should therefore be treated specifically. Continuing bisphosphonate treatment is not recommended in these cases [60]. Oral bisphosphonates may cause gastric irritation. Anemia was encountered in nearly one-third of patients who were treated with both zoledronic acid and denosumab [57]. Bisphosphonates are associated with an increased risk of cardiac arrhythmias, including atrial fibrillation and supraventricular tachycardia and stroke [61]. Pamidronate rarely may cause skin reaction and ototoxicity [60]. In osteoporosis trials, the incidence of infectious complications with denosumab was increased [62]. However, in cancer patients treated with denosumab or zoledronic acid, the incidence of infectious complications was similar [57].

Radionuclide Therapy for Breast Cancer Bone Metastasis

Radionuclides are used for the palliation of bone pain secondary to mainly osteoblastic bone metastasis of solid tumors. Radionuclide therapy is indicated in patients with multifocal bone metastasis. If external beam radiation is contraindicated or the patient suffers from severe pain despite adequate analgesia, radionuclide therapy is a reasonable palliative modality. Uncontrolled systemic disease, asymptomatic bone metastasis at fewer than three sites, pure osteolytic metastasis, poor bone marrow reserve, and less than 60 days of life expectancy are relative contraindications for radionuclide therapy. Absolute contraindications are spinal cord compression, a high risk of fracture or pathologic fracture of weight-bearing bones, renal failure, pregnancy, and breast feeding [63]. Strontium-89 hydrochloride

(Sr-89), samarium-153 lexidronam (Sm-153), and rhenium-186 hydroxyethylidene diphosphonate (Re-186) are approved radiopharmaceuticals for radionuclide therapy. Phosphorus-32 (P-32) is no longer used because of severe myelosuppression. After administration, radiopharmaceuticals incorporate into newly formed matrix, and the extent of incorporation is determined by osteoblastic activity. Therefore, painful metastatic sites should be visualized on bone scintigraphy before deciding upon radionuclide therapy. Strontium has similar properties to calcium; therefore, it directly incorporates into bone. Other isotopes are chelated to organic phosphates to facilitate incorporation into the bone. These radiopharmaceuticals deliver local radiation by emitting beta particles. Samarium and rhenium also emit gamma radiation, which enables imaging. Another important radiopharmaceutical is alpha-emitter radium 223 (Ra-223). It incorporates into the bone in the same way as strontium. Ra-223 treatment delays the time to first symptomatic SRE, prolongs overall survival, and is also a safe treatment modality in castration-resistant prostate carcinoma patients with only bone metastases [64]. The efficacy of Ra-223 in breast cancer bone metastasis has been shown in vivo and in a mouse model [65].

Most of the studies of radionuclides were performed on patients with prostate cancer [66–68]. Patients with breast cancer were also involved in some of the studies [69, 70]. The previously mentioned radiopharmaceuticals were found to be beneficial in palliating painful breast cancer bone metastasis in randomized clinical trials and in case series. In one study, 92 % of breast cancer bone metastasis patients that were refractory to conventional analgesia responded to Sr-89 therapy [69]. Generally, pain relief occurs 1–3 weeks after administration. One or 2 days after administration, a self-limited pain flare may be experienced. Re-186 provides earlier pain palliation, and the duration of myelosuppression is significantly shorter than with Sr-89 [71]. Repeated administration of these radiopharmaceuticals is also safe and effective in patients who benefited from the previous administration [72–74]. Transient myelosuppression is the most common toxicity. Generally,

thrombocytopenia is experienced, and significant neutropenia and anemia develop less frequently than thrombocytopenia [63].

Advances in the Treatment of Bone Metastasis

The current medical treatment of breast cancer bone metastasis is bisphosphonates and denosumab. However, numerous molecules that target this vicious cycle are being investigated. A nonreceptor tyrosine kinase, Src, plays an important role in breast cancer bone metastasis and osteoclastogenesis [75]. The Src inhibitor dasatinib, which has been used in chronic myelogenous leukemia, also inhibits osteoclastogenesis in vitro [76]. Another Src inhibitor, saracatinib, decreased bone resorption markers in a phase I study [77]. In two ongoing studies, dasatinib (NCT00566618) and saracatinib (NCT00558272) are still being investigated for the treatment of bone metastasis. In a randomized clinical trial, the cathepsin K inhibitor odanacatib suppressed bone resorption markers, in a manner similar to zoledronic acid, after 4 weeks of treatment and was well tolerated [78]. In the future, antibodies that block PTHrP, TGF-β antagonists, proteasome inhibitors, and many new molecules targeting this vicious cycle are being evaluated for the treatment of bone metastasis.

References

1. Coleman RE, Rubens RD. The clinical course of bone metastases from breast cancer. Br J Cancer. 1987;55(1):61–6.
2. Paget S. The distribution of secondary growths in cancer of the breast. 1889. Cancer Metastasis Rev. 1989;8(2):98–101.
3. Boyle WJ, Simonet WS, Lacey DL. Osteoclast differentiation and activation. Nature. 2003;423(6937):337–42.
4. Simonet WS, Lacey DL, Dunstan CR, Kelley M, Chang MS, Luthy R, et al. Osteoprotegerin: a novel secreted protein involved in the regulation of bone density. Cell. 1997;89(2):309–19.
5. Ohshiba T, Miyaura C, Ito A. Role of prostaglandin E produced by osteoblasts in osteolysis due to bone metastasis. Biochem Biophys Res Commun. 2003;300(4):957–64.

6. Kudo O, Sabokbar A, Pocock A, Itonaga I, Fujikawa Y, Athanasou NA. Interleukin-6 and interleukin-11 support human osteoclast formation by a RANKL-independent mechanism. Bone. 2003;32(1):1–7.

7. Kayamori K, Sakamoto K, Nakashima T, Takayanagi H, Morita K, Omura K, et al. Roles of interleukin-6 and parathyroid hormone-related peptide in osteoclast formation associated with oral cancers: significance of interleukin-6 synthesized by stromal cells in response to cancer cells. Am J Pathol. 2010;176(2):968–80.

8. Mazo IB, von Andrian UH. Adhesion and homing of blood-borne cells in bone marrow microvessels. J Leukoc Biol. 1999;66(1):25–32.

9. Bussard KM, Gay CV, Mastro AM. The bone microenvironment in metastasis; what is special about bone? Cancer Metastasis Rev. 2008;27(1):41–55.

10. van der P, Vloedgraven H, Papapoulos S, Lowick C, Grzesik W, Kerr J, et al. Attachment characteristics and involvement of integrins in adhesion of breast cancer cell lines to extracellular bone matrix components. Lab Inv J Tech Methods Pathol. 1997;77(6):665–75.

11. Pecheur I, Peyruchaud O, Serre CM, Guglielmi J, Voland C, Bourre F, et al. Integrin alpha(v)beta3 expression confers on tumor cells a greater propensity to metastasize to bone. FASEB J Off Publ Fed Am Soc Exp Biol. 2002;16(10):1266–8.

12. Pishvaian MJ, Feltes CM, Thompson P, Bussemakers MJ, Schalken JA, Byers SW. Cadherin-11 is expressed in invasive breast cancer cell lines. Cancer Res. 1999;59(4):947–52.

13. Guise TA. Parathyroid hormone-related protein and bone metastases. Cancer. 1997;80(8 Suppl):1572–80.

14. Hauschka PV, Mavrakos AE, Iafrati MD, Doleman SE, Klagsbrun M. Growth factors in bone matrix. Isolation of multiple types by affinity chromatography on heparin-Sepharose. J Biol Chem. 1986;261(27):12665–74.

15. Yoneda T, Hiraga T. Crosstalk between cancer cells and bone microenvironment in bone metastasis. Biochem Biophys Res Commun. 2005;328(3):679–87.

16. Russell RG, Watts NB, Ebetino FH, Rogers MJ. Mechanisms of action of bisphosphonates: similarities and differences and their potential influence on clinical efficacy. Osteoporos Int J Established Results Coop Eur Found Osteoporos Natl Osteoporos Found USA. 2008;19(6):733–59.

17. Russell RG. Bisphosphonates: the first 40 years. Bone. 2011;49(1):2–19.

18. Baron R, Ferrari S, Russell RG. Denosumab and bisphosphonates: different mechanisms of action and effects. Bone. 2011;48(4):677–92.

19. Frith JC, Monkkonen J, Auriola S, Monkkonen H, Rogers MJ. The molecular mechanism of action of the antiresorptive and antiinflammatory drug clodronate: evidence for the formation in vivo of a metabolite that inhibits bone resorption and causes osteoclast and macrophage apoptosis. Arthritis Rheum. 2001;44(9):2201–10.

20. Luckman SP, Hughes DE, Coxon FP, Graham R, Russell G, Rogers MJ. Nitrogen-containing bisphosphonates inhibit the mevalonate pathway and prevent post-translational prenylation of GTP-binding proteins, including Ras. J Bone Miner Res Off J Am Soc Bone and Miner Res. 1998;13(4):581–9.

21. van Holten-Verzantvoort AT, Bijvoet OL, Cleton FJ, Hermans J, Kroon HM, Harinck HI, et al. Reduced morbidity from skeletal metastases in breast cancer patients during long-term bisphosphonate (APD) treatment. Lancet. 1987;2(8566):983–5.

22. Elomaa I, Blomqvist C, Porkka L, Holmstrom T, Taube T, Lamberg-Allardt C, et al. Clodronate for osteolytic metastases due to breast cancer. Biomed Pharmacother Biomed Pharmacother. 1988;42(2):111–6.

23. Paterson AH, Powles TJ, Kanis JA, McCloskey E, Hanson J, Ashley S. Double-blind controlled trial of oral clodronate in patients with bone metastases from breast cancer. J Clin Oncol Off J Am Soc Clin Oncol. 1993;11(1):59–65.

24. Kristensen B, Ejlertsen B, Groenvold M, Hein S, Loft H, Mouridsen HT. Oral clodronate in breast cancer patients with bone metastases: a randomized study. J Intern Med. 1999;246(1):67–74.

25. Tubiana-Hulin M, Beuzeboc P, Mauriac L, Barbet N, Frenay M, Monnier A, et al. Double-blinded controlled study comparing clodronate versus placebo in patients with breast cancer bone metastases. Bull Cancer. 2001;88(7):701–7.

26. Hortobagyi GN, Theriault RL, Lipton A, Porter L, Blayney D, Sinoff C, et al. Long-term prevention of skeletal complications of metastatic breast cancer with pamidronate. Protocol 19 Aredia Breast Cancer Study Group. J Clin Oncol Off J Am Soc Clin Oncol. 1998;16(6):2038–44.

27. Theriault RL, Lipton A, Hortobagyi GN, Leff R, Gluck S, Stewart JF, et al. Pamidronate reduces skeletal morbidity in women with advanced breast cancer and lytic bone lesions: a randomized, placebo-controlled trial. Protocol 18 Aredia Breast Cancer Study Group. J Clin Oncol Off J Am Soc Clin Oncol. 1999;17(3):846–54.

28. Lipton A, Theriault RL, Hortobagyi GN, Simeone J, Knight RD, Mellars K, et al. Pamidronate prevents skeletal complications and is effective palliative treatment in women with breast carcinoma and osteolytic bone metastases: long term follow-up of two randomized, placebo-controlled trials. Cancer. 2000;88(5):1082–90.

29. Hultborn R, Gundersen S, Ryden S, Holmberg E, Carstensen J, Wallgren UB, et al. Efficacy of pamidronate in breast cancer with bone metastases: a randomized, double-blind placebo-controlled multicenter study. Anticancer Res. 1999;19(4c):3383–92.

30. Conte PF, Latreille J, Mauriac L, Calabresi F, Santos R, Campos D, et al. Delay in progression of bone metastases in breast cancer patients treated with intravenous pamidronate: results from a multinational randomized

controlled trial. The Aredia Multinational Cooperative Group. J Clin Oncol Off J Am Soc Clin Oncol. 1996;14(9):2552–9.

31. Rosen LS, Gordon D, Kaminski M, Howell A, Belch A, Mackey J, et al. Zoledronic acid versus pamidronate in the treatment of skeletal metastases in patients with breast cancer or osteolytic lesions of multiple myeloma: a phase III, double-blind, comparative trial. Cancer J (Sudbury Mass). 2001;7(5):377–87.

32. Rosen LS, Gordon DH, Dugan Jr W, Major P, Eisenberg PD, Provencher L, et al. Zoledronic acid is superior to pamidronate for the treatment of bone metastases in breast carcinoma patients with at least one osteolytic lesion. Cancer. 2004;100(1):36–43.

33. Rosen LS, Gordon D, Kaminski M, Howell A, Belch A, Mackey J, et al. Long-term efficacy and safety of zoledronic acid compared with pamidronate disodium in the treatment of skeletal complications in patients with advanced multiple myeloma or breast carcinoma: a randomized, double-blind, multicenter, comparative trial. Cancer. 2003;98(8):1735–44.

34. Body JJ, Diel IJ, Lichinitser MR, Kreuser ED, Dornoff W, Gorbunova VA, et al. Intravenous ibandronate reduces the incidence of skeletal complications in patients with breast cancer and bone metastases. Ann Oncol Off J Eur Soc Med Oncol ESMO. 2003;14(9):1399–405.

35. Heras P, Kritikos K, Hatzopoulos A, Georgopoulou AP. Efficacy of ibandronate for the treatment of skeletal events in patients with metastatic breast cancer. Eur J Cancer Care. 2009;18(6):653–6.

36. Body JJ, Diel IJ, Lichinitzer M, Lazarev A, Pecherstorfer M, Bell R, et al. Oral ibandronate reduces the risk of skeletal complications in breast cancer patients with metastatic bone disease: results from two randomised, placebo-controlled phase III studies. Br J Cancer. 2004;90(6):1133–7.

37. Palmieri C, Fullarton JR, Brown J. Comparative efficacy of bisphosphonates in metastatic breast and prostate cancer and multiple myeloma: a mixed-treatment meta-analysis. Clin Cancer Res Off J Am Assoc Cancer Res. 2013;19(24):6863–72.

38. Lipton A, Steger GG, Figueroa J, Alvarado C, Solal-Celigny P, Body JJ, et al. Randomized active-controlled phase II study of denosumab efficacy and safety in patients with breast cancer-related bone metastases. J Clin Oncol Off J Am Soc Clin Oncol. 2007;25(28):4431–7.

39. Stopeck AT, Lipton A, Body JJ, Steger GG, Tonkin K, de Boer RH, et al. Denosumab compared with zoledronic acid for the treatment of bone metastases in patients with advanced breast cancer: a randomized, double-blind study. J Clin Oncol Off J Am Soc Clin Oncol. 2010;28(35):5132–9.

40. Van Poznak CH, Temin S, Yee GC, Janjan NA, Barlow WE, Biermann JS, et al. American Society of Clinical Oncology executive summary of the clinical practice guideline update on the role of bone-modifying agents in metastatic breast cancer. J Clin Oncol Off J Am Soc Clin Oncol. 2011;29(9):1221–7.

41. Wong MH, Stockler MR, Pavlakis N. Bisphosphonates and other bone agents for breast cancer. Cochrane Database Syst Rev. 2012;2, Cd003474.

42. Morris PG, Lynch C, Feeney JN, Patil S, Howard J, Larson SM, et al. Integrated positron emission tomography/computed tomography may render bone scintigraphy unnecessary to investigate suspected metastatic breast cancer. J Clin Oncol Off J Am Soc Clin Oncol. 2010;28(19):3154–9.

43. Clemons M, Dranitsaris G, Ooi W, Cole DE. A phase II trial evaluating the palliative benefit of second-line oral ibandronate in breast cancer patients with either a skeletal related event (SRE) or progressive bone metastases (BM) despite standard bisphosphonate (BP) therapy. Breast Cancer Res Treat. 2008;108(1):79–85.

44. Clemons MJ, Dranitsaris G, Ooi WS, Yogendran G, Sukovic T, Wong BY, et al. Phase II trial evaluating the palliative benefit of second-line zoledronic acid in breast cancer patients with either a skeletal-related event or progressive bone metastases despite first-line bisphosphonate therapy. J Clin Oncol Off J Am Soc Clin Oncol. 2006;24(30):4895–900.

45. Fizazi K, Lipton A, Mariette X, Body JJ, Rahim Y, Gralow JR, et al. Randomized phase II trial of denosumab in patients with bone metastases from prostate cancer, breast cancer, or other neoplasms after intravenous bisphosphonates. J Clin Oncol Off J Am Soc Clin Oncol. 2009;27(10):1564–71.

46. Cleeland CS, Body JJ, Stopeck A, von Moos R, Fallowfield L, Mathias SD, et al. Pain outcomes in patients with advanced breast cancer and bone metastases: results from a randomized, double-blind study of denosumab and zoledronic acid. Cancer. 2013;119(4):832–8.

47. Hoff AO, Toth B, Hu M, Hortobagyi GN, Gagel RF. Epidemiology and risk factors for osteonecrosis of the jaw in cancer patients. Ann N Y Acad Sci. 2011;1218:47–54.

48. Hoff AO, Toth BB, Altundag K, Johnson MM, Warneke CL, Hu M, et al. Frequency and risk factors associated with osteonecrosis of the jaw in cancer patients treated with intravenous bisphosphonates. J Bone Miner Res Off J Am Soc Bone and Miner Res. 2008;23(6):826–36.

49. Saad F, Brown JE, Van Poznak C, Ibrahim T, Stemmer SM, Stopeck AT, et al. Incidence, risk factors, and outcomes of osteonecrosis of the jaw: integrated analysis from three blinded active-controlled phase III trials in cancer patients with bone metastases. Ann Oncol Off J Eur Soc Med Oncol ESMO. 2012;23(5):1341–7.

50. Hirschberg R. Renal complications from bisphosphonate treatment. Curr Opin Support Palliat Care. 2012;6(3):342–7.

51. Markowitz GS, Appel GB, Fine PL, Fenves AZ, Loon NR, Jagannath S, et al. Collapsing focal segmental

glomerulosclerosis following treatment with high-dose pamidronate. J Am Soc Nephrol JASN. 2001;12(6):1164–72.

52. Sauter M, Julg B, Porubsky S, Cohen C, Fischereder M, Sitter T, et al. Nephrotic-range proteinuria following pamidronate therapy in a patient with metastatic breast cancer: mitochondrial toxicity as a pathogenetic concept? Am J Kidney Dis Off J Natl Kidney Found. 2006;47(6):1075–80.

53. Berenson JR, Boccia R, Lopez T, Warsi GM, Argonza-Aviles E, Lake S, et al. Results of a multicenter open-label randomized trial evaluating infusion duration of zoledronic acid in multiple myeloma patients (the ZMAX trial). J Support Oncol. 2011;9(1):32–40.

54. Sun L, Yu S. Efficacy and safety of denosumab versus zoledronic acid in patients with bone metastases: a systematic review and meta-analysis. Am J Clin Oncol. 2013;36(4):399–403.

55. Peter R, Mishra V, Fraser WD. Severe hypocalcaemia after being given intravenous bisphosphonate. BMJ (Clin Res Ed). 2004;328(7435):335–6.

56. Chennuru S, Koduri J, Baumann MA. Risk factors for symptomatic hypocalcaemia complicating treatment with zoledronic acid. Intern Med J. 2008;38(8):635–7.

57. Lipton A, Fizazi K, Stopeck AT, Henry DH, Brown JE, Yardley DA, et al. Superiority of denosumab to zoledronic acid for prevention of skeletal-related events: a combined analysis of 3 pivotal, randomised, phase 3 trials. Eur J Cancer (Oxf Engl: 1990). 2012;48(16):3082–92.

58. Aapro M, Abrahamsson PA, Body JJ, Coleman RE, Colomer R, Costa L, et al. Guidance on the use of bisphosphonates in solid tumours: recommendations of an international expert panel. Ann Oncol Off J Eur Soc Med Oncol ESMO. 2008;19(3):420–32.

59. Pazianas M, Abrahamsen B. Safety of bisphosphonates. Bone. 2011;49(1):103–10.

60. Tanvetyanon T, Stiff PJ. Management of the adverse effects associated with intravenous bisphosphonates. Ann Oncol Off J Eur Soc Med Oncol ESMO. 2006;17(6):897–907.

61. Wilkinson GS, Baillargeon J, Kuo YF, Freeman JL, Goodwin JS. Atrial fibrillation and stroke associated with intravenous bisphosphonate therapy in older patients with cancer. J Clin Oncol Off J Am Soc Clin Oncol. 2010;28(33):4898–905.

62. Anastasilakis AD, Toulis KA, Goulis DG, Polyzos SA, Delaroudis S, Giomisi A, et al. Efficacy and safety of denosumab in postmenopausal women with osteopenia or osteoporosis: a systematic review and a meta-analysis. Horm Metab Res Hormon- und Stoffwechselforschung Horm Metab. 2009;41(10):721–9.

63. Tomblyn M. The role of bone-seeking radionuclides in the palliative treatment of patients with painful osteoblastic skeletal metastases. Cancer Control J Moffitt Cancer Cent. 2012;19(2):137–44.

64. Parker C, Nilsson S, Heinrich D, Helle SI, O'Sullivan JM, Fossa SD, et al. Alpha emitter radium-223 and survival in metastatic prostate cancer. N Engl J Med. 2013;369(3):213–23.

65. Suominen MI, Rissanen JP, Kakonen R, Fagerlund KM, Alhoniemi E, Mumberg D, et al. Survival benefit with radium-223 dichloride in a mouse model of breast cancer bone metastasis. J Natl Cancer Inst. 2013;105(12):908–16.

66. Tu SM, Millikan RE, Mengistu B, Delpassand ES, Amato RJ, Pagliaro LC, et al. Bone-targeted therapy for advanced androgen-independent carcinoma of the prostate: a randomised phase II trial. Lancet. 2001;357(9253):336–41.

67. Oosterhof GO, Roberts JT, de Reijke TM, Engelholm SA, Horenblas S, von der Maase H, et al. Strontium(89) chloride versus palliative local field radiotherapy in patients with hormonal escaped prostate cancer: a phase III study of the European Organisation for Research and Treatment of Cancer, Genitourinary Group. Eur Urol. 2003;44(5):519–26.

68. Sartor O, Reid RH, Hoskin PJ, Quick DP, Ell PJ, Coleman RE, et al. Samarium-153-Lexidronam complex for treatment of painful bone metastases in hormone-refractory prostate cancer. Urology. 2004;63(5):940–5.

69. Fuster D, Herranz D, Vidal-Sicart S, Munoz M, Conill C, Mateos JJ, et al. Usefulness of strontium-89 for bone pain palliation in metastatic breast cancer patients. Nucl Med Commun. 2000;21(7):623–6.

70. Baczyk M, Czepczynski R, Milecki P, Pisarek M, Oleksa R, Sowinski J. 89Sr versus 153Sm-EDTMP: comparison of treatment efficacy of painful bone metastases in prostate and breast carcinoma. Nucl Med Commun. 2007;28(4):245–50.

71. Sciuto R, Festa A, Pasqualoni R, Semprebene A, Rea S, Bergomi S, et al. Metastatic bone pain palliation with 89-Sr and 186-Re-HEDP in breast cancer patients. Breast Cancer Res Treat. 2001;66(2):101–9.

72. Kasalicky J, Krajska V. The effect of repeated strontium-89 chloride therapy on bone pain palliation in patients with skeletal cancer metastases. Eur J Nucl Med. 1998;25(10):1362–7.

73. Sartor O, Reid RH, Bushnell DL, Quick DP, Ell PJ. Safety and efficacy of repeat administration of samarium Sm-153 lexidronam to patients with metastatic bone pain. Cancer. 2007;109(3):637–42.

74. Englaro EE, Schroder LE, Thomas SR, Williams CC, Maxon 3rd HR. Safety and efficacy of repeated sequential administrations of Re-186(Sn)HEDP as palliative therapy for painful skeletal metastases. Initial case reports of two patients. Clin Nucl Med. 1992;17(1):41–4.

75. Hiscox S, Barrett-Lee P, Borley AC, Nicholson RI. Combining Src inhibitors and aromatase

inhibitors: a novel strategy for overcoming endocrine resistance and bone loss. Eur J Cancer (Oxf Engl: 1990). 2010;46(12):2187–95.

76. Vandyke K, Dewar AL, Farrugia AN, Fitter S, Bik To L, Hughes TP, et al. Therapeutic concentrations of dasatinib inhibit in vitro osteoclastogenesis. Leukemia. 2009;23(5):994–7.

77. Hannon RA, Finkelman RD, Clack G, Iacona RB, Rimmer M, Gossiel F, et al. Effects of Src kinase inhi-

bition by saracatinib (AZD0530) on bone turnover in advanced malignancy in a phase I study. Bone. 2012;50(4):885–92.

78. Jensen AB, Wynne C, Ramirez G, He W, Song Y, Berd Y, et al. The cathepsin K inhibitor odanacatib suppresses bone resorption in women with breast cancer and established bone metastases: results of a 4-week, double-blind, randomized, controlled trial. Clin Breast Cancer. 2010;10(6):452–8.

The Local Management of Bone Metastases

43

Levent Eralp and Halil Buldu

Abstract

Breast cancer is osteotropic, similar to prostate cancer; thus, breast cancer-related bone metastases are common. The local management of bone metastases is focused on pain control and the prevention or treatment of pathological fractures. In rare cases, the treatment may be definitive for the removal of isolated bone metastases, which may improve the patient's survival. All of these surgical treatment modalities are restricted by the patient's life expectancy and comorbidities. The major goal of the treatment is the improvement of the patient's quality of life. The treatment of bone metastases should be performed using a multidisciplinary team approach.

Keywords

Breast cancer • Bone metastases • PTH-rP • RANKL • Surgical treatment • Medical treatment • Metastases • Pathological fracture • Long bone • Vertebrae • Kyphoplasty • Vertebroplasty • M-CSF • PDGF • VEGF • Bone destruction • Bone production • Mirels score • Bisphosphonates • Hormone therapy • Tamoxifen • Polymethylmethacrylate • Impending fracture • Osteoarticular allografts • Intramedullary nail • Intercalary prosthesis • Kyphosis

L. Eralp, MD (✉)
Department of Orthopaedics and Traumatology,
University of Istanbul, Istanbul School of Medicine,
Hakki Yeten Cad. No: 14, Terrace Fulya Center 1 D:
83 Sisli, 34365 Istanbul, Turkey
e-mail: drleventeralp@gmail.com

H. Buldu, MD
Department of Orthopaedics and Traumatology,
Memorial Hospital, Istanbul, Turkey

Nişantaşi Hospital, Istanbul, Turkey
e-mail: halilb77@hotmail.com

Introduction

Metastatic disease is the most frequently observed malignant lesion of the bone [1]. Breast, kidney, thyroid, and lung cancers have high incidences of bone metastases [1, 2]. Approximately 70 % of patients who die of breast cancer have also had bone metastases [3]. Twenty percent of breast cancer bone metastases become symptomatic, and 17 % of these symptomatic cases require surgical

© Springer International Publishing Switzerland 2016
A. Aydiner et al. (eds.), *Breast Disease: Management and Therapies*,
DOI 10.1007/978-3-319-26012-9_43

treatment [4, 5]. Currently, the 5-year survival rate for metastatic breast cancer is 22 % [1].

There are two groups of breast cancer bone metastases with regard to the behavioral pattern of the bone cells. Osteolytic lesions, which are the most common form, lead to bone destruction and are a common cause of morbidity and mortality. Osteoblastic lesions lead to new bone formation. Bone metastases can exclusively comprise an osteolytic or osteoblastic phenotype but most likely simultaneously contain osteolytic and osteoblastic activities [2, 4, 6, 7].

Breast cancer bone metastases can lead to bone pain, pathological fractures, hypercalcemia, and spinal cord and other nerve compressions due to pathological fractures (osteolytic activity) or due to direct compression (osteoblastic activity).

Breast cancer patients with bone metastases and extensive bone destruction have significantly increased morbidity and markedly worse prognoses [8, 9].

Bone Metastasis Pathophysiology

The metastasis of breast cancer involves the progression through complex molecular and cellular stages. An understanding of these stages is very important for modifying therapeutic strategies.

Physiological bone architecture contains a unique microenvironment. The bone extracellular matrix comprises type 1 collagen and hydroxyapatite crystals. The cellular component contains three cell types: osteoblasts, osteocytes, and osteoclasts. These three cell types are controlled by many hormones and growth factors.

Bone is an active tissue that maintains mineral homeostasis through bone resorption via osteoclastic activity and bone formation via osteoblastic activity. Breast cancer cells disrupt this bone turnover.

The metastatic process begins by adhesion to the vessel endothelium and extravasation (via the activities of metalloproteinases and cathepsin K) into the bone tissue. Breast cancer cells produce parathyroid hormone-related peptide (PTH-rP); PTH-rP binds to the parathyroid hormone (PTH) receptor, which results in the expression of receptor

activator of nuclear factor κB ligand (RANKL) and macrophage colony-stimulating factor (M-CSF) by osteoblasts [2, 3]. RANKL binds to the RANK receptor on osteoclast precursors and induces the formation of mature osteoclasts. The excessive activity of osteoclasts due to RANKL and M-CSF results in bone degradation. Bone degradation is conducive to the release of IGF-1 and TGF-β (and possibly PDGF and BMP), which are stored in the bone [2, 3, 8].

IGF-1 stimulates DNA matrix synthesis, thereby stimulating breast cancer cell growth and migration into the bone (Fig. 43.1).

TGF-β potentiates DNA synthesis, inhibits type II collagen synthesis, and, in breast cancer cells, plays a key role in stimulating the secretion of PTH-rP. TGF-β also stimulates COX-2 expression in breast cancer cells, which causes increased PGE2 production [10].

Breast cancer cells produce several local factors such as tumor necrosis factor-alpha (TNF-α), IL-1, IL-6, IL-11, M-CSF, and prostaglandin E2. These cytokines activate osteoclastogenesis and suppress osteoblasts.

The hormone estrogen is a mitogenic factor for breast tumor cells; therefore, tumor cells express the estrogen receptor (ER). ER-positive tumors have a higher risk of developing bone metastases. Estrogen has been shown to regulate the level of PTH-rP in some tissues, but whether this regulation occurs in the bone microenvironment remains unclear [2, 11].

Increased blood flow is essential for the survival of metastatic cancer cells; therefore, tumor progression is critically dependent on angiogenesis. When osteoclasts resorb the bone matrix, platelet-derived growth factors (PDGF-1/PDGF-2) and platelet-derived endothelial cell growth factor (PD-ECGF), also known as thymidine phosphorylase (TP), are released. TP is the target of the chemotherapeutic agent 5-fluorouracil [12]. Breast cancer cells also express vascular endothelial growth factor (VEGF); VEGF is angiogenic and, furthermore, promotes osteoclastogenesis [2, 13].

Breast cancer cells induce angiogenesis through the chemotactic and mitogenic effects of PDGF, PD-ECGF, and VEGF on endothelial cells.

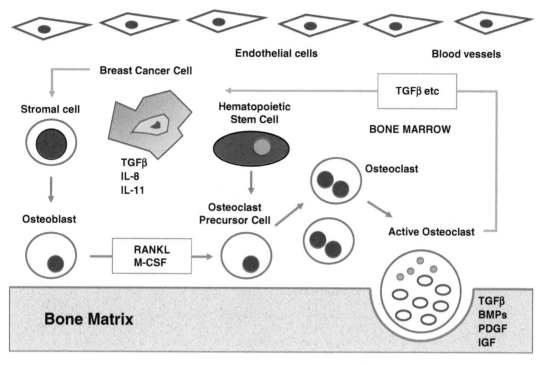

Fig. 43.1 NF-κB ligand (RANKL)/RANK pathway. Breast cancer cells activate osteoblasts with PTH-rP; RANKL is produced by osteoblasts. RANK receptor stimulation results in increasing the maturation of active osteoclasts

Long Bone Metastases

Metastatic bone disease usually causes significant pain and disability. Pain at rest and upon waking indicates a metastatic or primary bone tumor. If a patient with breast cancer has pain at rest in an extremity and a history of disability, a thorough examination, proper imaging, and clinical and pathological diagnoses are crucial.

Clinical Presentation, Evaluation, and Imaging

Patients with symptomatic osseous lesions note localized pain that does not resolve with rest or routine painkillers. The other ominous pain modality is observed only with weight bearing but does not resolve with rest and indicates a probable pathological fracture.

On physical examination, a visual inspection may reveal swelling, ulceration, venous changes, or deformity. Any restriction or pain with joint motion, local tenderness, pathological movement, crepitus, or lymphadenopathy may be established by palpation. Careful neurological and vascular assessments must be performed.

The radiographic evaluation should begin with two-plane X-rays of the affected extremity. When metastatic disease is present, one must determine the localization of the lesion, the relationship with the articular surface, and the distinction between the lesion and normal bone. As much as 50 % of the cortical bone must be lost to see plain radiographic evidence of a lytic lesion. The early stages of metastatic disease cannot be observed on plain X-rays. The radiographic appearance of a metastatic lesion may be osteolytic (the most common), osteoblastic, or mixed. The radiographic appearance depends on the balance of osteoclastic (bone destruction) and osteoblastic (bone production) activity levels.

If a patient has a solitary, isolated bone lesion with a history of breast cancer, the most probable diagnosis is metastatic bone disease; however, alternative diagnoses include multiple myeloma, a primary bone tumor, lymphoma, infection, Paget's sarcoma, and hyperparathyroidism. After a careful history has been taken, an examination, proper laboratory tests, and a radiologic evaluation should be performed. The laboratory tests should include the following: a complete blood count, serum protein electrophoresis, the serum calcium level, the prostate-specific antigen level, the C-reactive protein level, and the erythrocyte sedimentation rate (Fig. 43.2). The radiologic evaluation should include the following: two-plane X-rays of the entire long bone; contrast computed tomography (CT) of the chest, abdomen, and pelvis; and a whole body bone scan (although this scan may be negative in myeloma and metastatic renal cancer, a bone scan can detect multiple lesions, which are common in metastatic disease). A bone scan may miss early infiltration into the marrow; therefore, despite negative bone scan results in suspect cases, a magnetic resonance

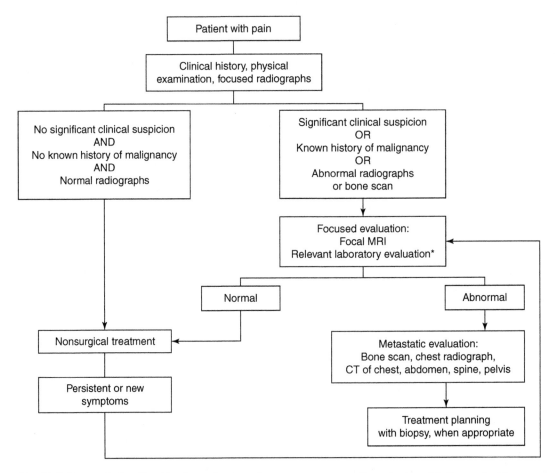

Fig. 43.2 Proposed algorithm for the evaluation of a patient for metastatic disease of the spine. *A relevant laboratory evaluation should include the following: a complete blood count, an erythrocyte sedimentation rate, and the level of C-reactive protein to evaluate reactive processes, as well as a basic metabolic panel with serum calcium level and, where appropriate, markers of specific disease, such as prostate-specific antigen, and serum/urine protein electrophoresis. *CT* computed tomography, *MRI* magnetic resonance imaging

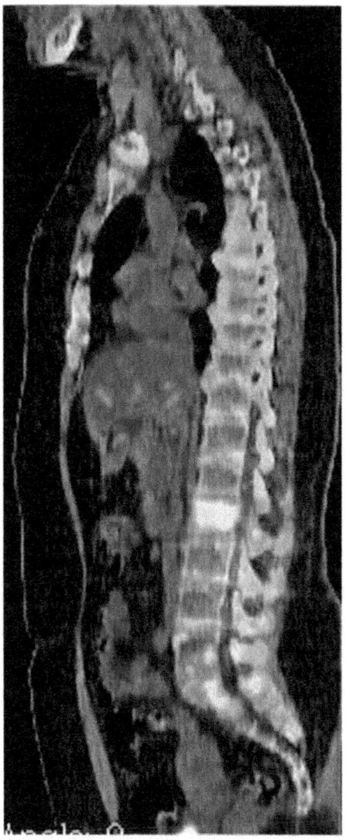

Fig. 43.3 A 55-year-old woman, PET-CT scan reveals a metastatic lesion from breast cancer on the L2 vertebrae and sacrum

imaging (MRI) scan should be performed to detect early-stage bone metastases (Fig. 43.3).

Guidelines

In 1973, Fidler suggested the prophylactic stabilization of long bones. His study indicates that prophylactic stabilization is necessary if long bone metastatic lesions have more than 50 % cortical bone destruction [14]. In 1982, Harrington considered three factors in the prophylactic stabilization of the femur: the lesion was ≥2.5 cm, the lesion involved >50 % cortical destruction, and the lesion caused persistent pain after a trial of radiotherapy [15].

In 1989, Mirels developed a scoring system according to the anatomic location of the metastatic lesion, the type of bone destruction (osteoblastic, osteolytic, or mixed), the size of the

defect, and the degree of pain [16] (Table 43.1). Prophylactic fixation is recommended for a score of ≥9 (33 % fracture risk within a year). A Mirels score of 12 indicates a fracture risk of 100 % within a year.

Indications

The major indication for prophylactic fixation is improving the quality of life. The purpose of the surgical treatment of a breast cancer patient with long bone metastases and no pathological fracture is to decrease pain, reduce the use of analgesics, restore skeletal stability, regain functional independence, and improve ambulatory and daily routine activity. However, the decision to proceed with surgical intervention is based on several factors and must be individualized. These factors include the following: histology of the primary lesion, the patient's comorbidities and expected lifespan, the severity of the symptoms, the location of the tumor, the expectations of the patient, and the efficacy of the intervention relative to alternative or adjuvant treatment modalities [17, 18].

The scoring systems are not conclusive and cannot predict all factors. For this reason, the operative decision should be based on both the scoring systems and the individual factors.

In a case where the patient has long bone metastases from breast cancer with a pathological long bone fracture, if the patient's life expectancy is ≥3 months, stabilization of the long bone is necessary for pain relief and for improving movement [18]. In a nonambulatory patient with a pathological long bone fracture, stabilization of the long bone can be performed for painless bed-to-chair transfer.

Asymptomatic lesions require clinical and radiological follow-up. These asymptomatic lesions can be effectively managed with medical treatment (such as bisphosphonate or hormonal therapy) and radiation [12, 18].

Prophylactic fixation results in decreased perioperative morbidity, shorter hospitalization (average of 2 days), fewer hardware complications,

Table 43.1 Mirels scoring system for assessing the risk of pathologic fracture in long bones

Score			
	1	2	3
Anatomic location	Upper limb	Lower limb	Peritrochanteric
Bone destruction type	Blastic	Mixed	Lytic
Size of the defect (as a proportion of shaft diameter)	<1/3	1/3–2/3	>2/3
Pain	Mild	Moderate	Functional

and improved survival compared with pathological fracture fixation.

The clear indication for long bone fixation is the presence of a pathological fracture in a weight-bearing long bone.

Medical Treatment

There are five different types of medical treatment: (1) hormone therapy, (2) chemotherapy, (3) bisphosphonates, (4) radiation therapy, and (5) external supports.

For hormone therapy, the response rate is closely related to the activity of the estrogen and progesterone receptors. The most commonly used agent is tamoxifen. Tamoxifen inhibits the effects of estrogen.

Chemotherapy is an effective treatment for bone metastases from breast cancer. For rapidly growing disease, hormonal therapy is ineffective, and chemotherapy use is indicated.

Bisphosphonates inhibit osteoclastic activity (bone resorption).

Upper Extremity Metastases

Twenty percent of breast cancer bone metastases involve the upper extremities, and 50 % occur in the humerus [19, 20].

Metastases in the upper extremities can result in the significant impairment of daily functions such as personal hygiene, eating, and the ability to use external aids.

Treatment strategies include both medical treatment (functional bracing, radiation, bisphosphonates, hormone therapy, and chemotherapy)

and surgical treatment (resection and reconstruction or stabilization).

Nonsurgical treatment options are usually chosen in cases of limited life expectancy, severe comorbidities, low-demand patients, small lesions, radiosensitive tumors, and asymptomatic lesions.

Lesions of the clavicle and scapula are generally treated nonsurgically with immobilization, radiation, or medical therapy. Nonetheless, destructive lesions of articular parts of the scapula and clavicle may require operative treatment.

A detailed preoperative assessment of the general medical condition is important to minimize complications. Hypercalcemia, sodium-potassium imbalance, anemia, renal and liver dysfunctions, and coagulopathy can be observed in these patients [20].

The cervical spine should be assessed for destructive lesions to avoid any cervical injury during anesthesia and positioning. The cervical spine should be evaluated with cervical X-rays or a bone scan to exclude any cervical metastases.

Surgical Treatment

Surgical treatment strategies include rigid and durable internal fixation for mechanical strength restoration, functional improvement, and pain relief. As a result, the upper extremity can be usable immediately after operation.

A variety of internal fixation or prosthetic devices can be utilized to maintain stable and durable fixation. Healing of the fracture should not be necessary to maintain functional stability.

Surgical treatment of the humerus is reviewed in detail below.

Humerus

Selection of the reconstruction device depends on the anatomic region and the amount of bone destruction. An intramedullary nail (IMN), a plate, hemiarthroplasty, a total shoulder replacement, an intercalary prosthesis, osteoarticular allografts (OAs), and polymethylmethacrylate (PMM) are potential reconstructive devices. PMM supplements poor bone quality when used with reconstruction devices.

Breast cancer metastases in the humerus can be divided into three anatomic regions: the proximal humerus, the humeral diaphysis, and the distal humerus.

Proximal Humerus

Pathological fractures of the proximal humerus usually occur with extensive destruction of the humeral head and metaphysis. A pathological fracture or impending fracture is usually treated with a humeral endoprosthesis. A total shoulder prosthesis is rarely used because intra-articular or glenoid involvement is rare. Resection and proximal humeral replacement achieve excellent pain relief but poor shoulder function [20, 21].

Osteoarticular allografts (OAs) for the reconstruction of the proximal humerus are not a good choice in the long term. The long-term results of OA have been unsatisfactory, and the recovery time is longer than with an endoprosthesis. Benjamin K. does not at all recommend the use of OAs at all due to the unacceptable complication rate [22].

A deltopectoral approach is used to remove the proximal humerus and to curettage all of the tumor tissue. All gross tumor tissue should be removed, but care must be taken not to remove periosteal tissue or the cortical shell. The diaphysis is prepared as the entire canal for the prosthetic stem. The application of the cement is extremely important, and the surgeon should avoid entering soft tissue. Cement extravasation can cause neurovascular injury.

Bos et al. reported the outcomes for 18 patients who underwent proximal humeral reconstruction;

10 underwent subluxation, which indicates a high instability rate [23]. Moeckel et al. reported the outcomes for 22 patients who had good results with proximal humerus reconstruction using a modular hemiarthroplasty; this design allows for an improved soft tissue balance [24].

In this region of the humerus, an intramedullary nail is not stable because of insufficient proximal fixation. Fixation with a plate is also insufficient and associated with extensive bone destruction because there is generally no location for stable screw fixation.

Diaphyseal Region

In the diaphyseal region, the best implant choice is intramedullary nailing (anterograde or retrograde) using a closed technique, and if tumor tissue resection was performed, using a polymethylmethacrylate support to maintain early stable fixation is advised (Fig. 43.4). The humerus has a very small intramedullary canal; thus, applying closed intramedullary nailing can be difficult.

An IMN has some advantages, including that the nail protects the long (almost entire diaphysis) segment of the humerus and that there is a low risk of implant failure and less soft tissue damage.

An anterograde IMN incision may damage the rotator cuff, which would require repair. Many patients complain of rotator cuff tendinitis and weakness. The tip of the nail can cause persistent symptoms.

IMN fixation can be used from between 2 and 3 cm below the greater tuberosity to 5 cm above the olecranon fossa [25]. Outside of these margins, an IMN can be made rigid with interlocking screws or with a polymethylmethacrylate support. To provide rigid fixation, there must be at least 4–5 cm of intramedullary nail on either side of the lesion with intact cortices [20]. However, after nail insertion, at least two locking screws, proximal and distal, are recommended to achieve stable fixation.

Redmond et al. reported 13 patients who underwent intramedullary nailing with the use of a closed technique to treat metastatic disease

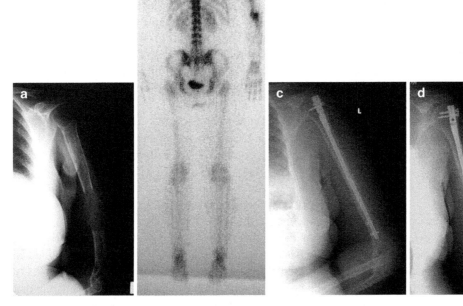

Fig. 43.4 A 59-year-old woman with metastatic breast cancer. (**a**) AP radiograph reveals lytic lesion on the shaft of the left humerus (impending fracture). (**b**) A bone scan with technetium 99 reveals increased uptake in the left humerus diaphysis. (**c**, **d**) Postoperative radiographs after curettage, cementation, and fixation with an intramedullary nail

[25]. As a result, the authors concluded that "interlocking intramedullary nailing of the humerus for pathological fractures provides immediate stability and can be accomplished with a closed technique, brief operative time, and minimum morbidity, with a resultant early return of function to the extremity."

Plate fixation is also a recommended method for impending and complete fractures of the diaphyseal region with some advantages and disadvantages. The major advantage of plate fixation is that the rotator cuff is not as affected as it is with anterograde intramedullary nailing and that fluoroscopy is usually not necessary. The disadvantages of plate usage include the following: extensive soft tissue damage, greater blood loss, possible radial nerve injury, a longer recovery period, and that the long segment is not as well controlled compared with intramedullary nailing. At least three screws should be placed in the normal cortical bone on either side of the fracture. For exposure for plate fixation, an anterolateral or posterior approach is usually used. Care must be taken when resecting the tumor tissue to avoid extensive removal of periosteal tissue or the cortical shell, which would hinder stable fixation in the remaining cortical bone and prolong the healing period.

Intercalary prostheses are suitable for dealing with extensive diaphyseal destruction, segmental defects, or a prior failed device. Intercalary prostheses offer a modular reconstruction option with a transition piece for the resection of large diaphyseal lesions.

Damron et al. reviewed the outcomes of 17 patients who had reconstructions with cemented modular intercalary prostheses; 88 % of the patients achieved immediate and stable humeral fixation, pain relief, and an early return of function [26]. Three radial nerve injuries, three implant failures, and two periprosthetic fractures were observed.

Distal Humerus

Metastatic lesions of the distal humerus are rare; breast cancer is one of the most common primary tumors that metastasizes to this location. Distal humeral metastases can be treated with bicondylar plate fixation, flexible intramedullary nails, resection, and prosthetic reconstruction. Additionally, PMM can be added to provide greater and immediate stability to this region. Because of the unique anatomy of this region and the thinning of the bone at the olecranon fossa, supracondylar pathologic fractures are particularly difficult to treat.

In cases of extensive bone destruction and in selected cases after resection of the elbow, arthroplasty provides marked pain relief and functional improvement.

After the prophylactic fixation or surgical treatment of pathological fractures, radiation therapy is recommended. The postoperative use of radiation therapy decreases bone destruction and minimizes the loosening of the fixation material.

Townsend et al. found that the addition of external beam radiation to surgery significantly improved functional outcomes.

Radiation therapy can be started 10 days after surgery. If the patient has previously received radiation, the sutures are left in place for approximately 4 weeks [20].

Lower Extremity Metastases

Metastatic lesions and pathological fractures are more common in the lower extremities than in the upper extremities. The result of a pathologic fracture in the lower extremity is more pronounced than that of a fracture occurring in the upper extremity (Fig. 43.5). Approximately two-thirds of all long bone pathological fractures occur in the femur [27]. The proximal femur (50 %) and the intertrochanteric region (20 %) are the most commonly involved areas.

Lower extremity metastases can result in significant impairments in daily functions due to the inability to walk. In addition, the inability to walk can cause emboli, lung problems, or infections.

Surgical Treatment

The aims of treatment for the lower extremity long bones are pain relief and ambulatory function restoration. If the life expectancy is longer than 3 months, surgical treatment is a possibility [1, 19, 27].

The surgeon should achieve stable fixation, and local tumor control can be achieved with radiation therapy, chemotherapy, and hormonal therapy. For breast cancer bone metastases, the local control of the tumor is usually provided with the aforementioned methods.

Femoral Head and Neck

For non-pathological fractures in the femoral head and neck region, there are high rates of nonunion and implant failure. For pathological fractures of the femoral neck, there is also a high risk of nonunion; thus, an endoprosthetic replacement is usually the treatment of choice. A long-stem prosthesis is recommended to prevent failure in the case of local tumor progression and to support the femoral shaft (Fig. 43.6). The surgeon should be mindful of the calcar area; when the tumor extends into this region, a special calcar replacement prosthesis should be chosen. When the acetabulum is not involved and there is no extensive degenerative joint disease, bipolar cups should be used for increased stability and less morbidity (Fig. 43.7).

Internal fixation with cement has an unacceptably high failure rate [27].

Lane et al. reported the results from 167 patients who were treated with prostheses for impending or complete pathological fractures of the hip [28]. All of the patients reported a dramatic relief of pain. The ambulatory status was significantly enhanced in those patients who

Fig. 43.5 A 41-year-old woman with a metastatic lesion from breast cancer on the subtrochanteric region. (**a**) AP view reveals an osteolytic lesion on the subtrochanteric region; note the lysis on the medial cortex of the femur; patient refused treatment. (**b**) Six months later, the impending fracture evolved to a pathologic fracture

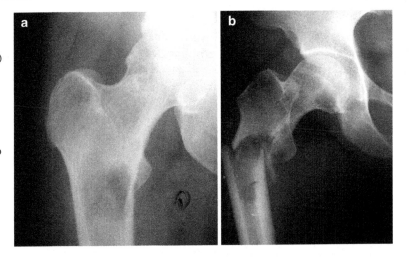

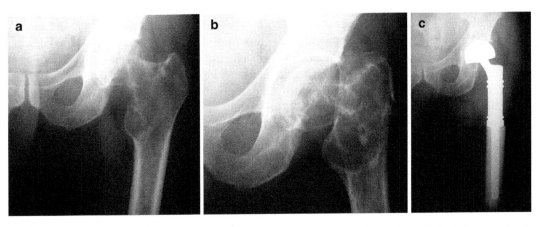

Fig. 43.6 A 61-year-old woman with breast carcinoma metastases to the proximal femur (**a**) AP view demonstrates a lytic lesion on the proximal femur; no pathologic fracture is present. (**b**) Patient received radiation therapy, but tumor progression and a pathologic fracture developed. (**c**) Radiograph of the hip after resection of the proximal femur and reconstruction with a bipolar cemented tumor prosthesis

were able to walk, but the ambulatory status of the gravely ill was not improved.

Intertrochanteric Region

An intramedullary nail (open or closed) should be chosen for most cases. If there is not extensive bone destruction or if there is enough bone stock to fix locking screws, an intramedullary nail is recommended. An intramedullary nail protects the entire femur.

If there is extensive bone destruction, particularly in the medial cortex of the femur, an intramedullary nail and plate-screw fixation cannot provide long-term durability. For better fixation, cement should be added to the osteosynthesis. An implant failure may occur due to high mechanical stress at this level or to femoral head necrosis after irradiation.

If the intertrochanteric region has extensive bone destruction, resection of the proximal femur and reconstruction with a cemented modular megaprosthesis are preferred for better pain relief and immediate ambulatory function. Megaprosthesis for the proximal femur should contain a modular system, be long stemmed and cemented, and have no intramedullary plug.

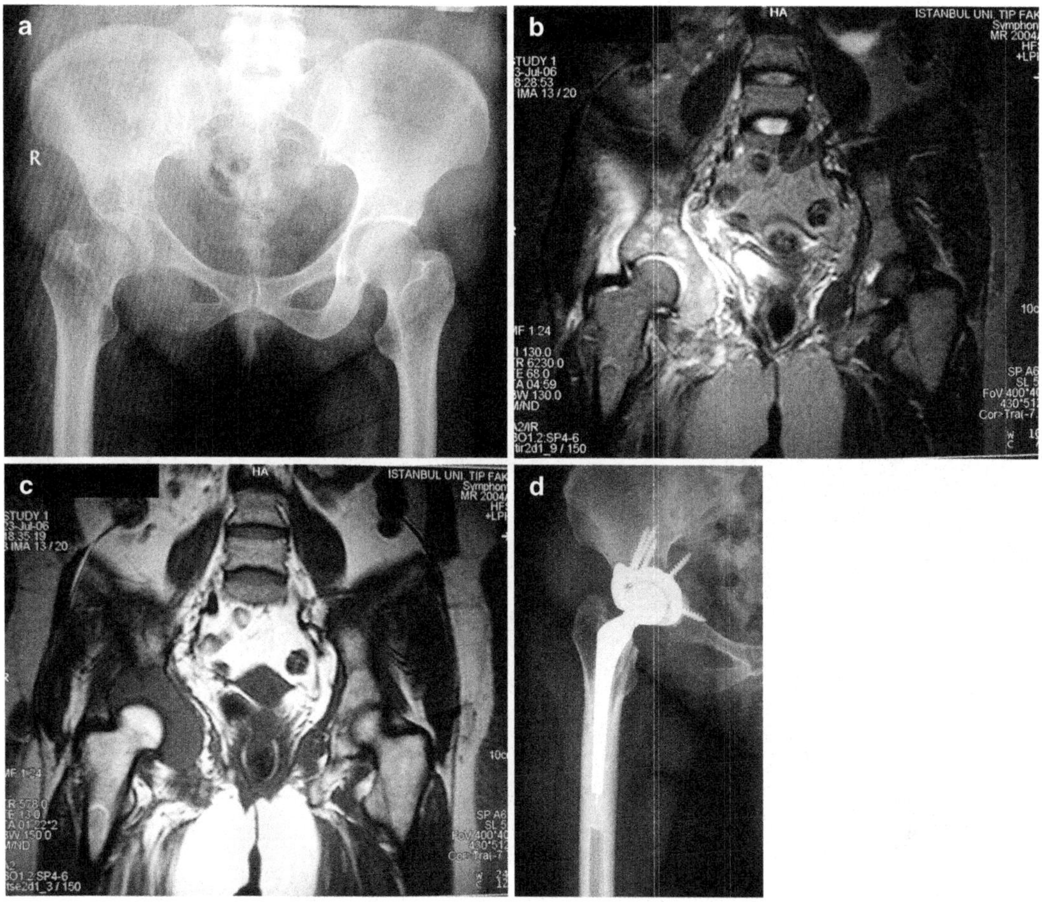

Fig. 43.7 A 41-year-old woman with breast carcinoma metastases to the acetabulum and femoral head. (**a**) AP pelvic radiograph reveals lytic metastatic lesions on the acetabulum, the inferior pubic ramus and the femoral head. (**b, c**) T2- and T1-weighted MRI images, respectively, show the metastatic lesion on the acetabulum. (**d**) Radiograph obtained after the resection of the acetabular metastasis and reconstruction with a cemented total hip arthroplasty, acetabulum reconstructed with an antiprotrusio cage

A calcar replacement prosthesis should be chosen for lesions with extensive bone destruction on the medial side of the proximal femur [27].

The cement acts as an adjuvant chemotherapeutic agent in the medullary canal. Cemented implants are less effective than non-cemented implants along with post- or preoperative irradiation.

Soft tissue coverage is important to avoid prosthetic luxation. A pelvic-hip abduction brace can be used to protect the muscle reattachment sutures during the 6 weeks of soft tissue healing [27].

Subtrochanteric Region

For subtrochanteric impending fractures or pathological fractures, the best treatment choice is an intramedullary nail (nearly the length of the entire femur) fixed with cement (Fig. 43.8). Compared with a plate-nail system (DHS), the nail shares the load and is resistant to bending stresses.

Zickel and Mouradian reported successful results in the treatment of 35 pathological fractures and 11 impending fractures in the subtrochanteric region with a specially designed intramedullary nail [29]. Early mobilization or

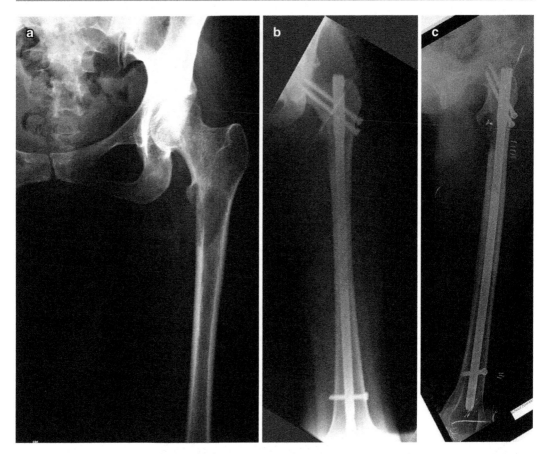

Fig. 43.8 Radiographs of the left femur of a 42-year-old woman with metastatic endometrial carcinoma. (**a**) AP view indicates an osteolytic lesion in the subtrochanteric region. (**b, c**) Biplanar radiographs of the entire femur; stabilization was achieved with an intramedullary reconstruction nail

ambulation was achieved in nearly all of the cases.

The surgeon should avoid creating new fractures during the process of reaming and placing the nail into the canal; for this reason, the nail diameter should be 2 mm smaller than the last reamer used. If there is not enough bone stock, locking screws should be supported with cement.

Proximal femur megaprostheses are potential approaches for lesions that are resistant to medical therapy and have extensive bone destruction of the head, neck, and peritrochanteric region and for which proximal locking screw fixation is not possible.

Diaphyseal Region

Pathological fractures or impending fractures of the shaft region should be treated with an intramedullary nail with or without cement. A plate-screw fixation also provides rigid fixation, but a nail fixation system has a greater long-term advantage.

Distal Femoral Region

Metastatic lesions of the distal femoral region are unusual and difficult to treat. The most common treatment option is open reduction, curettage, and plate fixation with cement.

Retrograde intramedullary nailing can be performed if there is not extensive bone destruction.

If there is extensive bone destruction, a constrained and cemented total knee prosthesis or modular-type distal femoral knee arthroplasty can achieve immediate stability and full weight bearing.

Tibia

Breast cancer metastases of the tibia are rarely observed and mostly occur in the metaphyseal region. The preferred method of treating metaphyseal region metastases is resection and the use of a cemented tibial prosthesis.

Spinal Metastases

Bone metastases of breast cancer are most commonly observed in the spine. Nearly 16–37 % of breast cancer patients develop spinal metastases. Symptomatic vertebral metastatic lesions occur in the thoracic (68–70 %), lumbosacral (16–22 %), and cervical (8–15 %) spine. Vertebrae are common target sites because of the highly vascular vertebral marrow and the extradural Batson's plexus [30, 31]. Some authors believe that the Batson's plexus is the route by which breast cancer cells metastasize to the thoracic spine. Prostate cancer cells similarly use Batson's plexus to metastasize to the lumbar spine.

There is a direct correlation between the vertebral body size and the influence of metastases.

An early diagnosis is essential to improve or preserve neurological function and maximize the quality of life. An early diagnosis is possible with clinical suspicion, and clinical suspicion begins with carefully listening to the patient's history and consequently conducting a detailed clinical examination (Fig. 43.2).

Clinical Presentation, Evaluation, and Imaging

Patients with spinal metastasis primarily complain about axial pain (85–96 %) [32]. The pain is characteristically nonmechanical and progressive, includes severe night pain, and does not resolve with routine painkillers. Extension of the tumor or collapse of the involved vertebra can cause neurologic symptoms. The neurological symptoms depend on which area of the medulla spinalis is involved. Nerve root compression leads to radicular pain, whereas spinal cord compression leads to myelopathy. A proper examination, which includes palpation for local tenderness and determining the limitation of motion and signs of nerve root or spinal cord compression and deformity, is critical. Kyphosis is the most common deformity due to vertebral compression fractures.

Plain radiographs must be obtained in two directions. A vertebral collapse and deformities can be easily observed, but at least 50 % of the bone must be lost to visualize a lesion in a plain radiograph.

Despite negative plain radiographs for a patient with a suspected or known malignancy, a bone scan is necessary. A bone scan can demonstrate skeletal metastases 3–18 months before their appearance on plain radiographs. A bone scan is a highly sensitive test but is not as specific as an MRI scan. MRI can differentiate between compression fractures resulting from osteoporosis and those caused by metastatic lesions [30, 33].

For evaluating spinal lesions, a CT-guided biopsy is safe and is an intervention with low morbidity. A transpedicular approach under fluoroscopic guidance, similar to that used for kyphoplasty, is also safe and associated with low morbidity. The diagnostic accuracy of CT-guided spinal biopsy ranges from 93 % for lytic lesions to 76 % for sclerotic lesions [34].

Indications

There are three indications for the surgical treatment of metastatic disease of the spine: a significant or progressive neurological deficit, deformity progression, and intractable pain. The risk factors for a progressive neurological deficit include osteolytic lesions and pedicle and posterior wall involvement. However, the decision to proceed with surgical intervention is not based on these three factors; the surgical decision must be individualized. Indeed, all treatment modalities for spinal metastasis are palliative, not curative; therefore, a general assessment of the patient's overall health, comorbidities, and life expectancy is important for the decision. The main goal is improving the quality of life, as is the case with other metastatic regions.

Most authors agree that a surgical treatment option is appropriate if the estimated life expectancy is longer than 3 months. Tokuhashi et al. published a scoring system for evaluating the prognosis of cancer patients with spinal metastases [35] (Table 43.2). This scoring system is widely acknowledged.

Kostuik et al. developed a system to evaluate the stability of spinal tumors based on the three-column classification of Denis [36]. This model divides each vertebral segment into two (left and

Table 43.2 Tokuhashi scoring system for preoperative evaluation of patients with a metastatic spine tumor [35]

Parameter	Score
General condition	
Poor	0
Moderate	1
Good	2
No. of extraspinal bone metastases	
≥3	0
1 or 2	1
0	2
No. of metastases in the spine	
≥3	0
2	1
1	2
Metastases to major internal organs	
Irremovable	0
Removable	1
No metastases	2
Primary site of cancer	
Lung, stomach	0
Kidney, liver, uterus, other	1
Thyroid, prostate, breast, rectum	2
Myelopathy	
Complete	0
Incomplete	1
None	2

right) anterior columns, two middle columns, and two posterior columns. The destruction of fewer than three columns is considered to be stable, whereas the destruction of five to six columns is considered to be markedly unstable.

Nonsurgical Treatment

Known metastatic lesions that are not painful and are not at risk of creating instability may be followed without any treatment.

Site-directed radiation, with or without chemotherapy, is the mainstay for treating painful metastatic lesions that do not compromise neural structures [30]. Breast cancer is moderately sensitive. A radiation oncologist should take care not to compromise potential surgical approaches. Additionally, hormone therapy can be used to support bone structure.

Surgical Treatment

The surgical options for treating spinal metastases include the following: an anterior vertebrectomy and stabilization, posterior decompression and stabilization, an anterior/posterior combination approach, vertebroplasty, and kyphoplasty.

Vertebroplasty and kyphoplasty are useful and minimally invasive procedures that can be applied to pathological vertebral compression fractures with minimal deformity, along with the percutaneous injection of bone cement to stabilize the vertebral body. An intact posterior wall and a lack of direct neural compression are important to reduce the risk of complications arising from the extrusion of cement. Furthermore, this procedure is contraindicated in the event that uncorrected coagulopathy is present. A tumor biopsy is often performed with this technique (Fig. 43.9). A study involving 97 cement augmentation procedures performed in 56 patients with various metastatic spinal tumors revealed that an improvement or complete relief of pain was achieved in 84 % of the procedures [37].

For an open surgery, the choice of approach depends on the location of the tumor and the goal of the operation; an anterior, posterior, or lateral approach or a combination of these approaches may be used. The majority of tumors invade the

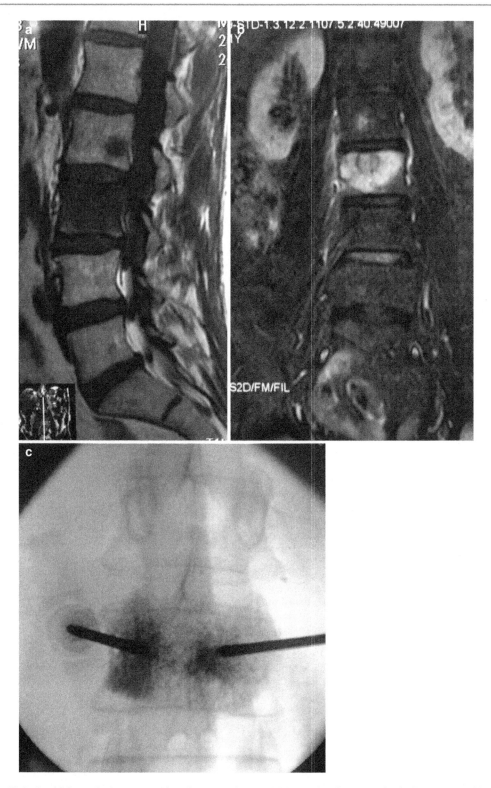

Fig. 43.9 (**a–c**) L3 vertebral metastases from breast carcinoma with impending fracture and pain. Percutaneous biopsy, frozen section, and vertebroplasty. Beware of intact posterior wall, no direct neural compression by the tumor

vertebral body; therefore, the anterior approach may often represent the most direct route to the lesion [37]. Kostuik et al. reported the return of neurological function in 40 % of posterior decompressions and 71 % of anterior decompressions [36]. The posterior approach can provide good visualization and allow persistent stabilization, but the anterior approach prevents excessive normal bone loss [21].

References

1. Jasmin C, Coleman RE, Coia LR, Capanna R, Molloy AP, Saillant G. Textbook of bone metastases. New York: Wiley; 2005.
2. Akhtari M, Mansuri J, Newman KA, Guise TM, Seth P. Biology of breast cancer bone metastasis. Cancer Biol Ther. 2008;7(1):3–9.
3. Theriault RL, Theriault RL. Biology of bone metastases. Cancer Control. 2012;19(2):92–101. Review.
4. Wegener B, Schlemmer M, Stemmler J, Jansson V, Dürr HR, Pietschmann MF. Analysis of orthopedic surgery of bone metastases in breast cancer patients. BMC Musculoskelet Disord. 2012;13(1):232.
5. Wedin R, Bauer HC, Rutqvist LE. Surgical treatment for skeletal breast cancer metastases: a population-based study of 641 patients. Cancer. 2001;92(2):257–62.
6. Boyce BF, Yoneda T, Guise TA. Factors regulating the growth of metastatic cancer in bone. Endocr Relat Cancer. 1999;6:333–47.
7. Mundy GR. Metastasis to bone: causes, consequences and therapeutic opportunities. Nat Rev Cancer. 2002;2:584–93.
8. Suva LJ, Griffin RJ, Makhoul I. Mechanisms of bone metastases of breast cancer. Endocr Relat Cancer. 2009;16(3):703–13.
9. Bhattacharyya S, Byrum S, Siegel ER, Suva LJ. Proteomic analysis of bone cancer: a review of current and future developments. Expert Rev Proteomics. 2007;4:371–8.
10. Hiraga T, Yoneda T. Stimulation of cyclooxygease-2 expression by TGF-β enhances bone metastases in breast cancer. J Bone Miner Res. 2004;19:S129.
11. Coleman RE, Rubens RD. The clinical course of bone metastases from breast cancer. Br J Cancer. 1987;55:61–6.
12. Petrut B, Trinkaus M, Simmons C, Clemons M. A primer of bone metastases management in breast cancer patients. Curr Oncol. 2008;15 Suppl 1:S50–7.
13. Aldridge SE, Lennard TWJ, Williams JR, Birch MA. Vascular endothelial growth factor acts as an osteolytic factor in breast cancer metastases to bone. Br J Cancer. 2005;92:1531–7.
14. Fidler M. Prophylactic internal fixation of secondary neoplastic deposits in long bones. Br Med J. 1973;1(5849):341–3.
15. Harrington KD. New trends in the management of lower extremity metastases. Clin Orthop Relat Res. 1982;169:53–61.
16. Mirels H. Metastatic disease in long bones. A proposed scoring system for diagnosing impending pathologic fractures. Clin Orthop Relat Res. 1989;249:256–64.
17. Katagiri H, Takahashi M, Wakai K, Sugiura H, Kataoka T, Nakanishi K. Prognostic factors and a scoring system for patients with skeletal metastasis. J Bone Joint Surg Br. 2005;87(5):698–703.
18. Attar S, Steffner RJ, Avedian R, Hussain WM. Surgical intervention of nonvertebral osseous metastasis. Cancer Control. 2012;19(2):113–21.
19. Mansel RE, Fodstad O, Jiang WG. Metastasis of breast cancer. Dordrecht: Springer; 2008.
20. Frassica FJ, Frassica DA. Metastatic bone disease of the humerus. J Am Acad Orthop Surg. 2003;11:282–8.
21. Singletary SE, Robb GL, Hortobagyi GN. Advanced therapy of breast disease. Hamilton, USA: BC Decker; 2004.
22. Potter BK, Adams SC, Pitcher Jr JD, Malinin TI, Temple HT. Proximal humerus reconstructions for tumors. Clin Orthop Relat Res. 2009;4:1035–41.
23. Bos G, Sim F, Pritchard D, Shives T, Rock M, Askew L, Chao E. Prosthetic replacement of the proximal humerus. Clin Orthop Relat Res. 1987;224:178–91.
24. Moeckel BH, Dines DM, Warren RF, Altchek DW. Modular hemiarthroplasty for fractures of the proximal part of the humerus. J Bone Joint Surg Am. 1992;74(6):884–9.
25. Redmond BJ, Biermann JS, Blasier RB. Interlocking intramedullary nailing of pathological fractures of the shaft of the humerus. J Bone Joint Surg Am. 1996;78(6):891–6.
26. Damron TA, Sim FH, Shives TC, An KN, Rock MG, Pritchard DJ. Intercalary spacers in the treatment of segmentally destructive diaphyseal humeral lesions in disseminated malignancies. Clin Orthop Relat Res. 1996;324:233–43.
27. Swanson KC, Pritchard DJ, Sim FH. Surgical treatment of metastatic disease of the femur. J Am Acad Orthop Surg. 2000;8(1):56–65.
28. Lane JM, Sculco TP, Zolan S. Treatment of pathological fractures of the hip by endoprosthetic replacement. J Bone Joint Surg Am. 1980;62(6):954–9.
29. Zickel RE, Mouradian WH. Intramedullary fixation of pathological fractures and lesions of the subtrochanteric region of the femur. J Bone Joint Surg Am. 1976;58(8):1061–6.
30. White AP, Kwon BK, Lindskog DM, Friedlaender GE, Grauer JN. Metastatic disease of the spine. J Am Acad Orthop Surg. 2006;14(11):587–98. Review.

31. Batson OV. The function of the vertebral veins and their role in the spread of metastases. Ann Surg. 1940;112(1):138–49.

32. Gilbert RW, Kim JH, Posner JB. Epidural spinal cord compression from metastatic tumor: diagnosis and treatment. Ann Neurol. 1978;3(1):40–51.

33. Chan JH, Peh WC, Tsui EY, Chau LF, Cheung KK, Chan KB, et al. Acute vertebral body compression fractures: discrimination between benign and malignant causes using apparent diffusion coefficients. Br J Radiol. 2002;75(891):207–14.

34. Lis E, Bilsky MH, Pisinski L, Boland P, Healey JH, O'malley B, Krol G. Percutaneous CT-guided biopsy of osseous lesion of the spine in patients with known or suspected malignancy. AJNR Am J Neuroradiol. 2004;25(9):1583–8.

35. Tokuhashi Y, Matsuzaki H, Toriyama S, Kawano H, Ohsaka S. Scoring system for the preoperative evaluation of metastatic spine tumor prognosis. Spine. 1990;15:1110–3.

36. Kostuik JP, Errico TJ, Gleason TF, Errico CC. Spinal stabilization of vertebral column tumors. Spine. 1988;13:250–6.

37. Fourney DR, Schomer DF, Nader R, Chlan-Fourney J, Suki D, Ahrar K, et al. Percutaneous vertebroplasty and kyphoplasty for painful vertebral body fractures in cancer patients. J Neurosurg. 2003; 98(1 Suppl):21–30.

Part VIII

Review of the Breast Cancer Management

A Review of Local and Systemic Therapy in Breast Cancer

44

Adnan Aydiner, Fatma Sen, Hasan Karanlik,
Isik Aslay, Maktav Dincer, and Abdullah İğci

Abstract

In breast cancer, the choice of treatment strategy is based on the features and biology of the tumor as well as on the age, general health status, and personal preferences of the patient. The clinical situations in which molecular tests have the greatest relevance for therapeutic decision-making are still being established; however, evidence is also increasing regarding the breast cancer types in which good predictions of prognosis can be obtained. One of the current challenges in treatment is the selection of the subset of patients who might preferentially benefit from therapy. Optimizing treatment to achieve the best clinical results while minimizing side effects of treatment is also imperative.

Keywords

Adjuvant • Metastatic • Surgery • Radiation treatment • Neoadjuvant • Endocrine treatment • HER2 • Estrogen receptor • Progesterone receptor • Contralateral mastectomy • Breast reconstruction • Skin-sparing mastectomy • Oncoplastic surgery • In situ disease • Invasive disease • Axillary staging • Radiotherapy techniques • Lobular carcinoma in situ • Ductal carcinoma in situ • Preoperative therapy • Triple negative

A. Aydiner, MD (✉) • F. Sen, MD
Department of Medical Oncology, Istanbul University
Istanbul Medical Faculty, Institute of Oncology,
Istanbul, Turkey
e-mail: adnanaydiner@superonline.com

H. Karanlik, MD
Department of Surgery, Istanbul University, Institute
of Oncology, Istanbul, Turkey

I. Aslay, MD
Department of Radiation Oncology, Acibadem
Hospital, Kozyatagi, Istanbul, Turkey

M. Dincer, MD
Department of Radiation Oncology, Florence
Nightingale Hospital, Gayrettepe, Istanbul, Turkey

A. İğci, MD, FRCS
Breast Unit, Department of General Surgery,
Istanbul University, Istanbul Medical Faculty,
Istanbul, Turkey

© Springer International Publishing Switzerland 2016
A. Aydiner et al. (eds.), *Breast Disease: Management and Therapies*,
DOI 10.1007/978-3-319-26012-9_44

731

Proposal levels	
Proposal 1	A full consensus is present based upon a high level of evidence
Proposal 2A	A full consensus is present based on clinical experience and a lower level of evidence
Proposal 2B	A consensus is present but not complete and is based upon a lower level of evidence, including clinical experience (however, there is no significant difference of opinion)

Carcinoma In Situ

The most common types of breast carcinoma in situ are lobular carcinoma in situ (LCIS) and ductal carcinoma in situ (DCIS). The workup for in situ carcinomas includes patient history, physical examination, bilateral mammography, and careful review of pathology. Estrogen receptor (ER) positivity should be assessed in DCIS, whereas it is not recommended in LCIS patients. Breast MRI is not currently a routine workup examination for in situ carcinomas, but may be useful for selected patients.

Lobular Carcinoma In Situ

If LCIS is not diagnosed based on excisional biopsy, surgical excision must be performed, and patients with pure LCIS should be counseled on risk-reduction strategies [1]. Pleomorphic LCIS and/or multifocal/multicentric LCIS may behave similarly to DCIS; thus, surgical excision with negative margins may be considered (Proposal 2A) [2].

Ductal Carcinoma In Situ

The standard treatment of ductal carcinoma in situ (DCIS) is breast-conserving lumpectomy with negative surgical margins (without axillary intervention) and whole-breast radiation (Proposal 1) [3]. If negative margins cannot be attained by breast-conserving surgery, mastectomy must be performed (Proposal 2A) [4].

Patients should be evaluated for hereditary breast cancer risk, and genetic counseling should be provided to DCIS patients with high-risk features (Proposal 2A).

Sentinel node biopsy should be routinely performed in patients with high-grade ductal carcinoma in situ who will undergo mastectomy or for whom breast-conserving surgery will not allow further sentinel node biopsy in the case of future recurrences (Proposal 2A) [5].

Re-excision is not required for surgical margins of 2–5 mm in DCIS (Proposal 2A). Multifocality and an increasing number of close or involved margins have been identified as predictive of additional disease on re-excision. These factors may be surrogate markers of an increased extent of disease. If the surgical margin is less than 1 mm at the skin or chest wall, boost radiation at a higher dose to the involved site should be provided instead of re-excision (Proposal 2B) [6]. Recent consensus guidelines issued jointly by the Society of Surgical Oncology and the American Society for Radiation Oncology, which recommend "no ink on tumor" as the standard for an adequate margin in invasive cancer, caution that these findings cannot be extrapolated to DCIS.

Radiotherapy

If total mastectomy is performed with negative margins, adjuvant irradiation is not required. If nipple-sparing mastectomy and reconstruction are performed, nipple-areola complex irradiation is not standard. Breast tissue that is inadvertently left under the skin flaps should not be an indication for postoperative radiotherapy.

In cases treated with lumpectomy, the use of adjuvant radiotherapy with partial breast irradiation (PBI) techniques is under investigation in randomized trials; according to the American Society for Radiation Oncology and other groups, such an approach should be considered "with caution" [7–10]. Lumpectomy without radiotherapy has been investigated in prospective and randomized trials in patients considered to be at low risk for local recurrence [11, 12]. In such low-risk DCIS patients, whole-breast radiotherapy should be considered in the decision-making process with the patient, accounting for age, comorbidities, radiation risks, patient preferences, and salvage options [13]. Radiotherapy following breast-conserving surgery is optional in DCIS patients with low-risk features (>60 years old, ER-positive, tumor diameter <1 cm, low grade, negative margins, no palpable mass) (Proposal 2B) [14]. For a patient to be considered a low-risk DCIS case, the following criteria must be present: mammographic detection, no palpable mass, small tumor, ER positivity, nuclear grade I or II, and clear surgical margins of at least 3 mm [13]. All other DCIS cases treated with lumpectomy are candidates for whole-breast irradiation (Proposal 1) [15–18].

The benefit of tamoxifen in ER-negative DCIS patients to reduce the risk of breast cancer recurrence after breast-conserving surgery and radiotherapy is uncertain, and tamoxifen should not be routinely recommended to ER-negative DCIS patients. Tamoxifen may be given to reduce the contralateral breast cancer risk in both premenopausal and postmenopausal patients with ER-positive DCIS after mastectomy (Proposal 2A) [19]. Anastrozole can be a safe and effective alternative endocrine therapy for postmenopausal women (particularly, in patients younger than 60 years old), with ER-positive or PR-positive DCIS [20].

Invasive Breast Cancer

Diagnosis

Personal and family histories; physical examination; complete blood count; blood biochemistry, including liver function tests and alkaline phosphatase levels; mammography; and pathology review, including receptor status determination, are the main components of a breast cancer workup.

For clinically early-stage disease (without N2 or T4 and with M0), screening for systemic metastasis in the absence of symptoms or signs of tumor spread should not be routinely performed before surgery in all patients (Proposal 2A). Only patients with symptomatic stage 1–2 disease should be screened for systemic metastasis. Before surgery, bone scintigraphy (Proposal 2B) and thoracoabdominal imaging methods such as CT or MRI (Proposal 2A) may be performed in patients with clinically stage IIIA disease (T3N1M0). Positron emission tomography (PET-CT) is not a routine diagnostic or screening test in stage IIIA (T3N1M0) disease unless standard staging tests cannot determine if metastasis is present (Proposal 2A).

Breast MRI is not a routine diagnostic test for all breast cancer patients, except under special conditions. Breast MRI may be performed to determine the multifocality/multicentricity of the tumor and to screen the contralateral breast for cancer when mammography and breast ultrasonography are inconclusive for malignancy (Proposal 2A) [21]. In patients with occult axillary involvement, breast MRI can be used to detect a primary breast tumor that was not diagnosed with routine diagnostic tests such as mammography and breast ultrasonography (Proposal 2A) [21]. In addition, in patients with Paget's disease who desire breast-conserving surgery, breast MRI may be performed to evaluate the breast for any additional invasive tumor (Proposal 2A). Patients with dense breast tissue should be routinely examined with breast MRI (Proposal 2B). Breast MRI must be performed only with breast coil-containing machines and must be evaluated by a radiologist with breast MRI expertise. For suspicious breast lesions, biopsy with wire localization should be performed if possible; otherwise, patients with suspicious lesions must be referred to centers that can provide further investigation (Proposal 2A).

Pathology

The pathology report must provide uniform information regarding the tumor and should include at least the parameters recommended in the ASCO-CAP guidelines (Proposal 2A). Ki67 should be included in all breast cancer pathology reports (Proposal 2B) [22].

For surgical margin evaluation, pins, inking or any other marking should be applied to the surgical specimen for orientation. In addition, the microscopic margin status and tumor type (DCIS or invasive carcinoma) near the surgical margin must be clearly defined (Proposal 2A) [23].

An extensive intraductal component can be defined as breast cancer if the DCIS volume is greater than 25 % of the invasive tumor volume and if the DCIS component is spreading to the normal breast parenchyma (Proposal 2A).

Molecular subtypes of breast cancer can be distinguished with common pathological variables, including ER, progesterone receptor (PR), HER2, and the Ki67 index (Proposal 2A). In HER2-negative breast cancer, the ER and PR statuses are not sufficient to distinguish "luminal A" subtype from "luminal B." However, by including the Ki67 proliferation index status, "luminal A" can be defined as ER+, PR+, HER2-, and low Ki67 proliferation index tumors (Proposal 2A) [24]. "Luminal B" can be defined as ER+, PR- (<20 % positive), HER2-, and/or high Ki67 proliferation index tumors (Proposal 2A) [24]. Tumors with Ki67 ≥20–29 should be accepted as having a high proliferation index, and tumors with Ki67 <15 should be accepted as having a low proliferation index, although the standardization of Ki67 tests between laboratories remains problematic (Proposal 2A).

"Basal-like/triple-negative breast cancer" may be CK5/6+ and/or EGFR+ (Proposal 2A). Chemotherapy should be included in adjuvant regimens according to the intrinsic tumor subtype (Proposal 2A). The decision regarding cytotoxic treatment (whether to use anthracycline, etc.) as an adjuvant regimen should not be planned based solely on the intrinsic tumor subtype (Proposal 2B).

Multigene expression array profiling is not required for subtype definition in all cases after clinicopathological assessment (Proposal 2A). In "luminal B" (HER2-negative) patients and lymph node-negative, ER+, and HER2- patients, multigene signature profiling may be performed (Proposal 2B), whereas in node-positive, ER+, and HER2- patients, multigene signature profiling is not required (Proposal 2B) [25]. However, the number of involved lymph nodes may change the decision regarding multigene signature [24].

The percentage of hormone receptor positivity required to designate a tumor as hormone receptor positive and, consequently, to initiate endocrine therapy should be 1 % (Proposal 2A).

In endocrine-responsive breast cancer patients, 21-gene RS should be used to select patients who might benefit from receiving adjuvant chemotherapy (Proposal 2B) [26]. The 70-gene signature may be used as an alternative to 21-gene RS for deciding whether to use adjuvant chemotherapy (Proposal 2B). Predicting chemotherapy response differs from predicting prognosis. Thus, the currently used 21-gene RS and 70-gene signature predict only the recurrence risk and thus should not be directly used to predict the chemotherapy response of a tumor.

In hormone receptor-positive tumors, in the case of inflammatory breast cancer, the involvement of ≥4 lymph nodes or a low ER% is an indication for adjuvant chemotherapy, and further molecular diagnostic tests can be omitted (Proposal 2A). Young age, grade 3 disease, one to three positive nodes, lymphovascular invasion, and large tumor size are not adequate features to omit molecular diagnostics in the decision to apply adjuvant chemotherapy [27]. However, in some patients, combinations of these features may be adequate in the decision to apply chemotherapy.

The data regarding the pathological characteristics of tumor stroma, such as immunocyte infiltration, microvascular density, or stromal p16 staining, are insufficient to influence therapy choice in routine clinical practice.

Determination of the tumor grade should be based on the invasive ductal component of mixed type or metaplastic breast cancer (Proposal 2A).

Heterogeneous HER2 overexpression, concomitant estrogen receptor expression, and polysomy 17, as well as the degree of tumor proliferation, should not affect the decision to apply anti-HER2 treatment.

Surgical Approach in Invasive Breast Cancer

The choice of treatment strategy is based on tumor features (location and size of the tumor, number of lesions, extent of lymph node involvement) and biology (pathology, including biomarkers and gene expression) and on the patient's age, general health status, and personal preferences. Patients should be actively involved in all management decisions. The possibility of hereditary cancer should be explored, and, if necessary, prophylactic procedures should be discussed following appropriate genetic counseling and testing of the patient. In younger premenopausal patients, possible fertility issues should be discussed, and guidance regarding fertility preservation techniques should be provided before treatment initiation [28–38].

Breast-conserving therapy, axillary lymph node dissection, and whole-breast irradiation are equivalent to mastectomy, with axillary lymph node dissection as the primary treatment for most women with stage I and stage II breast cancers (Proposal 1) [39–42].

Lumpectomy is contraindicated for patients who are pregnant and would require radiotherapy during pregnancy, who have diffuse disease that cannot be locally removed via a single incision with an acceptable cosmetic result, who have widespread suspicious or malignant-appearing microcalcifications on mammography, or who have positive pathological margins after surgery. Patients with pathologically positive margins generally should undergo re-excision to achieve negative pathological margins. If the margins remain positive after re-excision, mastectomy should be performed to achieve optimal local disease control.

Relative contraindications for lumpectomy include previous radiation therapy to the breast or chest wall, an active connective tissue disease involving the skin such as scleroderma and lupus, tumors larger than 5 cm (Proposal 2B), and focally positive pathological margins. Those patients with focally positive pathological margins who do not undergo re-excision should be considered for a higher radiation boost dose to the tumor bed. To adequately assess margins following lumpectomy, surgical specimens should be oriented, and the pathologist should provide descriptions of the gross and microscopic margin statuses and the distance, orientation, and type of tumor in relation to the closest margin. A careful histological assessment of resection margins is essential, with the requirement that no tumor be present at the inked margin [43]. Marking the tumor bed with clips facilitates accurate planning of the radiation boost field where appropriate. Acceptably low local recurrence rates remain the major quality assurance target. Current guidelines recommend that local recurrence rates after wide excision and radiotherapy should be <1 % per year (with a target of <0.5 %) and should not exceed 10 % overall.

Contralateral Mastectomy

Only limited data are available on the survival impact of contralateral mastectomy in unilateral breast cancer [44]. Women with breast cancer who are ≤35 years of age or premenopausal and carriers of a known BRCA1/2 mutation may be recommended additional risk-reduction strategies following appropriate risk assessment and counseling. The lifetime risk of breast cancer in a BRCA1 carrier is 80–85 %, with a 10-year actuarial risk of contralateral breast cancer ranging from 25 % to 31 %. With bilateral mastectomy, the risk of subsequent breast cancer incidence and mortality are both reduced by ~90–95 %. A decision should be made by a multidisciplinary team prior to surgery and should include a discussion of the risks associated with the development of contralateral breast cancer compared with the risks associated with recurrent disease from the primary cancer. Except as specifically outlined in some situations, prophylactic mastectomy of the breast contralateral to unilateral breast cancer treated with mastectomy is discouraged. The use of prophylactic mastectomy contralateral to the breast treated with breast-conserving surgery is very strongly discouraged in all patients.

Despite the overall trend toward breast conservation, increasing numbers of breast cancer patients are opting for bilateral mastectomy (incorporating contralateral risk-reducing surgery) over breast conservation and mammographic surveillance of the irradiated breast. These patients should be properly counseled and informed of the finding that patients with early-stage breast cancer may have a superior outcome after breast-conserving therapy compared with mastectomy.

Axillary Staging

Sentinel lymph node (SLN) mapping and surgical excision of clinically lymph node-negative axilla are recommended to evaluate the pathological status of the axillary lymph nodes (ALNs) in patients with stage I or stage II breast cancer (Proposal 2A) [45–51]. This recommendation is supported by the results of randomized clinical trials revealing decreased arm and shoulder morbidity such as pain, lymphedema, and sensory loss in patients with breast cancer undergoing SLN biopsy compared with patients undergoing standard ALN dissection [51, 52]. An experienced SLN team is required for SLN mapping and excision [53, 54]. With appropriate training in the dual radiocolloid/blue dye or indocyanine green fluorescence technique, acceptably low false-negative rates and favorable axillary recurrence rates following SLNB are achievable. Women with invasive breast cancer and without access to an experienced SLN team should be referred to an experienced SLN team for definitive surgical breast cancer treatment and ALN staging. Candidates for SLN mapping should have clinically negative ALNs or a negative fine-needle aspiration (FNA) biopsy of any clinically suspicious ALN. There is no consensus for the pathological assessment of SLNB. The significance of occult micrometastases in terms of surgical management and patient outcomes appears to be negligible. Thus, routine IHC or PCR is not recommended for the evaluation of sentinel

lymph nodes; treatment decisions should be made based on H&E staining [55].

Multiple attempts have been made to identify cohorts of women with SLN involvement at sufficiently low risk of non-SLN involvement. In these low risk patients complete axillary dissection might be avoided if the SLN is positive. None of the early studies identified a low-risk group of patients with positive SLN biopsies but consistently negative non-sentinel nodes [56–61]. Nonetheless, a randomized trial (ACOSOG Z0011) compared SLN resection alone to ALN dissection in women ≥18 years of age with T1/T2 tumors and fewer than 3 positive SLNs in women who were undergoing breast-conserving surgery and whole-breast irradiation. In this study, there was no difference in local recurrence, DFS, or OS between the two treatment groups. Only ER-negative status, age <50, and a lack of adjuvant systemic therapy were associated with decreased OS. At a median follow-up of 6.3 years, locoregional recurrences were noted in 4.1 % of patients in the ALN dissection group and 2.8 % of patients in the SLN dissection group ($p = 0.11$). The median OS was approximately 92 % in each group [62]. In addition to this study, the results of the IBCSG 23-01 trial indicate that further axillary treatment is not required when a sentinel node has micrometastasis (0.2–2 mm) [63]. Therefore, according to all of these results, patients with T1 or T2 tumors and one to two positive SLNs who are undergoing lumpectomy plus tangential breast irradiation may not require any further axillary procedure. However, these results must be confirmed and cannot be extended to patients with characteristics that differ from those of the patient population in the trial.

Level I or II axillary dissection should be recommended (1) in patients with clinically positive nodes confirmed by FNA or core biopsy at the time of diagnosis or (2) in patients in whom sentinel nodes are not identified. Traditional level I and level II ALN evaluation requires the removal of at least ten lymph nodes for pathological evaluation to accurately stage the axilla [64, 65]. Level III ALN dissection should be performed only if gross disease is apparent in the level II nodes. Level I–II lymph node dissection should include the tissue that is inferior to the axillary vein from the latissimus dorsi muscle and lateral to the medial border of the pectoralis minor muscle.

Furthermore, without definitive data demonstrating superior survival compared to ALN dissection or SLN resection, these procedures should be considered optional in patients with particularly favorable tumors, in patients for whom the selection of adjuvant systemic therapy will not be affected by the results of the procedure, in elderly patients, and in patients with serious comorbidities. Patients with SLN metastasis but no ALN dissection or irradiation are at increased risk of ipsilateral lymph node recurrence [66].

Surgical Approach After Primary Systemic Therapy

Primary systemic chemotherapy (preoperative chemotherapy) should be considered for women with large clinical stage IIA, stage IIB, and T3N1 tumors who meet the criteria for breast-conserving therapy except tumor size and who wish to undergo breast-conserving therapy. In patients who are anticipated to receive preoperative systemic therapy, a core biopsy of the breast tumor and the placement of an image-detectable marker should be considered to demarcate the tumor bed for any future post-chemotherapeutic surgical management. Clinically positive ALN should be sampled by FNA or core biopsy, and positive nodes must be removed following preoperative systemic therapy at the time of the definitive operation. Patients with clinically negative ALNs should undergo axillary ultrasound prior to neoadjuvant treatment. For those with clinically suspicious ALNs, core biopsy or FNA of these nodes is indicated [67]. If FNA or core biopsy indicates any positive nodes, these nodes should be removed following neoadjuvant therapy at the time of definitive surgery.

Sentinel lymph node biopsy or level I/II dissection can be performed as axillary staging after preoperative systemic therapy. Level I/II dissection should be performed when patients are proven node positive prior to neoadjuvant therapy (Proposal 2B). The false-negative rate of SLN biopsy in either the pre- or post-chemotherapy setting is low [50, 68–71]. However, a pathological complete response (pCR) following chemotherapy may occur in lymph node metastases previously undetected by clinical exam. An SLN excision can be considered before administering preoperative systemic therapy because it provides additional information to guide local and systemic treatment decisions. Close communication between members of the multidisciplinary team, including the pathologist, is particularly important when any treatment strategy involving preoperative systemic therapy is planned.

Because complete or near-complete clinical responses are common, the use of percutaneously placed clips into the breast under mammographic or ultrasound guidance aids in post-chemotherapeutic resection of the original tumor area and is encouraged. Breast conservation rates are higher following preoperative systemic therapy [72].

Local therapy following a complete or partial response to preoperative systemic therapy is generally lumpectomy, if possible, along with surgical axillary staging. If lumpectomy is not possible or if progressive disease is confirmed, mastectomy is performed along with surgical axillary staging with or without breast reconstruction. Surgical axillary staging may include SLN biopsy or level I/II dissection. If SLN biopsy was performed before administering preoperative systemic therapy and the findings were negative, then further ALN staging is not necessary. If an SLN procedure was performed before administering preoperative systemic therapy and the findings were positive, then a level I/II ALN dissection should be performed.

Patients with stage III disease may be further classified as (1) those for whom an initial surgical approach is unlikely to successfully remove all disease or to provide long-term local control and (2) those with disease for which a reasonable initial surgical approach is likely to achieve pathologically negative margins and provide long-term local control. Thus, stage IIIA patients are divided into those who have clinical T3N1 disease versus those who have clinical T any, N2, M0 disease, based on evaluation by a multidisciplinary team.

In patients with inoperable, locally advanced, non-inflammatory disease, anthracycline-based preoperative systemic therapy is the standard therapy. Local therapy following a clinical response to preoperative systemic therapy usually comprises mastectomy or lumpectomy with level I/II ALN dissection [72–74]. Delayed breast reconstruction can be considered in mastectomy patients.

Patients with a clinical/pathological diagnosis of inflammatory breast cancer (IBC) should always be treated with preoperative chemotherapy [75, 76]. Primary surgery and SLN dissection are not reliable approaches in patients with IBC [77].

The use of breast-conserving surgery in patients with IBC has been associated with poor cosmesis, and limited data suggest that local recurrence rates may be higher compared with mastectomy. Breast-conserving therapy is not recommended for patients with IBC.

Mastectomy with level I/II ALN dissection is the recommended surgical procedure for patients with IBC who respond to neoadjuvant chemotherapy. Delayed breast reconstruction is an option for patients with IBC who have undergone a modified radical mastectomy. Early/immediate reconstruction after mastectomy may compromise the postmastectomy radiotherapy outcomes [78].

For patients with IBC who do not respond to preoperative systemic therapy, mastectomy is not generally recommended. Additional systemic chemotherapy and/or preoperative radiation should be considered for these patients, and patients responding to this secondary therapy should undergo mastectomy and subsequent treatment as described above.

Breast Reconstruction

Breast reconstruction may be an option for any woman receiving surgical treatment for breast cancer. Therefore, all women undergoing breast cancer treatment should be educated about breast reconstructive options adapted to their individual clinical situation. However, breast reconstruction should not interfere with the appropriate surgical management of cancer.

The decision regarding the type of reconstruction includes the patient's preference, body habitus, smoking history, comorbidities, and plans for irradiation, as well as the reconstruction team's expertise and experience. Reconstruction is an optional procedure that does not impact the probability of recurrence or death but is associated with improved quality of life for many patients. It is sometimes necessary to perform surgery on the contralateral breast (e.g., breast reduction, implantation) to achieve optimal symmetry between the ipsilateral reconstructed breast and the contralateral breast.

The cosmetic, body image, and psychosocial issues caused by breast loss may be partially overcome by breast reconstruction. Reconstruction can be performed either immediately following mastectomy under the same anesthetic or in a delayed manner following mastectomy. Breast reconstruction usually involves a staged approach requiring more than one procedure.

Many factors must be considered in the decision-making process regarding breast reconstruction following mastectomy. Several different types of breast reconstruction, such as autogenous tissue use, implant use, or both, can be performed following mastectomy [79–81]. Reconstruction with implants can be performed either by immediately placing a permanent subpectoral implant or by initially placing a subpectoral expander and then replacing the expander with a permanent implant. Autogenous tissue reconstruction methods use various combinations of donor sites (e.g., abdomen, buttocks) that may be brought to the chest wall with their original blood supply or as free flaps with microvascular anastomoses to supply blood from the chest wall/thorax. Several procedures using autologous tissue are available, including transverse rectus abdominis myocutaneous flap, latissimus dorsi flap, and gluteus maximus myocutaneous flap reconstructions. Composite reconstruction techniques use implants in combination with autogenous tissue reconstruction to provide volume and symmetry. Patients with underlying diabetes or who smoke tobacco have increased rates of complications following autogenous tissue breast reconstruction, presumably due to underlying microvascular disease.

Skin-Sparing Mastectomy

Possible advantages of skin-sparing mastectomy include improvements in breast cosmesis, body image, and nipple sensation following mastectomy, although the impact of this procedure on these quality-of-life issues has not been well studied [82–84]. Limited data with short follow-up periods are available from surgical series suggesting that performance of nipple-areolar complex (NAC)-sparing mastectomy in selected patients is associated with low rates of occult NAC involvement in breast cancer and local disease recurrence. NAC-sparing procedures may be an option in patients who are carefully selected by experienced multidisciplinary teams. The assessment of retroareolar margins is mandatory in patients considering an NAC-sparing procedure [83, 85, 86]. Retrospective studies have validated the use of NAC-sparing procedures for breast cancer patients with low rates of nipple involvement and low rates of local recurrence due to early-stage, biologically favorable tumors located >2 cm away from the nipple [87, 88]. Contraindications for nipple preservation include findings of nipple involvement such as Paget's disease or bloody nipple discharge. Prospective trials to assess NAC-sparing mastectomy in the setting of malignancy are ongoing, and participation in these trials is encouraged.

Although no randomized studies have been performed, the results of several retrospective studies have indicated that the risk of local recurrence is not increased in patients receiving skin-sparing mastectomies compared to those undergoing non-skin-sparing procedures. However, strong selection biases almost certainly exist in the identification of patients who are appropriate for skin-sparing procedures [89–93].

NAC reconstruction may also be performed in a delayed fashion if desired by the patient. Reconstructed nipples are devoid of sensation. Skin-sparing mastectomy should be performed by an experienced breast surgery team working in a coordinated, multidisciplinary fashion to guide proper patient selection for skin-sparing mastectomy, determine optimal sequencing of the reconstructive procedure in relation to adjuvant therapies, and perform a resection that achieves appropriate surgical margins. Postmastectomy radiation should still be applied for patients treated by skin-sparing mastectomy, following the same selection criteria as for standard mastectomy.

Postmastectomy Radiation and Breast Reconstruction

The decision regarding postmastectomy radiation therapy can affect reconstruction strategies because of the increased risk of complications such as capsular contracture following implant irradiation. Postmastectomy radiation therapy may also have a negative impact on breast cosmesis when autologous tissue is used in immediate breast reconstruction [94, 95]. Some studies, however, have not achieved a significant compromise in reconstruction cosmesis following irradiation [96]. While some experienced breast cancer teams have employed protocols in which immediate tissue reconstructions are followed by radiation therapy, radiation therapy preceding placement of the autologous tissue is generally preferred because of the reported loss in reconstruction cosmesis (Proposal 2B).

When implant reconstruction is planned in a patient requiring radiation therapy, a two-staged approach with immediate tissue expander placement followed by implant placement is recommended. The exchange of tissue expanders with permanent implants can be performed prior to radiation or after the completion of radiation therapy. The expansion of irradiated skin can result in increased risks of malpositioning, capsular contracture, poor cosmesis, and implant exposure. The use of tissue expanders/implants is relatively contraindicated in patients who have been previously irradiated. Immediate implant placement in patients requiring postoperative radiation has an increased rate of complications such as capsular contracture, malpositioning, poor cosmesis, and implant exposure.

Breast Reconstruction Following Lumpectomy (Oncoplastic Approach)

The goal of optimizing the cosmetic and oncological outcomes of breast-conserving surgery has been addressed in recent years by the emergence of the field of oncoplastic surgery. The possible cosmetic outcome of lumpectomy should be evaluated prior to surgery. Oncoplastic techniques for breast conservation can extend breast-conserving surgical options in situations in which the resection itself would likely yield an unacceptable cosmetic outcome [97]. The definition of oncoplastic surgery has more recently been expanded to include a wide range of volume displacement or redistribution procedures performed by breast surgeons and general surgeons to optimize breast shape and volume following breast cancer surgery [98]. Oncoplastic volume displacement procedures combine the removal of generous regions of breast tissue with "mastopexy" techniques in which remaining breast tissues are shifted together within the breast envelope to fill the resulting surgical defect, thereby avoiding the creation of a significant breast deformity. Volume displacement techniques are generally performed in the same operative setting as the breast-conserving lumpectomy and by the same surgeon performing the cancer resection [97–99].

Oncoplastic volume displacement techniques are advantageous because they permit the removal of larger regions of breast tissue, thereby achieving wider surgical margins around the tumor while better preserving the natural shape and appearance of the breast compared to standard breast resections [100].

The limitations of oncoplastic volume displacement techniques include a lack of standardization among centers, restriction to a limited number of facilities, and the potential need for subsequent mastectomy if pathological margins are positive. Patients should be informed of the possibility of positive margins and the potential need for a secondary surgery, which could include re-excision segmental resection or mastectomy with or without nipple loss. Oncoplastic procedures can be combined with surgery on the contralateral unaffected breast to minimize long-term asymmetry.

The primary focus should be on treatment of the tumor, and such treatment should not be compromised when making decisions regarding breast reconstruction.

Adjuvant Systemic Treatment in Invasive Breast Cancer

Chemotherapy

All patients with invasive breast cancer should be evaluated for the need for adjuvant cytotoxic, trastuzumab, and/or endocrine therapy. When indicated, adjuvant cytotoxic chemotherapy should begin 2–8 weeks following surgery. If adjuvant endocrine (either tamoxifen or aromatase inhibitor (AI)) and cytotoxic therapy are indicated, chemotherapy should precede endocrine therapy.

Older age is not a contraindication for cytotoxic chemotherapy. Adjuvant treatment should be considered regardless of patient age (Proposal 1). The available data are insufficient to make specific recommendations for older age groups [101].

The positivity of any lymph node should not be the sole indication for adjuvant chemotherapy [27]. However, patients with more than three involved lymph nodes, low hormone receptor positivity, HER2-positive status, triple-negative status, a high 21-gene RS (e.g., >25), and a high-risk 70-gene score should receive adjuvant chemotherapy (Proposal 1–2A). A high Ki67 proliferation index and a histological grade 3 tumor are acceptable indications for adjuvant chemotherapy (Proposal 2A). Lymphovascular invasion without any other poor prognostic factor is not an indication for cytotoxic chemotherapy (Proposal 2B).

Breast cancers with a luminal A phenotype are less responsive to chemotherapy; patients with luminal A breast cancer may thus receive less intensive chemotherapy regimens, including four cycles of doxorubicin and cyclophosphamide (AC); six cycles of cyclophosphamide, methotrexate, and fluorouracil (CMF); or four cycles of docetaxel and cyclophosphamide (TC) (Proposal 2A) [101]. High tumor volume may be an indication for adjuvant chemotherapy (Proposal 2B) [102, 103].

A luminal B phenotype is an indication for adjuvant chemotherapy in most patients (Proposal 2B). If adjuvant chemotherapy is provided, patients with luminal B breast cancer should receive chemotherapy regimens containing at least six courses of anthracyclines and taxanes, rather than CMF (Proposal 2B). Patients with luminal B breast cancer may receive dose-dense chemotherapy (Proposal 2B) (Tables 44.1, 44.2, and 44.3).

There is no preferred adjuvant chemotherapy regimen for HER2+ early-stage breast cancer, but taxanes and/or anthracyclines must be part of the adjuvant chemotherapy regimen (Proposal 2A). HER2+ tumors with a diameter of less than 0.5 cm (T1a) may receive chemotherapy plus trastuzumab. HER2+ tumors with a diameter of 0.5–1.0 cm should be considered for adjuvant chemotherapy plus trastuzumab (Proposal 2A), and those larger than 1 cm (T1c-T4N0M0) require chemotherapy plus trastuzumab (Proposal 1). When chemotherapy is contraindicated, trastuzumab may be administered either alone or with endocrine therapy [104].

Trastuzumab should not be administered with anthracyclines, but should be provided concurrently with taxanes. ER positivity or negativity should not alter the decision regarding adjuvant trastuzumab, if otherwise indicated. The preferred duration of trastuzumab therapy is 1 year (Proposal 1) [104] (Tables 44.4, 44.5, 44.6, and 44.7).

Adjuvant chemotherapy is not recommended for patients with triple-negative invasive breast cancers with a diameter of less than 0.5 cm (T1aN0M0) (Proposal 2A). Patients with T1b and larger tumors should receive adjuvant cyto-

Table 44.1 Adjuvant or neoadjuvant systemic treatment in HER2-negative breast cancer – preferred

Regimen	Drug	Dosage (mg/m^2)	Frequency of cycles
4× dose-dense AC followed by 4× twoweekly paclitaxel			
AC[a]	Doxorubicin	60	Day 1
			Cycled every 14 days
	Cyclophosphamide	600	Day 1
			Cycled every 14 days
Paclitaxel[a]	Paclitaxel	175	Day 1
			Cycled every 14 days
4× dose-dense AC followed by 12× weekly paclitaxel			
AC[a]	Doxorubicin	60	Day 1
			Cycled every 14 days
	Cyclophosphamide	600	Day 1
			Cycled every 14 days
Paclitaxel	Paclitaxel	80	Day 1
			Cycled every 7 days
TC			
TC[a]	Docetaxel	75	Day 1
			Cycled every 21 days
	Cyclophosphamide	600	Day 1
			Cycled every 21 days

All drugs recommended in this table must be administered intravenously
[a]All cycles should be administered with lenograstim or filgrastim support

Table 44.2 Adjuvant or neoadjuvant anthracycline-based systemic treatment in HER2-negative breast cancer – others

Regimen	Drug	Dosage (mg/m²)	Frequency of cycles
4× dose-dense AC			
AC[a,c]	Doxorubicin	60	Day 1
			Cycled every 14 days
	Cyclophosphamide	600	Day 1
			Cycled every 14 days
4× AC			
AC[a]	Doxorubicin	60	Day 1
			Cycled every 21 days
	Cyclophosphamide	600	Day 1
			Cycled every 21 days
6× FAC			
FAC[a]	5-Fluorouracil	500	Days 1 and 8 or days 1 and 4
			Cycled every 21 days
	Doxorubicin	50	Day 1
			Cycled every 21 days
	Cyclophosphamide	500	Day 1
			Cycled every 21 days
6× CAF			
CAF	5-Fluorouracil[a]	500	Days 1 and 8
			Cycled every 28 days
	Doxorubicin[a]	30	Days 1 and 8
			Cycled every 28 days
	Cyclophosphamide[b]	100	Days 1–14
			Cycled every 28 days
8× EC			
EC[a]	Epirubicin	100	Day 1
			Cycled every 21 days
	Cyclophosphamide	830	Day 1
			Cycled every 21 days
6× CEF			
CEF	Cyclophosphamide[b]	75	Days 1–14
			Cycled every 28 days
	Epirubicin[a]	60	Days 1 and 8
			Cycled every 28 days
	5-Fluorouracil[a]	500	Days 1 and 8
			Cycled every 28 days
6× CMF			
CMF	Cyclophosphamide[b]	100	Once daily on days 1–14
			Cycled every 28 days
	Methotrexate[a]	40	Days 1 and 8
			Cycled every 28 days
	5-Fluorouracil[a]	600	Days 1 and 8
			Cycled every 28 days

[a]The drug(s) recommended must be administered intravenously
[b]The drug(s) recommended should be administered perorally
[c]All cycles should be administered with lenograstim or filgrastim support

Table 44.3 Adjuvant or neoadjuvant anthracycline plus taxane-based systemic treatment in HER2-negative breast cancer – others

Regimen	Drug	Dosage (mg/m²)	Frequency of cycles
4× AC followed by 4× docetaxel			
AC	Doxorubicin	60	Day 1
			Cycled every 21 days
	Cyclophosphamide	600	Day 1
			Cycled every 21 days
Docetaxel[a]	Docetaxel[a]	100	Day 1
			Cycled every 21 days
4× AC followed by 12× weekly paclitaxel			
AC	Doxorubicin	60	Day 1
			Cycled every 21 days
	Cyclophosphamide	600	Day 1
			Cycled every 21 days
Paclitaxel	Paclitaxel	80	Weekly
3× FEC followed by 3× docetaxel			
FEC[a]	5-Fluorouracil	500	Day 1
			Cycled every 21 days
	Epirubicin	100	Day 1
			Cycled every 21 days
	Cyclophosphamide	500	Day 1
			Cycled every 21 days
Docetaxel[a]	Docetaxel	100	Day 1
			Cycled every 21 days
4× FEC followed by 8× weekly paclitaxel			
FEC[a]	5-Fluorouracil	600	Day 1
			Cycled every 21 days
	Epirubicin	90	Day 1
			Cycled every 21 days
	Cyclophosphamide	600	Day 1
			Cycled every 21 days
Paclitaxel	Paclitaxel	100	Day 1
			Cycled every 7 days
6× FAC followed by 12× weekly paclitaxel			
FAC	5-Fluorouracil	500	Day 1
			Cycled every 21 days
	Doxorubicin	50	Day 1
			Cycled every 21 days
	Cyclophosphamide	500	Day 1
			Cycled every 21 days
Paclitaxel	Paclitaxel	80	Day 1
			Cycled every 7 days

(continued)

Table 44.3 (continued)

Regimen	Drug	Dosage (mg/m²)	Frequency of cycles
6× TAC			
TAC[a]	Docetaxel	75	Day 1
			Cycled every 21 days
	Doxorubicin	50	Day 1
			Cycled every 21 days
	Cyclophosphamide	500	Day 1
			Cycled every 21 days

All drugs recommended in this table must be administered intravenously
[a]All cycles should be administered with lenograstim or filgrastim support

Table 44.4 Adjuvant or neoadjuvant systemic treatment with trastuzumab in HER2-positive breast cancer – preferred

Regimen	Drug	Dosage	Frequency of cycles
4× AC followed by 12× weekly paclitaxel plus trastuzumab – trastuzumab for up to 1 year			
AC	Doxorubicin	60 mg/m²	Day 1
			Cycled every 21 days
	Cyclophosphamide	600 mg/m²	Day 1
			Cycled every 21 days
Paclitaxel plus trastuzumab	Paclitaxel	80 mg/m²	Weekly
	Trastuzumab	4 mg/kg on day 1 followed by 2 mg/kg	Weekly
Trastuzumab	Trastuzumab	After paclitaxel ended followed by 6 mg/kg	Day 1
			Cycled every 21 days
4× dose-dense AC followed by 4× paclitaxel plus trastuzumab – trastuzumab for up to 1 year			
AC[a]	Doxorubicin	60 mg/m²	Day 1
	Cyclophosphamide	600 mg/m²	Day 1
			Cycled every 14 days
Paclitaxel plus trastuzumab	Paclitaxel[a]	175 mg/m²	Day 1
			Cycled every 14 days
	Trastuzumab	4 mg/kg day followed by 2 mg/kg	Weekly
Trastuzumab	Trastuzumab	After paclitaxel ended followed by 6 mg/kg	Day 1
			Cycled every 21 days
6× TCH followed by trastuzumab for up to 1 year			
Docetaxel plus	Docetaxel	75 mg/m²	Day 1
			Cycled every 21 days
Carboplatin plus trastuzumab	Carboplatin	AUC 6	Day 1
			Cycled every 21 days
	Trastuzumab	4 mg/kg day 1 followed by 2 mg/kg	Weekly
Trastuzumab	Trastuzumab	After TC ended followed by 6 mg/kg	Day 1
			Cycled every 21 days

All drugs recommended in this table must be administered intravenously
[a]All cycles should be administered with lenograstim or filgrastim support

Table 44.5 Adjuvant or neoadjuvant systemic treatment with trastuzumab plus pertuzumab in HER2-positive breast cancer – preferred

Regimen	Drug	Dosage	Frequency of cycles
4× AC followed by 4× paclitaxel plus trastuzumab plus pertuzumab – trastuzumab for up to 1 year			
AC	Doxorubicin	60 mg/m^2	Day 1
			Cycled every 21 days
	Cyclophosphamide	600 mg/m^2	Day 1
			Cycled every 21 days
Paclitaxel plus trastuzumab Plus pertuzumab	Paclitaxel	80 mg/m^2	Days 1, 8, and 15
			Cycled every 21 days
	Trastuzumab	8 mg/kg day 1 followed by 6 mg/kg	Day 1
			Cycled every 21 days
	Pertuzumab	840 mg day 1 followed by 420 mg	Day 1
			Cycled every 21 days
Trastuzumab	Trastuzumab	After paclitaxel ended followed by 6 mg/kg	Day 1
			Cycled every 21 days
6× TCH plus pertuzumab followed by trastuzumab for up to 1 year			
Docetaxel plus Carboplatin plus Pertuzumab plus trastuzumab	Docetaxel	75 mg/m^2	Day 1
			Cycled every 21 days
	Carboplatin	AUC 6	Day 1
			Cycled every 21 days
	Pertuzumab	840 mg day 1 followed by 420 mg	Day 1
			Cycled every 21 days
	Trastuzumab	4 mg/kg day 1 followed by 2 mg/kg	Weekly
Trastuzumab	Trastuzumab	After TC ended followed by 6 mg/kg	Day 1
			Cycled every 21 days

All drugs recommended in this table must be administered intravenously

toxic therapy (Proposal 2A for T1b and Proposal 1 for T1c and larger tumors). The adjuvant chemotherapy regimen for triple-negative tumors should contain anthracyclines and taxanes (Proposal 2A) [27]. Platinum-based chemotherapy regimens are not standard, and the currently available data are insufficient to recommend these regimens as adjuvant chemotherapy in triple-negative breast cancer patients (Proposal 1). Platinum-based chemotherapy regimens may be an option in patients with BRCA mutations (Proposal 2B). The triple-negative phenotype may be an indication for dose-dense chemotherapy with growth factor support [27, 105].

For women desiring fertility preservation and patients with certain comorbidities such as cardiovascular disease and diabetic neuropathy, specific chemotherapy regimens may be preferred (Proposal 2A). Ovarian function suppression (OFS) with LHRH agonists can be performed during chemotherapy in patients with ER-negative tumors to preserve ovarian function. The intrinsic subtype or BRCA carrier status should not alter the type of adjuvant chemotherapy regimen chosen (Proposal 2A) [27].

Endocrine Therapy

Adjuvant endocrine therapy should be administered to patients with ER+ or PR+ invasive breast cancer regardless of the HER2 status, patient age, or the cytotoxic therapy provided [106]. Endocrine therapy can be initiated either with or after radiotherapy [104].

Tamoxifen is the standard adjuvant endocrine therapy in women who are premenopausal at the time of diagnosis. OFS might be added to

Table 44.6 Adjuvant or neoadjuvant cytotoxic therapy with trastuzumab in HER2-positive breast cancer – others

Regimen	Drug	Dosage	Frequency of cycles
4× AC followed by 4× docetaxel plus trastuzumab – trastuzumab for up to 1 year			
AC	Doxorubicin	60 mg/m²	Day 1
			Cycled every 21 days
	Cyclophosphamide	600 mg/m²	Day 1
			Cycled every 21 days
Docetaxel[a] plus trastuzumab	Docetaxel	100 mg/m²	Day 1
			Cycled every 21 days
	Trastuzumab	4 mg/kg day 1 followed by 2 mg/kg	Weekly
Trastuzumab	Trastuzumab	After docetaxel ended followed by 6 mg/kg	Day 1
			Cycled every 21 days
TC plus trastuzumab – trastuzumab for up to 1 year			
TC[a] plus trastuzumab	Docetaxel	75 mg/m²	Day 1
			Cycled every 21 days
	Cyclophosphamide	600 mg/m²	Day 1
			Cycled every 21 days
	Trastuzumab	4 mg/kg day 1 followed by 2 mg/kg	Weekly
Trastuzumab	Trastuzumab	After TC ended followed by 6 mg/kg	Day 1
			Cycled every 21 days
12× weekly paclitaxel plus trastuzumab – trastuzumab for up to 1 year			
Paclitaxel plus trastuzumab	Paclitaxel	80 mg/m²	Day 1
			Cycled every 7 days
	Trastuzumab	4 mg/kg day 1 followed by 2 mg/kg	Weekly
Trastuzumab	Trastuzumab	After paclitaxel ended followed by 6 mg/kg	Day 1
			Cycled every 21 days

All drugs recommended in this table must be administered intravenously

tamoxifen in some patients younger than 40 years (Proposal 2A). Factors supporting the inclusion of OFS include age ≤35 years, premenopausal estrogen levels following adjuvant chemotherapy, grade 3 disease, four or more involved lymph nodes, and adverse multigene test results [107]. In high-risk premenopausal patients with multiple poor prognostic factors, OFS plus AI may be a treatment option (Proposal 2A). The adjuvant tamoxifen treatment duration may be prolonged to 10 years in high-risk patients with axillary lymph node involvement, grade 3 disease or a high Ki67 proliferation index, and a multigene-based high risk of recurrence score [107–109]. Additionally, after 5 years of tamoxifen, if a patient becomes amenorrheic and if serial blood examinations reveal that follicle-stimulating hormone (FSH) and estradiol are at postmenopausal levels, endocrine therapy may be continued with AIs for an additional 5 years in patients, particularly those with positive lymph nodes, grade 3 disease, or high Ki67 (Proposal 1) [104].

In postmenopausal women, both tamoxifen and AIs may be valid endocrine therapy options. Some patients can be adequately treated with tamoxifen alone. Factors supporting the inclusion of an AI at some point include lymph node involvement, grade 3 disease or high Ki67, and HER2 positivity [107]. All AIs, including letrozole, anastrozole, and exemestane, can be used as adjuvant endocrine therapy in postmenopausal women. An AI provided for a total of 5 years, an AI provided for 2–3 years followed by tamoxifen to complete 5 years of adjuvant endocrine therapy, and tamoxifen provided for 2–3 years

Table 44.7 Adjuvant or neoadjuvant cytotoxic therapy with trastuzumab plus pertuzumab in HER2-positive breast cancer – others

Regimen	Drug	Dosage	Frequency of cycles
4× AC followed by 4× docetaxel plus trastuzumab plus pertuzumab – trastuzumab for up to 1 year			
AC	Doxorubicin	60 mg/m²	Day 1
			Cycled every 21 days
	Cyclophosphamide	600 mg/m²	Day 1
			Cycled every 21 days
Docetaxel plus trastuzumab Plus pertuzumab	Docetaxel	75–100 mg/m²	Day 1
			Cycled every 21 days
	Trastuzumab	8 mg/kg day 1 followed by 6 mg/kg	Day 1
			Cycled every 21 days
	Pertuzumab	840 mg day 1 followed by 420 mg	Day 1
			Cycled every 21 days
Trastuzumab	Trastuzumab	After docetaxel ended followed by 6 mg/kg	Day 1
			Cycled every 21 days
3× FEC followed by docetaxel plus trastuzumab plus pertuzumab followed by trastuzumab for up to 1 year			
FEC[a]	5-Fluorouracil	500 mg/m²	Day 1
			Cycled every 21 days
	Epirubicin	100 mg/m²	Day 1
			Cycled every 21 days
	Cyclophosphamide	500 mg/m²	Day 1
			Cycled every 21 days
Docetaxel plus trastuzumab Plus pertuzumab	Docetaxel	75–100 mg/m²	Day 1
			Cycled every 21 days
	Trastuzumab	8 mg/kg day 1 followed by 6 mg/kg	Day 1
			Cycled every 21 days
	Pertuzumab	840 mg day 1 followed by 420 mg	Day 1
			Cycled every 21 days
Trastuzumab	Trastuzumab	After docetaxel ended followed by 6 mg/kg	Day 1
			Cycled every 21 days
3× FEC followed by paclitaxel plus trastuzumab plus pertuzumab followed by trastuzumab for up to 1 year			
FEC[a]	5-Fluorouracil	500 mg/m²	Day 1
			Cycled every 21 days
	Epirubicin	100 mg/m²	Day 1
			Cycled every 21 days
	Cyclophosphamide	500 mg/m²	Day 1
			Cycled every 21 days
Paclitaxel plus trastuzumab Plus pertuzumab	Paclitaxel	80 mg/m²	Days 1, 8, and 15
			Cycled every 21 days
	Trastuzumab	8 mg/kg day 1 followed by 6 mg/kg	Day 1
			Cycled every 21 days
	Pertuzumab	840 mg day 1 followed by 420 mg	Day 1
			Cycled every 21 days
Trastuzumab	Trastuzumab	After paclitaxel ended followed by 6 mg/kg	Day 1
			Cycled every 21 days

(continued)

Table 44.7 (continued)

Regimen	Drug	Dosage	Frequency of cycles
4× paclitaxel plus trastuzumab plus pertuzumab followed by 3× FEC followed by trastuzumab for up to 1 year			
Paclitaxel plus trastuzumab Plus pertuzumab	Paclitaxel	80 mg/m^2	Days 1, 8, and 15
			Cycled every 21 days
	Trastuzumab	8 mg/kg day 1 followed by 6 mg/kg	Day 1
			Cycled every 21 days
	Pertuzumab	840 mg day 1 followed by 420 mg	Day 1
			Cycled every 21 days
FEC[a]	5-Fluorouracil	500 mg/m^2	Day 1
			Cycled every 21 days
	Epirubicin	100 mg/m^2	Day 1
			Cycled every 21 days
	Cyclophosphamide	500 mg/m^2	Day 1
			Cycled every 21 days
Trastuzumab	Trastuzumab	After chemotherapy ended followed by 6 mg/kg	Day 1
			Cycled every 21 days
4× docetaxel plus trastuzumab plus pertuzumab followed by 3x FEC followed by trastuzumab for up to 1 year			
Docetaxel plus trastuzumab Plus pertuzumab	Docetaxel	75–100 mg/m^2	Day 1
			Cycled every 21 days
	Trastuzumab	8 mg/kg day 1 followed by 6 mg/kg	Day 1
			Cycled every 21 days
	Pertuzumab	840 mg day 1 followed by 420 mg	Day 1
			Cycled every 21 days
FEC[a]	5-Fluorouracil	500 mg/m^2	Day 1
			Cycled every 21 days
	Epirubicin	90 mg/m^2	Day 1
			Cycled every 21 days
	Cyclophosphamide	600 mg/m^2	Day 1
			Cycled every 21 days
Trastuzumab	Trastuzumab	After docetaxel ended followed by 6 mg/kg	Day 1
			Cycled every 21 days

All drugs recommended in this table must be administered intravenously
[a]All cycles should be administered with lenograstim or filgrastim support

followed by an AI to complete 5 years of endocrine therapy are all Proposal 1 options [110, 111]. Tamoxifen for 4.5–6 years followed by 5 years of an AI or by tamoxifen for up to 10 years is also a Proposal 1 option [112]. Tamoxifen for 2–3 years followed by an AI for up to 5 years is a Proposal 2B option.

Extending AI treatment beyond 5 years in postmenopausal women cannot currently be recommended [107]. Tamoxifen might be considered as an additional adjuvant endocrine therapy for 5 years in patients who have already completed 5 years of AI treatment [107]. If the patient

has any contraindication to AI therapy or cannot tolerate AIs, tamoxifen for 5–10 years can be provided (Proposal 1).

Because favorable histologies such as tubular carcinoma and mucinous carcinoma are usually hormone receptor positive, the diagnosis of breast cancer with a favorable histology but without hormone receptor positivity should be reevaluated histologically to confirm that the histology or hormone receptor status is correct. Patients with hormone receptor-positive tubular or mucinous carcinoma and a tumor diameter of less than 1 cm should not receive adjuvant endocrine therapy. Patients with a tumor diameter ranging from 1 to 3 cm should be evaluated for adjuvant endocrine therapy. Tamoxifen with or without ovarian ablation therapy or AIs is indicated for primary tumors larger than 3 cm with or without axillary lymph node involvement. If lymph node involvement is pathologically confirmed, adjuvant chemotherapy may be administered according to patient and disease characteristics [104].

Preoperative Systemic Therapy

Preoperative systemic therapy is a commonly used therapeutic approach to treat locally advanced and operable, primarily non-operable, or inflammatory breast cancer. Preoperative systemic therapy should be an option for patients who would require adjuvant systemic therapy. The decision regarding neoadjuvant treatment should be made after discussing the patient's clinical, histological, and imaging characteristics by a multidisciplinary oncology board that includes surgical oncologists, medical oncologists, radiation oncologists, radiologists, and pathologists.

Neoadjuvant cytotoxic therapy should be discussed as an option in patients with luminal A- and B-like tumors if conservative surgery would not otherwise be feasible. Neoadjuvant endocrine therapy without cytotoxic agents is a reasonable option for postmenopausal patients with endocrine-responsive disease for a duration of at least 4–8 months or until a maximum response is achieved.

In patients with triple-negative breast cancer, the preoperative regimen should include anthracycline plus taxane. Nab-paclitaxel and alkylating agent-containing regimens such as CMF should not be employed in the neoadjuvant setting.

For patients with HER2-positive disease, the neoadjuvant regimen should include anthracycline plus taxane and an anti-HER2 agent. Trastuzumab±pertuzumab are the preferred anti-HER2 agents [104] (Tables 44.5 and 44.7).

Adjuvant Radiotherapy in Invasive Breast Cancer

Postmastectomy radiotherapy (PMRT) is the standard of care in patients with four or more involved lymph nodes with metastatic disease [113]. However, the benefit of PMRT in patients with one to three involved nodes was more controversial until recently. Although some trials from the 1990s indicated a benefit of PMRT in patients with one to three involved nodes, these studies were criticized for using substandard chemotherapy and having unusually high locoregional recurrence rates without PMRT compared with other studies [114–116]. A recent meta-analysis provided more evidence of the benefit of PMRT in patients with one to three involved nodes [40]. Indirect evidence from the preliminary results of another Canadian randomized trial also indicated the benefit of regional nodal irradiation in patients with less than three involved nodes [117]. PMRT does not provide any benefit in pathologically node-negative patients with negative surgical margins of at least 1 mm [40, 117, 118]. A collective analysis of NSABP trials revealed no benefit of PMRT in T3N0MX patients [119].

After lumpectomy, whole-breast radiotherapy remains the standard of care (Proposal 1) [41, 120–122]. A meta-analysis revealed a significant increase in in-breast control and a decrease in breast cancer-specific deaths [123]. Controversial results were obtained for partial-breast irradiation (PBI) in patients with a low local recurrence risk. Two large randomized (intraoperative) PBI trials observed higher in-breast recurrence rates in patients treated with PBI compared with whole-breast radiotherapy [124, 125]. Several different techniques such as external beam radiotherapy, intracavitary brachytherapy, interstitial brachytherapy, and intraoperative irradiation can be used to deliver PBI. Most likely, not all of these techniques will be capable of achieving adequate local control with low side effect rates [126, 127]. The results of large randomized trials are awaited before PBI can be considered standard in some patients [7, 8]. Data are accumulating to consider whether some elderly patients with low-risk disease (T1/T2N0M0), negative surgical margins, and hormone receptor-positive tumors can be followed without any postlumpectomy radiotherapy (Proposal 2A) [128, 129].

Techniques, Doses, and Fields

Chest Wall

If PMRT is indicated, the chest wall (CW) is always targeted as one of the radiotherapy fields because this is the most common site of locoregional recurrence. In cases with reconstruction, the CW is treated through tangential fields; without reconstruction, the CW can be treated through tangential fields or electron fields. Particularly in cases with a high risk of skin recurrence, the use of bolus material should be considered in at least part of the treatment. CT-based treatment planning should be performed to delineate target volumes and normal tissues to be protected (Proposal 1).

The PMRT adjuvant dose is 45.0–50.4 Gy in 25–28 fractions. In inflammatory cases, this dose could be increased to 60 Gy. Special consideration should be given to tolerance doses of the lungs, heart, and left coronary artery. In left-sided cases, breath-holding techniques could be used to better spare the heart. Targets include the ipsilateral CW, mastectomy scars, and, in advanced cases, drainage sites. Several guidelines for target delineation, including the ASTRO and ESTRO atlases, are available (www.guideline.gov, www.astro.org, www.estro.org).

Regional Lymph Nodes

In node-positive cases, medial axillary node and supraclavicular node treatment is considered even in cases with only a few (up to three) positive nodes. If axillary staging is performed according to the current standards, the irradiation of lower axillary levels (levels I and II) is not required unless remaining gross disease is suspected following surgery. Adjuvant internal mammary lymph node chain irradiation is considered in cases with central or medial tumors, axillary involvement, and/or detected drainage to

the parasternal nodes during an SLNB. The adjuvant dose provided to lymph node regions for subclinical disease is 45 Gy in 25 fractions (Proposal 2A).

Whole Breast

CT-based treatment planning should be used for target delineation. The most popular technique is tangential fields using forward planning (field-in-field) intensity-modulated radiation therapy (IMRT). The preferred dose homogeneity is ±7 %. For left-sided cases, breath-holding techniques are recommended. The classical dose provided to the whole breast is 45–50.4 Gy in 25–28 fractions, with an additional boost dose of 10–16 Gy in 2 Gy fractions to the tumor bed. In patients older than 50 years with T1/T2N0 disease and clear surgical margins, hypofractionated whole-breast irradiation at 42.5 Gy/16 fractions should be considered for both convenience and effectiveness.

Follow-Up

After primary treatment is completed in patients with early-stage disease, routine follow-up is required for all patients three to four times annually during the first 2–3 years following diagnosis and two times annually during the third to fifth years. No uniform consensus has been reached on monitoring complete blood counts or biochemistry or on scanning other than annual mammography. Physical examination and patient history collection should be routinely performed at all follow-up visits, and the chest, the abdominopelvic region, or any other body part should be scanned if any clinical indication is present. Premenopausal women should be educated regarding contraceptive techniques and should delay pregnancy until adjuvant therapy is completed. Patients on tamoxifen therapy should be referred to a gynecologist at least annually due to the possible risk of endometrial cancer. Bone mineral density should be initially assessed and then periodically evaluated in women who will receive AIs. The evaluation of possible recurrence sites by PET-CT should not be performed as a routine screening method.

Recurrent or Metastatic Disease

For recurrent or advanced breast cancer, less Proposal 1 evidence is available. The primary aim of treating advanced disease is prolonging disease-specific survival while improving the quality of life. Treatment should be tailored according to disease status and patient priorities as well as to any prior history of disease and to the patients' physical, functional, psychosocial, and spiritual characteristics.

Because elderly patients have several comorbidities that may preclude the initiation of some systemic agents or that may increase the overall toxicity, physicians may not provide a full course of therapy and occasionally may not treat elderly patients appropriately. Age may be an important factor during the treatment decision but should not be the sole guiding criterion in the treatment of breast cancer.

The workup of recurrent or metastatic breast cancer patients should include prior medical and breast cancer histories, physical examinations, complete blood counts, blood biochemistry measures comprising liver and renal functions, and chest and abdominopelvic CT (Proposal 2A). For symptomatic patients with central nervous system-related symptoms, brain MRI may be indicated; for patients with bone-related symptoms, bone scan or PET-CT may be indicated. Symptomatic bones and long, weight-bearing bones can be scanned with X-rays. FDG PET-CT should not be offered to all recurrent or metastatic patients unless the PET-CT results will radically change the treatment decision.

Patients with first disease recurrence and with distant metastasis should undergo a core biopsy of the site of recurrence or metastasis, which may provide new information regarding histology, hormone receptor status, HER2 status, and proliferation/grade [130]. The biopsy should be emphasized, particularly for patients who previously had hormone receptor-negative or HER2-negative breast cancer. If biopsy cannot be performed at the site of metastasis or recurrence, treatment should be planned according to the receptor status of the primary site or to previous pathological findings.

Major determinants of the treatment plan include the number of lesions, extent of visceral involvement, receptor status of the primary lesion, sites of recurrence and metastasis, previous response to anticancer agents, present function of organs, performance status of patients, and social support of patients.

In the absence of any contraindication, treatment with denosumab or a bisphosphonate, including zoledronic acid, ibandronic acid, and pamidronate, must be initiated along with other systemic therapies in patients with bone metastasis (Proposal 1) [131]. Calcium and vitamin D supplementation should also be added to bisphosphonates or denosumab [104]. Dental examinations and required interventions should be completed before these agents are initiated.

Systemic Treatment in Patients with Hormone Receptor-Positive±HER2-Positive Metastatic or Recurrent Breast Cancer

Premenopausal patients with recurrent or metastatic disease more than 1 year after completing tamoxifen treatment can be treated as "tamoxifen-naive" patients; tamoxifen can be restarted with an LHRH analogue, or an AI can be given with an LHRH analogue or with ovarian ablation therapy (Proposal 2A) [132]. Postmenopausal women with recurrent or metastatic disease more than 1 year after adjuvant AI completion can receive the previous AI, tamoxifen, other selective ER modulators (toremifene), or fulvestrant (Proposal 2A) [133–137]. Other options include switching AIs (e.g., if the previous AI was steroidal, nonsteroidal should be given and vice versa) (Proposal 2A) [138, 139].

Premenopausal patients with recurrent or metastatic disease within 1 year after tamoxifen completion or while receiving tamoxifen therapy should be accepted as "refractory or resistant to tamoxifen," and an AI or fulvestrant should be initiated with an LHRH analogue or ovarian ablation therapy (Proposal 2A) [104]. An AI of a different subgroup than the previously used AI (e.g., if the previous AI was steroidal, a nonsteroidal AI should be given and vice versa), tamoxifen, or another selective ER modulator or downregulator may be a choice for endocrine treatment for postmenopausal women with recurrent or metastatic disease within 1 year following adjuvant AI completion (Proposal 2A) [138, 139].

Palbociclib in combination with letrozole may be provided to patients with hormone receptor-positive and HER2-negative metastatic breast cancer as a first-line endocrine therapy (Proposal 2A) [140]. For patients receiving second-line endocrine therapy following disease progression on a nonsteroidal AI, within 12 months of a nonsteroidal AI, or at any time on tamoxifen, the combination of everolimus and exemestane represents an endocrine therapy option with Proposal 2A evidence [141].

For patients with HER2-positive and ER-positive/PR-positive breast cancer, clinicians may recommend either standard first-line therapy or, for selected patients, endocrine therapy plus HER2-targeted therapy or endocrine therapy alone [142]. Although no high-level evidence is available, if endocrine therapy is chosen as the initial systemic therapy instead of chemotherapy for patients with hormone

receptor- and HER2-positive advanced breast cancer, adding an anti-HER2 agent to the endocrine agent should be considered with the aim of increasing progression-free survival. Patients who have received anti-HER2 therapy with cytotoxic therapy and whose disease has stabilized may be considered for cytotoxic therapy termination and systemic treatment continuation with an anti-HER2 agent plus an endocrine agent. In the presence of any risk factor for subsequent organ failure, chemotherapy should be the first option for systemic treatment. The optimal duration of anti-HER2 treatment in the metastatic setting is not known (Tables 44.8, 44.9, 44.10, 44.11, and 44.12).

Systemic Treatment for Patients with Hormone Receptor-Negative or Endocrine-Refractory and HER2-Positive Metastatic or Recurrent Breast Cancer

All patients with HER2-positive recurrent or metastatic breast cancer and a previous history of adjuvant trastuzumab therapy should be evaluated for further anti-HER2 therapy in the absence of any contraindications. Trastuzumab alone or

Table 44.8 Combined usage of cytotoxic drugs with dual anti-HER2 inhibition for HER2-positive advanced breast cancer

Regimen	Drug	Dosage	Route of administration	Frequency of cycles
Trastuzumab plus pertuzumab with docetaxel	Trastuzumab	8 mg/kg IV day 1 followed by 6 mg/kg	Intravenous	Cycled every 21 days
	Pertuzumab	840 mg IV day 1 followed by 420 mg	Intravenous	Cycled every 21 days
	Docetaxel	75–100 mg/m^2	Intravenous	Day 1
				Cycled every 21 days
Trastuzumab plus pertuzumab with paclitaxel	Trastuzumab	8 mg/kg IV day 1 followed by 6 mg/kg	Intravenous	Cycled every 21 days
		4 mg/kg day 1 followed by 2 mg/kg	Intravenous	Weekly
	Pertuzumab	840 mg IV day 1 followed by 420 mg	Intravenous	Cycled every 21 days
	Paclitaxel	175 mg/m^2	Intravenous	Day 1
				Cycled every 21 days
	Paclitaxel	80–90 mg/m^2	Intravenous	Day 1
				Cycled every 7 days

Table 44.9 Combined usage of cytotoxic drugs with trastuzumab for HER2-positive advanced breast cancer

Regimen	Drug	Dosage	Route of administration	Frequency of cycles
Trastuzumab plus the following cytotoxic(s)	Trastuzumab	4 mg/kg day 1 followed by 2 mg/kg	Intravenous	Weekly
		8 mg/kg IV day 1 followed by 6 mg/kg	Intravenous	Cycled every 21 days
Paclitaxel/carboplatin	Carboplatin	AUC 6	Intravenous	Day 1
				Cycled every 21 days
	Paclitaxel	175 mg/m^2	Intravenous	Day 1
				Cycled every 21 days
Weekly paclitaxel/carboplatin	Carboplatin	AUC 2	Intravenous	Days 1, 8, and 15
				Cycled every 28 days
	Paclitaxel	80 mg/m^2	Intravenous	Days 1, 8, and 15
				Cycled every 28 days
Paclitaxel	Paclitaxel	175 mg/m^2	Intravenous	Day 1
				Cycled every 21 days
	Paclitaxel	80–90 mg/m^2	Intravenous	Day 1
				Cycled every 7 days
Docetaxel	Docetaxel	80–100 mg/m^2	Intravenous	Day 1
				Cycled every 21 days
	Docetaxel	35 mg/m^2	Intravenous	Day 1
				Cycled every week
Vinorelbine	Vinorelbine	25 mg/m^2	Intravenous	Day 1 weekly
				Cycled every 21 days
	Vinorelbine	30–35 mg/m^2	Intravenous	Days 1 and 8
				Cycled every 21 days
Capecitabine	Capecitabine	1000–1250 mg/m^2	Peroral	Twice daily days 1–14
				Cycled every 21 days

with chemotherapy (paclitaxel ± carboplatin, docetaxel, vinorelbine, capecitabine) (Proposal 2A) and trastuzumab in combination with pertuzumab and taxane (Proposal 1) (docetaxel or paclitaxel) are the preferred regimens in the first-line metastatic setting [143] (Tables 44.8, 44.9, and 44.10).

Pertuzumab-containing regimens may also be preferred in patients who have previously received trastuzumab as a part of adjuvant

Table 44.10 Systemic therapy for previously trastuzumab -treated HER2-positive advanced breast cancer patients

Regimen	Drug	Dosage	Route of administration	Frequency of cycles
(T-DM1)	Ado-trastuzumab emtansine	3.6 mg/kg	Intravenous	Day 1
				Cycled every 21 days
Lapatinib+capecitabine	Lapatinib PO daily	1250 mg	Peroral	Days 1–21
				Cycled every 21 days
	Capecitabine	1000 mg/m2	Peroral	Twice daily days 1–14
				Cycled every 21 days
Trastuzumab+capecitabine	Capecitabine	1000–1250 mg/m2	Peroral	Twice daily days 1–14
				Cycled every 21 days
	Trastuzumab	4 mg/kg day 1 followed by 2 mg/kg	Intravenous	Weekly
		8 mg/kg IV day 1 followed by 6 mg/kg	Intravenous	Cycled every 21 days
Trastuzumab+lapatinib (without cytotoxic therapy)	Lapatinib	1000 mg	Peroral	Days 1–21
				Cycled every 21 days
	Trastuzumab	4 mg/kg day 1 followed by 2 mg/kg	Intravenous	Weekly
		8 mg/kg IV day 1 followed by 6 mg/kg	Intravenous	Cycled every 21 days

systemic therapy, but not for recurrent or metastatic disease [143].

Patients whose disease progressed on a trastuzumab-containing regimen may again receive trastuzumab with lapatinib or another cytotoxic agent or may be considered for another anti-HER2 agent such as ado-trastuzumab emtansine or lapatinib with capecitabine (Proposal 2A) [144, 145]. However, following first-line trastuzumab-based systemic therapy, ado-trastuzumab emtansine should be chosen as the preferred second-line therapy due to its superiority over other anti-HER2 agents, including lapatinib+capecitabine or trastuzumab, as a post-progression strategy. Lapatinib-containing combination regimens should not be used as first-line systemic therapy in HER2-positive metastatic breast cancer patients.

The optimal duration of chemotherapy is at least 4–6 months or until a maximum response is reached, depending on toxicity and the absence of progression. HER2-targeted therapy must continue until progression or unacceptable toxicity

occurs [142]. The choice of anti-HER2 agent or agents should be planned according to the prior anti-HER2 therapy, relapse-free survival, and country-specific availability.

Systemic Treatment for Patients with Triple-Negative Metastatic or Recurrent Breast Cancer or at High Risk for a Visceral Crisis

Chemotherapy regimens, either single agent or combination, should be considered for patients with triple-negative metastatic or recurrent breast cancer or who are at high risk for a visceral crisis. No convincing data support the superiority of combination chemotherapy over single-agent chemotherapy. Although combination regimens may increase objective response rates, they also result in increased toxicity without any overall survival advantage.

The preferred single agents are paclitaxel, doxorubicin, pegylated liposomal doxorubicin,

Table 44.11 First-line single cytotoxic drugs for advanced breast cancer

Drug	Recommendation level	Dosage	Route of administration	Frequency of cycles
Anthracyclines				
Doxorubicin	Preferred	20 mg/m^2	Intravenous	Day 1, cycled weekly
	Preferred	60 mg/m^2	Intravenous	Day 1, cycled every 21 days
Pegylated liposomal doxorubicin	Preferred	50 mg/m^2	Intravenous	Day 1, cycled every 28 days
Epirubicin	Other	60–90 mg/m^2	Intravenous	Day 1, cycled every 21 days
Taxanes				
Paclitaxel	Preferred	80 mg/m^2	Intravenous	Day 1, cycled weekly
	Preferred	175 mg/m^2	Intravenous	Day 1, cycled every 21 days
Docetaxel	Other	60–100 mg/m^2	Intravenous	Day 1, cycled every 21 days
	Other	35 mg/m^2	Intravenous	Day 1, cycled weekly
Albumin-bound paclitaxel	Other	100 mg/m^2 or 150 mg/m^2	Intravenous	Days 1, 8, and 15, cycled every 28 days
	Other	260 mg/m^2	Intravenous	Day 1, cycled every 21 days
Other microtubule inhibitors				
Vinorelbine	Preferred	25 mg/m^2	Intravenous	Day 1, cycled weekly
Eribulin	Preferred	1.4 mg/m^2	Intravenous	Days 1 and 8, cycled every 21 days
Ixabepilone	Other	40 mg/m^2	Intravenous	Day 1, cycled every 21 days
Antimetabolites				
Capecitabine	Preferred	1000–1250 mg/m^2	Peroral	Twice daily from day 1 to 14, cycled every 21 days
Gemcitabine	Preferred	800–1200 mg/m^2	Intravenous	Days 1, 8, and 15, cycled every 28 days
Platinum compounds				
Cisplatin	Other	75 mg/m^2	Intravenous	Day 1, cycled every 21 days
Carboplatin	Other	AUC 6	Intravenous	Day 1, cycled every 21–28 days
Alkylating agents				
Cyclophosphamide	Other	50 mg	Peroral	Once daily on days 1–21, cycled every 28 days

Table 44.12 Combined usage of cytotoxic drugs for advanced breast cancer

Regimen	Drug	Dosage	Route of administration	Frequency of cycles
CAF	Cyclophosphamide	100 mg/m²	Peroral	Daily on days 1–14
	Doxorubicin	30 mg/m²	Intravenous	Days 1 and 8
	5-Fluorouracil	500 mg/m²	Intravenous	Days 1 and 8
				Cycled every 28 days
FAC	5-Fluorouracil	500 mg/m²	Intravenous	Days 1 and 8 or days 1 and 4
				Cycled every 28 days
	Doxorubicin	50 mg/m²	Intravenous	Day 1 or by 72 h continuous infusion
	Cyclophosphamide	500 mg/m²	Intravenous	Day 1
				Cycled every 21 days
FEC	5-Fluorouracil	500 mg/m²	Intravenous	Days 1 and 8
				Cycled every 28 days
	Epirubicin	50 mg/m²	Intravenous	Days 1 and 8
	Cyclophosphamide	400 mg/m²	Intravenous	Days 1 and 8
AC	Doxorubicin	60 mg/m²	Intravenous	Day 1
	Cyclophosphamide	600 mg/m²	Intravenous	Day 1
				Cycled every 21 days
EC	Epirubicin	75 mg/m²	Intravenous	Day 1
	Cyclophosphamide	600 mg/m²	Intravenous	Day 1
				Cycled every 21 days
CMF	Cyclophosphamide	100 mg/m²	Peroral	Once daily on days 1–14
				Cycled every 28 days
	Methotrexate	40 mg/m²	Intravenous	Days 1 and 8
				Cycled every 28 days
	5-Fluorouracil	600 mg/m²	Intravenous	Days 1 and 8
				Cycled every 28 days
Docetaxel/capecitabine	Docetaxel	75 mg/m²	Intravenous	Day 1
				Cycled every 21 days
	Capecitabine	950 mg/m²	Peroral	Twice daily from days 1–14, cycled every 21 days
GT	Paclitaxel IV day 1	175 mg/m²	Intravenous	Day 1
	Gemcitabine IV	1250 mg/m²	Intravenous	Days 1 and 8 (following paclitaxel on day 1)
				Cycled every 21 days
GC	Gemcitabine	1000 mg/m²	Intravenous	Days 1 and 8
	Carboplatin	AUC 2	Intravenous	Days 1 and 8
				Cycled every 21 days
Paclitaxel/bevacizumab	Paclitaxel	90 mg/m²	Intravenous	By 1 h days 1, 8, and 15
	Bevacizumab	10 mg/kg	Intravenous	Days 1 and 15
				Cycled every 28 days

capecitabine, gemcitabine, vinorelbine, and eribulin (Proposal 2A); other single agents provided in this situation include docetaxel, cisplatin, carboplatin, epirubicin, ixabepilone, cyclophosphamide, and albumin-bound paclitaxel (Proposal 2A). AC (doxorubicin and cyclophosphamide), EC (epirubicin and cyclophosphamide), FEC (fluorouracil and epirubicin and cyclophosphamide), FAC/CAF (fluorouracil and doxorubicin and cyclophosphamide), CMF (cyclophosphamide and methotrexate and fluorouracil), gemcitabine/paclitaxel, gemcitabine/carboplatin, and docetaxel/capecitabine are usually the preferred combination regimens (Proposal 2A) [104]. (Tables 44.11 and 44.12).

Patients who carry a BRCA mutation and have triple-negative or endocrine therapy-resistant metastatic breast cancer should be considered for platinum-based chemotherapy if they have received an anthracycline and a taxane in an adjuvant or metastatic setting (Proposal 2A). In the future, poly(ADP)-ribose polymerase (PARP) inhibitors may be an option for patients with BRCA mutations.

Surgery for Metastatic Breast Cancer

The primary treatment approach for women with metastatic breast cancer and an intact primary tumor is systemic therapy, with the consideration of surgery following initial systemic treatment in women requiring palliation of symptoms or with impending complications such as skin ulceration, bleeding, fungation, and pain [146]. Generally, such surgery should be performed only if complete local clearance of the tumor may be obtained and if other sites of disease are not immediately life threatening. Alternatively, radiation therapy may be considered as an alternative to surgery. Often, such surgery requires collaboration between the breast surgeon and the reconstructive surgeon to provide optimal cancer control and wound closure.

Retrospective studies suggest a potential survival benefit from complete excision of the primary tumor in select patients with metastatic breast cancer [147–150]. Substantial selection biases exist in all of these studies and are likely to confound the study results [151, 152]. Two recent prospective, randomized studies assessed whether surgery on the primary tumor in the breast is necessary for women who are diagnosed with metastatic breast cancer. The results from both studies presented at the 2013 San Antonio Breast Cancer Symposium were similar and revealed that surgical treatment of primary tumors in women presenting with stage IV disease does not produce an increase in OS in general [153, 154]. However, a survival advantage of primary tumor excision was observed only in patients with solitary bone metastasis in a Turkish study [154].

Randomized clinical trials that address the advantages and disadvantages of local therapy for patients with stage IV disease while eliminating selection biases are necessary. Patient enrollment in such trials is encouraged.

Conclusion

We have attempted to provide useful and explicit recommendations on management of breast cancer, but we must stress that these recommendations are subject to change. Some of the recommendations are controversial and the subject of ongoing clinical trials. The gold standard for breast cancer care includes an integrated multidisciplinary team approach, comprising pathologists, radiologists, surgical oncologists, medical oncologists, radiation oncologists, oncology nurses, and plastic surgeons.

References

1. O'Neil M, Madan R, Tawfik OW, Thomas PA, Fan F. Lobular carcinoma in situ/atypical lobular hyperplasia on breast needle biopsies: does it warrant surgical excisional biopsy? A study of 27 cases. Ann Diagn Pathol. 2010;14:251–5.
2. Anderson BO, Calhoun KE, Rosen EL. Evolving concepts in the management of lobular neoplasia. J Natl Compr Cancer Netw. 2006;4:511–22.
3. EORTC Breast Cancer Cooperative Group, EORTC Radiotherapy Group, Bijker N, Meijnen P, Peterse

JL, Bogaerts J, Van Hoorebeeck I, Julien JP, et al. Breast-conserving treatment with or without radiotherapy in ductal carcinoma-in-situ: ten-year results of European Organisation for Research and Treatment of Cancer randomized phase III trial 10853 – a study by the EORTC Breast Cancer Cooperative Group and EORTC Radiotherapy Group. J Clin Oncol. 2006;24:3381–7.

4. Vargas C, Kestin L, Go N, Krauss D, Chen P, Goldstein N, et al. Factors associated with local recurrence and cause-specific survival in patients with ductal carcinoma in situ of the breast treated with breast-conserving therapy or mastectomy. Int J Radiat Oncol Biol Phys. 2005;63:1514–21.

5. Cody 3rd HS, Van Zee KJ. Point: sentinel lymph node biopsy is indicated for patients with DCIS. J Natl Compr Cancer Netw. 2003;1:199–206.

6. Silverstein MJ, Lagios MD, Groshen S, Waisman JR, Lewinsky BS, Martino S, et al. The influence of margin width on local control of ductal carcinoma in situ of the breast. N Engl J Med. 1999;340:1455–61.

7. A randomized phase III study of conventional whole breast irradiation (WBI) versus partial breast irradiation (PBI) for women with stage 0, I, or II breast cancer. NCT00103181 https://clinicaltrials.gov/ct2/show/NCT00103181. Accessed 16 Jan 2015.

8. Smith BD, Arthur DW, Buchholz TA, Haffty BG, Hahn CA, Hardenbergh PH, et al. Accelerated partial breast irradiation consensus statement from the American Society for Radiation Oncology. Int J Radiat Oncol Biol Phys. 2009;74:987–1001.

9. ASBS: http://www.breastsurgeons.org/statements/APBI_statement_revised_100708.pdf.

10. ABS: http://www.americanbrachytherapy.org/recources/abs_breast_brachytherapy_taskgroup.pdf.

11. Hughes LL, Wang M, Page DL, Gray R, Solin LJ, Davidson NE, et al. Local excision alone without irradiation for ductal carcinoma in situ of the breast: a trial of the Eastern Cooperative Oncology Group. J Clin Oncol. 2009;27:5319–24.

12. McCormick B, Winter K, Hudis C, Kuerer HM, Rakovitch E, Smith BL, et al. RTOG 9804: a prospective randomized trial for good-risk ductal carcinoma in situ comparing radiotherapy with observation. J Clin Oncol. 2015. doi:10.1200/JCO.2014.57.9029.

13. Smith B. When is good enough really good enough? Defining the role of radiation in low-risk ductal carcinoma in situ. J Clin Oncol. 2015. doi:10.1200/JCO.2014.59.4259.

14. Lagios MD, Silverstein MJ. Ductal carcinoma in situ: recent history and areas of controversy. Breast J. 2015;21:21–6.

15. Fisher B, Dignam J, Wolmark N, Mamounas E, Costantino J, Poller W, et al. Lumpectomy and radiation therapy for the treatment of intraductal breast cancer: findings from the national surgical adjuvant breast and bowel project B-17. J Clin Oncol. 1998;16:441–52.

16. Julien JP, Bijker N, Fentiman IS, Peterse JL, Delledonne V, Rouanet P, et al. Radiotherapy in breast conserving treatment for ductal carcinoma in situ: first results of the EORTC randomized phase III trial 10853. Lancet. 2000;353:528–33.

17. UK Coordinating Committee on Cancer Research. Radiotherapy and tamoxifen in women with completely excised ductal carcinoma in situ of the breast in the UK, Australia, and New Zealand: randomized controlled trial. Lancet. 2003;362:95–102.

18. Fisher B, Land S, Mamounas E, Dignam J, Fisher ER, Wolmark N, et al. Prevention of invasive breast cancer in women with ductal carcinoma in situ: an update of the national surgical adjuvant breast and bowel project experience. Semin Oncol. 2001;28:400–18.

19. Staley H, McCallum I, Bruce J. Postoperative tamoxifen for ductal carcinoma in situ: Cochrane systematic review and meta-analysis. Breast. 2014;23:546–51.

20. Margolese RG, Cecchini RS, Julian TB, Ganz PA, Costantino JP, Vallow LA, et al. Anastrozole versus tamoxifen in postmenopausal women with ductal carcinoma in situ undergoing lumpectomy plus radiotherapy (NSABP B-35): a randomised, double-blind, phase 3 clinical trial. Lancet. 2015 Dec 10. pii: S0140-6736(15)01168-X. doi: 10.1016/S0140-6736(15)01168-X.

21. Lai HW, Chen DR, Wu YC, Chen CJ, Lee CW, Kuo SJ, et al. Comparison of the diagnostic accuracy of magnetic resonance imaging with sonography in the prediction of breast cancer tumor size: a concordance analysis with histopathologically determined tumor size. Ann Surg Oncol. 2015; 22(12):3816-23.

22. Ferguson NL, Bell J, Heidel R, Lee S, Vanmeter S, Duncan L, et al. Prognostic value of breast cancer subtypes, Ki-67 proliferation index, age, and pathologic tumor characteristics on breast cancer survival in Caucasian women. Breast J. 2013;19:22–30.

23. Wood WC. Close/positive margins after breast-conserving therapy: additional resection or no resection? Breast. 2013;22 Suppl 2:S115–7.

24. Maisonneuve P, Disalvatore D, Rotmensz N, Curigliano G, Colleoni M, Dellapasqua S, et al. Proposed new clinicopathological surrogate definitions of luminal A and luminal B (HER2-negative) intrinsic breast cancer subtypes. Breast Cancer Res. 2014;16:R65.

25. Oncotype DX in women and men with ER-positive, HER2-negative early stage breast cancer who are lymph node negative: a review of clinical effectiveness and guidelines [internet]. Ottawa: Canadian Agency for Drugs and Technologies in Health; 2014.

26. Guiu S, Michiels S, André F, Cortes J, Denkert C, Di Leo A, et al. Molecular subclasses of breast cancer: how do we define them? The IMPAKT 2012 Working Group Statement. Ann Oncol. 2012;23(12):2997–3006.

27. Untch M, Gerber B, Harbeck N, Jackisch C, Marschner N, Möbus V, et al. 13th St. Gallen international breast cancer conference 2013: primary therapy of early breast cancer evidence, controversies, consensus – opinion of a German Team of Experts (Zurich 2013). Breast Care. 2013;8:221–9.

28. Fourquet A, Campana F, Zafrani B, Mosseri V, Vielh P, Durand JC, et al. Prognostic factors of breast recurrence in the conservative management of early breast cancer: a 25-year follow-up. Int J Radiat Oncol Biol Phys. 1989;17:719–25.

29. Komoike Y, Akiyama F, Iino Y, Ikeda T, Akashi-Tanaka S, et al. Ipsilateral breast tumor recurrence (IBTR) after breast-conserving treatment for early breast cancer: risk factors and impact on distant metastases. Cancer. 2006;106:35–41.

30. Pierce LJ, Griffith KA, Buys S, Gaffney DK, Moran MS, Haffty BG, et al. Outcomes following breast conservation versus mastectomy in BRCA1/2 carriers with early-stage breast cancer [abstract]. J Clin Oncol. 2008;26(Suppl 15):Abstract 536.

31. Zhou P, Gautam S, Recht A. Factors affecting outcome for young women with early stage invasive breast cancer treated with breast- conserving therapy. Breast Cancer Res Treat. 2007;101:51–7.

32. Golshan M, Miron A, Nixon AJ, Garber JE, Cash EP, Iglehart JD, et al. The prevalence of germline BRCA1 and BRCA2 mutations in young women with breast cancer undergoing breast-conservation therapy. Am J Surg. 2006;192:58–62.

33. Kroman N, Holtveg H, Wohlfahrt J, Jensen MB, Mouridsen HT, Blichert-Toft M, et al. Effect of breast- conserving therapy versus radical mastectomy on prognosis for young women with breast carcinoma. Cancer. 2004;100:688–93.

34. Cruz MR, Prestes JC, Gimenes DL, Fanelli MF. Fertility preservation in women with breast cancer undergoing adjuvant chemotherapy: a systematic review. Fertil Steril. 2010;94:138–43.

35. Dunn L, Fox KR. Techniques for fertility preservation in patients with breast cancer. Curr Opin Obstet Gynecol. 2009;21:68–73.

36. Oktem O, Oktay K. Fertility preservation for breast cancer patients. Semin Reprod Med. 2009;27:486–92.

37. Redig AJ, Brannigan R, Stryker SJ, Woodruff TK, Jeruss JS. Incorporating fertility preservation into the care of young oncology patients. Cancer. 2011;117:4–10.

38. Lee S, Ozkavukcu S, Heytens E, Moy F, Oktay K. Value of early referral to fertility preservation in young women with breast cancer. J Clin Oncol. 2010;28:4683–6.

39. Arriagada R, Le MG, Rochard F, Contesso G. Conservative treatment versus mastectomy in early breast cancer: patterns of failure with 15 years of follow-up data. Institut Gustave-Roussy Breast Cancer Group. J Clin Oncol. 1996;14:1558–64.

40. McGale P, Taylor C, Correa C, Cutter D, Duane F, Ewertz M, et al. Effect of radiotherapy after mastectomy and axillary surgery on 10-year recurrence and 20-year breast cancer mortality: meta-analysis of individual patient data for 8135 women in 22 randomised trials.EBCTCG (Early Breast Cancer Trialists' Collaborative Group. Lancet. 2014;383:2127–35.

41. Fisher B, Anderson S, Bryant J, Margolese RG, Deutsch M, Fisher ER, et al. Twenty-year follow-up of a randomized trial comparing total mastectomy, lumpectomy, and lumpectomy plus irradiation for the treatment of invasive breast cancer. N Engl J Med. 2002;347:1233–41.

42. Veronesi U, Cascinelli N, Mariani L, Greco M, Saccozzi R, Luini A, et al. Twenty-year follow-up of a randomized study comparing breast-conserving surgery with radical mastectomy for early breast cancer. N Engl J Med. 2002;347:1227–32.

43. Cardoso F, Costa A, Norton L, Senkus E, Aapro M, André F, et al. ESO-ESMO 2nd international consensus guidelines for advanced breast cancer (ABC2). Ann Oncol. 2014;25(10):1871–88.

44. Recht A. Contralateral prophylactic mastectomy: caveat emptor. J Clin Oncol. 2009;27:1347–9.

45. Lyman GH, Giuliano AE, Somerfield MR, Benson 3rd AB, Bodurka DC, Burstein HJ, et al. American Society of Clinical Oncology guideline recommendations for sentinel lymph node biopsy in early-stage breast cancer. J Clin Oncol. 2005;23:7703–20.

46. Bass SS, Lyman GH, McCann CR, Ku NN, Berman C, Durand K, et al. Lymphatic mapping and sentinel lymph node biopsy. Breast J. 1999;5:288–95.

47. Cox CE, Nguyen K, Gray RJ, Salud C, Ku NN, Dupont E, et al. Importance of lymphatic mapping in ductal carcinoma in situ (DCIS): why map DCIS? Am Surg. 2001;67:513–9.

48. Krag D, Weaver D, Ashikaga T, Moffat F, Klimberg VS, Shriver C, et al. The sentinel node in breast cancer – a multicenter validation study. N Engl J Med. 1998;339:941–6.

49. Krag DN, Anderson SJ, Julian TB, Brown AM, Harlow SP, Costantino JP, et al. Sentinel-lymph-node resection compared with conventional axillary-lymph-node dissection in clinically node-negative patients with breast cancer: overall survival findings from the NSABP B-32 randomised phase 3 trial. Lancet Oncol. 2010;11:927–33.

50. Kuehn T, Vogl FD, Helms G, Pueckler SV, Schirrmeister H, Strueber R, et al. Sentinel-node biopsy for axillary staging in breast cancer: results from a large prospective German multi- institutional trial. Eur J Surg Oncol. 2004;30:252–9.

51. Veronesi U, Paganelli G, Viale G, Luini A, Zurrida S, Galimberti V, et al. A randomized comparison of sentinel-node biopsy with routine axillary dissection in breast cancer. N Engl J Med. 2003;349:546–53.

52. Mansel RE, Fallowfield L, Kissin M, Goyal A, Newcombe RG, Dixon JM, et al. Randomized multicenter trial of sentinel node biopsy versus standard axillary treatment in operable breast cancer: the ALMANAC Trial. J Natl Cancer Inst. 2006;98:599–609.

53. Cox CE, Salud CJ, Cantor A, Bass SS, Peltz ES, Ebert MD, et al. Learning curves for breast cancer sentinel lymph node mapping based on surgical volume analysis. J Am Coll Surg. 2001;193:593–600.

54. Dupont E, Cox C, Shivers S, Salud C, Nguyen K, Cantor A, et al. Learning curves and breast cancer

lymphatic mapping: institutional volume index. J Surg Res. 2001;97:92–6.

55. Giuliano AE, Hawes D, Ballman KV, Whitworth PW, Blumencranz PW, Reintgen DS, et al. Association of occult metastases in sentinel lymph nodes and bone marrow with survival among women with early-stage invasive breast cancer. JAMA. 2011;306:385–93.

56. Ozmen V, Karanlik H, Cabioglu N, Igci A, Kecer M, Asoglu O, et al. Factors predicting the sentinel and non-sentinel lymph node metastases in breast cancer. Breast Cancer Res Treat. 2006;95(1):1–6.

57. Houvenaeghel G, Nos C, Giard S, Mignotte H, Esterni B, Jacquemier J, et al. A nomogram predictive of non-sentinel lymph node involvement in breast cancer patients with a sentinel lymph node micrometastasis. Eur J Surg Oncol. 2009;35:690–5.

58. Katz A, Smith BL, Golshan M, Niemierko A, Kobayashi W, Raad RA, et al. Nomogram for the prediction of having four or more involved nodes for sentinel lymph node-positive breast cancer. J Clin Oncol. 2008;26:2093–8.

59. Scow JS, Degnim AC, Hoskin TL, Reynolds C, Boughey JC. Assessment of the performance of the Stanford Online Calculator for the prediction of nonsentinel lymph node metastasis in sentinel lymph node-positive breast cancer patients. Cancer. 2009;115:4064–70.

60. van la Parra RFD, Ernst MF, Bevilacqua JLB, Mol SJ, Van Zee KJ, Broekman JM, et al. Validation of a nomogram to predict the risk of nonsentinel lymph node metastases in breast cancer patients with a positive sentinel node biopsy: validation of the MSKCC breast nomogram. Ann Surg Oncol. 2009;16:1128–35.

61. Werkoff G, Lambaudie E, Fondrinier E, Levêque J, Marchal F, Uzan M, et al. Prospective multicenter comparison of models to predict four or more involved axillary lymph nodes in patients with breast cancer with one to three metastatic sentinel lymph nodes. J Clin Oncol. 2009;27:5707–12.

62. Giuliano AE, Hunt KK, Ballman KV, Beitsch PD, Whitworth PW, Blumencranz PW, et al. Axillary dissection vs no axillary dissection in women with invasive breast cancer and sentinel node metastasis: a randomized clinical trial. JAMA. 2011;305:569–75.

63. Galimberti V, Cole BF, Zurrida S, Viale G, Luini A, Veronesi P, et al. Axillary dissection versus no axillary dissection in patients with sentinel-node micrometastases (IBCSG 23-01): a phase 3 randomised controlled trial. Lancet Oncol. 2013;14:297–305.

64. Axelsson CK, Mouridsen HT, Zedeler K. Axillary dissection of level I and II lymph nodes is important in breast cancer classification. The Danish Breast Cancer Cooperative Group (DBCG). Eur J Cancer. 1992;28A:1415–8.

65. Kiricuta CI, Tausch J. A mathematical model of axillary lymph node involvement based on 1446 complete axillary dissections in patients with breast carcinoma. Cancer. 1992;69:2496–501.

66. Fisher B, Redmond C, Fisher ER, Bauer M, Wolmark N, Wickerham DL, et al. Ten-year results of a randomized clinical trial comparing radical mastectomy and total mastectomy with or without radiation. N Engl J Med. 1985;312:674–81.

67. Alkuwari E, Auger M. Accuracy of fine-needle aspiration cytology of axillary lymph nodes in breast cancer patients: a study of 115 cases with cytologic-histologic correlation. Cancer. 2008;114:89–93.

68. Classe JM, Bordes V, Campion L, Mignotte H, Dravet F, Leveque J, et al. Sentinel lymph node biopsy after neoadjuvant chemotherapy for advanced breast cancer: results of Ganglion Sentinelle et Chimiotherapie Neoadjuvante, a French prospective multicentric study. J Clin Oncol. 2009;27:726–32.

69. Hunt KK, Yi M, Mittendorf EA, Guerrero C, Babiera GV, Bedrosian I, et al. Sentinel lymph node surgery after neoadjuvant chemotherapy is accurate and reduces the need for axillary dissection in breast cancer patients. Ann Surg. 2009;250(4):558–66.

70. Kuehn T, Bauerfeind I, Fehm T, Fleige B, Hausschild M, Helms G, et al. Sentinel-lymph-node biopsy in patients with breast cancer before and after neoadjuvant chemotherapy (SENTINA): a prospective, multicentre cohort study. Lancet Oncol. 2013;14:609–18.

71. Boughey JC, Suman VJ, Mittendorf EA, Ahrendt GM, Wilke LG, Taback B, et al. Sentinel lymph node surgery after neoadjuvant chemotherapy in patients with node-positive breast cancer: the ACOSOG Z1071 (Alliance) clinical trial. JAMA. 2013;310:1455–61.

72. Fisher B, Bryant J, Wolmark N, Mamounas E, Brown A, Fisher ER, et al. Effect of preoperative chemotherapy on the outcome of women with operable breast cancer. J Clin Oncol. 1998;16:2672–85.

73. Bear HD, Anderson S, Smith RE, Geyer Jr CE, Mamounas EP, Fisher B, et al. Sequential preoperative or postoperative docetaxel added to preoperative doxorubicin plus cyclophosphamide for operable breast cancer: national surgical adjuvant breast and bowel project protocol B-27. J Clin Oncol. 2006;24: 2019–27.

74. Hudis C, Modi S. Preoperative chemotherapy for breast cancer: miracle or mirage? JAMA. 2007;298:2665–7.

75. Dawood S, Cristofanilli M. What progress have we made in managing inflammatory breast cancer? Oncology. 2007;21:673–9.

76. Kell MR, Morrow M. Surgical aspects of inflammatory breast cancer. Breast Dis. 2005;22:67–73.

77. Stearns V, Ewing CA, Slack R, Penannen MF, Hayes DF, Tsangaris TN. Sentinel lymphadenectomy after neoadjuvant chemotherapy for breast cancer may reliably represent the axilla except for inflammatory breast cancer. Ann Surg Oncol. 2002;9:235–42.

78. Motwani SB, Strom EA, Schechter NR, Butler CE, Lee GK, Langstein HN, et al. The impact of immediate breast reconstruction on the technical delivery of postmastectomy radiotherapy. Int J Radiat Oncol Biol Phys. 2006;66:76–82.

79. Ahmed S, Snelling A, Bains M, Whitworth IH. Breast reconstruction. BMJ. 2005;330:943–8.

80. Edlich RF, Winters KL, Faulkner BC, Bill TJ, Lin KY. Advances in breast reconstruction after mastectomy. J Long-Term Eff Med Implants. 2005;15:197–207.

81. Pennington DG. Breast reconstruction after mastectomy: current state of the art. ANZ J Surg. 2005;75:454–8.

82. Garcia-Etienne CA, Cody Iii HS, Disa JJ, Cordeiro P, Sacchini V. Nipple-sparing mastectomy: initial experience at the memorial sloan-kettering cancer center and a comprehensive review of literature. Breast J. 2009;15:440–9.

83. Petit JY, Veronesi U, Orecchia R, Rey P, Martella S, Didier F, et al. Nipple sparing mastectomy with nipple areola intraoperative radiotherapy: one thousand and one cases of a five years experience at the European institute of oncology of Milan (EIO). Breast Cancer Res Treat. 2009;117:333–8.

84. Yueh JH, Houlihan MJ, Slavin SA, Slavin SA, Lee BT, Pories SE, et al. Nipple-sparing mastectomy: evaluation of patient satisfaction, aesthetic results, and sensation. Ann Plast Surg. 2009;62:586–90.

85. Chung AP, Sacchini V. Nipple-sparing mastectomy: where are we now? Surg Oncol. 2008;17:261–6.

86. Gerber B, Krause A, Dieterich M, Kundt G, Reimer T. The oncological safety of skin sparing mastectomy with conservation of the nipple-areola complex and autologous reconstruction: an extended follow-up study. Ann Surg. 2009;249:461–8.

87. Piper M, Peled AW, Foster RD, Moore DH, Esserman LJ. Total skin-sparing mastectomy: a systematic review of oncologic outcomes and postoperative complications. Ann Plast Surg. 2013;70:435–7.

88. Mallon P, Feron JG, Couturaud B, Fitoussi A, Lemasurier P, Guihard T, et al. The role of nipple-sparing mastectomy in breast cancer: a comprehensive review of the literature. Plast Reconstr Surg. 2013;131:969–84.

89. Foster RD, Esserman LJ, Anthony JP, Hwang ES, Do H. Skin-sparing mastectomy and immediate breast reconstruction: a prospective cohort study for the treatment of advanced stages of breast carcinoma. Ann Surg Oncol. 2002;9:462–6.

90. Downes KJ, Glatt BS, Kanchwala SK, Mick R, Fraker DL, Fox KR, et al. Skin-sparing mastectomy and immediate reconstruction is an acceptable treatment option for patients with high-risk breast carcinoma. Cancer. 2005;103:906–13.

91. Carlson GW, Styblo TM, Lyles RH, Jones G, Murray DR, Staley CA, et al. The use of skin sparing mastectomy in the treatment of breast cancer: the Emory experience. Surg Oncol. 2003;12:265–9.

92. Newman LA, Kuerer HM, Hunt KK, Kroll SS, Ames FC, Ross MI, et al. Presentation, treatment, and outcome of local recurrence afterskin-sparing mastectomy and immediate breast reconstruction. Ann Surg Oncol. 1998;5:620–6.

93. Medina-Franco H, Vasconez LO, Fix RJ, Heslin MJ, Beenken SW, Bland KI, et al. Factors associated with local recurrence after skin-sparing mastectomy and immediate breast reconstruction for invasive breast cancer. Ann Surg. 2002;235:814–9.

94. Kronowitz SJ, Robb GL. Radiation therapy and breast reconstruction: a critical review of the literature. Plast Reconstr Surg. 2009;124:395–408.

95. Tran NV, Chang DW, Gupta A, Kroll SS, Robb GL. Comparison of immediate and delayed free TRAM flap breast reconstruction in patients receiving postmastectomy radiation therapy. Plast Reconstr Surg. 2001;108:78–82.

96. Mehta VK, Goffinet D. Postmastectomy radiation therapy after TRAM flap breast reconstruction. Breast J. 2004;10:118–22.

97. Clough KB, Kaufman GJ, Nos C, Buccimazza I, Sarfati IM. Improving breast cancer surgery: a classification and quadrant per quadrant atlas for oncoplastic surgery. Ann Surg Oncol. 2010;17:1375–91.

98. Anderson BO, Masetti R, Silverstein MJ. Oncoplastic approaches to partial mastectomy: an overview of volume-displacement techniques. Lancet Oncol. 2005;6:145–57.

99. Huemer GM, Schrenk P, Moser F, Wagner E, Wayand W. Oncoplastic techniques allow breast-conserving treatment in centrally located breast cancers. Plast Reconstr Surg. 2007;120:390–8.

100. Kaur N, Petit J-Y, Rietjens M, Maffini F, Luini A, Gatti G, et al. Comparative study of surgical margins in oncoplastic surgery and quadrantectomy in breast cancer. Ann Surg Oncol. 2005;12:539–45.

101. Early Breast Cancer Trialists' Collaborative Group. Effects of chemotherapy and hormonal therapy for early breast cancer on recurrence and 15-year survival: an overview of the randomised trials. Lancet. 2005;365:1687–717.

102. Jones S, Holmes FA, O'Shaughnessy J, et al. Docetaxel with cyclophosphamide is associated with an overall survival benefit compared with doxorubicin and cyclophosphamide: 7- year follow-up of US Oncology Research trial 9735. J Clin Oncol. 2009;27:1177–83.

103. Early Breast Cancer Trialists' Collaborative Group. Polychemotherapy for early breast cancer: an overview of the randomised trials. Lancet. 1998;352:930–42.

104. NCCN breast cancer guidelines. Version 2015.2.

105. Möbus V, et al. Intense dose-dense sequential chemotherapy with epirubicin, paclitaxel, and cyclophosphamide compared with conventionally scheduled chemotherapy in high-risk primary breast cancer: mature results of an AGO phase II study. JCO. 2010;28:2874–80.

106. Tamoxifen for early breast cancer: an overview of the randomised trials. Early breast cancer trialists' collaborative group. Lancet. 1998;351:1451–67.

107. St.Gallen breast cancer conference, Vienna, 2015.

108. Davies C, Pan H, Godwin J, Gray R, Arriagada R, Raina V, et al. Adjuvant Tamoxifen: Longer Against Shorter (ATLAS) Collaborative Group. Long-term effects of continuing adjuvant tamoxifen to 10 years versus stopping at 5 years after diagnosis of oestrogen receptor-positive breast cancer: ATLAS, a randomised trial. Lancet. 2013;381(9869):805–16.

109. Sestak I, Cuzick J, Dowsett M, Lopez-Knowles E, Filipits M, Dubsky P, Cowens JW, Ferree S, Schaper C, Fesl C, Gnant M. Prediction of late distant recurrence after 5 years of endocrine treatment: a combined analysis of patients from the Austrian Breast and Colorectal Cancer Study Group 8 and arimidex, tamoxifen alone or in combination randomized trials using the PAM50 risk of recurrence score. J Clin Oncol. 2015;33:916–22.

110. Coates AS, Keshaviah A, Thürlimann B, Mouridsen H, Mauriac L, Forbes JF, et al. Five years of letrozole compared with tamoxifen as initial adjuvant therapy for postmenopausal women with endocrine-responsive early breast cancer: update of study BIG 1-98. J Clin Oncol. 2007;25:486–92.

111. Howell A, Cuzick J, Baum M, Buzdar A, Dowsett M, Forbes JF, et al. Results of the ATAC (arimidex, tamoxifen, alone or in combination) trial after completion of 5 years' adjuvant treatment for breast cancer. Lancet. 2005;365:60–2.

112. Goss PE, Ingle JN, Martino S, Robert NJ, Muss HB, Piccart MJ, et al. Efficacy of letrozole extended adjuvant therapy according to estrogen receptor and progesterone receptor status of the primary tumor: National Cancer Institute of Canada Clinical Trials Group MA.17. J Clin Oncol. 2007;25:2006–11.

113. Harris JR, Halpin-Murphy P, McNeese M, Mendenhall NP, Morrow M, Robert NJ. Consensus statement on postmastectomy radiation therapy. Int J Radiat Oncol Biol Phys. 1999;44:989–90.

114. Overgaard M, Hansen PS, Overgaard J, Rose C, Andersson M, Bach F, et al. Postoperative radiotherapy in high-risk premenopausal women with breast cancer who receive adjuvant chemotherapy. N Engl J Med. 1997;337:949–55.

115. Overgaard M, Jensen MB, Overgaard J, Hansen PS, Rose C, Andersson M, et al. Postoperative radiotherapy in high-risk postmenopausal breast cancer patients given adjuvant tamoxifen: Danish Breast Cancer Cooperative Group DBCG 82c randomized trial. Lancet. 1999;353:1641–8.

116. Ragaz J, Jackson SM, Le N, Plenderleith IH, Spinelli JJ, Basco VE, et al. Adjuvant radiotherapy and chemotherapy in node-positive premenopausal women with breast cancer. N Engl J Med. 1997;337:956–62.

117. Whelan TJ, Olivotto I, Ackerman I, Chapman JW, Chua B, Nabid A, et al. NCIC-CTG MA.20: an intergroup trial of regional nodal irradiation in early breast cancer. Program and abstracts of the American Society of Clinical Oncology Annual Meeting; June 3-11, Chicago: LBA. 2011. 1003.

118. Taghian AG, Jeong JH, Mamounas EP, Parda DS, Deutsch M, Costantino JP, et al. Low locoregional recurrence rate among node-negative breast cancer patients with tumors 5 cm or larger treated by mastectomy, with or without adjuvant systemic therapy and without radiotherapy: results from five national surgical adjuvant breast and bowel project randomized clinical trials. J Clin Oncol. 2006;24:3927–32.

119. NCI: http//www.cancer.gov/cancertopics/pdq/treatment/breast/healthprofessional/page5#section_5.71.

120. Van Dongen JA, Voogd AC, Fentiman IS, Legrand C, Sylvester RJ, Tong D, et al. Long-term results of a randomized trial comparing breast-conserving therapy with mastectomy: European organization for research and treatment of cancer 10801 trial. J Natl Cancer Inst. 2000;92:1143–50.

121. Veronesi U, Marubini E, Marian L, Galimberti V, Luini A, Veronesi P, et al. Radiotherapy after breast-conserving surgery in small breast carcinoma: long-term results of a randomized trial. Ann Oncol. 2001;12:997–1003.

122. Veronesi U, Saccozzi R, Del Vecchio M, Banfi A, Clemente C, De Lena M, et al. Comparing radical mastectomy with quadrantectomy, axillary dissection, and radiotherapy in patients with small cancers of the breast. N Engl J Med. 1981;305:6–11.

123. Early Breast Cancer Trialists' Collaborative Group. Effect of radiotherapy after breast-conserving surgery on 10-year recurrence and 15-year breast cancer death: meta-analysis of individual patient data for 10,801 women in 17 randomised trials. Lancet. 2011;378:1707–16.

124. Vaidya JS, Joseph DJ, Tobias JS, Bulsara M, Wenz F, Saunders C, et al. Targeted intraoperative radiotherapy versus whole breast radiotherapy for breast cancer (TARGIT-A trial): an international, prospective, randomised, non-inferiority phase 3 trial. Lancet. 2010;276:91–102.

125. Veronesi U, Orecchia R, Maisonneuve, Viale G, Rotmensz N, Sangalli CP, et al. Intraoperative radiotherapy versus external radiotherapy for early breast cancer (ELIOT): a randomised controlled equivalence trial. Lancet Oncol. 2013;14:1269–77.

126. Smith GL, Xu Y, Buchholz TA, Giordano SH, Jiang J, Shih YC, et al. Association between treatment with brachytherapy vs whole-breast irradiation and subsequent mastectomy, complications, and survival among older women with invasive breast cancer. JAMA. 2012;307:1827–37.

127. Olivotto IA, Whelan TJ, Parpia S, Kim DH, Berrang T, Truong PT, et al. Interim cosmetic and toxicity results from RAPID: a randomized trial of accelerated partial breast irradiation using three-dimensional conformal external beam radiation therapy. J Clin Oncol. 2013;31:4038–45.

128. Kunkler I, Williams LJ, Jack WJL, Cameron DA, Dixon JM. Breast conserving surgery with or without irradiation in women aged 65 years or older

with early breast cancer (PRIME II): a randomised controlled trial. Lancet Oncol. 2015. doi:10.1016/S1470-2045(14)71221-5.

129. Hughes KS, Schnaper LA, Berry D, Cirrincione C, McCormick B, Shank B, et al. Lumpectomy plus tamoxifen with or without irradiation in women 70 years of age or older with early breast cancer. N Engl J Med. 2004;351:971–7.

130. Chang HJ, Han SW, Oh DY, Im SA, Jeon YK, Park IA, et al. Discordant human epidermal growth factor receptor 2 and hormone receptor status in primary and metastatic breast cancer and response to trastuzumab. Jpn J Clin Oncol. 2011;41:593–9.

131. Domschke C, Schuetz F. Side effects of bone-targeted therapies in advanced breast cancer. Breast Care (Basel). 2014;9:332–6.

132. Klijn JG, Blamey RW, Boccardo F, Tominaga T, Duchateau L, Sylvester R. Combined Hormone Agents Trialists' Group and the European Organization for Research and Treatment of Cancer. Combined tamoxifen and luteinizing hormone-releasing hormone (LHRH) agonist versus LHRH agonist alone in premenopausal advanced breast cancer: a meta-analysis of four randomized trials. J Clin Oncol. 2001;19:343–53.

133. Bonneterre J, Thurlimann B, Robertson JF, Krzakowski M, Mauriac L, Koralewski P, et al. Anastrozole versus tamoxifen as first-line therapy for advanced breast cancer in 668 postmenopausal women: results of the Tamoxifen or Arimidex Randomized Group Efficacy and Tolerability study. J Clin Oncol. 2000;18:3748–57.

134. Buzdar A, Douma J, Davidson N, Elledge R, Morgan M, Smith R, et al. Phase III, multicenter, double-blind, randomized study of letrozole, an AI, for advanced breast cancer versus megestrol acetate. J Clin Oncol. 2001;19:3357–66.

135. Nabholtz JM, Buzdar A, Pollak M, Harwin W, Burton G, Mangalik A, et al. Anastrozole is superior to tamoxifen as first-line therapy for advanced breast cancer in postmenopausal women: results of a North American multicenter randomized trial. Arimidex Study Group. J Clin Oncol. 2000;18:3758–67.

136. Paridaens RJ, Dirix LY, Beex LV, Nooij M, Cameron DA, Cufer T, et al. Phase III study comparing exemestane with tamoxifen as first-line hormonal treatment of MBC in postmenopausal women: the European Organisation for Research and Treatment of Cancer Breast Cancer Cooperative Group. J Clin Oncol. 2008;26:4883–90.

137. Mouridsen H, Gershanovich M, Sun Y, Perez-Carrion R, Boni C, Monnier A, et al. Phase III study of letrozole versus tamoxifen as first-line therapy of advanced breast cancer in postmenopausal women: analysis of survival and update of efficacy from the International Letrozole Breast Cancer Group. J Clin Oncol. 2003;21:2101–9.

138. Steele N, Zekri J, Coleman R, et al. Exemestane in metastatic breast cancer: effective therapy after third-generation non-steroidal aromatase inhibitor failure. Breast. 2006;15:430–6.

139. Bertelli G, Garrone O, Merlano M, et al. Sequential treatment with exemestane and non-steroidal aromatase inhibitors in advanced breast cancer. Oncology. 2005;69:471–7.

140. Finn RS, Crown JP, Lang I, Boer K, Bondarenko IM, Kulyk SO, et al. The cyclin-dependent kinase 4/6 inhibitor palbociclib in combination with letrozole versus letrozole alone as first-line treatment of oestrogen receptor-positive, HER2-negative, advanced breast cancer (PALOMA-1/TRIO-18): a randomised phase 2 study. Lancet Oncol. 2015;16: 25–35.

141. Piccart M, Hortobagyi GN, Campone M, Pritchard KI, Lebrun F, Ito Y, et al. Everolimus plus exemestane for hormone-receptor-positive, human epidermal growth factor receptor-2-negative advanced breast cancer: overall survival results from BOLERO-2†. Ann Oncol. 2014;25(12):2357–62.

142. Giordano SH, Temin S, Kirshner JJ, Chandarlapaty S, Crews JR, Davidson NE, et al. Systemic therapy for patients with advanced human epidermal growth factor receptor 2-positive breast cancer: American Society of Clinical Oncology clinical practice guideline. J Clin Oncol. 2014;32:2078–99.

143. Swain SM, Baselga J, Kim SB, Ro J, Semiglazov V, Campone M, CLEOPATRA Study Group, et al. Pertuzumab, trastuzumab, and docetaxel in HER2-positive metastatic breast cancer. N Engl J Med. 2015;372(8):724–34.

144. Geyer CE, Forster J, Lindquist D, Chan S, Romieu CG, Pienkowski T, et al. Lapatinib plus capecitabine for HER2-positive advanced breast cancer. N Engl J Med. 2006;355:2733–43.

145. Verma S, Miles D, Gianni L, Krop IE, Welslau M, Baselga J, EMILIA Study Group, et al. Trastuzumab emtansine for HER2-positive advanced breast cancer. N Engl J Med. 2012;367:1783–91.

146. Hortobagyi GN. Multidisciplinary management of advanced primary and metastatic breast cancer. Cancer. 1994;74:416–23.

147. Babiera GV, Rao R, Feng L, Meric-Bernstam F, Kuerer HM, Singletary SE, et al. Effect of primary tumor extirpation in breast cancer patients who present with stage IV disease and an intact primary tumor. Ann Surg Oncol. 2006;13:776–82.

148. Khan SA, Stewart AK, Morrow M. Does aggressive local therapy improve survival in metastatic breast cancer? Surgery. 2002;132:620–6.

149. Rao R, Feng L, Kuerer HM, Singletary SE, Bedrosian I, Hunt KK, et al. Timing of surgical intervention for the intact primary in stage IV breast cancer patients. Ann Surg Oncol. 2008;15:1696–702.

150. Rapiti E, Verkooijen HM, Vlastos G, Fioretta G, Neyroud-Caspar I, Sappino AP, et al. Complete excision of primary breast tumor improves survival of patients with metastatic breast cancer at diagnosis. J Clin Oncol. 2006;24:2743–9.

151. Morrow M, Goldstein L. Surgery of the primary tumor in metastatic breast cancer: closing the barn door after the horse has bolted? J Clin Oncol. 2006;24:2694–6.

152. Olson JA, Marcom PK. Benefit or bias? The role of surgery to remove the primary tumor in patients with metastatic breast cancer. Ann Surg. 2008;247:739–40.

153. Badwe R, Parmar V, Hawaldar R, Nair N, Kaushik R, Siddique S, et al. Surgical removal of primary breast tumor and axillary lymph nodes in women with metastatic breast cancer at first presentation: a randomized controlled trial. Presented at: 2013 [abstract]. San Antonio Breast Cancer Symposium 2013:Abstract S2-02.

154. Soran A, Ozmen V, Ozbas S, Karanlik H, Muslumanoglu M, Igci A, et al. Early follow up of a randomized trial evaluating resection of the primary breast tumor in women presenting with de novo stage IV breast cancer; Turkish study (protocol MF07-01) [abstract]. San Antonio Breast Cancer Symposium 2013:Abstract S2-03.

Decision Pathways in Breast Cancer Management

45

Adnan Aydiner, Fatma Sen, Hasan Karanlik,
Isik Aslay, Maktav Dincer, and Abdullah İğci

Abstract

This chapter is focused on providing a practical approach to the allocation of available diagnostic procedures and therapies to individual patients in the light of the most recent and reliable information from clinical trials and international guidelines. It reviewed substantial new evidence on locoregional and systemic therapies for early and advanced breast cancer and in situ carcinoma. In breast cancer, the choice of treatment strategy is based on the features and biology of the tumor as well as on the age, general health status, and personal preferences of the patient. The majority of breast cancer deaths now occur in less developed regions of the world. In these areas, less expensive pathology tests and treatment may be necessary. Economic considerations may require that less expensive and only marginally less effective therapies may be necessary in less-resourced areas. The gold standard for breast cancer care includes an integrated multidisciplinary team approach, comprising pathologists, radiologists, surgical oncologists, medical oncologists, radiation oncologists, oncology nurses, and plastic surgeons. This chapter comprises decision pathways outlining the step-by-step clinical decision-making process for patient management.

A. Aydiner, MD (✉)
Department of Medical Oncology, Istanbul University
Istanbul Medical Faculty, Institute of Oncology,
Istanbul, Turkey
e-mail: adnanaydiner@superonline.com

F. Sen, MD
Department of Medical Oncology, Istanbul University
Istanbul Medical Faculty, Institute of Oncology,
Istanbul, Turkey
e-mail: fkaragoz_2000@yahoo.com

H. Karanlik, MD
Department of Surgery, Istanbul University, Institute
of Oncology, Istanbul, Turkey
e-mail: hasankaranlik@yahoo.com

I. Aslay, MD
Department of Radiation Oncology, Acibadem
Hospital, Kozyatagi, Istanbul, Turkey
e-mail: isik.aslay@gmail.com

M. Dincer, MD
Department of Radiation Oncology, Florence
Nightingale Hospital, Istanbul, Turkey
e-mail: dincer@superonline.com

A. İğci, MD, FACS
Breast Unit, Department of General Surgery, Istanbul
University, Istanbul Medical Faculty, Istanbul, Turkey
e-mail: aiga@istanbul.edu.tr

© Springer International Publishing Switzerland 2016
A. Aydiner et al. (eds.), *Breast Disease: Management and Therapies*,
DOI 10.1007/978-3-319-26012-9_45

Keywords

Decision pathways • In situ carcinoma • Ductal carcinoma in situ (DCIS) •
Lobular carcinoma in situ (LCIS) • Invasive breast cancer (IBC) •
Noninflammatory breast cancer • Inflammatory breast cancer • Locally
advanced disease • Luminal A • Luminal B • Diagnosis • Staging • Axillary
staging • Locoregional treatment • Lumpectomy • Mastectomy • Radiotherapy
• Systemic therapy • Adjuvant • Neoadjuvant • Chemotherapy • Endocrine
therapy • Follow-up • Recurrence • Phylloides tumor • Paget disease •
Pregnancy • High-risk patients • Risk-reducing therapy • Ki 67 • Oncotype •
ER • PR • HER2 • Grade • Stage I • Stage II • Stage III • Stage IV

Introduction

The decision pathways are a comprehensive set
of guidelines detailing the sequential management decisions and interventions that currently
apply to breast cancer (BC) patients. The information in this chapter is not intended to cover
all possibilities, and all uses of the pathways are
subject to clinical judgment. Decision pathways
provide recommendations based on the best evidence available at the time of this book edition.

Because new data from randomized clinical
trials are published continuously, decision pathways must be subject to change. Several guidelines are continuously updated and revised to
reflect new data and clinical information that
may add to or alter current clinical practice
standards [1–16].

Proposal level	Description
Proposal 1	A consensus is present based upon a high level of evidence

Breast Disease: Management

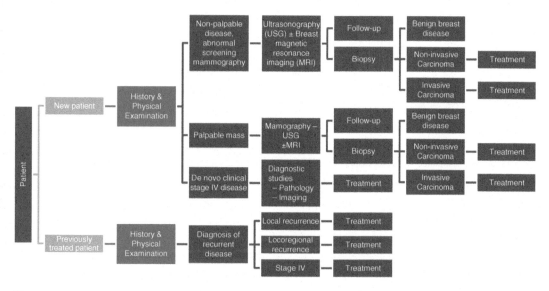

Fig. 45.1 Summary of the step-by-step clinical decision-making process for patient management (See Table 45.1)

Breast Disease: Approach for Benign Breast Disease

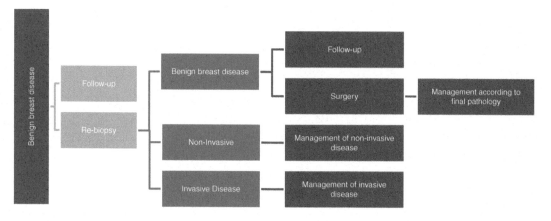

Fig. 45.2 Approach for benign breast disease after biopsy

Breast Disease: Diagnosis and Staging

Table 45.1 Diagnostic procedures of noninvasive (in situ) and invasive breast carcinoma

	In Situ Carcinoma	Invasive breast cancer		Inflammatory breast cancer
	Stage 0	Stage I, IIA, IIB, IIIA	Stage IIIA (N2), IIIB, IIIC	Stage T4d, N0-N3, M0
Medical history and physical examination	☑	☑	☑	☑
Mammography (MMG)	☑	☑	☑	☑
Ultrasonography (USG)		☑	If necessary ☑	If necessary ☑
Breast magnetic resonance imaging (MRI)	If necessary ☑	☑ Optional	☑ Optional	☑ Optional
Pathological evaluation	☑	☑	☑	☑
Hormone receptors (HR) [estrogen receptor (ER) and progesterone receptor (PR)] determination	☑	☑	☑	☑
Assessment of tumor HER2 status		☑	☑	☑
Genetic counseling for patients at high risk for hereditary breast cancer	☑	☑	☑	☑
If required, fertility counseling	☑	☑	☑	☑
Blood tests (complete blood count, liver function tests, renal function tests, alkaline phosphatase (ALP), calcium, glucose)		☑	☑	☑
Serum tumor markers: CEA, CA153			☑	☑
Serum tumor marker: Ca125 (for young patients)		☑	☑	☑
In the case of localized bone pain or high ALP: bone scintigraphy (if PET/CT scan is not necessary)		☑	☑	☑
In the presence of high ALP, abnormal liver function tests, abdominal symptoms, or abnormalities upon abdominopelvic physical examination: Abdomen ± pelvic computed tomography (CT) or MRI (or PET/CT scan)		☑	☑	☑
In the presence of pulmonary symptoms: chest CT		☑	☑	☑
FDG positron emission tomography (PET/CT)		☑ optional	☑	☑

Noninvasive Breast Cancer

In Situ Carcinoma

Stage 0 (Tis, N0, M0) (diagnosed with biopsy or surgical excision)

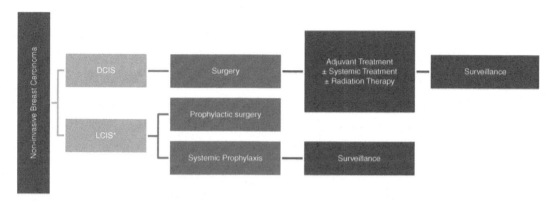

Fig. 45.3 Management of noninvasive breast carcinoma. * For the pleomorphic subtype of lobular carcinoma in situ (LCIS), ductal carcinoma in situ (DCIS) treatment alternatives should be administered

Ductal Carcinoma In Situ

Locoregional Therapy

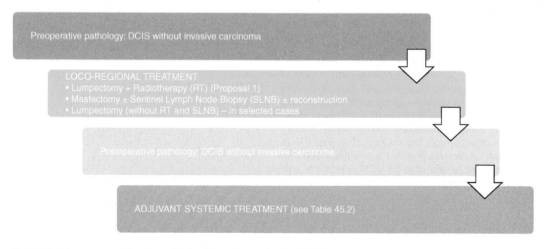

Fig. 45.4 Management of patient with ductal carcinoma in situ (DCIS)

Adjuvant Systemic Therapy

Table 45.2 Adjuvant systemic therapy of ductal carcinoma in situ (DCIS)

Post-breast conservation surgery
Risk-mitigating treatment for the ipsilateral breast
Tamoxifen for 5 years
For estrogen receptor (ER) or progesterone receptor (PR) positive patients who have undergone breast-conserving surgery (BCS) and radiotherapy (RT)
Benefit of tamoxifen is not definite for ER-negative patients
Patients treated with excision only
Anastrozole for 5 years[a]
For ER or PR positive postmenopausal patients who have undergone BCS and RT
Risk-mitigating treatment for the contralateral breast
Counseling for risk mitigation (see Figs. 45.38, 45.39, and 45.40 and Table 45.13)

[a]The primary endpoint of NSABP B-35, a phase III trial comparing anastrozole to tamoxifen, each given for 5 years, was breast cancer-free interval (BCFI), defined as the time from randomization to any breast cancer event including local, regional, or distant recurrence or contralateral disease, invasive or ductal carcinoma in situ (DCIS). Postmenopausal women with estrogen receptor (ER) or progesterone receptor (PR) positive (by IHC analysis) DCIS and no invasive BC who had undergone a lumpectomy with clear resection margins were randomly assigned. Stratification was by age (<60 v ≥60). There were 198 BCFI events, 114 in the tamoxifen group and 84 in the anastrozole group (hazard ratio, 0.73; $p=0.03$). There was a significant interaction between treatment and age group ($p=0.04$); benefit of anastrozole is only in women <60 years old. There were 63 cases of invasive breast cancer in the tamoxifen group and 39 in the anastrozole group (hazard ratio, 0.61; $p=0.02$). There was a non-significant trend for a reduction in breast second primary cancers with anastrozole (hazard ratio, 0.68; $p=0.07$). In conclusion, anastrozole provided a significant improvement compared to tamoxifen for BCFI, which was seen later in the study, primarily in women <60 years old [1]

Monitoring and Follow-Up

Table 45.3 DCIS – monitoring and follow-up

Medical history and physical examination
Every 6 months for 5 years
Once a year thereafter
Mammography
Once a year (if BCS is performed, at months 6–12 following RT)
If treated with tamoxifen monitor according to breast cancer risk mitigation guidelines

Lobular Carcinoma In Situ

Diagnosis and Management

Table 45.4 Diagnosis and management

Medical history
Physical examination
Mammography
Pathology: lobular carcinoma in situ (LCIS) (without DCIS or invasive carcinoma)[a]
Counseling for risk-mitigating approaches (see Figs. 45.38, 45.39, and 45.40)
Follow-up

[a]For the pleomorphic subtype of lobular carcinoma in situ, DCIS treatment alternatives should be administered

Invasive Breast Cancer (IBC)

Clinical Staging I, II, IIIA (T3N1M0)

Fig. 45.5 Clinical stages of invasive breast cancer

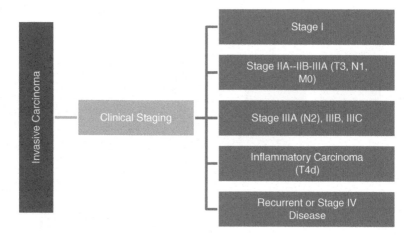

Axillary Evaluation

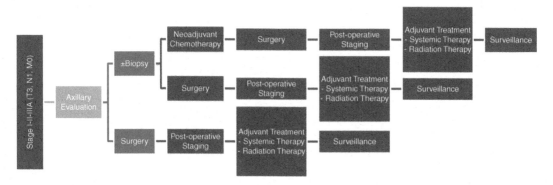

Fig. 45.6 Axillary evaluation and management of patients with clinical stages I, II, or IIIA (T3, N1, M0)

Surgical Axillary Staging and Management

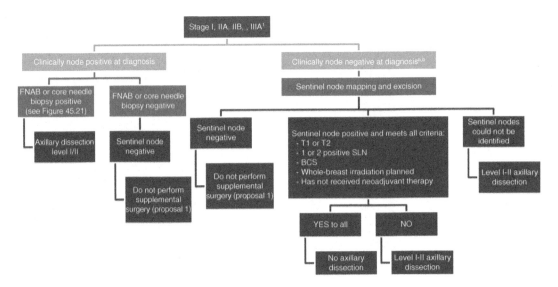

Fig. 45.7 Axillary management of patients with clinical stages I, II, or IIIA (T3, N1, M0) [3–6, 9–12]. [1]Stage I (T1, N0, M0); stage IIA (T0, N1, M0; T1, N1, M0; T2, N0, M0); stage IIB (T2, N1, M0; T3, N0, M0); stage IIIA (T3, N1, M0). [a]For breast conserving surgery (BCS): In patients with macro-metastases in 1–2 sentinel lymph nodes, complete axillary dissection can be safely omitted when "conservative resection with RT using high tangents to include the lower axilla" is performed [4, 9–12, 15, 16]. [b]For mastectomy: In patients with macro-metastases in 1–2 sentinel lymph nodes, complete axillary dissection must be performed when "no adjuvant RT is planned"; however, in patients for whom RT is planned, no consensus exists for omitting axillary dissection [4]

Surgical Approach

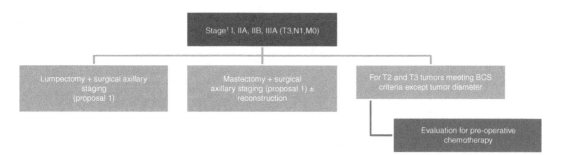

Fig. 45.8 Surgical treatment of patients with clinical stages I, II, or IIIA (T3N1M0) disease[a–e] [3–6]. [1]Stage IA (T1, N0, M0); stage IB (T0, N1mi; M0; T1, N1mi, M0); stage IIA (T0, N1, M0; T1, N1, M0; T2, N0, M0); stage IIB (T2, N1, M0; T3, N0, M0); stage IIIA (T3, N1, M0). [a]Absolute contraindications to breast-conserving surgery (BCS) include diffuse suspicious microcalcifications, widespread disease, and persistent positive pathological margins [3–6, 8]. Relative contraindications include tumor size >5 cm, prior radiation therapy, active connective tissue disease, focally positive margins, and a known or suspected genetic predisposition to breast cancer. According to St. Gallen 2015 consensus meeting, multifocal and multicentric (unilateral) tumors can be treated with BCS "provided that the margins are clear and that whole breast radiotherapy (RT) is planned" [4]. [b]In women undergoing BCS for invasive BC and proceeding to standard RT and adjuvant systemic therapy, the minimum acceptable surgical margin is "no ink on invasive tumor" [4, 8]. The tumor biology or patient age (<40) does not change the minimum acceptable surgical margins [4, 8]. [c]For BCS: In patients with macro-metastases in 1–2 sentinel lymph nodes, complete axillary dissection can be safely omitted when "conservative resection with RT using high tangents to include the lower axilla" is performed [4, 9]. [d]For mastectomy: In patients with macro-metastases in 1-2 sentinel nodes, complete axillary dissection must be performed if "no adjuvant RT is planned." In patients for whom RT is planned, no consensus has been reached for omitting axillary dissection [4]. [e]In a multidisciplinary consensus panel, margin widths and ipsilateral breast tumor recurrence (IBTR) were reviewed in 33 studies including 28,162 patients [8]. Positive margins (ink on invasive carcinoma or ductal carcinoma in situ) are associated with a twofold increase in the risk of IBTR compared with negative margins. This increased risk is not mitigated by favorable biology, endocrine therapy, or a radiation boost. More widely clear margins than no ink on tumor do not significantly decrease the rate of IBTR compared with no ink on tumor. No evidence indicates that more widely clear margins reduce IBTR in young patients or in those with unfavorable biology, lobular cancers, or cancers with an extensive intraductal component. The authors concluded that the use of no ink on tumor is the standard for adequate margins in invasive cancer but not in DCIS

Pathological Evaluation

Histology, Hormone-Receptor (HR) Status, HER2 Status, Intrinsic Subtype

Table 45.5 Ductal, lobular, mixed, metaplastic

ER positive and/or PR positive
HR-positive–HER2-positive disease treatment
HR-positive–HER2-negative disease treatment
ER negative and PR negative
HR-negative–HER2-positive disease treatment
HR-negative–HER2-negative disease treatment

Table 45.6 Tubular, mucinous histology

ER positive and/or PR positive (if ER-negative and PR-negative repeat assessment of tumor ER/PR status)

Table 45.7 Intrinsic subtype [4]

Intrinsic subtype	
Luminal A	Luminal A-like
Luminal B	Luminal B-like (HER2 negative)
	Luminal B-like (HER2 positive)
C-ERB B2 overexpression	HER2 positive (nonluminal)
Basal-like	Triple negative

Intrinsic Subtype: Luminal A-Like

Table 45.8 Recommendations for breast cancer depending on the intrinsic subtype and clinicopathological surrogate definitions [2–6]

Intrinsic subtype	Clinicopathological definition
Luminal A	*Luminal A-like*
	ER positive, PR positive[a], and HER2 negative, and Ki67 ≤14–19 %[b], and low recurrence risk with multigene tests

[a]More than 20 % positivity
[b]The minimum value of Ki67 required for "luminal B-like" is 20–29 %. Ki-67 scores should be interpreted in the light of local laboratory values: as an example, if a laboratory has a median Ki-67 score in receptor-positive disease of 20 %, values of 30 % or above could be considered clearly high; those of 10 % or less clearly low [4]

Intrinsic Subtype-Luminal B-Like

Table 45.9 Recommendations for breast cancer depending on the intrinsic subtype and clinicopathological surrogate definitions [2–6]

Intrinsic subtype	Clinicopathological definition
Luminal B	*Luminal B-like (HER2 negative)*
	ER positive, HER2 negative, and Ki67 ≥20–29 %[a] or PR low (<%20)/ negative or high recurrence risk according to multigene tests
	Luminal B-like (HER2 positive)
	ER and/or PR positive, and HER2 overexpression or amplification Any Ki-67

[a]The minimum value of Ki67 required for "luminal B-like" is 20–29 %. Ki-67 scores should be interpreted in the light of local laboratory values: as an example, if a laboratory has a median Ki-67 score in receptor-positive disease of 20 %, values of 30 % or above could be considered clearly high [4]

HER2 Testing

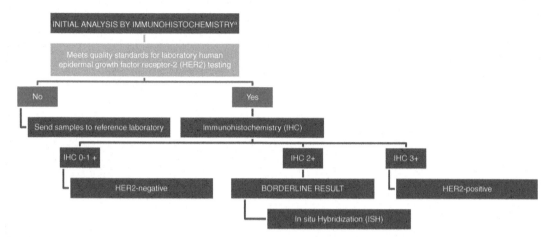

Fig. 45.9 Assessment of tumor HER2 status [2–6]. [a]Principles of HER 2 testing. The Update Committee of American Society of Clinical Oncology and College of American Pathologists (CAP) identified criteria and areas requiring clarification to improve the accuracy of HER2 testing by immunohistochemistry (IHC) or in situ hybridization (ISH). The committee recommended that the HER2 status (HER2 negative or positive) be determined in all patients with invasive (early-stage or recurrent) breast cancer based on one or more HER2 test results (negative, equivocal, or positive). Testing criteria define a HER2-positive status if (upon observing an area of the tumor representing >10 % contiguous and homogeneous tumor cells) there is evidence of protein overexpression (IHC) or gene amplification (HER2 copy number or HER2/CEP17 ratio by ISH based on counting at least 20 cells within the area). If the results are equivocal (revised criteria), reflex testing should be performed using an alternative assay (IHC or ISH). Repeat testing should be considered if the results appear to be discordant with other histopathological findings. Laboratories should demonstrate high concordance with a validated HER2 test on a sufficiently large and representative set of specimens. Testing must be performed in a laboratory accredited by the CAP or another accrediting entity [2–6]

Adjuvant Systemic Therapy

Luminal A-Like, Luminal B-Like, HER2-Positive, Triple Negative

Table 45.10 Recommendations for adjuvant treatment of breast cancer depending on intrinsic subtype and clinicopathological surrogate definitions [4–6]

Intrinsic subtype	Clinicopathological definition	Treatment	Special considerations
Luminal A	*Luminal A-like*		
	ER positive and PR positive[a] and HER2 negative and Kİ 67 ≤ (14–19 %)[b] and recurrence risk low with multigene tests	Endocrine therapy	Cytotoxics administered when; high gene RS (>25), 70-gene high-risk status, grade 3 disease, extensive lymphovascular invasion[c] ≥4 lymph node metastasis, young age (<35 years)[d]
Luminal B	*Luminal B-like (HER2 negative)*		
	ER positive and HER2 negative and Ki67 ≥(20–29 %)[b] or PR low/negative or recurrence risk high with multigene tests	Endocrine therapy for all, cytotoxics for most	
	Luminal B-like (HER2 positive)		
	ER and/or PR positive, and HER2 overexpressed or amplified any Ki-67	Cytotoxics and antiHER2 and endocrine therapy	
HER2 overexpression	*HER2 positive (nonluminal)*		
	HER2 overexpressed or amplified and ER and PR absent	Cytotoxics and antiHER2	
Basal-like	*Triple negative*		
	ER negative and PR negative HER2 negative	Cytotoxics	80 % overlap between triple negative and basal-like subtypes

[a]More than 20 % positivity
[b]St. Gallen 2015: the minimum value of Ki67 required for "luminal B-like" is 20–29 %. Ki-67 scores should be interpreted in the light of local laboratory values: as an example, if a laboratory has a median Ki-67 score in receptor-positive disease of 20 %, values of 30 % or above could be considered clearly high; those of 10 % or less clearly are low [4]
[c]Lymphovascular invasion without any other poor prognostic factor is not an indication for cytotoxic chemotherapy [4]
[d]The panel in St. Gallen was equally divided as to whether young age or per se was an indication for the addition of cytotoxics [4]

Ductal, Lobular, Mixed, Metaplastic Histology: Stage IA (T1N0M0) Disease

Hormone-Receptor-Positive or Hormone-Receptor-Negative and HER2-Positive Disease

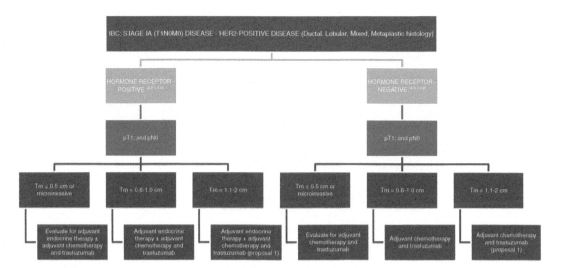

Fig. 45.10 Adjuvant systemic therapy for stage IA hormone-receptor-positive or hormone-receptor-negative and HER2-positive disease [3–7, 17, 18]. [a]There is no absolute age limit. Rather, treatment depends on the disease, the presence of comorbidities, the patient's life expectancy, and patient preferences. Treatment should be individualized for patients > 70 years of age [3–6]. [b]Chemotherapy and endocrine therapy use as adjuvant therapy should be given sequentially with endocrine therapy following chemotherapy. Available data suggest that sequential or concurrent endocrine therapy with radiation therapy is acceptable. [c]Assuming HER2 positivity is determined according to the ASCO/CAP guidelines, the majority of patients with T1b disease and all patients with T1c disease require anti-HER2 therapy [3, 4, 17, 18]. The chemotherapy regimen for these patients may contain anthracyclines. If provided in stage I and if the tumor diameter is <1 cm, the combination of paclitaxel and trastuzumab is the preferred regimen [18]. For patients in stage I with a tumor diameter >1 cm, anthracyclines followed by taxanes and trastuzumab may be preferred, although paclitaxel-trastuzumab may also be an option [4, 17, 18]. [d]Based on the eight eligible studies identified, a meta-analysis demonstrated a deleterious effect of the HER2-positive phenotype on disease-free survival (DFS; RR = 3.677, 95 % CI 2.606–5.189, $P<0.001$) and distant disease-free survival (DDFS; RR=3.824, 95 % CI 2.249-6.501, $P < 0.001$) compared with the HR-positive and HER2-negative subgroup [17]. However, a significant difference was not achieved in terms of any endpoint between HER2-positive breast cancer and triple-negative breast cancer (TNBC). Additionally, a marked improvement in DFS was observed with the addition of trastuzumab for HER2-positive pT1a-bN0M0 patients (RR=0.323, 95 % CI 0.191–0.547, $P < 0.001$). This meta-analysis suggested that the intrinsic subtype might be a reliable marker to predict the prognosis of pT1a-bN0M0 breast cancer. Additionally, adjuvant trastuzumab might yield a significant survival benefit, even for early-stage HER2-positive patients [17]. [e]In an uncontrolled, single-group, multicenter study of adjuvant paclitaxel and trastuzumab, 406 patients with tumors measuring up to 3 cm in the greatest dimension were included [18]. Patients received weekly treatment with paclitaxel and trastuzumab for 12 weeks, followed by 9 months of trastuzumab monotherapy. The median follow-up period was 4.0 years. The 3-year rate of survival free from invasive disease was 98.7 % (95 % confidence interval [CI], 97.6 to 99.8). Among women with predominantly stage I HER2-positive breast cancer, treatment with adjuvant paclitaxel plus trastuzumab was associated with a risk of early recurrence of approximately 2 %; 6 % of patients withdrew from the study due to protocol-specified adverse events [18]. [f]Fertility preservation (e.g., by ovarian tissue or oocyte conservation) should be offered to women <40 years of age. Ovarian function suppression with LHRHa during chemotherapy for hormone receptor-negative disease should be offered [3–6, 19]

Hormone-Receptor-Positive or Hormone-Receptor-Negative and HER2-Negative Disease

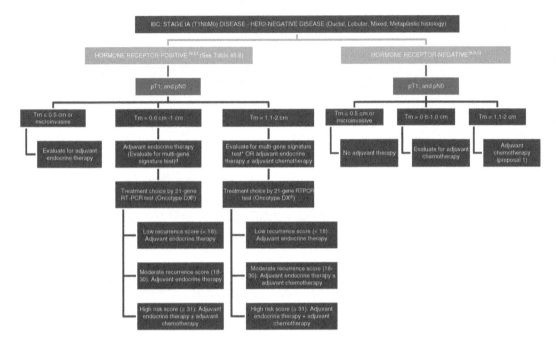

Fig. 45.11 Adjuvant systemic therapy for stage IA hormone-receptor (HR)-positive or HR-negative and HER2-negative disease [3–7]. *By multigene signature tests: chemotherapy may be omitted for patients with luminal B-like (HER2 negative) disease with a low Oncotype Dx® score, MammaPrint® low risk status, low PAM50 ROR score, or EndoPredict® low risk status [3–6]. [a]There is no absolute age limit. Rather, treatment depends on the disease, the presence of comorbidities, the patient's life expectancy, and patient preferences. Treatment should be individualized for patients > 70 years of age [3–6]. [b]Che- motherapy and endocrine therapy use as adjuvant therapy should be given sequentially with endocrine therapy following chemotherapy. Available data suggest that sequential or concurrent endocrine therapy with radiation therapy is acceptable. [c]Fertility preservation (e.g., by ovarian tissue or oocyte conservation) should be offered to women <40 years of age. Ovarian function suppression with LHRHa during chemotherapy for HR-negative disease should be offered [3–6, 19]. [d]Especially for Luminal B-like, high Ki67, and grade III tumors

Ductal, Lobular, Mixed, Metaplastic Histology: Stage IB–II–IIIA (T3N1M0) Disease

Hormone-Receptor-Positive and HER2-Positive Disease

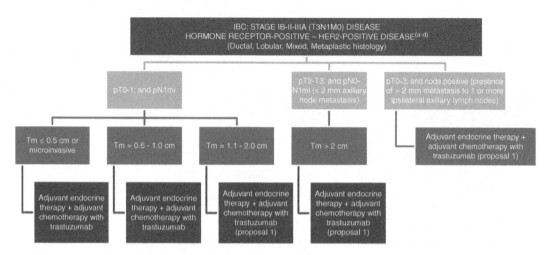

Fig. 45.12 Adjuvant systemic therapy for stages IB, II, and IIIA hormone-receptor-positive and HER2-positive disease [3–7]. [a]There is no absolute age limit. Rather, treatment depends on the disease, the presence of comorbidities, the patient's life expectancy, and patient preferences. Treatment should be individualized for patients >70 years of age [3–6]. [b]The version 1.0 2016 NCCN Guidelines recommend AC – paclitaxel and trastuzumab (± pertuzumab); TCH ± pertuzumab (pertuzumab given to patients with greater than or equal to T2 or greater than or equal to N1, HER2-positive early-stage breast cancer) [3]. Pending results from the ongoing APHINITY trial, the St. Gallen Consensus Panel did not support dual HER2 blockade by the addition of either pertuzumab or lapatinib to trastuzumab for postoperative adjuvant therapy [4]. [c]In high-risk premenopausal patients, "LHRH-agonist + exemestane" may be the preferred adjuvant endocrine therapy. In a randomized phase III study, a total of 3066 premenopausal women were stratified according to whether they previously received chemotherapy to receive 5 years of tamoxifen, tamoxifen plus ovarian suppression therapy, or exemestane plus ovarian suppression therapy [20]. After a median follow-up of 67 months, the estimated disease-free survival rate at 5 years was 86.6 % in the tamoxifen-ovarian suppression group and 84.7 % in the tamoxifen group (hazard ratio for disease recurrence, second invasive cancer, or death, 0.83; 95 % confidence interval [CI], 0.66 to 1.04; $P = 0.10$). At 5 years, the rate of freedom from breast cancer was 85.7 % in the exemestane-ovarian suppression group (hazard ratio for recurrence vs. tamoxifen, 0.65; 95 % CI, 0.49 to 0.87) [20]. In high-risk postmenopausal patients, aromatase inhibitors (AIs) may be preferred over tamoxifen [4]. [d]Chemotherapy and endocrine therapy use as adjuvant therapy should be given sequentially with endocrine therapy following chemotherapy. Available data suggest that sequential or concurrent endocrine therapy with radiation therapy is acceptable

Hormone-Receptor-Positive and HER2-Negative Disease

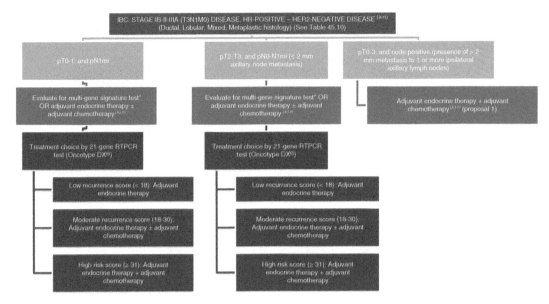

Fig. 45.13 Adjuvant systemic therapy for stages IB, II, and IIIA hormone-receptor-positive and HER2-negative disease [3–7]. * By multigene signature tests: Chemotherapy may be omitted for patients with luminal B-like (HER2 negative) disease with a low Oncotype Dx® score, MammaPrint® low risk status, low PAM50 ROR score, or EndoPredict® low risk status. ªThere is no absolute age limit. Rather, treatment depends on the disease, the presence of comorbidities, the patient's life expectancy, and patient preferences. For patients > 70 years of age, treatment should be individualized [3–6]. ᵇThe following factors are indications for including ovarian function suppression (OFS): age ≤ 35 years, premenopausal estrogen level following adjuvant chemotherapy, grade 3 disease, the involvement of 4 or more nodes, and adverse multigene test results [4]. ᶜIn high-risk premenopausal patients, "LHRH-agonist plus exemestane" may be the preferred adjuvant endocrine therapy [20]. The following factors are indications for the use of OFS plus aromatase inhibitor (AI) rather than OFS plus tamoxifen: age ≤ 35 years, grade 3 disease, the involvement of 4 or more nodes, adverse multigene test results [3, 4, 20]. ᵈIn patients with luminal A-like tumors and 1–3 positive lymph nodes (with the evaluation of other factors such as grade, age or multigene signature test results) "adjuvant endocrine therapy alone" may be an option (Table 45.10) [4]. ᵉSome patients may be adequately treated with tamoxifen alone. In high-risk postmenopausal patients, AIs may be preferred over tamoxifen [4]. The following factors argue for the inclusion of an AI at some point: lymph node involvement, grade 3 disease, high Ki67 proliferation index, or HER2 positivity. If an AI is used, it should be started upfront in patients at higher risk. The upfront AI can be switched to tamoxifen after 2 years in selected patients (e.g., those experiencing side effects of the AI) [3–7]. ᶠAfter 5 years of adjuvant tamoxifen, continued AI (to postmenopausal estrogen levels at baseline or to postmenopausal patients with premenopausal estrogen levels at baseline), or tamoxifen (to

premenopausal or postmenopausal patients) for up to 10 years should be recommended to patients with node-positive disease, grade 3 disease, or high Ki-67 [3–7]. ᵍAfter 5 years of adjuvant therapy involving a switch from tamoxifen to an AI (therefore assuming postmenopausal status at the 5-year time point and reasonable tolerance to endocrine therapy), patients may continue AI therapy for a cumulative total of 5 years. This subject requires clarification [3–7]. ʰAfter 5 years of continuous AI adjuvant therapy, we do not (yet) know whether to provide 3–5 years of tamoxifen, 3–5 years of AI, or no further endocrine treatment [3–7]. ⁱThe optimal duration of OFS may be 5 years but remains unclear [4]. ʲFactors that are relative indications for the inclusion of adjuvant cytotoxic chemotherapy include the following: histological grade 3 tumor, 4 or more positive nodes, high Ki67, extensive lymphovascular invasion, and low hormone receptor staining [3–6]. ᵏThe luminal A phenotype is less responsive to chemotherapy. In node-negative disease, chemotherapy should not be added based on the T size. A combination of the biological properties of the tumor (such as Ki67, LVI, grade, and multigene signature) must be used to assess whether to provide chemotherapy [3–6]. Chemotherapy should be added in high-risk patients based on the involvement of 4 or more lymph nodes (Table 45.10) [4–6]. ˡBy immunohistochemistry (IHC): in luminal B-like (HER2-negative) tumors, chemotherapy may be omitted in some low-risk patients (based on combinations of certain prognostic factors such as low tumor mass, low grade, low Ki67, an absence of LVI, older age) [4–6]. ᵐBy multigene signature tests: chemotherapy may be omitted for patients with luminal B-like (HER2-negative) disease with a low Oncotype Dx® score, MammaPrint® low risk status, low PAM50 ROR score or EndoPredict® low risk status [3–6]. ⁿFor Luminal B-like (HER2-negative) tumors, the regimen, if given, should contain anthracyclines and taxanes. A high-risk group might exist for which dose-dens therapy with G-CSF may also be preferred [3–6]

Hormone-Receptor-Negative and HER2-Positive Disease

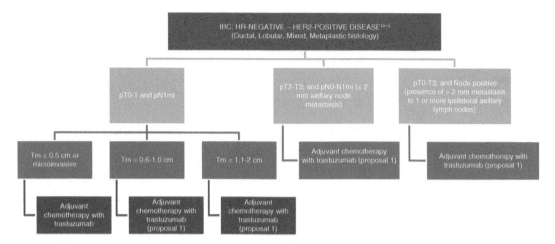

Fig. 45.14 Adjuvant systemic therapy for stages IB, II, and IIIA hormone-receptor-negative and HER2-positive disease [3–6]. [a]There is no absolute age limit. Rather, it depends on the disease, the presence of comorbidities, the patient's life expectancy, and patient preferences. For patients > 70 years of age, treatment should be individualized [3–6]. [b]The version 1.0 2016 NCCN Guidelines recommend AC – paclitaxel and trastuzumab (± pertuzumab); TCH ± pertuzumab (pertuzumab given to patients with greater than or equal to T2 or greater than or equal to N1, HER2-positive, early-stage breast cancer) [3]. In the St. Gallen 2015 guidelines, for patients requiring anti-HER2 therapy in the postoperative adjuvant setting for a T2 tumor with 4 involved nodes, both trastuzumab and pertuzumab were accepted by only 20 % of the panelists (79 % No) due to a lack of evidence [4]. [c]In patients with HER2-positive, stage 2 disease, chemotherapy should always be provided to patients who require anti-HER2 therapy. The chemotherapy regimen for these patients should preferably contain anthracyclines and taxanes. Anti-HER2 therapy should be initiated concurrently with taxane therapy [3–6]

Hormone-Receptor-Negative and HER2-Negative Disease

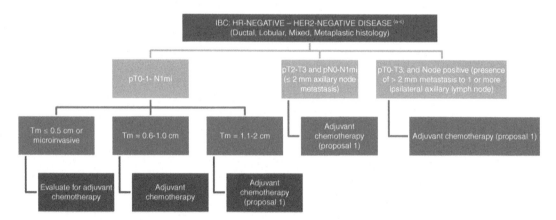

Fig. 45.15 Adjuvant systemic therapy for stages IB, II, and IIIA hormone-receptor-negative and HER2-negative disease [3–6]. [a]There is no absolute age limit. Rather, treatment depends on the disease, the presence of comorbidities, the patient's life expectancy, and patient preferences. For patients >70 years of age, treatment should be individualized [3–6]. [b]Fertility preservation (e.g., by ovarian tissue or oocyte conservation) should be offered to women <40 years of age. Ovarian function suppression with LHRHa during chemotherapy should be offered for receptor-negative disease [3–6, 19]. [c]In triple-negative breast cancer (TNBC), the regimen should include anthracyclines and taxanes. Although the data are insufficient, a platinum-based regimen may be considered only when a BRCA mutation has been identified. Anthracyclines followed by taxanes represent an acceptable regimen for BRCA-mutant TNBC. Dose-dense chemotherapy requiring growth factor support may also be an option [3–6]

Tubular-Mucinous CA: Stage I–II–III Disease

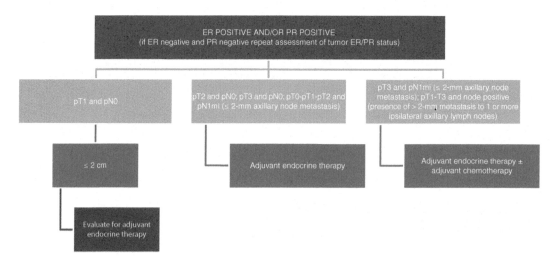

Fig. 45.16 Adjuvant systemic therapy for tubular and mucinous carcinoma [3–6]

Adjuvant Endocrine Therapy

Premenopause at Diagnosis

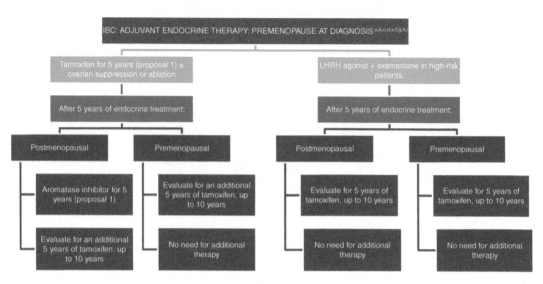

Fig. 45.17 Adjuvant endocrine therapy for premenopausal patients [3–7]. [a]The following factors are indications for including ovarian function suppression (OFS): age ≤ 35 years, premenopausal estrogen level following adjuvant chemotherapy, grade 3 disease, the involvement of 4 or more nodes, and adverse multigene test results [4]. [b]The optimal duration of OFS (with tamoxifen) may be 5 years but remains unclear [4]. [c]In high-risk premenopausal patients, 5 years of "LHRH-agonist plus exemestane" may be the preferred adjuvant endocrine therapy [20]. The following factors are indications for the use of OFS plus aromatase inhibitor (AI) rather than OFS plus tamoxifen: age ≤ 35 years, grade 3 disease, the involvement of 4 or more nodes, adverse multigene test results [3, 4, 20]. [d]After 5 years of continuous "LHRH-agonist plus exemestane" adjuvant therapy, we do not (yet) know whether to provide further endocrine treatment [3, 4, 20]. [e]In patients with luminal A-like tumors and 1–3 positive lymph nodes (with the evaluation of other factors such as grade, age or multigene signature test results) "adjuvant endocrine therapy alone" may be an option [4]. [f]After 5

years of adjuvant tamoxifen, continued AI (to postmenopausal patients with premenopausal estrogen levels at baseline), or tamoxifen for up to 10 years should be recommended to patients with node-positive disease, grade 3 disease, or high Ki-67 [3–7]. [g]After 5 years of adjuvant therapy involving a switch from tamoxifen to an AI (therefore assuming postmenopausal status at the 5-year time point and reasonable tolerance to endocrine therapy), patients may continue AI therapy for a cumulative total of 5 years. This subject requires clarification [3–7]. [h]By immunohistochemistry (IHC): In luminal B-like (HER2-negative) tumors, chemotherapy may be omitted in some low-risk patients (based on combinations of certain prognostic factors such as low tumor mass, low grade, low Ki67, an absence of LVI, older age) [4–7]. [i]By multigene signature tests: Chemotherapy may be omitted for patients with luminal B-like (HER2-negative) disease with a low Oncotype Dx® score, MammaPrint® low risk status, low PAM50 ROR score, or EndoPredict® low risk status [3–6]

Postmenopause at Diagnosis

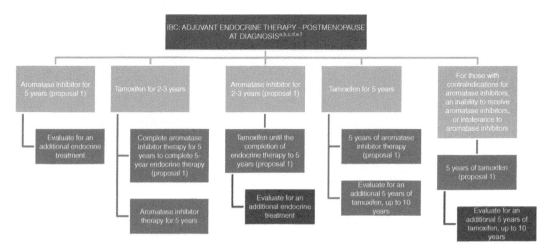

Fig. 45.18 Adjuvant endocrine therapy for postmenopausal patients [3–7]. [a]In patients with luminal A-like tumors and 1–3 positive lymph nodes (with the evaluation of other factors such as grade, age, or multigene signature test results) "adjuvant endocrine therapy alone" may be an option [4]. [b]Some patients may be adequately treated with tamoxifen alone. In high-risk postmenopausal patients, aromatase inhibitors (AIs) may be preferred over tamoxifen [4]. The following factors argue for the inclusion of an AI at some point: lymph node involvement, grade 3 disease, high Ki67 proliferation index, or HER2 positivity. If an AI is used, it should be started upfront in patients at higher risk. The upfront AI can be switched to tamoxifen after 2 years in selected patients (e.g., those experiencing side effects of the AI) [3–7]. [c]After 5 years of adjuvant tamoxifen, continued AI, or tamoxifen (for patients with intolerance to AI therapy) for up to 10 years should be recommended to patients with node-positive disease, grade 3 disease, or high Ki-67 [3–7]. [d]After 5 years of adjuvant therapy involving a switch from tamoxifen to an AI (therefore assuming postmenopausal status at the 5-year time point and reasonable tolerance to endocrine therapy), patients may continue AI therapy for a cumulative total of 5 years. This subject requires clarification [3–7]. [e]After 5 years of continuous AI adjuvant therapy, we do not (yet) know whether to provide 3–5 years of tamoxifen, 3–5 years of AI, or no further endocrine treatment [3–7]. [f]By multigene signature tests: chemotherapy may be omitted for patients with luminal B-like (HER2-negative) disease with a low Oncotype Dx® score, MammaPrint® low risk status, low PAM50 ROR score, or EndoPredict® low risk status [3–6]

Adjuvant Radiotherapy

Pathologic Stage I, II, IIIA, IIIB, IIIC

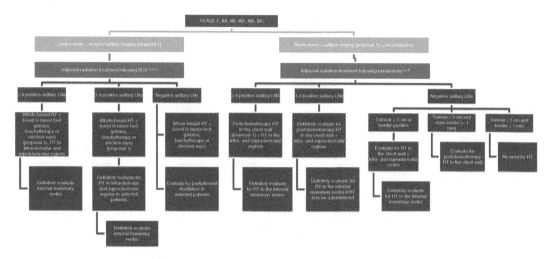

Fig. 45.19 Adjuvant radiotherapy after breast-conserving surgery or mastectomy [3–6, 13–16]. [1]Stage IA (T1, N0, M0); stage IB (T0, N1mi; M0; T1, N1mi, M0); stage IIA (T0, N1, M0; T1, N1, M0; T2, N0, M0); stage IIB (T2, N1, M0; T3, N0, M0); stage IIIA, IIIB, IIIC. [a]RT following chemotherapy if chemotherapy is indicated. [b]Following BCS, hypofractionated whole-breast irradiation may be used in patients without prior chemotherapy or axillary lymph node involvement, in patients 50 years of age or older (In St. Gallen 2015: Yes 89 %, No 2 %), and in patients < 50 years of age (In St. Gallen 2015: Yes 71 %, No 2 %) [4, 13, 16]. [c]Bane AL et al. attempted to assess whether tumor grade, molecular subtype and hypoxia status could predict the response to hypofractionated versus standard RT following BCS for node-negative breast cancer in a randomized controlled trial (RCT) [13]. In 989 patients, a central pathology review and tumor grade assessment using the Nottingham grading system was conducted. Tumors were classified by molecular subtype as luminal A, luminal B, HER2-enriched, basal-like, or unclassified using a six-biomarker panel: ER, PR, HER-2, Ki67, CK5/6, and EGFR. The median follow-up was 12 years. In the multivariable Cox model, molecular subtype was the only predictive factor for local recurrence; the 10-year cumulative incidence was 4.5 % for luminal A and basal-like, 7.9 % for luminal B, and 16.9 % for HER2-enriched tumors ($p < 0.01$) [13]. [d]Post-mastectomy RT is standard for patients who meet the following criteria: T size ≥ 5 cm (node negative); 1–3 nodes with adverse pathology [this is not the sole criterion in patients of a young age (<40); 4 or more positive axillary LNs; and positive sentinel lymph node biopsy with no axillary dissection [4]

Neoadjuvant Systemic Therapy: Clinical Stage II–IIIA (T3N1M0) Disease

General Treatment Approach

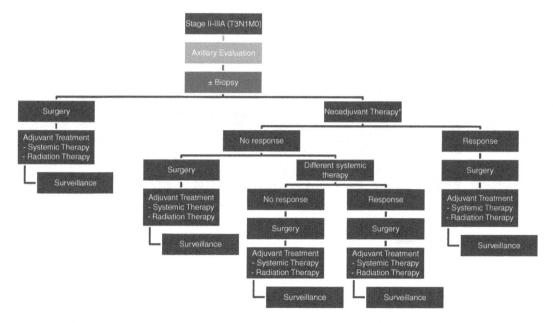

Fig. 45.20 Management of patients with neoadjuvant systemic therapy for stages II–IIIA (T3N1M0) breast cancer [3–6, 21]. *T2 and T3 tumors (N0-N1) meeting BCS criteria except tumor diameter

Axillary Evaluation Before Neoadjuvant Therapy

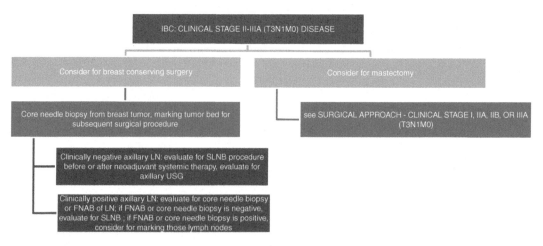

Fig. 45.21 Evaluation of axilla before neoadjuvant therapy [3–6, 21]

Response Evaluation and Surgical Treatment

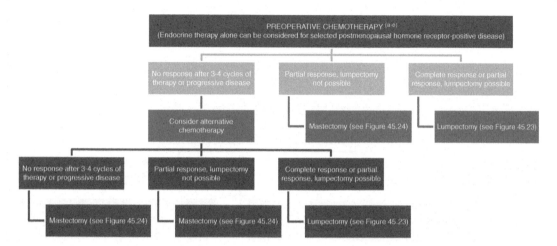

Fig. 45.22 Management of patients receiving neoadjuvant therapy for breast-conserving surgery (stage II or IIIA with N1) [3–6, 21]. [a]HER2-targeted therapy: According to the version 1.0 2016 NCCN Guidelines, patients with HER2-positive disease should receive trastuzumab plus chemotherapy in the neoadjuvant setting [3]. Pertuzumab can also be administered for tumors greater than or equal to T2 or greater than or equal to N1. Although the majority of the St. Gallen Panel supported dual anti-HER2 therapy with taxane, trastuzumab, and pertuzumab as "an acceptable regimen" for such patients, antracycline-taxane and anti-HER2 therapies were accepted as the best options [4]. [b]Stage II–III triple-negative disease: If provided to patients with triple-negative tumors, the preferred regimen should include an anthracycline and a taxane [4]. [c]Neoadjuvant cytotoxic therapy should be discussed as an option and often provided in patients with "luminal A-like" tumors, only if conservative surgery would not otherwise be feasible [4]. [d]Neoadjuvant endocrine therapy without cytotoxics represents a reasonable option for some selected postmenopausal patients with endocrine responsive disease. The duration of treatment must be at least 4 months, and treatment can be provided until a maximal response is reached [4]. [e]In triple-negative breast cancer (TNBC), the regimen should contain anthracyclines and taxanes. Although the available data are insufficient, a platinum-based regimen may be considered only in patients with a known BRCA mutation. Anthracyclines followed by taxanes is an acceptable regimen for BRCA-mutant TNBC. Dose-dense chemotherapy requiring growth factor support may also be an option [4]

Adjuvant Therapy After Lumpectomy

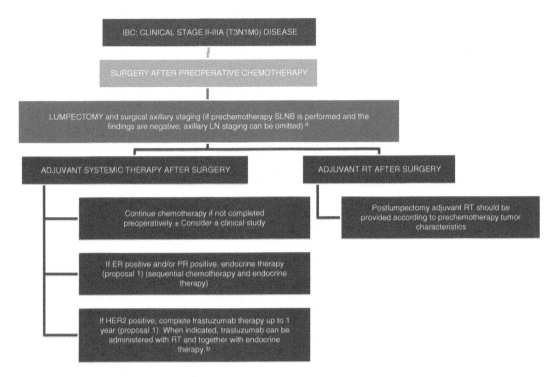

IBC: CLINICAL STAGE II-IIIA (T3N1M0) DISEASE

SURGERY AFTER PREOPERATIVE CHEMOTHERAPY

LUMPECTOMY and surgical axillary staging (if prechemotherapy SLNB is performed and the findings are negative, axillary LN staging can be omitted) [a]

ADJUVANT SYSTEMIC THERAPY AFTER SURGERY

ADJUVANT RT AFTER SURGERY

Continue chemotherapy if not completed preoperatively ± Consider a clinical study

Postlumpectomy adjuvant RT should be provided according to prechemotherapy tumor characteristics

If ER positive and/or PR positive, endocrine therapy (proposal 1) (sequential chemotherapy and endocrine therapy)

If HER2 positive, complete trastuzumab therapy up to 1 year (proposal 1). When indicated, trastuzumab can be administered with RT and together with endocrine therapy. [b]

Fig. 45.23 Locoregional and adjuvant systemic treatment after neoadjuvant therapy: lumpectomy [3–6, 21]. [a]In a patient who is clinically node positive at presentation and is downstaged after chemotherapy, sentinel lymph node (SLN) biopsy is appropriate. If 1 SLN is positive, axillary lymph node dissection must be performed. After downstaging, resecting the entire area of the original primary tumor is not necessary [4, 9, 11, 12]. [b]HER2-targeted therapy: According to the version 1.0 2016 NCCN Guidelines, in patients with HER2-positive disease who were not provided pertuzumab in the neoadjuvant setting, pertuzumab may be administered as additional adjuvant therapy [3]

Adjuvant Therapy After Mastectomy

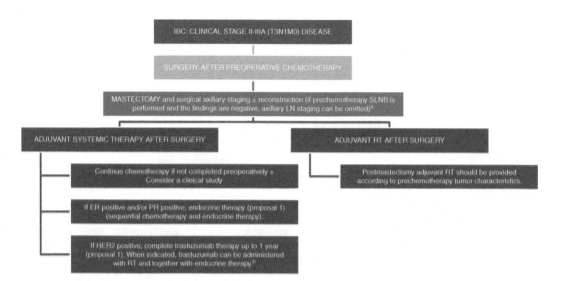

Fig. 45.24 Locoregional and adjuvant systemic treatment after neoadjuvant therapy: mastectomy [3–6]. [a]In a patient who is clinically node positive at presentation and is downstaged after chemotherapy, sentinel lymph node (SLN) biopsy is appropriate. If 1 SLN is positive, axillary lymph node dissection must be performed [4, 9, 11, 12].

[b]HER2-targeted therapy: According to the version 1.0 2016 NCCN Guidelines, in patients with HER2-positive disease who were not provided pertuzumab in the neoadjuvant setting, pertuzumab may be administered as additional adjuvant therapy [3]

Neoadjuvant Systemic Therapy: Clinical Stage IIIA (N2M0) – IIIB and IIIC (Non-inflammatory)

General Treatment Approach

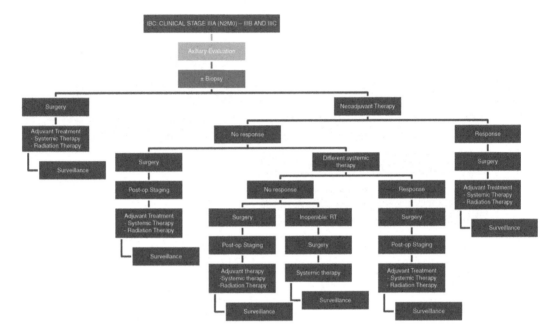

Fig. 45.25 Locoregional and adjuvant systemic treatment for clinical stages IIIA (N2M0), IIIB, and IIIC disease [3, 21]

Locoregional Treatment After Neoadjuvant Chemotherapy

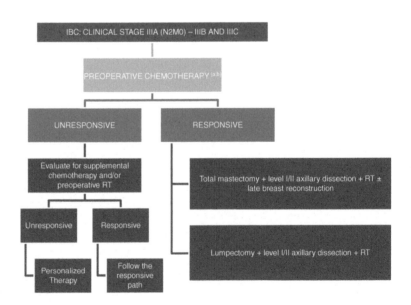

Fig. 45.26 Surgical approach after neoadjuvant systemic treatment for patients with clinical stages IIIA (N2M0), IIIB, and IIIC breast cancer [3, 21]

Adjuvant Therapy After Surgical Treatment

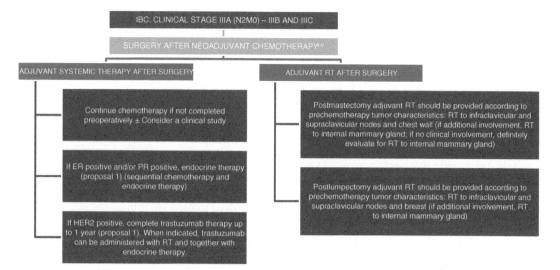

Fig. 45.27 Adjuvant treatment approach after neoadjuvant systemic treatment and surgery for patients with clinical stages IIIA (N2M0), IIIB, and IIIC breast cancer [3, 21]. [a]HER2-targeted therapy: Patients with HER2-positive disease should receive trastuzumab plus chemotherapy in the neoadjuvant setting. Pertuzumab can also be administered in tumors greater than or equal to T2 or greater than or equal to N1 [3, 4]. If pertuzumab is not administered in the neoadjuvant setting, pertuzumab may be administered as additional adjuvant therapy [3]. [b]For triple-negative breast cancer (TNBC), the regimen should contain anthracyclines and taxanes. Although the available data are insufficient, a platinum-based regimen may be considered only in patients with a known BRCA mutation. Anthracyclines followed by taxanes is an acceptable regimen for BRCA-mutant TNBC. Dose-dense chemotherapy requiring growth factor support may also be an option [3, 4]

Post-therapy Follow-Up

Table 45.11 Post-therapy follow-up of patients [3–6]

History and physical examination every 3–6 months in the first 3 years, every 6 months in the following 2 years, and then at 12-month intervals
Annual mammography (mammography can be performed in the 6th month in those undergoing RT after BCS)
Women receiving tamoxifen: if the uterus is present, annual gynecological examination
Women receiving an aromatase inhibitor or developing treatment-induced ovarian failure should be monitored for bone health by bone mineral density measurements at baseline and, later, periodically
Evaluate and encourage compliance with adjuvant endocrine therapy
Evidence suggests that maintaining an active lifestyle and reaching and maintaining an ideal body mass index (BMI 20–25) lead to optimal breast cancer outcomes. To reduce the risk of recurrence, an exercise regimen can be part of standard care. Weight loss and avoiding weight gain should be recommended
Pregnancy in breast cancer survivors: timing has no impact on prognosis. Considering pregnancy two years following the completion of therapy is better to allow for adequate ovarian recovery and to bypass the period of high risk of recurrence. Pregnancy is safe irrespective of the ER status of the tumor

Inflammatory Breast Cancer: Stage T4d, N0-N3, M0

General Treatment Approach

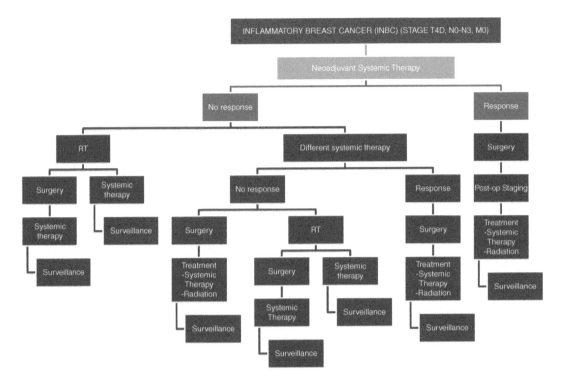

Fig. 45.28 Management of inflammatory breast cancer [3, 21, 22]

Locoregional and Systemic Therapy

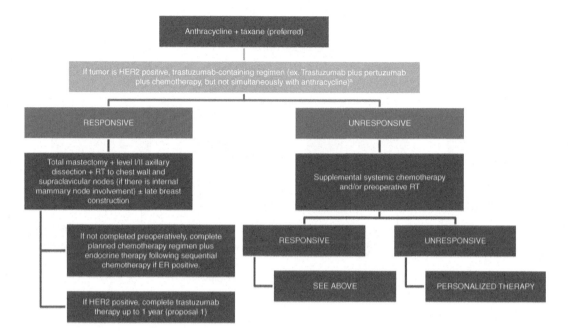

Fig. 45.29 Locoregional and systemic treatment of inflammatory breast cancer [3, 21, 22]. [a]HER2-targeted therapy: Patients with HER2-positive disease should receive trastuzumab plus chemotherapy in the neoadjuvant setting [3, 4]. Pertuzumab can also be administered. If pertuzumab was not administered in the neoadjuvant setting, pertuzumab may be given as additional adjuvant therapy [3]

Recurrent or Stage IV Disease

Diagnostic Procedures

Table 45.12 Diagnostic procedures

History and physical examination
Biopsy should be taken from the site of first disease recurrence. If not known, originally negative or not excessively expressed, determination of the tumor ER, PR, and HER2 status should be conducted
Blood tests, including tumor markers (CEA, Ca 153)
Thoracic diagnostic CT
Abdominopelvic diagnostic CT or MRI
If suspicious CNS symptoms, brain MRI
Bone scintigraphy or fluoride PET/CT
Evaluation of symptomatic bones and of long and weight-bearing bones appearing abnormal in bone scintigraphy
FDG PET/CT scan
Genetic counseling if at high risk for hereditary breast cancer

Recurrent Disease: Local Recurrence Only

General Treatment Approach

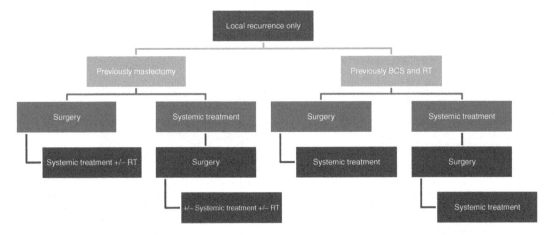

Fig. 45.30 Management of breast cancer patients with "local recurrence only"

Locoregional Treatment

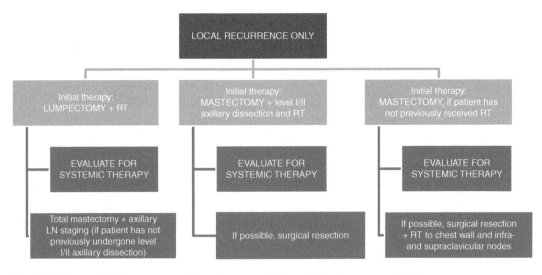

Fig. 45.31 Locoregional management of breast cancer patients with "local recurrence only"

Recurrent Disease: Locoregional Recurrence Only

General Treatment Approach

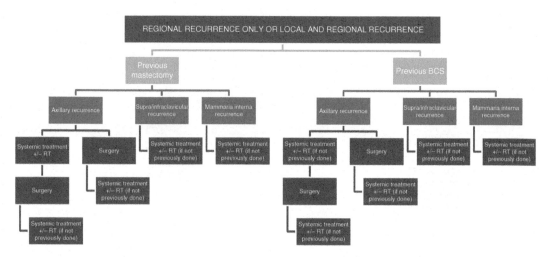

Fig. 45.32 Management of patients with "regional recurrence only" or "local and regional recurrence" [3, 23, 24]

Locoregional Treatment

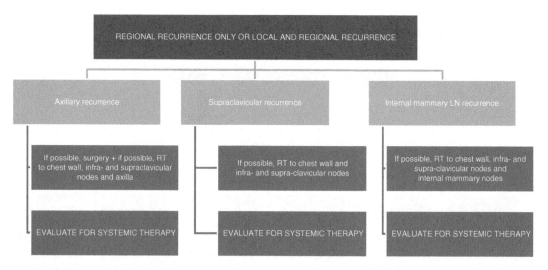

Fig. 45.33 Management of patients with regional recurrence [3, 23, 24]

Recurrent or Stage IV Disease

General Treatment Approach

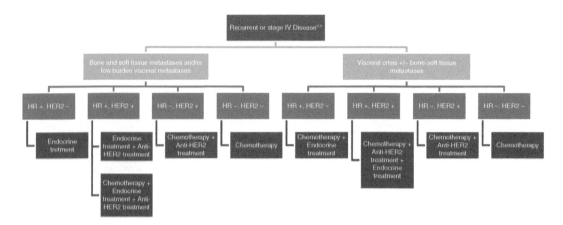

Fig. 45.34 Systemic treatment for recurrent or stage IV disease [3, 23, 24]. [a]The benefit of palliative local breast surgery to women presenting with stage IV disease remains unclear. This local therapy should be considered only after a response to initial systemic therapy. Notably, some studies suggest that surgery is only valuable if per-

formed with the same attention to detail (e.g., attaining clear margins and addressing disease in the axilla) as in patients with early-stage disease [3]. [b]If bone disease present: add denosumab, zoledronic acid, ibandronic acid, or pamidronate

Recurrent or Stage IV Disease: Systemic Treatment

HR Positive, HER2 Positive, or HER2 Negative

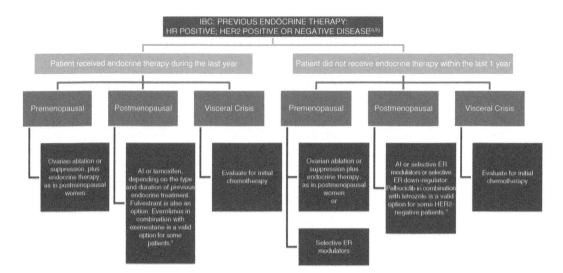

Fig. 45.35 Systemic treatment of recurrent stage IV hormone-receptor-positive disease [3, 23–27]. [a]Anti-her2 therapy must be added to HER2-positive patients [3, 24]. [b]If bone disease present: add denosumab, zoledronic acid, ibandronic acid, or pamidronate. [c]A combination of exemestane with everolimus can be considered for patients

who meet the eligibility criteria for BOLERO-2 (progressed within 12 months, on a nonsteroidal AI, or on tamoxifen at any time) [3, 25]. [d]Palbociclib in combination with letrozole may be considered as a treatment option for first-line therapy for postmenopausal patients with ER-positive, HER2-negative breast cancer [3, 26]

HER2 Negative, Hormone-Receptor-Negative, or Hormone-Receptor-Positive and Endocrine Refractory

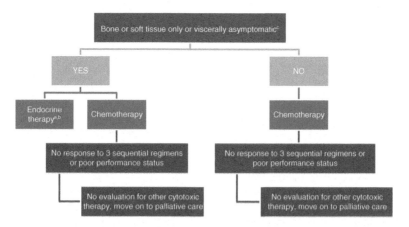

Fig. 45.36 Systemic therapy of patients with HER2-negative, HR-negative, or HR-positive and endocrine refractory disease [3, 23, 25, 27]. [a]A combination of exemestane with everolimus can be considered for patients who meet the eligibility criteria for BOLERO-2 (progressed within 12 months, on a nonsteroidal AI, or on tamoxifen at any time) [3, 25]. [b]Among patients with hormone-receptor–positive metastatic breast cancer who had progression of disease during prior endocrine therapy, palbociclib combined with fulvestrant resulted in longer PFS than fulvestrant alone (premenopausal or perimenopausal women also received goserelin) [27]. [c]If bone disease present: add denosumab, zoledronic acid, ibandronic acid, or pamidronate

HER2 Positive, Hormone-Receptor-Negative, or Hormone-Receptor-Positive and Endocrine Refractory

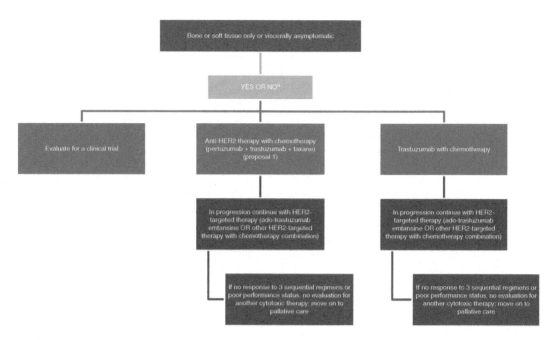

Fig. 45.37 Systemic therapy of patients with HER2-positive, HR-negative, or HR-positive and endocrine refractory disease [3, 24]. [a]If bone disease present: add denosumab, zoledronic acid, ibandronic acid, or pamidronate

Approach for High-Risk Patients: Genetic Risk Evaluation

Individuals with a Cancer Diagnosis

Table 45.13 Genetic risk evaluation for an individual with a cancer diagnosis [3, 4, 28]

Early onset of female breast cancer (<45 years of age)
Breast and ovarian/fallopian tube/primary peritoneal cancer in the same patient
2 primary breast cancers (ipsilateral or contralateral)
Breast cancer at any age and with at least one close blood relative with breast cancer at ≤50 years of age, ≥2 close blood relatives with breast cancer or pancreatic cancer at any age, or ≥1 close blood relative with invasive ovarian cancer at any age
The presence of one or more of the following together with breast cancer in the same side of the family: thyroid cancer, sarcoma, adrenocortical cancer, endometrial cancer, pancreatic cancer, brain tumor, diffuse gastric cancer, dermatological manifestations, and leukemia/lymphoma
A history of early-onset breast cancer and three or more of the following: thyroid cancer, sarcoma, adrenocortical cancer, endometrial cancer, pancreatic cancer, brain tumors, diffuse gastric cancer, dermatological manifestations, leukemia/lymphoma, prostate cancer (Gleason score ≥7), and hamartomatous polyps of the gastrointestinal tract
A known mutation in one family member in one of the genes with a tendency to cause breast cancer
Male breast cancer
Triple-negative (ER-, PR-, HER2-) breast cancer and ≤60 years of age
Ashkenazi Jew <60 years of age with breast cancer

Individuals with Family History of Breast/Ovarian Cancer

Table 45.14 Genetic risk evaluation for individuals without cancer but with a family history of breast/ovarian cancer [3, 4, 28]

Male breast cancer
First- or second-degree relative with breast cancer ≤45 years of age
≥2 individuals with primary breast cancer on the same side of the family
≥2 primary breast cancers in a single individual
≥1 primary invasive ovarian cancer
History of early onset and three or more of the following: thyroid cancer, sarcoma, adrenocortical cancer, endometrial cancer, pancreatic cancer, brain tumors, diffuse gastric cancer, dermatological manifestations, leukemia/lymphoma, prostate cancer (Gleason score ≥7), and hamartomatous polyps of the gastrointestinal tract
A known mutation in one family member in one of the genes with a tendency to cause breast cancer

Approach for High-Risk Patients: High-Risk Women Requesting Risk-Reducing Therapy

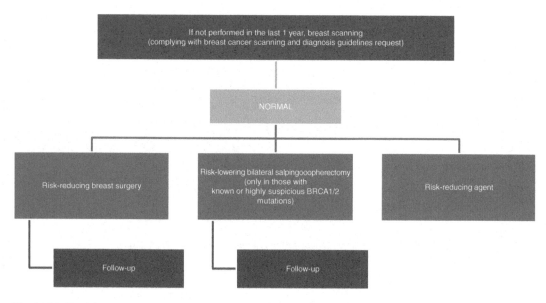

Fig. 45.38 Decision pathways for women requesting risk-reducing therapy [3, 4, 28]

Approach for High-Risk Patients: Risk-Reducing Agents

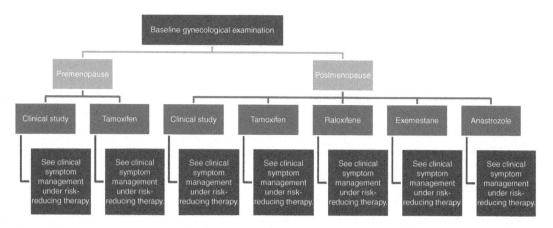

Fig. 45.39 Risk-reducing agents for premenopausal and postmenopausal women [3, 4, 28]

Approach for High-Risk Patients: Clinical Symptom Management Under Risk-Reducing Therapy

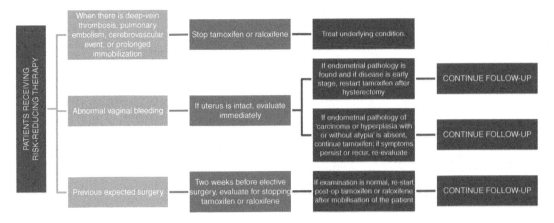

Fig. 45.40 Clinical symptom management of patients using risk-reducing therapy [3, 4, 28]

References

1. Margolese RG, Cecchini RS, Julian TB, Patricia A. Ganz PA, Costantino JP, et al. Primary results, NRG oncology/NSABP B-35: a clinical trial of anastrozole (A) versus tamoxifen (tam) in postmenopausal patients with DCIS undergoing lumpectomy plus radiotherapy. J Clin Oncol. 2015;33(Suppl; abstr LBA500).
2. Wolff AC, Hammond ME, Hicks DG, Dowsett M, McShane LM, Allison KH, et al. Recommendations for human epidermal growth factor receptor 2 testing in breast cancer: American Society of Clinical Oncology/College of American Pathologists clinical practice guideline update. J Clin Oncol. 2013;31:3997–4013.
3. NCCN guidelines for treatment of cancer by site. 1.0 2016 breast cancer. [Internet] Available from: www. NCCN.org.
4. Coates AS, Winer EP, Goldhirsch A, Gelber RD, Gnant M, Piccart-Gebhart M, et al. Tailoring therapies – improving the management of early breast cancer: St Gallen international expert consensus on the primary therapy of early breast cancer 2015. Ann Oncol Adv. Access published 4 May 2015.
5. Senkus E, Kyriakides S, Penault-Llorca F, Poortmans P, Thompson A, Zackrisson S, et al. Primary breast cancer: ESMO clinical practice guidelines for diagnosis, treatment and follow-up. Ann Oncol. 2013;24(Supplement 6):vi7–23.
6. Eisen A, Fletcher GG, Gandhi S, Mates M, Freedman OC, Dent SF, et al. Optimal systematic therapy for early female breast cancer, Program in Evidence-Based Care Evidence-Based Series, vol. 1–21.

Toronto: Cancer Care Ontario; 2014. 30 Sep 2014. Available from: http://www.cancercare.on.ca/.
7. Burstein HJ, Temin S, Anderson H, Buchholz TA, Davidson NE, Gelmon KE, et al. Adjuvant endocrine therapy for women with hormone receptor–positive breast cancer: American Society of Clinical Oncology clinical practice guideline focused update. J Clin Oncol. 2014;32:2255–69.
8. Lyman GH, Temin S, Edge SB, Newman LA, Turner RR, Weaver DL, et al. Sentinel lymph node biopsy for patients with early-stage breast cancer: American Society of Clinical Oncology clinical practice guideline update. J Clin Oncol. 2014;32:1365–83.
9. Moran MS, Schnitt SJ, Giuliano AE, Harris JR, Khan SA, Horton J, et al. Society of Surgical Oncology-American Society for Radiation Oncology consensus guideline on margins for breast-conserving surgery with whole-breast irradiation in stages I and II invasive breast cancer. Int J Radiat Oncol Biol Phys. 2014;88:553–64.
10. Giuliano AE, Mc Call LM, Beitsch PD, Whit PW, Morrow M, Blumencranz PW, et al. ACOSOGZ0011: a randomized trial of axillary node dissection in women with clinical T1-2 N0M0 breast cancer who have a positive sentinel node. J Clin Oncol. 2010;28(18). abstr CRA 506.
11. Boughey JC, Suman VJ, Mittendorf EA, Ahrendt GM, Wilke LG, Taback B, et al. Sentinel lymph node surgery after neoadjuvant chemotherapy in patients with node-positive breast cancer: the ACOSOG Z1071 (Alliance) clinical trial. JAMA. 2013;310: 1455–61.
12. Kuehn T, Bauerfeind I, Fehm T, Fleige B, Hausschild M, Helms G, et al. Sentinel-lymph-node biopsy in patients with breast cancer before and after neoadjuvant

chemotherapy (SENTINA): a prospective, multicentre cohort study. Lancet Oncology. 2013;14:609–18.

13. Bane AL, Whelan TJ, Pond GR, Parpia S, Gohla G, Fyles AW, et al. Tumor factors predictive of response to hypofractionated radiotherapy in a randomized trial following breast conserving therapy. Ann Oncol. 2014;25(5):992–8.

14. Marta GN, Macedo CR, Carvalho Hde A, Hanna SA, da Silva JL, Riera R. Accelerated partial irradiation for breast cancer: systematic review and meta-analysis of 8653 women in eight randomized trials. Radiother Oncol. 2015;114:42–9.

15. Budach W, Kammers K, Boelke E, Matuschek C. Adjuvant radiotherapy of regional lymph nodes in breast cancer – a meta-analysis of randomized trials. Radiat Oncol. 2013;8:267.

16. Bellon JR, Golshan M, Solin LJ. Controversies in radiation oncology for early-stage breast cancer. Ann Surg Oncol. 2015 [Epub ahead of print].

17. Zhou Q, Yin W, Du Y, Lu J. For or against adjuvant trastuzumab for pT1a-bN0M0 breast cancer patients with HER2-positive tumors: a meta-analysis of published literatures. PLoS One. 2014;9(1):e83646.

18. Tolaney SM, Barry WT, Dang CT, Yardley DA, Moy B, Marcom PK, et al. Adjuvant paclitaxel and trastuzumab for node-negative, HER2-positive breast cancer. N Engl J Med. 2015;372(2):134–41.

19. Gerber B, Ortmann O. Prevention of Early Menopause Study (POEMS): is it possible to preserve ovarian function by gonadotropin releasing hormone analogs (GnRHa)? Arch Gynecol Obstet. 2014;290:1051–3.

20. Francis PA, Regan MM, Fleming GF, Láng I, Ciruelos E, Bellet M, et al. Adjuvant ovarian suppression in premenopausal breast cancer. N Engl J Med. 2015;372:436–46.

21. PEBC Report Citation, Brackstone M, Fletcher GG, Dayes IS, Madarnas Y, SenGupta SK, Verma S. Locoregional therapy of locally advanced breast cancer (LABC), Program in Evidence-Based Care Evidence-Based, vol. 1–19. Toronto: Cancer Care Ontario; 2014. Available from: http://www.cancercare.on.ca/.

22. Dawood S, Merajver SD, Viens P, Vermeulen PB, Swain SM, Buchholz TA, et al. International expert panel on inflammatory breast cancer: consensus statement for standardized diagnosis and treatment. Ann Oncol. 2011;22(3):515–23.

23. Partridge AH, Rumble B, Carey LA, Come SE, Davidson NE, Leo AD, et al. Chemotherapy and targeted therapy for women with human epidermal growth factor receptor 2–negative (or unknown) advanced breast cancer: American Society of Clinical Oncology clinical practice guideline. J Clin Oncol. 2014;32:3307–29.

24. Giordano SH, Temin S, Kirshner JJ, Chandarlapaty S, Crews JR, Davidson NE, et al. Systemic therapy for patients with advanced human epidermal growth factor receptor 2–positive breast cancer: American Society of Clinical Oncology clinical practice guideline. J Clin Oncol. 2014;32:2078–99.

25. Piccart M, Hortobagyi GN, Campone M, Pritchard KI, Lebrun F, Ito Y, et al. Everolimus plus exemestane for hormone-receptor-positive, human epidermal growth factor receptor-2-negative advanced breast cancer: overall survival results from BOLERO-2†. Ann Oncol. 2014;25(12):2357–62.

26. Finn RS, Crown JP, Lang I, Boer K, Bondarenko IM, Kulyk SO, et al. The cyclin-dependent kinase 4/6 inhibitor palbociclib in combination with letrozole versus letrozole alone as first-line treatment of oestrogen receptor-positive, HER2-negative, advanced breast cancer (PALOMA-1/TRIO-18): a randomised phase 2 study. Lancet Oncol. 2015;16(1): 25–35.

27. Turner NC, Ro J, André F, Loi S, Verma S, Iwata H, et al. Palbociclib in hormone-receptor–positive advanced breast cancer. N Eng J Med. 2015. doi:10.1056/NEJMoa1505270.

28. Visvanathan K, Hurley P, Bantug E, Brown P, Col NF, Cuzick J, et al. Use of pharmacologic interventions for breast cancer risk reduction: American Society of Clinical Oncology clinical practice guideline. J Clin Oncol. 2013;31:2942–62.

Part IX

Supportive Care in Breast Cancer

Nursing Care and Management

46

Gulbeyaz Can

Abstract

Breast cancer is the most widespread type of cancer among women. Despite being associated with high morbidity and mortality, breast cancer can be diagnosed and treated early. Breast self-examination (BSE), clinical breast examination (CBE), and mammography are the most commonly known and used screening programs in the early diagnosis of this disease. Education about breast cancer and screening programs increases the awareness of the seriousness of the disease and increases compliance with early diagnostic practices. Nurses who provide health education about breast screening programs play an important role in the early diagnosis of breast cancer. Nurses improve the awareness and participation of women in breast screening programs. Specialist breast care nurses have training and expertise in the management, treatment, and follow-up of patients diagnosed with breast cancer and are important members of the multidisciplinary breast care team, providing a range of key interventions. These nurses routinely assess patients with breast cancer and provide information and emotional support while offering tailored information about emotional coping. Nurses also prepare patients for treatment and explain the prevention and management of treatment-related side effects, including lymphedema, neutropenia, fatigue, skin reaction, nausea, and vomiting. Furthermore, nurses provide contact with the medical team and other health professionals as required and refer patients to other services as needed, including liaison psychiatry, physiotherapy, algology, and other support services.

G. Can, RN, PhD
Department of Medical Nursing, Istanbul University
Florence Nightingale Nursing Faculty,
Abide-i Hürriyet Cad. Caglayan, Istanbul, Turkey
e-mail: gulbeyaz@istanbul.edu.tr

© Springer International Publishing Switzerland 2016
A. Aydiner et al. (eds.), *Breast Disease: Management and Therapies*,
DOI 10.1007/978-3-319-26012-9_46

805

Keywords

Nursing care • Breast cancer screening • Breast self-examination • BSE • Breast biopsy • Psychological support • Anxiety • Surgical treatment • Lymphedema • Systemic treatment • Fatigue • Neutropenia • Alopecia • Nausea and vomiting • Skin reaction • Neuropathy • Hot flashes • Pain • Complementary and alternative therapy

Roles and Responsibilities of Nurses in Breast Cancer Screening

Breast cancer is the second most common cancer in the world and by far the most frequent cancer among women, with an estimated 1.67 million new cancer cases diagnosed in 2012 (25 % of all cancers) [1]. Despite being associated with high morbidity and mortality, breast cancer can be diagnosed and treated early. Breast self-examination (BSE), clinical breast examination (CBE), and mammography are the most commonly known and used screening programs worldwide [2, 3]. The primary responsibilities of nurses at breast cancer screening centers are informing the public about cancer and screenings, teaching women how to perform breast self-examination (BSE), and performing age-appropriate cancer screening. Although BSE is not a part of the breast cancer screening recommendations in some Western countries due to the anxiety and unnecessary biopsies associated with BSE, BSE education is important for monitoring changes in breast tissue and for raising awareness. Education about breast cancer and BSE increases awareness of the seriousness of the disease and increases compliance with early diagnostic practices. Because many families in less-developed regions have low income and live in rural areas, many women do not receive mammograms and clinical breast examinations, which prevent the detection of the disease at early stages. Thus, the health education provided by nurses during cancer screening improves awareness about the early diagnosis of breast cancer and increases participation in screening programs [4–6]. However, nurses should understand the society they serve with respect to breast cancer risk factors, and they should determine the risk levels for each patient. To increase women's compliance with screening practices, nurses should know the health beliefs affecting the screening practices and should consider women's beliefs that affect screening practices (predisposition, seriousness, BSE benefits, BSE barriers, confidence, mammography benefits, mammography barriers, and health motivation) when planning breast health education. Nurses should encourage women to participate in screening programs that are appropriate for their age groups and should follow up with patients [3]. If any suspicious lesion is detected at screening, a biopsy should be taken from the suspicious lesion and the obtained material should be sent to a pathology unit for examination.

Nursing Care of Patients Undergoing Breast Biopsy

Many patients experience anxiety when a biopsy decision is made. The reason for the biopsy should be explained to the patient, and the necessary preparations before the procedure should be discussed. If the patient is taking drugs or dietary supplements that increase the risk of bleeding, such as nonsteroidal anti-inflammatory drugs or anticoagulants, the patient should be advised to cease taking the drugs to reduce the bleeding risk. Today, many biopsy procedures are performed under mild sedation or local anesthesia, and the patient is sent home as soon as she starts feeding by herself. After the procedure, before the patient is sent home, she should be informed about the potential complications and should be advised to report such complications to a health professional. Slight pain and ecchymosis over the biopsy region are normal, but the patient should be informed about the importance of seeing a health professional if edema, redness, or severe pain develops. The dressing over the biopsy area can be removed after 2 days, but female patients should be advised to wear bras for 3–7 days to limit movement of the breast and to reduce procedure-related tenderness. Paracetamol/acetaminophen can be offered to reduce procedure-related pain. Avoidance of activities requiring intense arm use should be advised. The patient should be sent home after planning the date of the follow-up visit when the pathology results will be available. The roles and responsibilities of the nurse will differ according to the result. If the result is negative, the patient is sent home after inspection of the biopsy region; however, if the result is positive, the nurse should provide psychological support to the patient upon the diagnosis of breast cancer and should inform her about the treatment process [7].

Approach to Patients Who Are Newly Diagnosed with Breast Cancer

When confronted with the breast cancer diagnosis, patients experience feelings of fear, shock, sadness, disbelief, or other psychosocial distress. Most patients, with or without psychosocial support, cope successfully with the psychological distress and adjust to their disease. However, some patients experience different psychological distress [8]. Some patients appear anxious and tend to ask an exhaustive number of questions regarding their diagnosis, prognosis, and treatments. This response is unsurprising, as many people still view cancer as a death sentence associated with pain and a lack of dignity. This view is particularly influenced by patients' past experiences and encounters with the disease, e.g., the death of a close relative. In view of the usually overwhelming emotional reactions to the diagnosis, the patient must be given time to absorb the significance of the diagnosis [7, 9].

Younger women worry about their work productivity and career advancement. They face many family concerns related to whether they will be able to have children, whether they will live to see their children grow, and whether their disease will recur and incapacitate them. Middle-aged women worry about their disease in relation to their family and work. They also worry about their aging parents and whether they will be able to care for them in the future. These women are increasingly concerned about their daughters' risk for breast cancer. Older women worry about whether they will have the resources to pay for medications [9, 10].

The need for information varies along with the patients' needs. It is important that the nurse assesses the individual need for information and provides it accordingly. It would be wrong, for example, to overload a patient in denial with an exhaustive amount of information, as this clearly does not allow the patient to utilize her own coping strategy. Equally, it would be wrong to not offer information to a patient who copes through active participation in her treatment [8].

Pathology results, screening results, previous treatments, and medical history can provide information that is an important component in developing an effective individualized treatment plan and can predict a response to a particular therapy and prognosis. Based on the results of these examinations, a nurse should plan the explanations of the disease and treatment process that she will provide to the patient at first meeting. During the explanations, positive survival results that are presented in the pathology report should be emphasized. For example, smaller tumors and negative lymph node status correlated with better prognosis. A smaller number of involved lymph nodes is better than a larger number. Patients with low recurrence risk benefit more from adjuvant chemotherapy. Emphasizing positive survival results during the interview reduces disease-related anxiety and increases compliance with treatment. Breast cancer can be divided into several groups based on histopathologic features: hormone receptor positive (ER and PR positive), triple negative (HER2 negative and ER and PR negative), and HER2 positive. Each subtype has different characteristics associated with different risks of recurrence, and these risks influence treatment choices. A negative hormone receptor status is associated with a less favorable prognosis. According to clinical stage HER2-positive tumors are associated with poorer survival. Additionally, the results of screening tests should also be considered during the patient explanation. Increased values on liver function tests may indicate possible liver metastasis. Increased calcium and alkaline phosphatase levels may indicate possible bone metastasis. Additional metastatic workup, including chest X-ray, bone scans, computed tomography (CT) scans, and positron emission tomography (PET)-CT scans, may indicate possible metastasis. Considering the low survival rates in metastasis, patients should not be given extra hope for recovery; information should focus on the effectiveness of the treatment. Misinforming these patients can adversely affect their trust in health professionals, generate anger toward health professionals, and lead patients to seek nonmedical treatments [7].

A nurse caring for a woman who has just received a diagnosis of breast cancer must be knowledgeable about current treatment options and be able to discuss them with the patient. Patients generally talk with their physician before talking with oncology nurses, and the doctor will have already provided the patient with a preliminary explanation regarding survival and future treatment based on the pathology report and screening test result. The nurse should be aware of the information that has been provided to the patient by the physician. The patient education concerning medications, the extent of treatment, the management of side effects, the possible reactions after treatment, the frequency and duration of treatment, and the treatment goals provided by the nurses must be similar to the physician's explanations. The amount and timing of the information provided are based on the patient's responses, coping ability, and readiness to learn [8].

Nursing Care During Breast Cancer Treatment

Most patients with breast cancer experience a complex course of care during the first year after diagnosis. These patients might undergo one or more procedures for diagnosis, multiple surgical consultations, one or more surgeries (including reconstruction), and multiple surgical follow-up visits. Most patients will consult radiation oncology and may undergo up to 6 weeks of daily radiation. Virtually all patients will discuss adjuvant (or neoadjuvant) systemic therapy with a medical oncologist. Those undergoing chemotherapy will be treated with 4–16 chemotherapy infusions depending on the regimen. The majority will also be treated with endocrine therapy and will undergo several follow-up visits within the first year [11]. The treatment duration can be longer in patients with advanced-stage breast cancer. Patients may receive numerous chemotherapy treatments to control the disease, and palliative care may need to be planned in patients with metastases.

The specialist breast care nurse must have training and expertise in the management, treatment, and follow-up of patients diagnosed with breast cancer. He or she is an important member of the multidisciplinary breast care team, providing a range of key interventions (e.g., psychosocial support, information, patient advocacy, and acting as a liaison among the various members of the healthcare team):

- Routinely assess and meet the patients' needs for information and support.
- Support the patient emotionally and offer tailored information about emotional coping.
- Prepare the patient for treatment and explain the prevention and management of treatment-related side effects such as lymphedema, neutropenia, fatigue, skin reaction, nausea and vomiting.
- Provide contact with the medical team and other health professionals as required.
- Refer patients to other services as needed, e.g., liaison psychiatry, physiotherapy, algology, and other support services [12].

Nursing Care in Surgical Treatment

The primary treatment approach in breast cancer is surgical excision and pathological examination of the tumor. Although the type of surgical intervention may vary depending on the clinical condition of the patient, risk factors, localization of the tumor, tumor size, clinical stage, and patient choice, the most frequent surgical treatment approaches are breast-conserving surgery and mastectomy. To determine the involvement of lymph nodes, sentinel lymph node biopsy (SLNB) and, if necessary, axillary lymph node dissection (ALND) can be performed during surgery. Although they depend on the type of surgery, the problems most frequently experienced by patients after surgical treatment are pain, infection, reduction in physical mobility, change in body image, and sexual dysfunction. Nurses in charge of patients who undergo surgery are responsible for preparing the patient for surgery, supporting the surgeon during procedures before surgery, monitoring the patient for operation-related complications and initiating appropriate treatment upon doctor request, and improving the quality of life of the patients [13].

Preoperative Patient Preparation

Nurses should ascertain whether the preoperative anesthesia exam and all other examinations are completed before the patient undergoing surgery is admitted to the unit. If there are any missing examinations, they should be completed. The patient should be informed about the procedure and possible postoperative complications. Informing the patient and her family about the procedures before surgery reduces the anxiety of the patient and patient's family and gives them the opportunity to obtain answers to any questions that might have arisen after the interview with the physician. During this explanation, the nurse should explain the purpose and risks of the surgery that is going to be performed [breast-conserving surgery, mastectomy, SLNB (sentinel lymph node biopsy), or ALND (axillary lymph node dissection)]. Drains that are likely to be placed during surgery and the site of the surgical incision should be explained to the patient. Nurses should educate the patient and demonstrate the shoulder and arm exercises and the coughing and breathing exercises that are necessary after the operation. If needed, the nurse should refer the patient to liaison psychiatry and

ensure that the patient receives psychological support as required [7, 9, 13].

Isosulfan and methylene blue, which are administered to patients during SLNB procedures, are excreted via bile and urine at rates of 90 % and 10 %, respectively; therefore, it should be explained to patients that there will be blue-green discoloration in their urine and feces for 24 h following biopsy. Some patients may experience allergic rashes against isosulfan blue on their neck, hands, and feet; in rare cases, hypotension may be observed. Following the procedure, the nurse should monitor the patient closely for allergic reactions, should educate the patient and her family about such reactions, and should inform the patient and family about the signs that should be reported to the nurse and physician [13].

Postoperative Patient Follow-Up and Nursing Care

The patient's vital signs and drainage status should be monitored for the first 12 h following the operation. Factors affecting wound healing should be evaluated, and drainage should be reported to the surgeon [13].

After the operation, the patient should lie down in a semi-Fowler's position, and drains should be emptied before they are full. The dressing and bedsheets should be checked for signs of leakage. The patient's arm should be elevated using a pillow, circulation of the arm should be checked, and loss of strength in the fingers, numbness of upper arm, and signs of swelling should be recorded. Blood pressure measurement, i.v. line placement, and other procedures should not be performed on the affected arm, and the patient should be informed about these precautions. The patient should be told to use the unaffected arm whenever she wants to turn in bed or sit up and to avoid tight clothes that could compress her arm. The presence of pain at the operated area should be evaluated, and if present, analgesics should be administered upon physician request [9, 13].

After mastectomy, the absence of a breast disturbs the patient emotionally and adversely affects self-respect and body image. Patients find it difficult to look at the operated area; it is better if the patient's first examination of the operated area is undertaken with the support of a nurse or another health professional. At that moment, patients should be encouraged to express their feelings. Sharing emotions is normal after breast surgery, and it relaxes the patient. A temporary breast prosthesis inside a bra can be offered at discharge to reduce the patient's embarrassment and increase her self-esteem. The patient can be informed about breast reconstruction and breast prostheses. When the patient and her partner are ready, the partner should also be invited to see the operated area [10, 13].

Discharge Education

The patient and her family should be informed about the postoperative period:

- It should be explained that mild redness, tenderness, and swelling over the operated area is normal.
- The patient should be informed about wound care, asepsis, drain care, signs and symptoms of infection, and frequency of dressing changes before discharge from the hospital. The patient should be educated on the following:
  - Checking the drain area for leakage
  - How to measure the drained volume and how to empty the drain and record it
  - The removal of the drains within approximately 7–10 days, when the drained volume is below 30 ml per 24 h
  - The importance of consulting the doctor if there are complaints such as bleeding, fever, and pain at disturbing levels
- Patients should be informed about the possibility of infection and edema at the operated area and should be educated on preventive measures against infection:
  - The patient should be advised to prevent skin damage by wearing gloves when gardening, avoiding exposure to sunlight, wearing a thimble when sewing, using electric shaving machines for axillary cleanup, and avoiding injections.
  - When there is damage to skin, the patient should understand the importance of

cleaning the area with soap and water, covering the area, and reporting any warmth or swelling over the area to a physician.
  - The patient should not wear tight accessories and should not lift heavy objects for extended periods.
- The patient should be informed about when the sutures will be removed.
- The patient should be told that numbness can occur over the operated area and arm, and its causes should be explained.
- It should be explained that the patient can use her arm normally after the drains are removed and that if limitations in the range of motion persist, she should elevate her arm for at least for 30 min every day.
- The starting date of additional exercise programs should be planned (generally 1 week later, with retrieval of sutures and drains), and the arm, wrist, and hand exercises that she has to perform (e.g., clenching a rubber ball, clenching and unclenching fingers, touching the shoulder with the hand and wrist movements) should be taught (Fig. 46.1).
  - The patient should be reminded to not abduct her arm as long as the drains are in place, as exercises that begin in the early period increase the risk of seroma formation; she can be told to start all exercises once wound healing is complete and drains are removed.
  - Until drains are retrieved, limited exercises such as hand and wrist extension can be started on postoperative days 1–3.
  - Arm and shoulder movements should start after drains are retrieved. Patients are advised to continue these exercises for 20 min, three times per day, until normal range of motion is obtained with these movements. The number of exercises can be increased in athletic women. Patients should be reminded that they can pause exercises if they experience pain during exercises and that they should continue the exercises for at least a year.
  - Patients should be encouraged to perform daily activities such as eating, combing hair, and washing their face.
  - It should be explained that both arms should be used during exercises to maintain the correct posture, that the patient should not

Exercise aimed at prevention of impaired posture

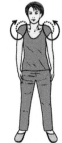
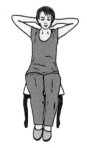
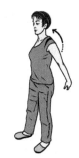

While standing, one shoulder is elevated and the other is depressed.

Both shoulders are moved backwards in circular motions.

While sitting on a chair, hands are clasped at back of the neck, and trunk is stretched upwards.

While standing, hands are clasped behind and shoulders are pulled backwards.

Strengthening chest muscles   **Strengthening arms**

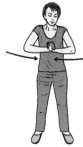
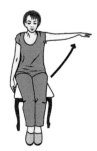
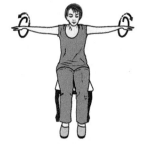

Hands are clasped at chest level, pushed towards each other, and then relaxed.

While sitting on a chair, arms are elevated to shoulder level and lowered back.

Arms are elevated to shoulder level, and small backwards circular motions are made with arms.

Working shoulder joints   **Prevention of lymphedema at arm**

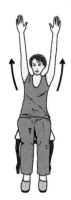
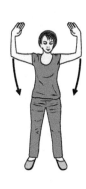
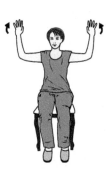
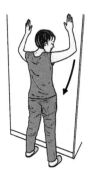

While sitting on a chair, hands are put on legs and then elevated and lowered back.

Arms are curled up from the elbows, and forearms are lowered and elevated, moving them from the elbow joint.

While sitting on a chair, upper arms are straight at shoulder level and forearms perpendicular to upper arms. Hands are clenched and unclenched 3-4 times. Arms are lowered and relaxed, and the exercise is repeated.

While close to and facing the wall, hands are placed on the wall and crawled upwards. If there is pain, exercise is paused.

Fig. 46.1 Shoulder and arm exercises after breast surgery

lift objects heavier than 2–3 kg with the affected arm, and that the patient should distribute weight evenly to both arms.

- It should be explained that the patient may start cycling or trekking as soon as she starts feeling well and that she may start driving once the drain is removed if she is not taking narcotic analgesics and if the range of motion is regained.

• Lymphedema can develop, especially in patients who undergo axillary dissection, due to the insufficiency of lymphatic drainage and the blockage of the outward motion of fluid and proteins from the interstitial space. Such patients should be informed about how lymphedema occurs, of the signs and symptoms of lymphedema, and of the preventive measures against it (Table 46.1).

• Patients should be informed that there is no harm in resuming sexual activities after discharge.

• The importance of prostheses should be explained to patients who undergo mastectomy, both to resolve cosmetic issues and to preserve spinal integrity; patients should be advised to start using prostheses approximately 6–7 weeks after surgery, once the operated area is healed.

• Patients should be advised to avoid creams and deodorants and to not shave their armpit for 2 weeks following surgery.

• Patients should be encouraged to talk about mastectomy, to express their feelings about the loss of a breast, and to communicate with their partners.

• Supporting relatives such as partners, family, and friends of the patients should be identified, and those people should be informed about the importance of the support they will provide to the patients [8, 10, 13, 14].

Monitoring and Management of Possible Complications

Various complications can be observed in patients after breast surgery, including lymphedema, transient edema, lymphangitis, hematoma, seroma, wound infection, and limitations in the range of shoulder and arm movements (frozen shoulder/contracture).

Table 46.1 Patient education for the prevention of lymphedema

Keep your affected arm above heart level while sitting for extended periods or while driving, lying down, or watching TV
Do not have injections made on the affected arm
Wear gloves when washing dishes or gardening
Protect your hand and arm from burns
Have your blood pressure measured from the unaffected arm
Use lanolin creams to avoid dryness of your hand and arm
In case of cuts and scratches, wash the area and apply antiseptics
Consult your doctor in case of signs or symptoms of infection
Elevate your arm from time to time during the day and while going to bed
Do not use underwire bras or heavy breast prostheses
Do not wear tight or elastic-sleeved clothes that could compress your arm
Do not wear tight watches, bracelets, or rings on your affected side
Do not lift heavy objects with your affected arm
Do not engage in activity that requires strength (rubbing, brushing, pushing, pulling, etc.) using your affected arm
You can have a professional manicure, but care should be taken when cutting cuticles to avoid any injury
Always wear a thimble when sewing to avoid needlestick
Do not stay outdoors for extended periods during hot weather
Avoid hot baths, hot showers, and saunas
Maintain your ideal weight with low-salt, fiber-rich foods
Avoid smoking and drinking alcohol
Partake in a diet rich in easily digestible proteins (fish and chicken)
Use a lymphedema bracelet
After the operation, regularly measure and record your hand circumference at the level of the thumb groove and your arm circumferences 10 cm above and 10 cm below the olecranon. If the measurement values differ by more than 2 cm between arms, consult your doctor for an evaluation of lymphedema

Transient Edema

Following ALND, collateral circulation takes on the function of lymphatic circulation; therefore, some patients may experience transient edema. It should be explained to patients that transient edema is not lymphedema, and they should be advised to keep their arm above heart level until collateral circulation develops.

Lymphangitis

Lymphangitis, which is the infection of lymphatic vessels, causes rash, itchiness, swelling, local heat, pain in the arm, fever, and tremor. Antibiotic treatment should be initiated in those patients upon physician request; body temperature and leukocyte counts should be monitored. The affected arm should be elevated, and no invasive procedures should be performed on this arm.

Hematoma

Hematoma, which is the collection of blood in the operated area, can develop during the first 12 h following either mastectomy or breast-conserving surgeries. Swelling, tenderness, pain, and ecchymosis in the skin can occur at the operated area due to hematoma, and the amount of drained bloody discharge may increase. These signs should be reported to the surgeon, and compression dressings should be applied as required for approximately 12 h [13].

Seroma

Seroma is collection of serous fluid under the breast incision or in the axillary region following mastectomy or BCS. The risk of seroma increases with modified radical mastectomy, greater volumes of drainage during the first 3 days, and being overweight, so such patients should be closely monitored for signs and symptoms of seroma, such as swelling, pain, and dullness at the incision area or axillary region; necessary treatment should be initiated as required, upon physician request [13].

Limitation in Range of Shoulder and Arm Movements

Limitations in the range of shoulder and arm movements can occur due to surgical procedures and radiotherapy. Patients should be advised to practice arm-shoulder exercises regularly and should be referred to physical therapy as required [7, 13].

In conclusion, the surgery specialist nurse should get to know the patient and her family upon the surgery decision, determine the care needs of the patient, and plan individual interventions. Additionally, as a member of a multidisciplinary team, the nurse should take on an active role in the coordination of care and complete preoperative preparations, monitor operation-related complications after surgery, report complications to the doctor at an early stage, and manage such complications. The nurse should educate the patient on an exercise program for the prevention of lymphedema (Fig. 46.1), drain care, and other preventive measures after surgery, and the nurse should support patients who experience altered body image and refer such patients to liaison psychiatry as required [8–10, 14].

Nursing Care During Radiation Therapy

Although it has been used as a treatment modality for years, many patients experience anxiety concerning radiotherapy. Information regarding the radiotherapy process is important for patients to experience effective therapy. Information facilitates patient participation in treatment decisions, reduces anxiety, and increases compliance with treatment [15]. Moreover, if the need for information is not satisfied, patients may continue to experience treatment-related anxiety and may even misbehave, requiring significantly more time from health professionals [16].

Patient education is one of the main responsibilities of radiotherapy specialist nurses. There are many studies in the nursing field that have evaluated the effect of education on patient satisfaction and the appropriate education content [16]. It is emphasized in these studies that patient education should not be generic but should be specifically planned for breast radiotherapy. Furthermore, patient education should focus on the process and effect of breast radiotherapy, the purpose of therapy, reactions likely to occur during therapy (preventive measures and prevention), examinations that should be performed during treatment, and control visits in general. Although there is not a defined standard with respect to when to inform the patient about radiotherapy, it is important to begin patient education during the first meeting with a health professional and to continue the education process during each weekly control visit to increase its effectiveness. Moreover, it is best that a standard education on the treatment process is planned ahead specifically for each week based on the needs of the patient [16–18].

The education nurse first should explain the purpose of radiation therapy and describe how it will affect the disease of the patient. Subsequently, the following topics must be explained to the patient before treatment:

- To define the area of external radiotherapy, the therapy area will be marked with lines at the first meeting, and these lines should not be erased during the duration of the treatment.
- Therapy will continue every weekday for approximately 6 weeks, and each session will last approximately 1–3 min.
- The patient will be alone in the room during therapy, but she will be closely monitored by a radiotherapist and can talk to the radiotherapist via a closed-circuit system.
- Radiation will pass through her body, and it will not cause any pain.
- Patients should maintain the position directed by the radiotherapist (arm under the head). This position may be uncomfortable, especially during the initial therapy sessions. Therefore, the patient should continue arm exercises and can take analgesics 1 h before the therapy as required.
- The patient will not be radioactive after external radiotherapy.
- Patients should not fast during therapy, and it is best if patients eat a little before therapy.
- Because it can adversely affect the therapy, the patient should not take a multivitamin supplement unless recommended by the physician.
- It is important to attend therapy on time every day.

Patients may experience many physical, psychological, and psychosocial problems during radiotherapy, affecting both themselves and their family relationships. Skin changes, fatigue, pain related to nerve or pectoral muscle inflammation, edema of the breast tissue, and tenderness are the most frequently reported problems. However, every individual is affected at different levels. Some patients continue their daily lives unaffected, whereas others find it difficult because of the symptoms related to the treatment [17].

Today, because there is not a widely accepted standard regarding the prevention and management of skin reactions, patients should be advised to not apply any moisturizing lotion, hot or cold applications, or bandages before therapy unless recommended by the radiotherapist. Patients should be advised to avoid tight, irritating clothes during treatment and to wear comfortable cotton clothes. The patients should be informed about the importance of avoiding skin exposure to direct sunlight and to use sunscreen (30 SPF minimum) when going outdoors. Patients should be advised not to swim in pools and not to visit saunas during therapy [18–20]. For patients experiencing itchiness due to dry desquamation, an appropriate moisturizer and corticosteroid lotion can be recommended to provide comfort for the patient, upon the recommendation of doctor. Dressings can be applied to control wet desquamations with bleeding and discharge. Hyaluronic acid pomades can be initiated upon recommendation of the radiotherapist [18]. Furthermore, because smoking increases the severity of skin reactions, patients should be advised not to smoke during radiotherapy and should be encouraged to quit smoking [21].

In the past, patients were advised to not take baths and to not use deodorants if the axilla was included in the therapy area. However, studies have failed to demonstrate the effectiveness of this approach in the management of skin reactions, and avoiding bathing for the duration of therapy can discomfort patients. Today, it is stated that there is no harm in washing the therapy area with water and soap, and patients are encouraged to wash their skin with soap and water without irritating it and to dry their skin completely with a soft towel applying tapotement [22]. Other than deodorants containing aluminum chlorohydrate, there is no harm in using deodorants during therapy unless skin integrity is damaged. Aluminum chlorohydrate-containing deodorants increase the dose in the skin via the bolus effect, so they are not recommended. However, the utilization of deodorants during therapy is not a well-studied topic [18]. In a study performed in 2009 that included 84 women receiving breast radiotherapy, Theberge et al. reported higher levels of skin reactions in women using deodorants not containing aluminum chlorohydrate than in women not using deodorant [23].

Various studies have stated that the utilization of *Calendula officinalis* can be beneficial for the prevention of skin reactions in patients receiving breast radiotherapy and may be recommended for this purpose [18, 24].

Because the evidence is insufficient to determine the best application in the management of radiation dermatitis today, there is significant diversity in clinical applications. A widely accepted standard preventive method has not yet been established [18, 19]. In Turkey, radiotherapy units follow their own specific skin care protocols.

Another problem that is frequently experienced by patients receiving breast radiotherapy is fatigue. Fatigue related to radiotherapy can adversely affect patients' quality of life both during the treatment period and long after the treatment. Fatigue can be caused by anemia, sleeplessness, poor nutrition, hypothyroidism, depression, previous chemotherapy administration, and pain. The primary approach for management is the treatment of the cause (management of anemia, depression, etc.). Additionally, non-pharmacological approaches that have been shown to be effective in the management of fatigue, such as education, exercise, cognitive behavioral therapies, massage, and Reiki, are also recommended. With respect to education, focused education including the causes of fatigue and coping strategies has been shown to be beneficial [25]. In a recent meta-analysis, 20–30 min of aerobic exercise three times per week and participation in regular exercise programs during the posttreatment period were determined to be beneficial for the management of fatigue in breast patients [26]. As one of the most studied subjects in oncology, the effectiveness of exercise on fatigue has been reported in many studies; quality of life is better and the level of fatigue is lower in breast patients participating in regular exercise programs, and exercise is regarded as a care standard in the management of fatigue, unless there is spinal or bone metastasis [26, 27].

In conclusion, the radiotherapy specialist nurse should get to know the patient and her family from the moment the radiotherapy decision is made and should determine the care needs of the patient and plan the individual interventions. Furthermore, as a member of a multidisciplinary team, the nurse should take an active role in the coordination of the care and provide the patient with a safe care service. Nurses should support patients in returning to their normal lives once treatment is over.

Nursing Care in Systemic Treatment

Treatment protocols that include combinations of various drugs (Adriamycin, paclitaxel, docetaxel, Herceptin, etc.) are used in the treatment of breast cancer depending on the prognostic factors and the patient's response to treatment. Depending on the protocol used, various side effects can develop during treatment, including nausea/vomiting, fatigue, hair loss, weight gain, loss of appetite, joint and muscle pain, and constipation, which can cause the patient to refuse treatment. The purpose of care for these patients is to improve their quality of life by preventing or controlling treatment-related symptoms. Most of the symptoms caused by systemic treatment are multidimensional, complicated, and subjective, reflecting changes in the biopsychosocial functions of the patient. Therefore, symptom management is important for these patients and constitutes an important part of nursing applications in oncology. Cancer patients generally prefer pharmacological approaches (72.5 %) for controlling these symptoms. Moreover, fewer patients benefit from non-pharmacological approaches such as resting (38.2 %) and sleeping (12.9 %) for controlling fatigue, staying hydrated (9 %) and maintaining mouth care (15.9 %) for dryness of the mouth, and resting (6.5 %) and exercising (1.5 %) for dealing with psychological symptoms [28]. Although pharmacological approaches are offered to patients, different non-pharmacological approaches can also be recommended for preventing and controlling different symptoms [29].

To control nausea and vomiting, which are observed frequently in Adriamycin-based treatments in breast patients, acupuncture, acupressure, music therapy, progressive muscle relaxation exercises, and diet changes can be suggested. Meals should be prepared in a different environment from the patient, and the patient should be encouraged to eat in small amounts and more frequently, increasing the number of meals from 3 to 5–6. Furthermore, because they are tolerated better than hot food, cold-served foods such as sandwiches, cheese, fat-free toast, and mashed potatoes should be offered; apple juices, cranberry juice, lemonade, and mint tea can be recommended in small sips. Patients are advised to not eat sweet, fat, salty, spicy, and smelly foods because they can increase nausea. Furthermore, because they can decrease appetite, patients should avoid their favorite foods if they experience nausea/vomiting. Based on the emetic effect of the patient's chemotherapy protocol, upon physician request, appropriate antiemetic agents should be recommended for at least 3 days [30, 31]. Although acupressure application in chemotherapy patients has been reported to reduce the intensity of acute nausea, it is not effective for acute vomiting or for late complaints. Nonetheless, the use of an acupressure band can be recommended to some patients who experience high levels of nausea and vomiting [31].

Myelosuppression or a decrease in blood counts is one of the most important side effects during treatment and can lead to a reduction in treatment dosage or postponement of treatment. This side effect is most commonly observed in breast cancer patients receiving doxorubicin, cyclophosphamide, or paclitaxel. Age, previous radiotherapy administration, bone metastases, insufficient renal function, high therapy doses, and long-term therapy can increase the risk for myelosuppression; the selected treatment protocol can also contribute to level of myelosuppression. The most important problem in myelosuppression is neutropenia. In neutropenia, leukocyte counts fall and predispose the patient to infections. These patients should be advised to avoid infected people and to take extra care with their personal hygiene (particularly for the mouth

and perineal region) for the following week after therapy. Additionally, the patient should be educated on measuring body temperature, and it should be explained that if her fever rises above 38 °C, she must report it to her physician and follow the physician's recommendations [32].

Fatigue is a multidimensional symptom affecting breast cancer patients in different ways. Fatigue can be caused by decreased hemoglobin levels, pain, depression, or the effects of drugs. Fatigue is especially frequent in patients receiving the taxane group of drugs. Exercise, psychosocial interventions, and other approaches are reported to be effective in the management of fatigue [25]. Most researchers have focused on the effect of exercise on quality of life, physical function, emotional well-being, and fatigue, and studies have examined health-related outcomes, such as cardiovascular fitness, muscular strength, and objective physical functioning [33]. McNeely and colleagues conducted a systematic review and meta-analysis of 14 RCTs involving exercise interventions in 717 breast cancer survivors aged 35–72 years. Pooled data from 156 patients in these trials revealed significant positive effects of exercise on quality of life, cardiorespiratory fitness, and cardiovascular fitness. The pooled data also demonstrated a statistically significant impact on fatigue reduction but only during the survivorship phase [26, 33]. In two studies performed by Yates et al. (2005) and Ream et al. (2006), psychosocial education provided by the nurses decreased the frequency, intensity, and effect of fatigue [34, 35]. Preventive treatment related to the management of fatigue in cancer patients is generally theoretical, and medical approaches focus on the treatment of the symptoms that cause fatigue. For example, patients experiencing fatigue due to pain are given analgesics, patients experiencing fatigue due to anemia are given erythrocyte suspension or Fe^{++}, and patients experiencing fatigue due to depression are given antidepressants and psychostimulants [25].

Although not frequent, oral mucositis is a side effect reported by patients, particularly when leukocyte counts fall 1 week after treatment. For this reason, it is important to review blood counts in patients developing oral mucositis and plan treatment aimed at the cause (e.g., antiseptics, antifungal agents, topical analgesics, or growth factors). Regular application of mouth care protocols and holding ice in the mouth (cryotherapy) for patients receiving bolus 5-fluorouracil can be beneficial for the prevention of this problem [36]. In meta-analyses on this subject, traditional Chinese medicines, cryotherapy, mouth care protocols, and honey are effective for decreasing the prevalence and intensity of oral mucositis [36] but not effective in treating it [36, 37].

Alopecia can be defined as transient or partial hair loss caused by chemotherapy. Although the extent of hair loss depends on the type, dose, and duration of administration of the selected drug, it is generally transient. Methotrexate or 5-fluorouracil causes a small extent of hair loss, whereas complete hair loss is observed in patients receiving doxorubicin, cyclophosphamide, or paclitaxel. Although alopecia is not a side effect that necessitates lowering the treatment dosage, it adversely affects patient quality of life by negatively altering body image, sexual life, and self-respect through effects on individual physical appearance. Hair loss generally begins 2 weeks following treatment, and hair starts to grow again within 8 weeks after treatment is over; it is important to inform the patient of this timeline [38].

Neurotoxicity is a problem during taxane-based treatments. This side effect affects the nervous system, manifesting as paresthesia of the hands and feet and the development of constipation. Paresthesia of the hands and feet is a frequent problem in patients receiving taxane-based treatments. Although this problem is temporary in most patients, some patients can experience symptoms of longer duration, which may require lowering the dose of the administered drug or its discontinuation [39].

For constipation problems, the use of laxatives, a fiber-rich diet, and increased fluid intake can be recommended to the patient [40].

Menopause-like symptoms such as hot flashes or vaginal dryness occur due to the effects of drugs on the hormonal system. The use of water-based lubricants and vaginal dilators during sexual intercourse can be recommended to patients to prevent vaginal dryness. For hot flashes, wearing light clothes, avoidance of synthetic and woolly clothes, reducing smoking, reducing tea and coffee consumption, practicing relaxing exercises, and having a warm shower before bed can be recommended [41].

Nursing Care in the Terminal Period

Upon diagnosis of cancer, the patient is confronted with many questions and problems from diagnosis to treatment and the posttreatment period, such as accepting the diagnosis, dealing with disease- and treatment-related symptoms, continuing treatment, dealing with social problems, and fulfilling familial responsibilities. However, approaching the terminal phase, problems such as psychological issues, pain, nausea/vomiting, fatigue, dyspnea, anorexia, cachexia, constipation, and delirium constitute the focus of palliative care.

Psychological problems coalesce as the disease advances and disturb the patient's quality of life; the patient and her family can manifest different emotional reactions based on their personalities and previous experiences. Patients should be supported at this stage and during the later stages of the disease to address psychosocial problems and to use their coping skills effectively. Specialists working in liaison psychiatry should be consulted as required, and appropriate treatment modalities such as cognitive behavioral therapies and pharmacological treatment should be initiated. Patients should be encouraged to take active roles in decisions about their treatment and to keep diaries reflecting their mood changes, and they should be encouraged to share their emotions with the people they love [12].

One of the symptoms that are generally difficult to control in the terminal period is pain. Pain is significantly more frequent in patients with bone metastasis. Psychoeducation, supportive psychotherapy, and behavioral cognitive interventions are non-pharmacological approaches shown to be effective in pain control. Additionally, as a part of the multidisciplinary approach, mind-body therapies are recommended for controlling chronic pain and improving quality of life [29, 42]. Listening to music reduces pain levels and the need for opiates, but its benefit is small, and its clinical importance is not clear [43]. For pharmacological treatment of cancer pain, two key concepts, "by the clock" and "ladder method," are very important for the effective management of pain. Whichever drug or method is used for cancer pain, the administration of drugs with certain intervals based on the duration of action should be adopted ("drugs by the clock"). Additionally, the recommendations of the WHO for cancer pain should be considered, and analgesic drugs should be added to treatment step by step, according to their potency. In this approach, non-opioids (paracetamol, aspirin, and nonsteroidal anti-inflammatory drugs) and adjuvant analgesics should be used for mild pain as the first step. In the second step, weak opioids (codeine and tramadol) should be added to the first-step drugs for moderate pain that cannot be controlled with non-opioids. In the third step, strong opioids (morphine and fentanyl) should be initiated for patients experiencing intense pain that is uncontrollable with weak opioids ("ladder method") [42].

Chronic fatigue can be an important problem for many patients. In these patients, fatigue is a multidimensional concept that affects patients differently. The cause of pain can be the disease itself, treatments, nutritional status, drugs, pain, activity level, sleeping problems, infections, or psychosocial problems such as anxiety and depression. Therefore, prevention related to the management of fatigue in cancer patients is generally theoretical, and medical approaches focus on the treatment of symptoms that cause fatigue. For example, patients experiencing fatigue due to pain are given analgesics, and patients experiencing fatigue due to depression are given antidepressants and psychostimulants. Additionally, studies have demonstrated that various approaches, including exercise, psychosocial interventions, decreasing energy consumption, nutrition, and acupuncture, are effective in the management of fatigue [25].

Anorexia and cachexia can also be observed in terminal-phase patient. Their causes can be the local and systemic effects of cancer, chemotherapy and radiotherapy, alterations in the sense of taste, stomatitis, dryness of the mouth, nausea/vomiting, and depression. To manage anorexia and cachexia, nutritional status should be improved with frequent meals in small amounts, and nutritional support should be provided as required. Nutritional balance should be maintained with a high-calorie diet. Progesterone preparations (medroxyprogesterone acetate, etc.), corticosteroids, and prokinetic agents (metoclopramide, etc.) can be used for this purpose. It should be noted that steroids cause a negative nitrogen balance [13].

Utilization of Complementary Approaches in Breast Cancer

After diagnosis, many women with breast cancer want to know, in addition to conventional therapies, what proactive steps they can take to positively impact their prognosis. Most patients make lifestyle changes, and some begin to use different forms of complementary and alternative therapies (CAM), many hoping for a cure. However, complementary methods are not administered to cure such diseases; rather, they may help control symptoms and improve wellbeing [44]. However, it should be noted that, although studies have demonstrated the safety and efficacy of some CAM approaches, the reliability and effectiveness of most of the methods used by our patients have not yet been proved, results related to their effectiveness are limited, and poorly informed utilization can do more harm than good. Therefore, upon diagnosis, all breast cancer patients should be questioned regarding their use of CAM and informed about CAM utilization by health professionals. Furthermore, because the most correct way for the patient to obtain informed about the interaction of these approaches with her treatment is to discuss the issue with health professionals, one of our primary responsibilities is to guide the patient in this respect to complete a successful course of treatment [45].

References

1. GLOBOCAN 2012: Estimated incidence, mortality and prevalence worldwide in 2012. http://globocan.iarc.fr/Pages/fact_sheets_cancer.aspx. Accessed 27 Mar 2015.

2. Ozmen V. Breast cancer screening: current controversies. J Breast Health. 2011;7:1–4.

3. Yilmaz D, Bebis H, Ortabag T. Determining the awareness of and compliance with breast cancer screening among Turkish residential women. Asian Pac J Cancer Prev. 2013;14(5):3281–8.

4. Avci AI, Atasoy A, Sabah E. The Effect on women's beliefs knowledge and practices regarding breast self examination of education with video. IUFN Hem Derg. 2007;60:119–28.

5. Secginli S, Nahcivan NO. Factor associated with breast cancer screening behaviours in a sample of Turkish Women: a questionnaire survey. Int J Nurs Stud. 2006;43:161–71.

6. Koc Z, Saglam S. Determination of the knowledge and the practice of female patients about breast cancer, preventive measures and breast self examination and effectiveness of education. J Breast Health. 2009;5:25–33.

7. Breast Conditions. In: Nettina, Sandra M, editors. Lippincott Manual of Nursing Practice. 9th ed. Philadelphia, USA: Walter Kluver; 2010.

8. Liao MN, Chen SC, Lin YC, Chen MF, Wang CH, Jane SW. Education and psychological support meet the supportive care needs of Taiwanese women three months after surgery for newly diagnosed breast cancer: a non-randomised quasi-experimental study. Int J Nurs Stud. 2014;51(3):390–9.

9. Stephens PA, Osowski M, Fidale MS, Spagnoli C. Identifying the educational needs and concerns of newly diagnosed patients with breast cancer after surgery. Clin J Oncol Nurs. 2008;12(2):253–8.

10. Dawe DE, Bennett LR, Kearney A, Westera D. Emotional and informational needs of women experiencing outpatient surgery for breast cancer. Can Oncol Nurs J. 2014;24(1):20–30.

11. Peppercorn J. Need to improve communication in breast cancer care. J Clin Oncol. 2012;30(15):1744–6.

12. Watts K, Meiser B, Conlon H, Rovelli S, Tiller K, Zorbas H, et al. A specialist breast care nurse role for women with metastatic breast cancer: enhancing supportive care. Oncol Nurs Forum. 2011;38(6):627–31.

13. Foxon SB, Lattimer JG, Felder B. Breast cancer. In: Yarbro HC, Wujcik D, Gobel HB, editors. Cancer nursing: principles and practice. 7th ed. Sudbury: Jones and Bartlett Publishers; 2011.

14. Fu MR, Deng J, Armer JM. Putting evidence into practice: cancer-related lymphedema. Clin J Oncol Nurs. 2014;18(Suppl):68–79.

15. Halkett GK, Short M, Kristjanson LJ. How do radiation oncology health professionals inform breast cancer patients about the medical and technical aspects of their treatment? Radiother Oncol. 2009;90(1):153–9.

16. Halkett GKB, Kristjanson LJ, Lobb E, O'Driscoll C, Taylor M, Spry N. Meeting breast cancer patients' information needs during radiotherapy: what can we do to improve the information and support that is currently provided? Eur J Cancer Care. 2010;19:538–47.

17. Sjövall K, Strömbeck G, Löfgren A, Bendahl PO, Gunnars B. Adjuvant radiotherapy of women with breast cancer – information, support and side-effects. Eur J Oncol Nurs. 2010;14(2):147–53.

18. Poirier P. Nursing-led management of side effects of radiation: evidence-based recommendations for practice. Nurs Res Rev. 2013;3:47–57.

19. McQuestion M. Evidence-based skin care management in radiation therapy: clinical update. Semin Oncol Nurs. 2011;27(2):E1–17.

20. Ruppert R. Radiation therapy 101. What you need to know to help cancer patients understand their treatment and cope with side effects. Am Nurs Today. 2011;6(1):24–9.

21. Kraus-Tiefenbacher U, Sfintizky A, Welzel G, Simeonova A, Sperk E, Siebenlist K, et al. Factors of influence on acute skin toxicity of breast cancer patients treated with standard three-dimensional conformal radiotherapy (3D-CRT) after breast conserving surgery (BCS). Radiat Oncol. 2012;7:217.

22. deAndrade M, Clapis MJ, doNascimento TG, Gozzo TO, de Almeida AM. Prevention of skin reactions due to teletherapy in women with breast cancer: a comprehensive review. Rev Latino-Am Enfermagem. 2012;20(3):604–11.

23. Theberge V, Harel F, Dagnault A. Use of axillary deodorant and effect on acute skin toxicity during radiotherapy for breast cancer: a prospective randomized noninferiority trial. Int J Radiat Oncol Biol Phys. 2009;75(4):1048–52.

24. Pommier P, Gomez R, Sunyach MP, D'Hombres A, Carrie C, Montbarbon X. Phase III randomized trial of Calendula officinalis compared with trolamine for the prevention of acute dermatitis during irradiation for breast cancer. J Clin Oncol. 2004;22(8):1447–53.

25. NCCN Clinical Practice Guidelines in Oncology-Cancer Related Fatigue, Version 1.2015. Accessed date 29 Mar 2015.

26. Velthuis MJ, Agasi-Idenburg SC, Aufdemkampe G, Wittink HM. The effect of physical exercise on cancer-related fatigue during cancer treatment: a meta-analysis of randomised controlled trials. Clin Oncol. 2010;22(3):208–21.

27. Lee H, Lim Y, Yoo MS, Kim Y. Effects of a nurse-led cognitive-behavior therapy on fatigue and quality of life of patients with breast cancer undergoing radiotherapy: an exploratory study. Cancer Nurs. 2011;34(6):E22–30.

28. Can G, Erol O, Aydiner A, Topuz E. Non-pharmacological interventions used by cancer patients during chemotherapy in Turkey. Eur J Oncol Nurs. 2011;15:178–84.

29. Blaes AH, Kreitzer MJ, Torkelson C, Haddad T. Nonpharmacologic complementary therapies in

symptom management for breast cancer survivors. Semin Oncol. 2011;38(3):394–402.

30. Tipton JM, McDaniel RW, Barbour L, Johnston MP, Kayne M, LeRoy P, et al. Putting evidence into practice: evidence-based interventions to prevent, manage and treat chemotherapy-induced nausea and vomiting. Clin J Oncol Nurs. 2007;11(1):69–78.

31. Ezzo JM, Richardson MA, Vickers A, Allen C, Dibble SL, Issell BF, et al. Acupuncture-point stimulation for chemotherapy-induced nausea or vomiting. Cochrane Database Syst Rev. 2006;2, CD002285.

32. National Comprehensive Cancer Network (NCCN). Prevention and treatment of cancer-related infections. 2015. http://www.nccn.org. Accessed 28 Mar 2015.

33. McNeely ML, Campbell KL, Rowe BH, Klassen TP, Mackey JR, Courneya KS. Effects of exercise on breast cancer patients and survivors: a systematic review and meta-analysis. CMAJ. 2006;175:34–41.

34. Yates P, Aranda S, Hargraves M, Mirolo B, Clavarino A, McLachlan S, et al. Randomised controlled trial of an educational intervention for managing fatigue in women receiving adjuvant chemotherapy for early-stage breast cancer. J Clin Oncol. 2005;23(25): 6027–36.

35. Ream E, Richardson A, Alexander-Dann C. Supportive intervention for fatigue in patients undergoing chemotherapy: a randomized controlled trial. J Pain Symptom Manag. 2006;31(2):148–61.

36. Worthington HV, Clarkson JE, Eden TOB. Interventions for preventing oral mucositis for patients with cancer receiving treatment. Cochrane Database Syst Rev. 2007;3, CD000978.

37. Clarkson JE, Worthington HV, Eden TOB. Interventions for treating oral mucositis for patients with cancer receiving treatment. Cochrane Database Syst Rev. 2007;1, CD001973.

38. van den Hurk CJ, Winstanley J, Young A, Boyle F. Measurement of chemotherapy-induced alopecia-time to change. Support Care Cancer. 2015;23: 1197–9.

39. Hershman DL, Lacchetti C, Dworkin RH, Lavoie Smith EM, Bleeker J, Cavaletti G, et al. Prevention and management of chemotherapy-induced peripheral neuropathy in survivors of adult cancers: American Society of Clinical Oncology Clinical Practice Guideline. J Clin Oncol. 2014;32(18):1941–67.

40. Fritz D, Pitlick M. Evidence about the prevention and management of constipation: implications for comfort part 1. Home Healthc Nurs. 2012;30(9):533–40.

41. Boutet G. Management of hot flushes for breast cancer survivors. Gynecol Obstet Fertil. 2012;40(4): 241–54.

42. Satija A, Ahmed SM, Gupta R, Ahmed A, Rana SP, Singh SP, et al. Breast cancer pain management – a review of current & novel therapies. Indian J Med Res. 2014;139(2):216–25.

43. Cepeda MS, Carr DB, Lau J, Alvarez H. Music for pain relief. Cochrane Database Syst Rev. 2006;19(2), CDO04843.

44. Wanchai A, Armer JM, Stewart BR. Complementary and alternative medicine use among women with breast cancer: a systematic review. Clin J Oncol Nurs. 2010;14(4):E45–55.

45. Deng GE, Frenkel M, Cohen L, Cassileth BR, Abrams DI, Capodice JL, et al. Evidence-based clinical practice guidelines for integrative oncology: complementary therapies and botanicals. J Soc Integr Oncol. 2009;7(3):85–120.

Psychosocial Adaptation During and After Breast Cancer

47

Mine Özkan

Abstract

Cancer is a chronic, life-threatening disease that greatly impacts all spheres of life. Cancer patients develop various and differing emotional, mental, and behavioral reactions regarding their illness during diagnosis, treatment, and the palliative period. Some of these reactions are normal and may even tend toward adaptation in some cases. The treatment team must understand such reactions and support them. Disordered or maladaptive reactions, however, require psychiatric evaluation and treatment.

A breast cancer diagnosis can be devastating and trigger emotional reactions such as chaos, uncertainty, anxiety, hopelessness, and despair. Psychological distress, such as depression, anxiety, and difficulty concentrating, is common. Breast cancer and mastectomy are perceived to be as much of a threat to physical integrity and the sense of femininity as they are to life. The side effects from surgery, chemotherapy, and radiotherapy can be significantly disfiguring, including deformation and/or breast loss, visible scarring, skin changes related to radiotherapy, hair loss due to chemotherapy, and lymphedema.

The disease profoundly disrupts a woman's emotional equilibrium and quality of life. Health-related quality of life represents the functional effects of an illness and its treatment on the patients and thus is an important indicator of the psychosocial and psychological burden of the illness.

It is essential to encourage the patient to express her feelings, to support the patient, and to provide her with security. Healthcare professionals

M. Özkan, MD
Department of Psychosocial Oncology, Institute of
Oncology, University of Istanbul, Çapa, Istanbul,
Turkey

Department of Consultation Liaison Psychiatry,
University of Istanbul, Istanbul Faculty of Medicine,
Çapa, Istanbul, Turkey
e-mail: mineozkan_klp@yahoo.com

© Springer International Publishing Switzerland 2016
A. Aydiner et al. (eds.), *Breast Disease: Management and Therapies*,
DOI 10.1007/978-3-319-26012-9_47

should be aware of and respect women's coping strategies and encourage them to use these strategies to reduce psychological symptoms. They should also make family members and friends aware of their role in supporting and encouraging coping strategies.

This chapter clearly documents that an interdisciplinary approach combining oncologic and psychiatric treatments is required for decreasing the emotional, physiological, and social burdens of breast cancer.

Keywords

Psychosocial oncology • Breast cancer intervention • Psychotherapy of cancer patients • Psychological distress • Coping • Distress • Coping strategies • Adaptive or maladaptive coping • Radiotherapy effects • Chemotherapy effects • Quality of life • Psychological response • Depression in cancer patients • Anxiety in cancer patients • Breast cancer • Body image • Self-esteem • Marital adjustment • Cancer • Psychooncology • Social support • Sexual problems • Liaison psychiatry • Cognitive dysfunction • Stress • PTSD • Posttraumatic growth • Breast reconstruction • Cognitive impairment • Adaptation • Family of cancer patient

Psychosocial Reaction During and After Cancer

From a medical perspective, cancer involves pathophysiological, organic processes; from the patient's point of view, it is a crisis of life, identity, and existence as well as a multidimensional issue that implicates biological, mental, social, environmental, familial, psychosocial, and psychosexual elements. In modern medicine, it is necessary to create solutions for diseases in conceptual and clinical terms by addressing the biological, mental, and social components in concert. We cannot understand the disease and the reactions without understanding the patient as a whole.

In general medical practices, physical diseases are accompanied by organic, mental, psychophysiological, psychopathological, behavioral, and psychosocial morbidity. The psychological-behavioral state is instrumental in the susceptibility to physical diseases, the progression and course of the medical illness, the adaptation of the patient, the response of the patient to treatment, and patient care and survival as a whole. Physical diseases and their complications induce a crisis in the patient and affect the mental state.

While providing treatment and care for the patient, it is essential for medical treatment and care to go hand in hand with mental treatment and care in a coordinated and systematic approach [1, 2].

Cancer is a chronic, life-threatening disease that greatly impacts all spheres of life. During the initial phase, the patients experience feelings of disbelief, shock, panic, and a sense of hopelessness. Anger, hostility, and the feeling of losing control over one's life are also common reactions to cancer. Over time, cancer patients and their families and friends face several difficult situations such as making sense of complex medical information, making difficult treatment decisions, dealing with treatment side effects, living with the fear of recurrence, and, for some, facing the unfortunate possibility of impending death, which further disrupts the quality of life [3].

A series of medical, psychical, and psychosocial factors play roles in the adaptation of the cancer patient. These factors are listed below:

• The patient herself—her experiences and opinions regarding medical diseases; the patient's illness; the type, symptoms, signs, and course of the illness; and the organ affected by the illness.

- The age period in which the patient became ill and the level of threat her illness poses to the goals and projects that the patient had at the time (work, family, age period).
- The support systems surrounding the patient and the cultural and social approaches to the illness.

Cancer patients develop various differing emotional, mental, and behavioral reactions regarding their illness during diagnosis, treatment, and the palliative period. Some of these reactions are normal and may even tend toward adaptation. The treatment team must understand such reactions and support them as well. Disordered or maladaptive reactions, however, require psychiatric evaluation and treatment [2].

People react to cancer in numerous ways. In the first stage, the most common reactions are shock and disbelief. Immediate denial of the truth is a defense mechanism against the anxiety, panic, and desperation caused by the truth; these reactions are often very difficult to endure and even impossible for some people to withstand. In a sense, the patient protects herself against unbearable anxiety by refusing to accept the truth and pretending that it does not exist; therefore, it may be more advisable to prepare the patient psychologically by providing her with environmental, social, and emotional support and gently informing her of her condition. Subsequently, anger and depression develop. The patient's inability to express her anger and her feelings of rebellion increases the risk of developing depression. Specialists working in oncology services must be aware that such patients might project their anxiety, overreactions, and anger to their families and treatment team. States such as anxiety, not eating or drinking, distractibility, and uneasiness are normal during this period. Feelings of rage and rebellion entailing the question "why me?" can also be experienced.

Bolund has defined the cancer crisis as a four-phase process:

1. State of shock
2. Reaction phase
3. Resistance
4. Adaptation

Due to the catastrophic associations it brings about, a cancer diagnosis creates a reaction of shock in the first phase. The person becomes estranged to her own body and feels that her future investments are threatened. She enters into a life crisis. The most common adaptation style in this phase is denial. Denial is an effort to keep an unendurable truth from entering consciousness and to protect the integrity of the self. Psychological defense reactions such as disaggregation and projection frequently develop. The person appears to be unable to hear what is being said or to comprehend the truth. This state may extend from a few hours to a few days or even to a few weeks, depending on the person. The patient must be given time and positive messages that may inspire hope. Additionally, probabilities and options regarding treatment must be explained to her, and she should receive family support.

Reactions are excessive during the second phase. The person tends to accept the truth and shows emotional reactions to it. The main type of reaction is anxiety. The threat of extinction, the perception of loss, thoughts of separation and death, and the feeling of becoming estranged from one's own body are the main elements of this anxiety. A state of anxiety manifests itself through varying symptoms.

The third phase is the adaptation phase, in which the patient accepts the truth and directs her mental strength to her new life. This is the phase in which the patient learns to live with her illness. Specifying treatment options and presenting a treatment program helps to facilitate acceptance. In this phase, the person starts reinterpreting her life—past, future, and existence. She questions her identity, her purpose in life, her own narcissistic aims, and her life choices. She seeks security and balance.

Elizabeth Kübler Ross has defined the psychological phases of cancer in five phases, starting from the phase specifying how the patient reacts to the cancer diagnosis and continuing on to the processes involving the following reactions:

1. Denial
2. Anger
3. Bargaining
4. Depression
5. Acceptance

Green et al. have designed the Mental Adjustment to Cancer and listed adaptation mechanisms as follows:

1. Fighting spirit
2. Helplessness/hopelessness
3. Anxious preoccupation
4. Fatalism
5. Avoidance and denial

It is the incontestable and fundamental right of every person to learn the truth about one's self. Empathy, understanding, support, and sympathy are essential in conveying the diagnosis to the patient. The patient must be informed in a way that keeps her from losing hope and enables her to accept and continue her treatment. The patient should be told of her situation in a mode, period, and process that she can tolerate. Optionally, this might also be achieved in multiple sessions. Another important factor regarding this issue is that the diagnosis should be explained by the responsible, authorized oncologist or specialist who has been directly involved in the treatment. Liaison psychiatry aids in evaluating the patient and can occasionally be utilized to inform the patient of the diagnosis. It also helps to evaluate and treat the psychopathology that develops afterward.

Interestingly, most patients develop selective denial. In other words, they accept the truth to an extent that they are able to tolerate and adapt without resorting to reactions such as refusing treatment or feeling that treatment is unnecessary. These patients accept the truth up to a degree that they can tolerate. In such cases, it is best to inform the patient of the diagnosis after presenting treatment options and clinical and social support opportunities.

Once it is definitive, the diagnosis must be told with sympathy, directness, and realistic hopefulness. It is best if it is told by including treatment and care options and in a way that enables the patient to understand and that keeps her from denying the situation [1, 2].

Breast Cancer and Psychosocial Responses

Breast cancer is the most common tumor in women and is one of the leading causes of death from cancer. Breast cancer comprises 29 % of all cancers observed in women in the USA. Breast cancer comprises 24.9 % of all cases of cancer in women in Turkey [4]. The incidence in eastern regions is 20/100,000, whereas in western regions, it is 40–50/100,000 [5]. Although the incidence and prognosis vary geographically, the incidence of breast cancer in Turkey has increased by 1.5 % annually [4]. Breast cancer is the most prevalent tumor among women and is one of the main reasons for fatalities from cancer. Unfortunately, the prevalence of breast cancer is increasing every year, and the use of breast self-examination and mammography remains low [3].

Research conducted on breast cancer patients focuses on the following:

- The predispositional role of a premorbid personality in the development of breast cancer
- Stressful life events and breast cancer
- Psychological reactions to breast cancer diagnosis and treatment
- Psychiatric disorders (anxiety, depression, delirium, etc.)
- Lifestyle changes (as a result of problems associated with physical discomfort, marital relations or difficulties experienced in sexual relations, and changes in activity levels)
- The relationship between defense mechanisms, psychological disorders, and personality types
- The impact of organ loss on body image and self-esteem

- Psychiatric disorders in the postsurgical period and the factors affecting them
- Spirituality
- Quality-of-life issues
- Treatment side effects
- The effects of psychological interventions

Breast cancer is a disease that threatens an organ associated with self-respect, sexuality, and femininity. Developments in treatment methods have significantly altered the socio-cultural climate for women struggling with breast cancer. The difficulties that women encounter today are different from those that women faced 15–20 years ago. Nevertheless, while the emotional problems they experience today may be different, they are equally challenging [3]. These psychosocial stresses can be summarized as follows:

- Fear of death due to "malignant disease"
- Worries related to uncertainty about the future
- Dread that the illness will reoccur
- Separation anxiety
- The worry that one will lose her self-sufficiency, control over her own body, autonomy, and fundamental functions
- The worry that body parts and organs will be harmed
- Change and deterioration in appearance
- Fears of disfigurement and loss of sexual attractiveness
- Fear of losing love, sympathy, and support
- Feelings of inadequacy and fear of being dependent on others
- Fear of not being able to take care of children
- Fears concerning fertility
- Worry about painful, appearance-altering conditions such as aches and hair loss and worries associated with guilt and punishment
- Confusion about the disease etiology
- Uncertainty about the effects and the effectiveness of treatment regimens
- Fears of recurrence and metastasis [2, 6] that are common among breast cancer patients

A diagnosis of breast cancer can be devastating and can trigger emotional reactions such as chaos, uncertainty, anxiety, hopelessness, and despair. Psychological distress such as depression and difficulty concentrating is common. The breast cancer diagnosis places extraordinary demands on a woman's coping abilities. Women must therefore adapt to being breast cancer patients and redefine their lives and themselves accordingly. Thus, the task for patients is to incorporate the diagnosis (and all that comes with it) into their existing beliefs of meaning in life. They either rework the diagnosis to make it fit existing beliefs or revise their beliefs to better match their experience [6].

Psychosocial Adaptation in Breast Cancer

The term "adjustment to cancer" is used to describe the processes of adaptation that occur during the illness. "Mental adjustment" to cancer has been defined as a person's cognitive and behavioral responses to a cancer diagnosis. The adaptation process requires the patient to accommodate the changes that the cancer introduced into a multitude of dimensions of their lives [7]. To measure the adaptation of these types of changes, the quality of life (QoL) is used as the main instrument. The QoL is considered a multidimensional concept defined as a subjective assessment of physical, functional, emotional, and social well-being [8].

Various models have been proposed to explain the process of adaptation after a personal crisis. According to the transactional theory [9], the process of dealing with a stressor comprises antecedent, mediating, and outcome variables. The outcome is the individual's more-or-less successful adaptation to stress; environmental and personal variables are causal antecedents of the adaptation to stress. The effect of these antecedent variables is mediated by the person's appraisal and coping. Hobfoll's [10] theory of the conservation of resources underscores the importance of personal and coping resources as predictors of positive long-term adaptation. According to social cognitive theory [11], perceived self-efficacy strongly influences behavior and is positively associated with adjustment.

A woman who receives a diagnosis of breast cancer must adjust to the transition from being healthy to having a life-threatening disease. The patient's coping styles and perception of the illness are crucial factors in this adjustment process. Diagnosis and treatment are commonly affected by psychological stress. Coping styles and social support have an impact on the distress experienced by the patient [8, 12]. Psychological, behavioral, emotional, and physical adjustments are unique for every patient and are related to a number of factors. Factors that contribute to the psychological responses of women to breast cancer can be grouped as follows:

1. Medical factors (stage of cancer at diagnosis and treatments received)
2. Sociocultural context, treatment options, and decision making
3. Psychological and psychosocial factors

The age at the onset of cancer, premorbid emotional balance (personality and coping style), attitudes toward illness, attitudes toward breast cancer in particular, prior psychiatric history, and the existence and accessibility of interpersonal support have been reported to be important variables in psychosocial adjustment [2].

Factors Affecting Psychosocial Adaptation in Breast Cancer

Life Cycle or Age

The life cycle during which breast cancer arises is important because the disease threatens to undermine or altogether curtail the social responsibilities women have at different times in their lives. Studies have consistently shown that younger women (<age 50) report greater psychological morbidity following a breast cancer diagnosis than older women [13–15]. Several investigations have also found that younger women with breast cancer report significantly worse quality of life than older women, particularly in the emotional and social domains [13, 16]. From a developmental perspective, younger women face unique issues

such as premature onset of menopause, which may lead to infertility; sudden onset of vasomotor symptoms; long-term consequences of ovarian decline; concern about future pregnancies; changes in relationships with partners and/or children; multiple role demands of parenthood and work; career and work concerns related to productivity, job security, and career interruption; and greater concerns about body image and sexuality [13, 15]. Studies have shown that being married was associated with better adjustment, including better quality of life and possibly even increased survival. Married women have also been found to have less distress and to show better adjustment compared with unmarried women [17].

Coping and Personality

Other variables that affect adjustment are personality and coping styles. Every woman has her own coping style that she uses to adjust to stress. Coping can be defined as constantly changing cognitive and behavioral efforts to manage specific external and/or internal demands that are appreciated as a stressor, according to Lazarus. Coping strategies are classified as "problem-focused coping," behavior directed at solving the problem or situations, and "emotion-focused coping," behavior directed at changing the emotional reactions to the problem or situations. The latter also covers various defensive and avoidance strategies. Coping is independent of the outcome, and defense is regarded as a specific form of coping behavior [18]. The five most significant styles for adjusting to cancer have been summarized as fighting spirit, fatalism, cognitive avoidance, anxious preoccupation, and helplessness/hopelessness [19].

In a longitudinal study of 101 breast cancer patients [20], the latent construct of perceived control, which included measures of fighting spirit, helplessness/hopelessness, and self-efficacy, predicted less psychological distress. In a sample of 55 breast cancer patients, cognitive avoidance was associated with worse psychological adjustment 3 years later [21]. A study of coping patterns and distress showed that women with breast cancer who used emotion-focused engagement coping, i.e., acceptance or emotional expression combined with social support, experienced less distress 3 months later than women with breast cancer who had not used any emotion-focused engagement coping [22]. In a study investigating the correlation between coping responses and psychological adjustment in women with breast cancer, a significant correlation was found between poor adjustment and cognitive avoidance and minimal use of approach-based coping responses [21].

Every individual has a subjective way of perceiving and coping with stress shaped by culture. The most effective coping strategies in the management of breast cancer stress were defined by Penman (1980). According to Penman, women who use more avoidant and passive ways of coping experience higher levels of difficulties adjusting than women who use direct and active coping strategies. Furthermore, women who have a sense of control over the experience take a more active role within their treatment phases. Pessimistic reactions reflect insufficient psychological coping. Therefore, educational level and socioeconomic status are important in ensuring better adjustment. As cited from Baider (2004), in a study that examined the possible predictors of adjustment to breast cancer, the most consistent predictor of psychological distress at 1 and 4 months after diagnosis was avoidant coping: women who reported more avoidant coping were more distressed. However, some authors have suggested that avoidant coping facilitates adjustment and decreases emotional distress. For example, in a literature review, it was concluded that avoidant coping could be especially beneficial during active treatment [3].

Several studies have looked at coping strategies employed over time in women with breast cancer. One short-term study found a significant decrease in active behavioral and cognitive coping strategies and no change in the use of avoidance over a 4-month period [23]. Women with early-stage breast cancer were followed for a year and found that some coping strategies such as active coping, planning, denial, and religious coping were used more frequently at the time of diagnosis and rapidly decreased, whereas other coping strategies such as the use of social support, self-distraction, restraint, and suppression of competing activities remained relatively constant or dropped off more slowly. Acceptance was the most frequently employed coping strategy and increased over the year following diagnosis [24]. A longitudinal study that followed women for up to 5 years found that variability in coping strategies was observed at the times of greatest stress (treatment, recurrence, terminal phase of cancer) and suggested that changes in coping strategies may be linked more to "illness stages" than to any specific length of time since diagnosis [25].

Coping strategies used during the diagnostic phases of breast cancer have been found to be indicators of psychological adjustment after surgery. Active acceptance at diagnosis predicts better adjustment through the first year. Defensive strategies reduce distress at 3 months but increase fear of cancer recurrence at 1 year. Defensive avoidance-oriented coping, which is a helplessness/hopelessness coping style combined with pessimism or passive acceptance and resignation, predicts poor psychological adaptation 1–3 years later [26].

Research suggests that optimism plays an important role in coping and adaptation to breast cancer and is thus included as a covariate. Healthcare professionals should be aware of and respect women's coping strategies and encourage their use to reduce the psychological symptoms. They should also make family members and friends aware of their role in supporting and encouraging coping strategies.

Social Support

Social support is a complex construct that has long been suggested to have direct and buffering effects on well-being and emotional adjustment in cancer. Although the literature on the ameliorative effects of social support in cancer progression appear to be more convincing than in cancer onset [27], conclusive evidence is missing. Interesting and relevant questions include whether social support plays a prognostic role in cancer and whether the quantity or quality of this support is important. The inconsistent findings on social support and cancer progression can be broadly attributed to varying operational definitions of the term social support, the use of its various measures across studies, and the inclusion of various types of cancer and insufficient control for confounding variables in analyses [28].

Social interdependence, having good friends and relationships, and having no other serious family problems were contributing factors. Several researchers have documented the importance of social support when facing breast cancer and have shown that a cancer diagnosis is harder to handle for those with other personal or family problems [29].

It is not possible to separate the experience of the breast cancer patient from the patient's family. The diagnosis of cancer is a traumatic experience for the entire family. The shock due to the diagnosis of cancer can change the relationship and communication between the patient, the family, and the other members. During this period, some patients could form closer relationships with others, whereas other patients could escape from interpersonal relationships. Feelings of fear and uncertainty usually lead to an increase in patients' need for social support. However, during the long intervention period, patients usually have difficulties finding energy to continue their social relationships and may not have the necessary support when they need it most. Supportive family relationships are particularly important to cancer patients due to the fear and uncertainty associated with cancer. Related studies suggest that adjustment to cancer is better in a family environment characterized by cohesiveness, open expression of feelings, and the absence of family conflict. Nevertheless, the fear of cancer, which leads cancer patients to need more support from their families, also may interfere with the amount of support that family members are likely to provide [30].

There is a reciprocal relationship between the partners' reactions and adjustment and the patients' reactions and adjustment. The severity of depressive symptoms experienced by a woman with breast cancer may be influenced by her appraisal of the adequacy of support available from her partner [31]. Quite often, a spouse or significant other is confused about the prospective effects of the illness and thus hides these feelings from the patient.

This type of behavior is more prevalent after mastectomy because the woman experiences a loss. In addition, husbands displayed similar psychological reactions and distress as their spouses did throughout the course of treatment, showing that the experience of breast cancer is a shared experience for couples. Importantly, husbands who had an active role in the decision-making process had better psychological adjustment. In a recent case study in Turkey, husbands of young women with cancer, especially gynecological and breast cancer, perceived the situation as highly traumatic; thus, the marital relationship was negatively affected [32]. Literature on the subject clearly indicates that the partner relationship is unique and that additional social support cannot overcome the negative effect of a distant husband on the female patient's emotional well-being [31].

Children can also experience different fear and anxiety problems according to their development level and can easily be affected during this difficult period. Another anxiety faced by family members is fear of inheriting this illness. Because of the genetic association of breast cancer, family members could have fear and anxiety regarding the risk of having breast cancer.

On one hand, people without cancer could become distant toward people with cancer due to a fear of cancer or death. On the other hand, family and friends could escape from interactions and arguments with the patients because of feelings of shock and uncertainty and feeling uncomfortable for not knowing how to behave. A stigmatizing attitude toward cancer could lead to inconsistent and confused attitudes of the patient and destructive feedback for them. Breast cancer leads to fundamental problems for women's jobs or careers, working environment, and economic status. These problems generally include having no health insurance, being unable to work again, having to change working activities, changing their priorities, and experiencing stigmatization and discrimination about work [33].

Prior Psychiatric History

The risk of anxiety and adjustment difficulties are greater in women with a history of psychiatric illness prior to breast cancer. Adjustment to the diagnosis of breast cancer is also related to a family history of breast cancer. Adjustment is also closely related to the reactions and behaviors of one's social and familial environment. The attitudes of spouses or partners, families, and friends have a great impact on both how a patient perceives the situation and how she copes with the disease [13].

Psychosocial adjustment to cancer varies during the illness, specifically during the treatment time. It is useful for health professionals, nurses, and physicians to know of these changes in patients with cancer to detect and respond to a patient's psychological distress more effectively. The early detection of psychological morbidity may allow for an early intervention, thus reducing distress experienced by the patients.

Psychiatric Morbidity in Breast Cancer Patients

Researchers investigating the impact of breast cancer report high levels of depression and anxiety in breast cancer patients. In a study by Kissane et al. (1998) of women with breast cancer, the prevalence of psychiatric disorders was reported as 45 % [34]. One of the most comprehensive reviews on the prevalence of depression in breast cancer patients was conducted by Rowland and Massie [35]. The review included 17 studies, and the percentage of depression in breast cancer patients in these studies changed from 1.5 % to 50 % depending on the number of patients, the definition of depression, and the evaluation tool used [35]. Some studies have indicated that approximately 20–41 % of breast cancer patients confront clinically significant psychological distress [36, 37]. Loscalzo et al. [38] reported that approximately 30 % of cancer patients have psychological problems, although only approximately 6 % of these patients seek help from family or medical staff. This indicates that medical professionals must be proactively involved in the psychological treatment of breast cancer patients.

Psychological discomfort among breast cancer patients is associated with depressive disorders, anxiety disorders, anger, low self-esteem, and little emotional support [2]. The prevalence of depression in patients with breast cancer is estimated at approximately 10–25 %, but there is no definitive meta-analysis of depression prevalence data [39].

We evaluated pre-intervention and post-intervention anxiety, depression, and quality of life in breast cancer patients and found that from the stage of diagnosis, the risk of depression was high and continued throughout the first year. In this study, we analyzed the patients' risk rates of anxiety (33.3 %, 35.7 %, 28.6 %) and depression (40.5 %, 42.9 %, 44 %) in three stages and found that patients were under psychological risk beginning from the stage of diagnosis [40].

In a study including women with breast cancer who were evaluated six times within the first 5 years following diagnosis, it was found that the depression rate (48 %) was highest at least 1 year after the diagnosis [37]. In another study, it was found that although the average reported anxiety and depression scores decreased over time, the anxiety rate was 38.4 %, and the depression rate was 32.3 % in the 18th month [41]. Four of every ten women were found to have severe depression and anxiety [42]. Morasso et al. [43] tried to detect depression among 132 breast cancer patients in stages I–III of the disease. Using screening tools for detecting mood disorders, they found a prevalence of psychiatric disorders of approximately 38 %, with a classical rate of depression (major episode, adjustment disorder) of approximately 25.9 %. Major depressive disorder was found in 8 % of patients during the follow-up; 10.6 % had adjustment disorders along with depressed mood, and 4.5 % had adjustment disorders with mixed anxiety and depressed mood.

Depressive symptoms are typically higher in the period surrounding diagnosis and active treatment and decline over time as patients learn to cope with the disease. Studies have found the depressive symptoms of long-term breast cancer survivors to be comparable to those of the general population [44]. The occurrence of depression in breast cancer patients is more strongly influenced by the patients' psychosocial environment and personality than by factors associated with the diagnosis and treatment regimen.

The prevalence of depression among women with early-stage breast cancer is twice that observed in the general female population, especially during the first year after diagnosis [37]. One of the most consistent findings is that the rate of depression diagnosis is the third highest in breast cancer, after pancreatic and oropharyngeal cancers [45]. The high rate of depression in patients with breast cancer highlights why it is important to identify it and to then provide appropriate resources and treatment.

To diagnose depression among this specific population, several parameters must be taken into account, such as the diagnostic system used, which means determining the type of criteria that might be more relevant regarding the nosography used, and the time of evaluation, which is an important factor because psychological disturbance changes over time [46]. Moreover, the incidence of depression appears to be dependent on the following parameters: the disease severity and the patient's disability and physical impairment levels, performance status, and past history of depression [47]. Paradoxically, major depression and depressive symptoms are underrated and undertreated in women with breast cancer. One explanation could be that women with breast cancer are generally reluctant to disclose their affective concern. Another reason could be that oncologists are not familiar with screening for depressive symptoms. The failure to diagnose mood disorders can be problematic because depression and its associated symptoms decrease the quality of life, affect compliance with medical therapies, and might reduce survival [48]. In addition to the classical clinical symptomatology of depression, such as sadness, anhedonia, guilt, helplessness, hopelessness, and suicidal ideation, the following risk factors of depression among breast cancer patients must be looked for:

- Past history of psychiatric illness
- The nature of the illness and cancer-related concerns (e.g., pain)
- A lack of confiding relationship
- A personality characterized by neuroticism
- Cognitive attitudes of helplessness/ hopelessness
- Racial or ethnic minority status [49]

Greater demands at work or from parenting may make cancer treatment more stressful for younger women. Furthermore, previous psychiatric illness or depression, poorer socioeconomic status, lower levels of social support, and lower levels of education are risk factors for depressive symptoms. In terms of clinical characteristics, several studies on depressive disorder suggest that patients with advanced disease are more likely to report depressive symptoms. In addition, poorer performance status, more severe physical symptoms, and higher disability and physical impairment levels are associated with higher levels of depressive symptoms [50].

The correlation between depression levels with coping styles and cognitive errors in women treated for breast cancer was examined by a study performed at the University of Istanbul. Breast cancer outpatients who had undergone surgery at least 6 months previously, had completed adjuvant cancer treatment, and had not experienced metastasis or recurrent lesions were evaluated. Higher cognitive errors and automatic thought scores were found in the depression group. A fighting spirit was found to be the primary coping style used in the non-depression group, whereas helplessness/hopelessness, anxiousness/preoccupation, and fatalism were the coping styles used most in the depression group. No associations among depression and sociodemographic (except for educational level) and cancer-related variables were detected. However, it was found that automatic thoughts, cognitive errors, education level, fighting spirit, and anxiousness/preoccupation are important indicators of depression in our sample. A causal relationship exists between depression and a patient's cognitive patterns and accompanying anxiety [51].

In another study conducted at our department, the effects of illness perception on depression in patients with breast cancer were evaluated. Depression scores were positively associated with scores of identity and perceived serious consequences and were negatively associated with scores of illness coherence and treatment control. In breast cancer patients, the recognition of the relationship between illness perception and psychiatric factors may provide better recognition of the maladaptive reactions of patients to illness and treatment according to patients' visions [52].

Could depression be a risk factor for breast cancer evolution? In the literature, there are some positive arguments supporting this possibility. First, major depression decreases motivation and reduces compliance with treatments such as chemotherapy. Second, major depression could be an important predictor of late-stage breast cancer diagnosis because patients will delay seeking a medical consultation after finding a lump. Third, considering the two previous points, major depression might have a detrimental effect on the outcome in breast cancer patients. Could depression be considered a possible prognostic factor for breast cancer mortality? The answer to that question remains unclear [49]. Some studies suggest a link between depression and breast cancer mortality. Watson et al. [53] in a prospective study among 578 early breast cancer patients found that depressive symptoms and hopelessness are linked with a significantly reduced chance of survival at 5-year follow-up. Hjerl et al. [54] analyzed data from breast cancer central registers in a study of a retrospective Danish cohort comparing early-stage and late-stage disease. In this study, they found that breast cancer with depression had a modestly but significantly higher risk of mortality depending on the stage of cancer and the time of depression. When women are confronted with advanced or even palliative or terminal stage cancer, they can experience suicidal ideation or can even attempt suicide to hasten death [55].

Certainly, in terms of suicidality, depression claims lives and represents a considerable risk factor for suicide. The risk for suicide is high among cancer patients compared with the general population. The relative risk for suicide is two times higher in the patient population. Suicide is possible when depression and desperation are comorbid with advanced stages of cancer and with the occurrence of uncontrollable symptoms such as severe pain. Risk factors for cancer patients include a previous history of psychiatric disorders, previous depression, a previous suicide attempt, a recent loss, alcohol or drug abuse, being male, a family history of depression or suicide, inadequate social support, and unemployment. Delirium, dysfunctional judgment, and impulse control disorder could lead to an unpredictable suicide attempt [56]. Although most of the women with breast cancer can adapt well to the situation, being single and having a low socioeconomic status are risk factors for suicide [55].

Anxiety is a normal response to unpleasant stimuli and can promote adaptive responses to new demands. However, it is detrimental when it is excessive and affects one's ability to cope with stress. Many patients diagnosed with breast cancer face extensive uncertainty about the future, concern over potential metastasis, fear of physical suffering, and overwhelming anxiety. Anxiety is one of the most dominant psychological challenges associated with cancer, with rates ranging from 10 % to 50 %. Research conducted in the USA and the UK has shown that anxiety prevails throughout the spectrum of treatment and recovery for female patients with breast cancer, even among disease-free breast cancer survivors [57]. In another study, moderate-to-severe anxiety was found in 27 % of breast cancer patients [58].

A review was conducted of studies discussing the level of anxiety among women with breast cancer who were undergoing cancer treatment(s) and on the factor(s) contributing to anxiety in various treatment modalities between 1990 and 2010. Anxiety appears to be ubiquitous, presenting itself in all treatment types for breast cancer. The anxiety levels in women who underwent chemotherapy were highest, particularly before the first chemotherapy infusion, and were mediated by age and trait anxiety. Radiotherapy regimens did not affect anxiety levels in radiotherapy-treated patients, and most research concluded that anxiety levels were higher among women who underwent mastectomy than those who underwent breast-conserving therapy [57].

Anxiety has also been shown to have a physiological impact, influencing the neuroendocrine and immune systems [59]. Anxiety is negatively correlated with the treatment outcome. It was also reported that anxiety in breast cancer has a detrimental effect on the QoL of female patients, affecting their physical, medical, and sexual QoL indicators [37]. Factors that contribute to anxiety in patients with breast cancer can be broadly classified into physical, psychological, social, and environmental causes. Physical factors include age, treatment side effects, hormonal changes, and issues surrounding fertility. Psychological factors encompass their perception about change in body image and positive and negative feelings about the disease. Social factors include social support, decreased sexual interest, and sexual dysfunction, whereas environmental factors include multiple hospital visits, which adversely affect daily routine and work life, and stress pertaining to the financial situation [15, 60]. When comparing treatment modalities, women receiving radiotherapy or chemotherapy tended to exhibit a higher anxiety score over time compared with those undergoing surgery alone [60]. The level of anxiety is also reported to be higher in patients undergoing chemotherapy compared with radiotherapy, and a higher level of anxiety at the start of chemotherapy has an inverse relationship with the QoL score [61]. Thus, different cancer treatment modalities have a variable impact on the anxiety experienced by patients and should neither be negated nor combined as one single issue to address. Healthcare professionals should pay greater attention to identify signs of anxiety in patients and to design interventions to help alleviate anxiety earlier.

Because breast cancer was acknowledged as a possible traumatic stressor, researchers have documented that dealing with breast cancer could result in poor psychological outcomes such as posttraumatic stress disorder (PTSD) or in positive personal changes and an enhanced appreciation of life, known as posttraumatic growth (PTG). The rate of PTSD in breast cancer patients and survivors was relatively low, varying from 2.4 % to 19 %. PTSD appears to be related to younger age at diagnosis, lower educational level, and lower socioeconomic status. PTSD was related to disease severity, to perceiving the disease as more stressful and threatening, and to stressful or poor adjustment to the diagnosis. Chemotherapy was also associated with increased symptoms of hyperarousal, which is requisite for identifying PTSD, whereas a longer hospital stay was positively associated with PTSD [62, 63].

Tokgüz et al. [64] reported the prevalence of PTSD in cancer patients as 19 %. It is supposed that chemotherapy is a situation that reminds the patient of trauma and could thus lead to continuous problems of traumatic stress; thus, patients receiving chemotherapy require more intense and effective psychological approaches.

The reported prevalence of sleep disorders in cancer patients is approximately 50 %; they are found more in women than in men and are also prevalent among breast cancer patients [64]. A sleep disorder is usually severe for cancer patients; however, it is often assumed to be a normal reaction for cancer or is not reported by patients. Thus, sleep disorder is a frequent but neglected problem. Studies found that associations exist between poor sleep quality and fatigue, difficulty sleeping and maintaining sleep, perceiving less sleep adequacy, and experiencing restless sleep. Therefore, treating one complaint could affect another. Cancer-related fatigue and sleep disturbances are reported to have a common etiology, and these two situations are related to pain, depression, concentration, and cognitive functional loss [22].

Psychiatric Effects of Breast Cancer Treatment

Surgery: Mastectomy

As in all physical illnesses and surgical procedures, mastectomy is a stressful event that causes psychosocial crises in patients. The psychiatric approach toward mastectomy has created a model for the psychiatric complications brought on by surgical interventions as a whole [1, 2]. Generally, mastectomy has the potential to unleash psychological reactions that are observed in other physical illnesses—concerns over the underlying illness and the narcissistic damage associated with surgical interventions and unique concerns related to the symbolic connection of the breast to femininity and sexuality.

Mastectomy not only creates a heightened sense of loss but also impacts a person's functions, body image and perception, psychological state, and relations with those around her. Moreover, it may engender various concerns and fears, including anxiety over separation from friends and relatives, the loss of love, attention, support, and approval stemming from aesthetic concerns, and the loss of fundamental functions and control over one's body. Feelings of guilt and the fear of punishment due to premorbid lifestyle (smoking and alcohol consumption) may also be observed. Another major worry associated with breast cancer and mastectomy is related to disease recurrence. Various behavioral and emotional reactions such as distress, anxiety, depression, anger, denial, hostility, projection, pathological dependence, angry resistance, and psychological stress may develop in a patient with these types of concerns [20].

Changes in physical appearance greatly impact a woman's quality of life, self-esteem, sexuality, social roles, and relationships. The psychological effects of the surgical treatment of breast cancer on body image and sexuality include embarrassment of exposing one's body, discomfort showing scars, overall bodily changes, lack of sexual interest, problems with sexual relationships, concerns about the resumption of sexual activity and the frequency, and difficulties with becoming sexually aroused [3].

Research on mastectomy has created a model for the psychiatric complications of surgical interventions. The first study on the psychological reactions associated with mastectomy was performed in 1952 by Renneker and Cutler. This pioneering clinical study drew attention to the existence of a grief state and the prevalence of the form of grief defined by "depression, anxiety, insomnia, guilt" and defined the relationship

between this state and organ loss. During the same period, Sutherland (1955) reported a similar psychological syndrome but stated that fear of death was fundamental and that the psychological state related to organ loss was not common. After the 1970s, these studies gained momentum. The current research indicates that psychiatric morbidity develops after cancer surgeries. Cancer surgery brings anxiety and problems regarding both the surgical intervention and the underlying disease. In other words, the practice of mastectomy has become a significant area of research for understanding the relationship and interaction between cancer, organ loss, and psychopathology [2, 3].

According to the results of a prospective study involving 42 mastectomy cases conducted by Özkan et al. in 1992 [65] on the characteristics and prevalence of psychiatric disorders arising post-op and the factors that impact adjustment, mild depression was found to be present in 32 % of the patients during the pre-op period, in 52 % in the first week and first month post-op, and in 11 % 1 year later. Depression was more severe in patients from 20 to 40 years of age, in single individuals, in less educated persons, and in persons who did not know their diagnosis. Anxiety was experienced by 28 % of the patients in the pre-op period and 64 % of the patients in the early post-op period (the first week after surgery). Anxiety is significantly less common at the first year post-op but is still higher than in the pre-op period. In other words, the highest levels of anxiety and depression are observed in the first week and month post-op, but these levels drop by the end of the first year.

According to the findings from the thesis of Özkan, which was prepared in 1993 to define the effectiveness of the liaison model in patients who underwent mastectomy at the University Hospital of Istanbul, 26.2 % of the patients were found to have depressive disorder in general, and 13.8 % were found to have major depression during the period before mastectomy. After the operation, adaptation difficulties were frequently observed in these cases, especially during the first 6 months [2, 3].

Research has indicated that preoperative experiences and coping methods for breast cancer have postoperative impacts [26]. Previous studies of women's experiences of coping in the period between diagnosis and surgery do not provide an in-depth understanding of their experiences. In addition, most studies of women's coping in the preoperative period have been conducted retrospectively. Retrospective investigations have disadvantages such as recall bias and the repression of unpleasant memories, as well as the fact that the outcome of the surgery may color the memories [6].

Acceptance and humor were negatively correlated with distress, whereas denial and emotional expression were positively correlated with distress after surgery and 3 months later. The relationships between coping patterns and distress were also examined. Specifically, participants who used emotion-focused engagement coping presurgery, i.e., acceptance or emotional expression combined with social support, experienced less distress 3 months later than participants who did not use any emotion-focused engagement coping. Finally, flexibility, defined as the use of multiple coping strategies, was found to negatively predict distress. These results indicate that the presurgical use of emotion-focused engagement coping can be adaptive and that the adaptiveness of each strategy may vary as the stressor evolves [22].

Anxiety in patients treated by surgery was high; thus, surgery was a physical factor that contributed to anxiety. However, there was no unanimous conclusion on whether the type of surgery served as a moderating factor for anxiety in these patients, as shown by the differing conclusions drawn from the included articles. Nevertheless, all of the included articles illustrated that the level of anxiety preoperatively, if present, was higher in the mastectomy group, although some levels were not statistically significant [57].

For women with breast cancer, recurrence anxiety is reported to be the most common form of anxiety. One year after total mastectomy, relapse anxiety is ranked as number one. The intensity declines over the years; however, the anxiety remains. According to the findings of a study conducted in Turkey, a negative correlation

exists between the fear of relapse and the date of surgery. However, according to western sources, in this stage, concerns regarding femininity and sexuality are more emphasized than relapse. As a second important concern, needing someone and being unable to meet their own needs are reported. This type of anxiety was reported by 33 % in the study, whereas according to studies in the East and Far East, the rate is much lower, 10–11 % [65].

Secondary problems such as pain, sensation loss, and arm swelling are common among mastectomy patients, resulting in further disability in daily life. Several studies have found that lymphedema negatively affects psychosocial well-being, although few of these studies report the specific impact on body image. Lymphedema (potentially exacerbated by weight gain and additional treatment, including radiation therapy) could manifest at a later time and may therefore be more likely to affect body image in the long term [66].

Women weigh multiple factors when deciding which surgical treatment is appropriate and should thus be informed of the potential for greater image concerns associated with more radical surgery. For the majority of women who have a choice regarding the type of breast surgery they receive, awareness that body image might be more compromised by mastectomy than by lumpectomy in the months following surgery may be an important part of the decision-making process. Future research evaluating surgical decision-making in young women and associated body image and psychosocial outcomes is clearly warranted, particularly given the increase in bilateral mastectomies in recent years in this population [66].

Related literature involves studies that compare the effects of radical mastectomy and partial mastectomy on body image, psychosocial adjustment, sex life, and recurrence anxiety. The findings indicate that the body image of women who underwent lumpectomy or partial mastectomies was more positive and that the fear of nudity was less prevalent. The effects of different surgical approaches on psychological adjustment and quality of life have also been extensively examined. A recent meta-analysis of 40 investigations examined postsurgical adjustment in women who underwent partial or radical mastectomy. After controlling for unpublished negative findings, body/self-image was the only factor that significantly differed between the treatment groups, with women who underwent partial mastectomy reporting better body/self-image [67]. Yılmazer et al. [68] conducted a study to compare body image, self-esteem, and social support. The women in the partial mastectomy group had more positive body images. The two groups showed a negligible difference with respect to self-esteem and social support. Furthermore, a negative correlation was found between body image and social support.

Al-Ghazal et al. [69] conducted a study about psychological effects and satisfaction depending on different types of surgery and found that mastectomy has negative effects on body image, self-esteem, and marital adjustment. According to a study of approximately 204 women's problems regarding breast cancer, the main problems were feeling discomfort due to changes in the body and having problems in their relationships with spouses [70]. According to a study by Sertöz et al. [71] which was conducted in Turkey with women with breast cancer, mastectomy has negative effects on body image and self-esteem but not on marital adjustment. Studies comparing different types of surgery and breast cancer reported that mastectomy has negative effects on body image [72].

Several studies have reported that women who had breast-conserving surgery continue to report fewer body image concerns compared with women who underwent more radical surgery in a longer follow-up [69, 70, 72]. Other studies, however, have found no differences between surgical groups in the years following treatment [73]. Both mastectomy and breast-conserving surgery are associated with a poorer body image, which may result in depressive symptoms. However, the type of surgery is not associated with the level of depressive symptoms [49].

With the aim of establishing the demographic, medical, and psychological factors associated with the breast cancer patient's decision-making process and of assessing their satisfaction with the type of surgery received, Noyan et al. [74] assessed patients with breast cancer who had only mastectomy and women who had mastectomy and breast reconstruction surgery. The authors reported that in both groups, women with a low income and less education were more likely to experience decision regret or low satisfaction. Moreover, patients who only underwent total mastectomy had lower self-esteem compared with reconstructive surgery patients and healthy women. According to the authors, Turkish breast cancer patients may be more concerned with surviving the dreadful cancer diagnosis than the presentation of their feminine form and may therefore be less likely to be interested in breast reconstruction.

One important assumption derived from earlier studies is that a major contributor to psychopathology is the cancer diagnosis itself. Our clinical experience based on liaison with the breast surgery unit and research findings supports this assumption and shows that the primary factors leading to psychopathology in mastectomy patients are related more to the fears and perceptions regarding the underlying illness (cancer) and less to organ loss [1].

Similarly, findings of the thesis studies conducted at the Psychosocial Oncology Department in Istanbul University indicate that in breast cancer patients who had undergone mastectomy, the main basis for distress was the cancer itself; aesthetic concerns and the effects of cancer on the quality of life were secondary. Thus, patients require more information and psychological support regarding their illnesses. It was found that adjustment to mastectomy lasted approximately 6 months and that marital relationships became stronger after the operation. Findings regarding the effects of cancer on sexual life indicated that in addition to the negative effects of the treatment and surgery, misinformation, fear, depression, guilt, and low self-esteem were found to have a significant negative impact on sexual life [3].

The best approach to patients with breast cancer would be to consider psychosocial aspects and the concerns regarding quality of life when deciding on the type of surgery and postoperative treatment modalities. Preoperative psychological preparation and support reduce post-op medical and behavioral complications and hasten psychosocial adjustment. Psychological preparation facilitates the ability of the patient to cope with the difficulties of surgical intervention. This preparation makes it easier for the patient to accept reality and improves her cooperation. It also encourages the patient to assume responsibility and promotes a sense of being in control of her own life. Pre-op psychological preparation and support should be provided with the general knowledge and training of the surgeon. Getting the patient to express her anxieties and fears, providing emotional support and trust, improving her motivation, and promoting a fighting spirit in her are essential to enable the patient to take responsibility, to have the courage to act, and to ameliorate possible catastrophic conditions. Short-term psychotherapy, relaxation, and stress-coping techniques are among the methods used for this purpose [2].

Postmastectomy Reconstructive Surgery

Breast reconstruction is a common option for women undergoing mastectomy. Breast reconstruction can occur at the time of the mastectomy or can be delayed. Reconstruction is cited as the most commonly performed surgery because women have "the psychological desire to feel 'whole' again" and because surgeons want to "restore self-image and self-confidence and improve quality of life" [75].

As presented above, breast cancer and mastectomy experiences are perceived as threats to life, to the wholeness of the body, and to femininity. Although there is a slight increase in the number of women preferring breast reconstruction in Turkey, the number remains low compared with other western countries [74]. However, the exact percentage is unknown because the data on the rate of breast reconstruction are insufficient.

As indicated above, breast cancer and mastectomy are perceived to be as much a threat to physical integrity and to the sense of femininity as they are to life. In recent years, there has been an increase in the number of women undergoing plastic surgery and breast reconstruction. There are many studies demonstrating the favorable impacts of breast reconstruction on the mental health of women who have undergone mastectomies. This intervention plays a major role in attenuating the sense of loss experienced through surgery, and it improves women's psychological, social, and sexual functionality. It has been reported that post-op plastic and breast reconstruction surgeries improve body image [74].

However, it is difficult to show that the use of prostheses enhances a woman's sexual desire and feelings of attractiveness and sexual satisfaction. It appears that the overall emotional adjustment of women, the satisfaction that they obtain from sexual relations, and the quality of their pre-illness sexual life have a much greater impact on post-op sexual adjustment and satisfaction. Some authors have indicated that chemotherapy and radiotherapy have even greater negative effects on sexual desire [35].

Self-esteem is the sum total of the feelings a person has about herself, the importance that she places on those feelings, the judgments that she makes about herself, and how she values herself. Low self-esteem can undermine a person's body image. A person's contentment with her own body is not simply a physical phenomenon; rather, it is a reflection of her psychology.

The use of prostheses enhances a woman's feeling of wholeness and her quality of life. The positive impacts of this type of surgery are multifold:

- Enhances relationships and social interactions
- Improves body image
- Supports mental health
- Improves self-confidence
- Improves mood and satisfaction with body and social functions

Janz et al. [76] reported that body image is the poorest among women who underwent a mastectomy with reconstructive surgery. Collins et al. [77] found that at 6 months post surgery, women who had undergone reconstruction had worse body images compared with those who only had a mastectomy; however, this difference was no longer apparent 1 year after surgery. In a study by Fobair et al. [78], women who were considering or had already undergone reconstruction had the most body image concerns during the first few months following diagnosis. As the majority of the women included in these prior studies were older than 40, it is important to consider that the divergent findings regarding the impact of reconstruction might reflect differences in body image perceptions in young women versus older women.

Our study aimed to investigate the relationship between body image and psychological problems following mastectomy and the attitudes of Turkish women toward breast reconstruction. It was found that 46.7 % of the cases had high depression scores, that 20 % had high anxiety scores, and that cases with high depression scores had negative body images. Additionally, 23.3 % of the patients were willing to undergo breast reconstruction surgery. For these patients, the psychological effects of breast loss, such as abstention from looking in the mirror, excess mental involvement regarding breast loss, the inability to dress down near a partner, and lessened feelings of femininity and attractiveness, were found to be significant. In patients under 45 years old whose surgeries were performed <2 years prior, the desire to undergo breast reconstruction surgery was high. There were no significant differences between the two groups in terms of depression or anxiety [79].

Adjuvant Therapies

Chemotherapy

The side effects and limitations of adjuvant radiotherapy, chemotherapy, and hormone therapy add to the challenges faced by these women [3]. In general, more complex or toxic treatment regimens are predictors of depressive symptoms. Patients who receive chemotherapy have a higher risk of depressive symptoms, which are associated with the onset of premature menopause, as well as other physical adverse effects of chemotherapy. Some studies indicate that receiving hormonal therapy increases the levels of depressive symptoms, but the results are inconclusive and further research is warranted on this matter [39].

Some studies have suggested that body image may be adversely affected in women undergoing chemotherapy. This is generally attributed to alopecia, a common side effect of many chemotherapeutic regimens [76, 78]. Although chemotherapy itself was not a significant factor, other sequelae often associated with adjuvant treatment were associated with body image, including fatigue, which is consistent with findings from a recent study in which fatigue was negatively correlated with body image [80]. Similarly, weight gain is a well-documented side effect of adjuvant treatment [81]. Although Fobair et al. [78] found that concern with either weight gain or weight loss was associated with poorer body image, most studies in breast cancer survivors have focused exclusively on perceptions of weight gain, which occurs much more commonly than weight loss in this population [82].

Breast cancer treatments potentially confer additional psychiatric risk beyond the risk of depression in a patient with breast cancer. Increased levels of depression are found in perimenopausal patients and in women taking antiestrogen treatments such as tamoxifen; antiestrogens may induce a menopausal state and may contribute to increased levels of depression. Hormonal shifts related to either chemical or surgical menopause may affect mood [83].

Studies identified both age (physical factor) and trait anxiety (psychological factor) as being predictive of anxiety in female patients with breast cancer who were undergoing chemotherapy acutely (when chemotherapy was initiated), chronically (in subsequent chemotherapy infusions), or 2 years after diagnosis, in the form of needle anxiety [84].

In a recently performed systematic review, it was confirmed that anxiety is prevalent in women with breast cancer who are undergoing treatment, especially those being given chemotherapy. Specifically, women of younger age and with higher trait anxiety were more anxious during chemotherapy [57]. Healthcare professionals must thus pay greater attention to younger patients commencing chemotherapy—especially those who exhibit a more anxious personality—and initiate psychiatric help earlier, if necessary.

Central nervous system toxicity caused by chemotherapy or combination radiotherapy and chemotherapy is not fully understood. It can be observed in 3–11 % of cases, depending on whether methotrexate is used. Toxic effects can be observed immediately after the treatment or in the future as cognitive and neurological disorders (changes in consciousness, leukoencephalopathy, seizures, cerebral infarction, paralysis, neuropathy, ototoxicity). The initial responses to steroids are euphoria and irritability. Some other effects are feeling good and increased appetite and weight gain, whereas insomnia, restlessness, hyperactivity, muscle weakness, fatigue, and depression can also be observed. With a sudden increase, decrease, or cessation of the steroid dose, hallucinations or delusions can sometimes be observed. Tamoxifen rarely causes depression or delusional disorder. Most chemotherapy agents can cause depression, hallucinations, or delirium [85]. Patients receiving chemotherapy frequently complain about changes in their cognitive functions. This situation can be designated as chemo brain; some examples of complaints include forgetfulness, drowsiness, and the inability to focus on daily tasks [86].

Fitch et al. [87] interviewed 32 cancer survivors (including 15 breast cancer survivors) who had started chemotherapy within the last 6 months and found that the most common cognitive changes reported were problems with memory, comprehension, and concentration. More recently, Myers [88] interviewed 18 breast cancer survivors who were 6–12 months post-chemotherapy and found that most women reported problems with short-term memory, focusing, word finding, reading, and driving. As part of a larger symptom management survey, Boykoff et al. [89] interviewed breast cancer survivors who were at least 1 year posttreatment and identified cognitive impairment as a side effect of their treatment. Problems with memory, reading, comprehension, and processing speed were described. Cognitive changes in this study were also associated with

significant negative outcomes such as decreased quality of life and ability to work.

Cognitive dysfunction in cancer patients is multifactorial and occurs as a result of the interaction between the cancer, the individual (host) factors such as genetic susceptibility and immune reactivity, and the effect of specific treatments. In addition, the real-life impact of cognitive dysfunction on cancer patients is dependent on their pre-illness level of function, the type of work they do, their developmental stage of life (e.g., working parents with small children vs. retired persons), and their overall ability to manage and cope with changing life circumstances [90].

Radiotherapy

A recent study evaluated changes in depressive symptoms from the initiation of radiotherapy (RT) and for 6 months thereafter and investigated whether specific demographic, clinical, symptomatic, and psychological adjustment characteristics predicted the initial levels and trajectories of depressive symptoms. Approximately one-fourth of patients had clinically meaningful levels of depressive symptoms prior to RT, but the trajectory of depressive symptoms improved over time. Women who had less education, children living at home, a higher level of sleep disturbance, worry about disease outcome, less meaning in life, and less support from family and friends had higher levels of depressive symptoms prior to RT [50].

Consistent with previous research [91, 92], women with breast cancer experience higher levels of depressive symptoms prior to and during RT, and these symptoms then decline following the completion of RT. In a recent review, Stiegelis and colleagues [93] summarized findings from several studies that investigated psychological functioning in cancer patients who received RT. Although the results are inconsistent, depressive symptoms were more common during and at the completion of RT than in the period prior to treatment. In addition, psychological functioning improved following the completion of RT.

Previous longitudinal studies were identified that specifically evaluated depressive symptoms in breast cancer patients who underwent RT [91, 92].

Consistent with the review mentioned above, these studies reported higher levels of depressive symptoms during and immediately after RT, followed by a decrease over time. In addition to understanding the trajectories of depressive symptoms during and after RT, it is important to determine patient characteristics associated with higher levels of depressive symptoms. In addition, younger women with breast cancer often require adjuvant treatment, which results in premature menopause and alterations in sexual functioning [15].

Despite the identification of several risk factors, it is difficult to identify a set of predictors that are consistently linked with depressive symptoms in breast cancer patients because of the predictors' potential associations with specific factors such as the treatment type. Most studies that aim to identify predictors of depressive symptoms are cross-sectional and examine different populations of breast cancer patients [94]. Among the studies of depressive symptoms in breast cancer patients receiving RT [92], several predictors associated with demographic, clinical, and treatment characteristics were evaluated. Except for one study [91] in which fatigue was assessed, none of these studies evaluated the impact of physical symptoms on depressive symptoms. In addition, none of these studies examined the impact of physical functioning (e.g., comorbidities and performance status) on patients' levels of depressive symptoms.

Effects on Body Image

Body image is conceptualized as a multifaceted construct, defined as the mental representation of one's body; thoughts and feelings about one's physical appearance, attractiveness, and competence; and one's perceived state of overall health, wholeness, functioning, and sexuality. Body image is a dynamic interaction between this personal expression of being and the social world [95]. One of the most difficult and often persistent challenges facing breast cancer survivors is coping with the various changes to their physical appearance and function resulting from treatment. Side effects from surgery, chemotherapy, and radiotherapy can be significantly disfiguring,

including deformation and/or loss of the breast(s), visible scarring, skin changes due to radiotherapy, hair loss due to chemotherapy, and lymphedema. The universal experience of breast cancer survivors is one of profound loss of their body's physical integrity and function, perceived femininity, self-esteem, and confidence [78]. These considerable physical and physiological alterations can dramatically affect a woman's body image. For many breast cancer survivors, dissatisfaction with one's "new" body has detrimental influences on many psychosocial domains. Body image disturbance following treatment has been consistently associated with mental distress, anxiety, reduced physical health, sexual dysfunction, and impaired quality of life [96].

Body image is an important component of a cancer patient's quality of life and plays an important role in adjustment to the disease. Women with better body image perceptions had higher levels of self-confidence in coping with breast cancer [97]. On the other hand, poorer body image is associated with poorer self-rated health, chronic fatigue, mental distress, and poorer generic and disease-related quality of life [96]. Therefore, body image is an important component of the quality-of-life assessment, but a review of the literature revealed the lack of a suitable scale to measure body image in cancer patients, particularly in the clinical trial setting.

Satisfaction with the body is not only a physical concept but also a psychological experience. In mastectomy applications, body image is one of the important components of the experienced distress and requirement for further adjustment. The formation of body image is a process that starts in infancy and develops throughout life. Self-esteem, however, is the sum of perceptions of how one feels about herself and about values attributed to the self. Body image is one of the main factors of general self-esteem and personality development. The process of body image development is not only related to the general appearance of one's body but also shaped by cognitive functions and environmental messages. Body image involves a sense of wholeness and functionality. Women who consider body image to be a major part of their sense of self-worth, attractiveness, or wholeness are clearly at an increased risk of poor psychosocial adjustment following breast cancer surgery [3].

The lack of change with regard to body image must be considered and compared with studies that have demonstrated improved body image over time, especially in women who have undergone mastectomy, likely due to increased skills in coping with body image impairment. Women with breast reconstruction (BR) and breast-conserving surgery (BCS) scored no differently on the body concern domain of body image. However, women undergoing BR had a significantly worse score on the body stigma domain of body image than women receiving BCS. Women with BR had a better body image score than women who underwent mastectomy. Women who are satisfied with their body shape may still perceive deficiencies because of the stigma of mastectomy and its effect on body image [98].

Effects on Sexuality

Breast cancer patients also often receive chemotherapy, radiotherapy, hormone therapy, or a combination of these treatments. All of the treatments have varying impacts on sexual functioning [70]. Surgery can impact a patient's body image, which may in turn affect sexual functioning. Women receiving breast-conserving surgery or reconstruction report greater satisfaction with their sex lives compared with women receiving mastectomy [99].

Poor adjustment was related to unsatisfactory or unfavorable sexual experiences, a strong emotional attachment to breasts, body image problems, and difficulty in discussing personal problems. Some women who place great importance on their bodies may not be able to tolerate even the idea of damage to or loss of their breast. The risk of these women having problems in adjustment after treatment is also high. Adjustment also depends on the responses of significant others such as spouses or partners, family, and friends [35].

A sizable proportion of women describe mastectomy as a mutilating and disfiguring experience. Approximately one-fourth of these women describe negative effects on sexual adjustment, including a decreased frequency of intercourse, decreased sexual satisfaction, and more difficulty in achieving an orgasm. Research suggests that although sexual issues may not be a patient's main concerns during treatment, they are still important issues. Although any cancer diagnosis can cause sexual problems, breast cancer is a unique case in that the breast, although not directly a sex organ, is observed as a symbol of femininity and plays a role in pleasure and stimulation. Female sexual functioning disorders can be classified into the following categories: sexual desire, sexual arousal, and orgasmic and sexual pain. Avoidance and noncommunication in sexual relationships were the most frequent sexual dysfunctions observed among breast cancer survivors. Sexual problems can be difficult to diagnose. Many women experience sexual problems as a result of a breast cancer diagnosis and its treatment. They can only be identified if sexual functioning is reported using a patient-reported outcome questionnaire [100].

Fatigue, nausea, and alopecia (i.e., hair loss), side effects from chemotherapy and other agents, are often related to reduced sexual desire [101]. Emotionally, a cancer diagnosis can affect sexuality through associated stress, anxiety, depression, body image changes due to surgical scars or damage to sexual organs or other body parts, and feelings of loss of femininity that can arise due to hormonal therapies. In the interpersonal or social realm, changes in a couple's relationship from equal partners to a patient/caregiver relationship create threats to established sexual roles and sexual interest. Moreover, many couples who avoid sexual activity during treatment may find it more challenging to resume sex once the treatment is completed. Although the whole range of cancer types can impact sexuality, breast cancer has a number of unique consequences because of the status of the breast as a signifier of feminine sexuality and its role as a source of erotic pleasure and stimulation. This suggests that clinicians should be particularly sensitive to the consequences of breast cancer for women's sexuality and body image and to the consequences for the women's partners [102].

Quality of Life

Breast cancer thus profoundly disrupts women's emotional equilibrium and quality of life. Health-related quality of life represents the functional effects of an illness and its treatment on the patients and is thus an important indicator of the psychosocial and psychological burden of the illness.

Improvement in the early detection and treatment of breast cancer has led to longer survival of these patients. Breast cancer also affects women's identities; therefore, studying quality of life in women who lose their breasts is vital. In addition, it is believed that women play an important role in families. When a woman develops breast cancer, all of her family members may develop some sort of illness. Thus, the issue of "survivorship" has now become an important topic in breast cancer care that demands the investigation of the long-term effects of a breast cancer diagnosis and its treatment. The time of diagnosis, the initial stages of an adjuvant treatment course, and the months immediately following the end of adjuvant treatment are transition times associated with poor adjustment and decreased quality of life in breast cancer patients [103]. Studies have shown that decreased health-related quality of life as a result of chemotherapy side effects may predict early treatment discontinuation in patients with breast cancer [104]. However, studies on the posttreatment adjustment of breast cancer survivors demonstrated that breast cancer patients might experience a good quality of life [105].

The major concerns were fatigue, aches and pains, sleep problems, psychological distress from cancer diagnosis and treatment, fear of recurrence, family distress, sexuality issues, family burden, and uncertainty, all of which had a negative impact on overall QoL [106]. Helgeson et al. [107] indicated difficulties in physical functioning in disease-free breast cancer survivors. The results showed that they had a high incidence of symptoms related to depression and trait anxiety, resulting in lower QoL. Certain demographic variables, including being of older age at cancer diagnosis, a longer time lapse since diagnosis, being ethnically non-Hispanic white, being more

educated, and being employed, predicted lower psychosocial distress. The younger age at diagnosis group showed poorer outcomes in the social aspect, with major concerns regarding changes in self-esteem and appearance. Women who received adjuvant systemic therapy had poorer QoL outcomes in the physical, psychosocial, and sexual aspects compared with women who did not receive systemic adjuvant therapy. Women who had a mastectomy reported more physical concerns compared with women who had breast-conserving therapy. Moreover, the presence of breast-related symptoms such as pain, swelling, and numbness resulted in poor QoL [106].

A study conducted by Uzun et al. [108] that included a sample with a significant proportion of Turkish women examined the quality of life of Turkish women with breast cancer. The findings showed that the educational level, employment status, and degree of pain affected the quality of life to varying degrees. According to the authors, these findings have many implications. The authors stated that patient education should focus on factors that affect quality of life and that supportive interventions should be adapted to the needs of illiterate and literate unemployed surgical patients.

A number of studies have investigated improvements in the psychological status, the QoL following the completion of treatment [105], or the QoL among long-term breast cancer survivors. Some studies have reported certain restrictions in the QoL not only by patients in the first 2 years after initial treatment but also by patients with a survival time longer than 5 years at follow-up [109], whereas gradual improvements in well-being have been observed 5 years after diagnosis. It has been argued that most aspects of health-related QoL during breast cancer treatment or its residual effects vary depending on the type of cancer treatment. However, other studies have indicated that the cognitive variables had a more significant effect on QoL and distress than the type of cancer treatment [110]. Although it was assumed that symptom distress was inversely related to QoL, a previous study performed among a Spanish-speaking population found a significant negative effect of psychological distress on the QoL [111]. Several minor studies have specifically concentrated on longitudinal analysis of the QoL over the illness continuum, whereas other studies have shown that psychological distress impaired the QoL over a 6-month treatment period [112]. Psychological adjustment was a significant predictor of better QoL 1 year after the initial diagnosis of breast cancer [113].

Some studies have described long-term impairment of QoL, impaired functioning, and continuing symptoms, as well as a high percentage of distress in breast cancer survivors [114], whereas others have reported an improving QoL over time [115]. Arndt et al. [114] compared breast cancer patients with reference data from the general population. Three years after diagnosis, breast cancer patients had poorer role functioning and poorer emotional, cognitive, and social functioning, as well as more symptoms of insomnia, fatigue, and dyspnea, especially at younger ages.

We found that patients' physical, psychological, social relationships, general quality of life, and perceived health quality of life decrease to the greatest extent immediately after the operation, whereas the scores of other parts, except the social relationship part, increase later after the operation. However, we reported that the first-year scores were lower compared with the pre-operation scores and that patients were under psychological risk beginning at the time of diagnosis [40]. Schou et al. [116] claimed that breast cancer patients' emotional, cognitive, and social functioning is affected beginning at the time of diagnosis and that their cognitive and social functioning slowly recovers.

The impact of breast cancer diagnosis and its treatment on the quality of life of women with breast cancer was examined longitudinally. Although there were deteriorations in patients' scores for body image and sexual functioning, there were significant improvements for breast symptoms, systematic therapy side effects, and patients' future perspectives. The findings suggest that overall, breast cancer patients perceived benefits from their cancer treatment in the long term. However, patients reported problems with global quality of life, pain, arm symptoms, and

body image even 18 months following their treatments. In addition, most of the functional scores did not improve. The results showed that physical functioning was improved 1 year after the completion of breast cancer treatment and later [117]. In our study, patients reported poor social functioning following the completion of breast cancer treatment. Similarly, studies have found that breast cancer survivors suffer from poor social functioning [116].

A 5-year prospective study showed that with the exceptions of body image, sexual functioning, and deterioration in the patient's way of life, the other areas improve over time (within the first 2 years), and there are no fundamental changes observed in the quality-of-life scores in the second, third, and fourth years [72].

Hartl [118] investigated changes in the quality of life (QoL) and body image among breast cancer patients over 2 years and different predictive factors for the QoL 2 years after the primary operation. The overall QoL and most of the functional and symptom scales improved during the 2-year period. The greatest changes in health-related QoL, functioning, and symptoms were observed during the first 6 months. However, cognitive functioning, body image, and the three symptom scales of insomnia, constipation, and diarrhea did not change during the follow-up period. At the time of diagnosis and primary surgery, being confronted with breast cancer as a life-threatening disease has a negative impact on well-being and the QoL. Because most patients are likely to have recovered from the shock of diagnosis, surgery, and hospitalization after 6 months and will have completed radiotherapy and cytotoxic therapy, an improvement in their QoL would be expected. Interestingly, after 12, 18, and 24 months, there were only minor changes in the QoL. The lack of change in cognitive functioning, which is in line with previous studies [116], has been under discussion as a long-lasting neuropsychological effect of chemotherapy.

According to some studies monitoring breast cancer patients' quality of life at different times [72, 115, 118], many aspects of quality of life recover; however, other studies [114] reported that these aspects do not recover in the long term. Studies about this subject generally include the postsurgical treatment period; few studies have evaluated patients' quality of life before the diagnosis.

Risk factors of depression such as fatigue, a past history or recent episode of depression after the onset of breast cancer, and cognitive attitudes of helplessness/hopelessness and resignation might impair the quality of life [49]. During breast cancer diagnosis, the quality of information delivered by doctors and communication about disease concerns and feelings are two important parameters to preserve the quality of life. Many studies have clearly demonstrated that depression and its associated symptoms, such as dysphoria, decrease the quality of life, affect compliance with medical therapies, and reduce survival. This decrease occurs because depression affects interpersonal relationships, occupational performance, stress, and perceptions of health and physical symptoms. Therefore, depression impacts patients' overall quality of life [33, 48]. Two studies [113, 119] found that depression is correlated with lower quality of life. Weitzner et al. [119] studied 60 long-term stage I–III breast cancer survivors (disease-free for 5 years) versus 93 low-risk breast cancer screening patients. In both groups, increased depression is correlated with lower quality of life functioning, except for family functioning.

The quality of life among the breast cancer population requires assessment and subsequent treatment of mood disorders. In a population of 691 older women (>65 years old) with breast cancer, Ganz et al. [113] assessed psychosocial adjustment 15 months after surgery. They showed a decline in mental health scores of the MHI-5 (Mental Health Inventory) and noticed that physical, emotional, and social dimensions impact their quality of life but that cancer-specific psychosocial quality of life improved over time (15 months). The quality of life can be impaired by a number of stressful life events, body image problems, problems with sexual intercourse, financial problems, anxious preoccupations, and, of course, depression. The burden of depression, which has a negative impact, influences the severity and the number of side effects from medical treatment (surgery, chemotherapy, radiotherapy, hormonal therapy) by increasing digestive inconveniences (nausea) and the sense of fatigue and by decreasing cognitive function (difficulty concentrating), all of which can lower the quality of life. However, medical variables such as the tumor stage or sociodemographic data (education, marital status), with the exception of younger age, do not have an adverse impact on the quality of life [120]. Breast cancer treatment can be traumatic for women who can subsequently develop different patterns of depression that might worsen the quality of life [121].

The quality of life and psychological distress during breast cancer treatment were assessed in a longitudinal study. Anxiety symptoms are prevalent at the time of diagnosis, at the beginning of treatment, and in the middle of treatment, whereas women did not report elevated levels of anxiety at the end of treatment. Psychosocial factors were consistently related to the QoL. The women suffering from probable significant distress can be considered as having high anxiety at pretreatment and during treatment, independently of the treatment combination type. This increase in distress could be explained by the uncertainty and fears that patients have during the first stage of cancer treatment. Longitudinal studies can greatly aid in our understanding of the treatment's impact on the patient's quality of life because occasional changes could be identified. Psychosocial adjustment to breast cancer was dependent on the distinct stages of the illness. The efforts to detect a patient's psychological distress at the early stage of treatment may be the key factor to improve their QoL [8].

A study examined coping strategies over time and the reciprocal relationship between coping strategies and the QoL among younger women with breast cancer within 6 months of diagnosis. Positive cognitive restructuring was the most frequently used strategy. Over time, seeking social support, spirituality, and wishful thinking declined, whereas detachment increased. Prior QoL predicted three subsequent coping strategies (seeking social support, keeping feelings to self, wishful thinking). Coping strategies were minimally associated with the subsequent QoL. Coping strategies and the QoL are dynamic processes. The QoL may predict coping strategies as well as or more than vice versa [13]. Numerous studies have shown a relationship between coping strategies and the QoL among women with breast cancer [23, 120, 121]. Better QoL was associated with the use of more active coping strategies [18, 23, 120, 121]. Despite the unique issues and difficulties experienced by younger women with breast cancer, their coping strategies do not appear to differ from those of the group of all female breast cancer patients [23, 24]. In fact, two studies have shown that coping strategies play a more important role than medical or treatment factors in predicting the QoL [120, 121]. Previous cross-sectional findings suggest that women with breast cancer who use strategies such as positive cognitive restructuring (also known as positive reappraisal), acceptance, emotional processing, or emotional expression have better QoL than those who use more passive coping strategies such as avoidance or minimizing the importance of their cancer [18, 23, 120, 121]. Longitudinal studies have shown similar results. In a short-term 4-month longitudinal study of women with breast cancer, the use of avoidant coping strategies was associated with poorer QoL concurrently but not prospectively [23]. Another study of women with breast cancer found that high use of acceptance within 5 months of treatment was related to better QoL 3 months later. This study also found that emotionally expressive coping was associated with improved QoL, but only for those women who perceived their social context as being highly receptive to their discussion of cancer [122].

Breast Cancer Survivorship

Although the incidence of the most commonly diagnosed cancer in women is on the rise worldwide, breast cancer mortality rates have been stable or have decreased over the past 25 years. Better breast screening procedures have led to the earlier detection of breast cancer, and advances in

treatment have also reduced mortality. Europe has geographical variation regarding countries' performance in managing cancer. These differences might be related to the evolving organization of healthcare systems and cultures. Breast cancer is one of the most prevalent tumors in women but also constitutes the largest group of cancer survivors [15]. Despite the increasing 5-year survival rate, survivors remain at high risk for developing psychological problems [123].

We found that the most common symptoms affecting breast cancer survivors were fatigue, insomnia, depression, cognitive dysfunction, reproductive and menopausal symptoms, and lymphedema. Some of these symptoms have even been the objective of randomized controlled trials, but consistent data are missing [124].

Depression substantially impairs the QoL and is associated with poorer adherence to medical regimens. Furthermore, depression may be associated with the progression of cancer or with decreased survival [123]. Dalton et al. [125] have observed an elevated risk of first hospitalization for depression for up to 10 years after breast cancer diagnosis. Furthermore, breast cancer survivors may still experience some specific problems such as lymphedema and sexual dysfunction [101].

The psychological and social problems for cancer survivors include depression, anxiety, distress, fear of recurrence, and impacts on social support/function, family and relationships, and the quality of life. A substantial minority of people surviving cancer experience depression, anxiety, distress, or fear associated with recurrence or follow-up. Receiving treatment for the disease, self-monitoring the symptoms and signs of the disease, attending control appointments, and awaiting laboratory results led people to repeatedly experience the same emotions, including fear and uncertainty. There is some indication that social support is positively associated with better outcomes. The quality of life for cancer survivors appears generally good for most people, but an important minority experiences a reduction in the quality of life, especially those with more advanced disease and reduced social and economic resources. The majority of research knowledge is based on women with breast cancer [126].

One psychosocial factor that is believed to influence body image is the gender role socialization of "standards" regarding physical appearance and behavior. Direct and indirect communications from various influential sources (media, family, and friends/peers) indoctrinate and more importantly, reinforce present-day cultural normative ideals of attractiveness and the roles that women are encouraged to adopt to gain societal approval. Research has shown that an important influential factor is not the bombardment of media messages per se but rather the extent that an individual internalizes the societal ideals, which then become part of one's self-concept [127]. The impact of gender role socialization on body image disturbances in breast cancer survivors, particularly with respect to adjusting and integrating a "new" body and to changed self-identity and role functioning, has yet to be elucidated.

Women with breast cancer who were more invested in their physical appearance exhibited greater difficulty adjusting after treatment and reported more body dissatisfaction and poorer mental health than those who were less invested [128].

Findings indicate that survivors who demonstrated greater internalization of gender role beliefs, engaged in greater self-surveillance, and reported greater levels of body shame showed greater body image disturbance post treatment. Greater body image disturbance was also significantly associated with poorer quality of life. Increasing awareness of cultural forces shaping gender role expectations and behaviors may be an important element in psychosocial interventions for breast cancer. Psychosocial interventions that help women redefine personal standards of beauty, femininity, and role functioning that are realistic, achievable, and less focused on societal expectations might facilitate flexibility in perceptions and diminish potential negative self-evaluation after treatment, thus promoting adjustment and survivor well-being [95].

The majority of studies show a significant relationship between psychosocial factors and survival, but the actual psychosocial variables related to survival are not consistently measured across studies, and the associations of many of the psychosocial variables with survival/recurrence are not consistent across studies. In particular, more research is likely warranted regarding the role of social support, marriage, minimizing, denial, depression, and emotional constraint on breast cancer survival. Adequately powered multicenter studies using valid assessment tools and meta-analytical approaches may be necessary to show the potential roles of various psychosocial factors in breast cancer outcomes.

Posttraumatic Growth

The adjustment to cancer is not always negative. A healthy adjustment without psychological morbidity may combine with an active psychosocial process to facilitate personal growth [8].

Regarding the effect of cancer on the perception of life, Öner et al. [129] reported optimistic findings. In the study, 80 % of the cases reported that cancer had a great impact on their lives, and 48 % evaluated the impact as a positive, life-enhancing experience. Patients reported that experiencing cancer has been a power forcing them to see their lives more positively, giving them a chance to restructure their lives and to change their perspective toward people and the world.

The authors reviewed 24 studies published from 1990 to 2010 that measured posttraumatic stress disorder and posttraumatic growth in women with breast cancer in terms of frequency rates, factors associated with posttraumatic stress disorder and posttraumatic growth, and their interrelationships. A relatively small percentage of women experienced posttraumatic stress disorder, whereas the majority reported posttraumatic growth. Age, education, economic status, subjective appraisal of the threat of the disease, treatment, support from significant others, and positive coping strategies were among the most frequently reported factors associated with these phenomena [130].

Breast cancer, due to its severity and traumatic nature, can shatter the patient's core assumptions about the world, and in struggling to rebuild them, he or she may experience positive changes within five aspects (personal strength, new possibilities, relating to others, appreciation of life, and spiritual changes), which constitute PTG [131]. Thus, breast cancer may also be a cathartic and transformative experience for the individual. Clearly, PTG and PTSD represent two different outcomes of the breast cancer experience that have some common parameters, indicating that a relationship exists between them. First, both PTG and PTSD proportionally increase to the level of the perceived threat from the experience. Second, both result from the cognitive struggle of the individual to reconcile the shock from breast cancer diagnosis and treatment with core beliefs about life, justice, and the world. Furthermore, both depend on time passing; according to the stress evaporation theory [132], PTSD diminishes over time, whereas Tedeschi and Calhoun [131] have stated that PTG appears in the weeks, months, or years after trauma. Finally, both PTG and PTSD are connected to social support. According to the social cognitive processing model [133], the existence of an unsupportive social network raises the likelihood of PTSD and simultaneously does not allow growth to occur.

Regardless of their design, studies have concluded that a majority of patients with breast cancer experienced PTG after their diagnosis. For example, in the study by Sears et al. [134] 83 % of breast cancer survivors experienced positive changes after their disease, whereas Weiss [135] found that 98 % of patients reported PTG.

The thesis of Bayraktar (2008) was conducted at our department and was titled "Post traumatic growth in cancer patients and related factors." The main aim of this study was to address positive transformations that occur after the diagnosis and the experience of cancer in a set period of time. Half of the patients were breast cancer patients. Sociodemographic and illness-related factors and the impact of coping and illness perceptions on posttraumatic growth were evaluated. The results showed that cancer patients in this sample have higher posttraumatic growth levels compared with the mean. The time since diagnosis and the sufficiency of information

regarding the illness and treatment variables are correlated with posttraumatic growth. The results for posttraumatic growth and coping revealed a relationship between posttraumatic growth and confrontive coping, self-controlling, accepting responsibility, escape-avoidance, intentional problem solving, positive reappraisal, and seeking social support. The ways of coping and perceptions of illness were important variables affecting posttraumatic growth.

Parry and Chesler [136] intended to explain the possible positive psychosocial consequences of cancer such as development in their qualitative study. The results showed that coping processes and creating meaning and spiritual-moral development are especially associated with long-term psychosocial well-being.

Principles of Medical Psychotherapy

Psychological treatment undertakings in cancer are systematic efforts that are intended to develop behaviors to cope with cancer via consultancy, training, or psychotherapeutic methods. The main goal of these efforts is to raise morale, increase self-confidence and coping abilities, and decrease distress and mental problems. The principal targets in these undertakings are developing the individual's sense of control as she struggles with a disease; enabling her to bring practical solutions to the problems she faces; ensuring that her emotions and reactions such as anger, rage, and guilt are freely expressed; encouraging her to voice her thoughts about the disease; improving her quality of life by providing psychological and social adaptation; and strengthening her interactions with her family and with others [2].

General Approaches in Psychotherapy

It is essential to encourage the patient to express her feelings about the disease; to support the patient and provide her with security regarding the disease; to reveal the factors that affect her responses by discovering connections between her past and current states; to shed light on emotions, behaviors, and defenses by psychodynamic methods; to examine methods for coping with the uncertainty of the future and existence; and to inquire about sources of distress outside of the disease. Furthermore, investigating the effect of the disease on the family members might encourage the sharing of emotions by bringing the patient and her family together.

A therapist who works in this field must prioritize knowing the medical condition of the patient, evaluating the progression of the disease, and explaining the complications and side effects regarding the medical condition and its treatment to the patient. Understanding psychological problems begins with comprehending how the patient perceives her condition and disease. It is essential to inform the patient without causing her to lose hope, to ensure that she goes through a realistic acceptance process, to explain the treatment possibilities and options to her, and to correct her wrong attitudes and knowledge. The possible catastrophic interpretations that a patient may have must be rectified. The therapist must examine the psychological dynamics of the patient, interpret her defense mechanisms, and aid her in developing more effective positive defense mechanisms. The therapist must also encourage the patient to express her normal psychological and emotional reactions. During periods in which feelings of anxiety and desperation are at their highest, the therapist should apply crisis intervention treatment. It would also help to discuss the patient's current daily problems and to evaluate sources of anxiety regarding family, work, and social environment. In patients who are going through the terminal period, the main subjective experiences of these patients must be discussed, and the focus points in their lives must be addressed during therapy. Bringing together patients who have similar diseases and problems would doubtlessly help the patients to develop empathy. The state of being in a group decreases the feeling of loneliness and facilitates the development of positive defense mechanisms [2].

Psychological Treatment

After the patient has been evaluated, interventions that are in accordance with the aims specified below are planned and applied. The aims of psychological treatment can be summarized as follows:

- Correcting and decreasing psychic morbidity
- Decreasing psychological pain
- Improving the quality of life by providing the patient with psychological and social adaptations
- Resolving psychiatric symptoms such as anxiety, depression, and catastrophic reactions
- Enhancing the fighting spirit and will to live and strengthening the mental-behavioral adaptation to cancer
- Developing and increasing the patient's feeling that she has control over her disease and life and ensuring active participation of the patient in the cancer treatment
- Ensuring that the patient can cope with physical and psychological problems regarding cancer, helping the patient develop effective methods and approaches
- Encouraging the patient to freely express emotions and reactions such as rage, anger, and guilt and to voice her thoughts on the disease
- Enhancing communication between the patient and her family and enhancing other elements of social interaction
- Examining the ways of coping with the uncertainty regarding the future and existence

The interpretations, perceptions, and evaluations of the patient as an individual are crucial elements in her emotional and behavioral reactions. When the cancer is perceived as a loss of physical strength, role, expectations, and future, the patient will have a depressive reaction. When it is perceived as a threat to life, independence, and autonomy, anxiety and panic disorders are more prevalent. If the patient perceives her disease as an injustice and a consequence of other people's faults, anger and rage come to the forefront. From a medical perspective, the disease is a biomedical and pathophysiological fact.

However, for the patient, it goes beyond that and becomes a (bio)psychosocial condition with mental, familial, social, and psychosexual meaning and significance.

The psychiatrist must be in close contact with the specialist who treats the patient to facilitate information exchange and cooperation. We can summarize the methods pertaining to the constituents of this treatment process as follows:

- Biopsychosocial formulation
- Reduction and treatment of symptoms
- Free expression of emotions
- Identification of problem areas
- Examination of perceptual scope
- Examination of wrong, negative, and automatic thoughts, attitudes, views, and interpretations within the perceptual scope
- Informing the patient
- Correction of the cognitive style that causes adjustment disorders and emotional reactions
- Ensuring natural, daily maintenance of life
- Examination of automatic thoughts and cognitive coping methods and reconstruction of perceptual style
- Conducting appropriate and indicated behavior techniques
- Ensuring family communication
- Encouraging new areas of interest and investment
- Improving the quality of life [1, 2].

To care for breast cancer patients with depressive disorders, pharmacological treatment must be combined with psychosocial interventions. Psychosocial interventions improve the well-being of cancer patients by decreasing emotional distress and depression in women diagnosed with breast cancer but do not necessarily impact survival [137]. Many psychotherapeutic interventions for this particular population can be implemented such as individual psychosocial support, adjuvant psychological therapy, cancer support groups, online support for adjuvant psychological treatment, and cognitive-behavioral stress management intervention. All of these psychosocial interventions can be used to treat depression and can also improve the range of coping strategies and, therefore, the quality of life.

Conclusion

A biopsychosocial approach and integrated treatment for cancer patients is very important. A multidisciplinary team and interdisciplinary approach is required for the optimal care of breast cancer patients. The periods of diagnosis, treatment, and recurrence of breast cancer represent a high burden and are highly distressful for the patients. Psychological distress and depression affect the quality of life of the patients, the progression of the disease, and the response to treatment. Thus, the management of distress is one of the vital issues in survivorship.

References

1. Özkan S. Psikiyatrik tıp: Konsültasyon liyezon psikiyatrisi. İstanbul: Roche, İÜ Basimevi; 1993.
2. Özkan S. Meme kanserli hastaya psikolojik yaklaşım, yaşam kalitesi. In: Topuz E, Aydıner A, Dinçer Mİ, editors. Meme kanseri. İstanbul: Nobel Tip Kitapevleri; 2003. p. 681–90.
3. Özkan S, Özkan M, Armay Z. The burden of mastectomy. In: Preedy VR, Watson RR, editors. Handbook of disease burdens and quality of life measures. New York: Springer; 2010.
4. Hamzaoglu O, Ozcan U. Health statistics for Turkey. Turk Med Assoc Publ. 2006;1:60–1.
5. Ozmen V. Breast cancer in the world and Turkey. J Breast Health. 2008;4:1–4.
6. Drageset S, Lindstrøm TC, Underlid K. Coping with breast cancer: between diagnosis and surgery. J Adv Nurs. 2010;66(1):149–58.
7. Brennan J. Adjustment to cancer–coping or personal transition? Psychooncology. 2001;10:1–18.
8. Costa-Requena G, Rodríguez A, Fernández-Ortega P. Longitudinal assessment of distress and quality of life in the early stages of breast cancer treatment. Scand J Caring Sci. 2013;27(1):77–83.
9. Lazarus RS, Folkman S. Transactional theory and research on emotions and coping. Eur J Personal. 1987;1(3):141–69.
10. Hobfoll SE. Conservation of resources—a new attempt at conceptualizing stress. Am Psychol. 1989;44(3):513–24.
11. Bandura A. Self-efficacy: the exercise of control. New York: Freeman; 1997.
12. Ozkan S, Alcalar N. Psychological reactions to the surgical treatment of breast cancer. J Breast Health. 2009;5:60–4.
13. Danhauer SC, Crawford SL, Farmer DF, Avis NE. A longitudinal investigation of coping strategies and quality of life among younger women with breast cancer. J Behav Med. 2009;32(4):371–9.

14. Avis NE, Deimling GT. Cancer survivorship and aging. Cancer. 2008;15:3519–29.
15. Mosher CE, Danoff-Burg S. A review of age differences in psychological adjustment to breast cancer. J Psychosoc Oncol. 2005;23:101–14.
16. Arndt V, Merx H, Sturmer T, Stegmaier C, Ziegler H, Brenner H. Age-specific detriments to quality of life among breast cancer patients one year after diagnosis. Eur J Cancer. 2004;40:673–80.
17. Broeckel JA, Jacobsen PB, Balducci L, Horton J, Lyman GH. Quality of life after adjuvant chemotherapy for breast cancer. Breast Cancer Res Treat. 2000;62(2):141–50.
18. Lazarus RS, Folkman S. Stress, appraisal, and coping. New York: Springer; 1984.
19. Greer S, Watson M. Mental adjustment to cancer: its measurement and prognostic importance. Cancer Surv. 1987;6(3):439–53.
20. Barez M, Blasco T, Fernandez-Castro J, Viladrich C. Perceived control and psychological distress in women with breast cancer: a longitudinal study. J Behav Med. 2009;32(2):187–96.
21. Hack TF, Degner LF. Coping responses following breast cancer diagnosis predict psychological adjustment three years later. Psychooncology. 2004;13:235–47.
22. Roussi P, Krikeli V, Hatzidimitriou C, Koutri I. Patterns of coping, flexibility in coping and psychological distress in women diagnosed with breast cancer. Cogn Ther Res. 2007;31:97–109.
23. McCaul KD, Sandgren AK, King B, O'Donnell S, Branstetter A, Foreman G. Coping and adjustment to breast cancer. Psycho-Oncology. 1999;8:230–6.
24. Carver CS, Pozo C, Harris SD, Noriega V, Scheier MF, Robinson DS, et al. How coping mediates the effect of optimism on distress: a study of women with early stage breast cancer. J Pers Soc Psychol. 1993;65:375–90.
25. Heim E, Valach L, Schaffner L. Coping and psychosocial adaptation: longitudinal effects over time and stages in breast cancer. Psychosom Med. 1997;59:408–18.
26. Stanton AL, Danoff-Burg S, Huggins ME. The first year after breast cancer diagnosis: hope and coping strategies as predictors of adjustment. Psycho-Oncology. 2002;11(2):93–102.
27. Garssen B, Goodkin K. On the role of immunological factors as mediators between psychosocial factors and cancer progression. Psychiatry Res. 1999;85:51–61.
28. Nausheen B, Gidron Y, Peveler R, Moss-Morris R. Social support and cancer progression: a systematic review. J Psychosom Res. 2009;67(5):403–15.
29. Liao MN, Chen MF, Chen SC, Chen PL. Healthcare and support needs of women with suspected breast cancer. J Adv Nurs. 2007;60(3):289–98.
30. Friedman LC, Baer PE, Nelson DV, Lane M, Smith FE, Dworkin RJ. Women with breast cancer: perception of family functioning and adjustment to illness. Psychosom Med. 1988;50:529–40.
31. Baider L, Andritsch E, Goldzweig G. Changes in psychological distress of women with breast cancer in long-term remission and their husbands. Psychosomatics. 2004;45:58–68.
32. Hocaoğlu Ç, Kandemir G, Civil F. Meme kanserinin aile ilişkilerine etkileri. Meme Sağlığı Derg. 2007;3(3):163–6.
33. Rustoen T, Begnum S. Quality of life in women with breast cancer. Cancer Nurs. 2000;23(6):416–21.
34. Kissane DW, Clarke DM, Ikin J, Bloch S, Smith GC, Vitetta L, McKenzie DP. Psychooncological morbidity and quality of life in Australian women with early stage breast cancer: a cross sectional survey. Med J Aust. 1998;169:192–6.
35. Rowland JH, Massie MJ. Breast cancer. In: Holland JC, editor. Psycho-oncology. New York: Oxford University Press; 1998.
36. Hegel MT, Moore CP, Collins ED, Kearing S, Gillock KL, Riggs RL, et al. Distress, psychiatric syndromes and impairment of function in women with newly diagnosed breast cancer. Cancer. 2006;107(12):2924–31.
37. Burgess C, Cornelius V, Love S, Graham J, Richards M, Ramirez A. Depression and anxiety in women with early breast cancer; five year observational cohort study. Br Med J. 2005;330:702–6.
38. Loscalzo M, Clarl KL. Problem-related distress in cancer patients drives requests for help: a prospective study. Oncology (Williston Park). 2007;21(9):1133–8.
39. Weinberger T, Forrester A, Markov D, Chism K, Kunkel EJ. Women at a dangerous intersection:diagnosis and treatment of depression and related disorders in patients with breast cancer. Psychiatr Clin N Am. 2010;33(2):409–22.
40. Kocaman Yıldırım N, Özkan M, Özkan S, Özçınar B, Güler SA, Özmen V. Meme kanserli hastaların tedavi öncesi ve sonrası anksiyete, depresyon ve yaşam kalitesi: Bir yıllık prospektif değerlendirme sonuçları. Arch Neuropsychiatr. 2009;46(4):175–81.
41. Vahdaninia M, Omidvari S, Montazeri A. What do predict anxiety and depression in breast cancer patients? A follow-up study. Soc Psychiatry Psychiatr Epidemiol. 2010;45(3):355–61.
42. Gallagher J, Parle M, Cairns D. Appraisal and psychological distress six months after diagnosis of breast cancer. Br J Health Psychol. 2002;7:365–76.
43. Morasso G, Costantini M, Viterbori P, Bonci F, Del Mastro L, Musso M, et al. Predicting mood disorders in breast cancer patients. Eur J Cancer. 2001;37:216–23.
44. Ganz PA, Rowland JH, Desmond K, Meyerowitz BE, Wyatt GE. Life after breast cancer: understanding women's health-related quality of life and sexual functioning. J Clin Oncol. 1998;16(2):501–14.
45. Massie MJ. Prevalence of depression in patients with cancer. J Natl Cancer Instgr. 2004;32:57–71.
46. Kathol RG, Mutgi A, Williams J, Clamon G, Noyes Jr R. Diagnosis of major depression in cancer patients according to four sets of criteria. Am J Psychiatry. 1990;147:1021–4.
47. Massie MJ, Holland JC. Depression and the cancer patient. J Clin Psychiatry. 1990;51(7):12–7.

48. Somerset W, Stout SC, Miller AH. Breast cancer and depression. Oncology (Williston Park). 2004;18(8):1021–34.

49. Reich M, Lesur A, Perdrizet-Chevallier C. Depression, quality of life and breast cancer: a review of the literature. Breast Cancer Res Treat. 2008;110(1):9–17.

50. Lindviksmoen G, Hofsø K, Paul SM, Miaskowski C, Rustøen T. Predictors of initial levels and trajectories of depressive symptoms in women with breast cancer undergoing radiation therapy. Cancer Nurs. 2012;36(6):34–43.

51. Alcalar N, Ozkan S, Kucucuk S, Aslay I, Ozkan M. Association of coping style, cognitive errors and cancer-related variables with depression in women treated for breast cancer. Jpn J Clin Oncol. 2012;42(10):940–7.

52. Oflaz S, Anuk D, Kocaman Yıldırım N, Yaci Ö, Sen F, Güveli M, Özkan S. The relationship between the illness perception and depression in patients with breast cancer. Psycho-Oncology. 2011;20(2):246.

53. Watson M, Haviland JS, Greer S, Davidson J, Bliss JM. Influence of psychological response on survival in breast cancer: a population-based cohort study. Lancet. 1999;354:1331–6.

54. Hjerl K, Andersen EW, Keiding N, Mouridsen HT, Mortensen PB, Jorgensen T. Depression as a prognostic factor for breast cancer mortality. Psychosomatics. 2003;44(1):24–30.

55. Schairer C, Brown LM, Chen BE, Howard R, Lynch CF, Hall P, et al. Suicide after breast cancer: an international population-based study of 723,810 women. J Natl Cancer Inst. 2006;98(19):1416–9.

56. Breitbart W. Suicide risk and pain in cancer and AIDS patient. In: Chapman CR, Foley KM, editors. Current and emerging issues in cancer pain: research and practice. New York: Raven; 1993.

57. Lim CC, Devi MK, Ang E. Anxiety in women with breast cancer undergoing treatment: a systematic review. Int J Evid Based Healthc. 2011;9(3):215–35.

58. Noyes JR, Holt CS, Massie MJ. Anxiety disorders. In: Holland JC, editor. Psycho-oncology. New York: Oxford University Press; 1998.

59. McGregor BA, Antoni MH. Psychological intervention and health outcomes among women treated for breast cancer: a review of stress pathways and biological mediators. Brain Behav Immun. 2009;23:159–66.

60. Schwarz R, Krauss O, Höckel M, Meyer A, Zenger M, Hinz A. The course of anxiety and depression in patients with breast cancer and gynaecological cancer. Breast Care (Basel). 2008;3:417–22.

61. Schreier AM, Williams SA. Anxiety and quality of life of women who receive radiation or chemotherapy for breast cancer. Oncol Nurs Forum. 2004;31:127–30.

62. Mehnert A, Koch U. Prevalence of acute and post-traumatic stress disorder and comorbid mental disorders in breast cancer patients during primary cancer care: a prospective study. Psycho-Oncology. 2007;16:181–8.

63. Jacobsen PB, Widows MR, Hann DM, Andrykowski MA, Kronish LE, Fields KK. Posttraumatic stress disorder symptoms after bone marrow transplantation for breast cancer. Psychosom Med. 1998;60:366–71.

64. Tokgöz G, Yaluğ İ, Özdemir S, Yazıcı A, Uygun K, Aker T. Kanserli hastalarda travma sonrası stres bozukluğunun yaygınlığı ve ruhsal gelişim. Yeni Symp. 1998;46:51–61.

65. Özkan S, Turgay M. Mastektomi olgularında psikiyatrik morbidite psikoosyal uyum ve kanser-organ kaybı-psikopatoloji ilişkisi. Nöro Psikiyatri Arşivi. 1992;29(4):207–15.

66. Rosenberg SM, Tamimi RM, Gelber S, Ruddy KJ, Kereakoglow S, Borges VF, et al. Body image in recently diagnosed young women with early breast cancer. Psychooncology. 2013;22(8):1849–55.

67. Cohen L, Hack TF, de Moor C, Katz J, Goss PE. The effects of type of surgery and time on psychological adjustment in women after breast cancer treatment. Ann Surg Oncol. 2000;7(6):427–34.

68. Yılmazer N, Aydıner A, Özkan S, Aslay I, Bilge N. A comparison of body image, self-esteem and social support in total mastectomy and breast-conserving therapy in Turkish women. Support Care Cancer. 1994;2(4):238–41.

69. Al-Ghazal SK, Fallowfield L, Blamey RW. Comparison of psychological aspects and patient satisfaction following breast conserving surgery, simple mastectomy and breast reconstruction. Eur J Cancer. 2000;36(15):1938–43.

70. Avıs N, Crawford S, Manuel J. Psychosocial problems among younger women with breast cancer. Psycho-Oncology. 2004;13(5):295–308.

71. Sertöz O, Elbi HM, Noyan A, Alper M, Kapkac M. Effects of surgery type on body image, sexuality, self-esteem, and marital adjustment in breast cancer: a controlled study. Türk Psikiyatri Derg. 2004;15(4):264–75.

72. Engel J, Kerr J, Schlesinger-Raab A, Sauer H, Holzel D. Quality of life following breast-conserving therapy or mastectomy: results of a 5-year prospective study. Breast J. 2004;10(3):223–31.

73. Schover LR, Yetman RJ, Tuason LJ, Meisler E, Esselstyn CB, Hermann RE, et al. Partial mastectomy and breast reconstruction. A comparison of their effects on psychosocial adjustment, body image, and sexuality. Cancer. 1995;75:54–64.

74. Noyan A, Sertöz OO, Elbi H, Kayar R, Yılmaz R. Variables affecting patient satisfaction in breast surgery: a cross-sectional sample of Turkish women with breast cancer. Int J Psychiatry Med. 2006;36(3):299–313.

75. Clugston P, Warren R. Reconstructive surgery. In: Glegg C, editor. Intelligent patient guide to breast cancer: all you need to know to take an active part in your treatment. 3rd ed. Vancouver: Gordon Soules Book Publishers Ltd; 2001. p. 232–43.

76. Janz NK, Mujahid M, Lantz PM, Fagerlin A, Salem B, Morrow M, et al. Population-based study of the relationship of treatment and sociodemographics on

quality of life for early stage breast cancer. Qual Life Res. 2005;14:1467–79.

77. Collins KK, Liu Y, Schootman M, et al. Effects of breast cancer surgery and surgical side effects on body image over time. Breast Cancer Res Treat. 2011;126:167–76.

78. Fobair P, Stewart SL, Chang S, D'Onofrio C, Banks PJ, Bloom JR. Body image and sexual problems in young women with breast cancer. Psycho-Oncology. 2006;15:579–94.

79. Özkan M, Anuk D, Özkan S, Kurul S. Anxiety, depression and body image in women following mastectomy and attitude towards breast reconstructions. The 6th Annual Scientific Meeting of the European Association of Consultation and Liaison Psychiatry and Psychosomatics (EACLPP) Abstract Book, Zaragosa. 2003. p. 19.

80. Cantarero-Villanueva I, Fernandez-Lao C, Fernandez DEL-PC. Associations among musculoskeletal impairments, depression, body image and fatigue in breast cancer survivors within the first year after treatment. Eur J Cancer Care. 2011;20(5):632–9.

81. Helms R, O'Hea EL, Corso M. Body image issues in women with breast cancer. Psychol Health Med. 2008;13:313–25.

82. Howard-Anderson J, Ganz PA, Bower JE, Stanton AL. Quality of life, fertility concerns, and behavioral health outcomes in younger breast cancer survivors: a systematic review. J Natl Cancer Inst. 2012;5:386–405.

83. Navari RM, Brenner MC, Wilson MN. Treatment of depressive symptoms in patients with early stage breast cancer undergoing adjuvant therapy. Breast Cancer Res Treat. 2008;112:197–201.

84. Cox AC, Fallowfield LJ. After going through chemotherapy. I can't see another needle. Eur J Oncol Nurs. 2007;11:43–8.

85. Twombly R. Decades after cancer, suicide risk remains high. J Natl Cancer Inst. 2006;98:1356–8.

86. Hess LM, Insel KC. Chemotherapy-related change in cognitive function: a conceptual model. Oncol Nurs Forum. 2007;34:981–94.

87. Fitch MI, Armstrong J, Tsang S. Patients' experiences with cognitive changes after chemotherapy. Can Oncol Nurs J. 2008;18(4):180–92.

88. Myers JS. Chemotherapy-related cognitive impairment: the breast cancer experience. Oncol Nurs Forum. 2012;39(1):31–40.

89. Boykoff N, Moieni M, Subramanian SK. Confronting chemobrain: an in-depth look at survivors' reports of impact on work, social networks, and health care response. J Cancer Survivorship. 2009;3(4):223–32.

90. Meyers CA. Cognitive complaints after breast cancer treatments: patient report and objective evidence. J Natl Cancer Inst. 2013;105(11):761–2.

91. Noal S, Levy C, Hardouin A, Rieux C, Heutte N, Ségura C, et al. One-year longitudinal study of fatigue, cognitive functions, and quality of life after adjuvant radiotherapy for breast cancer. Int J Radiat Oncol Biol Phys. 2011;81(3):795–803.

92. Hopwood P, Sumo G, Mills J, Haviland J, Bliss JM. The course of anxiety and depression over 5 years of follow-up and risk factors in women with early breast cancer: results from the UK Standardisation of Radiotherapy Trials (START). Breast. 2010;19(2):84–91.

93. Stiegelis HE, Ranchor AV, Sanderman R. Psychological functioning in cancer patients treated with radiotherapy. Patient Educ Couns. 2004;52(2):131–41.

94. Bardwell WA, Natarajan L, Dimsdale JE, Rock CL, Mortimer JE, Hollenbach K, et al. Objective cancer-related variables are not associated with depressive symptoms in women treated for early-stage breast cancer. J Clin Oncol. 2006;24(16):2420–7.

95. Boquiren VM, Esplen MJ, Wong J, Toner B, Warner E. Exploring the influence of gender role socialization and objectified body consciousness on body image disturbance in breast cancer survivors. Psychooncology. 2013;22(10):2177–85.

96. Falk Dahl CA, Reinertsen KV, Nesvold IL, Fosså SD, Dahl AA. A study of body image in long-term breast cancer survivors. Cancer. 2010;116:3549–57.

97. Khang D, Rim HD, Woo J. The korean version of the body image scale-reliability and validity in a sample of breast cancer patients. Psychiatry Investig. 2013;10(1):26–33.

98. Fang SY, Shu BC, Chang YJ. The effect of breast reconstruction surgery on body image among women after mastectomy: a meta-analysis. Breast Cancer Res Treat. 2013;137(1):13–21.

99. Markopoulos C, Tsaroucha AK, Kouskos E, Mantas D, Antonopoulou Z, Karvelis S. Impact of breast cancer surgery on the self-esteem and sexual life of female patients. J Int Med Res. 2009;37:182–8.

100. Taylor S, Harley C, Ziegler L, Brown J, Velikova G. Interventions for sexual problems following treatment for breast cancer: a systematic review. Breast Cancer Res Treat. 2011;130(3):711–24.

101. Alder J, Zanetti R, Wight E, Urech C, Fink N, Bitzer J. Sexual dysfunction after premenopausal stage I and II breast cancer: do androgens play a role? J Sex Med. 2008;5(8):1898–906.

102. Emilee G, Ussher JM, Perz J. Sexuality after breast cancer: a review. Maturitas. 2010;66:397–407.

103. Schnipper HH. Life after breast cancer. J Clin Oncol. 2001;19:3581–4.

104. Richardson LC, Wang W, Hartzema AG, Wagner S. The role of health-related quality of life in early discontinuation of chemotherapy for breast cancer. Breast J. 2007;13:581–7.

105. Costanzo ES, Lutgendorf SK, Mattes ML, Trehan S, Robinson CB, Tewfik F, Roman SL. Adjusting to life after treatment: distress and quality of life following treatment for breast cancer. Br J Cancer. 2007;97:1625–31.

106. Chopra I, Kamal KM. A systematic review of quality of life instruments in long-term breast cancer survivors. Health Qual Life Outcomes. 2012;10:14.

107. Helgeson VS, Tomich PL. Surviving cancer: a comparison of 5-year disease-free breast cancer survivors with healthy women. Psychooncology. 2005;14:307–17.

108. Uzun Ö, Aslan FE, Selimen D, Koç M. Quality of life in women with breast cancer in Turkey. J Nurs Scholarsh. 2004;36(3):207–14.

109. Holzner B, Kemmler G, Kopp M, Moschen R, Schweigkofler H, Du¨ nser M, Margreiter R, Fleischhacker WW, Sperner-Unterweger B. Quality of life in breast cancer patients-not enough attention for long-term survivors? Psychosomatics. 2001;42:117–23.

110. Hack TF, Pickles T, Ruether JD, Weir L, Bultz BD, Mackey J, Degner LF. Predictors of distress and quality of life in patients undergoing cancer therapy: impact of treatment type and decisional role. Psychooncology. 2010;19:606–16.

111. Dapueto JJ, Servente L, Francolino C, Hahn EA. Determinants of quality of life in patients with cancer. Cancer. 2005;103:1072–81.

112. Wong WS, Fielding R. Change in quality of life in Chinese women with breast cancer: changes in psychological distress as a predictor. Support Care Cancer. 2007;15:1223–30.

113. Ganz PA, Guadagnoli E, Landrum MB, Lash TL, Rakowski W, Silliman RA. Breast cancer in older women: quality of life and psychosocial adjustment in the 15 months after diagnosis. J Clin Oncol. 2003;21:4027–33.

114. Arndt V, Merx H, Stegmaier C, Ziegler H, Brenner H. Persistence of restrictions in quality of life from the first to the third year after diagnosis in women with breast cancer. J Clin Oncol. 2005;23:4945–53.

115. Bloom JR, Stewart SL, Chang S, Banks PJ. Then, and now: quality of life of young breast cancer survivors. Psychooncology. 2004;13:147–60.

116. Schou I, Ekeberg O, Sandvik L, Hjermstad MJ, Ruland CM. Multiple predictors of health-related quality of life in early stage breast cancer. Data from a year follow-up study compared with the general population. Qual Life Res. 2005;14:1813–23.

117. Montazeri A, Vahdaninia M, Harirchi I, Ebrahimi M, Khaleghi F, Jarvandi S. Quality of life in patients with breast cancer before and after diagnosis: an eighteen months follow-up study. BMC Cancer. 2008;8:330.

118. Hartl K, Engel J, Herschbach P, Reinecker H, Sommer H, Friese K. Personality traits and psychosocial stress: quality of life over 2 years following breast cancer diagnosis and psychological impact factors. Psychooncology. 2009;19(2):160–9.

119. Weitzner MA, Meyers CA, Stuebing KK, Saleeba AK. Relationship between quality of life and mood in long-term survivors of breast cancer treated with mastectomy. Support Care Cancer. 1997;5:241–8.

120. Avis NE, Crawford S, Manuel J. Quality of life among younger women with breast cancer. J Clin Oncol. 2005;23:3322–30.

121. Sears SR, Stanton AL, Danoff–Burg S. The yellow brick road and the emerald city: benefit finding, positive reappraisal coping and posttraumatic growth in women with early-stage breast cancer. Health Psychol. 2003;22:487–97.

122. Stanton AL, Danoff-Burg S, Cameron CL, Bishop M, Collins CA, Kirk SB, et al. Emotionally expressive coping predicts psychological and physical adjustment to breast cancer. J Consult Clin Psychol. 2000;68:875–82.

123. Jang JE, Kim SW, Kim SY, Kim JM, Park MH, Yoon JH, et al. Religiosity, depression, and quality of life in Korean patients with breast cancer: a 1-year prospective longitudinal study. Psychooncology. 2013;22(4):922–9.

124. Pinto AC, de Azambuja E. Improving quality of life after breast cancer: dealing with symptoms. Maturitas. 2011;70(4):343–8.

125. Dalton SO, Laursen TM, Ross L, Mortensen PB, Johansen C. Risk for hospitalization with depression after a cancer diagnosis: a nationwide, population-based study of cancer patients in Denmark from 1973 to 2003. J Clin Oncol. 2009;27(9):1440–5.

126. Jarrett N, Scott I, Addington-Hall J, Amir Z, Brearley S, Hodges L, et al. Informing future research priorities into the psychological and social problems faced by cancer survivors: a rapid review and synthesis of the literature. Eur J Oncol Nurs. 2013; 17(5):510–20.

127. Bessenoff GR, Snow D. Absorbing society's influence: body image self-discrepancy and internalized shame. Sex Roles. 2006;54:727–31.

128. Petronis VM, Carver CS, Antoni MH, Weiss S. Investment in body image and psychosocial well-being among women treated for early stage breast cancer: partial replication and extension. Psychol Health. 2003;18:1–13.

129. Öner H, İmamoğlu O. Meme kanseri olan Türk kadınlarının hastalıklarına ve uyumlarına ilişkin yargılar. Kriz Derg. 1994;2(1):261–8.

130. Koutrouli N, Anagnostopoulos F, Potamianos G. Posttraumatic stress disorder and posttraumatic growth in breast cancer patients: a systematic review. Women Health. 2012;52(5):503–16.

131. Tedeschi RG, Calhoun LG. The foundations of post-traumatic growth: new considerations. Psychol Inq. 2004;15:1–18.

132. Figley CR. Stress disorders among Vietnam veterans. New York: Brunner/Mazel; 1978.

133. Lepore SJ. A social cognitive processing model of emotional adjustment to cancer. In: Baum A, Andersen BL, editors. Psychosocial interventions for cancer. Washington, DC: American Psychological Association; 2001. p. 99–116.

134. Sears SR, Stanton AL, Danoff-Burg S. The yellow brick road and the emerald city: benefit finding, positive reappraisal coping, and post-traumatic growth in women with early-stage breast cancer. Health Psychology. 2003;22(5):487–97.

135. Weiss T. Posttraumatic growth in women with breast cancer and their husbands: an intersubjective validation study. J Psychosoc Oncol. 2002;20:65–80.

136. Parry C, Chesler MA. Thematic evidence of psychosocial thriving in childhood cancer survivors. Qual Health Res. 2005;15(8):1055–73.

137. Chow E, Tsao MN, Harth T. Does psychosocial intervention improve survival in cancer? A meta-analysis. Palliat Med. 2004;18(1):25–31.

Breast Cancer-Related Lymphedema (BCRL)

48

Atilla Soran, Ayfer Kamali Polat,
and Lisa Groen Mager

Abstract

After undergoing treatment for breast cancer, many patients endure life-long problems, such as lymphedema (LE), musculoskeletal problems, and psychosocial problems. Every patient with breast cancer-related LE (BCRL) should be assessed thoroughly for physical and psychological needs by a multidisciplinary team. In recent years, there has been increasing awareness of the diagnosis and treatment of BCRL. BCRL will be discussed in detail in this chapter.

Keywords

Lymphedema • Breast • Prevention • Diagnosis • Treatment

A. Soran, MD, MPH, FACS (✉)
Department of Surgery, Division of Surgical Oncology, Magee-Womens Hospital, University of Pittsburgh Medical Center, Pittsburgh, PA, USA
e-mail: asoran@upmc.edu, asoran65@gmail.com

A.K. Polat, MD, FACS
Department of Surgery, Division of Surgical Oncology, University of Pittsburgh Medical Center, Pittsburgh, PA, USA

General Surgery Department, Ondokuz Mayis University, Kurupelit, Samsun 55139, Turkey
e-mail: ayferkp@yahoo.com

L.G. Mager, MPT, CLT-LANA, WCS
Physical Therapy, UPMC Lemieux Sports Complex, 8000 Cranberry Springs Drive. Suite 100, Cranberry Twp, PA 16066, USA

University of Pittsburgh Medical Center, Pittsburgh, PA, USA
e-mail: lgroen@upmc.edu

© Springer International Publishing Switzerland 2016
A. Aydiner et al. (eds.), *Breast Disease: Management and Therapies*,
DOI 10.1007/978-3-319-26012-9_48

Description, Incidence, and Stages of LE

The lymphatic vessels travel parallel to the veins. The lymphatic circulatory system consists of superficial and deep vessels that drain the skin and the skeletal muscle, respectively. Small superficial lymph vessels are referred to as lymph capillaries and lie near blood capillaries in the interstitial space. These lymphatic capillaries form larger vessels called pre-collectors and collectors, which possess one-way valves that prevent the backflow of lymph. The lymphatic system has its own circulation of fluid and cells (mainly lymphocytes) from the blood stream, through the interstitial spaces, through the lymph vessels and nodes, and back to the blood stream. The lymphatic system has no single pump; fluid is forwarded via contraction of smooth muscle in the walls of the lymph vessels. Lymphatic fluid then drains into the lymph nodes, which function as a filtering system. Lymph nodes have an outer fibrous capsule and inner collection of immunologically active cells. Foreign substances such as bacteria and toxins are filtered and destroyed in the nodes. The lymph vessels finally open into large ducts—the thoracic duct and right lymphatic duct—and then drain into the neck veins [1–4].

The lymphatic system interacts with other circulatory and immune systems in the body. This collective circulation of the lymphatic system is responsible for transporting immune chemicals and cells and for monitoring the body for any cell or substance (microorganisms or toxins, mutated or cancerous cells) that is recognized as foreign by immunosurveillance. This interaction is the primary reason why people with lymphatic system impairment, such as LE, are predisposed to infection. Additionally, fats and fat-soluble vitamins are absorbed from the digestive system via the lymphatic system and transported to the venous circulation. The lymphatic system also helps maintain fluid balance and macromolecular homeostasis within the body.

LE is defined as blockage of the lymphatic fluid circulation, and it causes swelling of a part of the body. LE may occur if there is an interruption of the lymphatic system or if there is failure of normal capillary-lymph exchange. These interruptions of the lymphatic system can occur with surgery after breast cancer, parasites, bacterial infection, cancer, or fibrotic tissue growth after radiation therapy. Accumulation of lymph fluid containing protein and cell debris causes swelling in the affected area of the body. LE is multifactorial and has been described as one of the most significant survivorship problems after breast cancer treatment, causing functional and psychological issues. Women are restricted in their daily productive life activities (e.g., work, housework, and hobbies such as gardening and knitting). The debilitating pain, anguish, suffering, and disfiguring swelling of LE can cause physical and emotional distress. Women who develop LE face a lifetime of treatment [2–5]. BCRL symptoms can develop any time after breast cancer treatment. However, BCRL is commonly seen within the first 3 years following the surgical procedure. Initially, lymphedema may be asymptomatic. Unfortunately, lymphedema is chronic and progressive, and it advances slowly. Chronic inflammation, infection, and fibrosis of the skin result in further lymph vessel damage and progression to more severe stages of edema. Minor physical traumas, including cuts, burns, tight jewelry, or other injuries to the fingers or hands, may transform a latent condition into active LE that requires treatment [3]. The initial symptoms may be reversible, but over time, LE becomes irreversible and adversely impacts the survivor's quality of life. Early detection allows intervention to prevent the progression of LE to the more severe stages. Progressive LE is complicated by recurrent infections, nonhealing wounds, discomfort or pain, difficulty with daily tasks, and emotional and social distress.

Breast cancer survivors have significant physical, functional, quality of life, and economic consequences. In a prospective cohort study, Cormier et al. assessed limb volume change (LVC) and quality of life in breast cancer survivors and found that even a small increase in volume was associated with a significant decrease in quality of life [2].

Although BCRL has largely been neglected by healthcare professionals, there have recently been significant improvements in the awareness, clinical diagnosis, and management of BCRL [4–7].

Clinical Definitions of LE

Typically, patients report heaviness or swelling sometime in the past year. The diagnostic criteria for BCRL are based on limb volumes measured in different ways: volume increase greater than or equal to 200 mL as detected by water displacement, volume difference greater than 3 % between limbs, or 2 cm in circumferential increase.

The consensus of the Clinical Resource Efficiency Support Team (CREST) LE group is that a 5 % or greater increase in circumferential measurement indicates LE. It is recommended that limbs be measured prior to surgery, radiotherapy, or other possible risks of LE. Measurement changes from the baseline or between limbs may be used to detect LE [6].

Staging of LE

The *International Society of Lymphology* (ISL) has established a staging system for identifying the severity and progression of BCRL. This staging system is based on the amount of swelling and the condition of the skin and tissues at each stage. The system also allows the identification of the progression and success of treatments. Currently, there are four stages in the ISL LE staging system [7].

Stage 0 LE (Latent or Pre-Clinical)

At this stage, there is no apparent swelling or visible evidence of impaired lymph transport. Non-pitting edema may exist, and patients may report "heaviness." Although patients in stage 0 are at risk of LE, the appearance of more severe signs of LE may take months or years. Slower flow may be detected by lymphoscintigraphy or with bioimpedance spectroscopy or perometry, and it is possible to identify changes in the at-risk limb before they become visible. When changes develop, if specialized treatment is started immediately, it may be possible to prevent the development of further stages of LE.

Stage 1 LE (Spontaneously Reversible, Acute Phase)

Extracellular accumulation of fluid with high protein content is present in stage 1 LE. There is visible mild swelling consisting of protein-rich lymph. The volume increase does not exceed 20 %. Edema is reversible and can be temporarily reduced with elevation of the limb. The swelling makes the tissues soft and doughy. Mild pitting edema is present. There is little or no tissue fibrosis. Stage 1 LE is detectable with all techniques. Lymph flow as detected by lymphoscintigraphy is slow and reveals initial dermal backflow. The diagnosis can be made by classical measurement techniques. As soon as LE signs are detected, effective treatment should begin. At this stage, LE can often be controlled by prompt treatment so that the condition does not become more severe.

Stage 2 LE (Not Spontaneously Reversible, Chronic Phase)

Swelling is remarkable and irreversible at stage 2 LE. Swelling is mild to moderate, and the volume increase is 20–40 %. Excess accumulation of extracellular fluid is seen. There is no reduction of swelling upon elevation of the limb. Changes in the tissues are mostly due to *fibrosis*, the formation of fine scar-like structures within the tissues that make the tissues harder. The extracellular fluid compartment is expanded. Thickening of the soft tissues continues progressively. A slight indentation is seen with pressure, and pitting becomes more difficult (non-pitting). There is minimal or no decrease with elevation. Stage 2 LE can usually be improved with intense treatment. Stemmer's sign is positive. This stage is too late for prevention; lifelong physiotherapy is needed. Stemmer's Sign; is positive; when thickened skin fold at the dorsum of the fingers or toes cannot be lifted or is difficult to lift.

Stage 3 LE (Lymphostatic Elephantiasis)

Stage 3 LE is also known as lymphostatic elephantiasis. At this stage, the tissue becomes extremely swollen and thickened due to a blockage in the flow of lymph. Swelling is remarkable and irreversible. There is no reduction of swelling with elevation of the limb, and the volume increases more than 50 %. No pitting is seen with pressure. There are irreversible structural changes and smooth muscle cell atrophy at the lymphatic vessels. The tissues become hardened and sclerotic. Fibrosis and fat have replaced most of the fluid accumulated in the tissue. Stemmer's sign is positive. The skin has lost its elasticity and may change color. Hyperkeratosis, lymphangiomata, papillomatosis, and fungal infections can be seen. Intensive therapy can prevent stage 3 LE from worsening, but response to CDT is limited. Stage 3 LE is rarely reversed back to the earlier stage. Surgical debulking may be performed to reduce the size of the limb. However, morbidity after this surgery is high, and the hardened skin, hanging folds, and deep creases persist. These areas are at increased risk for fungal infections and open wounds because of the increased risk of breaks in the skin. Acute lymphostasis may progress to chronic fibrosis more than 5 years post-treatment, and soft tissue contractures may occur.

Stemmer's Sign

After long-standing chronic LE, patients may develop lymphangiosarcoma, also known as Stewart-Treves syndrome, a rare, deadly cutaneous angiosarcoma.

Risk Factors of LE

Reports of LE risk factors vary in reliability because detection methods, follow-ups, and treatments are not standardized, and current knowledge is largely based on patient's self-reports. BCRL has been the most-studied cause of secondary LE, but LE can occur as a result of other cancers, including melanoma, gynecologic cancer, head and neck cancer, and sarcoma. The average risk of BCRL is 25 %. There are an estimated 2.3 million US survivors of breast cancer who are affected by LE; of those, approximately 19–33 % develop LE following axillary lymph node dissection (ALND) and radiation therapy (RT), and 3.5–24 % develop LE following sentinel node (SLN) biopsy and RT. The reported incidence of lymphedema after breast cancer treatment varies from 6 % to 63 %, depending on the study [1–3]. The incidence of LE ranges from 7 % to 77 % of patients who undergo ALND. Several cooperative group trials have indicated that LE occurs at 0–23 % with SLN biopsy alone and 21–51 % after axillary radiation therapy and lymph node surgery [8–10]. The

5-year cumulative incidence of lymphedema is 42 %, and lymphedema first occurs within 2 years of diagnosis in 80 % of patients and within 3 years in 89 % of patients [9].

The risk factors of LE include the following:

- Surgery (incision, types of mastectomies, axillary surgery [SLNB, AD], reconstruction surgery)
- Number of lymph nodes removed
- Radiotherapy: multi-field irradiation
- Tumor-related factors (size, stage, location of tumor)
- Chemotherapy
- Age
- Postoperative seroma and/or infection
- Venous obstruction
- Obesity and higher body mass index
- Delays in the return of shoulder motion
- Sedentary life
- Trauma-induced infection
- Excessive sun exposure, which may be an inflammatory stimulus to the impaired lymphatic system that results in recurrent LE

The onset of BCRL is commonly observed within the first 3 years following the definitive surgical procedure. Even conservative techniques for the breast or axilla do not guarantee a complete elimination of the disorder. Once the condition develops, the possibility of progression to more severe stages of edema increases. Recurrent infections, nonhealing wounds, discomfort or pain, difficulty with daily tasks, and emotional and social distress may complicate LE. Most commonly, minor physical traumas, including cuts, burns, tight jewelry, or other injuries to the fingers or hands, may transform a latent condition into active LE.

Due to their lifelong risk of LE, breast cancer survivors must be diligent with daily skin care to prevent and detect cellulitis as well as to prevent LE onset or exacerbation [3].

Diagnosis of BCRL

The diagnosis of BCRL remains a challenge for many women whose BCRL remains undiagnosed until the condition causes significant morbidity. The treatment of LE is based on the correct diagnosis and ruling out differential diagnoses. Not every condition that causes swelling (edema) is LE, and LE can coexist with other issues such as chronic venous insufficiency (CVI) or lipedema. The correct diagnosis of LE requires specialized diagnostic testing.

Clinical History and Physical Examination

History and physical examination is important for all patients with suspected LE and must be performed by experienced healthcare providers. The age at onset, location of swelling, pain and other symptoms, medications, progression, and factors associated with swelling, such as cancer, injury, or infection, should be reviewed. A family history is important to the diagnosis of inherited forms of LE. The physical examination includes skin and soft tissues in the swollen body part, palpation of lymph nodes, and evaluation of the vascular system. To make a correct diagnosis, diagnostic tests and imaging must be performed with the guidance of findings from the history and physical examination [3, 6, 9, 10]. Self-scored symptoms include the following: swollen appearance or feeling (tightness of rings and bracelets), heaviness, tightness, discomfort, fullness or numbness, redness, tenderness, pain, weakness, and restricted movements. A common technique for assessing BCRL is patient self-assessment. Patients may also be asked questions regarding hand dominance, social constraints, performance loss at work, body image, anxiety, depression, adaptation problems, and social and sexual issues focusing on quality of life.

Clinical Findings

- Asymmetry of arms
- Skin folds are lost in areas relevant for anatomical structures such as tendons, bone projection, and veins
- Pitting of the skin with digital compression
- Skin hypertrophy, skin tension, and stiffness
- Sensory disturbance and joint stiffness in the hands and feet
- Recurrent soft tissue infection
- Chronic fibrosis and soft tissue contractures

Measures of volume: Traditional techniques for diagnosis and monitoring of BCRL are circumference-based measurements and the water displacement method. Perometry is now being used and can detect volume differences of as little as 3 % between limbs.

Circumferential volume measurement: Calculation of limb volume from circumferential measurements is the most widely used and easily accessible method. This method is noninvasive and inexpensive and has a sensitivity of 35–91 % and moderate specificity. The limb circumference is measured with a tape at fixed anatomical points with repeated 4 cm measurements. These circumferential measurements are entered into a computer program for automatic calculation of limb volume. This technique has been confirmed by some studies, including the NSABP B-04 trial [11], but it has some limitations such as there are no standard points of measurement, and interobserver variability is a major problem. As another example, McLaughlin et al. [12] performed circumferential measurements at 10 cm above and 5 cm below the olecranon process in both arms preoperatively. Measurements were taken at the same points during follow-up visits. This technique can be accurate if it is performed in precisely the same way each time and is most accurate when the same person takes the measurements each time.

The conical frustum method is used for volume calculation. It is based on the formula for a truncated cone. $V = 1/3x \cdot \pi x h x \left(r_1^2 + r_2^2 + r_1^2 x r_2^2 \right)$. *The frustum of a cone is shaped by removing the apex of a cone by a plane parallel to the base.*

The water displacement method is considered the gold standard for assessing limb volume, especially for hands and feet. The underlying principle is that an object displaces a volume of water equal to its own volume. The body part is plunged into a large cylinder full of water. The difference in the water level with and without the body part in place reflects the volume of the body part. This method is effective and accurate when performed properly. However, hygiene issues and practicality are limitations of this method and may discourage its use. Additionally, this procedure cannot distinguish LE from other types of edema and changes in muscle, adipose, or extracellular fluid volume or identify localized areas of swelling. It is also not advisable in patients with wounds or infections associated with BCRL [6].

Perometry (optoelectronic volumetry) uses an infrared optical electronic scanner consisting of arrays of optoelectronic sensors to measure limb volume at each 4 mm distance. The calculated volume measures size excluding extracellular fluid. Perometry can measure limb volume quickly and accurately if the body part is in the same position each time and the machine is calibrated properly. In breast cancer survivors, perometry can detect changes in limb volume of as little as 3 %. Currently, there is no standard cutoff in various volumetric analyses. Although circumferential increases of 2 cm or greater and volume increases of 200 mL have been increasingly used in the literature, these parameters have not been standardized in the clinic. Because this device is relatively large and requires significant space, its usage is limited in clinical settings [6, 13].

Changes in Electrical Conductance: Bioimpedance Spectroscopy (BIS)

BIS measures extracellular fluid based on the impedance to the flow of an imperceptible, low-level electric current. BIS measures impedance to an alternating current over a range of frequencies (4–1,000 kHz). BIS is performed by passing a small, painless electrical current through the limb and measuring the resistance (impedance). The machine uses certain current frequencies to determine whether more fluid exists than in the contralateral limb. BIS accurately measures extracellular fluid volume differences between the arms to aid in the clinical assessment of unilateral LE. The method does this by comparing the difference in electrical resistance of interstitial fluid to that of intracellular fluid. BIS currently is performed on the whole limb because the resistance to current flow in the standard technique is calculated with respect to the length of the body part. The higher the water content in the interstitial tissue, the lower the resistance. The device is portable, and it is easy to position the patient. BIS measures skin texture and resistance quantitatively. As fluid accumulates in the at-risk arm, the L-Dex value increases. The L-Dex number provides an easy means for clinicians to track extracellular fluid changes in the patient's arm over time. An increase of ten L-Dex units from a patient's baseline value represents a change of three standard deviations. BIS has been used for many years for fitness and weight loss purposes to assess the total water content of the body and body composition. BIS is now available to measure interstitial fluid as a component of the LE diagnosis [3, 6]. Cornish et al. used limb impedance ratios and compared the affected and unaffected limbs, finding that an increase of greater than three standard deviations in the affected arm compared with the contralateral arm was clinically relevant to the early assessment of LE. Further, recent data suggest that BIS represents an improvement in sensitivity over traditional assessment tools, with an average detection of 4 months earlier and in some cases up to 10 months earlier [14]. This is important because data from the National Institutes of Health (NIH) have confirmed that the management of patients with subclinical BCRL can be achieved simply and effectively with minimal long-term morbidity, making it imperative to diagnose BCRL at the subclinical stage to improve outcomes [15]. An L-Dex measurement greater than 10 and a difference from the baseline or subsequent measurement greater than 10 are considered the early stage (stage 0) of LE.

In their study, Cornish et al. reported the sensitivity and specificity of BIS as 100 % and 98 %, respectively [14]. Subsequently, Hayes et al. used BIS as the criterion standard to calculate the sensitivity and specificity of self-reported assessment of BCRL [16]. There are limitations in detecting non-pitting later-stage edema, at which point fluid increases have been replaced by adipose tissue and/or fibrotic tissue. Similarly, in patients with chronic BCRL, irreversible tissue changes can develop, and extracellular fluid differences alone no longer represent the true nature of the disease [14–16]. Soran et al. investigated the role of monitoring with BIS on the detection and early treatment of subclinical LE in patients who had ALND. In their prospective

Monitoring lymphedema

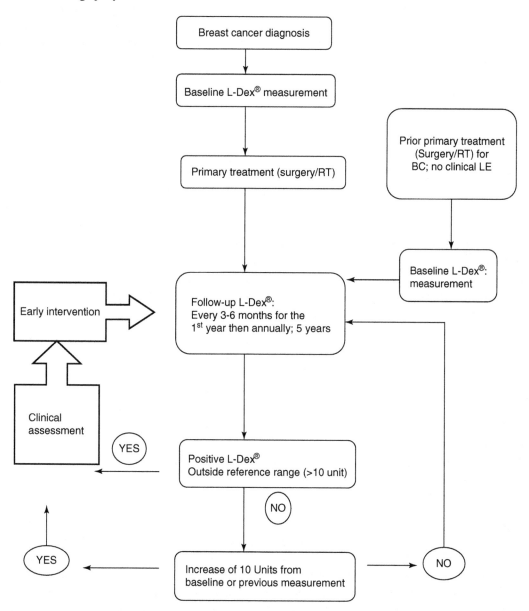

Fig. 48.1 Clinical practice pathways (Figure reprinted with permission from *Lymphatic Research and Biology* Vol. 12, 2014, pp. 289–294, published by Mary Ann Liebert, Inc., New Rochelle, NY [17])

observational study, the incidence of any LE was 33.8 %. One-third of women required early intervention, and only 4.4 % progressed to clinical LE. After a 2-year follow-up with early diagnosis and intervention, the authors reported a 32 % reduction in the rate of clinical LE [17] (Fig. 48.1).

Changes in Biomechanical Properties: Tonometry (Dielectric Constant and Tonometry)

In addition to increasing limb volume, LE causes inflammation and fibrosis of the skin and subcutaneous tissues, and the skin texture of the affected area becomes progressively harder. These skin changes are reported as features of tissue texture, edema, inflammation, pitting, enlarged skin folds, or other dermatologic conditions such as wounds or papillomas found by physical examination. The tissue dielectric constant and tonometry are quantitative methods for measuring skin texture and resistance [3]. The tissue dielectric constant measures tissue water content. This test is performed with a device that passes an electrical current of a specific frequency to one location of the skin and measures the reflected wave that returns. The reflected waveform indicates the amount of water present in the tissue [18]. Tonometry measures the amount of force required to indent a certain amount of tissue. Tonometry yields a value reflecting the level of dermal compliance, induration, and fibrosis. The compressibility of skin is correlated to the LE volume. However, due to some technical difficulties related to the use of tonometry devices, environmental factors, and operator differences, the results obtained may vary [19, 20].

Soft Tissue Imaging

Magnetic resonance imaging (MRI), computed tomography (CT), and ultrasound (US) can demonstrate the presence of extra fluid in the tissues. However, these imaging techniques should be used in conjunction with clinical history, physical examination, and other imaging tests to explain the causes of edema. Other conditions such as heart failure or low proteins in the blood from liver disease or malnutrition can cause fluid to build up in the tissues. These imaging modalities are especially helpful if there is a concern that the LE is related to cancer diagnosis [6]. Ultrasonic skin thickness measurement can be used for monitoring LE [21–25]. Ultrasound scans, particularly high-resolution Doppler, can help to differentiate LE from lipedema and may also be helpful in the detection of LE of the head and neck. MRI of the skin can reveal thickening of the dermis in LE. The subcutaneous tissue may exhibit a honeycomb pattern or a reticular pattern

if edema is marked. MRI scans of lower limb LE have been performed using gadodiamide as a contrast agent given intradermally to facilitate visualization of the lymphatic pathways [26].

A newer technique for improving the clinical assessment of BCRL is dual-energy X-ray absorptiometry (DEXA). DEXA scans measure fat, lean muscle, and bone mineral content in the region of interest extending from the glenohumeral joint to the fingertips. A recent study found that DEXA was superior to circumferential measurements and water displacement with respect to the reproducibility of measurements of the affected and contralateral arms [27]. Skin viscoelasticity and dual-beam absorptiometry are other techniques used for detection of LE [28, 29].

Lymph Vessel and Lymph Node Imaging: Lymphoscintigraphy

Lymphoscintigraphy is beneficial in limb swelling where the diagnosis is unclear [6]. Many studies of lymphoscintigraphy are in the area of BCRL, where it can detect early LE with 73 % sensitivity and 100 % specificity. However, in some patients with LE, lymphoscintigraphy is negative [30–32]. There is no standard protocol, with international differences in the colloid used, injection site (dermal or subcutaneous), and exercise protocol. There is debate as to whether lymphoscintigraphy should be quantitative or qualitative and whether epifascial as well as subfascial lymphatic vessels should be imaged. Typically, a technetium-labeled sulfur colloid is used. Lymphoscintigraphy is accurate for detecting abnormalities of the lymphatic system in the extremities regardless of the cause. Lymphoscintigraphy demonstrates slow or absent lymph flow and areas of reflux (backflow). It can reveal abnormalities of lymph uptake in lymph nodes with some forms of LE and can predict response to treatment. Lymphoscintigraphy reveals the main, larger lymph vessels and nodes and the basic architecture of the peripheral lymphatic system but does not show the deep transport lymph vessels carrying lymph from the nodes back to the blood circulation.

Lymphoscintigraphy identifies lymphatic abnormalities at late stages, after LE has occurred. Lymphoscintigraphy, in combination with other vascular studies, can differentiate venous edema from LE. Lymphoscintigraphy may not be necessary in some forms of secondary LE where the diagnosis is clear from the history and physical examination or from other imaging. The specific tests needed are determined by a specialist in LE. The type of lymphoscintigraphy performed for the diagnosis of LE is not available at all radiology departments. Most radiology departments, however, can perform a type of lymphoscintigraphy used to identify the sentinel lymph node for cancers such as breast and melanoma. These studies for the sentinel lymph node are different from the lymphoscintigraphy studies performed for diagnosis of LE. Before undergoing a lymphoscintigraphy study, the patient should inquire whether the radiologist performing and reading the study has a large amount of experience with lymphoscintigraphy studies specifically for the diagnosis of LE.

Other Vascular Imaging: Lymphangiography and Near-Infrared Fluorescence (NIR) Imaging

Lymphangiography: MR angiography involves the direct administration of an iodinated contrast agent into a cannulated lymph vessel for radiography or CT. Lymph vessel architecture, lymph nodes, collateral vessels, and dermal back flow can be clearly visualized by MR (indirect) lymphangiography [33].

Near-infrared fluorescence imaging (NIR) is a new technique for imaging lymph vessels using a substance known as indocyanine green (ICG). ICG is a green dye that has been used safely in other areas of the body, such as the liver and eyes, and it can be used in very small amounts to image the lymphatic vessels. ICG is injected into the skin and immediately imaged with a dynamic (real-time) infrared fluorescence camera. With NIR-ICG, even very small lymphatic vessels can be visualized. Because the study is dynamic, the actual function of the lymphatic vessels can be

analyzed. Diseased lymphatic vessels that do not contract (or pulse) normally can be seen with NIR-ICG. NIR-ICG can diagnose LE and identify abnormalities at an early stage, possibly before swelling is obvious. Although this technique shows promise for the diagnosis of LE, it is currently available at very few centers, most of which are involved in research [33, 34].

Differential Diagnosis

There is no blood test for LE. Other medical conditions such as hypothyroidism (myxedema) or low protein (hypoproteinemia) can cause edema and must be considered as part of a complete evaluation of swelling. Standard plain X-rays may be ordered for some inherited LEs to evaluate the presence of orthopedic conditions. Edema can be caused by diseases of the cardiovascular system (heart, arteries, and veins), such as cardiac failure, chronic venous insufficiency (CVI), or related lipedema. The most common condition, CVI, is a condition in which the veins of the legs do not efficiently return blood to the heart. Reduced capacity of the venous system caused by damage to the veins increases the workload for the lymphatic system in the affected area. If the diagnosis is primary LE, it is important to evaluate the patient for the presence of other vascular abnormalities. Edema secondary to cardiac failure is generally bilateral, symmetrical, and markedly pitting.

Lipedema and LipoLE are also misdiagnosed as LE. Lipedema is a bilateral, symmetrical, fatty swelling that consists of adipose tissue deposition. The exact cause of lipedema is not well known. LipoLE is a form of swelling combining lipedema and LE. LipoLE may also present with edema related to CVI and other vascular diseases.

To properly treat edema, detailed clinical examination and some imaging studies of the heart, veins, or arteries are needed to obtain a complete and accurate diagnosis of the main cause. The most common cardiovascular studies ordered for the evaluation of complex edemas are echocardiogram, venous ultrasound, and arterial ultrasound with ankle-brachial index (ABI). Alternatively, more advanced imaging, such as computed tomography venograms or arteriograms, may be recommended.

Early Diagnosis and Monitoring

Traditional measurement procedures have significant limitations and there are no standard points of measurements. Inter-observer and inter-measurement variabilities and failure to measure the extracellular space can be observed. Using traditional measures, only clinically apparent LE is easily diagnosed, and subclinical disease is detected with relatively low sensitivity compared with newer techniques. Hutson et al. examined the operator variability of traditional measurements and found variation using circumferential and volume measurements. Recent studies have reported that newer assessment procedures are able to detect BCRL on average 4–10 months earlier than traditional methods [14–17]. Early management has been found to improve outcomes in BCRL. Newer tools provide increased diagnostic accuracy and can directly measure the extracellular volume as well. The most appropriate methods and tools to identify the early versus late stages of LE are BIS and perometry. The L-Dex monitoring protocol and nomogram integrated care delivery model are considered part of preoperative assessment and are performed every 3 months. Every patient with LE should have access to established effective treatment for this condition.

The treatment for LE is most effective when the disease is diagnosed at the earliest stage, with no irreversible changes such as fibrosis. Early physiotherapy is an effective intervention for the prevention of secondary LE after breast cancer surgery, and it improves quality of life [35]. However, Maria Torres Lacomba et al. reported in 2010 that physiotherapy for every patient after breast cancer surgery may not be feasible in terms of both cost effectiveness and patient and physician compliance [36]. A minority of patients develop severe, long-term physi-

cal impairments. In this study, among 116 women, therapeutic benefits were observed in 4 (7 %) patients in the early physiotherapy group who were treated by a physiotherapist with a program including manual lymph drainage, scar tissue mobilization, and progressive active and action-assisted shoulder exercises. This group also received an educational strategy. The control group received the educational strategy only. Of the control patients, 14 (25 %) had secondary LE (intervention/control, hazard ratio 0.26, 95 % confidence interval 0.09–0.79), and LE occurred four times sooner in the control group ($P=0.01$) [36].

Components of LE Monitoring

Protocol with BIS: An L-Dex measurement greater than 10 and a difference from the baseline or inter-measurement greater than 10 represents stage 0 LE. This permits early detection and effective early treatment. Preoperative assessment is followed by postsurgical assessments at months 1, 3, 6, 9, and 12. Every 3 months, surveillance care is compared to baseline measurements as needed [17, 37]. A 5-year study funded by the National Institutes of Health assessed LE (with perometry) in breast cancer patients: 196 patients were assessed preoperatively and then again at 1, 3, 6, 9, and 12 months post surgery. Of these patients, 43 (22 %) were identified with subclinical LE. Intervention with a compression sleeve resulted in reversal of symptoms in all patients [38].

Prediction of high-risk patients: The Cleveland Clinic published a questionnaire study based on the formation of a nomogram as a risk prediction assessment tool (http://www.LErisk.com). The 5-year cumulative incidence of LE was 30.3 %. Independent risk factors for LE included age, body mass index, ipsilateral arm chemotherapy infusions, level of ALND, location of radiotherapy field, development of postoperative seroma, infection, and early edema. The proposal of the study was that nomograms could help predict the 5-year probability of LE after ALND for breast cancer [39].

Management of LE

The current standard management for BCRL consists of physiotherapy based on complete decongestive therapy. The procedures of lymphedema management are listed below.

Physiotherapy

The comprehensive goals for the effective management of all patients with BCRL are as follows:

(a) Facilitation of functional independence, including musculoskeletal function and correct posture
(b) Infection prevention
(c) Providing control of limb volume and shape
(d) Improving lymph drainage in affected areas and minimizing fibrosis
(e) Maximize psychological support
(f) Promoting self-management with education of patients

Complete Decongestive Therapy (CDT)

The goals of CDT are to decrease swelling, increase lymph drainage from the congested areas, reduce skin fibrosis, improve skin condition, enhance the patient's functional status, relieve discomfort, improve quality of life, and reduce the risk of cellulitis and Stewart-Treves Syndrome, a rare form of angiosarcoma-related LE. Complete decongestive therapy is also described as combined, complex, or comprehensive decongestive therapy or as multimodal physical therapy [3, 6]. CDT is the "gold standard" of the conservative management of LE; it has been shown to be safe and effective [37, 40]. CDT consists of two phases: the initial intensive decongestive phase (Phase I) and maintenance (Phase II). In Phase I, the main goals are reducing the size of the limb and improving the skin condition. Acute management generally occurs in an outpatient clinic setting. On average, management consists of a 4-week program of manual lymphatic drainage, short-stretch compression bandaging, exercise, and proper skin and nail care. Daily treatment is performed on up to 5 days per week (up to 6 weeks) by LE therapists skilled in CDT. Phase I should lead directly into Phase II, which involves individualized self-management for the long-term maintenance of Phase I reductions. During Phase II, the maintenance of care transfers to the patient, who is encouraged to continue lifetime regular checkups or further intensive treatment. The self-management program consists of self-performed manual lymph drainage (also referred to as simple lymphatic drainage), home lymphatic exercises, skin care, and independent application of compression garments or bandages. Phase II maintenance must be monitored and adjusted periodically, just as with treatment for any other chronic medical condition. Compression garments must be replaced every 4–6 months to be effective. Specialized equipment requires maintenance and replacement according to manufacturers' guidelines. Phase II CDT and periodic medical monitoring are essential to the long-term success of LE treatment. These measures may include garments with Velcro, specialized foam construction garments, and pneumatic compression devices. For the therapy to be successful, all the components of CDT must be performed in a combination. When performed properly, CDT is currently the most effective treatment for LE. The literature is conflicting on some points regarding the effectiveness of certain CDT components. CDT may sometimes need to be modified in the presence of complex comorbidities or according to the patient's preference, such as for elderly patients living alone who are not able to manage daily visits or intensive treatment as planned. The reasons for modifying the treatment should be clearly explained for each patient's treatment plan. Treatment options are discussed with the patient to formulate an individualized protocol. Many trials confirm the efficacy of CDT. One of the largest studies was performed by Vignes et al. who evaluated 537 patients undergoing CDT and found that the mean volume of lymphedema was $1,054 \pm 633$ mL prior to CDT and 647 ± 351 mL after intensive decongestive physiotherapy [41].

Components of CDT

Manual Lymphatic Drainage (MLD)

Manual lymph drainage is an essential part of CDT. MLD is a special manual (hands-on) technique that stimulates superficial lymphatic vessels to remove excess interstitial fluid [3, 6]. MLD moves the fluid through subdermal (under the skin) fluid channels that form when lymphatic vessels are damaged. MLD is a type of massage, but it differs from the commonly known types of muscle or myofascial massage. MLD is the use of specific massage techniques (based on the knowledge of lymphatic anatomy and physiology) that mobilize the skin and stimulate the lymphatic system. MLD is a gentle skin technique performed by certified LE therapists. MLD moves the lymphatic fluid stream into the venous circulation by using existing lymphovenous anastomoses and lymph vessels/lymph nodes that are properly functioning instead of those from edematous areas with damaged lymphatic vessels. MLD is most effective when combined with compression bandaging, skin care, and exercise. Evidence supporting MLD is insufficient in the literature. However, international expert opinion has reached a consensus that MLD is a primary component of CDT, as MLD is the only technique to move fluid away from the congested areas.

Contraindications for MLD

In addition to all general contraindications, MLD contraindications include pregnancy, menstruation, recent abdominal surgery, radiation fibrosis/colitis/cystitis, history of DVT in the pelvic veins, inflammatory bowel disease, diverticulitis, cirrhosis of the liver, abdominal aortic aneurysm, unexplained pain, and ileus.

Compression Bandaging: LE Bandaging Multilayer LE Bandaging (MLLB)

Compression therapy includes compression bandages, compression garments, gradient compression devices, and pneumatic compression devices to mobilize the lymph fluid.

Compression bandaging is used to create safe and effective compression by applying multiple layers of several materials. Compression bandaging is always a part of Phase I CDT. The components of compression bandaging are as follows: a skin protection layer (non-compression), a padding layer (may be foam or layered wool, polyester, cotton, or foam under-cast padding), short-stretch compression bandages, tubular bandage lining, and digit bandages. Multiple layers of short-stretch bandages with 50 % overlap and 50 % stretch to cover the entire limb are recommended. In some patients, it may be necessary to use polyurethane foam in various densities and configurations within the bandaging system. Short-stretch bandages have limited stretching capacity when pulled. They can stretch 40–60 % from resting length, whereas long-stretch bandages stretch by greater than 140 % of resting length. To achieve an effective compression gradient, short-stretch bandages must be strategically applied with low to moderate tension using more layers at the distal ends of the extremities than proximally. Pressure within the short-stretch bandages is low when the patient is resting ("resting pressure"). As muscles expand within the limited space of the short-stretch bandages, muscle contractions increase interstitial fluid circulation ("working pressure") to help the fluid to move out of congested areas. The cycling between low resting and high working pressures in the interstitial fluid within the compression bandage creates an internal pumping action. The short-stretch bandages increase the drainage of congested interstitial fluid into the vascular circulation and prevent reaccumulation of the fluid into the tissues. These bandages can also reduce areas of fibrosis and reshape the limb.

In the maintenance phase, patients may need to perform nocturnal self-bandaging to supplement compression garments. Incorrect bandaging techniques may cause additional damage.

Contraindications for Multilayer Bandaging

Absolute contraindications: Cardiac edema, peripheral arterial disease, ankle-brachial index (ABI) <0.5, and acute infection

Relative contraindications: Arterial high blood pressure, cardiac arrhythmia, scleroderma, chronic polyarthritis, Sudeck's atrophy, malignant LE, ABI 0.6–0.8, and specialist consideration

Compression Garments

Following the success of maximal volume reduction with Phase I CDT, patients should be fitted with a compression garment [3]. Garments may be sleeves, bras, face or neck compression wear, or other garments. The patient should receive two garments at a time for each affected body part: one to wear and one to wash and dry. Having two garments ensures that the patient does not wear a dirty or wet garment, which would promote bacterial or fungal infection. Manufacturer instructions must be followed for washing and drying to prolong the life of the garment.

Properly fitted garments are essential for the long-term control of LE. Garment style and compression strength should be prescribed according to the patient's ability to manage the garment and maintain the best volume control and skin health. Compression garments are commonly used, deliver 20–60 mmHg of pressure, and can be worn for a few hours per day or all day. Ready-made garments come in a variety of sizes and can be fitted to many individuals. Custom garments are specifically sewn or created for the individual who cannot fit a ready-made garment. Such garments are more expensive than ready-made garments and may be required for patients with irregularly shaped limb(s) or body parts, wounds, lack of sensation, or difficulty with hand dexterity. Custom garments allow for options including special linings to reduce the risk of skin breakdown, as well as fastening devices that may assist the patient in donning and doffing the garment.

Garments should be washed daily to ensure that the garment lasts as long as possible and does not lose its compression strength. For optimal results, the garments should be fitted by trained personnel and be replaced every 6 months or when the tension from the elasticity decreases. Most daily garments must be replaced every 4–6 months to maintain compression strength. The efficacy of compression garments is controversial, yet they continue to be used frequently in patients with early stage or limited BCRL. Providing correctly fitting garments for each individual patient is essential. Non-fitting garments can be harmful, causing the edema to worsen and further permanent damage. In addition to the day garments used in Phase II, some patients with more severe forms of LE will need night garments or advanced day garments to maintain the reductions obtained in Phase I. These include VELCRO® brand closure garments and specialized foam compression garments [3–5].

In choosing garments, the clinician should consider the following:

- Limb shape and size/distribution of swelling
- Presence of skin folds
- LE status (stage I–III)—texture of skin
- Skin sensitivity
- Overall status of underlying disease, e.g., cancer, arterial disease, or diabetes
- Patient's functional ability
- Patient's choice regarding material, color, texture, and fabric
- Patient's compliance
- Some garments have additional attachments, including shoulder attachments, separate handpieces, and waist attachments. In the maintenance phase of treatment reassessment, it is important for a trained clinician to reassess garment choice. Garments should only be assessed by a trained clinician. All patients should be provided with accurate contact details of local LE services in case they require further advice [3, 6].

Vignes et al. reported a total lymphedema volume reduction of 33 %. Intensive phase CDT for 11 days resulted in significantly greater volume reduction in breast cancer-related lymphedema than did 4 days of CDT [42].

Data from the NIH have demonstrated that use of compression sleeves in patients with subclinical LE leads to excellent results with minimal morbidity [43].

Absolute contraindications for compression garments: Uncontrolled heart failure, risk of increased cardiac edema, acute deep vein thrombosis (DVT), risk of dislodging the clot, acute ineffective episode (cellulitis, erysipelas), superior vena cava obstruction (SVCO), and acute renal failure.

Relative contraindication: Malignancy (risk of spread of active cancer).

Intermittent Pneumatic Compression Therapy (IPCT)

IPCT, also known as compression pump therapy, can be useful in some patients as an adjunct to Phase I CDT or as a necessary component of a successful home program (Phase II CDT) [3, 6]. Intermittent pneumatic compression (IPCT) uses compression pumps daily for anywhere from 30 min to several hours and should only be used in conjunction with manual treatments. IPCT is contraindicated in patients with congestive heart failure, active infection, or deep venous thrombosis. Single-chamber pumps are no longer used for LE. Single-chamber pumps can cause fluid to move in both directions, which may allow additional fluid to accumulate in the swollen area. Furthermore, the pressure in single-chamber pumps does not stimulate lymphatic flow as well as sequential pumps. Acceptable pumps should have appliances (pump garments) that deliver sequential pressure through multiple chambers in a pattern tailored to each patient, depending on the diagnosis and pattern of LE. LE is a condition involving a quadrant of the body (upper or lower trunk, chest, and abdomen), not only the limb with the edema, and many patients who require IPCT will need a pump that treats both the trunk of the body and the edematous limb. Recommended pump pressures generally range from 20 to 60 mmHg, although lower or higher pressures may be indicated. The pressure displayed on the pump may not accurately reflect what is delivered to the skin surface. This is a significant concern because if the pressures applied in therapy are too high, the superficial structures may be harmed. In general, lower pressures are considered safer, but the pressure has to be individualized to the patient's diagnosis and skin condition. Typically, treatment takes one hour. IPCT is utilized along with standard CDT to maintain control of LE at home as part of Phase II management. To control edema, a compression garment or short-stretch bandages should be worn between pump treatments and also when IPCT therapy is discontinued. It is important to select the proper device and protocol for IPCT. The prescription must include the intensity of pressure and the pattern of pressure needed, considering several aspects of the patient's situation. The treating physician must consider the possible need for programmable pressure to treat fibrotic areas, address the treatment of ulcers, and adjust for the patient's level of pain and skin sensitivity. If trunk, chest, or genital swelling is present, the physician must determine whether a pump that provides appliances to treat those areas is necessary or whether the patient can manage the trunk swelling through self-MLD or garments. If a pump with only extremity attachments is used, there should be close monitoring to detect any increase in edema or fibrotic tissue, called a fibrosclerotic ring, above the device sleeve. If this occurs, consideration should be given to using a device that treats the trunk in addition to the extremities. Furthermore, the physician or healthcare provider must evaluate the impact of various other medical conditions that are usually considered contraindications for pneumatic compression therapy, including acute infection, severe arterial vascular disease, acute superficial or deep vein phlebitis (inflammation or clot), recurrent cancer in the affected area, or uncompensated congestive heart failure [37, 40–43].

Documented results with IPCT are limited [44]. IPCT was compared with manual lymphatic drainage in patients using compression sleeves and did not exhibit advantages in BCRL; The advanced IPCT devices "new generation" pumps that provide custom treatment to address individual patient needs. IPCT is essential for long term care, provides good quality of life, provides independence, saves money by reducing office visits and reduce use of resources. It should be remembered that in some areas IPCT is the only daily available lymphedema treatment and works very well stand-alone. In additional, older or disabled patients who have difficulty with self-bandaging or application of gradient elastic garments may easily use IPCT and it can be adjusted by patient's medical condition [45].

Ridner et al. reported favorable data about the Flexitouch. The Flexitouch system is an advanced, programmable pneumatic compression device that is cleared by the US Food and Drug Administration for home use. This device is designed to emulate the therapeutic techniques of MLD. The Flexitouch system for upper extremities consists of three compressive garments for the trunk, chest, and arm [46, 47].

Modifications and Individualization of CDT

CDT programs should be individualized based on the presence of other medical conditions and the patient's abilities. Patients with wounds, scars, or musculoskeletal conditions, palliative care patients, and patients with postradiation fibrosis may require adaptations of CDT. If there is limited mobility of the body part with or near the swelling, the patient may require other therapies, such as scar mobilization or myofascial therapy, in addition to CDT, to benefit from CDT.

Exercise (Therapeutic Exercises Including Lymphatic "Remedial Exercise")

Remedial exercise refers to exercises that aid lymph flow through repeated contraction and relaxation of muscles. These exercises should be individualized and should be performed while the edematous arm is bandaged. Ideally, these exercises are initiated by well-trained therapists and then continued at home. Therapeutic exercise and manual lymphatic drainage (MLD) are two treatment options that often represent a bridge between compression sleeves and CDT. Exercise significantly improves tissue resistance and symptomatic heaviness. More recent data has found that active exercise further reduces limb volume along with standard therapy. MLD, while commonly used, has shown limited benefit compared with standard treatments. Analysis of MLD as a single treatment has indicated volume reductions of 100–150 mL with reductions in limb heaviness. Recently, some data has supported MLD, with a crossover trial finding that MLD showed a trend for decreased arm volumes in 31 patients receiving MLD (10 % vs. 4 %, $p = 0.053$) [15]. With LE, individualized exercise is beneficial for all patients. Although heavy activity may temporarily increase fluid load, appropriate exercise enables the patient with LE to resume activity while minimizing the risk of increased swelling. For people with LE, compression garments or compression bandages must be worn during exercise (except in aqua therapy) to reduce the buildup of interstitial fluid [37, 43]. Because exercise has been shown to have significant positive effects during and after cancer treatment, safe exercise must be a goal for all cancer-related LE. People with or at risk for LE are encouraged to work with an LE specialist to incorporate an individualized exercise program into their LE management. Remedial exercises are performed in the intensive phase of treatment in conjunction with multilayer bandages and in the maintenance phase with a compression garment. The aim is to enhance the efficiency of the muscle pump, thus increasing lymph circulation. Patients are given an individually tailored exercise program suited to their particular requirements and abilities.

Summary of CDT Treatment of LE

Treatment of LE should be performed only by experienced practitioners after completion of the diagnostic evaluation according to accepted guidelines. The current international standard of care for managing LE is CDT. CDT has been shown to be effective in a large number of case studies. Limb volume reductions of 50–70 % or more, improved appearance of the limb, reduced symptoms, improved quality of life, and fewer infections were demonstrated after CDT treatment. Even patients with progressive LE for 30 years or more before starting CDT have been shown to respond. CDT adaptations or other LE treatments should be used as individualized treatments to improve patient adherence and should be applied under the supervision of a healthcare provider (physician, nurse, physician assistant, or therapist) who is experienced in LE management. IPCT is a demonstrated effective adjunct to CDT. The main goals must include reducing and maintaining the volume reduction, preventing medical complications, improving skin condition, reducing infection, and improving patient comfort, adherence, and quality of life for all interventions of LE [48]. Trained therapists providing CDT should have completed at least 135 hours of training as recommended by the Lymphology Association of North America® [43].

Patient Education

Patient education: LE is a lifelong condition; therefore, patient education in self-management is mandatory. All patients with LE or at risk for LE should be instructed in essential self-care. Risk-reduction practices, self-lymph drainage, skin care, signs and symptoms of infection, proper fit and care of garments, and the importance of good nutrition, exercise, and weight control are important areas of education.

Skin and nail care: Good skin care is essential in the management of LE to maintain skin integrity against traumas such as cuts and punctures and to reduce risk of infection. Meticulous hygiene is important to decrease the amount of fungus and bacteria on the skin. Using low pH emollients is recommended to keep skin from drying and cracking, which provides entry points for bacteria and fungus. Cuts and abrasions should be monitored for signs of infection [43]. Skin infections or cellulitis (or erysipelas) requires antibiotic treatment. For more complex skin conditions such as psoriasis or eczema, the patient should be referred to a local dermatology department to optimize the outcome of their LE treatment [49, 50]. Similarly, patients with complex wounds/ulcers should be assessed.

Weight loss: LE risk increases with obesity; therefore, weight management is an integral part of LE treatment as well as the maintenance of optimal weight in normal-weight individuals. An increased body mass index (BMI), especially >30, is noted as a significant risk factor. Patients with high BMI should be referred to dietetic services. LE treatment is more effective when combined with a weight-loss program. LE volume measurements completed in therapy must be correlated with BMI [48, 51, 52].

Exercise: For at risk BCRL patients who followed the same 90 minute exercise program, LE development at one year follow up was significantly less (70 %).

Comorbidities: Having significant comorbid conditions is generally thought to add to the risk of developing LE. Elevated blood pressure has also been cited as a risk factor. Cellulitis is both a risk factor and cause of LE.

Surgical Treatment of LE

Although surgery for LE is not performed with curative intent, it has been used for the control of severe conditions in specific circumstances. Surgery may be considered for reducing the weight of the affected limb, improving the cosmetic appearance/shape of the limb, minimizing the frequency of inflammatory attacks, or fitting the limb into garments. The risks and benefits of surgical procedures must be balanced according to the personalized needs of the patient and the experience of the surgical team. Surgery is usually performed if all usual treatment methods have failed or in very early stage of lymphedema. Nonetheless, surgery for LE must be performed in conjunction with CDT and should not be performed alone. Both treatment modalities interact positively with each other [6, 48, 53–56].

There are several types of LE surgery procedures available:

(a) Excisional operations, including debulking and liposuction
(b) Vascularized lymph node transfer: tissue transfers
(c) Microsurgical lymphatic reconstruction

There are very few surgeons who perform the above-listed procedures. It is important that patients with lymphedema are treated by qualified physicians. Working with a certified LE therapist for ongoing care after surgery is also important for successful outcomes.

Debulking

Debulking surgery removes the fibrotic connective tissue and any large folds of fatty tissue associated with the LE. The risks associated with debulking include prolonged hospitalization, high morbidity, poor wound healing, nerve damage or loss, significant scarring, risk of destruction of the remaining lymphatic vessels, loss/or decreased limb function, recurrence of swelling, poor cosmetic results, and decrease in quality of life. Lifelong compression garments are necessary postoperatively for the maintenance of the limb due to the lymphatic scarring from these surgeries and lymphatic insufficiency.

Liposuction

Liposuction surgery of the limb is the circumferential removal of fatty tissue deposits of the affected part by LE. Liposuction performed for LE is similar but not identical to cosmetic liposuction. Tubular suction devices are inserted into many small incisions, and fat tissues break up, liquefy, and are removed. Patients with lymphedema require bandaging postoperatively to stop the bleeding. Lifelong compression garments are generally needed to prevent LE recurrence due to the scarring of lymph vessels that may occur after the procedure. The risks of liposuction include bleeding, infection, skin loss, abnormal sensations such as numbness and tingling, and the return of LE.

Vascularized Lymph Node Transfer: Tissue Transfers

Tissue transfers (grafts) are performed to relocate lymph vessels into a congested area to remove excess interstitial fluid. There are few studies of the long-term effectiveness of tissue transfers for LE. Published articles are either outdated, performed on animals, or are insufficient to demonstrate lymph vessel function in breast reconstruction flaps [53–57].

Microsurgical Lymphatic Reconstruction

Microsurgical and supramicrosurgical techniques have been developed to relocate lymphatic vessels to congested areas in an attempt to improve lymphatic drainage. The surgical procedure involves the anastomosis of lymph vessels and veins, lymph nodes and veins, or lymph vessels to lymph vessels. Although there are no long-term studies of the effectiveness of these techniques, there are several preliminary studies reporting reductions in limb volume [53–55]. Surgical treatments in general are associated with significant risks and morbidities, but the outcomes are promising. However, it is difficult to predict the length of time required for LE to reduce postsurgically. The surgical management of LE should be undertaken in conjunction with a CDT protocol. CDT and adjunctive therapies (advanced garments and IPCT) can usually produce excellent management in compliant patients, and surgery is rarely a necessary consideration.

Pharmaceutical Approaches, Natural Supplements, and Complementary Medicines

Pharmacological interventions for BCRL have included benzopyrones, flavonoids, diuretics, hyaluronidase, pantothenic acid, and selenium. Benzopyrones have been used widely in Europe to treat BCRL; however, benzopyrones are not approved by the US Food and Drug Administration because of its serious side effects. Casley-Smith et al. reported a randomized, double-blind, placebo-controlled study in which benzo-[alpha]-pyrone was administered. Thirty-one patients with BCRL were treated with 400 mg of 5,6-benzo-[alpha]-pyrone (18 patients) or placebo (13 patients) for 6 months. The authors observed a significant decrease in the amount of edema in the upper extremities, with reduction of pain, tightness, and acute inflammation among those patients given 5,6-benzo-[alpha]-pyrone [58]. However, Loprinzi et al. found no significant difference in arm volumes at 6 and 12 months in 140 patients with BCRL who were treated with 200 mg of oral coumarin twice daily for 6 months [59]. Selenium, a free radical scavenger, has been shown to be effective in improving radiation-induced secondary LE in the head and neck region. Micke et al. confirmed that volume decrease was observed in 83 % of patients (10 of 12) after the administration of selenium. Although nausea, vomiting, diarrhea, and tachycardia are documented as adverse effects, no toxicities were observed with selenium use in this setting [60]. Diuretics are ineffective for the removal of interstitial fluid from tissues. Excess diuretic use can lead to dehydration, electrolyte imbalance, and tissue damage. However, diuretics may be medically indicated in patients with high blood pressure and heart disease. Therefore, diuretic use must be assessed on a case-by-case basis. Some drugs such as coumarin and diosmin have been investigated for LE but have not been found to be effective for LE and produce adverse side effects.

Natural Supplements

There is limited evidence on the use of natural supplements for treating LE. Studies have demonstrated that American horse chestnut may help venous edema but not LE. Selenium has been reported to improve LE in head and neck cancer. Bromelain, a substance found in pineapple, exhibits anti-inflammatory, anticoagulant, enzymatic, and diuretic effects. Some have wondered whether there might be a benefit of bromelain use with LE, but no studies have been undertaken. Due to potential interactions with prescription drugs and other negative side effects, patients should check with their physician or healthcare provider before taking any natural supplement [43].

Complementary and Alternative Treatments

Some promising treatments have been reported, but they have not yet been subjected to sufficient research to be recommended as the standard of care. These treatments include cold laser, electrical stimulation, vibratory therapy, oscillation therapy, and aqua lymphatic therapy. All of these techniques are performed in combination with components of CDT. In particular, acupuncture has shown benefits for some symptoms of cancer and cancer treatment, including fatigue, hot flashes, muscular or joint pain, neuropathy, and nausea. There are no evidence-based studies on using acupuncture for treating LE or using acupuncture on LE extremities [43]. Cold/infrared lasers known as "low-power laser or low-level laser therapy (LLLT)" are typically between 5 and 500 mW, use nonthermal mechanisms (photochemical reactions), and can be used to deliver energy to tissues for a wide variety of rehabilitation purposes. Cold lasers can be applied either by handheld units (contact or noncontact devices) using spot application to specific anatomical surfaces or by scanning units in which LLLT is applied over a larger region. The nonthermal effects of LLLT include the stimulation of adenosine triphosphate production, the promotion of ribonucleic acid and collagen production, the modulation of inflammatory cytokines, the inhibition of bacterial growth, the promotion of vasodilatation and endothelial regeneration, the stimulation of fibroblast activity, the alteration of nerve conduction velocity, and the promotion of neural regeneration. LLLT was found to decrease the expression of pro-fibrotic transforming growth factor and type I collagen deposition in the rat tibialis anterior muscle after muscle lesion, suggesting that LLLT may be helpful in preventing tissue fibrosis. These data suggest that LLLT may provide benefit to patients with LE by increasing lymphatic flow through the encouragement of lymphangiogenesis, the stimulation of lymphatic motoricity, and the prevention of tissue fibrosis that could potentially further disrupt lymphatic function. Evidence suggests that a dose of 1–2 J/cm^2 per point applied to several points covering the fibrotic area can reduce limb volume following BCRL [61–63].

Risk Reduction and Guidelines

Physical activity (NCCN general principles):

- All cancer survivors should be encouraged to avoid inactivity or a sedentary lifestyle and to return to daily activities as soon as possible. Patients who are able should be encouraged to engage in daily physical activity.
- Physical activity and exercise recommendations should be tailored to the individual survivor's abilities and preferences.
- General recommendations for cancer survivors: The overall volume of weekly activity should be at least 150 min of moderate-intensity activity or 75 min of vigorous-intensity activity or an equivalent combination.
- Survivors should perform two to three sessions per week of strength training that includes major muscle groups.
- Major muscle groups should be stretched on days exercises are performed [48].

Recent studies in weight lifting, exercise, and weight loss have demonstrated benefits in the prevention of LE in at-risk patients and in patients with LE. A trial in which 154 breast cancer patients without BCRL were randomly assigned either a progressive weight lifting regimen or no activity found that significantly fewer patients developed BCRL in the lifting group (11 % v. 17 %, $p = 0.04$). These data have been confirmed by a randomized trial that found no increase in BCRL when patients (with lymphedema) began progressive weight lifting compared with no activity. Breast cancer survivors (at risk for lymphedema) who performed slowly progressive weight lifting twice weekly for 1 year were less likely to experience clinically significant increases in arm swelling than women in the control group. One study of LE onset among survivors at risk for BCRL compared a 1-year trial of slowly progressing weight lifting (the intervention) with no exercise (the control). The weight lifting did not result in an increased incidence of LE [64].

Physical Activity and LE (PAL) Trial

The PAL trial was a randomized controlled intervention study involving 295 women who had previously been treated for breast cancer. The trial evaluated the effect of twice-weekly progressive weight lifting during a 12-month period on LE status [65]. Four diagnostic methods were used to evaluate LE outcomes: (i) interlimb volume difference through water displacement, (ii) interlimb size difference through sum of arm circumferences, (iii) interlimb impedance ratio using bioimpedance spectroscopy, and (iv) a validated self-report survey. For the 71 women in the weight lifting group and the 70 women in the control group defined as having LE according to the PAL trial definition, the median time since LE diagnosis was 45 (1, 183) and 56 (2, 170) months, respectively. Approximately 40 % of these women had LE for between 1 and 3 years, whereas approximately 60 % had LE for more than 3 years [65]. Progressive weight lifting was shown to be safe for women following breast cancer, even for those at risk for or with LE.

Reducing Risk of BCRL

SLNB versus ALND: The incidence of BCRL is less after sentinel lymph node biopsy (SLNB) than after axillary lymph node dissection (ALND). The NSABP B-32 trial compared 3-year postsurgical morbidity levels of patients with negative SLNB alone and those with negative SLNB and ALND and reported that arm volume differences of more than 10 % at 36 months were evident for the ALND (14 %) and SLNB (8 %) groups ($P < 0.05$) [66]. IBCSG 23-01 is a randomized trial of axillary dissection vs. no axillary dissection for patients with clinically node-negative breast cancer and micrometastases in the sentinel node, and in this study, BCRL was 13 % after ALND and 3 % after SLNB at a median follow-up of 5.0 years [67]. A retrospective study evaluated the rates of lymphedema in mastectomy patients who received SLNB with RT relative to ALND with or without RT. Six hundred twenty-seven breast cancer patients who underwent mastectomies between 2005 and 2013 were prospectively screened for lymphedema with a median 22.8 months of follow-up (range 3.0–86.9). The 2-year cumulative lymphedema incidence was 10.0 % (95 % CI 2.6–34.4 %) for SLNB + RT compared with 19.3 % (95 % CI 10.8–33.1 %) for ALND-no RT and 30.1 % (95 % CI 23.7–37.8 %) for ALND + RT. The lowest cumulative incidence was 2.19 % (95 % CI 0.88–5.40 %) for SLNB-no RT. Multivariate analysis showed that factors significantly associated with increased LE risk included RT ($p = 0.0017$), ALND ($p = 0.0001$), and the number of lymph nodes removed ($p = 0.0006$) [68].

In the EORTC 10981-22023 AMAROS trial from Europe (a randomized, multicenter, open-label, phase 3 non-inferiority trial) patients were randomly assigned by a computer-generated allocation schedule to receive either ALND or axillary RT in the case of a positive SLNB.

Information on LE and arm circumference increases were collected from 98 % of 1,265 patients at baseline, 820 (65 %) of 1,255 patients at 1 year, 714 (62 %) of 1,154 patients at 3 years, and 614 (69 %) of 895 patients at 5 years. LE was noted significantly more often after ALND than after axillary RT at every measured timepoint. An increase in arm circumference of at least 10 % was reported in a numerically greater proportion of patients in the ALND group compared with the axillary RT group; however, the difference was only significant at 5 years. LE was significantly more frequently reported in this subgroup compared with patients who were treated with ALND or axillary RT only (13 % vs. 6 %, respectively) [69].

Axillary reverse mapping (ARM) is a new concept. The ARM technique has been developed to map and preserve arm lymphatic drainage during ALND and/or SLNB and to minimize arm LE. The arm and breast lymphatic drainage patterns can be visualized using blue dye or radioisotopes or with subdermal injection of indocyanine green (ICG) via photodynamic eye (Hamamatsu Photonics, Hamamatsu, Japan). This technique protects the lymphatic channels draining the upper extremity during ALND or SLNB via removal of only the breast lymphatic vessels. The hypothesis of the ARM procedure is based on mapping the lymphatic pathways of both the arm and breast and preserving the arm lymphatic drainage during ALND and/or SLNB. However, there are important drawbacks to the ARM procedure; the ARM nodes may be involved with metastatic foci in patients with extensive axillary lymph node metastases, or the SLNB draining of the breast may be the same as the ARM node draining of the upper extremity in a minority of patients. The success of ARM in reducing LE has not yet been determined, and ARM is not a standard procedure in the surgical management of breast cancer. Further, there are practical issues concerning the ARM procedure that remain to be resolved: (a) insufficient identification rates of the ARM nodes and/or lymphatic vessels as well as a persistent blue stain at the site of injection; (b) the ARM nodes may be involved with metastatic foci in patients with axillary lymph node metastases; and (c) the SLNB draining of the breast may be the same as the ARM node draining of the upper extremity in a minority of patients. Therefore, further studies are needed before this technology can be included as a standard procedure in breast cancer surgical management [8, 70].

Challenges and Conclusion

There is significant heterogeneity in the literature regarding the incidence, diagnosis, and management of BCRL. Diagnosis, treatment, and the level of awareness of BCRL are not standard among either patients or healthcare providers. There is varying information available regarding the risk factors of lymphedema. Treatments applied in breast cancer, patient records, and follow-up are not standardized (the extent and type of surgery: BCT, MRM, oncoplastic, AD, SLNB, RT ±), and even though there are many reported suggestions in the literature, there are no studies on universal recommendations. Recommendations are based on basic pathophysiological information but not on any prospective randomized study. During the decision-making process for each surgical, radiation, and chemotherapeutic procedure, the incidence of BCRL should be assessed. Newer diagnosis techniques, such as DEXA and BIS, demonstrate significant improvements relative to traditional techniques by providing additional quantitative standardized cutoffs values without observer variability, which increase the sensitivity of the detection of subclinical patients and accurately measure the extracellular fluid space. Treatment paradigms have evolved over the last decade. There is increasing support in the literature for the use of compression sleeves for subclinical disease, demonstrating excellent outcomes with minimal morbidity, and for the use of CDT in more advanced cases of BCRL. Long-term outcomes with treatment strategies are limited. Risk-reduction strategies need to incorporate treatment and individual patient risk factors that increase BCRL. These strategies must include proper surveillance and diagnosis to increase the number of patients diagnosed at early subclinical stages. Awareness is important to reduce the factors that affect lymphedema. Long-term research studies are required to investigate risk factors for the development of lymphedema in patients undergoing surgical or radiotherapy treatment. Relevant healthcare professionals, particularly within primary care and the specialties of oncology, palliative care, vascular surgery, genetics, and dermatology, as well as patients, should be aware of the signs and symptoms of LE. After diagnosis, appropriate referral pathways should be constructed for all relevant healthcare professionals with an adequate level of education regarding lymphological disorders and correct treatment.

Conclusion

The main objectives are reducing lymph production and preventing the blockage of lymph flow:

- Subclinical monitoring for early diagnosis and early initiation of therapy and prevention of transition to advanced stages.
- Supporting lymph flow: arm and shoulder exercises, massage, and elevation and avoiding bandages and clothing that are excessively tight.
- Guarding against infection: keep skin moist, avoid excessive sun and extreme cold, and avoid injury that disrupts the skin integrity.

Current findings:

- Early diagnosis and intervention prevents from advanced stage lymphedema.
- Exercise, massage, elevation and avoid tight clothing are important for lymph flow.
- Controlling weight: maintain normal healthy weight and perform regular exercise.
- Development of LE affects general well-being and patient quality of life.
- Exercise does not lead to an increase in LE but improves the quality of life due to the positive functional effect.
- Starting shoulder exercises is more effective in the first 48 h than after 7 days.
- Monitoring for LE with BIS and early physiotherapy: education and increased exercise programs.
- Physical therapy programs: manual lymphatic massage produces improvements.
- Scar tissue massage produces improvements.
- Relaxation therapy combined with exercise produces improvements.

Suggestions for preventing BCRL:

- Protection from sunburn.
- Infection prevention (manicures, skin incisions).
- Skin care and moisturizing.
- Avoiding heavy exercise, which may increase the blood flow in the arm and therefore the production of lymph.
- Avoiding tight clothing, which can disrupt the flow of lymph.
- Any compression garment must be provided by an experienced therapist. Otherwise, it may trigger LE through a tourniquet effect.
- Although there is no consensus regarding the prophylactic use of compression garments, their use for high-risk situations such as air travel is recommended.

References

1. Smoot BJ, Wong JF, Dodd MJ. Comparison of diagnostic accuracy of clinical measures of breast cancer-related lymphedema: area under the curve. Arch Phys Med Rehabil. 2011;92:603–10.
2. Cormier JN, Askew RL, Mungovan KS, Xing Y, Ross MI, Armer JM. Lymphedema beyond breast cancer: a systematic review and meta-analysis of cancer-related secondary lymphedema. Cancer. 2010;116:5138–49.
3. Hurlbert M, Hutchison NA, McGarvey CL, Rockson SG, Schonholz S, Vicini FA. White paper: recent advances in breast cancer related lymphedema. Proceedings from April 2011 Expert Panel. Accessed http://www.avonfoundation.org/assets/le-white-paper.pdf, 2/2/2015.
4. Tam EK, Shen L, Munneke JR, Ackerson LM, Partee PN, Somkin CP, et al. Clinician awareness and knowledge of breast cancer-related lymphedema in a large, integrated health care delivery setting. Breast Cancer Res Treat. 2012;131:1029–38.
5. Tsai RJ, Dennis LK, Lynch CF, Snetselaar LG, Zamba GK, Scott-Conner C. The risk of developing arm lymphedema among breast cancer survivors: a meta-analysis of treatment factors. Ann Surg Oncol. 2009;16:1959–72.
6. Guidelines for the diagnosis, assessment and management of lymphedema. Clinical Resource Efficacy Support Team (CREST), Feb 2008. www.crestni.org.uk (public domain) 2015.
7. International Society of Lymphology. The diagnosis and treatment of peripheral lymphedema: 2013 Consensus Document of the International Society of Lymphology. Lymphology. 2013;46:1–11.

8. Noguchi M. Axillary reverse mapping for breast cancer. Breast Cancer Res Treat. 2010;119:529–35.

9. Norman SA, Localio AR, Potashnik SL, Simoes Torpey HA, Kallan MJ, Weber AL, et al. Lymphedema in breast cancer survivors: incidence, degree, time course, treatment, and symptoms. J Clin Oncol. 2009;27:390–7.

10. Kwan ML, Darbinian J, Schmitz KH, Citron R, Partee P, Kutner SE, et al. Risk factors for lymphedema in a prospective breast cancer survivorship study: the Pathways Study. Arch Surg. 2010;145:1055–63.

11. Deutsch M, Land S, Begovic M, Sharif S. The incidence of arm edema in women with breast cancer randomized on the National Surgical Adjuvant Breast and Bowel Project study B-04 to radical mastectomy versus total mastectomy and radiotherapy versus total mastectomy alone. Int J Radiat Oncol Biol Phys. 2008;70:1020–4.

12. McLaughlin SA. Lymphedema: separating fact from fiction. Oncology (Williston Park). 2012;26:242–9.

13. Armer JM, Stewart BR. A comparison of four diagnostic criteria for lymphedema in a post-breast cancer population. Lymphat Res Biol. 2005;3:208–17.

14. Cornish BH, Chapman M, Hirst C, Mirolo B, Bunce IH, Ward LC, et al. Early diagnosis of lymphedema using multiple frequency bioimpedance. Lymphology. 2001;34:2–11.

15. Shah C, Vicini F, Beitsch P, Laidley A, Anglin B, Ridner SH, et al. The use of bioimpedance spectroscopy to monitor therapeutic intervention in patients treated for breast cancer related lymphedema. Lymphology. 2013;46:184–92.

16. Hayes SC, Janda M, Cornish B, Battistutta D, Newman B. Lymphedema after breast cancer: incidence, risk factors, and effect on upper body function. J Clin Oncol. 2008;26:3536–42.

17. Soran A, Ozmen T, McGuire KP, Diego EJ, McAuliffe PF, Bonaventura M, et al. The importance of detection of subclinical lymphedema for the prevention of breast cancer-related clinical lymphedema after axillary lymph node dissection; a prospective observational study. Lymphat Res Biol. 2014;12:289–94.

18. Mayrovitz HN, Davey S, Shapiro E. Local tissue water changes assessed by tissue dielectric constant: single measurements versus averaging of multiple measurements. Lymphology. 2008;41:186–8.

19. Clodius L, Deak L, Piller NB. A new instrument for the evaluation of tissue tonicity in lymphoedema. Lymphology. 1976;9:1–5.

20. Nuutinen J, Ikäheimo R, Lahtinen T. Validation of a new dielectric device to assess changes of tissue water in skin and subcutaneous fat. Physiol Meas. 2004;25:447–54.

21. Shukla HS, Gravelle IH, Hughes LE, Newcombe RG, Williams S. Mammary skin oedema: a new prognostic indicator for breast cancer. Br Med J (Clin Res Ed). 1984;288:1338–41.

22. Warszawski A, Röttinger EM, Vogel R, Warszawski N. 20 MHz ultrasonic imaging for quantitative assessment and documentation of early and late postradiation skin reactions in breast cancer patients. Radiother Oncol. 1998;47:241–7.

23. Mellor RH, Bush NL, Stanton AW, Bamber JC, Levick JR, Mortimer PS. Dual-frequency ultrasound examination of skin and subcutis thickness in breast cancer-related lymphedema. Breast J. 2004;10: 496–503.

24. Rönkä RH, Pamilo MS, von Smitten KA, Leidenius MH. Breast lymphedema after breast conserving treatment. Acta Oncol. 2004;43:551–7.

25. Devoogdt N, Pans S, De Groef A, Geraerts I, Christiaens MR, Neven P, et al. Postoperative evolution of thickness and echogenicity of cutis and subcutis of patients with and without breast cancer-related lymphedema. Lymphat Res Biol. 2014;12:23–31.

26. Idy-Peretti I, Bittoun J, Alliot FA, Richard SB, Querleux BG, Cluzan RV. Lymphedematous skin and subcutis: in vivo high resolution magnetic resonance imaging evaluation. J Invest Dermatol. 1998;110: 782–7.

27. Newman AL, Rosenthall L, Towers A, Hodgson P, Shay CA, Tidhar D, et al. Determining the precision of dual energy x-ray absorptiometry and bioelectric impedance spectroscopy in the assessment of breast cancer-related lymphedema. Lymphat Res Biol. 2013;11:104–9.

28. Clancy NT, Nilsson GE, Anderson CD, Leahy MJ. A new device for assessing changes in skin viscoelasticity using indentation and optical measurement. Skin Res Technol. 2010;16:210–28.

29. Marcenaro M, Sacco S, Pentimalli S, Berretta L, Andretta V, Grasso R, et al. Measures of late effects in conservative treatment of breast cancer with standard or hypofractionated radiotherapy. Tumori. 2004;90: 586–91.

30. Boccardo F, Casabona F, DeCian F, Friedman D, Murelli F, Puglisi M, et al. Lymphatic microsurgical preventing healing approach (LYMPHA) for primary surgical prevention of breast cancer-related lymphedema: over 4 years follow-up. Microsurgery. 2014; 34:421–4.

31. Weissleder H, Weissleder R. Lymphedema: evaluation of qualitative and quantitative lymphoscintigraphy in 238 patients. Radiology. 1988;167:729–35.

32. Szuba A, Shin WS, Strauss HW, Rockson S. The third circulation: radionuclide lymphoscintigraphy in the evaluation of lymphedema. J Nucl Med. 2003;44: 43–57.

33. Sharma R, Wendt JA, Rasmussen JC, Adams KE, Marshall MV, Sevick-Muraca EM. New horizons for imaging lymphatic function. Ann N Y Acad Sci. 2008;1131:13–36.

34. Aldrich MB, Guilliod R, Fife CE, Maus EA, Smith L, Rasmussen JC, et al. Lymphatic abnormalities in the normal contralateral arms of subjects with breast cancer-related lymphedema as assessed by near-infrared fluorescent imaging. Biomed Opt Express. 2012;3:1256–65.

35. Binkley JM, Harris SR, Levangie PK, Pearl M, Guglielmino J, Kraus V, et al. Patient perspectives on breast cancer treatment side effects and the prospective surveillance model for physical rehabilitation for women with breast cancer. Cancer. 2012;118: 2207–16.

36. Torres Lacomba M, Yuste Sánchez MJ, Zapico Goñi A, Prieto Merino D, Mayoral del Moral O, Cerezo Téllez E, et al. Effectiveness of early physiotherapy to prevent lymphoedema after surgery for breast cancer: randomised, single blinded, clinical trial. BMJ. 2010;340:b5396.

37. Ostby PL, Armer JM, Dale PS, Van Loo MJ, Wilbanks CL, Stewart BR. Surveillance recommendations in reducing risk of and optimally managing breast cancer-related lymphedema. J Personalized Med. 2014;4:424–47.

38. Stout Gergich NL, Pfalzer LA, McGarvey C, Springer B, Gerber LH, Soballe P. Preoperative assessment enables the early diagnosis and successful treatment of lymphedema. Cancer. 2008;112(12):2809–19.

39. Bevilacqua JL, Kattan MW, Changhong Y, Koifman S, Mattos IE, Koifman RJ, et al. Nomograms for predicting the risk of arm lymphedema after axillary dissection in breast cancer. Ann Surg Oncol. 2012;19:2580–9.

40. Tambour M, Tange B, Christensen R, Gram B. Effect of physical therapy on breast cancer related lymphedema: protocol for a multicenter, randomized, single-blind, equivalence trial. BMC Cancer. 2014;14:239.

41. Vignes S, Porcher R, Arrault M, Dupuy A. Long-term management of breast cancer-related lymphedema after intensive decongestive physiotherapy. Breast Cancer Res Treat. 2007;101:285–90.

42. Vignes S, Blanchard M, Arrault M, Porcher R. Intensive complete decongestive physiotherapy for cancer-related upper-limb lymphedema: 11 days achieved greater volume reduction than 4. Gynecol Oncol. 2013;131:127–30.

43. Screening and measurement for early detection of breast cancer related lymphedema. National Lymphedema Network (NLN) Position paper http://www.lymphnet.org/pdfDocs/nlnBCLE.pdf.

44. Shao Y, Qi K, Zhou QH, Zhong DS. Intermittent pneumatic compression pump for breast cancer-related lymphedema: a systematic review and meta-analysis of randomized controlled trials. Oncol Res Treat. 2014;37:170–4.

45. Uzkeser H, Karatay S, Erdemci B, Koc M, Senel K. Efficacy of manual lymphatic drainage and intermittent pneumatic compression pump use in the treatment of lymphedema after mastectomy: a randomized controlled trial. Breast Cancer. 2015;22(3):300–7.

46. Ridner SH, Murphy B, Deng J, Kidd N, Galford E, Bonner C, et al. A randomized clinical trial comparing advanced pneumatic truncal, chest, and arm treatment to arm treatment only in self-care of arm lymphedema. Breast Cancer Res Treat. 2012;131:147–58.

47. Ridner SH, Murphy B, Deng J, Kidd N, Galford E, Dietrich MS. Advanced pneumatic therapy in self-care of chronic lymphedema of the trunk. Lymphat Res Biol. 2010;8:209–15.

48. NCCN Guidelines for Supportive Care; Survivorship: http://www.nccn.org/professionals/physician_gls/pdf/survivorship.pdf. Accessed on 2 Feb 2015.

49. Baddour LM. Breast cellulitis complicating breast conservation therapy. J Intern Med. 1999;245:5–9.

50. Zippel D, Siegelmann-Danieli N, Ayalon S, Kaufman B, Pfeffer R, Zvi Papa M. Delayed breast cellulitis following breast conserving operation. Eur J Surg Oncol. 2003;29:327–30.

51. Dominick SA, Madlensky L, Natarajan L, Pierce JP. Risk factors associated with breast cancer-related lymphedema in the WHEL study. J Cancer Surviv. 2013;7:115–23.

52. Stigant A. Tackling obesity as part of a lymphoedema management programme. Br J Community Nurs. 2009;14:9–14.

53. Campisi C, Bellini C, Campisi C, Accogli S, Bonioli E, Boccardo F. Microsurgery for lymphedema: clinical research and long-term results. Microsurgery. 2010;30:256–60.

54. Campisi C, Davini D, Bellini C, Taddei G, Villa G, Fulcheri E, et al. Is there a role for microsurgery in the prevention of arm lymphedema secondary to breast cancer treatment? Microsurgery. 2006;26:70–2.

55. Patel KM, Lin CY, Cheng MH. A prospective evaluation of lymphedema-specific quality-of-life outcomes following vascularized lymph node transfer. Ann Surg Oncol. 2015;22(7):2424–30.

56. Aschen SZ, Farias-Eisner G, Cuzzone DA, Albano NJ, Ghanta S, Weitman ES, et al. Lymph node transplantation results in spontaneous lymphatic reconnection and restoration of lymphatic flow. Plast Reconstr Surg. 2014;133(2):301–10.

57. Viitanen TP, Visuri MT, Hartiala P, Mäki MT, Seppänen MP, Suominen EA, et al. Lymphatic vessel function and lymphatic growth factor secretion after microvascular lymph node transfer in lymphedema patients. Plast Reconstr Surg Glob Open. 2013;1:1–9.

58. Casley-Smith JR, Morgan RG, Piller NB. Treatment of lymphedema of the arms and legs with 5,6-benzo-[alpha]-pyrone. N Engl J Med. 1993;329:1158–63.

59. Loprinzi CL, Kugler JW, Sloan JA, Rooke TW, Quella SK, Novotny P, et al. Lack of effect of coumarin in women with lymphedema after treatment for breast cancer. N Engl J Med. 1999;340:346–50.

60. Micke O, Bruns F, Mücke R, Schäfer U, Glatzel M, DeVries AF, et al. Selenium in the treatment of radiation-associated secondary lymphedema. Int J Radiat Oncol Biol Phys. 2003;56:40–9.

61. Omar MT, Shaheen AA, Zafar H. A systematic review of the effect of low-level laser therapy in the management of breast cancer-related lymphedema. Support Care Cancer. 2012;20:2977–84.

62. Smoot B, Chiavola-Larson L, Lee J, Manibusan H, Allen DD. Effect of low-level laser therapy on pain

and swelling in women with breast cancer-related lymphedema: a systematic review and meta-analysis. J Cancer Surviv. 2015;9(2):287–304.

63. Dirican A, Andacoglu O, Johnson R, McGuire K, Mager L, Soran A. The short-term effects of low-level laser therapy in the management of breast-cancer-related lymphedema. Support Care Cancer. 2011;19:685–90.

64. Schmitz KH, Ahmed RL, Troxel AB, Cheville A, Lewis-Grant L, Smith R, et al. Weight-lifting for women at risk for breast cancer-related lymphedema: a randomized trial. JAMA. 2010;304:2699–705.

65. Hayes SC, Speck RM, Reimet E, Stark A, Schmitz KH. Does the effect of weight-lifting on lymphedema following breast cancer differ by diagnostic method: results from a randomized controlled trial. Breast Cancer Res Treat. 2011;130:227–34.

66. Ashikaga T, Krag DN, Land SR, Julian TB, Anderson SJ, Brown AM, National Surgical Adjuvant Breast, Bowel Project, et al. Morbidity results from the NSABP B-32 trial comparing sentinel lymph node dissection versus axillary dissection. J Surg Oncol. 2010;102:111–8.

67. Galimberti V, Cole BF, Zurrida S. Axillary dissection versus no axillary dissection in patients with sentinel-node micrometastases (IBCSG 23-01): a phase 3 randomised controlled trial. Lancet Oncol. 2013;14: 297–305.

68. Miller CL, Specht MC, Skolny MN. Risk of lymphedema after mastectomy: potential benefit of applying ACOSOG Z0011 protocol to mastectomy patients. Breast Cancer Res Treat. 2014;144:71–7.

69. Donker M, van Tienhoven G, Straver ME, Meijnen P, van de Velde CJ, Mansel RE, et al. Radiotherapy or surgery of the axilla after a positive sentinel node in breast cancer (EORTC 10981-22023 AMAROS): a randomised, multicentre, open-label, phase 3 non-inferiority trial. Lancet Oncol. 2014;15:1303–10.

70. Ochoa D, Korourian S, Boneti C, Adkins L, Badgwell B, Klimberg VS. Axillary reverse mapping: five-year experience. Surgery. 2014;156:1261–8.

Reproductive Issues in Breast Cancer

49

Ercan Bastu and Faruk Buyru

Abstract

In this chapter, our aim is to present associations between the risk of developing breast cancer and reproductive issues, breast cancer treatment and fetal effects during pregnancy, and finally evidence regarding the effect of breast cancer treatments on fertility and potential fertility preservation methods. Strong evidence regarding reproductive risks exists for hormone (estrogen and/or progesterone) receptor-positive (HR+) breast cancers. Specifically, plausible data in the literature suggest significant associations between HR-positive breast cancers and nulliparity, current hormone use, and age at first birth. If breast cancer is detected during pregnancy, termination of the pregnancy does not necessarily improve the cancer prognosis. Breast cancer during pregnancy must be managed with a multidisciplinary approach that should follow standard protocols for nonpregnant patients as much as possible while considering the safety of the fetus. Various assisted reproductive technology (ART) approaches are available for breast cancer patients who wish to preserve fertility after cancer treatment. These approaches can be utilized before or after the initiation of adjuvant breast cancer treatment. Hence, adequate counseling should be provided to premenopausal breast cancer patients prior to cancer treatment. If the patient wishes to preserve her fertility, her chances must be optimized by providing the most suitable ART treatment via a multidisciplinary approach.

E. Bastu, MD • F. Buyru, MD (✉)
Department of Obstetrics and Gynecology,
Istanbul University School of Medicine,
Capa, Istanbul 34093, Turkey
e-mail: dr.ercanbastu@yahoo.com;
farukbuyru@gmail.com

© Springer International Publishing Switzerland 2016
A. Aydiner et al. (eds.), *Breast Disease: Management and Therapies*,
DOI 10.1007/978-3-319-26012-9_49

Keywords

Reproduction • Breast cancer • Hormone receptor positive • Human epidermal receptor 2 protein • Triple-negative breast cancer • Parity • Breastfeeding • Menstruation • Hormone use • Ovulation induction • Infertility • Assisted reproductive technologies • Fertility drugs • In vitro fertilization • In vitro maturation • BRCA mutation • Preimplantation genetic diagnosis • Pregnancy • Cytotoxic treatment • Chemotherapy • Radiotherapy • Bisphosphonates • Trastuzumab • Bevacizumab • Oocyte cryopreservation • Oocyte tissue cryopreservation • Embryo cryopreservation • Fertility preservation • Oncofertility

Introduction

Of the 805,500 women diagnosed with cancer in 2013, 20–30 % were younger than 45 years of age [1]. Generally, cancer can have detrimental effects on the future fertility and pregnancies of women in adolescence or their reproductive years.

In addition to the age and family history of the patient, developing breast cancer is also associated with reproductive issues, which can be characterized as the exposure to sex hormones. When a patient is diagnosed with breast cancer during pregnancy, treatment is possible. However, treatment should be administered using a multidisciplinary approach. In the developed world, there is a trend toward delaying childbirth to later years of reproductive age. Infertility is a risk faced by breast cancer patients undergoing cancer treatment. Hence, preservation of the fertility of breast cancer survivors of reproductive age has become an important factory in their quality of life after cancer.

In this chapter, our aim is to present associations between the risk of developing breast cancer and reproductive issues, breast cancer treatment and fetal effects during pregnancy, evidence regarding the effect of breast cancer treatments on fertility and potential fertility preservation methods.

Reproductive Risk Factors in Breast Cancers

Given recent advances in medical technology, it is now possible to perform molecular testing to subcategorize breast tumors to personalize the cancer treatment regimen according to the specific needs of the patients. Hence, the associations in the chapter will be covered according to the breast tumor subtypes. The subtypes will be evaluated in three main categories: (1) breast tumors that are hormone (estrogen and/or progesterone) receptor positive (HR+); (2) breast tumors that overexpress the human epidermal receptor 2 protein (HER2+); and (3) breast tumors that lack three markers (estrogen, progesterone, HER2+), which is also referred to as triple-negative breast cancer (TNBC). Evaluating potential associations at the subtype level is vital to advance the understanding of breast cancer's etiology and enable clinicians to establish personalized breast cancer treatment regimens.

Reproductive Risks in HR-Positive Breast Cancers

Parity

According to the currently available literature, the risk of developing HR-positive breast cancers exhibits the strongest association with parity [2–18]. In TNBC, the evidence is not as strong as that observed in HR-positive breast cancers because only few studies have reported a potential association [16, 19, 20]. The literature on HER-positive breast cancers is even more limited. One cohort study documented that women with at least one child exhibited a decreased risk of developing HER-positive breast cancers compared with women with no children [16].

Breastfeeding

Data on the association between the risk of developing HR-positive breast cancers and lactation history are more limited compared with parity. Nevertheless, a few studies indicated a significant, inverse association between the risk of developing HR-positive breast cancers and lactation history [2, 13, 14, 16].

Menstruation

Menstruation characteristics are associated with the risk of developing HR-positive breast cancer, especially for patients with a younger age at menarche [2, 3, 11–14, 16, 17, 21, 22]. Menopause at an older age is only associated with risk of developing HR-positive breast cancer in a few studies [2, 18, 22].

Hormone Use

Related literature suggests that current hormone usage is associated with an increased risk of developing HR-positive breast cancer [12, 22, 23]. Previous hormone usage does not have a similar strong association; only one study to date has reported a significant association [2].

Reproductive Risks in HER2-Positive Breast Cancers

Current literature on reproductive risks in HER2-positive breast cancers is somewhat limited. One study argued that women who had a single child exhibited a significantly decreased risk of developing HER2-positive breast cancers compared

with nulliparous women [16]. The same study suggested that breastfeeding was inversely associated with the risk of developing HER2-positive breast cancers. Another case-control study confirmed this finding [13]. The literature on hormone use and HER2-positive breast cancers is inconclusive [8, 22, 24].

Reproductive Risks in Triple-Negative Breast Cancer

Similar to HER2-positive breast cancers, the literature on reproductive risks in TNBCs is limited. Whereas several studies indicated a strong inverse relationship between parity and risk of developing HR-positive breast cancers, only a few studies indicated such a relationship in TNBCs [19, 20]. Breastfeeding was inversely associated with the risk of developing TNBCs [4, 5, 13, 16, 22]. Likewise, age at menarche has an inverse association with the risk of developing HER2-positive breast cancers [13, 18, 19]. Regarding hormone use, only one study documented a significant association with current use and not previous use [22].

Infertility Treatments and Breast Cancer

Some studies have evaluated whether assisted reproductive technology (ART) treatments increase the risk of breast cancer as well as other types of cancers. In one multicenter case-control study, the use of fertility drugs did not increase the risk of developing breast cancer, with the exception of long-term use of human menopausal gonadotropin (hMG) [25]. In a Swedish cohort study on 24,058 women who underwent in vitro fertilization (IVF) of whom 1,279 also had a diagnosis of cancer, a reduced risk of developing breast cancer was noted, and this result was even more significant in participants with a history of multiple birth delivery [26]. In a Danish cohort study of

54,362 women who commonly used clomiphene as an ovulation induction agent, a significant association was not noted between developing breast cancer and ovulation-inducing agents [27]. In a meta-analysis that included 22 studies, a significant association between developing breast cancer and ovulation-inducting agents was not documented [28].

Pregnancy During Breast Cancer

Similar to nonpregnant women, breast cancer in pregnant women presents as a palpable mass, changes in skin, and/or bloody nipple discharge. However, these symptoms are occasionally confused with the physiological changes experienced during pregnancy [29, 30]. As more women participate in the workforce and obtain an education, they tend to defer childbearing, especially in developed countries. Because the incidence of several cancers increases with age, facing breast and other cancers during pregnancy has become a more frequent occurrence.

Treatment of Breast Cancer During Pregnancy

Breast cancer treatment strategies during pregnancy depend on several factors, such as the tumor biology and stage, gestational week, and the goals of the mother and the father. Because this condition is a complex issue, counseling is imperative. A multidisciplinary approach to counseling is beneficial. Such a team might include obstetrics, oncological, psychological, and pediatric specialists.

Termination of Pregnancy

When a patient is diagnosed with breast cancer during pregnancy, her choices determine the course of action to continue the pregnancy [31]. The patient and her partner should be well informed regarding potential treatment options, and it should be noted that the termination of pregnancy does not necessarily improve the maternal outcome [32]. However, the continuation or termination of pregnancy is the decision of the patient.

A few studies in the literature have documented that the survival rate is decreased for a patient who chooses pregnancy termination compared with a patient who chooses to continue the pregnancy [33, 34]. However, in both studies, the cancer stage was not matched between the termination and continuation groups, thus creating a clear bias. Clinicians are likely more inclined to recommend pregnancy termination to patients with poor prognosis, which might serve as a possible explanation for the bias.

Breast Cancer Surgery During Pregnancy

If breast cancer surgery is chosen as the treatment approach, the use of anesthetic agents is safe for the fetus at any gestational age [35–37]. However, a multidisciplinary approach is beneficial. Such a team should consist of surgeons, obstetricians, pediatricians, and anesthesiologists. Some potential concerns include infections, hypotension, hypoglycemia, thrombosis, or hypoxia because these factors may have detrimental effects on the fetus. It is advisable for surgeons to utilize fetal heart rate monitoring to monitor fetal distress. If the patient feels pain, it can trigger preterm labor. Hence, adequate usage of analgesia is of the utmost importance. Tocometry can be performed postoperatively to evaluate uterine activity that was potentially masked by analgesia [29]. Given the risk of thrombosis, a low molecular weight heparin for thromboprophylaxis should be considered.

In a study that included 67 breast cancer surgeries during pregnancy, only a few complications were documented [38]. If the patient wants breast reconstruction, reconstruction should be considered after the delivery due to physiological changes during and after pregnancy [39].

Lymph node staging appears to be safe during pregnancy [40–43]. The absorbed doses of sulfur colloid into the breast are estimated to be 0.00045 Gy [44], which is considerably less than the fetal threshold of 0.1–0.2 Gy [41, 43]. However, the use of dye may result in an anaphylactic maternal reaction that can cause distress to the fetus; thus, dyes should be not be used during the pregnancy [45]. For lymph node biopsies during pregnancy, technetium-based identification has been used with success [40]. Instead of a 2-day protocol, a low-dose 1-day protocol may be preferred.

Cytotoxic Treatment During Pregnancy

The administration of cytotoxic treatments during pregnancy has varying effects depending on the gestational age of the patient. If treatment is undertaken during the period of fertilization and implantation, it will most likely be an "all-or-nothing" event. Depending on how many omnipotent stem cells survive, a healthy embryo will develop, or a miscarriage will occur. During organogenesis, congenital malformations may occur in the fetus. During the second and third trimesters of pregnancy, fetal anomalies will likely not occur during fetal maturation and growth. However, growth restriction, prematurity, and intrauterine death may occur during these trimesters [46]. The long-term outcome of cytotoxic exposure is not reported in the literature. However, genetic anomalies, carcinogenesis, and neurodevelopmental problems may theoretically occur [42, 46].

Chemotherapy is typically utilized in breast cancer patients, especially in young patients. If the patient is pregnant, the gestational age should be considered along with the timing of surgery and the potential requirement of radiotherapy. It is preferable to utilize chemotherapy after the first trimester. Adjuvant or neoadjuvant therapy may be used. Various clinicians have used weekly epirubicin given its fetal safety [47]. However, epirubicin is not a standard chemotherapy for the treatment of breast cancer. Dose-intensified chemotherapy treatments are beneficial to TNBC patients with increased disease-free rates [48]. TNBC is frequently observed in pregnant women. However, the literature regarding the use of dose-intensified chemotherapy during pregnancy is lacking. Regardless of the treatment used, it is prudent to calculate the drug dosage based on the current weight and constantly modify the dose as the weight of the patient increases during the pregnancy [29].

For the safety of the fetus, chemotherapy is not indicated until week 10 of gestation. The short-term outcomes of such exposure, including congenital malformations, appear to be safe [32, 47, 49–56]. Fetal growth restriction has been documented as a result of chemotherapy exposure due to cancer in general [46]. However, in studies that focused on breast cancer treatment during pregnancy, this growth restriction was not identified [55].

Only a few studies regarding the long-term outcomes of exposure to chemotherapy are available. In one study with a follow-up period of 19 years, no congenital or neurological anomalies were identified [57]. In another study, only 2 of 57 children experienced developmental problems [53]. In a study of 70 children exposed to chemotherapy, their general health was similar to the age-matched population [58]. In this study, prematurity was frequently documented. Hence, iatrogenic preterm delivery should be avoided whenever possible.

Bisphosphonates and Hormonal Agents During Pregnancy

In premenopausal breast cancer patients, the use of bisphosphonates combined with endocrine therapy appears to be effective [59]. However, bisphosphonates have not been utilized in pregnant breast cancer patients to date. In pregnant animal studies, maternal toxicity, skeletal retardation, fetal underdevelopment, and hypocalcemia have been documented [60]. Hence, the use of bisphosphonates is not indicated during pregnancy. The US Food and Drug Administration (FDA) has rated bisphosphonates as a category C pregnancy risk.

Bisphosphonates can remain in mineralized bone for many years. Thus, if patients use these agents before conception and/or during pregnancy, a teratogenic risk is possible. However, studies on breast cancer patients who received bisphosphonates prior to conception and during pregnancy did not document a significant increase in the risk of forming malformations or changes in fetal bone modeling [61]. If the breast cancer patient uses bisphosphonates during pregnancy, hypocalcemia should be avoided if possible because it can negatively affect uterine contractility.

Any hormonal agents (e.g., selective estrogen receptor modulators) should not be utilized during the pregnancy because they can potentially alter the hormonal environment. According to the available evidence, tamoxifen may cause fetal harm, including ambiguous genitalia, craniofacial malformations, and fetal death [62]. Hence, its usage should be avoided during pregnancy. Similarly, aromatase inhibitors should not be used in premenopausal patients who are pregnant.

Targeted Therapy During Pregnancy

Because HER2 is expressed in the fetal renal epithelium [63], long-term administration of trastuzumab may cause renal failure or fetal death in HER2-positive breast cancer patients [64]. Hence, the use of trastuzumab is not recommended in pregnant HER2-positive breast cancer patients. However, short-term usage of trastuzumab appears to be less toxic because renal function is recovered upon the withdrawal of the drug in the children who survive [29]. More recent breast cancer treatment agents, such as tyrosine and bevacizumab kinase inhibitors, have not been adequately studied in pregnant patient groups. Their usage in the pregnant women with breast cancer may be considered after the results of an adequate number of well-designed studies are available.

Fertility After Breast Cancer

Premenopausal patients with breast cancer who have delayed pregnancy or want more children in the future may want to preserve their ovarian function after breast cancer treatment or be curious as to how treatment will affect their fertility. These concerns are valid because the treatment of breast cancer may increase the risk of infertility in several patients.

Per clinical routine, premenopausal patients who are diagnosed with breast cancer currently receive an adjuvant therapy. This therapy consists of cytotoxic chemotherapy; (surgical, irradiation, and chemical) all describe ovarian suppression, antiestrogen therapy, or a combination of the abovementioned therapies. The use of adjuvant

therapy with the abovementioned approaches significantly improves the survival rate of premenopausal breast cancer patients. However, patients must also address toxicity, which can cause early menopause and infertility. For example, cytotoxic chemotherapy agents may have detrimental effects on the germ cells of the ovary, which can lead to premature ovarian failure (POF) in premenopausal patients with breast cancer [65–68]. Hence, the preservation of fertility has become an important aspect of the quality of life after cancer in premenopausal patients who have survived breast cancer. Fertility preservation in cancer survivors of reproductive age has created a new subfield in reproductive medicine [69], which is referred to as "oncofertility" by some researchers.

Fertility Preservation Options in Breast Cancer Patients

For patients who have survived breast cancer or were recently diagnosed with breast cancer, the American Society of Clinical Oncology recommends exploring fertility outcomes and obtaining a referral to an infertility subspecialist [70]. The fertility preservation approach will depend on the age of the patient and the urgency of the adjuvant treatment for the recently diagnosed patient [71, 72].

With the introduction of more effective adjuvant treatments in the field of oncology, more patients with breast cancer are surviving. Hence, the desire to become pregnant after surviving cancer has become a real concern for many premenopausal breast cancer patients. Based on the current clinical routine, various options are available that can preserve fertility in premenopausal breast cancer patients who must address potential POF. These options include ART, such as IVF, in vitro maturation (IVM), and oocyte or ovarian tissue or embryo cryopreservation [73–89].

In 1992, a patient who was infertile due to radical mastectomy for breast cancer gave birth to a healthy baby via ovarian stimulation and IVF [78]. However, because increased levels of estrogen may trigger dissemination and proliferation of breast cancer cells, several oncologists do not recommend ovarian stimulation protocols for breast cancer survivors [85]. By foregoing ovarian stimulation, natural cycle IVF treatment along with embryo cryopreservation has been the preferred approach in breast cancer patients who have a partner at the time of the treatment. Interestingly, tamoxifen, an agent that is frequently used in breast cancer patients, has been utilized in infertile patients who are anovulatory as well [80]. However, tamoxifen is not regularly used in ovarian stimulation protocols in IVF. In a study of breast cancer patients, ovarian stimulation with tamoxifen was compared with natural cycle for IVF treatment [81]. The number of embryos achieved in the group that received tamoxifen was significantly increased compared with the group in which the natural cycle was utilized. Ovarian stimulation with tamoxifen increased estradiol levels. However, because tamoxifen has suppressive effects, this agent may reduce the risk of breast cancer. In another study by the same researchers [82], breast cancer patients were divided into three groups: one group received tamoxifen alone, a second group received tamoxifen with a low-dose follicle-stimulating hormone (FSH), and the final group received tamoxifen with low-dose FSH and an aromatase inhibitor (letrozole). The researchers reported that tamoxifen in combination with FSH and/or FSH in combination with letrozole significantly increased the number of embryos. However, the researchers argued that tamoxifen alone might be the preferred protocol because it leads to a lower increase in estrogen levels. In a more recent study, the usage of short-term gonadotropins and aromatase inhibitors as ovarian stimulation agents is safe in breast cancer patients prior to the administration of adjuvant treatment for breast cancer [86].

If IVF will be utilized after the breast cancer patient has received adjuvant treatment, the safety period remains poorly established. Various studies have documented no significant increase in congenital malformations using IVF after adjuvant therapies in breast cancer survivors [90, 91]. However, until a safety period is well defined, it would be prudent to evaluate all fetuses cytogenetically. However, embryo cryopreservation before receiving adjuvant treatments appears to be the most preferred fertility preservation approach in premenopausal breast cancer patients. Oocyte and/or oocyte tissue cryopreservation may be an option for breast cancer patients who do not have a partner at the time of treatment or who do not wish to use a sperm donor or cannot use a sperm donor due to legal issues in the country in which she resides. Evidence suggests that embryo and/or oocyte cryopreservation after ovarian stimulation provides the best chance for fertility preservation [92]. Ovarian tissue cryopreservation may be an option for breast cancer patients who do not want to receive ovarian stimulation or have limited time before the initiation of adjuvant treatment because ovarian stimulation typically requires 10–14 days. A live birth was documented after orthotopic autotransplantation of cryopreserved ovarian tissue in one study [76]. A more recent study argued that the transplantation of cryopreserved ovarian tissue should no longer be regarded as an experimental treatment [77]. Especially in young breast cancer patients who will receive adjuvant treatment, ovarian tissue cryopreservation serves as an interesting option. In addition, IVM is also a promising option in such groups because it significantly improves the oocyte outcome [83]. The use of IVM before oocyte or embryo cryopreservation achieved pregnancy rates of 3.8 % and 8.1 %, respectively, in one study [93]. Another recent approach involves the use of ovarian tissue cryopreservation in combination with immature oocyte collection from the tissue followed by oocyte vitrification via IVM in fertility preservation, specifically in younger breast cancer patients [74]. However, the risk of cryopreserving malignant cells that can be potentially transferred back to the patient during reimplantation is always a concern. Hence, it would be prudent to develop screening using immunohistochemical markers. Leukemia is an example of a cancer with a high risk of malignant cell reimplantation. Hence, it is vital to screen for residual disease before ovarian tissue re-transplantation, especially in patients with hematologic cancers [75].

Recent advances in the fields of oncology and reproductive medicine have created several options for breast cancer patients who wish to preserve their fertility. However, hurdles must still be overcome. For example, the management of patients with BRCA mutations remains a challenge. Preimplantation genetic diagnosis during IVF treatment can serve as one alternative to prevent the transmittance of the mutation to the offspring in such patients [87]. Moreover, prenatal diagnosis after implantation can be performed. Consequently, a patient may decide to continue the pregnancy if the fetus is not a carrier of the mutation. Of course, there is an ongoing debate on the ethical concerns and wishes of the patients regarding the usage of such methods [94–96].

Summary of Findings

Strong evidence on reproductive risks exists for HR-positive breast cancers. Specifically, plausible data suggest significant associations between HR-positive breast cancers and nulliparity, current hormone use, and age at first birth. The limited data on HER-positive breast cancers do not reveal a strong association with any potential reproductive risk. There is also limited literature available on TNBCs compared with HR-positive breast cancers. The most consistent finding from these studies involves the inverse association between breastfeeding and the risk of developing TNBCs. Because the TNBC subtype is aggressive in nature, there is a definite need for studies to better characterize this subtype.

If breast cancer is detected during pregnancy, termination of pregnancy does not necessarily improve the prognosis of the cancer. Breast cancer during pregnancy must be managed with a multidisciplinary approach that should follow standard protocols for nonpregnant patients as much as possible while considering the safety of the fetus. Several clinicians suggest that the usage of chemotherapy and radiotherapy is safe during pregnancy in breast cancer patients. However, studies that focus on the long-term outcome of children exposed to such treatments are urgently needed to confirm such recommendations. Premature birth will lead to a negative outcome and should be avoided as much as possible in breast cancer patients.

Various ART approaches are available for breast cancer patients who wish to their preserve fertility after cancer treatment. These approaches can be utilized before or after the initiation of adjuvant treatment for breast cancer. Hence, adequate counseling should be provided to premenopausal breast cancer patients prior to cancer treatment. If the patient wishes to preserve her fertility, her chances must be optimized by providing the most suitable ART treatment for her via a multidisciplinary approach.

References

1. Siegel R, Naishadham D, Jemal A. Cancer statistics, 2013. CA Cancer J Clin. 2013;63:11–30.
2. Bao PP, Shu XO, Gao YT, Zheng Y, Cai H, Deming SL, et al. Association of hormone-related characteristics and breast cancer risk by estrogen receptor/progesterone receptor status in the shanghai breast cancer study. Am J Epidemiol. 2011;174:661–71.
3. Chung S, Park SK, Sung H, Song N, Han W, Noh DY, et al. Association between chronological change of reproductive factors and breast cancer risk defined by hormone receptor status: results from the Seoul Breast Cancer Study. Breast Cancer Res Treat. 2013;140:557–65.
4. Gaudet MM, Press MF, Haile RW, Lynch CF, Glaser SL, Schildkraut J, et al. Risk factors by molecular subtypes of breast cancer across a population-based study of women 56 years or younger. Breast Cancer Res Treat. 2011;130:587–97.
5. Li CI, Beaber EF, Tang MT, Porter PL, Daling JR, Malone KE. Reproductive factors and risk of estrogen receptor positive, triple-negative, and HER2-neu overexpressing breast cancer among women 20–44 years of age. Breast Cancer Res Treat. 2013;137:579–87.
6. Li CI, Malone KE, Daling JR, Potter JD, Bernstein L, Marchbanks PA, et al. Timing of menarche and first full-term birth in relation to breast cancer risk. Am J Epidemiol. 2008;167:230–9.
7. Ma H, Bernstein L, Pike MC, Ursin G. Reproductive factors and breast cancer risk according to joint estrogen and progesterone receptor status: a meta-analysis of epidemiological studies. Breast Cancer Res BCR. 2006;8:R43.
8. Ma H, Henderson KD, Sullivan-Halley J, Duan L, Marshall SF, Ursin G, et al. Pregnancy-related factors and the risk of breast carcinoma in situ and invasive breast cancer among postmenopausal women in the California Teachers Study cohort. Breast Cancer Res BCR. 2010;12:R35.
9. Palmer JR, Boggs DA, Wise LA, Ambrosone CB, Adams-Campbell LL, Rosenberg L. Parity and lactation

in relation to estrogen receptor negative breast cancer in African American women. Cancer Epidemiol Biomark Prev Publ Am Assoc Cancer Res Cosponsored Am Soc Prev Oncol. 2011;20:1883–91.

10. Phipps AI, Buist DS, Malone KE, Barlow WE, Porter PL, Kerlikowske K, et al. Reproductive history and risk of three breast cancer subtypes defined by three biomarkers. Cancer Causes Control CCC. 2011;22:399–405.

11. Ritte R, Tikk K, Lukanova A, Tjonneland A, Olsen A, Overvad K, et al. Reproductive factors and risk of hormone receptor positive and negative breast cancer: a cohort study. BMC Cancer. 2013;13:584.

12. Setiawan VW, Monroe KR, Wilkens LR, Kolonel LN, Pike MC, Henderson BE. Breast cancer risk factors defined by estrogen and progesterone receptor status: the multiethnic cohort study. Am J Epidemiol. 2009;169:1251–9.

13. Trivers KF, Lund MJ, Porter PL, Liff JM, Flagg EW, Coates RJ, et al. The epidemiology of triple-negative breast cancer, including race. Cancer Causes Control CCC. 2009;20:1071–82.

14. Warner ET, Colditz GA, Palmer JR, Partridge AH, Rosner BA, Tamimi RM. Reproductive factors and risk of premenopausal breast cancer by age at diagnosis: are there differences before and after age 40? Breast Cancer Res Treat. 2013;142:165–75.

15. Warner ET, Tamimi RM, Boggs DA, Rosner B, Rosenberg L, Colditz GA, et al. Estrogen receptor positive tumors: do reproductive factors explain differences in incidence between black and white women? Cancer Causes Control CCC. 2013;24:731–9.

16. Xing P, Li J, Jin F. A case-control study of reproductive factors associated with subtypes of breast cancer in Northeast China. Med Oncol. 2010;27:926–31.

17. Yang XR, Chang-Claude J, Goode EL, Couch FJ, Nevanlinna H, Milne RL, et al. Associations of breast cancer risk factors with tumor subtypes: a pooled analysis from the Breast Cancer Association Consortium studies. J Natl Cancer Inst. 2011;103:250–63.

18. Yang XR, Sherman ME, Rimm DL, Lissowska J, Brinton LA, Peplonska B, et al. Differences in risk factors for breast cancer molecular subtypes in a population-based study. Cancer Epidemiol Biomark Prev Publ Am Assoc Cancer Res Cosponsored Am Soc Prev Oncol. 2007;16:439–43.

19. Millikan RC, Newman B, Tse CK, Moorman PG, Conway K, Dressler LG, et al. Epidemiology of basal-like breast cancer. Breast Cancer Res Treat. 2008;109:123–39.

20. Phipps AI, Chlebowski RT, Prentice R, McTiernan A, Wactawski-Wende J, Kuller LH, et al. Reproductive history and oral contraceptive use in relation to risk of triple-negative breast cancer. J Natl Cancer Inst. 2011;103:470–7.

21. Islam T, Matsuo K, Ito H, Hosono S, Watanabe M, Iwata H, et al. Reproductive and hormonal risk factors for luminal, HER2-overexpressing, and triple-negative breast cancer in Japanese women. Ann Oncol Off J Eur Soc Med Oncol/ESMO. 2012;23:2435–41.

22. Tamimi RM, Colditz GA, Hazra A, Baer HJ, Hankinson SE, Rosner B, et al. Traditional breast cancer risk factors in relation to molecular subtypes of breast cancer. Breast Cancer Res Treat. 2012;131:159–67.

23. Ritte R, Lukanova A, Berrino F, Dossus L, Tjonneland A, Olsen A, et al. Adiposity, hormone replacement therapy use and breast cancer risk by age and hormone receptor status: a large prospective cohort study. Breast Cancer Res BCR. 2012;14:R76.

24. Dolle JM, Daling JR, White E, Brinton LA, Doody DR, Porter PL, et al. Risk factors for triple-negative breast cancer in women under the age of 45 years. Cancer Epidemiol Biomark Prev Publ Am Assoc Cancer Res Cosponsored Am Soc Prev Oncol. 2009;18:1157–66.

25. Burkman RT, Tang MT, Malone KE, Marchbanks PA, McDonald JA, Folger SG, et al. Infertility drugs and the risk of breast cancer: findings from the National Institute of Child Health and Human Development Women's Contraceptive and Reproductive Experiences Study. Fertil Steril. 2003;79:844–51.

26. Kallen B, Finnstrom O, Lindam A, Nilsson E, Nygren KG, Olausson PO. Malignancies among women who gave birth after in vitro fertilization. Hum Reprod. 2011;26:253–8.

27. Jensen A, Sharif H, Svare EI, Frederiksen K, Kjaer SK. Risk of breast cancer after exposure to fertility drugs: results from a large Danish cohort study. Cancer Epidemiol Biomark Prev Publ Am Assoc Cancer Res Cosponsored Am Soc Prev Oncol. 2007;16:1400–7.

28. Zreik TG, Mazloom A, Chen Y, Vannucci M, Pinnix CC, Fulton S, et al. Fertility drugs and the risk of breast cancer: a meta-analysis and review. Breast Cancer Res Treat. 2010;124:13–26.

29. Amant F, Deckers S, Van Calsteren K, Loibl S, Halaska M, Brepoels L, et al. Breast cancer in pregnancy: recommendations of an international consensus meeting. Eur J Cancer. 2010;46:3158–68.

30. Sorosky JI, Scott-Conner CE. Breast disease complicating pregnancy. Obstet Gynecol Clin North Am. 1998;25:353–63.

31. Ives A, Musiello T, Saunders C. The experience of pregnancy and early motherhood in women diagnosed with gestational breast cancer. Psychooncology. 2012;21:754–61.

32. Cardonick E, Dougherty R, Grana G, Gilmandyar D, Ghaffar S, Usmani A. Breast cancer during pregnancy: maternal and fetal outcomes. Cancer J. 2010;16:76–82.

33. Nugent P, O'Connell TX. Breast cancer and pregnancy. Arch Surg. 1985;120:1221–4.

34. Zemlickis D, Lishner M, Degendorfer P, Panzarella T, Burke B, Sutcliffe SB, et al. Maternal and fetal outcome after breast cancer in pregnancy. Am J Obstet Gynecol. 1992;166:781–7.

35. Cohen-Kerem R, Railton C, Oren D, Lishner M, Koren G. Pregnancy outcome following non-obstetric surgical intervention. Am J Surg. 2005;190:467–73.

36. Moran BJ, Yano H, Al Zahir N, Farquharson M. Conflicting priorities in surgical intervention for cancer in pregnancy. Lancet Oncol. 2007;8:536–44.

37. Ni Mhuireachtaigh R, O'Gorman DA. Anesthesia in pregnant patients for nonobstetric surgery. J Clin Anesth. 2006;18:60–6.

38. Dominici LS, Kuerer HM, Babiera G, Hahn KM, Perkins G, Middleton L, et al. Wound complications from surgery in pregnancy-associated breast cancer (PABC). Breast Dis. 2010;31:1–5.

39. Gumus N. Severe influence of early pregnancy on newly reconstructed breast. Breast. 2008;17:429–31.

40. Gentilini O, Cremonesi M, Toesca A, Colombo N, Peccatori F, Sironi R, et al. Sentinel lymph node biopsy in pregnant patients with breast cancer. Eur J Nucl Med Mol Imaging. 2010;37:78–83.

41. Gentilini O, Cremonesi M, Trifiro G, Ferrari M, Baio SM, Caracciolo M, et al. Safety of sentinel node biopsy in pregnant patients with breast cancer. Ann Oncol Off J Eur Soc Med Oncol/ESMO. 2004;15:1348–51.

42. Kal HB, Struikmans H. Radiotherapy during pregnancy: fact and fiction. Lancet Oncol. 2005;6:328–33.

43. Keleher A, Wendt 3rd R, Delpassand E, Stachowiak AM, Kuerer HM. The safety of lymphatic mapping in pregnant breast cancer patients using Tc-99m sulfur colloid. Breast J. 2004;10:492–5.

44. Ellner SJ, Hoh CK, Vera DR, Darrah DD, Schulteis G, Wallace AM. Dose-dependent biodistribution of [(99m)Tc]DTPA-mannosyl-dextran for breast cancer sentinel lymph node mapping. Nucl Med Biol. 2003;30:805–10.

45. Khera SY, Kiluk JV, Hasson DM, Meade TL, Meyers MP, Dupont EL, et al. Pregnancy-associated breast cancer patients can safely undergo lymphatic mapping. Breast J. 2008;14:250–4.

46. Cardonick E, Iacobucci A. Use of chemotherapy during human pregnancy. Lancet Oncol. 2004;5:283–91.

47. Peccatori FA, Azim Jr HA, Scarfone G, Gadducci A, Bonazzi C, Gentilini O, et al. Weekly epirubicin in the treatment of gestational breast cancer (GBC). Breast Cancer Res Treat. 2009;115:591–4.

48. Bonilla L, Ben-Aharon I, Vidal L, Gafter-Gvili A, Leibovici L, Stemmer SM. Dose-dense chemotherapy in nonmetastatic breast cancer: a systematic review and meta-analysis of randomized controlled trials. J Natl Cancer Inst. 2010;102:1845–54.

49. Berry DL, Theriault RL, Holmes FA, Parisi VM, Booser DJ, Singletary SE, et al. Management of breast cancer during pregnancy using a standardized protocol. J Clin Oncol Off J Am Soc Clin Oncol. 1999;17:855–61.

50. Ebert U, Loffler H, Kirch W. Cytotoxic therapy and pregnancy. Pharmacol Ther. 1997;74:207–20.

51. Garcia-Manero M, Royo MP, Espinos J, Pina L, Alcazar JL, Lopez G. Pregnancy associated breast cancer. Eur J Surg Oncol J Eur Soc Surg Oncol Br Assoc Surg Oncol. 2009;35:215–8.

52. Giacalone PL, Laffargue F, Benos P. Chemotherapy for breast carcinoma during pregnancy: a French national survey. Cancer. 1999;86:2266–72.

53. Hahn KM, Johnson PH, Gordon N, Kuerer H, Middleton L, Ramirez M, et al. Treatment of pregnant breast cancer patients and outcomes of children exposed to chemotherapy in utero. Cancer. 2006;107:1219–26.

54. Mir O, Berveiller P, Goffinet F, Treluyer JM, Serreau R, Goldwasser F, et al. Taxanes for breast cancer during pregnancy: a systematic review. Ann Oncol Off J Eur Soc Med Oncol/ESMO. 2010;21:425–6.

55. Ring AE, Smith IE, Jones A, Shannon C, Galani E, Ellis PA. Chemotherapy for breast cancer during pregnancy: an 18-year experience from five London teaching hospitals. J Clin Oncol Off J Am Soc Clin Oncol. 2005;23:4192–7.

56. Van Calsteren K, Heyns L, De Smet F, Van Eycken L, Gziri MM, Van Gemert W, et al. Cancer during pregnancy: an analysis of 215 patients emphasizing the obstetrical and the neonatal outcomes. J Clin Oncol Off J Am Soc Clin Oncol. 2010;28:683–9.

57. Aviles A, Neri N. Hematological malignancies and pregnancy: a final report of 84 children who received chemotherapy in utero. Clin Lymphoma. 2001;2:173–7.

58. Amant F, Van Calsteren K, Halaska MJ, Gziri MM, Hui W, Lagae L, et al. Long-term cognitive and cardiac outcomes after prenatal exposure to chemotherapy in children aged 18 months or older: an observational study. Lancet Oncol. 2012;13:256–64.

59. Gnant M, Mlineritsch B, Schippinger W, Luschin-Ebengreuth G, Postlberger S, Menzel C, et al. Endocrine therapy plus zoledronic acid in premenopausal breast cancer. N Engl J Med. 2009;360:679–91.

60. Minsker DH, Manson JM, Peter CP. Effects of the bisphosphonate, alendronate, on parturition in the rat. Toxicol Appl Pharmacol. 1993;121:217–23.

61. Levy S, Fayez I, Taguchi N, Han JY, Aiello J, Matsui D, et al. Pregnancy outcome following in utero exposure to bisphosphonates. Bone. 2009;44:428–30.

62. Isaacs RJ, Hunter W, Clark K. Tamoxifen as systemic treatment of advanced breast cancer during pregnancy – case report and literature review. Gynecol Oncol. 2001;80:405–8.

63. Press MF, Cordon-Cardo C, Slamon DJ. Expression of the HER-2/neu proto-oncogene in normal human adult and fetal tissues. Oncogene. 1990;5:953–62.

64. Azim Jr HA, Azim H, Peccatori FA. Treatment of cancer during pregnancy with monoclonal antibodies:

a real challenge. Expert Rev Clin Immunol. 2010;6:821–6.

65. Arriagada R, Le MG, Contesso G, Guinebretiere JM, Rochard F, Spielmann M. Predictive factors for local recurrence in 2006 patients with surgically resected small breast cancer. Ann Oncol Off J Eur Soc Med Oncol/ESMO. 2002;13:1404–13.

66. Emens LA, Davidson NE. Adjuvant hormonal therapy for premenopausal women with breast cancer. Clin Cancer Res Off J Am Assoc Cancer Res. 2003;9:486S–94.

67. Kalantaridou SN, Davis SR, Nelson LM. Premature ovarian failure. Endocrinol Metab Clin North Am. 1998;27:989–1006.

68. Malamos NA, Stathopoulos GP, Keramopoulos A, Papadiamantis J, Vassilaros S. Pregnancy and offspring after the appearance of breast cancer. Oncology. 1996;53:471–5.

69. Oktem O, Oktay K. Fertility preservation for breast cancer patients. Semin Reprod Med. 2009;27:486–92.

70. Loren AW, Mangu PB, Beck LN, Brennan L, Magdalinski AJ, Partridge AH, et al. Fertility preservation for patients with cancer: American Society of Clinical Oncology clinical practice guideline update. J Clin Oncol Off J Am Soc Clin Oncol. 2013;31:2500–10.

71. Del Mastro L, Boni L, Michelotti A, Gamucci T, Olmeo N, Gori S, et al. Effect of the gonadotropin-releasing hormone analogue triptorelin on the occurrence of chemotherapy-induced early menopause in premenopausal women with breast cancer: a randomized trial. JAMA. 2011;306:269–76.

72. McLaren JF, Bates GW. Fertility preservation in women of reproductive age with cancer. Am J Obstet Gynecol. 2012;207:455–62.

73. Barcroft J, Dayoub N, Thong KJ. Fifteen year follow-up of embryos cryopreserved in cancer patients for fertility preservation. J Assist Reprod Genet. 2013;30:1407–13.

74. Chian RC, Uzelac PS, Nargund G. In vitro maturation of human immature oocytes for fertility preservation. Fertil Steril. 2013;99:1173–81.

75. Dolmans MM, Luyckx V, Donnez J, Andersen CY, Greve T. Risk of transferring malignant cells with transplanted frozen-thawed ovarian tissue. Fertil Steril. 2013;99:1514–22.

76. Donnez J, Dolmans MM, Demylle D, Jadoul P, Pirard C, Squifflet J, et al. Live birth after orthotopic transplantation of cryopreserved ovarian tissue. Lancet. 2004;364:1405–10.

77. Donnez J, Dolmans MM, Pellicer A, Diaz-Garcia C, Sanchez Serrano M, Schmidt KT, et al. Restoration of ovarian activity and pregnancy after transplantation of cryopreserved ovarian tissue: a review of 60 cases of reimplantation. Fertil Steril. 2013;99:1503–13.

78. el Hussein E, Tan SL. Successful in vitro fertilization and embryo transfer after treatment of invasive carcinoma of the breast. Fertil Steril. 1992;58:194–6.

79. Garcia-Velasco JA, Domingo J, Cobo A, Martinez M, Carmona L, Pellicer A. Five years' experience using oocyte vitrification to preserve fertility for medical and nonmedical indications. Fertil Steril. 2013;99:1994–9.

80. Mourits MJ, De Vries EG, Willemse PH, Ten Hoor KA, Hollema H, Van der Zee AG. Tamoxifen treatment and gynecologic side effects: a review. Obstet Gynecol. 2001;97:855–66.

81. Oktay K, Buyuk E, Davis O, Yermakova I, Veeck L, Rosenwaks Z. Fertility preservation in breast cancer patients: IVF and embryo cryopreservation after ovarian stimulation with tamoxifen. Hum Reprod. 2003;18:90–5.

82. Oktay K, Buyuk E, Libertella N, Akar M, Rosenwaks Z. Fertility preservation in breast cancer patients: a prospective controlled comparison of ovarian stimulation with tamoxifen and letrozole for embryo cryopreservation. J Clin Oncol Off J Am Soc Clin Oncol. 2005;23:4347–53.

83. Oktay K, Buyuk E, Rodriguez-Wallberg KA, Sahin G. In vitro maturation improves oocyte or embryo cryopreservation outcome in breast cancer patients undergoing ovarian stimulation for fertility preservation. Reprod Biomed Online. 2010;20:634–8.

84. Oktay K, Oktem O. Ovarian cryopreservation and transplantation for fertility preservation for medical indications: report of an ongoing experience. Fertil Steril. 2010;93:762–8.

85. Prest SJ, May FE, Westley BR. The estrogen-regulated protein, TFF1, stimulates migration of human breast cancer cells. FASEB J Off Publ Fed Am Soc Exp Biol. 2002;16:592–4.

86. Reddy J, Oktay K. Ovarian stimulation and fertility preservation with the use of aromatase inhibitors in women with breast cancer. Fertil Steril. 2012;98:1363–9.

87. Rodriguez-Wallberg KA, Oktay K. Fertility preservation and pregnancy in women with and without BRCA mutation-positive breast cancer. Oncologist. 2012;17:1409–17.

88. Surbone A, Petrek JA. Childbearing issues in breast carcinoma survivors. Cancer. 1997;79:1271–8.

89. Titus S, Li F, Stobezki R, Akula K, Unsal E, Jeong K, et al. Impairment of BRCA1-related DNA double-strand break repair leads to ovarian aging in mice and humans. Sci Transl Med. 2013;5:172ra21.

90. Doll DC, Ringenberg QS, Yarbro JW. Antineoplastic agents and pregnancy. Semin Oncol. 1989;16:337–46.

91. Sutton R, Buzdar AU, Hortobagyi GN. Pregnancy and offspring after adjuvant chemotherapy in breast cancer patients. Cancer. 1990;65:847–50.

92. Decanter C, Gligorov J. Oocyte/embryo cryopreservation before chemotherapy for breast cancer. Gynecol Obstet Fertil. 2011;39:501–3.

93. Shalom-Paz E, Almog B, Shehata F, Huang J, Holzer H, Chian RC, et al. Fertility preservation for breast-cancer patients using IVM followed by oocyte or embryo vitrification. Reprod Biomed Online. 2010;21:566–71.

94. Menon U, Harper J, Sharma A, Fraser L, Burnell M, ElMasry K, et al. Views of BRCA gene mutation carriers on preimplantation genetic diagnosis as a reproductive option for hereditary breast and ovarian cancer. Hum Reprod. 2007;22:1573–7.

95. Sagi M, Weinberg N, Eilat A, Aizenman E, Werner M, Girsh E, et al. Preimplantation genetic diagnosis for BRCA1/2 – a novel clinical experience. Prenat Diagn. 2009;29:508–13.

96. Wang CW, Hui EC. Ethical, legal and social implications of prenatal and preimplantation genetic testing for cancer susceptibility. Reprod Biomed Online. 2009;19 Suppl 2:23–33.

Onco-cardiology for Breast Cancer

Ozlem Soran

Abstract

The purpose of this chapter is to underline the importance of cardiotoxicity, to identify the patients at risk for cardiotoxicity, and to outline strategies for the management of cardiac adverse events in patients with breast cancer undergoing systemic therapy. Several trials have suggested that regular assessment of cardiac function and parameters, including serum lipids that might be affected by adjuvant therapy, the management of hypertension, and weight control are important to minimize cardiovascular risks, especially in women aged >65 years, who constitute >50 % of the breast cancer population. The decision to use one specific cancer treatment regime should depend on its toxicity and efficacy profile. Reducing the severity and frequency of adverse cardiac events may improve the quality of life for patients undergoing systemic therapy for breast cancer and offer continuation of the well-documented and beneficial therapies. Management approaches should consider risk management plans to support the use of life-saving systemic therapeutics agents and avoid the interruption of their use due to the mismanagement of side effects. Cancer patients are vulnerable to many conditions; they can be protected from adverse events with better therapy regimens and regular assessment.

Keywords

Cardiotoxicity • Breast cancer • Adverse cardiovascular effects • Cardio-oncology

Introduction

Over the last decade, the breast cancer mortality rate has significantly decreased, and the perception of breast cancer has consequently dramatically changed from a mortal disease to a chronic

O. Soran, MD, MPH, FACC, FESC
Heart and Vascular Institute, University of Pittsburgh, 200 Lothrop Street, Pittsburgh, PA 15213, USA
e-mail: zos1@pitt.edu; osoran@lycos.com

© Springer International Publishing Switzerland 2016
A. Aydiner et al. (eds.), *Breast Disease: Management and Therapies*,
DOI 10.1007/978-3-319-26012-9_50

disease. Similar to all chronic diseases, breast cancer patients face different health challenging problems in addition to cancer-related problems.

Breast cancer is the most often diagnosed cancer and the second leading cause of cancer mortality following lung cancer. Breast cancer is a common health problem in the Western world, comprising approximately one-third of all cancers in women [1]. The breast cancer incidence increased approximately 0.2 % annually between 1997 and 2000; during the same time, mortality due to breast cancer was reduced by 2.3 % per year. Women with early-stage breast cancer are now surviving longer by means of improved outcomes with chemo- and hormone therapy; one disadvantage of this improvement is the risk of adverse cardiovascular effects from breast cancer therapy, also known as cardiotoxicity. The National Cancer Institute generally defines cardiotoxicity as "toxicity that affects the heart" [2]. This definition embraces a variety of side effects affecting both the heart and circulation: valvular injury, dysrhythmias, changes in blood pressure, arterial/venous thrombosis, or impairment in myocardial contraction or relaxation (i.e., systolic and diastolic dysfunction) [3]. In fact, the recognition of cardiotoxicity goes back at least to the classic report by von Hoff and colleagues in the mid-1970s that outlined the relationship between the severity of heart failure and the dosage of doxorubicin. By the mid-1980s, the concept of cardio-oncology or oncologic cardiology became a recognized speciality [4, 5]. From a clinical standpoint, drug-related cardiotoxicity was defined by the Cardiac Review and Evaluation Committee, which supervised trastuzumab clinical trials, as one or more of the following: (a) cardiomyopathy in terms of a reduction in left ventricular ejection fraction (LVEF), either global or more severe in the septum; (b) symptoms associated with congestive heart failure (CHF); (c) signs associated with CHF (e.g., tachycardia); and (d) reduction in LVEF from baseline that is in the range of less than or equal to 5 % to less than 55 % with accompanying signs or symptoms of heart failure or a reduction in LVEF in the range of equal to or greater than 10 % to less than 55 %, without

accompanying signs or symptoms [6]. Notably, the severity of these cardiovascular toxicities may range from asymptomatic subclinical abnormalities, such as LVEF decline, to life-threatening events, such as acute ischemia [3].

Figure 50.1 summarizes the most common cardiovascular side effects of the chemotherapeutics drugs used in breast cancer treatment (Fig. 50.1). Breast cancer survivors now actually have a higher risk of developing cardiovascular disease than recurrent cancer. Heart failure has become the most common side effect. Many patients who will be cured of their cancer will suffer from heart failure. In fact, the American College of Cardiology and American Heart Association's staging classification for heart failure categorize cardiotoxic chemotherapy as stage A. This classification suggests that exposure to certain chemotherapeutic drugs is considered a high-risk factor for developing heart failure [7, 8].

Heart failure is a syndrome of epidemic proportions in the USA, affecting more than five million patients. The syndrome is the end result of multiple etiologies, including coronary artery disease, diabetes, hypertension, exposure to chemotherapeutic drugs, family history of cardiomyopathy, previous myocardial infarction (MI), and asymptomatic valvular disease [9, 10]. Heart failure is a clinical syndrome caused by systolic or diastolic left ventricular dysfunction or a combination of both. Beta-blockers, angiotensin-converting enzyme (ACE) inhibitors (ACE-i), and diuretics are the choices of asymptomatic and symptomatic left ventricular dysfunction management. Systolic function is measured via the LVEF,

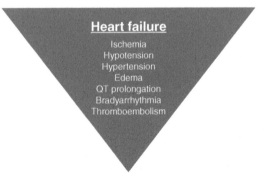

Fig. 50.1 Common cardiovascular manifestations

which represents the percentage of blood expelled from the resting left ventricle with each systolic contraction. The normal LVEF is 50 % or greater. Diastolic dysfunction is defined as left ventricular dysfunction with normal LVEF, and diastolic heart failure occurs when diastolic dysfunction is accompanied with dyspnea, fatigue, and fluid retention. Left ventricular dysfunction occurs in patients with both decreased and normal ejection. Once heart failure is diagnosed, the survival rate is significantly reduced. Awareness of cardiac sequelae will help oncologists manage patient care and seek cardiac assistance to continue their life-saving treatments [10].

This chapter reviews the cardiotoxic effects of commonly used systemic therapeutic agents in patients with breast cancer and offers advice for effective patient management. Terms "onco-cardiology", "cardio-oncology", and "oncologic cardiology" are used interchangeably throughout the chapter.

Anthracyclines

Anthracycline-based regimens, including epirubicin or doxorubicin, have been the mainstream of breast cancer chemotherapy in both adjuvant and metastatic settings [11]. However, the recognition of cardiac dysfunction as a consequence of these treatments has significantly affected their use [12]. The most common manifestation of anthracycline-induced cardiotoxicity is left ventricular dysfunction.

Although anthracycline-related cardiotoxicity is a well-known adverse effect, its underlying mechanism remains uncharacterized. A well-known hypothesis draws attention to the role of oxygen free radicals that could lead to irreversible damage in cardiomyocytes. However, this hypothesis has been questioned in the last decade because it does not appear to explain the complete mechanism [12]. Recently, a molecular hypothesis suggested that anthracycline impairs DNA repair pathways via interacting with the topoisomerase-II-beta enzyme in myocytes [13]. Anthracycline-related cardiac toxicities are known as type I chemotherapy-related cardiac

dysfunction [14]. This type of toxicity causes irreversible damage. A recent meta-analysis revealed a fivefold increased risk of clinical cardiotoxicity, a sixfold increased risk of subclinical cardiotoxicity, and a fivefold increased risk of cardiac death among cancer patients treated with anthracyclines compared with those treated with non-anthracycline-based regimens [15].

Several risk factors have been associated with the increased risk for anthracycline-related cardiac toxicity. One such risk factor is the cumulative dose [16]. For doxorubicin, the estimated percentage of patients with doxorubicin-related heart failure is 5.0 % at a cumulative dose of 400 mg/m^2, 26.0 % at 550 mg/m^2, and 48.0 % at 700 mg/m^2 [17]. Likewise for epirubicin, the risk of cardiotoxicity increased from 1.9 % at a dose of 800 mg/m2 to 4.3 % at a dose of 900 mg/m^2 and 15.0 % at a dose of 1,000 mg/m^2 [18]. These observations have led to the adoption of thresholds regarding the accepted cumulative dose of anthracyclines in treated patients. These thresholds differ for epirubicin and doxorubicin because epirubicin is less cardiotoxic than doxorubicin at equimolar doses. In addition, epirubicin produces lower levels of secondary alcohol metabolites [19]. In the previously mentioned meta-analysis, the authors found that the use of epirubicin significantly decreased the risks of both clinical and subclinical cardiotoxicity [15]. However, recent evidence indicates that anthracycline-related cardiotoxicity may occur even in lower cumulative doses, especially among patients with preexisting cardiovascular risk factors. Therefore, no safe threshold exists. Consequently, in patients receiving anthracycline-based therapy, other classical risk factors for cardiac toxicity should be considered. These risk factors include the following [20]:

1. The age at the time of drug exposure
2. Concomitant administration of other cardiotoxic chemotherapeutic agents (e.g., trastuzumab)
3. Concurrent or prior chest irradiation
4. Preexisting coronary artery disease
5. Preexisting hypertension
6. Preexisting peripheral vascular disease
7. Preexisting diabetes

Because the abovementioned risk factors have been recognized for anthracycline-related cardiotoxicity, a variety of approaches have been suggested to decrease the risk of cardiotoxicity while maintaining efficacy. These following suggestions have been proposed [21, 22]:

1. Alterations in schedules of drug administration
2. Limiting the total cumulative dose
3. Administration of non-anthracycline-based chemotherapy without jeopardizing survival
4. Modifications of the anthracycline molecule (e.g., liposomal anthracyclines)
5. The use of adjunctive cardioprotective treatment with dexrazoxane

Several investigators suggest that bolus administration of anthracyclines may increase the incidence of cardiotoxicity compared with infusional administration. A Cochrane review of five randomized controlled trials found that continuous infusion for 6 h or longer significantly reduced the risk of clinical heart failure (and likely also subclinical cardiac damage) compared with infusions for 1 h or less [21]. No evidence suggests that continuous infusion reduces response rate or survival. Therefore, per the currently available data, the infusional administration of anthracyclines for greater than 6 h may serve as the correct approach to decrease the incidence of cardiotoxicity; however, the need for hospitalization and central venous catheters and its questionable cost-effectiveness limit its clinical use.

The encapsulation of doxorubicin into liposomes significantly reduces its distribution volume, diminishing its diffusion and consequently its toxicity in healthy tissues [23]. In a metaanalysis, liposomal compared with conventional doxorubicin significantly decreased the risk of clinical and subclinical cardiotoxicity [15]. However, all the studies included in the meta-analysis investigated the role of liposomal doxorubicin in patients with metastatic breast cancer, and the role of liposomal doxorubicin in the adjuvant setting is currently unknown and under investigation. Early phase II trials demonstrated that liposomal doxorubicin appears to be a feasible option for elderly patients and can be concurrently administered with trastuzumab as an adjuvant treatment [23, 24]. Several ongoing randomized trials are investigating the efficacy and safety of liposomal doxorubicin in elderly early breast cancer populations. With the use of cross-linked multilamellar liposomes, advances in the liposome formulation have been recently published, and in vivo experiments have demonstrated reduced systemic toxicity and improved anticancer activity compared with currently available liposomal doxorubicin [25]. This new formulation incorporates two different chemotherapeutic agents into the same liposome (doxorubicin and paclitaxel) to reduce the toxicity and increase the synergistic effect. Further studies on this new liposome formulation are warranted [26, 27].

The iron-chelating agent *dexrazoxane* may decrease the cardiotoxic effect of doxorubicin. This drug effectively inhibits the generation of free radicals. Dexrazoxane administered with either doxorubicin or epirubicin significantly reduced the incidence of clinical and subclinical cardiotoxicity in a meta-analysis of six randomized trials, of which only three examined dexrazoxane use in a homogenous breast cancer population that had received initial anthracyclinebased therapy. However, a nonsignificant trend toward lower response rates among those who received anthracycline plus dexrazoxane was noted [21]. Dexrazoxane is not recommended for use in early breast cancer because of the lack of clinical data on dexrazoxane in the adjuvant setting and the concerns about potential impact on antitumor efficacy.

Another approach to reduce cardiotoxicity involves the avoidance of anthracycline-based chemotherapy in the adjuvant setting. Recently, the docetaxel–carboplatin–trastuzumab triple combination was proven to be as effective as the anthracycline- and taxane-based standard of care chemotherapies with less cardiac events. This regime offers a worthwhile alternative in patients with human epidermal growth factor 2 (HER2)-positive early breast cancer [28].

Taxanes

Taxanes were originally identified as the natural product paclitaxel derived from the bark of the Pacific yew tree. Taxane agents include paclitaxel and docetaxel. Docetaxel is a semisynthetic analog of paclitaxel, whereas taxane was originally referred to as taxol. Taxanes prevent the separation of chromosomes during anaphase of cell division [29]. Compared with non-taxane combination chemotherapy, taxane chemotherapy as first-line or a second-line treatment is more effective against breast cancer, especially in patients who had been previously treated with anthracyclines. Taxanes decreases cancer progression (i.e., slows down the development of cancer). However, serious arrhythmias, such as bradycardia, ventricular tachycardia, and MI, have been reported in patients with breast cancer who have undergone taxane therapy [29]. According to a study performed by Arbuck et al., paclitaxel caused acute asymptomatic bradycardia in up to 30 % of patients [30]. An early series reported a 5 % incidence of serious arrhythmias and MI, including ventricular tachycardia in 5 of 140 patients (3.6 %) [31]. However, a larger database found that only 0.1 % of patients suffered from serious bradycardias and could not confirm that taxanes increased the frequency of ventricular tachycardia or MI [30]. At high cumulative anthracycline doses, taxanes interfere with the metabolism and excretion of anthracyclines and potentiate anthracycline-induced cardiotoxicity. Excess chemotherapy-related cardiac dysfunction has been noted among patients with cumulative doxorubicin doses that exceed 360 mg/m^2 who also received short paclitaxel infusions shortly after doxorubicin treatment [32].

What Can Be Done to Reduce Cardiotoxicity in the Setting of Taxane Therapy?

Slow infusion of paclitaxel and doxorubicin or increased time (24 h) between doxorubicin and paclitaxel treatments could potentially decrease cardiotoxicity [33, 34]. When combined with paclitaxel, the cumulative doxorubicin dose should not exceed 360 mg/m^2, and doxorubicin should be administered before paclitaxel [32]. Combination treatments with epirubicin and taxane may be less cardiotoxic [35, 36]. A cumulative epirubicin dose limit of 990 mg/m^2 in combination treatments with paclitaxel has been proposed [36]. In clinical trials, docetaxel is associated with increased cardiotoxicity when combined with doxorubicin or epirubicin. Modern adjuvant regimens of taxanes do not increase anthracycline cardiotoxicity. A trial comparing doxorubicin (75 mg/m^2) followed by CMF with the combination of paclitaxel and doxorubicin (60 mg/m^2) followed by CMF found that the incidences of symptomatic cardiac events at 31 months were similar between arms with (0.3 % of patients) and without (0.5 %) paclitaxel [37]. In a randomized controlled trial of three cycles of dose-dense epirubicin followed by three cycles of paclitaxel then CMF compared with three cycles of dose-dense epirubicin followed by CMF, no severe cardiotoxicity was observed in either arm [38].

Nanoparticle albumin-bound paclitaxel is a newer paclitaxel formulation that may cause less anthracycline cardiotoxicity [39]. Thus, cardiotoxicity may be minimized by carefully choosing agents and regimens [40].

Trastuzumab

Patients with HER2-positive breast cancer exhibited the worst prognosis among breast cancer patients until 1998, when trastuzumab, a humanized anti-HER2 monoclonal antibody, was first approved for the treatment of HER2-positive metastatic breast cancer. In the adjuvant setting, 1-year treatment with trastuzumab offers substantial benefit in terms of both disease-free and overall survival [41, 42].

In the early pivotal trials in the metastatic setting, cardiac dysfunction was recognized as a potential toxicity of trastuzumab, and the rates of cardiac dysfunction ranged from 8 % to the unacceptably high rate of 30 % in cases of concomitant administration of trastuzumab with anthracyclines [6]. These findings had a significant impact on the design of adjuvant trials. Treatment schedules with the sequential use of anthracyclines and trastuzumab instead of concomitant administration were followed. Strict cardiac exclusion criteria, such as monitoring cardiac function and interim cardiac safety analyses, were adopted [43]. As a consequence, the cardiotoxicity rates in adjuvant randomized trials were reduced compared with metastatic cases (symptomatic CHF rate ranged from 0.8 % to 14.2 %) [43]. However, a significantly increased risk for both reduced LVEF and CHF was observed in the trastuzumab-treated arm [44]. In the real-world setting, where cardiac exclusion criteria are not as strict as those applied in randomized controlled trials, the rate of cardiac toxicity is similar to that observed in randomized clinical trials [45, 46].

Although trastuzumab-related cardiotoxicity is a well-known adverse effect, its underlying mechanism remains largely uncharacterized. Preclinical data have suggested an important role for the HER2 signaling pathway in cardiac physiology because both HER receptors and their ligands are expressed in cardiomyocytes [47]. The mechanisms of trastuzumab-induced cardiotoxicity differ from those of anthracyclines. Although anthracycline-induced cardiotoxicity is dose dependent, trastuzumab-induced cardiotoxicity is not. An important characteristic of trastuzumab-induced cardiotoxicity is that cardiac dysfunction is reversible upon therapy withdrawal, and the drug can be safely readministered after the recovery of cardiac function [14]. This type of reversible cardiac toxicity is classified as type II chemotherapy-related cardiac dysfunction [14]. One potential mechanism of cardiotoxicity involves the inactivation of a HER ligand-mediated pathway that leads to cell survival in cases of adverse hemodynamics or other stressors [48]. This proposed mechanism could explain both the increased risk for cardiotoxicity when trastuzumab and anthracyclines are combined (the stress and damage caused by anthracyclines is increased) and the reversibility of cardiotoxicity with trastuzumab withdrawal (the pathway becomes functional again) [48].

Investigators have identified several risk factors for trastuzumab-induced cardiotoxicity. These risk factors are as follows [49–55]:

1. Concomitant administration with anthracyclines
2. Advanced age
3. Antihypertensive medications
4. Borderline cardiac function at baseline
5. A history of heart disease
6. Certain polymorphisms in the HER2 gene

The most critical risk factor for trastuzumab-induced cardiotoxicity is concomitant administration with anthracyclines. The association between cumulative anthracycline doses and trastuzumab-induced cardiotoxicity has been clearly demonstrated [49, 56, 57]. In the neoadjuvant setting, the concomitant administration of anthracyclines and trastuzumab was not correlated with an increased risk for cardiac adverse events compared with sequential administration [58–60]. Due to the absence of any difference in pathologic complete remission with the concurrent administration of trastuzumab and epirubicin, this approach is not recommended as a standard of care [58]. In addition, limited follow-up for cardiac events is reported in these studies, which is an important concern [60].

Some efforts have been made to identify certain polymorphisms in the HER2 gene that could trigger cardiotoxicity. The I655V polymorphism in the HER2 gene is associated with cardiac toxicity in three different research groups [53–55]. With the help of genome-wide association studies, pharmacogenomics may play a pivotal role in identifying patients who are at high risk for trastuzumab-induced cardiac toxicity.

In addition to trastuzumab, two additional anti-HER2 agents have been developed and approved for the treatment of HER2-positive breast cancer: the tyrosine kinase inhibitor lapatinib is approved in the metastatic setting, and the monoclonal antibody pertuzumab is approved in the neoadjuvant and metastatic setting [56–58]. The combination of two anti-HER2 agents has been evaluated as a new treatment option for patients with HER2-positive breast cancers. Lapatinib in combination with trastuzumab exhibits promising results as neoadjuvant and metastatic treatments, whereas pertuzumab is approved only in combination with trastuzumab for neoadjuvant and metastatic treatments [59, 60]. Both of these agents have cardiotoxicity risk [56–58]. This increased risk for cardiac adverse events is a concern regarding the potential risk when two anti-HER2 agents that both increase cardiac toxicity are combined. However, a recent meta-analysis did not reveal an increased risk for cardiac toxicity with any of the combinations compared with anti-HER2 monotherapy [61]. Randomized trials investigating the role of dual anti-HER2 blockade in the adjuvant setting are needed.

Endocrine Therapy for Postmenopausal Women with BC

Cardiovascular disease is a major health problem in many developed countries, with 42.7 million cases in 2005 and 459,000 deaths in 2004 in the USA [62]. In addition, cardiovascular disease constitutes an important health concern in older, postmenopausal women independent of BC [62, 63]. Endocrine treatment remains the mainstay of adjuvant therapy for postmenopausal women with hormone-responsive BC.

Historically, tamoxifen was the standard adjuvant endocrine therapy for postmenopausal women with BC, resulting in a reduction in BC recurrence by 40 % and death by 26 % after 5 years [64]. In women with estrogen receptor (ER)-positive (or ER unknown) disease, treatment with tamoxifen for 5 years after definitive surgery reduces the annual recurrence rate by 41 % and BC mortality by 34 %, translating into a 9.2 % absolute reduction in patients dying from BC at 15 years [65]. Meta-analysis results revealed that tamoxifen produces lipid-lowering effects; a potential cardioprotective effect of the drug was observed in which the rate of death from serious cardiovascular events, such as MI, was reduced during active treatment [65–68]. However, tamoxifen is associated with some potential and occasionally life-threatening side effects due to its partial estrogen-agonist activity.

These side effects include an increased incidence of endometrial cancer and thromboembolic events related to the duration of drug exposure [65, 69, 70]. Cancer Research Network results have demonstrated that third-generation AIs have been replacing tamoxifen as adjuvant endocrine therapy for postmenopausal women with early BC since 2000 [71].

Third-generation AIs are highly selective for the aromatase enzyme and substantially well tolerated. Currently, three third-generation AIs are being used clinically in the USA. All third-generation AIs reduce systemic estrogen levels by 98 % [72]. A review of 25 studies reported that AIs demonstrate a significant survival benefit in the treatment of metastatic BC compared with other endocrine therapies [73]. AIs are between 15 % and 25 % more effective than tamoxifen in reducing the relative risk of recurrence [74–76]. Both anastrozole and letrozole improved 5-year disease-free survival but not overall survival compared with tamoxifen. A meta-analysis of first-line and sequential strategies endorsed the recommendation that AIs should be included in adjuvant therapy for postmenopausal women with endocrine-responsive BC [77–79].

Women with BC live longer due to effective therapies; most may not suffer BC recurrence even though they are all vulnerable to toxicities. Therefore, these women are at increased risk of both cardiovascular disease and the cardiovascular side effects of BC treatments [40, 80]. Cardiovascular disease will remain as a potential cause of death in these patients. In the USA, as many as 2.3 million women live with such risk [80].

The risk of cardiovascular disease increases after menopause and is the greatest cause of morbidity and mortality in postmenopausal women. Estrogen is an independent risk factor for coronary heart disease in symptomatic women [81]. The effects of estrogen in cardiovascular disease are under investigation. However, estrogen contributes to the cardiovascular system via numerous mechanisms, affecting endothelial integrity, inflammation, thrombosis, and lipids [82]. Whether the increasing rate of cardiovascular events observed with AIs compared with tamoxifen results from direct AI cardiac toxicity or is due to the cardioprotective effect of tamoxifen remains under investigation.

Given the incidence of cardiovascular disease that is mostly unrecognized in women and the potential BC therapy-related adverse effects of cardiovascular disease, it is important to assess cardiovascular risk factors in postmenopausal women administered with adjuvant treatment for BC. An updated analysis of the BIG 1-98 trial demonstrated increased rates of cardiac events in the letrozole-treated arm compared with the tamoxifen-treated arm, particularly for women between 65 and 74 years of age [83]. Recent data suggest that women with early BC are more likely to die of heart disease than recurrent cancer [84].

The Effect of Estrogen on Cardiovascular Disease

Estrogen protects against cardiovascular disease in premenopausal women compared with age-matched men, but these advantages in women disappear with increasing age and decreasing estrogen levels due to menopause [85]. The classical ERs ER-α and ER-β affect the cardiovascular system via intracellular interactions. Estrogen promotes endothelial progenitor cell mobilization, increases mesenchymal stem cell-mediated vascular endothelial growth factor (VEGF) release, and improves endothelial and myocardial function after ischemia [86–88]. A new membrane-bound and G protein-coupled estrogen receptor (GPR30) was recently described. Ischemic reperfusion injury was reduced and cardiac function was preserved via activation of the GPR30 receptor in the heart. The decreasing effect of estrogen is related to increased methylation of the ER promoter with age in menopausal women. ER expression in the arterial wall diminishes sharply with menopause [89, 90].

Clinical Studies with Tamoxifen and Aromatase Inhibitors

Two approaches are available for the treatment of hormone receptor-positive BC, namely, inhibi-

tion of estrogen synthesis or its action. Several prospective studies compared the effects of various AIs (e.g., anastrozole, exemestane, and letrozole) with tamoxifen. These studies examined the effects of these approaches on behalf of their therapeutic effects in postmenopausal women with hormone receptor-positive BC. The third-generation AIs exhibited enhanced efficacy compared with tamoxifen in regard to improvement in disease-free survival and possibly overall survival rate in women with BC [76, 91–93].

Nonsteroidal Aromatase Inhibitors

Anastrozole

Anastrozole, a nonsteroidal AI, binds reversibly to the heme group of the aromatase enzyme. The Arimidex, Tamoxifen, Alone or in Combination (ATAC) trial compared the efficacy and safety of the third-generation AIs anastrozole (1 mg) with tamoxifen (20 mg). Both drugs were administered orally every day for 5 years as first-line adjuvant endocrine treatment for postmenopausal women with hormone receptor-positive early BC. This trial compared anastrozole with tamoxifen in 9,366 women with newly diagnosed early-stage BC, and 84 % of these women were hormone-receptor positive. This trial failed to note significant differences in cardiac events between anastrozole and tamoxifen therapies. However, the trial's definition of cardiovascular events was limited to ischemic heart disease. The event rate was 4.1 % and 3.4 % in the anastrozole and tamoxifen groups, respectively ($P=0.1$) [75]. ATAC was the first trial to reveal that an AI is more effective and has fewer serious adverse effects than tamoxifen in adjuvant treatment. The ATAC trial recently published data from 120 months of follow-up [94]. The highest relative reduction in time to recurrence, contralateral BC, and disease-free survival was observed in the anastrozole group compared with the tamoxifen group in the first 2 years of the active treatment. These differences were maintained throughout the follow-up period, including after treatment completion between treatment groups. The absolute reduction of recurrence for the anastrozole group was 2.7 % at 5 years and 4.3 % at 10 years of follow-up compared with tamoxifen in hormone receptor-positive BC patients [94]. Tamoxifen exhibits a carryover benefit for recurrence in the first 5 years after treatment but not thereafter [65]. The carryover effect for recurrence was more prolonged for anastrozole than tamoxifen in the present study and remained significant for the 10-year follow-up period.

Generally, treatment-related serious adverse events were reduced in the anastrozole group compared with the tamoxifen group (OR 0.84, 95 % CI 0.60–1.19; $P = 0.3$), but a similar number of events were noted after completion of treatment (OR 0.84, 95 % CI 0.60–1.19; $P = 0.3$) [94]. Of note, the increased fracture rate associated with anastrozole during treatment did not continue after treatment because this short-term effect could be managed with dual-energy x-ray absorptiometry scans and bisphosphonates when needed [75, 95, 96]. Because the study's definition of cardiovascular events was limited to ischemic heart disease, the 68-month follow-up did not provide safety data on all cardiovascular diseases. At the 68-month follow-up, the incidence of ischemic heart disease was not significantly increased with anastrozole compared with tamoxifen (4.1 % versus 3.4 %, $P = 0.10$) (Table 50.1). Angina pectoris was slightly increased in the anastrozole group compared with the tamoxifen group, but the difference was not significant (2 % versus 1.5 %, respectively; $P = 0.07$). The MI rate was similar (1 %) in both treatment arms both during treatment and after its completion; when only serious events were analyzed at 68 months, there was 34 (0.27) and 33 (0.27) events on treatment, and there was 26 (0.28) and 28 (0.30) off-treatment until 100 months of follow-up. The incidence of both vascular and thrombotic events was significantly reduced with anastrozole versus tamoxifen overall (2.8 % versus 4.5 %, respectively; $P = 0.0004$), and the incidence of thromboembolic events at 100 months of follow-up was similar to that at 68 months of follow-up [75, 80]. Serious cerebrovascular events were less common in patients administered with anastrozole during treatment (OR 0.59 (0.32–1.05), $P = 0.056$) but not afterward (OR

1.10 (0.57–2.13), $P = 0.75$) [96]. Additionally, the number of cardiovascular deaths was similar between the anastrozole and tamoxifen groups (49 versus 46 at 68 months of follow-up, 2 % versus 2 % at 100 months of follow-up, and 2.9 % versus 3.0 % at 120 months of follow-up, respectively). Fewer cardiovascular deaths were noted in the anastrozole group. This finding has been verified in several studies with AIs [77, 97].

Additionally, trials in which tamoxifen was switched to anastrozole in women with BC have been conducted. In the ARNO-95/ABCSG-8 trials (in which patients were switched to anastrozole after 2–3 years of tamoxifen), the incidence of MI was reduced in both the anastrozole and the tamoxifen groups (Table 50.1). The Italian Tamoxifen Arimidex (ITA) trial compared continued tamoxifen therapy to switching to anastrozole after 2–3 years. Overall, the serious adverse event rate was similar (40 versus 37, respectively; $P = 0.7$); additionally, no difference in cardiovascular event rates was noted between the two arms (14 versus 16, $P = 0.4$ in the preliminary data; 14 versus 17, respectively; $P = 0.6$ at update).

Letrozole

Letrozole is another nonsteroidal AI that binds reversibly to the heme group of the aromatase enzyme and displays a longer half-life at 96 h. The BIG 1-98 trial is the only study with a four-arm design comparing the 5-year sequence of either tamoxifen followed by letrozole or the inverse (letrozole followed by tamoxifen) over 5 years. The BIG 1-98 trial was designed to gather the potential effects of letrozole on cardiac risk. These effects included any cardiac adverse effects, ischemic heart disease, cardiac failure, hypertension, peripheral atherosclerosis, thromboembolic events, and other cardiovascular adverse effects. Specific adverse events were graded according to the Common Toxicity Criteria of the National Cancer Institute (version 2) at each study visit during treatment [98]. All data were collected separately on adverse effects of any grade, especially grade 3–5 effects. The safety data, with a median 30.1 months of follow-up, revealed that the incidence of cardiovascular events was similarly low in both the letrozole and

Table 50.1 Anastrozole: reversible, third-generation nonsteroidal aromatase inhibitor

	ATAC (Arimidex, Tamoxifen, Alone or in Combination) Tamoxifen for 5 years vs anastrozole for 5 years (tamoxifen+anastrozole arm was discontinued at 47 months)									ITA (The Italian Tamoxifen Anastrozole Trial) Tamoxifen for 5 years vs tamoxifen for 2–3 years followed by anastrozole			ABCSG8/ARNO 95 (The Austrian Breast and Colorectal Study Group/Arimidex-Nolvadex 95) Tamoxifen for 5 years vs tamoxifen for 2–3 years followed by anastrozole		
Design	First-line adjuvant									Combined adjuvant			Combined adjuvant		
Median follow-up	68 months			100 months			120 months (overall)			64 months			28 months		
	ANA	TAM	P value	ANA	TAM	P value	ANA	TAM	P value	ANA	TAM	P value	ANA	TAM	P value
Number of patients	3125	3116								223	225		1618	1606	
Median age	64.1 years (+5.7 years)			72 years			+13 months			63 years			62 years		
Disease-free survival	HR: 0.83 (0.73–0.94)		P=0.005	HR: 0.85 (0.76–0.94)		P=0.003	HR: 0.86 (0.78–0.95)		P=0.003	**HR: 0.42 (A>T)		P=0.001	HR: 0.42 (A>T)		P=0.0001
Time to distant recurrence	HR: 0.84 (0.70–1.00)		P=0.06	HR: 0.84 (0.72–0.97)		P=0.022	HR: 0.85 (0.73–0.98)		P=0.02						
Time to recurrence	HR: 0.74 (0.64–0.87)		P=0.0002	HR: 0.76 (0.67–0.87)		P=0.0001	HR: 0.79 (0.70–0.89)		P=0.0002	NA			NA		
Overall survival	HR: 0.97 (0.85–1.12)		P=0.7	HR: 0.97 (0.86–1.11)		P=0.7	HR: 0.95 (0.84–1.06)		P=0.4	HR: 0.56 (0.28–1.15)		P=0.1	HR: 0.7 (A>T)		P=0.038
Ischemic cardiovascular events	127 (4.1%)	104 (3.4%)	P=0.10	NA			NA			NA			NA		
Myocardial infarction	37 (1.0%)	34 (1.0%)	P=0.5	60 (1.9%)	61 (1.9%)		NA			NA			3 (<1%)	2 (<1%)	P=1
Angina	71 (2.0%)	51 (1.5%)	P=0.07	NA			NA			NA			NA		

Cerebrovascular events	62 (2.0%)	88 (3.0%)	P=0.03	64	91	P=0.03	NA	NA	NA	2 (<1%)	9 (<1%)	P=0.064
Thromboembolic disease	87 (2.8%)	140 (4.5%)	P=0.0004	NA			NA	NA	NA	3 (<1%)	12 (<1%)	P=0.034
All cardiac events	NA	NA		NA			NA	NA	All cardiovascular disease A: 7.6%, T: 6.2%	P=0.6	NA	
Cardiovascular deaths	49 (2%)	46 (1%)		67 (2%)	66 (2%)		91 (2.9%)	95 (3.0%)				
Cerebrovascular deaths	14 (<1%)	22 (1%)	P=NS	25 (0.8)	29 (0.9)		33 (1.1%)	36 (1.2%)				

ATAC results from ATAC study were obtained from the HR+ group, *NA* not available, *HR* hazard ratio

**36 months of follow-up

tamoxifen arms, whereas letrozole was associated with significantly more peripheral atherosclerosis and other cardiovascular events of any grade [98]. When all events were reassessed for grade 3–5 adverse effects, tamoxifen resulted in more grade 3–5 thromboembolic events, and letrozole resulted in significantly more grade 3–5 cardiac events of any type, especially cardiac failure (2.4 % versus 1.4 %, respectively; $P = 0.001$). However, the event rate was relatively low in both arms [98].

The incidence of ischemic heart disease was increased with letrozole compared with tamoxifen, but results did not achieve significance (1.1 % versus 0.7 %, respectively; $P = 0.06$) [98]. At 51 months of follow-up, no significant differences in cardiac events overall (5.5 % versus 5.0 %), ischemic heart disease (2.2 % versus 1.7 %), and cardiac failure (1 % versus 0.6 %) were noted between the letrozole and tamoxifen monotherapy groups, respectively, even though letrozole is associated with increased cardiac events in each grade compared with tamoxifen [99] (Table 50.2). Although the number of events was minimal in each arm, an increase in the incidence of grade 3–5 cardiac events was noted with letrozole (Fisher exact test, $P < 0.001$) [99]. At a median follow-up of 71 months after randomization, the incidence of any type or grade of cardiac events was similar between women who were treated with one of the regimens that included letrozole and women who were treated with tamoxifen monotherapy (6.1–7.0 % and 5.7 %, respectively; $P = 0.45$) [97]. The incidence of thromboembolic events was significantly reduced with letrozole compared with tamoxifen before switching tamoxifen to letrozole (1.5 % versus 3.5 %, $P < 0.001$) or vice versa (1.7 % versus 3.9 %, $P < 0.001$ at 25.8 months; Table 50.2) [74]. Furthermore, the reduction in thromboembolic events with letrozole remained significant (versus tamoxifen) after switching the monotherapy arms at 51 months and 74 months (2 % versus 3.8 %, respectively; $P < 0.001$ at 51 months, 2.6 % versus 4.3 %, respectively; $P < 0.001$ at 74 months of follow-up) [99, 100]. Hence, the reduction in letrozole monotherapy remained significant compared with one of the regimens that included

tamoxifen at a median follow-up of 71 months ($P < 0.001$) [97].

Letrozole has a similar incidence of cerebrovascular accidents/transient ischemic attacks (CVA/TIA) as tamoxifen before switching tamoxifen to letrozole or vice versa (Table 50.2) [98]. Additionally, the incidence of CVA/TIA remained similar after 51 months and 74 months of follow-up (1.8 % and 1.6 %, respectively). Furthermore, similar rates of patients with previous CVA/TIA were assigned to one of the regimens that included tamoxifen and letrozole monotherapy [97].

The MA.17 trial was designed to evaluate the impact of letrozole on lipid parameters compared with placebo in postmenopausal women who were previously subjected to 5 years adjuvant tamoxifen treatment for early-stage BC [101]. The incidence of cardiovascular disease was similar between the letrozole group and the placebo group at 2.5 years of follow-up [101]. MI was noted in <1 % of patients for both groups.

Steroidal Aromatase Inhibitors

Exemestane

Exemestane is a third-generation steroidal AI that is orally active and binds irreversibly to the substrate-binding pocket of the aromatase enzyme. Exemestane is indicated as an adjuvant treatment for hormone receptor-positive early-stage BC after 2–3 years of tamoxifen treatment in postmenopausal women. When exemestane is used as a first-line adjuvant treatment in patients who were not previously exposed to AIs, increases in the response rate (from 31 % to 46 %) and progression-free survival (from 5.8 to 9.9 months) were noted compared with tamoxifen [102]. Three trials are currently evaluating the use of exemestane as an adjuvant treatment in postmenopausal women with early-stage BC, including IES (Intergroup Exemestane Study), TEAM (Tamoxifen, Exemestane, Adjuvant, Multicenter), and NSABP (National Surgical Adjuvant Breast and Bowel Project) B-33 [103].

The IES study has randomized 4,724 postmenopausal patients with unilateral invasive,

Table 50.2 Letrozole: reversible, third-generation nonsteroidal aromatase inhibitor

	BIG 1-98												MA.17		
	Adjuvant Endocrine Therapy for Early Breast Cancer Using Letrozole of Tamoxifen (four-arm trial comparing 5 years of monotherapy with tamoxifen or with letrozole with sequences of 2 years of one of these agents followed by 3 years of the other)												Letrozole vs placebo after 5 years of tamoxifen treatment		
Design	First-line adjuvant												Extended adjuvant		
Median follow-up	25.8 months			30.1 months			51 months**			74 months**			30 months		
	LET	TAM	P value	LET	TAM	P value	LET	TAM	P value	LET	TAM	P value	LET	TAM	P value
Number of patients	4003	4007		3975	3988		2448	2447		2448	2447		2583	2587	
Median age	61 years			61 years			61 years			61 years			62 years		
Disease-free survival	HR: 0.81 (0.70–0.93)		P=0.003	NA			HR: 0.88 (0.71–0.95)		P=0.007	HR: 0.83 (0.74–0.94)		P=0.03	HR: 0.58 (0.45–0.76)		P<0.01
TTR	HR: 0.72 (0.61–0.86)		P<0.001	NA			231 (0.65)	291 (0.92)	P=0.004	NA			NA		
TTDR	HR: 0.73 (0.60–0.88)		P=0.001	NA			HR: 0.81 (0.67–0.98)		P=0.03	HR: 0.80 (0.67–0.94)		P=0.05	HR: 0.60 (0.43–0.84)		P=0.002
Overall survival	HR: 0.86 (0.70–1.06)		P=0.16	NA			HR: 0.91 (0.75–1.11)		P=0.35	HR: 0.82 (0.70–0.95)		P=0.08	HR: 0.82 (0.57–1.19)		P=0.3
Cardiac events	162 (4.1)	153 (3.8)	P=0.61	191 (4.8)	188 (4.7)	P=0.87	134 (5.5)	122 (5.0)	P=0.48	169 (6.9)	152 (6.2)	P=0.36	NA		
Grade 3–5	85 (2.1)	44 (1.1)	P<0.001	96 (2.4)	57 (1.4)	P=0.001	74 (3.0)	45 (1.8)	P<0.001	93 (3.8)	51 (2.1)		NA		
Ischemic heart disease	57 (1.4)	46 (1.2)	P=0.28	68 (1.7)	60 (1.5)	P=0.48	54 (2.2)	41 (1.7)	P=0.21	69 (2.8)	49 (2.0)	P=0.08	NA		
Myocardial infarction	NA			NA			NA			NA			9 (0.3)	11 (0.4)	NS
Angina	NA			NA			NA			NA			31 (1.2)	23 (0.9)	NS
Cardiac failure	31 (0.8)	14 (0.4)	P=0.01	40 (1.0)	29 (0.7)	P=0.19	24 (1.0)	14 (0.6)	P=0.14	30 (1.2)	25 (1.0)	P=0.59			

(continued)

Table 50.2 (continued)

	BIG 1-98												MA.17		
Other cardiovascular events	19 (0.5)	8 (0.2)	P=0.04	26 (0.7)	11 (0.3)	P=0.01	19 (0.8)	6 (0.2)	P=0.014	24 (1.0)	13 (0.5)	P=0.10	100 (3.9)	95 (3.7)	NS
CVA/TIA	39 (1.0)	41 (1.0)	P=0.91	47 (1.2)	49 (1.2)	P=0.92	34 (1.4)	35 (1.4)	P=0.90	45 (1.8)	38 (1.6)	P=0.51	17 (0.7)	15 (0.6)	NS
Thromboembolism	61 (1.5)	140 (3.5)	P<0.001	68 (1.7)	154 (3.9)	P<0.001	50 (2.0)	94 (3.8)	P<0.001	63 (2.6)	104 (4.3)	P<0.001	11 (0.4)	6 (0.2)	NS
Cardiac death	13 (0.3)	6 (0.2)		NA			12 (0.5)	7 (0.3)		NA			5*	5*	
Cerebrovascular death	7 (0.2)	1 (0.03)		NA			8 (0.3)	3 (0.1)		NA			2*	1*	

TTDR time to distant recurrence, *TTR* time to recurrence, *NA* not available, *NS* not significance, *HR* hazard ratio

*Lymph node-negative patients

**Results from monotherapy arms

ER-positive (or unknown) BC who were disease-free after 2–3 years of tamoxifen treatment to switch to exemestane ($n=2,352$) or to continue tamoxifen ($n=2,372$). With a median follow-up of 55.7 months, exemestane exhibited a 3.3 % absolute benefit by the end of the treatment. When ER-negative patients were excluded, the hazard ratio (HR) was 0.75 (0.65–0.87; $P=0.0001$), and the absolute benefit was 3.5 %. Furthermore, a plausible difference in overall survival was noted, reaching significance with an HR of 0.83 (0.69–1.00) [76]. An updated analysis was reported at the 2009 San Antonio Cancer Symposium [104]. These data verified the significant improvement in overall survival with an HR of 0.86 (0.75–0.99, $P=0.04$), translating into an absolute survival benefit of 2.4 % after 8 years of randomization.

The IES trial compared the toxicity profile of exemestane with tamoxifen in patients who previously received adjuvant tamoxifen for 2–3 years before randomization with women with early-stage BC. Cardiac events were defined as ischemic and other events. Results from the trial revealed that the overall rates of ischemic events were 9.9 % in the exemestane group and 8.6 % in the tamoxifen group. In addition, the MI rates were 1.3 % for exemestane and 0.8 % for tamoxifen, and the angina rates were 7.1 % for exemestane and 6.5 % for tamoxifen. Although the overall rates were increased in the exemestane group compared with the tamoxifen group, none of these increases were significant [105]. At 55.7 months of follow-up, the incidence of cardiovascular events did not differ between the exemestane and tamoxifen groups either during treatment (16.5 % and 15 %, respectively) or posttreatment [76]. The incidence of ischemic cardiovascular disease was comparable between the two arms: 8 % for the exemestane group and 6.9 % for the tamoxifen group ($P=0.17$). Significance was not achieved in terms of MI (1.3 % versus 0.8 %, respectively; $P=0.08$). However, patients in the exemestane arm who experienced an MI had more severe histories of hypertension compared with patients in the tamoxifen arm (71.1 % versus 31.6 %, respectively). These findings emphasize the importance of blood pressure monitoring for patients administered with adjuvant exemestane

[76]. The incidence of venous thromboembolic events was 1.2 % in patients who switched to exemestane and 2.3 % in patients who remained on tamoxifen ($P=0.004$), and similar results were observed in the overall study ($P=0.01$) (Table 50.3). The incidence of cerebrovascular events occurred in similar proportion between exemestane and tamoxifen in the IES (2.5 % versus 2.4 %, respectively; $P=0.89$). Consequently, the number of cardiovascular deaths was very low in both treatment groups.

The TEAM phase 3-trial was primarily designed to evaluate the efficacy and safety of 5 years of adjuvant exemestane compared with 5 years of tamoxifen in postmenopausal women with early-stage BC. Although results were in favor of the exemestane group during that period, a recent update analyzing 5 years of disease-free survival revealed similar rates between the groups (85.7 % versus 85.4 %, respectively) randomized to up-front exemestane or sequential treatment with tamoxifen followed by exemestane, and no differences in time to recurrence or overall survival were noted [106]. The incidence of hypertension was increased in the exemestane arm compared with the sequential arm but the difference not significant (4 % versus 3 %, respectively; $p=0.38$). The frequency of arrhythmia was 4 % versus 3 % for the exemestane arm versus the sequential arm, respectively ($P=0.038$). The frequency of myocardial ischemia or infarction was 2 % versus 1 %, respectively ($P=0.171$); the frequency of cardiac failure was 1 % versus <1 %, respectively ($P=0.009$). Although the overall incidence of cardiovascular events was increased in the exemestane group compared with the sequential arm, none of these results achieved significance. The benefit of AI on tamoxifen in terms of reducing vascular thrombotic events was evident in women with previous exposure to tamoxifen. In the TEAM study, vascular thrombotic events occurred in 2 % of patients who switched to exemestane compared with <1 % of patients who were exclusively exposed to exemestane ($P=0.0001$).

Cardiovascular deaths were increased with exemestane compared with sequential treatment; however, this difference was not significant

Table 50.3 Exemestane: irreversible, third-generation steroidal aromatase inhibitor

	IES (Intergroup Exemestane Study)			TEAM (The Tamoxifen Exemestane Adjuvant Multicenter)		
	Tamoxifen vs exemestane after 2–3 years of tamoxifen (total of 5 years)			Exemestane vs exemestane after 2–3 years of tamoxifen (total of 5 years)		
Design	Combined adjuvant			First-line adjuvant		
Median follow-up	55.7 months			5.1 years		
	TAM-EXE	TAM	P value	TAM-EXE	EXE	P value
Number of patients	2352	2372		4868	4898	
Median age	<60: 32.4 %, 60–69: 42.7 %	<60: 32.0 %, 60–69: 42.8 %		64 years		
Disease-free survival	HR: 0.75 (0.64–0.88)		P=0.0003	HR: 0.97 (0.88–1.08)		P=0.60
TTDR	HR: 0.83 (0.70–0.98)		P=0.03	HR: 0.93 (0.81–1.07)		P=0.30
Overall survival	HR: 0.83 (0.69–0.99)		P=0.04	HR: 1.00 (0.89–1.14)		P>0.99
All cardiac events	483 (20.8)	441 (18.9)	P=0.09	NA	NA	
Cardiac events	NA	NA		NA	NA	
Ischemic heart disease	229 (9.9)	200 (8.6)	P=0.12	NA	NA	
MI or ischemia	31 (1.3)	19 (0.8)	P=0.08	64 (1%)	82 (2%)	P=0.171
Angina	7.1%	6.5%	P=0.44	NA	NA	
Cardiac failure	1.8%	1.8%	P=0.94	26 (<1%)	50 (1%)	
Other cardiovascular events	261 (11.3)	262 (11.2)	P=0.96	73 (2%)	77 (2%)	P=0.843
CVA/TIA	2.5%	2.4%	P=0.89	60 (1%)	87 (2%)	P=0.035
Thromboembolism	45 (1.9)	572 (3.1)	P=0.01	99 (2%)	47 (<1%)	P=0.0001
Venous thrombosis				28 (<1%)	43 (<1%)	
Cardiac death	14	13		14 (<1%)	19 (<1%)	P=0.11
Cerebral related						
Vascular related	17	11		3 (<1%)	4 (<1%)	

IES HR+ group, *TEAM* Phase 3, HR+ group. *MI* myocardial infarction, *NA* not available, *HR* hazard ratio, *TTDR* time to distant recurrence

(<1 %). Depending on the differences between exemestane monotherapy and sequential treatment in terms of adverse events, the safety of these treatment strategies might play an important role in treatment decisions. It is important to consider the impact of patient age on cardiovascular health because the prevalence of comorbid illness among newly diagnosed BC patients increases with age; the most common comorbid illness is cardiovascular disease. History of hypertension was a significant predictor of ischemic heart disease, CVA/TIA, and thromboembolism. Hypercholesterolemia was associated with any adverse cardiac events, especially ischemic heart disease [85].

Comparison of AIs Versus Tamoxifen in Lowering the Incidence of Common Serious Events

Current treatments for BC, which is the most common malignancy among women, involve the adjuvant use of endocrine therapy for hormone receptor-positive BC after surgery (Table 50.4) [107, 108]. AIs are more effective and safer than tamoxifen in adjuvant endocrine strategies for either early or advanced stage hormone receptor-positive BC in postmenopausal women [73, 109–114]. As an endocrine therapy, increasing the use of AIs either sequentially or instead of tamoxifen appears to be beneficial in reducing the incidence of common serious events, such as thromboembolism and stroke, which are increased with tamoxifen treatment. The molecular differences between third-generation AIs affect not only selectivity for aromatase binding but also adverse cardiovascular events via binding to cardiovascular receptors or causing small alterations in serum lipid levels. However, evidence from large clinical trials indicates no major differences with respect to overall cardiovascular safety among AIs [40, 115]. Anastrozole is primarily specific to the aromatase enzyme and has fewer interactions with other enzymes. Hence, anastrozole is emerging as one plausible standard adjuvant treatment for hormone-sensitive early BC [116]. A recently published 10-year

analysis of the ATAC trial confirmed the previously reported efficacy and tolerability benefits of anastrozole as an initial adjuvant therapy for hormone-sensitive BC. Treatment-related serious adverse events were reduced in the anastrozole arm compared with the tamoxifen arm ($P < 0.0001$); however, rates were similar in the posttreatment period ($P = 0.3$) [94]. Although deaths without recurrence were increased with anastrozole (10.8 % versus 9.8 %, respectively; P = NS), cardiovascular deaths were less common with anastrozole compared with tamoxifen (2.9 % versus 3.0 %, respectively). Additionally, the incidence of cardiovascular deaths may have decreased with anastrozole in the off-treatment period compared with tamoxifen (Table 50.1). Although the median age was 72 years and tamoxifen exerts a cardioprotective effect, the decrease observed with anastrozole is considered remarkable. Regarding the reduction in distant recurrence, the decreased cardiovascular mortality observed with anastrozole might become significantly lower than that observed with tamoxifen in the future. At the 100-month follow-up, fewer CVAs were reported in patients receiving anastrozole ($P = 0.056$) but not in the off-treatment period ($P = 0.75$) [96]. After publishing 74 months of BIG 1-98 follow-up data, the incidence of cardiac and thromboembolic events was proportionately consistent during follow-up. Ischemic heart disease was increased in the letrozole arm compared with the tamoxifen arm, despite overall similar cardiac events (Table 50.2). An increase in the incidence of grade 3–5 cardiac events with letrozole remained evident with 74 months of follow-up; however, the number of events was minimal in each arm (3.8 % versus 2.1 % in the tamoxifen arm). In the BIG 1-98 trial, the incidence of heart failure was similar at 74 months of median follow-up between the letrozole and tamoxifen monotherapy groups (1.2 % versus 1.0 %, respectively); however, the results were significantly different at 25.8 months of follow-up (0.8 % versus 0.4 %, respectively; $P = 0.01$). The incidence of heart failure was reduced after cessation of letrozole treatment compared with the active treatment period.

Table 50.4 Comparing 5 years follow-up of aromatase inhibitors

	ATAC			BIG 1-98			IES			TEAM		
	Tamoxifen for 5 years vs anastrozole for 5 years (tamoxifen + anastrozole arm was discontinued at 47 months)			Four-arm trial; 5 tamoxifen vs letrozole or sequences of 2 years of one of these agents followed by 3 years of the other			Tamoxifen vs exemestane after 2–3 years tamoxifen (total of 5 years)			Exemestane vs exemestane after 2–3 years tamoxifen (total of 5 years)		
Median follow-up	68 months			74 months			55.7 months			5.1 years		
	ANA	TAM	P value	LET	TAM	P value	TAM-EXE	TAM	P value	TAM-EXE	EXE	P value
Number of patients	3125	3116		2448	2447		2352	2372		4868	4898	
Median age	64.1 years			61 years						64 years		
Disease-free survival	HR: 0.83 (0.73–0.94)		P=0.005	HR: 0.83 (0.74–0.94)		P=0.03	HR: 0.75 (0.64–0.88)		P=0.0003	HR: 0.97 (0.88–1.08)		P=0.60
Time to distant recurrence	HR: 0.84 (0.70–1.00)		P=0.06	HR: 0.80 (0.67–0.94)		P=0.05	HR: 0.83 (0.70–0.98)		P=0.03	HR: 0.93 (0.81–1.07)		P=0.30
Overall survival	HR: 0.97 (0.85–1.12)		P=0.7	HR: 0.82 (0.70–0.95)		P=0.08	HR: 0.83 (0.69–0.99)		P=0.04	HR: 1.00 (0.89–1.14)		P>0.99
All cardiac events	NA						483 (20.8)	441 (18.9)	P=0.09	NA		
Cardiac events	NA			169 (6.9)	152 (6.2)	P=0.36				NA		
Ischemic heart disease				69 (2.8)	49 (2.0)	P=0.08	229 (9.9)	200 (8.6)	P=0.12	NA		
Ischemic CV events	127 (4 %)	104 (3 %)	P=0.10							NA		
Myocardial infarction	37 (1.0%)	34 (1.0%)	P=0.5				31 (1.3)	19 (0.8)	P=0.08	64 (1 %)	82 (2 %)	P=0.171
Angina	71 (2.0%)	51 (2%)	P=0.07				7.1 %	6.5 %	P=0.44	NA		
Cardiac failure				30 (1.2)	25 (1.0)	P=0.59	1.8 %	1.8 %	P=0.94	26 (<1%)	50 (1%)	
Other CV events				24 (1.0)	13 (0.5)	P=0.10	261 (11.3)	262 (11.2)	P=0.96	73 (2%)	77 (2%)	P=0.843
Thromboembolism	87 (2.8%)	140 (4.5 %)	P=0.0004	63 (2.6)	104 (4.3)	P<0.001	45 (1.9)	572 (3.1)	P=0.01			
Cerebrovascular events	62 (2.0%)	88 (3.0%)	P=0.03	45 (1.8)	38 (1.6)	P=0.51	2.5 %	2.4 %	P=0.89			
Cardiovascular deaths	49 (2%)	46 (1%)								28 (<1 %)	43 (<1 %)	P=0.11
Cerebrovascular deaths	14 (<1%)	22 (1%)	P=NS							14 (<1 %)	19 (<1 %)	
										3 (<1 %)	4 (<1 %)	

NA not available, *NS* not significance, *HR* hazard ratio, *CV* cardiovascular events

In the IES, the frequency MI was very low in both treatment groups at 55.7 months of follow-up even though the patients comprised a population at risk for adverse cardiac events given their age [76]. Most patients who experienced MI in the exemestane group had a history of hypertension (71.1 %) compared with the tamoxifen group (31.6 %). The importance of blood pressure monitoring should be stressed [76]. Disregarding the other cardiovascular risk factors, advanced age and uncontrolled blood pressure are potentially related to these cardiac events. In the TEAM trial, no significant differences were reported between the exemestane and sequential groups in terms of disease-free survival ($P=0.60$) and overall survival ($P>0.99$) at a median 5.1 years of follow-up [64]. Data on disease-free survival were consistent with those from the BIG 1-98 trial, in which tamoxifen followed by letrozole or the reverse sequence versus letrozole alone was not associated with significant differences in efficacy after a median 71 months of follow-up [97]. Cardiac-related deaths were not significantly different in these treatment groups; however, the number of events was increased with exemestane compared with the sequential group ($P=0.11$). The incidence of cardiac failure was significantly increased in the exemestane monotherapy group compared with the sequential group ($P=0.009$). This result did not emerge previously in AI monotherapy trials. However, the result may be evident in the next follow-up because approximately 20 % of patients were still undergoing the trial treatment. Consequently, treatment compliance appears suboptimum, particularly in the sequence group (47 % of patients in the sequence group and 19 % of patients in the exemestane group discontinued treatment before 5 years for reasons other than disease-free survival).

The lipid-lowering effect of tamoxifen may explain the increased lipid levels with AIs versus tamoxifen [117, 118]. Whether AIs have long-term detrimental effects on lipids is unknown despite the findings that significantly more patients had hypercholesterolemia in the aromatase group compared with the tamoxifen group in the ATAC and BIG 1-98 trials [74, 75]. Although a steroidal AI (exemestane) was thought to have beneficial effects on lipid metabolism, all third-generation AIs have similar effects on lipids [119]. Additionally, cardiovascular events were similar between the letrozole and placebo groups after 5 years of tamoxifen treatment in the MA.17 trial.

All studies comparing the safety of AIs with tamoxifen have demonstrated an overall decreased risk of thromboembolic events in patients administered with AIs versus tamoxifen; however, postmenopausal women administered with endocrine therapy for BC live longer with their disease and remain at risk for such adverse events [65]. Because AIs carry a risk for cardiovascular events, these patients should be evaluated more carefully than age-matched individuals to minimize cardiovascular events during therapy [85].

Cardiac Monitoring

Several recommendations and guidelines are available for the assessment and monitoring of cardiac toxicity during and after breast cancer treatment [120–125]. These recommendations are mainly based on expert consensus due to the paucity of available high-level evidence.

Two of the basic concepts that are common in all the guidelines include the value of a careful case-by-case baseline evaluation of preexisting risk factors for cardiac adverse events and the need for appropriate and well-structured cardiac monitoring during and after cancer therapy to identify patients with asymptomatic cardiac dysfunction such that breast cancer treatments can be modified and cardiac medication can be initiated.

Table 50.1 presents a summary of recommendations and areas of active research regarding the assessment, monitoring, and treatment of cardiac toxicity due to cancer therapy in patients with early breast cancer.

Baseline Assessment/Evaluation

The purpose of the baseline evaluation is to identify patients at high risk for cardiac toxicity due to cancer therapy. We previously discussed in this chapter several risk factors for cardiac toxicity during anticancer therapy that has been identified. However, it is difficult to incorporate the baseline assessment in an algorithm for cardiac monitoring given the lack of evidence regarding the strength of each risk factor in the estimation of cardiac risk. The only available cardiac risk score has been developed by investigators from the NSABP B-31 trial (trastuzumab versus no trastuzumab in the adjuvant setting) to predict the absolute risk of heart failure in individual patients who received trastuzumab as adjuvant therapy [126]. However, the lack of independent validation of the model limits its clinical use to date.

The baseline evaluation also includes a cardiac imaging test for the evaluation of cardiac structure and function [120–125]. Some guidelines recognize the practical difficulty of performing baseline imaging evaluation on all breast cancer patients before adjuvant treatment and recommend exclusively evaluating women with risk factors for cardiac toxicities or those who plan to receive high cumulative doses of anthracyclines or at least two therapies that could influence heart function [91]. However, baseline imaging is mandatory for all patients who plan to receive trastuzumab without any exceptions [121, 122].

At present, the most frequently used modality for detecting cardiotoxicity is the measurement of LVEF via either echocardiography or multi-gated acquisition scanning (MUGA). Echocardiography is generally preferred over MUGA given its widespread availability, the ability to investigate diastolic function, and the absence of radiation exposure [95]. However, echocardiography depends on the expertise and interpretation of echocardiographers, whereas MUGA offers a more objective and reliable calculation of LVEF [127].

The major shortcoming in measuring LVEF is that the technique is insensitive to slight changes in myocardial function [5]. As a consequence, a decrease in LVEF occurs when a critical amount of myocardial damage, which might be irreversible, has already occurred [128, 129]. Moreover, LVEF is a measurement of systolic cardiac function and does not provide any assessment of other measurements, such as diastolic function or valvular structure and function. Novel ultrasound imaging techniques, including tissue

Doppler imaging (TDI) and 3D and contrast echocardiography, overcome some of the shortcomings of conventional echocardiography. Contrast and 3D echocardiography offer a more accurate calculation of LVEF compared with standard 2D echocardiography [130, 131]. In addition, 3D echocardiography might provide a tool for earlier identification of subclinical myocardial damages [132]. TDI is a relatively new echocardiographic technique that uses Doppler principles to measure the velocity of myocardial motion, deformation (strain), and the rate of deformation (strain rate). Clinical studies have reported that TDI measurements detect preclinical changes in systolic function that occur prior to conventional changes in LVEF regardless of the cancer therapy (e.g., anthracyclines radiotherapy, trastuzumab) that was responsible for the cardiac toxicity [133–136].

Recently, studies on the general population found that the coronary artery score, as assessed by computed tomography, could serve as an additional marker for the prediction of coronary artery disease [137]. Whether this marker can be used in the baseline assessment of breast cancer patients before adjuvant therapy is unknown. Further studies are necessary to identify the predictive value of these imaging modalities.

Cardiac magnetic resonance imaging is considered the gold standard for LVEF assessment as well as volume and mass measurements. Early studies in cancer patients allow accurate assessments of subclinical or established cardiotoxicity from cancer therapy [138]. However, its lack of availability and high cost limit its routine use. Based on the current data of cost and availability of the method, the authors of a recent review concluded that magnetic resonance imaging is an important complement to the current algorithms of cardiac assessment and monitoring rather than a screening tool for all patients treated with cardiotoxic cancer therapies [138]. In addition to imaging modalities, a new approach based on biochemical cardiac markers (troponins T and I, B-type natriuretic peptide (BNP), and N-terminal pro-BNP (NT-proBNP)) has emerged as a tool for both baseline assessment and monitoring during cancer therapy. In patients treated with anthracyclines, an early elevation of troponin appears to identify patients who are at risk for cardiac toxicity, which allows the individualization of monitoring and the adoption of preventive strategies in selected patients [139, 140]. Similarly, in patients treated with trastuzumab, elevation of troponin during therapy could identify a group of patients who are at high risk for cardiac toxicity and have a reduced likelihood of recovery of cardiac function [141–143]. However, others have failed to detect any clinical value of cardiac troponins during or following cancer therapy [136, 144].

The family of natriuretic peptides (BNP and NT-proBNP) has also been investigated as markers of early cardiac damage during cancer therapy with less reliable and consistent results compared with troponin. Some studies have reported an association between BNP or NT-proBNP elevation and increased risk for cardiac toxicity, whereas others did not identify any correlation [145–150].

A number of barriers in cardiac biomarker studies limit their widespread application as early markers of cancer therapy-induced cardiac toxicity. First, the timing of biomarker assessment varies among studies, which may partially explain the inconsistent results. Thus, the optimal timing remains uncharacterized. Moreover, an optimal assay and a widely acceptable cutoff value are not available. In addition, most of the available studies are small with heterogeneous cancer populations who received multiple types of cancer therapy. As a result, the utility of cardiac biomarkers as diagnostic and predictive tools for cardiac dysfunction in patients with potential cardiotoxic cancer therapy must be clarified using results from larger ongoing studies. Despite these caveats, some guidelines have included the measurements of cardiac biomarkers in their suggested algorithms [121, 122].

Guidelines on Cardiac Monitoring

The same imaging modalities and cardiac biomarkers that were discussed earlier as methods for baseline assessment and evaluation are also available for cardiac monitoring during cancer therapy. Echocardiography or MUGA for the calculation of LVEF is the backbone of all the current guidelines regarding cardiac monitoring during cancer therapy [120–125].

The ESMO guidelines recommend serial monitoring of cardiac function with echocardiography or MUGA at baseline; 3, 6, and 9 months during treatment (anthracyclines and/or trastuzumab); and 12 and 18 months after the initiation of treatment [89]. The authors also discuss the possibility of using repeated measurements of cardiac biomarkers as an additional monitoring technique [121]. However, they recognize the need for further data by classifying this recommendation as B with a level of evidence III. No recommendations are available regarding the assessment and monitoring of breast cancer patients treated with radiotherapy in the ESMO guidelines [121].

The American Society of Echocardiography (ASE) and the European Association of Cardiovascular Imaging (EACVI) use guidelines that are largely similar to the ESMO guidelines concerning time intervals in cardiac monitoring during trastuzumab therapy and the potential value of cardiac biomarkers in the baseline assessment and monitoring [122]. However, some differences are noted in some recommendations. The ASE/EACVI guidelines recommend cardiac monitoring 6 months after completion of trastuzumab therapy only in patients who previously received a type I cardiotoxic agent (i.e., anthracyclines). In addition to cardiac biomarkers, the ASE/EACVI guidelines recommend (with the same grade of recommendation) the use of an additional echocardiographic parameter, namely, global longitudinal strain. The ASE/EACVI guidelines recommend that cardiac monitoring during anthracycline-based chemotherapy is performed at baseline, treatment completion, and 6 months after treatment completion.

The same societies (ASE/EACVI) currently released the first guidelines regarding assessment and cardiac monitoring in adult patients with cancer treated with radiotherapy that will result in a radiation dose to the heart [120]. The authors recommend baseline assessment of cardiovascular risk factors and baseline echocardiography to identify any cardiac abnormalities for all patients before radiotherapy. During follow-up, a yearly history and physical examination with close attention to symptoms and signs of heart disease is recommended. In asymptomatic patients, screening echocardiography is recommended 10 years after treatment (or 5 years in case of high-risk populations, namely, those who received left-side chest radiotherapy or those with at least one risk factor for RIHD) and every 5 years after the initial 10-year echocardiographic screening examination. In high-risk populations, noninvasive stress imaging to screen for coronary artery disease should be considered given the increased risk of coronary events 5–10 years after radiotherapy [27].

Prevention and Management of Cardiac Toxicity in BC Survivors

Strategies to Prevent Cardiac Toxicity

The interest in the use of standard cardiovascular medications to prevent cardiac toxicity due to cancer therapy in breast cancer patients is growing. HMG-CoA reductase inhibitors (statins) attenuate doxorubicin-induced cardiomyocyte cell death and radiation-induced cell apoptosis in preclinical studies. One retrospective study (201 patients) and one small randomized trial (40 patients) support the potential role of statins in reducing heart failure and maintaining cardiac function in breast cancer patients treated with anthracyclines [151–154]. No clinical data on the potential protective effect of statins in radiation-induced cardiac toxicity are available. Several studies that investigate the use of statins to prevent cancer therapy-associated cardiac toxicity in breast cancer patients are ongoing, and the results will enlighten their role as cardioprotective agents.

Beta-blockers have also been studied as preventive agents against cardiac toxicity in breast cancer patients. Although the exact mechanism of cardioprotection from beta-blockers remains unclear, several mechanisms have been proposed based on preclinical data, including mitigation of oxidative stress and preservation of β-adrenergic receptor recruitment of β-arrestin, which is an

endogenous protective agent [155, 156]. In the only published randomized trial dedicated to breast cancer patients, the administration of nebivolol ($n=27$) with anthracycline-based chemotherapy was associated with a reduced risk of LVEF decline at 6 months compared with the placebo arm ($n=18$) [157]. Similar data were observed in two additional randomized trials: a small trial with 50 patients treated with anthracycline-based chemotherapy (34 of 50 patients had breast cancer) wherein carvedilol was compared with placebo and a larger trial of 90 patients with hematologic malignancies in which the combination of enalapril and carvedilol was compared with nonintervention [158, 159]. This latter trial (OVERCOME trial) is the first randomized trial to investigate the protective effect of cardiovascular medication in cancer treatment-related cardiotoxicity that presented not only data on surrogate outcomes of cardiac toxicity but also clinically relevant outcomes, such as symptomatic heart failure and death. Interestingly, patients in the intervention group exhibited a reduced incidence of the combined event of death or heart failure compared with the nonintervention group [159]. In contrast with beta-blockers and anthracycline-based cardiotoxicity, limited clinical evidence regarding the role of beta-blockers in trastuzumab-associated cardiotoxicity is available. Two retrospective studies have found that the combination of beta-blockers and ACE-i lead to an increased possibility of LVEF recovery [160, 161]. As noted for the statins, several randomized trials are ongoing and will hopefully definitively define the role of beta-blockers as cardioprotective agents in anthracycline- and trastuzumab-associated cardiac toxicity.

The third category of cardiovascular medication with potential benefit as a cardioprotective agent for cancer therapy-related cardiotoxicity includes ACE-i/angiotensin II receptor blockers (ARB). Several mechanisms that could mediate this cardioprotective effect have been proposed based on preclinical data: reduction in interstitial fibrosis, attenuation of oxidative stress, and down-regulation of the actions of the NRG-1/ErbB system [162–164]. Several small randomized trials have reported that the administration of ACE-i/

ARB during anthracycline-based chemotherapy reduces the risk for cardiac dysfunction, as measured by conventional cardiac imaging modalities [165–167]. In addition, in the previously mentioned OVERCOME trial, the combination of beta-blockers and ACE-i reduced the risk of clinically relevant outcomes [159]. The study of Cardinale et al. is unique in its design because the authors used a biomarker (troponin I) to guide treatment [167]. The authors used the elevation of troponin I, which was measured soon after high-dose chemotherapy, to select 114 patients with various malignancies for randomization to placebo versus 20 mg enalapril daily for 1 year. The incidence of a 10 % LVEF decline was significantly increased in the control arm (43 %) compared with the ACE-i-treated arm (0 %) [167]. Only preclinical data are available; no clinical evidence is available on the potential cardioprotective effect of ACE-i/ARB with trastuzumab or radiation therapy [168]. However, this potential cardioprotective effect is an area of active investigation.

In addition to pharmacological interventions, some preclinical data suggest that even non-pharmacological interventions may prevent cardiac toxicity. Aerobic exercise attenuates doxorubicin-induced cardiotoxicity in animal models [169]. However, a small study in patients treated with trastuzumab found that exercise training was not effective in preventing adverse left ventricular remodeling [170]. Whether aerobic exercise is a protective intervention against anthracycline- or trastuzumab-related cardiac toxicity in breast cancer patients must be studied in randomized trials. The only medication that has been approved by the US Food and Drug Administration for the prevention of anthracycline-related cardiotoxicity is dexrazoxane. Its mechanism of action and clinical evidence for its use were described earlier in this chapter.

Management of Cardiac Toxicity

In the general population, the guidelines suggest the use of beta-blockers and ACE-i/ARBs in patients with asymptomatic LVEF decline [171]. A similar treatment strategy, namely, the initia-tion of appropriate medication promptly after the detection of asymptomatic cardiac dysfunction, should be pursued in patients with cardiac dysfunction due to cancer therapy [121]. However, the evidence behind this treatment strategy for cancer patients is obtained from relatively small prospective studies, and further studies, preferably randomized trials, are still needed [167, 172]. In trastuzumab-treated patients, the evidence that supports the use of ACE-i/ARBs with or without beta-blockers in asymptomatic cardiac dysfunction (LVEF, 40 % or between 40 % and 50 % in some guidelines) is limited to small case series, but this strategy is generally accepted [121, 122, 124]. Two additional parameters that should be considered in trastuzumab-induced cardiac toxicity include the need to withhold trastuzumab according to specific criteria (LVEF 44 % or LVEF 45–49 % and 10 % from baseline) with reevaluation after 3–4 weeks and the fact that the therapeutic target of cardiovascular medications should be achieved faster compared with the general population to readminister trastuzumab [121, 173–175].

In cases of symptomatic heart failure due to cancer therapy, the recommended treatment strategy does not differ from the treatment of heart failure patients in general and includes the routine use of either ACE-i or ARB and beta-blockers with diuretics added for symptomatic congestion. In trastuzumab-induced heart failure, the LVEF should be reevaluated after adequate dose titrations of cardiovascular medication. If the LVEF returns to baseline, trastuzumab can be restarted in combination with cardiovascular medications [121, 173]. If the LVEF remains persistently low or further declines or if heart failure symptoms recur, the treating oncologist should discuss the risks and benefits of discontinuation of trastuzumab with the patient [121, 173]. Patients with radiation-induced heart diseases should be treated as non-radiation-related patients [121].

Recent advancements in curative-intent therapies have led to significant improvements in BC survival, but these advancements have come at the direct expense of increased risks of cardiovascular event or injury. It is important to recognize cardiac toxicity and to attempt to mitigate its onset not only by selecting appropriate patients for adjuvant therapy but also by selecting appropriate therapy based on patient risk factors and risk of recurrence. Increasing awareness and educating patients about cardiac toxicity is crucial. Overall, women with BC exhibit a notably worse cardiovascular risk profile compared with age-matched controls [176, 177]. Adjuvant therapies are selected on the basis of a complex schema, including patient factors (age, comorbid illness, and patient preference) and tumor factors (grade, size, lymph node involvement, ER and HER-2) [178].

Women diagnosed with BC are already at risk for cardiovascular disease, and almost all adjuvant therapies are associated with unique and varying degrees of cardiovascular injury. When selecting a treatment regimen, these patients are subjected to a series of sequential cardiovascular injury risks coupled with lifestyle perturbations that leave patients with obvious or subclinical cardiovascular disease. Unfortunately, each of the chemotherapeutic agents used in BC treatment has identically acute and long-term cardiac complications. Ischemic heart disease (e.g., MI, angina pectoris), cardiac failure, hypertension, peripheral atherosclerosis, and thromboembolic events are the major adverse events associated with these agents. The mechanism of chemotherapy-associated cardiac dysfunction or injury remains uncharacterized [85].

Measurement of the LVEF by echocardiography is a frequently used, effective approach to monitor cardiac function and its impairment by chemotherapy. LVEF is one of the most important predictors of prognosis because patients with significantly reduced ejection fractions typically exhibit poorer prognoses. However, current imaging techniques (echocardiography, coronary angiography, etc.) have limited ability to detect early cardiac damage [40]. The use of sensitive monitoring modalities (e.g., magnetic resonance imaging, exercise, or dobutamine stress testing) and biochemical markers (e.g., troponin I, BNP) permits more accurate detection and quantification of subclinical cardiac damage [179]. Increased troponin I levels are a significant predictor of left ventricular dysfunction after chemotherapy among cancer patients [139].

Decreases in physical activity with a diagnosis of BC may trigger increases in body weight and body fat, which may lead to a worse cancer prognosis [180, 181]. A greater decrease in physical activity has been observed among obese BC patients compared with normal weight and overweight patients ($P < 0.05$), suggesting a potential weight gain among already obese women [180, 181]. Furthermore, obesity is significantly associated with an increased recurrence risk in BC patients without any association with age or menopausal status [182, 183]. Results from one weight gain study reported that 84 % of 535 BC patients gained weight (mean 1.6 kg) in the first year after diagnosis, and the Women's Healthy Eating and Living (WHEL) study reported that 60 % of 1,116 women gained weight (mean 2.7 kg) from 1 year before diagnosis to up to 4 years after diagnosis [184, 185]. The effects of weight gain on BC are unclear. Although some studies report an association between weight gain and an earlier disease recurrence, others have failed to produce similar results [184, 186–192]. One study in which 646 patients were followed for a median of 6.6 years found that premenopausal women who gained more than 5.9 kg were 1.5-fold more likely to relapse and 1.6-fold more likely to die from BC than those who were gaining less weight [187]. Although it is unknown whether post-diagnosis weight gain influences the risk for progressive disease, weight gain unfavorably affects risks of cardiovascular disease, hypertension, and diabetes [193–195].

Several strategies have been advised to prevent or reduce cardiac toxicity. One of these strategies involves ACE inhibition, which results in a significant reduction in LV dysfunction in patients with increased troponin I levels soon after chemotherapy [167]. The management of risk factors in patients with BC is crucial. Recommendations for the treatment of these risk factors include either pharmacotherapy or lifestyle modification. Beta-blockers and ACE-i are primarily suggested as initial therapies for hypertension with the subsequent addition of other agents (e.g., thiazides). In cases of hypercholesterolemia, statins are recommended to reduce low-density lipoprotein cholesterol to less than 100 mg/dl. Furthermore, statins are associated with a reduced incidence of thromboembolism in patients with cancer [196]. Additionally, diabetes mellitus management is related to cardiovascular disease given the utility of using biguanides or sulfonylurea for women with type II diabetes to achieve a 7 % glycosylated hemoglobin (HbA1c) [197]. Exercise training may be favorable with regard to its demonstrated effects on cardiovascular reserve, individual risk factors, and overall reductions in cardiovascular mortality [198, 199]. A meta-analysis reported that exercise training resulted in a significant increase in exercise capacity among women with early BC, whereas epidemiologic data suggest that greater physical activity after therapy is related to a reduction in all causes of mortality, including BC-specific causes [200].

Of note, data on the adverse cardiovascular effects of AIs must be interpreted with caution in conjunction with baseline cardiovascular disease, LVEF, and cardiac risk factors. All of the safety analyses were conducted via comparisons with tamoxifen, whereas the mechanisms of cardiovascular events have not been clearly elucidated. It is difficult to know how to apply the results of these safety analyses to patients with an elevated risk of cardiovascular disease without analyzing baseline cardiovascular risk factors. Given this weak evidence regarding cardiovascular toxicity and short-term follow-up, no consensus is available regarding the management of cardiovascular toxicity and its consequences [85].

Further research is required to anticipate the relative portion of cardiovascular morbidity and mortality attributable to either lifestyle modification or adjuvant therapy among women with BC.

Conclusion

Exciting new cancer therapies are being discovered; however, to maximize their potential, cardiac toxicities must be identified and addressed up front. Although recent clinical experience has demonstrated significant cardiotoxicity posttrial with cancer therapies, we have also observed the resolution of toxicity using evidence-based cardiology guidelines. For continued success in making cancer history, cardiology and oncology must align their clinical and translational research goals. Cardiologists should also collaborate with oncologists in trial designs.

References

1. Jemal A, Thomas A, Murray T, Thun M. Cancer statistics, 2002. CA Cancer J Clin. 2002;52:23–47.
2. NCI Dictionary of Cancer Terms http://www.cancer.gov/dictionary
3. Raschi E, Ponti FD. Cardiovascular toxicity of anticancer-targeted therapy: emerging issues in the era of cardio-oncology. Intern Emerg Med. 2012;7:113–31.
4. Von Hoff DD, Layard MW, Basa P, Davis Jr HL, Von Hoff AL, Rozencweig M, Muggia FM. Risk factors for doxorubicin-induced congestive heart failure. Ann Intern Med. 1979;91:710–7.
5. Ewer MS, Ali MK, Mackay B, Wallace S, Valdivieso M, Legha SS, et al. A comparison of cardiac biopsy grades and ejection fraction estimations in patients receiving Adriamycin. J Clin Oncol. 1984;2:112–7.
6. Seidman A, Hudis C, Pierri MK, Shak S, Paton V, Ashby M, et al. Cardiac dysfunction in the trastuzumab clinical trials experience. J Clin Oncol. 2002;20:1215–21.
7. Jessup M, Abraham WT, Casey DE. 2009 focused update ACCF/AHA guidelines for the diagnosis and management of heart failure in adults. J Am Coll Cardiol. 2009;53:1343–82.
8. Yancy, et al. ACCF/AHA heart failure guideline. Circulation. 2013;128:e240–327.
9. Soran OZ, Piña IL, Lamas GA, Kelsey SF, Selzer F, Pilotte J, Lave JR, Feldman AM. A randomized clinical trial of the clinical effects of enhanced heart failure monitoring using a computer-based telephonic monitoring system in older minorities and women. J Card Fail. 2008;14:711–7.
10. Soran O, Vargo JA, Polat AV, Soran A, Sumkin J, Beriwal S. No association between left-breast radiation therapy or breast arterial calcification and long-term cardiac events in patients with breast cancer. J Women's Health (Larchmt). 2014;23:1005–111.
11. Kaklamani VG, Gradishar WJ. Epirubicin versus doxorubicin: which is the anthracycline of choice for the treatment of breast cancer? Clin Breast Cancer. 2003;4 Suppl 1:S26–33.
12. Singal PK, Iliskovic N. Doxorubicin-induced cardiomyopathy. N Engl J Med. 1998;339:900–5.
13. Lyu YL, Kerrigan JE, Lin CP, Azarova AM, Tsai YC, Ban Y, Liu LF. Topoisomerase II beta mediated DNA double-strand breaks: implications in doxorubicin cardiotoxicity and prevention by dexrazoxane. Cancer Res. 2007;67:8839–46.

14. Ewer MS, Lippman SM. Type II chemotherapy-related cardiac dysfunction: time to recognize a new entity. J Clin Oncol. 2005;23:2900–2.

15. Smith LA, Cornelius VR, Plummer CJ, Levitt G, Verrill M, Canney P, Jones A. Cardiotoxicity of anthracycline agents for the treatment of cancer: systematic review and meta-analysis of randomised controlled trials. BMC Cancer. 2010;10:337.

16. Lotrionte M, Biondi-Zoccai G, Abbate A, Lanzetta G, D'Ascenzo F, Malavasi V, et al. Review and meta-analysis of incidence and clinical predictors of anthracycline cardiotoxicity. Am J Cardiol. 2013;112:1980–4.

17. Swain SM, Whaley FS, Ewer MS. Congestive heart failure in patients treated with doxorubicin: a retrospective analysis of three trials. Cancer. 2003;97:2869–79.

18. Ryberg M, Nielsen D, Skovsgaard T, Hansen J, Jensen BV, Dombernowsky P. Epirubicin cardiotoxicity: an analysis of 469 patients with metastatic breast cancer. J Clin Oncol. 1998;16:3502–8.

19. Minotti G, Licata S, Saponiero A, Menna P, Calafiore AM, Di Giammarco G, et al. Anthracycline metabolism and toxicity in human myocardium: comparisons between doxorubicin, epirubicin, and a novel disaccharide analogue with a reduced level of formation and (4Fe-4S) reactivity of its secondary alcohol metabolite. Chem Res Toxicol. 2000;13:1336–41.

20. Ryberg M, Nielsen D, Cortese G, Nielsen G, Skovsgaard T, Andersen PK. New insight into epirubicin cardiac toxicity: competing risks analysis of 1097 breast cancer patients. J Natl Cancer Inst. 2008;100:1058–67.

21. van Dalen EC, van der Pal HJ, Caron HN, Kremer LC. Different dosage schedules for reducing cardiotoxicity in cancer patients receiving anthracycline chemotherapy. Cochrane Database Syst Rev. 2006;4, CD005008.

22. Giotta F, Lorusso V, Maiello E, Filippelli G, Valerio MR, Caruso M, et al. Liposomal-encapsulated doxorubicin plus cyclophosphamide as first-line therapy in metastatic breast cancer: a phase II multicentric study. Ann Oncol. 2007;18 Suppl 6:vi66–9.

23. Brain EG, Mertens C, Girre V, Rousseau F, Blot E, Abadie S, et al. Impact of liposomal doxorubicin-based adjuvant chemotherapy on autonomy in women over 70 with hormone-receptor-negative breast carcinoma: a French Geriatric Oncology Group (GERICO) phase II multicentre trial. Crit Rev Oncol Hematol. 2011;80:160–70.

24. Rayson D, Suter TM, Jackisch C, van der Vegt S, Bermejo B, van den Bosch J, et al. Cardiac safety of adjuvant pegylated liposomal doxorubicin with concurrent trastuzumab: a randomized phase II trial. Ann Oncol. 2012;23(7):1780–8.

25. Joo KI, Xiao L, Liu S, Liu Y, Lee CL, Conti PS, et al. Crosslinked multilamellar liposomes for controlled delivery of anticancer drugs. Biomaterials. 2013;34: 3098–109.

26. Liu Y, Fang J, Kim YJ, Wong MK, Wang P. Codelivery of doxorubicin and paclitaxel by cross-linked multilamellar liposome enables synergistic antitumor activity. Mol Pharm. 2014;11:1651–61.

27. Valachis A, Nilsson C. Cardiac risk in the treatment of breast cancer: assessment and management. Breast Cancer Targets Ther. 2015;7:21–35.

28. Slamon D, Eiermann W, Robert N, Pienkowski T, Martin M, Press M, et al. Adjuvant trastuzumab in HER2-positive breast cancer. N Engl J Med. 2011;365:1273–83.

29. Sparano JA. Taxanes for breast cancer: an evidence-based review of randomized phase II and phase III trials. Clin Breast Cancer. 2000;1(1):32–40.

30. Arbuck SG, Strauss H, Rowinsky E, Christian M, Suffness M, Adams J, et al. A reassessment of cardiac toxicity associated with taxol. J Natl Cancer Inst Monogr. 1993;15:117–30.

31. Rowinsky EK, McGuire WP, Guarnieri T, Fisherman JS, Christian MC, Donehower RC, et al. Cardiac disturbances during the administration of taxol. J Clin Oncol. 1991;9:1704–12.

32. Giordano SH, Booser DJ, Murray JL, Ibrahim NK, Rahman ZU, Valero V, et al. A detailed evaluation of cardiac toxicity: a phase II study of doxorubicin and one- or three-hour-infusion paclitaxel in patients with metastatic breast cancer. Clin Cancer Res. 2002;8:3360–8.

33. Holmes FA, Valero V, Walters RS, Theriault RL, Booser DJ, Gibbs H, et al. Paclitaxel by 24-hour infusion with doxorubicin by 48-hour infusion as initial therapy for metastatic breast cancer: phase I results. Ann Oncol. 1999;10:403–11.

34. Jassem J, Pienkowski, Pluzanska A, Jelic S, Gorbunova V, Berzins J, et al. Doxorubicin and paclitaxel versus fluorouracil, doxorubicin, and cyclophosphamide as first-line therapy for women with metastatic breast cancer: final results of a randomized phase III multicenter trial. J Clin Oncol. 2001;19:1707–15.

35. Grasselli G, Vigano L, Capri G, Locatelli A, Tarenzi E, Spreafico C, et al. Clinical and pharmacologic study of the epirubicin and paclitaxel combination in women with metastatic breast cancer. J Clin Oncol. 2001;19:2222–36.

36. Gennari A, Salvadori B, Donati S, Bengala C, Orlandini C, Danesi R, et al. Cardiotoxicity of epirubicin/paclitaxel-containing regimens: role of cardiac risk factors. J Clin Oncol. 1999;17:3596–602.

37. Gianni L, Baselga J, Eiermann W, Guillem Porta V, Semiglazov V, et al. Feasibility and tolerability of sequential doxorubicin/paclitaxel followed by cyclophosphamide, methotrexate, and fluorouracil and its effects on tumor response as preoperative therapy. Clin Cancer Res. 2005;11:8715–21.

38. Fountzilas G, Skarlos D, Dafni U, Gogas H, Briasoulis E, Pectasides D, et al. Postoperative dose-dense sequential chemotherapy with epirubicin, followed by

CMF with or without paclitaxel, in patients with high-risk operable breast cancer: a randomized phase III study conducted by the Hellenic Cooperative Oncol Group. Ann Oncol. 2005;16:1762–71.

39. Nyman DW, Campbell KJ, Hersh E, Long K, Richardson K, Trieu V, et al. Phase I and pharmacokinetics trial of ABI-007, a novel nanoparticle formulation of paclitaxel in patients with advanced nonhematologic malignancies. J Natl Cancer Inst. 2005;23:7785–93.

40. Brian RJ, Bird H, Swain SM. Cardiac toxicity in breast cancer survivors: review of potential cardiac problems. Clin Cancer Res. 2008;14:14–23.

41. Dawood S, Broglio K, Buzdar AU, Hortobagyi GN, Giordano SH. Prognosis of women with metastatic breast cancer by HER2 status and trastuzumab treatment: an institutional-based review. J Clin Oncol. 2010;28:92–8.

42. Viani GA, Afonso SL, Stefano EJ, De Fendi LI, Soares FV. Adjuvant trastuzumab in the treatment of her-2-positive early breast cancer: a meta-analysis of published randomized trials. BMC Cancer. 2007; 7:153.

43. Onitilo AA, Engel JM, Stankowski RV. Cardiovascular toxicity associated with adjuvant trastuzumab therapy: prevalence, patient characteristics, and risk factors. Ther Adv Drug Saf. 2014;5:154–66.

44. Moja L, Tagliabue L, Balduzzi S, Parmelli E, Pistotti V, Guarneri V, et al. Trastuzumab containing regimens for early breast cancer. Cochrane Database Syst Rev. 2012;4:CD006243.

45. Bowles EJ, Wellman R, Feigelson HS, Onitilo AA, Freedman AN, Delate T, et al. Risk of heart failure in breast cancer patients after anthracycline and trastuzumab treatment: a retrospective cohort study. J Natl Cancer Inst. 2012;104:1293–305.

46. Naumann D, Rusius V, Margiotta C, Nevill A, Carmichael A, Rea D, et al. Factors predicting trastuzumab-related cardiotoxicity in a real-world population of women with HER2+ breast cancer. Anticancer Res. 2013;33:1717–20.

47. Zhao YY, Sawyer DR, Baliga RR, Opel DJ, Han X, Marchionni MA, et al. Neuregulins promote survival and growth of cardiac myocytes. Persistence of ErbB2 and ErbB4 expression in neonatal and adult ventricular myocytes. J Biol Chem. 1998;273: 10261–9.

48. De Keulenaer GW, Doggen K, Lemmens K. The vulnerability of the heart as a pluricellular paracrine organ: lessons from unexpected triggers of heart failure in targeted erbb2 anticancer therapy. Circ Res. 2010;106:35–46.

49. Russo G, Cioffi G, Di Lenarda A, Tuccia F, Bovelli D, Di Tano G, et al. Role of renal function on the development of cardiotoxicity associated with trastuzumab-based adjuvant chemotherapy for early breast cancer. Intern Emerg Med. 2012;7:439–46.

50. Perez EA, Suman VJ, Davidson NE, Gralow JR, Kaufman PA, Visscher DW, et al. Cardiac safety analysis of doxorubicin and cyclophosphamide followed by paclitaxel with or without trastuzumab in the North Central Cancer Treatment Group N9831 adjuvant breast cancer trial. J Clin Oncol. 2008;26: 1231–8.

51. Chen J, Long JB, Hurria A, Owusu C, Steingart RM, Gross CP. Incidence of heart failure or cardiomyopathy after adjuvant trastuzumab therapy for breast cancer. J Am Coll Cardiol. 2012;60:2504–12.

52. Serrano C, Cortés J, De Mattos-Arruda L, Bellet M, Gómez P, Saura C, et al. Trastuzumab-related cardiotoxicity in the elderly: a role for cardiovascular risk factors. Ann Oncol. 2012;23:897–902.

53. Beauclair S, Formento P, Fischel JL, Lescaut W, Largillier R, Chamorey E, et al. Role of the HER2 (Ile655Val) genetic polymorphism in tumorogenesis and in the risk of trastuzumab-related cardiotoxicity. Ann Oncol. 2007;18:1335–41.

54. Lemieux J, Diorio C, Côté MA, Provencher L, Barabé F, Jacob S, et al. Alcohol and HER2 polymorphisms as risk factor for cardiotoxicity in breast cancer treated with trastuzumab. Anticancer Res. 2013;33:2569–76.

55. Roca L, Diéras V, Roché H, Lappartient E, Kerbrat P, Cany L, et al. Correlation of HER2, FCGR2A, and FCGR3A gene polymorphisms with trastuzumab related cardiac toxicity and efficacy in a subgroup of patients from UNICANCER-PACS 04 trial. Breast Cancer Res Treat. 2013;139:789–800.

56. Geyer CE, Forster J, Lindquist D, Chan S, Romieu CG, Pienkowski T, et al. Lapatinib plus capecitabine for HER2-positive advanced breast cancer. N Engl J Med. 2006;355:2733–43.

57. Baselga J, Cortés J, Kim SB, Im SA, Hegg R, Im YH, et al. Pertuzumab plus trastuzumab plus docetaxel for metastatic breast cancer. N Engl J Med. 2012;366:109–19.

58. Gianni L, Pienkowski T, Im YH, Roman L, Tseng LM, Liu MC, et al. Efficacy and safety of neoadjuvant pertuzumab and trastuzumab in women with locally advanced, inflammatory, or early HER2-positive breast cancer (NeoSphere): a randomised multicentre, open-label, phase 2 trial. Lancet Oncol. 2012;13:25–32.

59. Valachis A, Nearchou A, Lind P, Mauri D. Lapatinib, trastuzumab or the combination added to preoperative chemotherapy for breast cancer: a meta-analysis of randomized evidence. Breast Cancer Res Treat. 2012;135:655–62.

60. Blackwell KL, Burstein HJ, Storniolo AM, Rugo H, Sledge G, Koehler M, et al. Overall survival benefit with lapatinib in combination with trastuzumab for patients with human epidermal growth factor receptor 2-positive metastatic breast cancer: final results from the EGF104900 Study. J Clin Oncol. 2012;30:2585–92.

61. Valachis A, Nearchou A, Polyzos NP, Lind P. Cardiac toxicity in breast cancer patients treated with dual HER2 blockade. Int J Cancer. 2013;133:2245–52.

62. Rosamond W, Flegal K, Furie K, Go A, Greenlund K, Haase N, et al. Heart disease and stroke statistics – 2008 update: a report from the American Heart Association Statistics Committee and Stroke Statistics Subcommittee. Circulation. 2008;117: e25–146.

63. British Heart Foundation. European cardiovascular disease statistics. London: British Heart Foundation; 2005.

64. van de Velde CJ, Rea D, Seynaeve C, Putter H, Hasenburg A, Vannetzel JM, et al. Adjuvant tamoxifen and exemestane in early breast cancer (TEAM): a randomised phase 3 trial. Lancet. 2011;377:321–31.

65. Early Breast Cancer Trialists' Collaborative Group (EBCTCG). Effects of chemotherapy and hormonal therapy for early breast cancer on recurrence and 15-year survival: an overview of the randomised trials. Lancet. 2005;365:1687–717.

66. Braithwaite RS, Chlebowski RT, Lau J, George S, Hess R, Col NF, et al. Meta-analysis of vascular and neoplastic events associated with tamoxifen. J Gen Intern Med. 2003;18:937–47.

67. McDonald CC, Alexander FE, Whyte BW, Forrest AP, Stewart HJ, et al. Cardiac and vascular morbidity in women receiving adjuvant tamoxifen for breast cancer in a randomised trial. The Scottish Cancer Trials Breast Group. BMJ. 1995;311:977–80.

68. Herrington DM, Klein KP. Cardiovascular trials of estrogen replacement therapy. Ann N Y Acad Sci. 2001;949:153–62.

69. Wysowski DK, Honig SF, Beitz J. Uterine sarcoma associated with tamoxifen use. N Engl J Med. 2002;346:1832–3.

70. Fisher B, Dignam J, Bryant J, Wolmark N. Five versus more than five years of tamoxifen therapy for breast cancer patients with negative lymph nodes and estrogen receptor-positive tumors. J Natl Cancer Inst. 1996;88:1529–42.

71. Aiello EJ, Buist DS, Wagner EH, Tuzzio L, Greene SM, Lamerato LE, et al. Diffusion of AIs for breast cancer therapy between 1996 and 2003 in the Cancer Research Network. Breast Cancer Res Treat. 2008;107:397–403.

72. Janicke F. Are all AIs the same? A review of the current evidence. Breast. 2004;13 Suppl 1:S10–8.

73. Gibson LJ, Dawson CK, Lawrence DH, Bliss JM. AIs for treatment of advanced breast cancer in postmenopausal women. Cochrane Database Syst Rev. 2007;(1):CD003370.

74. Thurlimann B, Keshaviah A, Coates AS, Mouridsen H, Mauriac L, Forbes JF, et al. A comparison of letrozole and tamoxifen in postmenopausal women with early breast cancer. N Engl J Med. 2005;353:2747–57.

75. Howell A, Cuzick J, Baum M, Buzdar A, Dowsett M, Forbes JF, et al. Results of the ATAC (Arimidex, Tamoxifen, Alone or in Combination) trial after completion of 5 years' adjuvant treatment for breast cancer. Lancet. 2005;365:60–2.

76. Coombes RC, Kilburn LS, Snowdon CF, Paridaens R, Coleman RE, Jones SE, et al. Survival and safety of exemestane versus tamoxifen after 2–3 years' tamoxifen treatment (Intergroup Exemestane Study): a randomised controlled trial. Lancet. 2007;369: 559–70.

77. Dowsett M, Cuzick J, Ingle J, Coates A, Forbes J, Bliss J, et al. Meta-analysis of breast cancer outcomes in adjuvant trials of AIs versus tamoxifen. J Clin Oncol. 2010;28:509–18.

78. Winer EP, Hudis C, Burstein HJ, Wolff AC, Pritchard KI, Ingle JN, et al. American Society of Clinical Oncology technology assessment on the use of AIs as adjuvant therapy for postmenopausal women with hormone receptor-positive breast cancer: status report 2004. J Clin Oncol. 2005;23:619–29.

79. Goldhirsch A, Wood WC, Gelber RD, Coates AS, Thürlimann B, Senn HJ. Progress and promise: highlights of the international expert consensus on the primary therapy of early breast cancer 2007. Ann Oncol. 2007;18:1133–44.

80. Jones LW, Haykowsky MJ, Swartz JJ, Douglas PS, Mackey JR. Early breast cancer therapy and cardiovascular injury. J Am Coll Cardiol. 2007;50: 1435–41.

81. Esteva FJ, Hortobagyi GN. Comparative assessment of lipid effects of endocrine therapy for breast cancer: implications for cardiovascular disease prevention in postmenopausal women. Breast. 2006;15:301–12.

82. Walsh BW, Schiff I, Rosner B, Greenberg L, Ravnikar V, Sacks FM. Effects of postmenopausal estrogen replacement on the concentrations and metabolism of plasma lipoproteins. N Engl J Med. 1991;325:1196–204.

83. Crivellari D, Sun Z, Coates AS, Price KN, Thürlimann B, Mouridsen H, et al. Letrozole compared with tamoxifen for elderly patients with endocrine-responsive early breast cancer: the BIG 1-98 trial. J Clin Oncol. 2008;26:1972–9.

84. Hanrahan EO, Gonzalez-Angulo AM, Giordano SH, Price KN, Thürlimann B, Mouridsen H, et al. Overall survival and cause-specific mortality of patients with stage T1a, bN0M0 breast carcinoma. J Clin Oncol. 2007;25:4952–60.

85. Cuglan B, Soran O. Cardiovascular adverse effects of aromatase inhibitors in postmenopausal patients diagnosed with breast cancer. Int Heart Vasc Dis J. 2013;1:30–43.

86. Erwin GS, Crisostomo PR, Wang Y, Wang M, Markel TA, Guzman M, et al. Estradiol-treated mesenchymal stem cells improve myocardial recovery after ischemia. J Surg Res. 2009;152:319–24.

87. Bolego C, Rossoni G, Fadini GP, Vegeto E, Pinna C, Albiero M, et al. Selective estrogen receptor-alpha agonist provides widespread heart and vascular protection with enhanced endothelial progenitor cell

mobilization in the absence of uterotrophic action. FASEB J. 2010;24:2262–72.

88. Baruscotti I, Barchiesi F, Jackson EK, Imthurn B, Stiller R, Kim JH, et al. Estradiol stimulates capillary formation by human endothelial progenitor cells: role of estrogen receptor-{alpha}/{beta}, heme oxygenase 1, and tyrosine kinase. Hypertension. 2010;56:397–404.

89. Post WS, Goldschmidt-Clermont PJ, Wilhide CC, Heldman AW, Sussman MS, Ouyang P, et al. Methylation of the estrogen receptor gene is associated with aging and atherosclerosis in the cardiovascular system. Cardiovasc Res. 1999;43:985–91.

90. Kim J, Kim JY, Song KS, Lee YH, Seo JS, Jelinek J, et al. Epigenetic changes in estrogen receptor beta gene in atherosclerotic cardiovascular tissues and in-vitro vascular senescence. Biochim Biophys Acta. 2007;1772:72–80.

91. Brufsky A, Bundred N, Coleman R, Lambert-Falls R, Mena R, Hadji P, et al. Integrated analysis of zoledronic acid for prevention of AI-associated bone loss in postmenopausal women with early breast cancer receiving adjuvant letrozole. Oncologist. 2008;13: 503–14.

92. Boccardo F, Rubagotti A, Aldrighetti D, Buzzi F, Cruciani G, Farris A, et al. Switching to an AI provides mortality benefit in early breast carcinoma: pooled analysis of 2 consecutive trials. Cancer. 2007;109:1060–7.

93. Brown SA, Guise TA. Cancer treatment-related bone disease. Crit Rev Eukaryot Gene Expr. 2009;19: 47–60.

94. Cuzick J, Sestak I, Baum M, Buzdar A, Howell A, Dowsett M, et al. Effect of anastrozole and tamoxifen as adjuvant treatment for early-stage breast cancer: 10-year analysis of the ATAC trial. Lancet Oncol. 2010;11:1135–41.

95. Baum M, Buzdar A, Cuzick J, Forbes J, Houghton J, Howell A, et al. Anastrozole alone or in combination with tamoxifen versus tamoxifen alone for adjuvant treatment of postmenopausal women with early-stage breast cancer: results of the ATAC (Arimidex, Tamoxifen Alone or in Combination) trial efficacy and safety update analyses. Cancer. 2003;98:1802–10.

96. Forbes JF, Cuzick J, Buzdar A, et al. Effect of anastrozole and tamoxifen as adjuvant treatment for early-stage breast cancer: 100-month analysis of the ATAC trial. Lancet Oncol. 2008;9:45–53.

97. Mouridsen H, Giobbie-Hurder A, Goldhirsch A, Thürlimann B, Paridaens R, Smith I, et al. Letrozole therapy alone or in sequence with tamoxifen in women with breast cancer. N Engl J Med. 2009; 361:766–76.

98. Mouridsen H, Keshaviah A, Coates AS, Rabaglio M, Castiglione-Gertsch M, Sun Z, et al. Cardiovascular adverse events during adjuvant endocrine therapy for early breast cancer using letrozole or tamoxifen: safety analysis of BIG 1-98 trial. J Clin Oncol. 2007;25:5715–22.

99. Coates AS, Keshaviah A, Thürlimann B, Mouridsen H, Mauriac L, Forbes JF, Paridaens R, et al. Five years of letrozole compared with tamoxifen as initial adjuvant therapy for postmenopausal women with endocrine-responsive early breast cancer: update of study BIG 1-98. J Clin Oncol. 2007;25:486–92.

100. Colleoni M, Giobbie-Hurder A, Regan MM, Thürlimann B, Mouridsen H, Mauriac L, et al. Analyses adjusting for selective crossover show improved overall survival with adjuvant letrozole compared with tamoxifen in the BIG 1-98 study. J Clin Oncol. 2011;29:1117–24.

101. Goss PE, Ingle JN, Martino S, Robert NJ, Muss HB, Piccart MJ, et al. Randomized trial of letrozole following tamoxifen as extended adjuvant therapy in receptor-positive breast cancer: updated findings from NCIC CTG MA.17. J Natl Cancer Inst. 2005;97:1262–71.

102. Paridaens RJ, Dirix LY, Beex LV, Nooij M, Cameron DA, Cufer T, et al. Phase III study comparing exemestane with tamoxifen as first-line hormonal treatment of metastatic breast cancer in postmenopausal women: the European Organisation for Research and Treatment of Cancer Breast Cancer Cooperative Group. J Clin Oncol. 2008;26: 4883–90.

103. Robinson A. A review of the use of exemestane in early breast cancer. Ther Clin Risk Manag. 2009;5: 91–8.

104. Bliss JM, Kilburn LS, Coleman RE, Forbes JF, Coates AS, Jones SE, et al. Disease-related outcomes with long-term follow-up: an updated analysis of the intergroup exemestane study. J Clin Oncol. 2012;30:709–17.

105. Coombes RC, Paridaens R, Jassem J. First mature analysis of the Intergroup Exemestane Study. J Clin Oncol. 2006;24(9s suppl; abstr LBA527)

106. Rea D, Hasenburg A, Seynaeve C. Five years of exemestane as initial therapy compared to 5 years of tamoxifen followed by exemestane: the TEAM trial, a prospective, randomized, phase III trial in postmenopausal women with hormone-sensitive early breast cancer. Cancer Res. 2009;69(24 Suppl 3): Abstract 11.

107. Parkin DM, Bray F, Ferlay J, Pisani P. Global cancer statistics, 2002. CA Cancer J Clin. 2005;55:74–108.

108. Ingle JN. Adjuvant endocrine therapy for postmenopausal women with early breast cancer. Clin Cancer Res. 2006;12:1031s–6.

109. Mauri D, Pavlidis N, Polyzos NP, Ioannidis JP. Survival with AIs and inactivators versus standard hormonal therapy in advanced breast cancer: meta-analysis. J Natl Cancer Inst. 2006;98: 1285–91.

110. Mouridsen HT, Robert NJ. The role of AIs as adjuvant therapy for early breast cancer in postmenopausal women. Eur J Cancer. 2005;41:1678–89.

111. Morandi P, Rouzier R, Altundag K, Buzdar AU, Theriault RL, Hortobagyi G. The role of AIs in the adjuvant treatment of breast carcinoma: the M. D.

Anderson Cancer Center evidence-based approach. Cancer. 2004;101:1482–9.

112. Henderson IC, Piccart-Gebhart MJ. The evolving role of AIs in adjuvant breast cancer therapy. Clin Breast Cancer. 2005;6:206–15.

113. Goss PE. Emerging role of AIs in the adjuvant setting. Am J Clin Oncol. 2003;26:S27–33.

114. Buzdar A, Chlebowski R, Cuzick J, Duffy S, Forbes J, Jonat W, Ravdin P. Defining the role of AIs in the adjuvant endocrine treatment of early breast cancer. Curr Med Res Opin. 2006;22:1575–85.

115. Boccardo F, Rubagotti A, Guglielmini P, Fini A, Paladini G, Mesiti M, et al. Switching to anastrozole versus continued tamoxifen treatment of early breast cancer. Updated results of the Italian tamoxifen anastrozole (ITA) trial. Ann Oncol. 2006;17 Suppl 7:vii10–4.

116. Buzdar A. Anastrozole as adjuvant therapy for early-stage breast cancer: implications of the ATAC trial. Clin Breast Cancer. 2003;4 Suppl 1:S42–8.

117. Wasan KM, Goss PE, Pritchard PH, Shepherd L, Palmer MJ, Liu S, et al. The influence of letrozole on serum lipid concentrations in postmenopausal women with primary breast cancer who have completed 5 years of adjuvant tamoxifen (NCIC CTG MA.17L). Ann Oncol. 2005;16:707–15.

118. Gandhi S, Verma S. AIs and cardiac toxicity: getting to the heart of the matter. Breast Cancer Res Treat. 2007;106:1–9.

119. McCloskey EV, Hannon RA, Lakner G, Fraser WD, Clack G, Miyamoto A, et al. Effects of third generation AIs on bone health and other safety parameters: results of an open, randomised, multi-centre study of letrozole, exemestane and anastrozole in healthy postmenopausal women. Eur J Cancer. 2007;43: 2523–31.

120. Lancellotti P, Nkomo VT, Badano LP, Bergler-Klein J, Bogaert J, Davin L, et al. Expert consensus for multi-modality imaging evaluation of cardiovascular complications of radiotherapy in adults: a report from the European Association of Cardiovascular Imaging and the American Society of Echocardiography. Eur Heart J Cardiovasc Imaging. 2013;14:721–40.

121. Curigliano G, Cardinale D, Suter T, Platanioti G, de Azambuja E, Sandri MT, et al. Cardiovascular toxicity induced by chemotherapy, targeted agents and radiotherapy: ESMO Clinical Practice Guidelines. Ann Oncol. 2012;23 Suppl 7:vii155–66.

122. Plana JC, Galderisi M, Barac A, Ewer MS, Ky B, Scherrer-Crosbie M, et al. Expert consensus for multimodality imaging evaluation of adult patients during and after cancer therapy: a report from the American Society of Echocardiography and the European Association of Cardiovascular Imaging. Eur Heart J Cardiovasc Imaging. 2014;15:1063–93.

123. Floyd J, Morgan JP. Cardiotoxicity of anthracycline-like chemotherapy agents. In: www.UpToDate, Savarese DFM, editors. Waltham: UpToDate. Accessed on 8 Sept 2014.

124. Perez EA, Morgan JP. Cardiotoxicity of trastuzumab and other HER2-targeted agents. In: www. UpToDate, Savarese DFM, editors. Waltham: UpToDate. Accessed on 15 Sept 2014.

125. Marks LB, Constine LS, Jacob Adams M. Cardiotoxicity of radiation therapy for malignancy. In: UpToDate, Ross ME, editors. Waltham: www.UpToDate. Accessed on 1 Sept 2014.

126. Romond EH, Jeong JH, Rastogi P, Swain SM, Geyer Jr CE, Ewer MS, et al. Seven-year follow-up assessment of cardiac function in NSABP B-31, a randomized trial comparing doxorubicin and cyclophosphamide followed by paclitaxel (ACP) with ACP plus trastuzumab as adjuvant therapy for patients with node-positive, human epidermal growth factor receptor 2-positive breast cancer. J Clin Oncol. 2012;30:3792–9.

127. Altena R, Perik PJ, van Veldhuisen DJ, de Vries EG, Gietema JA. Cardiovascular toxicity caused by cancer treatment: strategies for early detection. Lancet Oncol. 2009;10:391–9.

128. Jensen BV, Skovsgaard T, Nielsen SL. Functional monitoring of anthracycline cardiotoxicity: a prospective, blinded, long-term observational study of outcome in 120 patients. Ann Oncol. 2002;13: 699–709.

129. Ewer MS, Lenihan DJ. Left ventricular ejection fraction and cardiotoxicity: is our ear really to the ground? J Clin Oncol. 2008;26:1201–3.

130. Thavendiranathan P, Grant AD, Negishi T, Plana JC, Popović ZB, Marwick TH. Reproducibility of echocardiographic techniques for sequential assessment of left ventricular ejection fraction and volumes: application to patients undergoing cancer chemotherapy. J Am Coll Cardiol. 2013;61:77–84.

131. Lang RM, Mor-Avi V, Dent JM, Kramer CM. Three-dimensional echocardiography: is it ready for everyday clinical use? JACC Cardiovasc Imaging. 2009; 2:114–7.

132. Lorenzini C, Corsi C, Aquilina M. Early detection of cardiotoxicity in chemotherapy-treated patients from real-time 3D echocardiography. Computing in Cardiology Conference (CinC). 2013. p. 249–52.

133. Jurcut R, Wildiers H, Ganame J, D'hooge J, De Backer J, Denys H, et al. Strain rate imaging detects early cardiac effects of pegylated liposomal doxorubicin as adjuvant therapy in elderly patients with breast cancer. J Am Soc Echocardiogr. 2008;21:1283–9.

134. Hare JL, Brown JK, Leano R, Jenkins C, Woodward N, Marwick TH. Use of myocardial deformation imaging to detect preclinical myocardial dysfunction before conventional measures in patients undergoing breast cancer treatment with trastuzumab. Am Heart J. 2009;158:294–301.

135. Fallah-Rad N, Walker JR, Wassef A, Lytwyn M, Bohonis S, Fang T, et al. The utility of cardiac biomarkers, tissue velocity and strain imaging, and cardiac magnetic resonance imaging in predicting early left ventricular dysfunction in patients with human

epidermal growth factor receptor II-positive breast cancer treated with adjuvant trastuzumab therapy. J Am Coll Cardiol. 2011;57:2263–70.

136. Erven K, Jurcut R, Weltens C, Giusca S, Ector J, Wildiers H, et al. Acute radiation effects on cardiac function detected by strain rate imaging in breast cancer patients. Int J Radiat Oncol Biol Phys. 2011;79:1444–51.

137. Kavousi M, Elias-Smale S, Rutten JH, Leening MJ, Vliegenthart R, Verwoert GC, et al. Evaluation of newer risk markers for coronary heart disease risk classification: a cohort study. Ann Intern Med. 2012;156:438–44.

138. Thavendiranathan P, Wintersperger BJ, Flamm SD, Marwick TH. Cardiac MRI in the assessment of cardiac injury and toxicity from cancer chemotherapy: a systematic review. Circ Cardiovasc Imaging. 2013;6:1080–91.

139. Cardinale D, Sandri MT, Colombo A, Colombo N, Boeri M, Lamantia G, et al. Prognostic value of troponin I in cardiac risk stratification of cancer patients undergoing high-dose chemotherapy. Circulation. 2004;109:2749–54.

140. Sawaya H, Sebag IA, Plana JC, Januzzi JL, Ky B, Cohen V, et al. Early detection and prediction of cardiotoxicity in chemotherapy-treated patients. Am J Cardiol. 2011;107:1375–80.

141. Cardinale D, Colombo A, Torrisi R, et al. Trastuzumab-induced cardiotoxicity: clinical and prognostic implications of troponin I evaluation. J Clin Oncol. 2010;28:3910–6.

142. Sawaya H, Sebag IA, Plana JC, Januzzi JL, Ky B, Tan TC, et al. Assessment of echocardiography and biomarkers for the extended prediction of cardiotoxicity in patients treated with anthracyclines, taxanes, and trastuzumab. Circ Cardiovasc Imaging. 2012;5: 596–603.

143. Kutteh LA, Hobday T, Jaffe A. A correlative study of cardiac biomarkers and left ventricular ejection fraction (LVEF) from N9831, a phase III randomized trial of chemotherapy and trastuzumab as adjuvant therapy for HER2-positive breast cancer. J Clin Oncol. 2007;25(18S):579.

144. Raderer M, Kornek G, Weinländer G, Kastner J. Serum troponin T levels in adults undergoing anthracycline therapy. J Natl Cancer Inst. 1997; 89(2):171.

145. Lenihan DJ, Massey MR, Baysinger KB. Superior detection of cardiotoxicity during chemotherapy using biomarkers. J Card Fail. 2007;13:S151.

146. Romano S, Fratini S, Ricevuto E, Procaccini V, Stifano G, Mancini M, et al. Serial measurements of NT-proBNP are predictive of not-high-dose anthracycline cardiotoxicity in breast cancer patients. Br J Cancer. 2011;105:1663–8.

147. Skovgaard D, Hasbak P, Kjaer A. BNP predicts chemotherapy-related cardiotoxicity and death: comparison with gated equilibrium radionuclide ventriculography. PLoS One. 2014;9:e96736.

148. Dodos F, Halbsguth T, Erdmann E, Hoppe UC. Usefulness of myocardial performance index and biochemical markers for early detection of anthracycline-induced cardiotoxicity in adults. Clin Res Cardiol. 2008;97:318–26.

149. Knobloch K, Tepe J, Lichtinghagen R, Luck HJ, Vogt PM. Monitoring of cardiotoxicity during immunotherapy with Herceptin using simultaneous continuous wave Doppler depending on N-terminal pro-brain natriuretic peptide. Clin Med. 2007;7:88–9.

150. Knobloch K, Tepe J, Rossner D, et al. Combined NT-pro-BNP and CW-Doppler ultrasound cardiac output monitoring (USCOM) in epirubicin and liposomal doxorubicin therapy. Int J Cardiol. 2008;128:316–25.

151. Damrot J, Nubel T, Epe B, Roos WP, Kaina B, Fritz G. Lovastatin protects human endothelial cells from the genotoxic and cytotoxic effects of the anticancer drugs doxorubicin and etoposide. Br J Pharmacol. 2006;149:988–97.

152. Ran XZ, Ran X, Zong ZW, Liu DQ, Xiang GM, Su YP, et al. Protective effect of atorvastatin on radiation-induced vascular endothelial cell injury in vitro. J Radiat Res. 2010;51:527–33.

153. Seicean S, Seicean A, Plana JC, Budd GT, Marwick TH. Effect of statin therapy on the risk for incident heart failure in patients with breast cancer receiving anthracycline chemotherapy: an observational clinical cohort study. J Am Coll Cardiol. 2012;60: 2384–90.

154. Acar Z, Kale A, Turgut M, Demircan S, Durna K, Demir S, et al. Efficiency of atorvastatin in the protection of anthracycline-induced cardiomyopathy. J Am Coll Cardiol. 2011;58:988–9.

155. Asanuma H, Minamino T, Sanada S, Takashima S, Ogita H, Ogai A, et al. Beta-adrenoceptor blocker carvedilol provides cardioprotection via an adenosine-dependent mechanism in ischemic canine hearts. Circulation. 2004;109:2773–9.

156. Kim IM, Tilley DG, Chen J, Salazar NC, Whalen EJ, Violin JD, et al. Beta-blockers alprenolol and carvedilol stimulate beta-arrestin-mediated EGFR transactivation. Proc Natl Acad Sci U S A. 2008;105:14555–60.

157. Kaya MG, Ozkan M, Gunebakmaz O, Akkaya H, Kaya EG, Akpek M, et al. Protective effects of nebivolol against anthracycline-induced cardiomyopathy: a randomized control study. Int J Cardiol. 2013;167:2306–10.

158. Kalay N, Basar E, Ozdogru I, Er O, Cetinkaya Y, Dogan A, et al. Protective effects of carvedilol against anthracycline-induced cardiomyopathy. J Am Coll Cardiol. 2006;48:2258–62.

159. Bosch X, Rovira M, Sitges M, Domènech A, Ortiz-Pérez JT, de Caralt TM, et al. Enalapril and carvedilol for preventing chemotherapy-induced left ventricular systolic dysfunction in patients with malignant hemopathies: the OVERCOME trial (prevention of left ventricular dysfunction with enalapril and carvedilol in patients submitted to intensive chemo-

therapy for the treatment of malignant hemopathies). J Am Coll Cardiol. 2013;61:2355–62.

160. Ewer MS, Vooletich MT, Durand JB, Woods ML, Davis JR, Valero V, et al. Reversibility of trastuzumab-related cardiotoxicity: new insights based on clinical course and response to medical treatment. J Clin Oncol. 2005;23:7820–6.

161. Oliva S, Cioffi G, Frattini S, Simoncini EL, Faggiano P, Boccardi L, Italian Cardio-Oncological Network, et al. Administration of angiotensin-converting enzyme inhibitors and β-blockers during adjuvant trastuzumab chemotherapy for nonmetastatic breast cancer: marker of risk or cardioprotection in the real world? Oncologist. 2012;17:917–24.

162. Tokudome T, Mizushige K, Noma T, Manabe K, Murakami K, Tsuji T, et al. Prevention of doxorubicin (adriamycin)-induced cardiomyopathy by simultaneous administration of angiotensin-converting enzyme inhibitor assessed by acoustic densitometry. J Cardiovasc Pharmacol. 2000;36:361–8.

163. Abd El-Aziz MA, Othman AI, Amer M, El-Missiry MA. Potential protective role of angiotensin-converting enzyme inhibitors captopril and enalapril against adriamycin-induced acute cardiac and hepatic toxicity in rats. J Appl Toxicol. 2001;21:469–73.

164. Lemmens K, Segers VF, Demolder M, De Keulenaer GW. Role of neuregulin-1/ErbB2 signaling in endothelium-cardiomyocyte cross-talk. J Biol Chem. 2006;281:19469–77.

165. Nakamae H, Tsumura K, Terada Y, Nakane T, Nakamae M, Ohta K, et al. Notable effects of angiotensin II receptor blocker, valsartan, on acute cardiotoxic changes after standard chemotherapy with cyclophosphamide, doxorubicin, vincristine, and prednisolone. Cancer. 2005;104:2492–8.

166. Dessì M, Madeddu C, Piras A, Cadeddu C, Deidda M, Massa E, et al. Long-term, up to 18 months, protective effects of the angiotensin II receptor blocker telmisartan on Epirubicin-induced inflammation and oxidative stress assessed by serial strain rate. Springerplus. 2013;2:198.

167. Cardinale D, Colombo A, Sandri MT, Lamantia G, Colombo N, Civelli M, et al. Prevention of high-dose chemotherapy-induced cardiotoxicity in high-risk patients by angiotensin-converting enzyme inhibition. Circulation. 2006;114:2474–81.

168. Tofield A. ACE inhibitor reduces radiation injury to myocardium. Eur Heart J. 2013;34:2023–4.

169. Scott JM, Khakoo A, Mackey JR, Haykowsky MJ, Douglas PS, Jones LW. Modulation of anthracycline-induced cardiotoxicity by aerobic exercise in breast cancer: current evidence and underlying mechanisms. Circulation. 2011;124:642–50.

170. Haykowsky MJ, Mackey JR, Thompson RB, Jones LW, Paterson DI. Adjuvant trastuzumab induces ventricular remodeling despite aerobic exercise training. Clin Cancer Res. 2009;15:4963–7.

171. Hunt SA, Abraham WT, Chin MH, Feldman AM, Francis GS, Ganiats TG, et al. 2009 focused update incorporated into the ACC/AHA 2005 Guidelines for the Diagnosis and Management of Heart Failure in Adults a report of the American College of Cardiology Foundation/American Heart Association Task Force on Practice Guidelines developed in collaboration with the International Society for Heart and Lung Transplantation. J Am Coll Cardiol. 2009;53:e1–90.

172. Cardinale D, Colombo A, Lamantia G, Colombo N, Civelli M, De Giacomi G, et al. Anthracycline-induced cardiomyopathy: clinical relevance and response to pharmacologic therapy. J Am Coll Cardiol. 2010;55:213–20.

173. Tocchetti CG, Ragone G, Coppola C, Rea D, Piscopo G, Scala S, et al. Detection, monitoring, and management of trastuzumab-induced left ventricular dysfunction: an actual challenge. Eur J Heart Fail. 2012;14:130–7.

174. Suter TM, Procter M, van Veldhuisen DJ, Muscholl M, Bergh J, Carlomagno C, et al. Trastuzumab-associated cardiac adverse effects in the herceptin adjuvant trial. J Clin Oncol. 2007;25:3859–65.

175. Mackey JR, Clemons M, Coté MA, Delgado D, Dent S, Paterson A, et al. Cardiac management during adjuvant trastuzumab therapy: recommendations of the Canadian Trastuzumab Working Group. Curr Oncol. 2008;15:24–35.

176. Jones LW, Haykowsky M, Peddle CJ, Joy AA, Pituskin EN, Tkachuk LM, et al. Cardiovascular risk profile of patients with HER2/neu-positive breast cancer treated with anthracycline-taxane-containing adjuvant chemotherapy and/or trastuzumab. Cancer Epidemiol Biomarkers Prev. 2007;16:1026–231.

177. Jones LW, Haykowsky M, Pituskin EN, Jendzjowsky NG, Tomczak CR, Haennel RG, et al. Cardiovascular reserve and risk profile of postmenopausal women after chemoendocrine therapy for hormone receptor – positive operable breast cancer. Oncologist. 2007;12:1156–64.

178. Carlson RW, Hudis CA, Pritchard KI. Adjuvant endocrine therapy in hormone receptor-positive postmenopausal breast cancer: evolution of NCCN, ASCO, and St Gallen recommendations. J Natl Compr Cancer Netw. 2006;4:971–9.

179. McCrohon JA, Moon JC, Prasad SK, McKenna WJ, Lorenz CH, Coats AJ, et al. Differentiation of heart failure related to dilated cardiomyopathy and coronary artery disease using gadolinium-enhanced cardiovascular magnetic resonance. Circulation. 2003;108:54–9.

180. Demark-Wahnefried W, Rimer BK, Winer EP. Weight gain in women diagnosed with breast cancer. J Am Diet Assoc. 1997;97:519–26, 29; quiz 27–8.

181. Goodwin P, Esplen MJ, Butler K, Winocur J, Pritchard K, Brazel S, et al. Multidisciplinary weight management in locoregional breast cancer: results of a phase II study. Breast Cancer Res Treat. 1998;48:53–64.

182. Holmberg L, Lund E, Bergstrom R, Adami HO, Meirik O. Oral contraceptives and prognosis in

breast cancer: effects of duration, latency, recency, age at first use and relation to parity and body mass index in young women with breast cancer. Eur J Cancer. 1994;30A:351–4.

183. Lethaby AE, Mason BH, Harvey VJ, Holdaway IM. Survival of women with node negative breast cancer in the Auckland region. N Z Med J. 1996;109:330–3.

184. Goodwin PJ, Ennis M, Pritchard KI, McCready D, Koo J, Sidlofsky S, et al. Adjuvant treatment and onset of menopause predict weight gain after breast cancer diagnosis. J Clin Oncol. 1999;17:120–9.

185. Rock CL, Flatt SW, Newman V, Caan BJ, Haan MN, Stefanick ML, et al. Factors associated with weight gain in women after diagnosis of breast cancer. Women's Healthy Eating and Living Study Group. J Am Diet Assoc. 1999;99:1212–21.

186. Chlebowski RT, Weiner JM, Reynolds R, Luce J, Bulcavage L, Bateman JR. Long-term survival following relapse after 5-FU but not CMF adjuvant breast cancer therapy. Breast Cancer Res Treat. 1986;7:23–30.

187. Camoriano JK, Loprinzi CL, Ingle JN, Therneau TM, Krook JE, Veeder MH. Weight change in women treated with adjuvant therapy or observed following mastectomy for node-positive breast cancer. J Clin Oncol. 1990;8:1327–34.

188. Bonomi P, Bunting N, Fishman D, et al. Weight gain during adjuvant chemotherapy or hormone-chemotherapy for stage II breast cancer evaluated in relation to disease free survival. BCRT. 1985;4:339.(abstr)

189. Levine EG, Raczynski JM, Carpenter JT. Weight gain with breast cancer adjuvant treatment. Cancer. 1991;67:1954–9.

190. Heasman KZ, Sutherland HJ, Campbell JA, Elhakim T, Boyd NF. Weight gain during adjuvant chemotherapy for breast cancer. Breast Cancer Res Treat. 1985;5:195–200.

191. Goodwin PJ, Panzarella T, Boyd NF. Weight gain in women with localized breast cancer – a descriptive study. Breast Cancer Res Treat. 1988;11:59–66.

192. Costa LJ, Varella PC, del Giglio A. Weight changes during chemotherapy for breast cancer. Sao Paulo Med J. 2002;120:113–7.

193. Willett WC, Manson JE, Stampfer MJ, Colditz GA, Rosner B, Speizer FE, et al. Weight, weight change, and coronary heart disease in women. Risk within the 'normal' weight range. JAMA. 1995;273:461–5.

194. Calle EE, Thun MJ, Petrelli JM, Rodriguez C, Heath Jr CW. Body-mass index and mortality in a prospective cohort of U.S. adults. N Engl J Med. 1999;341:1097–105.

195. Kopelman PG. Obesity as a medical problem. Nature. 2000;404:635–43.

196. Khemasuwan D, Divietro ML, Tangdhanakanond K, Pomerantz SC, Eiger G, et al. Statins decrease the occurrence of venous thromboembolism in patients with cancer. Am J Med. 2010;123:60–5.

197. Mosca L, Banka CL, Benjamin EJ, Berra K, Bushnell C, Dolor RJ, et al. Evidence-based guidelines for cardiovascular disease prevention in women: 2007 update. J Am Coll Cardiol. 2007;49:1230–50.

198. Gulati M, Pandey DK, Arnsdorf MF, Lauderdale DS, Thisted RA, Wicklund RH, et al. Exercise capacity and the risk of death in women: the St James Women Take Heart Project. Circulation. 2003;108:1554–9.

199. Manson JE, Greenland P, LaCroix AZ, Stefanick ML, Mouton CP, Oberman A, et al. Walking compared with vigorous exercise for the prevention of cardiovascular events in women. N Engl J Med. 2002;347:716–25.

200. Holmes MD, Chen WY, Feskanich D, Kroenke CH, Colditz GA, et al. Physical activity and survival after breast cancer diagnosis. JAMA. 2005;293: 2479–86.

Index

© Springer International Publishing Switzerland 2016
A. Aydiner et al. (eds.), *Breast Disease: Management and Therapies*,
DOI 10.1007/978-3-319-26012-9

Printed by Printforce, the Netherlands